Nadas'
Pediatric
Cardiology

Nadas' Pediatric Cardiology

Edited by

Donald C. Fyler, M.D.

Professor Emeritus of Pediatrics
Harvard Medical School
Associate Chief of Cardiology Emeritus
Children's Hospital
Boston, Massachusetts

HANLEY & BELFUS, INC./Philadelphia
MOSBY – YEAR BOOK, INC./St. Louis • Baltimore • Boston • Chicago • London
  Philadelphia • Sydney • Toronto

Publisher: HANLEY & BELFUS, INC.
210 S. 13th Street
Philadelphia, PA 19107
(215) 546-7293

North American and worldwide sales and distribution:

MOSBY-YEAR BOOK, INC.
11830 Westline Industrial Drive
St. Louis, MO 63146

In Canada: THE C.V. MOSBY COMPANY, LTD.
5240 Finch Avenue East
Unit 1
Scarborough, Ontario M1S 5A2
Canada

Nadas' Pediatric Cardiology   ISBN 0-932883-94-X

Library of Congress Catalog Card Number 91-72312

Last digit is the print number: 9 8 7 6 5 4 3 2

CONTENTS

SECTION I: HISTORICAL PERSPECTIVE

1 The Nadas Years: 1949–1982 .... **1**
Donald C. Fyler, M.D.

SECTION II: DEVELOPMENTAL ANATOMY

2 Embryology **5**
Richard Van Praagh, M.D.

3 Morphologic Anatomy **17**
Richard Van Praagh, M.D., and Stella Van Praagh, M.D.

4 Segmental Approach to Diagnosis **27**
Richard Van Praagh, M.D.

SECTION III: DYSMORPHOLOGY

5 Dysmorphology **37**
Ronald V. Lacro, M.D.

SECTION IV: NORMAL CIRCULATORY PHYSIOLOGY

6 Fetal and Transitional Circulation **57**
Michael D. Freed, M.D.

SECTION V: PROBLEMS CAUSED BY HEART DISEASE

7 Congestive Heart Failure **63**
Michael D. Freed, M.D.

8 Hypoxemia **73**
Alexander S. Nadas, M.D.

9 Central Nervous System Sequelae of Congenital Heart Disease **77**
Jane W. Newburger, M.D., M.P.H.

10 Pulmonary Hypertension... **83**
Thomas J. Kulik, M.D.

SECTION VI: TOOLS OF DIAGNOSIS

11 History, Physical Examination, and Laboratory Tests **101**
Donald C. Fyler, M.D., and Alexander S. Nadas, M.D.

12 Electrocardiography and Introduction to Electrophysiologic Techniques **117**
    Edward P. Walsh, M.D.

13 Echocardiography.. **159**
    Stephen P. Sanders, M.D.

14 Cardiac Catheterization **187**
    James E. Lock, M.D., John F. Keane, M.D., Valerie S. Mandell, M.D.,
    and Stanton B. Perry, M.D.

15 Assessment of Ventricular and Myocardial Performance **225**
    Steven D. Colan, M.D.

16 Exercise Testing... **249**
    Steven D. Colan, M.D.

17 Computing.. **265**
    Donald C. Fyler, M.D.

SECTION VII: PREVALENCE

18 Trends **273**
    Donald C. Fyler, M.D.

SECTION VIII: ACQUIRED HEART DISEASE

19 Innocent Murmurs **281**
    Jane W. Newburger, M.D., M.P.H.

20 Dyslipidemia in Childhood and Adolescence................................ **285**
    Jane W. Newburger, M.D., M.P.H.

21 Systemic Arterial Hypertension **295**
    J.R. Ingelfinger, M.D.

22 Rheumatic Fever.. **305**
    Donald C. Fyler, M.D.

23 Kawasaki Syndrome... **319**
    Jane W. Newburger, M.D., M.P.H.

24 Cardiomyopathies... **329**
    Steven D. Colan, M.D., Philip J. Spevak, M.D., Ira A. Parness, M.D.,
    and Alexander S. Nadas, M.D.

25 Pericardial Disease.. **363**
    Donald C. Fyler, M.D.

26 Infective Endocarditis **369**
    Jane W. Newburger, M.D., M.P.H.

27 Cardiac Arrhythmias **377**
    Edward P. Walsh, M.D., and J. Philip Saul, M.D.

SECTION IX: CONGENITAL HEART DISEASE

28 Ventricular Septal Defect **435**
Donald C. Fyler, M.D.

29 Pulmonary Stenosis **459**
Donald C. Fyler, M.D.

30 Tetralogy of Fallot.. **471**
Donald C. Fyler, M.D.

31 Aortic Outflow Abnormalities.. **493**
Donald C. Fyler, M.D.

32 Atrial Septal Defect Secundum... **513**
Donald C. Fyler, M.D.

33 Patent Ductus Arteriosus **525**
Donald C. Fyler, M.D.

34 Coarctation of the Aorta **535**
Donald C. Fyler, M.D.

35 D-Transposition of the Great Arteries **557**
Donald C. Fyler, M.D.

36 Endocardial Cushion Defects **577**
Donald C. Fyler, M.D.

37 Cardiac Malpositions with Special Emphasis on Visceral Heterotaxy
(Asplenia and Polysplenia Syndromes) **589**
Stella Van Praagh, M.D., Francesco Santini, M.D., and Stephen P. Sanders, M.D

38 Mitral Valve and Left Atrial Lesions **609**
Donald C. Fyler, M.D.

39 Hypoplastic Left Heart Syndrome, Mitral Atresia, and Aortic Atresia **623**
Peter Lang, M.D., and Donald C. Fyler, M.D.

40 Pulmonary Atresia with Intact Ventricular Septum **635**
Donald C. Fyler, M.D.

41 Double-Outlet Right Ventricle **643**
Donald C. Fyler, M.D.

42 Single Ventricle **649**
Donald C. Fyler, M.D.

43 Tricuspid Atresia **659**
Donald C. Fyler, M.D.

44 Tricuspid Valve Problems **669**
    Donald C. Fyler, M.D.

45 Truncus Arteriosus **675**
    Donald C. Fyler, M.D

46 Total Anomalous Pulmonary Venous Return **683**
    Donald C. Fyler, M.D.

47 Aortopulmonary Window **693**
    Donald C. Fyler, M.D.

48 Origin of a Right Pulmonary Artery from the Aorta (Hemitruncus) **697**
    Donald C. Fyler, M.D.

49 "Corrected" Transposition of the Great Arteries **701**
    Donald C. Fyler, M.D.

50 Congenital Vascular Fistulas **707**
    Donald C. Fyler, M.D.

51 Anomalous Origin of the Left Coronary Artery **715**
    Donald C. Fyler, M.D.

52 Vascular Rings and Slings **719**
    Valerie S. Mandell, M.D., and Richard M. Braverman, M.D.

53 Cardiac Tumors **727**
    Donald C. Fyler, M.D.

SECTION X: SURGICAL CONSIDERATIONS

54 Surgery for Infants with Congenital Heart Disease **731**
    Aldo R. Castaneda, M.D., Richard A. Jonas, M.D., and John E. Mayer, Jr., M.D.

SECTION XI: THE FUTURE

55 A Cellular and Molecular Approach to Pediatric Cardiology **747**
    Bernardo Nadal-Ginard, M.D., Ph.D., and Vijak Mahdavi, Ph.D.

Appendix: Principal Drugs Used in Pediatric Cardiology **760**

Index **769**

CONTRIBUTORS

RICHARD M. BRAVERMAN, M.D.
Clinical Fellow in Radiology, Harvard Medical
School; Assistant in Radiology, Children's
Hospital, Boston, Massachusetts

ALDO R. CASTANEDA, M.D. Ph.D.
William E. Ladd Professor of Surgery, Harvard
Medical School; Surgeon-in-Chief, Children's
Hospital, Boston, Massachusetts

STEVEN D. COLAN, M.D.
Associate Professor of Pediatrics, Harvard
Medical School; Senior Associate in Cardiology,
Children's Hospital, Boston, Massachusetts

MICHAEL D. FREED, M.D.
Associate Professor of Pediatrics, Harvard
Medical School; Senior Associate in Cardiology,
and Director, Inpatient Cardiovascular Service,
Children's Hospital, Boston, Massachusetts

DONALD C. FYLER, M.D.
Professor Emeritus of Pediatrics, Harvard
Medical School; Associate Chief of Cardiology
Emeritus, Children's Hospital, Boston,
Massachusetts

JULIE R. INGELFINGER, M.D.
Associate Professor of Pediatrics, Harvard
Medical School; Co-Chief, Pediatric
Nephrology, Massachusetts General Hospital,
Boston, Massachusetts

RICHARD A. JONAS, M.D.
Associate Professor of Surgery, Harvard
Medical School; Senior Associate in Cardiac
Surgery, Children's Hospital, Boston,
Massachusetts

JOHN F. KEANE, M.D.
Associate Professor of Pediatrics, Harvard
Medical School; Senior Associate in Cardiology
and Director, Cardiac Catheterization
Laboratories, Children's Hospital, Boston,
Massachusetts

THOMAS J. KULIK, M.D.
Assistant Professor of Pediatrics, Harvard
Medical School; Associate in Cardiology,
Children's Hospital, Boston, Massachusetts

RONALD V. LACRO, M.D.
Instructor in Pediatrics, Harvard Medical
School; Assistant in Cardiology, Children's
Hospital, Boston, Massachusetts

PETER LANG, M.D.
Associate Professor of Pediatrics, Harvard
Medical School; Chief of Pediatric Cardiology,
Children's Hospital, Boston Massachusetts

JAMES E. LOCK, M.D.
Associate Professor of Pediatrics, Harvard
Medical School; Chief of Clinical Cardiology and
Director of Invasive Cardiology, Children's
Hospital, Boston, Massachusetts

VIJAK MAHDAVI, Ph.D.
Associate Professor of Pediatrics, Harvard
Medical School; Senior Associate in Cardiology,
Children's Hospital, Boston, Massachusetts

VALERIE S. MANDELL, M.D.
Assistant Professor of Radiology, Harvard
Medical School; Staff Radiologist, Children's
Hospital, Boston, Massachusetts

JOHN E. MAYER, JR., M.D.
Associate Professor of Surgery, Harvard
Medical School; Senior Associate in
Cardiovascular Surgery, Children's Hospital,
Boston, Massachusetts

BERNARDO NADAL-GINARD, M.D., Ph.D.
Alexander S. Nadas Professor of Pediatrics,
Professor of Cellular and Molecular
Physiology, Harvard Medical School and
Howard Hughes Medical Institute;
Chairman, Department of Cardiology, and
Cardiologist-in-Chief, Children's Hospital;
Boston, Massachusetts

ALEXANDER S. NADAS, M.D.
Professor Emeritus of Pediatrics, Harvard
Medical School; Chairman Emeritus,
Department of Cardiology, Children's Hospital,
Boston, Massachusetts

JANE W. NEWBURGER, M.D., M.P.H.
Associate Professor of Pediatrics, Harvard
Medical School; Director of Outpatient Services
and Preventive Cardiology, Senior Associate in
Cardiology, Children's Hospital, Boston,
Massachusetts

IRA ALLEN PARNESS, M.D.
Assistant Professor of Pediatrics, Harvard
Medical School; Associate in Cardiology,
Children's Hospital, Boston, Massachusetts

STANTON B. PERRY, M.D.
Assistant Professor of Pediatrics, Harvard
Medical School; Associate in Cardiology,
Children's Hospital, Boston, Massachusetts

STEPHEN P. SANDERS, M.D.
Associate Professor of Pediatrics, Harvard
Medical School; Senior Associate in Cardiology,
and Director, Noninvasive Laboratories,
Children's Hospital, Boston, Massachusetts

FRANCESCO SANTINI, M.D.
Research Fellow in Cardiac Pathology, Harvard
Medical School and Children's Hospital, Boston,
Massachusetts; present address: University of
Padova Medical School, Padova, Italy

J. PHILIP SAUL, M.D.
Assistant Professor of Pediatrics, Harvard
Medical School; Associate in Cardiology,
Children's Hospital, Boston, Massachusetts

PHILIP J. SPEVAK, M.D.
Assistant Professor of Pediatrics, Harvard
Medical School; Associate in Cardiology,
Children's Hospital, Boston, Massachusetts

RICHARD VAN PRAAGH, M.D.
Professor of Pathology, Harvard Medical
School; Director of the Cardiac Registry,
Research Associate in Cardiology, and Research
Associate in Cardiac Surgery, Children's
Hospital, Boston, Massachusetts

STELLA VAN PRAAGH, M.D.
Assistant Professor of Pathology, Harvard
Medical School; Associate in Cardiology,
Children's Hospital, Boston, Massachusetts

EDWARD P. WALSH, M.D.
Assistant Professor of Pediatrics, Harvard
Medical School; Director, Electrophysiologic
Laboratories, Children's Hospital, Boston,
Massachusetts

PREFACE

This book was written to honor Dr. Alexander S. Nadas, the Chief of Cardiology at Children's Hospital in Boston from 1949–1982. He was the Chief to most of the contributors to this volume and a mentor and a colleague to all. It seemed fitting to revise the textbook *Pediatric Cardiology* that he so successfully carried through three editions.

It would be impossible to provide the lucidity and charm of the Nadas texts or, given the magnitude of modern knowledge, for one author to rewrite the original text. Still, the present book is to some extent based on the concepts of his text. In an attempt to provide some of the consistency that characterized the Nadas texts, the clinical sections have been largely written by one person. The more technical chapters are written by local experts.

The Nadas texts were intended as a handbook for pediatricians, general practitioners, and medical students, but were designed to contain enough associated science and technology to whet the interest. In 1991 there is more information available to pediatric cardiologists than can be presented in a single volume. In response to this fact, this book has a somewhat narrower focus. Once again, the science and technology important to pediatric cardiology are presented, albeit with a Boston bias. This book is not intended to be a reference work covering all details of clinical cardiology or the basic sciences underpinning modern cardiology. Each chapter emphasizes local experience and opinions as a starting point and provides references for further study. With some exceptions, references published in the past 10 years have been favored.

For years it has been apparent that, when conducting clinical studies in pediatric cardiology, legitimate scientific criteria chosen for a particular study exclude some patients who do not appear in any other study. Often these omitted patients have the most difficult problems and, for various reasons, do not get discussed under any heading. In this book an attempt was made to present all case material encountered in a 15-year period. The goal is to account for every patient in some category. Forcing patients into familiar categories is easier said than done and carries some dangers. The possibility exists that the categories selected include unusual material and thereby slant the results in an unexpected way. This does not seem to have happened and the reader can at least be assured that no group of patients exists that is not mentioned someplace in the text. This idea is untried, at least on this scale, and, of necessity, is based on a somewhat unfamiliar hierarchical classification, but, in the editor's opinion, is preferable to statements of "personal clinical experience."

This approach would not have been possible but for the power of modern computing. Fortunately, the cardiology department of Children's Hospital in Boston has systematically computerized its data for 20 years. Unfortunately, this has been an evolving process and data computed in 1973 are not directly comparable to data recorded in 1987. Even today, techniques for output from such a system are primitive. In several chapters (i.e., Myocardial Diseases, Arrhythmias, and Malpositions), recent major changes in classification have limited the usefulness of such an approach.

In 1991, at the time of this writing, the Cardiology Department of Children's Hospital in Boston has grown to include over 75 MDs and PhDs. These individuals are invaluable resources, and have been tapped shamelessly. Our Chief, Dr. Bernardo Nadal-Ginard, and his administrative assistant, Jackie Yarian, have been consistently supportive of the whimseys of a retiring member of the department and his desire to punctuate the end of a career with a textbook honoring his long-time chief. Dr. Stephen Sanders has been a superb resource for information about echocardiography and produced most of the material on this topic. Dr. Richard Van Praagh has served as the oracle in matters anatomic and pathologic. The cooperation and willingness of all contributors to make time for this enterprise have been gratifying.

Marcia Lawson, who contributed to all the previous Nadas texts, once again provided excellent editorial and organizational expertise. Most departmental secretaries contributed, with Diane MacKinnon taking the brunt of secretarial and reference material labor. Frank Kulash solved programming questions. Emily MacIntosh Flynn produced illustrations. Marc Regnier made most of the electrocardiographic figures. Amy Itzkovitz handled correspondence related to gathering permissions. Finally, without the unfailing support of Linda Belfus, our publisher, we would have given up long ago.

DONALD C. FYLER, M.D.
Boston, Massachusetts

FOREWORD

The late Clement Andrew Smith, Professor of Pediatrics at the Harvard Medical School, founder of Neonatology and my friend and mentor, traced the evolution of pediatric cardiology at Harvard Medical School and Children's Hospital in the Foreword to the first edition of Pediatric Cardiology in 1957. A great deal of progress has been made since then. It may be worthwhile to retrace the evolution back to the source. The intellectual origins of pediatric cardiology in this century, within the English speaking world, go back to Maude Abbott, a Canadian; James Brown, an Englishman; and Helen Taussig, an American. The impetus for the development of the subspecialty, in my view, came from the epoch-making surgical accomplishment of the first successful division of a patent ductus arteriosus by Robert Edward Gross in August 1938. Organizationally, the majority of pediatric cardiologists come from Pediatrics, not from Cardiology. By contrast, Pediatric Cardiologist Surgeons, with notable exceptions, come from Cardiac Surgery, not Pediatric Surgery. Since the establishment of the Sub-board of Cardiology of the Board of Pediatrics in 1961, there are by now close to 900 Diplomates of the Sub-board.

As we are approaching the end of the century, Pediatric Cardiology Departments nationwide have many subdivisions: Surgery, Medicine, Diagnostic Catheterization, Invasive Cardiology, Radiology, Echocardiology, Electrophysiology, Epidemiology, Pathology, and, within the past 10 years or so, Molecular Cardiology. All these disciplines work together to the benefit of the patients and of research. All of these divisions are well represented in this volume by contributions by the present staff of Children's Hospital in Boston. This is an intramural multi-author text edited by Donald C. Fyler. As I said in the preface to the third edition in 1972, "Now he can worry about the next edition." And worry he did!

Finally, more personally, I wish to express my gratitude to this country, to Children's Hospital, and to Harvard Medical School for allowing me to grow; to my wife Elizabeth, who helped me and put up with me through 50 years of marriage; and to my father, a writer and journalist back in Hungary at the turn of the century, who decided that I should become a physician in America. The emblem of his magazine of a running courier appears below, as it did in previous editions.

ALEXANDER S. NADAS, M.D.
Boston, Massachusetts

Section I
Historical Perspective

Chapter 1

THE NADAS YEARS: 1949–1982

Donald C. Fyler, M.D.

This textbook, in earlier editions called *Pediatric Cardiology*, was renamed in this edition to honor Dr. Alexander Sandor Nadas. This was done to recognize Dr. Nadas' influence on the field of pediatric cardiology. While he was chief of cardiology at the Children's Hospital in Boston, he trained over 150 pediatric cardiologists, published many scientific papers, influenced the course of pediatric cardiology through professional organizations, headed several major special studies, and, perhaps most important, was a persuasive spokesman for the field. Most of the authors in this text are his trainees and all consider him to be a mentor. It is appropriate to begin this book with an outline of his career and to pay tribute to his accomplishments.

Alexander Nadas was born in Hungary. His father was a writer and journalist, his mother a prominent milliner in Budapest and in later years on Madison Ave in New York City. He attended the University of Budapest. At that time a large number of outstanding Hungarian scientists escaped to the West as the Nazi influence spread in their direction. In 1938, having completed medical training, Nadas joined the exodus, the next 6 months being spent in London pursuing his special interest in cardiology under Paul Wood. This must have been a powerful experience because Paul Wood served as the model cardiologist for Nadas for the rest of his career. At about the same time in the United States, Gross performed the first successful ligation of a patent ductus arteriosus in a child,[11] galvanizing the field of cardiac surgery. A decade later Nadas and Gross would comprise the cardiac medical and cardiac surgical teams at the Boston Children's Hospital.

Nadas left London by ship. The details of the trip were memorable at this impressionable time of life and form the basis of many of his stories. One story has the young Nadas entrusting a sizeable amount of money to a shipboard acquaintance. He was despondent when the money was not returned after docking in New York and gave up any thought of its return. Some days later the American stranger found him and returned the money, much to the surprise of the Hungarian.

One has to wonder whether the difficulties of getting started as an "F.M.G." (foreign medical graduate, later one of his favorite terms) in the U.S. was appreciated by Nadas. Whether or not, he soon found out that the medical profession in the U.S. was not patiently awaiting his arrival. Years later, Nadas was asked on many occasions to advise young immigrant physicians seeking entry into American medicine. He always painted a rather dark picture, emphasizing the necessity to become familiar with American culture and nuances of language before trying to manage a position in an American teaching hospital. He always stressed starting in a position with minimal demands and working up, as he had.

After 3–4 years in various roles, he joined the house staff at the Children's Hospital in Boston. Here he found his calling. Dr. Clement Smith reported that late on a hot and busy 1942 night on Infants Upper, surrounded by his charges, all of them at last asleep, asked, "How do you feel?" Nadas responded, "Like God!"[30]

At the completion of his pediatric training, he joined Dr. Smith at the Children's Hospital in Detroit for a brief period before settling down in a small New England town to practice pediatrics.

1

In 1949 the new professor of pediatrics, Charles A. Janeway, aware of Nadas' success as a house officer and his former interest in cardiology, invited him to leave his country practice to develop pediatric cardiology at the Boston Children's Hospital. Nadas accepted, surely not because of the meager salary, the cramped space, or the almost nonexistent financial support. It can be supposed that he understood the potential of this appointment, but neither man could have anticipated the ultimate success of this venture, begun on a shoestring. Perhaps this was the first evidence of a characteristic that marks Nadas' career. He has shown an uncanny ability to select the right course of action, to select the right person for the job, to be on the winning side. After all, according to Nadas, a Hungarian may be defined as a person who enters the revolving door after you and comes out ahead.

It is difficult to remember the primitive state of pediatric cardiology in the late 1940s and early 1950s. It seemed that all one needed to know was that pink children with congenital heart disease should be sent to Boston and blue ones to Baltimore. Gross' daring ligation of a patent ductus arteriosus[11] and Taussig and Blalock's inventive aorto-pulmonary shunt[2] showed that children with congenital heart disease can be greatly improved with surgery. For years Nadas has enjoyed reminding his fellows that while one of these operations removed a ductus arteriosus, the other created one, the upshot being that the number of ductus in the world remained constant.

At this time Cournand and Richards were on their way to the Nobel prize and, with Janet Baldwin, were in the process of demonstrating that cardiac catheterization could be used to diagnose congenital heart disease. Taussig had carried cardiac diagnosis by fluoroscopy to its limits. Castellanos[3] was still in Havana, but his idea of cardiac diagnosis by angiography had reached the mainland, and ways to make it safe were being sought. The means to make the diagnosis and to help the patient with surgery were at hand. Furthermore, the development of a pump-oxygenator that would allow surgical approaches to the inside of the heart was under way. It was in this time of ferment that Janeway asked Nadas to become a cardiologist, in effect to develop the field of pediatric cardiology in Boston.

Nadas spent one year studying adult cardiology under the tutelage of Samuel A. Levine and Lewis Dexter at the Bent Brigham Hospital. In 1950, at the Children's Hospital, he set about establishing the fundamental facts of pediatric cardiology as they could be measured at that time. Data from normal children were accumulated to use as a basis for interpretation of electrocardiogram.[1] This was the beginning of an absorbing interest in the electrocardiogram. For over 15 years Nadas read every tracing. The transition to vectorcardiograms in pediatrics actually preceded application of the technique in adult cardiology in Boston.[13,14] Ellison and Restieaux's textbook of vectorcardiography[6] was published while they were fellows in Nadas' department.

Nadas was strongly influenced by the auscultatory skills of Sam Levine. To strengthen his auscultation, Nadas examined each patient the night before cardiac catheterization. The details were dictated on the readily-found pink consultation sheets in the patients' charts. Within a few years confirmation of auscultation using phonocardiography was possible, and a fruitful association with Maurice Rappaport, an engineer interested in medical instrumentation, developed and put the art of auscultation in pediatrics on a scientific basis.[23,26]

Nadas' auscultatory observations, as recorded on the pink sheets, formed the basis of many papers and culminated in his best-selling textbook published in three editions, 1957, 1962, 1972, and Ongley and Nadas' monograph, *Heart Sounds and Murmurs*.[23] Nadas' interest in auscultation continues to the present with his weekly stethoscope rounds.

In that era it was gospel that the presence of a diastolic rumble indicated mitral stenosis. Many children were erroneously diagnosed as having mitral valve disease until Nadas collected enough observations in children with left-to-right shunting lesions to dispel "The Myth of Lutembacher's Syndrome."[18] The observations recorded at the nightly documentation sessions were reviewed and a diagnosis recorded. At first these diagnostic impressions were more often wrong than right!

From the beginning in 1950 Nadas held a weekly conference initially reviewing patients seen in clinic the preceding week and later adding the discussion of patients scheduled to have surgery. His wit and caustic comments in these sessions are legendary ("I don't get ulcers; I give them!"), and, without doubt, much that is presented in this book arose from these vigorous discussions. His humor and jokes tempered the discussion, stimulating the students and fellows to new knowledge. No one slept! These sessions continue to the present time; the repartee is still entertaining.

Rounds on the cardiac division were equally provocative, and memorable episodes are cherished by most who participated. Once when confronted with students and house staff, all of whom came from different countries, he announced that while they seemed to be a version of the United Nations, they were, at the risk of his wrath, going to function better. He was virtually the only visiting physician for many years, and, even when others were nominally in charge, he was aware of all that went on Division 35, dropping in unexpectedly at odd times and maintaining frequent telephone contact, even on weekends.

Despite a remarkable command of the American version of the English language, Nadas never lost his Hungarian accent or his European manners. One fellow watching him charm a visiting lady physician was heard to mumble "Oh, to be Continental!" The charm, wit, and ability to see the answer to difficult problems resulted in an appointment to the Board of Trustees of the hospital in later years. To this date, long after "retiring," he is still sought to give opinions on matters of importance to the Children's Hospital. A year ago the grateful Board endowed the Alexander Nadas Chair in Pediatric Cardiology at the Harvard Medical School and the Children's Hospital.

There are 222 publications listed in his bibliography. Using the recorded notes from the pink sheets in the hospital record, Nadas put together the basic diagnostic and natural history facts for most major pediatric cardiac problems, for example: paroxysmal atrial tachycardia,[19] pulmonary stenosis,[29] ventricular septal defects,[8] total anomalous pulmonary venous drainage,[12] patent ductus in infancy,[28] hypoplastic left heart syndrome,[21] congenital complete heart block,[24] aortic stenosis,[22] transposition of the great arteries,[20,25] and many others in the same vein of clinical description. The modern understanding of many congenital heart lesions began with these papers. The coauthors now hold positions of responsibility around the U.S.

Early, he became interested in the possibility of diagnosis without the need for cardiac catheterization using estimations of ventricular pressure by electrocardiographic, vectorcardiographic, and phonocardiographic methods in patients with pulmonary stenosis or aortic stenosis.[4,9,13,15,29] This interest presaged by many years the present-day trend of avoiding cardiac catheterization.

In the 1960s Nadas became involved in the multicentered Natural History Study of Congenital Heart Defects, a study designed to provide the data needed to plan treatment for several of the more common defects. The success of the project is evident in the American Heart Association monograph,[17] edited by Nadas, which documents the results. The study has been revived, and the course of these patients has been followed to the present time,[31] over 30 years after its inception.

Nadas encouraged Abraham Rudolph, one of his early fellows, to study physiology at the Harvard Medical School. When Rudolph returned, he assumed responsibility for the cardiac catheterization laboratory at the Children's Hospital; since then, physiology has been a major focus of Nadas' department. In the early 1960s Rudolph and Nadas studied the role of a patent ductus arteriosus in the respiratory distress syndrome.[27] Thus began an interest that resulted in a multicenter study, headed by Nadas, to evaluate the effect of indomethacin on patent ductus arteriosus in premature infants,[5,10] an effect that had been pointed out earlier.[16]

Nadas readily grasped the complexities of delivery of medical care to children with heart disease. The New England Regional Infant Cardiac Program[7] was a successful model for the integration of medical services for infants with critical congenital heart disease. This program encompassed all hospitals in New England providing tertiary care to infants critically ill with heart disease and continued for over a decade. During this time the mortality for these babies fell by over 20%. This organization of pediatric care has been adopted in various modifications in several countries.

Although not a technological person, Nadas has recognized the value of new instrumentation as it became available and echocardiography was no exception. With his encouragement, three of his fellow taught themselves echocardiography in much the same way Nadas learned cardiology and have recently published a textbook on pediatric cardiac echocardiography (Williams, Bierman, Sanders[32]).

While Nadas' influence on the development of pediatric cardiology is easily documented, his imprint on the field through his fellows will be his greatest legacy. There are currently over 150 graduates of his fellowship program in virtually every major pediatric cardiac center in the U.S. as well as in many foreign countries.

Because of rapid growth, the cardiology group at the Children's Hospital was declared a Division of the Department of Medicine (1966), and later, an independent Department of Cardiology (1969). In 1950, there was a secretary, a technician, a new Sanborn ECG machine, one cardiac clinic a week, and the services of a catheterization team from the Peter Bent Brigham Hospital one day a week. Fifty cardiac catheterizations were carried out. By 1982 when Nadas "retired" (he still comes to the hospital several days a week), there were 20 staff physicians and over 100 personnel involved in the department. There were 500 catheterizations, some thousands of electrocardiograms, echocardiograms, and several hundred operations performed yearly. There was a cardiac ward, a cardiac intensive care unit, and cardiac clinics every day in the week, sometimes twice a day. At the present time (1991) the number of professional personnel, procedures, and patients has doubled again (see chapter 18, Trends).

One of Nadas' outstanding qualities has been his ability to select the right person at the right time. Most of the physicians appointed to his staff later went on to influential positions in pediatric cardiology elsewhere. Most of the major cities in the United States have at least one of his graduates. While only partly Nadas' responsibility, the appointment of Aldo Castaneda as Chief of Cardiovascular Surgery and the appointment of Bernardo Nadal-Ginard to be Nadas' successor as Chief of

Cardiology have been notably successful. Under their direction the Nadas' legacy has mushroomed and will be a permanent feature of the Boston Children's Hospital and the field of pediatric cardiology for many years to come.

In this brief review, I have attempted to highlight Alexander Nadas' career. If this man's career is to be summed up, the one feature that describes his phenomenal success is his ability to choose the right course, to choose the right person to do the job, and to convince everyone involved through wit and charm that he was right—to see the solution! Few physicians have this talent.

All of us are grateful to have been exposed to this remarkable man and take this occasion to honor him by naming this book *Nadas' Pediatric Cardiology*.

REFERENCES

1. Alimurung MM, Joseph LG, Nadas AS, et al: Unipolar precordial and extremity electrocardiogram in normal infants and children. Circulation 4:420–429, 1951.
2. Blalock A, Taussig HB: The surgical treatment of malformations of the heart. JAMA 128:189–202, 1945.
3. Castellanos A, Pereires R, Garcia A: La angio-cardiografia radio-opaca. Arch Soc Estud Clin Habana 31:9–10, 1937.
4. Cayler GG, Ongley PA, Nadas AS: Relation of systolic pressure in the right ventricle to the electrocardiogram. N Engl J Med 258:979–982, 1958.
5. Ellison RE, Nadas AS: Indomethacin and patent ductus arteriosus in premature infants: Report from the collaborative study in the United States. Pediatr Cardiol 4(Suppl 2):93–97, 1983.
6. Ellison RC, Restieaux NJ: Vectorcardiography in Congenital Heart Disease: A Method of Estimating Severity. Philadelphia, W.B. Saunders, 1972.
7. Fyler DC, Buckley LP, Hellenbrand WE, et al: Report of the New England Regional Infant Cardiac Program. Pediatrics 65:375–461, 1980.
8. Fyler DC, Rudolph AM, Wittenborg MH, et al: Ventricular septal defect in infants and children: A correlation of clinical, physiological, and autopsy data. Circulation 18:833–851, 1958.
9. Gamboa R, Hugenholtz PG, Nadas AS: Comparison of electrocardiogram and vectorcardiogram in congenital aortic stenosis. Br Heart J 27:344–354, 1965.
10. Gersony WM, Peckham GJ, Ellison RE, et al: Effects of indomethacin in premature infants with patent ductus arteriosus. J Pediatr 102:895–906, 1983.
11. Gross RE, Hubbard JP: Surgical ligation of a patent ductus arteriosus: Report of first successful case. JAMA 112:729–731, 1939.
12. Guntheroth WG, Nadas AS, Gross RE: Transposition of the pulmonary veins. Circulation 31:117–137, 1958.
13. Hugenholtz PG, Liebman J: The normal orthogonal vectorcardiogram in 100 normal children (Frank system) and comparative data recorded by the cube system. Circulation 26:891–901, 1962.
14. Liebman J, Nadas AS: The vectorcardiogram in the differential diagnosis of atrial septal defect. Circulation 22:956–975, 1960.
15. Lees MH, Hauck AJ, Starkey GWB, et al: Congenital aortic stenosis: Operative indications and surgical results. Br Heart J 24:31–38, 1962.
16. Nadas AS: Patent ductus revisited. (Editorial commenting on two articles in same issue concerning pharmacologic closure of patent ductus arteriosus.) N Engl J Med 295:563–565, 1976.
17. Nadas AS (ed): Report of the joint study on the natural history of congenital heart defects. PS, AS, VSD: Clinical course and indirect assessment. Circulation 56(suppl 1):1–87, 1987.
18. Nadas AS, Alimurung MM: Apical diastolic murmurs in congenital heart disease: The myth of Lutembacher's syndrome. Am Heart J 42:691–706, 1952.
19. Nadas AS, Daeschner CW, Roth A, et al: Paroxysmal tachycardia in infants and children. Study of 41 cases. Pediatrics 9:167–181, 1952.
20. Noonan JA, Nadas AS, Rudolph AM, et al: Transposition of the great arteries: A correlation of clinical, physiologic and autopsy data. N Engl J Med 263:593–596, 637–642, 684–692, 739–744, 1960.
21. Noonan JA, Nadas AS: The hypoplastic left heart syndrome: An analysis of 101 cases. Pediatr Clin North Am 5:1029–1056, 1958.
22. Ongley PA, Nadas AS, Paul MH, et al: Aortic stenosis in infants and children. Pediatrics 21:207–221, 1958.
23. Ongley PA, Sprague HB, Rappaport MH, et al: Heart Sounds and Murmurs: A Clinical and Phonocardiographic Study. New York, Grune & Stratton, 1960.
24. Paul MH, Rudolph AM, Nadas AS: Congenital complete atrioventricular block: Problems of clinical assessment. Circulation 18:183–190, 1958.
25. Plauth WH, Nadas AS, Bernhard WF, et al: Changing hemodynamics in patients with transposition of the great arteries. Circulation 42:131–142, 1970.
26. Rappaport MB, Sprague HB: Physiologic and physical laws that govern auscultation and their clinical application. Am Heart J 21:257–318, 1941.
27. Rudolph AM, Drorbaugh JE, Auld PAM, et al: Studies on the circulation in the neonatal period: The circulation in the respiratory distress syndrome. Pediatrics 27:551, 1961.
28. Rudolph AM, Mayer FE, Nadas AS, et al: Patent ductus arteriosus: A clinical and hemodynamic study of 23 patients in the first year of life. Pediatrics 22:892–904, 1958.
29. Silverman BK, Nadas AS, Wittenborg MH, et al: Pulmonary stenosis with intact ventricular septum: Correlation of clinical and physiologic data, with operative results. Am J Med 20:53–64, 1956.
30. Smith CA: The Children's Hospital of Boston: "Built Better Than They Knew". Boston, Little, Brown, 1983, p. 121.
31. Weidman W, et al: Natural history study of congenital heart defects III. To be published fall 1991.
32. Williams RE, Bierman FZ, Sanders SP: Echocardiographic Diagnosis of Cardiac Malformations. Boston, Little, Brown, 1986.

Section II
Developmental Anatomy

Chapter 2

EMBRYOLOGY*

Richard Van Praagh, M.D.

Embryology is important to pediatric cardiology as a means of understanding. Embryology makes possible the comprehension of complex congenital heart disease, which in turn facilitates its accurate clinical diagnosis. Embryology also helps to clarify both the morphogenesis (pathogenesis) and the etiology (basic causes) of cardiac malformations.

DEFINITION

In man, embryology may be defined as developmental biology from conception to the end of the second month of life, i.e., from conception to the end of the 8th week.

THE FIRST WEEK OF LIFE

The salient events of the first week of life from 0 to 7 days (Fig. 1) are (1) ovulation, (2) fertilization, (3) segmentation, (4) blastocyst formation, and (5) the beginning of implantation.

THE SECOND WEEK OF LIFE

The principal developments of the second week of life, from 8 to 14 days, (Fig. 2) are (1) completion of implantation, (2) bilaminar disc formation, consisting of ectoderm and endoderm, (3) develop-

*This chapter is based on the personal study of embryos from the following sources: the Minot Collection, Harvard Medical School, Boston; the Carnegie Collection, Carnegie Institution, Baltimore; chick embryology, morphologic and experimental, the Carnegie Institution, Baltimore, and The Children's Hospital, Boston; *iv/iv* mouse embryology, Dartmouth Medical School, Hanover, New Hampshire; and the literature.

ment of the amniotic cavity, (4) appearance of the yolk sac, and (5) the elaboration of primitive villi of the developing placenta. It is noteworthy that during the first two weeks of life, man has no heart and no vascular system.

THE THIRD WEEK OF LIFE

From the cardiovascular standpoint, the main events of the third week of life, from 15–21 days, may be summarized as follows (Figs. 3–5):

1. In man, the **mesoderm** develops from the ectoderm on the 15th day of life (Fig. 3). It is from the mesoderm that the cardiovascular system is formed.

2. The **cardiogenic crescent** of precardiac mesoderm, the immediate precursor of the heart, appears on the 18th day of life (Fig. 4A).

3. The **intra-embryonic celom** also develops on the 18th day of life (Fig. 5). Cavitation of the mesoderm forms the intra-embryonic celom, from which are derived all of the body cavities—pericardial, pleural, and peritoneal.

4. The **straight heart tube**, or preloop stage, normally develops by 20 days of age (Fig. 4B). By analogy with chick embryos, the heart beat in man probably begins at the straight tube stage, or at the early D-loop or L-loop stage (Fig. 4C and D).

5. **Cardiac loop formation**, normally to the right (D-loop formation) and abnormally to the left (L-loop formation), begins by 21 days of age (Fig. 4C and D).

THE FOURTH WEEK OF LIFE

The main features of cardiovascular development from 22–28 days are the following:

5

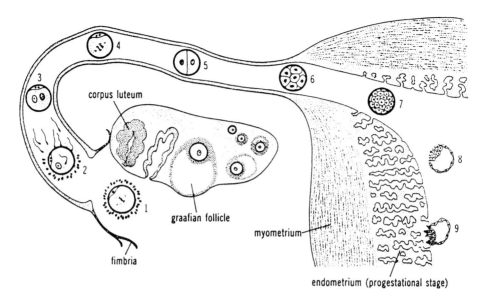

Figure 1. Schematic representation of the events taking place during the first week of human development. (1) Oocyte immediately after ovulation. (2) Fertilization approximately 12–24 hours after ovulation. (3) Stage of the male and female pronuclei. (4) Spindle of the first mitotic division. (5) Two-cell stage (approximately 30 hours of age). (6) Morula containing 12–16 blastomeres (approximately 3 days of age). (7) Advanced morula stage reaching the uterine lumen (approximately 4 days of age). (8) Early blastocyst stage (approximately 4½ days of age). The zona pellucida has now disappeared. (9) Early phase of implantation (blastocyst approximately 6 days of age). The ovary shows the stages of the transformation between a primary follicle and a graafian follicle as well as a corpus luteum. The uterine endometrium is depicted in the progestational stage. (From Langman J: Medical Embryology, 4th ed. Baltimore, Williams & Wilkins, 1981, with permission.)

1. Normally, D-loop formation is completed (Fig. 6, horizon XI).

2. The development of the morphologically left ventricle and of the morphologically right ventricle begins (Fig. 6, horizon XIII).

3. The circulation commences.

4. Cardiovascular septation is initiated.

5. The evolution of the aortic arches begins (Figs. 7–9).

Streeter's **horizons** (Fig. 10) are indicated by Roman numerals in Figure 6. Each horizon is a two-day time interval. In order to obtain the approximate age of the embryo, double the horizon number. For example, horizon XI indicates a time interval that begins on day 22. Because each horizon is two days long, horizon XI extends from days 22–24 (Fig. 10). Embryonic lengths (in mm) are also given in Figure 10, and it is readily possible to convert the length of a normal human embryo into both the developmental stage (horizon) and approximate age.

Both the left and the right ventricles develop by evagination or outpouching from the primary heart tube, beginning at 22–24 days (horizon XI, Fig. 6, left). By 26–28 days (horizon XIII, Fig. 6, right), development of the left ventricle is more advanced than that of the right (Fig. 6, right).

True circulation (as opposed to ebb and flow) is thought to begin in man at this stage (26–28 days, horizon XIII, Fig. 6, right). This is known as the "in-series circulation" because the blood goes from the morphologically right atrium to the morphologically left atrium, to the left ventricle, to the right ventricle, and to the truncus arteriosus (arterial trunk) (Fig. 6, right). The in-series circulation is similar to that which persists in tricuspid atresia.

At the beginning of the fourth week, the first pair of aortic arches has formed (Fig. 7). At this stage, the ventricle (future left ventricle) of the D-bulboventricular loop is ventral (anterior) to the proximal bulbus cordis (future right ventricle) (Fig. 7, right). Thus, early in D-loop formation, the left ventricle is anterior to (ventral to) the right ventricle. Hence, among children with congenital heart disease, the anterior ventricle is not necessarily the right ventricle, although usually it is.

By the 26th day of life, the first pair of aortic arches (earlier mandibular arteries) have involuted completely, or nearly completely (Fig. 8). The second and third aortic arches have formed, and the fourth and sixth aortic arches are beginning to form (Fig. 8). A large communication between the respiratory and gastrointestinal tracts is present, i.e., a large tracheoesophageal "fistula" is normal at this stage (Fig. 8, right).

By the end of the fourth week (28 days, Fig. 9), aortic arches 1 and 2 have involuted. Aortic arches 3 and 4 are present (Fig. 9). Aortic arches 5 are incomplete bilaterally. Aortic arches 6 are in the

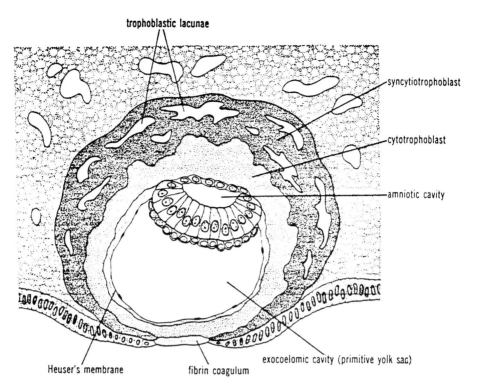

Figure 2. The second week of life: the implanted bilaminar disc consisting of ectoderm and endoderm, prior to the appearance of the mesoderm. (From Langman J: Medical Embryology, 4th ed. Baltimore, Williams & Wilkins, 1981, with permission.)

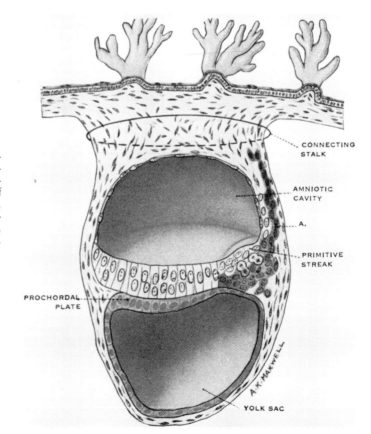

Figure 3. The appearance of the mesoderm, from which the cardiovascular system will arise, at 15 days of age. The mesoderm (meaning "middle skin") buds off from the ectoderm. (From Hamilton WJ, Mossman HW: Human Embryology: Prenatal Development of Form and Function, 4th ed. Baltimore, Williams & Wilkins, 1972, with permission.)

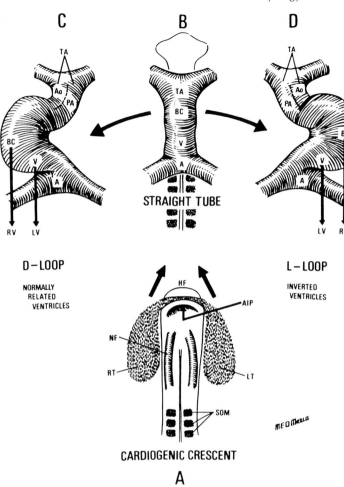

Figure 4. Cardiac loop formation: **A,** Cardiogenic crescent of precardiac mesoderm. **B,** Straight heart tube or preloop stage. **C,** D-loop, with solitus (noninverted) ventricles. **D,** L-loop with inverted (mirror-image) ventricles. A, atrium; AIP, anterior intestinal portal; Ao, aorta; BC, bulbus cordis; HF, head fold; LT, left; LV, morphologically left ventricle; NF, neural fold; PA, (main) pulmonary artery; RT, right; RV, morphologically right ventricle; SOM, somites; TA, truncus arteriosus. (From Van Praagh R, Weinberg PM, Matsuoka R, et al: Malpositions of the heart. In Adams FH, Emmanouilides GC (eds): Heart Disease in Infants, Children and Adolescents, 4th ed. Baltimore, Williams & Wilkins, 1983, with permission.)

process of forming (complete on the right and incomplete on the left, Fig. 9). Both pulmonary artery branches are present, as is the common pulmonary vein (Fig. 9, left).

THE FIFTH WEEK OF LIFE

The major cardiovascular developments between days 29 and 35 may be summarized as follows:

1. The left ventricle, right ventricle, and ventricular septum continue to grow and develop (Fig. 11).

2. There is approximation of the aorta to the interventricular foramen, mitral valve, and left ventricle (Figs. 11 and 12).

3. Separation of the ascending aorta and main pulmonary artery occurs (Fig. 12, horizon XVIa, i.e., days 32–33).

4. Separation of the mitral and tricuspid valves is accomplished (Fig. 12, horizon XVII, i.e., days 34–36).

5. The right ventricle enlarges (compare Fig. 11, left, with Fig. 11, right).

6. In association with right ventricular enlargement, the muscular ventricular septum moves from right to left beneath the atrioventricular canal (compare Fig. 11, left, with Fig. 11, right).

7. The tricuspid valve now opens into the right ventricle (Fig. 11, right, and Fig. 12, horizon XVII).

8. The ostium primum is closed by tissue from the endocardial cushions of the atrioventricular canal (Fig. 13), thereby separating the atria.

9. The ventricular apex swings horizontally leftward.

10. From days 30–36, the pulmonary valve moves from posterior and to the left of the developing aortic valve (30–32 days, horizon XV, Fig. 12), to a position beside and to the left of the aortic valve (days 32–33, horizon XVIa, Fig. 12), then somewhat anterior and to the left of the aortic valve (days 33–34, horizon XVIb, Fig. 12), and finally to its normal anterior position to the left of the aortic valve (days 34–36, horizon XVII, Fig. 12).

Text continues on page 14.

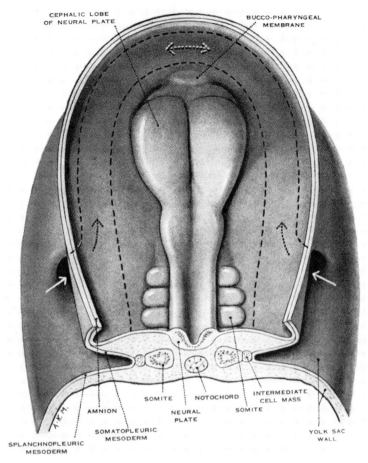

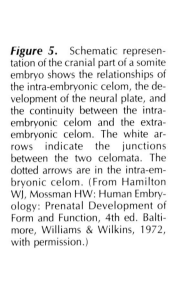

Figure 5. Schematic representation of the cranial part of a somite embryo shows the relationships of the intra-embryonic celom, the development of the neural plate, and the continuity between the intra-embryonic celom and the extra-embryonic celom. The white arrows indicate the junctions between the two celomata. The dotted arrows are in the intra-embryonic celom. (From Hamilton WJ, Mossman HW: Human Embryology: Prenatal Development of Form and Function, 4th ed. Baltimore, Williams & Wilkins, 1972, with permission.)

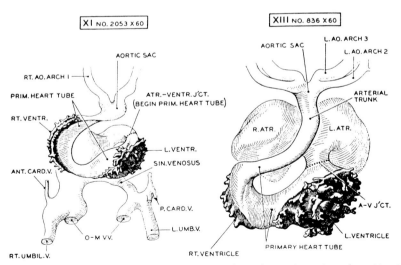

Figure 6. Formation of the ventricles. **Left,** Horizon XI, 22–24 days of age. Carnegie embryo No. 2053, original reconstruction of cardiovascular lumen × 60 magnification. **Right,** Horizon XIII, 26–28 days of age, Carnegie embryo No. 836, original reconstruction of cardiovascular lumen × 60 magnification. ANT. CARD. V., anterior cardinal vein; ATR.-VENTR. J'CT., atrioventricular junction; L. ATR., morphologically left atrium; LT. Ao. ARCH, left aortic arch; L. UMB. V., left umbilical vein; L. VENTR., morphologically left ventricle; O-M VV., omphalomesenteric veins; P. CARD. V., posterior cardinal vein; PRIM., primitive; RT. AO., right aorta; R. ATR., morphologically right atrium; RT. VENTR., morphologically right ventricle; RT. UMBIL. V., right umbilical vein; SIN. VENOSUS, sinus venosus. (From Streeter GL: Developmental horizons in human embryos, age groups XI to XXIII. Embryology Reprint. Washington, D.C., Carnegie Institution, Vol. II, 1951, with permission.)

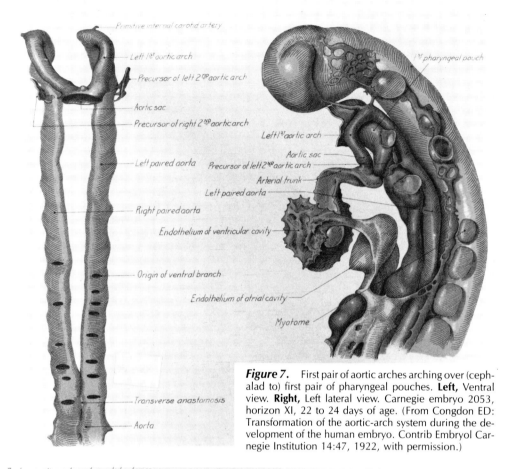

Figure 7. First pair of aortic arches arching over (cephalad to) first pair of pharyngeal pouches. **Left,** Ventral view. **Right,** Left lateral view. Carnegie embryo 2053, horizon XI, 22 to 24 days of age. (From Congdon ED: Transformation of the aortic-arch system during the development of the human embryo. Contrib Embryol Carnegie Institution 14:47, 1922, with permission.)

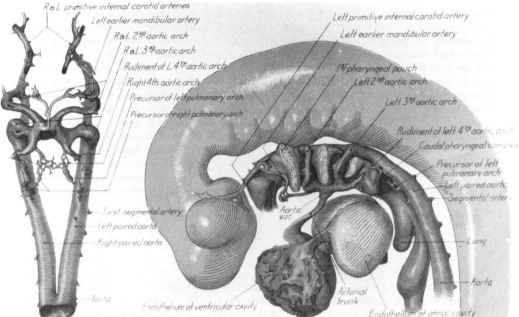

Figure 8. Second and third pairs of aortic arches. **Left,** Ventral view. **Right,** Left lateral view. Carnegie embryo 836, early horizon XIII, 26 days of age. Each aortic arch passes cephalad to its pharyngeal pouch. Arches 1 are involuting. Arches 4 and 6 are just forming. (From Congdon ED: Transformation of the aortic-arch system during the development of the human embryo. Contrib Embryol Carnegie Institution 14:47, 1922, with permission.)

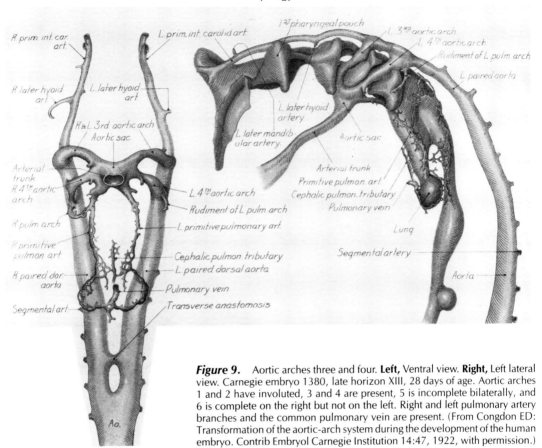

Figure 9. Aortic arches three and four. **Left,** Ventral view. **Right,** Left lateral view. Carnegie embryo 1380, late horizon XIII, 28 days of age. Aortic arches 1 and 2 have involuted, 3 and 4 are present, 5 is incomplete bilaterally, and 6 is complete on the right but not on the left. Right and left pulmonary artery branches and the common pulmonary vein are present. (From Congdon ED: Transformation of the aortic-arch system during the development of the human embryo. Contrib Embryol Carnegie Institution 14:47, 1922, with permission.)

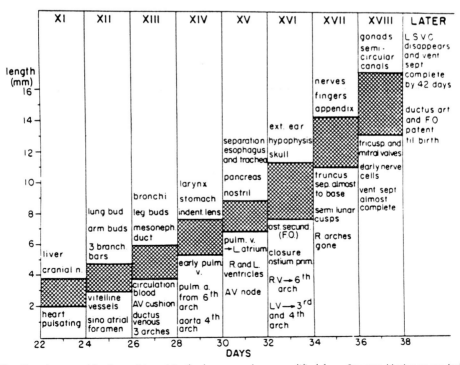

Figure 10. Developmental horizons (stages) in the human embryo, modified from Streeter. Horizons are indicated at the top in Roman numerals. Embryonic ages are shown at the bottom in days. Embryonic lengths are given at the left in millimeters (mm). Salient features of each horizon are indicated. (From Neill CA: Development of the pulmonary veins with reference to the embryology of anomalies of pulmonary venous return. Pediatrics 18:880, 1956, with permission.)

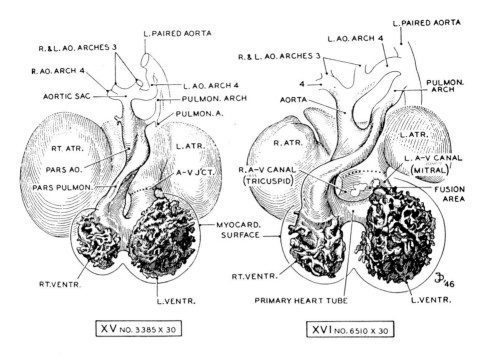

Figure 11. Fifth week of life. **Left,** Horizon XV, 30–32 days of age, Carnegie embryo 3385, original reconstruction of cardiovascular lumen × 30. **Right,** Horizon XVI, Carnegie embryo 6510, original reconstruction of cardiovascular lumen × 30. Abbreviations as in previous figures. (From Streeter GL: Developmental horizons in human embryos, age groups XI to XXIII. Embryology Reprint. Washington, D.C., Carnegie Institution, Vol. II, 1951, with permission.)

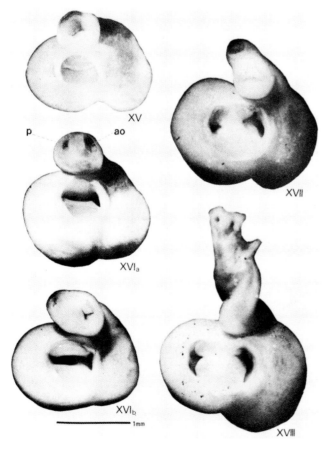

Figure 12. Dissections of human embryonic hearts, viewed from above (dorsal aspect), to show positional changes of pulmonary valve (p) relative to aortic valve (ao) from horizons XV to XVIII. Top of figure is ventral (anterior), bottom of figure is dorsal (posterior), the developing pulmonary valve (p) is to the embryo's left, and the developing aortic valve (ao) is to the embryo's right. The atria have been removed to show partitioning of the atrioventricular canal. At the conotruncal junction, the major part of the movement takes place on the pulmonary side of the outlet (p). The aortic valve (ao) keeps on facing the anteriorly migrating pulmonary valve (p), but otherwise the aortic valve moves only slightly. (From Asami I: Partitioning of the arterial end of the embryonic heart. In Van Praagh R, Takao A (eds): Etiology and Morphogenesis of Congenital Heart Disease. Mount Kisco, NY, Futura Publishing Co., 1980, p. 51, with permission.)

Figure 13. Closure of ostium primum by tissue from the endocardial cushions of the atrioventricular (AV) canal, horizon XVI, 33 days of age, Harvard embryo 736, sagittal section number 138, borax carmine and Lyons blue stain, original magnification × 130, right lateral view. Tissue of the superior cushion (SC) and inferior cushion (IC) of the atrioventricular canal has fused with the atrial septum, which is composed of venous or sinus venosus tissue (SVT), this fusion closing the ostium primum. CoS, coronary sinus; CPV, common pulmonary vein; E, esophagus; LA, left atrium; T, trachea. (From Van Praagh R, Corsini I: Cor triatriatum: pathologic anatomy and consideration of morphogenesis based on 13 postmortem cases and a study of normal development of the pulmonary vein and atrial septum in 83 human embryos. Am Heart J 78:379–405, 1969, with permission.)

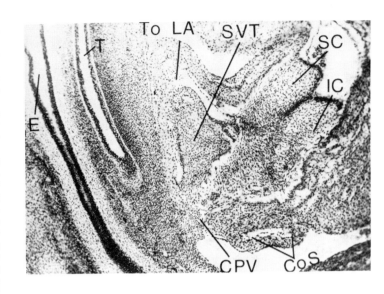

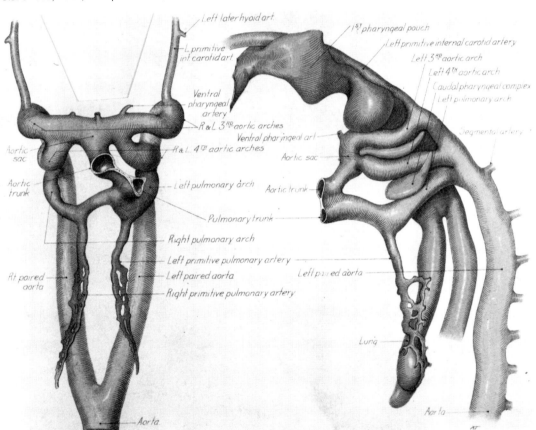

Figure 14. Aortic arches 3, 4, and 6. **Left,** Ventral view. **Right,** Left lateral view. Carnegie embryo 1121, horizon XVII, 34–36 days of age. Distal aortopulmonary septation is well seen (left). Both ductus arteriosi (sixth arches) and both dorsal aortae are still intact. (From Congdon ED: Transformation of the aortic-arch system during the development of the human embryo. Contrib Embryol Carnegie Institution 14:47, 1922, with permission.)

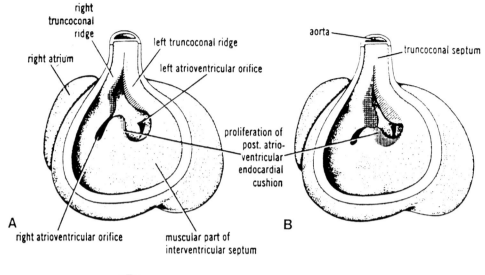

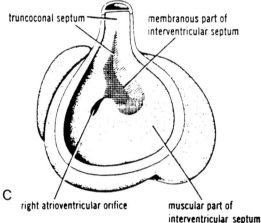

Figure 15. Closure of the conal (infundibular) septum and the interventricular foramen. **A,** 6 weeks. **B,** Beginning of seventh week. **C,** End of seventh week. (From Langman J: Medical Embryology, 4th ed. Baltimore, Williams & Wilkins, 1981, with permission.)

Hence, the morphogenetic movement of the pulmonary valve is from posterior to anterior, to the left of the aortic valve (Fig. 12). The aortic valve moves virtually not at all, except that it keeps on facing the anteriorly moving pulmonary valve (Fig. 12). It is thought that the reason for the normal anterior morphogenetic movement of the pulmonary valve is the normal growth and development of the subpulmonary infundibulum, which carries the pulmonary valve superiorly and anteriorly. Conversely, the normal lack of morphogenetic movement of the aortic valve appears to be due to the normal lack of growth and development of the subaortic conus.

The semilunar interrelationship at 30–32 days in the human embryo is very similar to that of **D-transposition of the great arteries** (horizon XV, Fig. 12). At days 32–33, the semilunar interrelationship is side-by-side, similar to that of the **Taussig-Bing malformation** (horizon XVIa, Fig. 12). At days 33–34, the semilunar interrelationship is very similar to that of **tetralogy of Fallot** (horizon XVIb,

Fig. 12). Because the pulmonary valve has been carried from posterior to anterior on the left-hand side of the ascending aorta, the pulmonary artery must pass in the opposite direction—from anterior to posterior on the left of the ascending aorta—as it passes from the pulmonary valve, proximally, to the pulmonary bifurcation, distally (horizon XVIII, Fig. 12). This anterior-to-posterior course of the main pulmonary artery makes it look as though normally related great arteries twist around each other. However, it is thought that the great arteries really are passively **untwisting** about each other as the pulmonary artery passes from the anterior pulmonary valve to the posterior pulmonary bifurcation (horizon XVIII, Fig. 12).

Thus, the fifth week is when the primitive, single, in-series circulation—that suffices for water-"breathing" fish—is converted into the definitive, double, in-parallel circulations that characterize air-breathing mammals. Cardiovascular septation is nearly completed. However, the interventricular foramen (ventricular septal defect) is still patent.

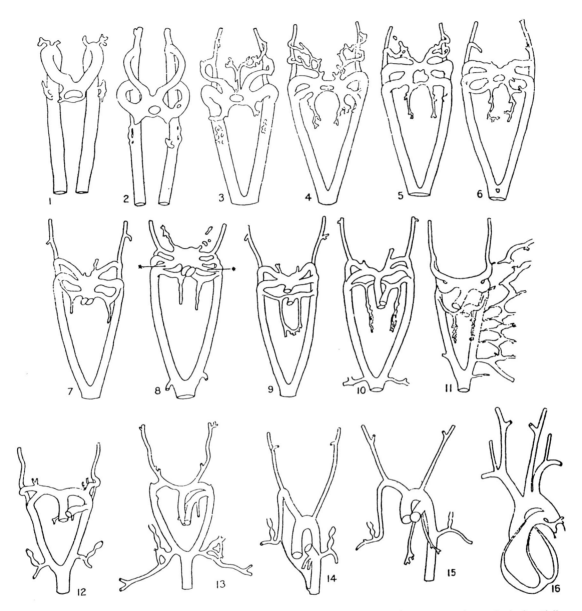

Figure 16. Development of the aortic arches. In the earliest stage, only the first arch is present, whereas in the last (full-term fetus), the vessels have acquired nearly their adult form. (From Congdon ED: Transformation of the aortic-arch system during the development of the human embryo. Contrib Embryol Carnegie Institution 14:47, 1922, with permission.)

By the end of the fifth week, aortic arches 3, 4, and 6 are present (Fig. 14). Both ductus arteriosi and both dorsal aortae are still intact.

THE SIXTH AND SEVENTH WEEKS OF LIFE

The main cardiovascular developments between the 36th and the 49th days of life are (1) closure of the conal (infundibular) septum and (2) closure of the membranous part of the ventricular septum (Fig. 15). The ventricular septum usually is closed between 38 and 45 days of age. Closure of the

interventricular foramen can be delayed until after birth, when it is known as spontaneous (i.e., surgically unassisted) ventricular septal defect closure.

DEVELOPMENT OF THE AORTIC ARCHES

The evolution of the aortic arches is summarized in Figure 16. This diagram is helpful for the understanding of **vascular rings**.

In diagram 8 (Fig. 16), the asterisks indicate the presence of **fifth arches** bilaterally; these are present in about a third of embryos at this stage.

There are **four normal interruptions** of the aortic arch system: (1) involution of the right ductus arteriosus or 6th arch (diagram 12, Fig. 16); (2) and (3) involution of the ductus caroticus bilaterally, i.e., involution of the dorsal aortae between arches 3 and 4, bilaterally (diagram 13, Fig. 16); and (4) involution of the right dorsal aorta distal to the seventh intersegmental artery (part of the embryonic right subclavian artery), resulting in a left aortic arch (diagram 14, Fig. 16).

What determines whether one has a left aortic arch or a right aortic arch? The answer is: whichever **dorsal aorta** persists. If the left dorsal aorta persists, one has a left aortic arch. If the right dorsal aorta persists and the left involutes, one has a right aortic arch. If both dorsal aortae persist, a **double aortic arch** results.

If the right dorsal aorta involutes proximal or cephalad to the seventh intersegmental artery (instead of distal to this artery), the result is an **aberrant right subclavian artery**, which arises as the last brachiocephalic artery from the top of the descending thoracic aorta.

It has often been said (erroneously) that whichever aortic arch is present depends on which fourth aortic arch (left or right) persists. Therefore, it is helpful to know that **both** fourth aortic arches (left and right) normally always persist (Fig. 16), no matter whether a left or a right aortic arch is present. Thus, which aortic arch is present is determined not by the fourth or aortic arches *per se*, but by which dorsal aorta persists and which involutes (diagram 14, Fig. 16).

SUMMARY

Cardiogenesis begins on the 18th day of life with the formation of the cardiogenic crescent or pre-cardiac mesoderm (Fig. 4A), and normally is completed by the 45th day of life, with the formation of the membranous part of the ventricular septum (Fig. 15). Cardiovascular maturation continues until well after birth.

REFERENCES

1. Asami I: Partitioning of the arterial end of the embryonic heart. In Van Praagh R, Takao A (eds): Etiology and Morphogenesis of Congenital Heart Disease. Mount Kisco, NY, Futura Publishing Co., 1980, p. 51.
2. Congdon ED: Transformation of the aortic-arch system during the development of the human embryo. Contrib Embryol Carnegie Institution 14:47, 1922.
3. Hamilton WJ, Mossman HW: Human Embryology: Prenatal Development of Form and Function, 4th ed. Baltimore, Williams & Wilkins, 1972.
4. Langman J: Human development—normal and abnormal. In Medical Embryology, 4th ed. Baltimore, Williams & Wilkins, 1981.
5. Neill CA: Development of the pulmonary veins with reference to the embryology of anomalies of pulmonary venous return. Pediatrics 18:880, 1956.
6. Streeter GL: Developmental horizons in human embryos, age groups XI to XXIII. Embryology Reprint. Washington, D.C., Carnegie Institute, Vol. II, 1951.
7. Van Praagh R, Corsini I: Cor triatriatum: pathologic anatomy and consideration of morphogenesis based on 13 postmortem cases and a study of normal development of the pulmonary vein and atrial septum in 83 human embryos. Am Heart J 78:379–405, 1969.
8. Van Praagh R, Weinberg PM, Matsuoka R, et al: Malpositions of the heart. In Adams FH, Emmanouilides GC (eds): Heart Disease in Infants, Children and Adolescents, 4th ed. Baltimore, Williams & Wilkins, 1983, pp. 530–580.

Chapter 3

MORPHOLOGIC ANATOMY

Richard Van Praagh, M.D., and Stella Van Praagh, M.D.

An understanding of normal morphologic anatomy is basic to the accurate diagnosis of congenital heart disease. One of the diagnostic problems posed by congenital heart disease is that any cardiac chamber, valve, or vessel can be virtually "anywhere." This means that the diagnostic identification of the cardiac chambers cannot be based on relative position (right-sided or left-sided) or function (venous or arterial, pulmonary or systemic), because position and function are variables in congenital heart disease. A ventricle may be described as left-sided and arterial, but the question then arises, which ventricle is it—the morphologically left or the morphologically right? The diagnostic problem is that a **positionally** left ventricle may be a **morphologically** left ventricle or a **morphologically** right ventricle. Morphologic anatomic identification is the cornerstone of accurate diagnosis.

THE ATRIA

The anatomic features of the morphologically right atrium and the morphologically left atrium are presented in Figures 1 to 4, and their morphologic anatomic features are summarized in Table 1.

The Morphologically Right Atrium

The **external appearance** of the right atrium is highly characteristic (Fig. 1). The appendage is broad or triangular. It resembles "Snoopy, looking to his left" (Fig. 1). The "bridge of Snoopy's nose" is formed by the tinea sagittalis (see p. 18). Normally, the inferior vena cava and the superior vena cava are also visible externally, returning to the right atrium.

The **internal appearance** of the right atrium is pathognomonic (Fig. 2). The **inferior vena cava** connects with the venous (sinus venosus) portion of the right atrium inferiorly, the **superior vena cava** connects with the venous portion superiorly, and the **coronary sinus** opens into the venous portion medially (Fig. 2).

The right atrium is that atrium which on its septal surface displays the **septum secundum** (Fig. 2). The septum secundum is also known as the **limbic ledge,** immediately beneath which a cardiac catheter may be passed into the left atrium, either through a patent foramen ovale or a secundum type of atrial septal defect, or through the septum primum if the fossa ovalis is sealed. Septum secundum's superior limbic band is also called the **crista dividens,** because this is the muscular crest on which the oxygenated blood returning from the placenta up the inferior vena cava in prenatal life

Table 1. Morphologic Anatomic Features of Right Atrium and Left Atrium

Anatomic Features	Right Atrium	Left Atrium
Veins	Inferior vena cava, constant Superior vena cava, variable Coronary sinus, variable appendage	Pulmonary veins, variable
Appendage	Broad, triangular	Narrow, finger-like
Musculi pectinati	Many	Few
Crista terminalis	Present	Absent
Tinea sagittalis	Present	Absent
Septal surface	Septum secundum	Septum primum
Conduction system	Sinoatrial node Atrioventricular node and bundle	None

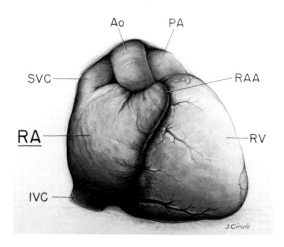

Figure 1. Exterior of the morphologically right atrium (RA) (see Table 1). RA, right atrium; RAA, right atrial appendage; Ao, aorta; IVC, inferior vena cava; PA, pulmonary artery; RV, morphologically right ventricle; SVC, superior vena cava. (From Van Praagh R, Vlad P: Dextrocardia, mesocardia, and levocardia. The segmental approach to diagnosis in congenital heart disease. In Keith JD, Rowe RD, Vlad P (eds): Heart Disease in Infancy and Childhood, 3rd ed. New York, Macmillan, 1978, pp. 638–695, with permission.)

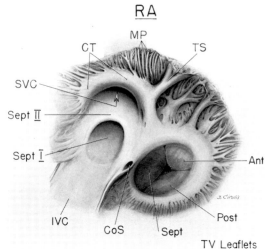

Figure 2. Interior of the morphologically right atrium (RA) (see Table 1). Ant, anterior; CoS, coronary sinus; CT, crista terminalis; IVC, inferior vena cava; MP, musculi pectinati; Post, posterior; Sept, septal; Sept I, septum primum; Sept II, septum secundum; SVC, superior vena cava; TS, tinea sagittalis; TV, tricuspid valve. (From Van Praagh R, Vlad P: Dextrocardia, mesocardia, and levocardia. The segmental approach to diagnosis in congenital heart disease. In Keith JD, Rowe RD, Vlad P (eds): Heart Disease in Infancy and Childhood, 3rd ed. New York, Macmillan, 1978, pp. 638–695, with permission.)

divides into two streams, the **via sinistra** flowing into the left heart, and the **via dextra** passing into the right heart. The superior limbic band of the septum secundum is a muscular structure, the **anterior interatrial plica** (fold), which normally lies directly behind the aortic root (Fig. 1). It is **medial** to the entry of the superior vena cava (Fig. 2).

The **crista terminalis** is a muscular crest that lies **lateral** to the entry of the superior vena cava (Fig. 2). The crista terminalis corresponds internally to the **sulcus terminalis** externally, at the sinoatrial junction, where the **sinoatrial node** (the pacemaker of the heart) is located. The crista terminalis marks the termination of the medial sinus venosus or venous part of the right atrium and the beginning of the muscular or primitive atrium component of the right atrium. Surgical sutures sunk deeply into the crista terminalis can lead to thrombosis of the artery to the sinoatrial node, resulting in sinoatrial nodal infarction and the sick sinus syndrome. The sinoatrial nodal artery runs through the sinoatrial node like a shishkabob skewer.

The **musculi pectinati** form approximately parallel ridges that do not crisscross; instead, they are like the bellows of an accordion. The **tinea sagittalis** (Fig. 1) intersects the crista terminalis at an approximate right angle (Fig. 2). The tip of a cardiac catheter may get lodged behind the tinea sagittalis, leading to perforation of the right atrium.

The **atrioventricular node and bundle** are not grossly visible; hence, it is necessary to know where these structures are, in order to avoid surgically induced heart block. The atrioventricular

node is located directly in front of the ostium of the coronary sinus. If one mentally draws a line between the ostium of the coronary sinus and the commissure between the anterior and the septal leaflets of the tricuspid valve (Fig. 2), this is where the atrioventricular node and the bundle of His are located. The **pars membranacea septi** (membranous part of the septum) is just medial to the commissure between the anterior and septal leaflets of the tricuspid valve. The membranous septum has an **atrioventricular portion** between the right atrium and the left ventricle, and an **interventricular portion** between the right and left ventricles. The atrioventricular bundle penetrates just behind the membranous septum to pass from the atrial to the ventricular level, this portion being known as the **penetrating bundle.** The atrioventricular node and bundle consist of specialized muscle (not nerve tissue). The atrioventricular node and bundle are located within the **triangle of Koch.** The sides of this triangle are formed by the origin of the septal leaflet of the tricuspid valve, the thebesian valve of the coronary sinus, and the tendon of Todaro. The tendon of Todaro is formed by the anterior prolongations of the eustachian valve of the inferior vena cava and the thebesian valve of the coronary sinus, which fuse and run anteriorly as one tendon beneath the right atrial endocardial surface. Thus, although well seen histologically, the tendon of Todaro is not visible grossly. Moreover, the thebesian valve of the coronary sinus is quite a variable structure. Consequently, the most practical way to localize the invisible atrioventricular node and bundle is to draw a line mentally between the ostium of the coronary sinus and the membranous septum at the anteroseptal commissure of the tricuspid valve (Fig. 2).

The Morphologically Left Atrium

The **external appearance** of the left atrium is highly characteristic because the left atrial appendage is relatively narrow and long (Fig. 3). When straight, the left atrial appendage resembles a pointing finger, or a windsock; when bent or crooked, the appendage vaguely resembles a map of Central America. The left atrial appendage remains an appendix to the cavity of the left atrium because the primitive atrial component (the appendage) does not become incorporated into the main cavity of the left atrium (Fig. 3), whereas the right atrial appendage does (Figs. 1 and 2). This is why the shapes of the right and left atrial appendages are so distinctive and so different. The **pulmonary veins** normally connect with the left atrium (Fig. 3); however, the pulmonary venous connections are variable, as totally anomalous pulmonary venous connection makes clear.

The **internal appearance** of the left atrium is pathognomonic (Fig. 4). The left atrium is that atrium which displays on its septal surface the **septum primum** (Fig. 4), which is the flap valve of the foramen ovale. In situs solitus of the atria, the septum primum lies to the **left** of the septum secun-

dum (Fig. 5), whereas in visceroatrial situs inversus, the septum primum lies to the **right** of the septum secundum (Fig. 5).

A comparison of the morphologically right and left atria (Figs. 1 to 4) is summarized in Table 1. The right and left atria are a study in contrasts, virtually all details being distinctive and different. This is why, from the diagnostic standpoint, it is readily possible to recognize the morphologically right atrium as opposed to the morphologically left, no matter where either may be located.

Developmentally, each atrium consists of three main components: (1) venous portion, (2) primitive atrium, and (3) atrioventricular canal. The venous component of the morphologically right atrium is the sinus venosus, consisting of the smooth venous component medially formed by the entry and confluence of the inferior vena cava, the superior vena cava, and the coronary sinus.

The venous component of the morphologically left atrium consists of the common pulmonary vein, which normally is incorporated up to the primary division of each pulmonary venous branch.

The primitive atrium component of both atria consists of the appendages, with their characteristic musculi pectinati (pectinate muscles).

The atrioventricular canal component of both atria is composed of the atrioventricular valves and the septum of the atrioventricular canal (the atrioventricular septum).

Is it always possible to identify the morphologically right atrium and the morphologically left atrium? Contrary to what has often been said, the

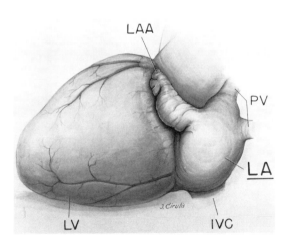

Figure 3. Exterior of the morphologically left atrium (LA) (see Table 1). IVC, inferior vena cava (connecting with the right atrium); LAA, left atrial appendage; LV, morphologically left ventricle; PV, pulmonary veins. (From Van Praagh R, Vlad P: Dextrocardia, mesocardia, and levocardia. The segmental approach to diagnosis in congenital heart disease. In Keith JD, Rowe RD, Vlad P (eds): Heart Disease in Infancy and Childhood, 3rd ed. New York, Macmillan, 1978, pp. 638–695, with permission.)

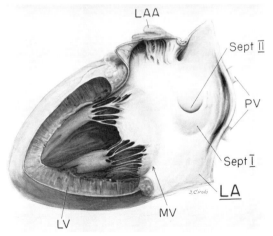

Figure 4. Interior of morphologically left atrium (LA) (see Table 1). LAA, left atrial appendage; LV, morphologically left ventricle; MV, mitral valve; PV, pulmonary vein; Sept I, septum primum; Sept II, septum secundum. (From Van Praagh R, Vlad P: Dextrocardia, mesocardia, and levocardia. The segmental approach to diagnosis in congenital heart disease. In Keith JD, Rowe RD, Vlad P (eds): Heart Disease in Infancy and Childhood, 3rd ed. New York, Macmillan, 1978, pp. 638–695, with permission.)

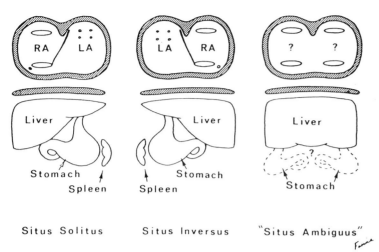

Figure 5. The two types of viscero-atrial situs, important diagnostically for atrial localization. In so-called situs ambiguus, the atrial situs is undiagnosed (?). LA, morphologically left atrium; RA, morphologically right atrium. (From Van Praagh R: The segmental approach to diagnosis in congenital heart disease. In Bergsma D (ed): March of Dimes Birth Defects: OAS 8:4–23, 1972, with permission.)

authors now believe that the correct answer is "Yes." The single most highly reliable diagnostic feature of the right atrium[1] is the suprahepatic segment of the inferior vena cava. That atrium with which the inferior vena cava connects almost always is the right atrium (Figs. 1 and 2), apparent exceptions being very rare. The inferior vena cava rarely can open into an unroofed coronary sinus, i.e., into a coronary sinus with a large coronary sinus septal defect. This creates the impression that the inferior vena cava is connecting with the left atrium. However, the authors believe that, in fact, the inferior vena cava is connecting with the coronary sinus, which normally would drain into the right atrium if the coronary sinus septum were normally formed.[6] Although the inferior vena cava **connects** with the coronary sinus, the inferior vena cava **drains** into the left atrium because of the co-existence of a large coronary sinus septal defect.*

Often in the **polysplenia syndrome,** the renal-to-hepatic segment of the inferior vena cava is absent and there is an enlarged azygos vein to the superior vena cava. In such cases, with "absence" (i.e., interruption) of the inferior vena cava, the suprahepatic segment of the inferior vena cava serves as an accurate diagnostic marker of the right atrium, because, essentially, the suprahepatic portion of the inferior vena cava is always present.

Even in so-called **situs ambiguus** of the viscera and atria (Fig. 5, right), which typically is associated with the asplenia and the polysplenia syndromes, recent evidence indicates that the connection of the inferior vena cava identifies the sinus venosus and, hence, the right atrium with accuracy. Typically, the inferior vena cava leads **directly** to the right atrium. Occasionally, the inferior vena cava opens into an "unroofed" coronary sinus, which in turn leads **indirectly** to the right atrium.

*Whenever the terms **right** or **left** are applied to the atria or the ventricles without further qualification, **morphologically right** or **morphologically left** is understood.

This means that the inferior vena caval connection makes it possible to diagnose the atrial situs in so-called situs ambiguus.[6]

Typically, the appendage of the morphologically right atrium is larger and more anterior than is the appendage of the morphologically left atrium. Thus, both the venous component (the inferior vena cava and the coronary sinus) and the primitive atrial component (the appendage) are helpful in the diagnostic localization of the morphologically right atrium.

The concept of **atrial isomerism** is erroneous, i.e., the concept of right atrial isomerism with the asplenia syndrome, and left atrial isomerism with the polysplenia syndrome. Bilateral morphologically right atria and bilateral morphologically left atria have never been documented. For example, a heart with left atrial appendages bilaterally, with a septum primum on both septal surfaces, and with four pulmonary veins bilaterally has never been documented; therefore, to the best of our knowledge, bilateral left atria do not exist. Similarly, a heart with right atrial appendages bilaterally, bilateral inferior and superior venae cavae, coronary sinus entering bilaterally, and having a septum secundum on each septal surface also has never been documented; therefore, bilateral right atria also do not exist. Just as each individual has only one right ventricle and one left ventricle, so too each individual really has only one right atrium and one left atrium. Even though atrial isomerism does not exist, the appearance suggestive of **isomeric atrial appendages** should certainly make one think of the visceral heterotaxy syndromes: the asplenia syndrome (right "isomerism" of the atrial appendages) or the polysplenia syndrome (left "isomerism" of the atrial appendages).

It follows that there are really only two types of atrial situs: (1) **situs solitus,** the usual or normal type of atrial arrangement in which the right atrium lies to the right and the left atrium lies to the left; and (2) **situs inversus,** the mirror-image type of atrial arrangement in which the morphologically right atrium is left-sided and the morphologically left atrium is right-sided.

The authors now believe that so-called **situs ambiguus** of the atria indicates those cases in which the atrial situs (solitus or inversus) is undiagnosed. There are really only two types of atrial situs (patterns of anatomic organization), not three.

THE VENTRICLES

The anatomic features of the morphologically right ventricle and the morphologically left ventricle are presented in Figures 6 to 12 and are summarized in Table 2.

The Morphologically Right Ventricle

The **external appearance** of the right ventricle is distinctive (Fig. 6). Like the right atrium, the right ventricle also is triangular in shape. The angle between the anterior and diaphragmatic surfaces is typically an acute angle, somewhat less than 90 degrees. Hence, the junction between the anterior and diaphragmatic surfaces of the right ventricle is known as the **acute margin.** The epicardial branches of the **coronary arteries** are highly characteristic, consisting of conal or preventricular branches and of the acute marginal branch of the right coronary artery (Fig. 6).

The **internal appearance** of the morphologically right ventricle is pathognomonic (Figs. 7 to 9). The **trabeculae carneae** (muscular trabeculations) are relatively coarse, few, and straight, tending to parallel the right ventricular inflow and outflow tracts. The **papillary muscles** of the right ventricle are relatively small (making right ventriculotomy readily possible) and numerous, and they attach both to the septal and to the free wall surfaces. Because

of its numerous attachments to the right ventricular septal surface (mostly to the posteroinferior margin of the septal band), the tricuspid valve may be described as "septophilic" (Figs. 7 to 9).

The number of leaflets of the **tricuspid valve** varies from two in infancy (parietal and septal), to four in old age (anterior, posterior, septal, infundibular). However, throughout most of life, the majority of persons have three leaflets (anterior, posterior, septal). Nonetheless, in view of the above-mentioned variations, one cannot reliably identify the tricuspid valve by counting its leaflets.

What, then, may be used to distinguish the tricuspid valve from the mitral? The tricuspid leaflets all tend to be approximately the same depth (Figs. 7 to 9), although the anterior leaflet often is somewhat deeper than the other two (but without nearly as great a difference in leaflet depth as normally exists in the mitral valve). The tricuspid valve is an **inflow valve only,** whereas (as will be seen) the mitral valve is both an inflow and an outflow valve, i.e., forming part of both the ventricular inflow and outflow tracts.

The normal definitive right ventricle has a large infundibular or conal component making up its outflow tract (Figs. 7 to 10). The **infundibulum,** or **conus arteriosus,** is incorporated mainly into the right ventricle, where it forms a **conal ring** consisting of three components: (1) the **distal conal septum** (Fig. 10, component 4), which extends on to the parietal or free wall, forming the **parietal band** (Figs. 7 to 9); (2) the **septal band,** or **proximal conal septum** (Figs. 7 to 9, and Fig. 10, component 3); and (3) the **moderator band** (Figs. 7 and 9).

The definitive right ventricle consists of **four anatomic components** (Fig. 10): (1) the atrioventricular canal, or junction (Fig. 10, component 1); (2) the right ventricular sinus, or body—the pumping portion of the right ventricle (Fig. 10, component

Table 2.   Morphologic Anatomic Features of the Right Ventricle and Left Ventricle

Anatomic Features	Right Ventricle	Left Ventricle
Trabeculae carneae	Coarse Few Straight	Fine Numerous Oblique
Papillary muscles	Numerous Small Septal and free wall	Two Large Free wall origins only
Atrioventricular valve leaflets	Three Approximately equal depth	Two Very unequal depths
Infundibulum	Well developed	Absent
Semilunar-atrioventricular fibrous continuity	Absent	Present
Coronaries	One (right coronary artery)	Two (left anterior descending and circumflex branch of left coronary)
Conduction system radiations	One	Two

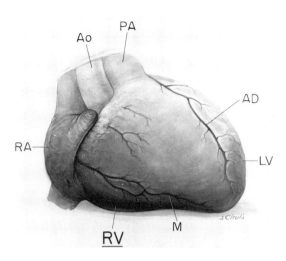

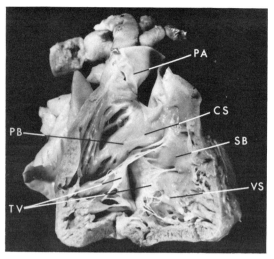

Figure 6. Exterior of morphologically right ventricle (RV). AD, anterior descending coronary artery; Ao, aorta; LV, morphologically left ventricle; M, acute marginal branch of the right coronary artery; PA, main pulmonary artery; RA, morphologically right atrium. (From Van Praagh R, Vlad P: Dextrocardia, mesocardia, and levocardia. The segmental approach to diagnosis in congenital heart disease. In Keith JD, Rowe RD, Vlad P (eds): Heart Disease in Infancy and Childhood, 3rd ed. New York, Macmillan, 1978, pp. 638–695, with permission.)

Figure 8. Photograph of interior of morphologically right ventricle of young patient (2 months of age). Note the "suture" between the crista supraventricularis (CS) of the parietal band (PB) and the septal band (SB). This junction between the parietal band and the septal band, visible in young patients with thin endocardium, is where the parietal band and the septal band dissociate or separate in conotruncal anomalies. VS is the ventricular septum. Other abbreviations are as in Figure 7. (From Van Praagh R, Vlad P: Dextrocardia, mesocardia, and levocardia. The segmental approach to diagnosis in congenital heart disease. In Keith JD, Rowe RD, Vlad P (eds): Heart Disease in Infancy and Childhood, 3rd ed. New York, Macmillan, 1978, pp. 638–695, with permission.)

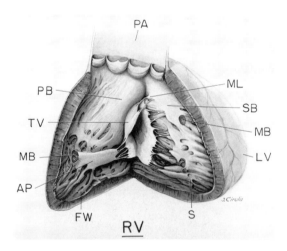

Figure 7. Interior of morphologically right ventricle (RV) (see Table 2). AP, anterior papillary muscle; FW, free wall; LV, morphologically left ventricle; MB, moderator band; ML, muscle of Lancisi; PA, main pulmonary artery; PB, parietal band; S, septum; SB, septal band; TV, tricuspid valve. (From Van Praagh R, Vlad P: Dextrocardia, mesocardia, and levocardia. The segmental approach to diagnosis in congenital heart disease. In Keith JD, Rowe RD, Vlad P (eds): Heart Disease in Infancy and Childhood, 3rd ed. New York, Macmillan, 1978, pp. 638–695, with permission.)

2); (3) the septal band, or proximal conus (Fig. 10, component 3); and (4) the parietal band, or distal conus (Fig. 10, component 4).

The **right ventricular inflow tract** consists of the atrioventricular canal component and the right ventricular sinus (components 1 and 2, Fig. 10).

The **right ventricular outflow tract,** or conus, consists of the septal band and the parietal band (components 3 and 4, Fig. 10).

The apex of the right ventricular sinus lies proximal to the moderator band (Fig. 9), while the apex of the infundibulum or conus lies distal to the moderator band (Fig. 9). Hence, the right ventricle has two apices, proximal and distal to the moderator band.

For the sake of understanding, it is important to appreciate that the **infundibulum (conus)** consists not only of the parietal band (component 4, Fig. 10), but also of the septal and moderator bands (component 3, Fig. 10). The septal and moderator bands are also known as the trabecula septomarginalis. An understanding of the four components of the interventricular septum (Fig. 10) helps to make **ventricular septal defects** comprehensible.

The right ventricle may be described as a one-coronary ventricle, being perfused by the **right coronary artery** and its branches (Fig. 6). However, it should be understood that the right cor-

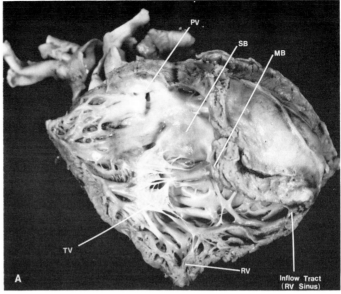

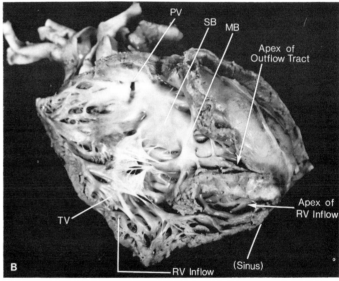

Figure 9. Photograph of interior of opened right ventricle and infundibulum. The right ventricular sinus lies inferior and posterior to a ring of infundibular myocardium formed by the parietal band, septal band (SB), and moderator band (MB). The infundibulum (conus) extends from the infundibular ring to the semilunar valve, normally the pulmonary valve (PV). The apex of the right ventricular sinus is proximal to and inferior to the septal band and moderator band (Panel A). The apex of the infundibulum or outflow tract is distal to and superior to the septal and moderator bands (Panel B). The septal band and moderator band belong to the proximal, or apical, or "septal band part" of the infundibulum. The parietal band is part of the distal, or subsemilunar, or "parietal band part" of the infundibulum. Abbreviations are the same as in previous figures. (From Van Praagh R, Plett JA, Van Praagh S: Single ventricle: pathology, embryology, terminology, and classification. Herz 4:113–150, 1979, with permission.)

onary artery is really the fusion of two arteries: (1) the conus coronary to the conus arteriosus; and (2) the right coronary to the right ventricular sinus.

The **conduction system** of the right ventricle, i.e., the right bundle branch, represents the superior radiation. The right bundle emerges just beneath the papillary muscle of the conus (muscle of Lancisi) and runs down the septal band close to its posterior margin and then crosses via the moderator band to the base of the anterior papillary muscle and, thence, to the right ventricular free wall (Fig. 7). The anterior papillary muscle is the only relatively large papillary muscle in the right ventricle, the others being little more than trabeculae carneae (Fig. 7). The conduction system

of the right ventricle has no posterior radiation, perhaps because of the absence of a sizable posterior papillary muscle in this ventricle.

The Morphologically Left Ventricle

The **external appearance** of the left ventricle is reminiscent of that of a bullet or a torpedo (Fig. 11). Because its external contour is rounded, the left ventricle is said to have an **obtuse margin**. In addition to the anterior descending branch of the **left coronary artery,** which externally marks the location of the anterior (ventral) portion of the interventricular septum (Figs. 6 and 11), anterior and

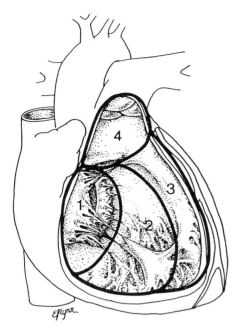

Figure 10. The four main anatomic and developmental components of the interventricular septum, right ventricular view: 1, septum of the atrioventricular canal; 2, muscular ventricular septum, or sinus septum; 3, septal band or proximal conal septum; 4, parietal band or distal conal septum. (Reprinted with permission from the American College of Cardiology, Journal of the American College of Cardiology 14:1298–1299, 1989.)

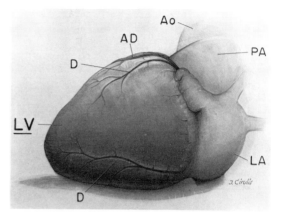

Figure 11. Exterior of morphologically left ventricle (LV). AD, anterior descending coronary artery; Ao, aorta; D, diagonal or obtuse marginal coronary artery branches; LA, morphologically left atrium; PA, main pulmonary artery. (From Van Praagh R, Vlad P: Dextrocardia, mesocardia, and levocardia. The segmental approach to diagnosis in congenital heart disease. In Keith JD, Rowe RD, Vlad P (eds): Heart Disease in Infancy and Childhood, 3rd ed. New York, Macmillan, 1978, pp. 638–695, with permission.)

posterior obtuse marginal branches of the left coronary artery course across the left ventricular free wall (Fig. 11). Also known as diagonals, these branches supply the large papillary muscles and the adjacent left ventricular free wall.

The **interior of the left ventricle** is shown in Figures 12 to 14. The superior portion of the left ventricular septal surface is smooth (nontrabeculated). The inferior portion displays numerous, fine, oblique trabeculae carneae that form a lattice-like mesh. Hence, the **trabeculation** of the left ventricle is fine, very different from the coarse trabeculation of the right ventricle (Figs. 7 to 9).

The **papillary muscles** of the left ventricle are two: the anterolateral and the posteromedial. The anterolateral is superior and relatively far from the interventricular septum, whereas the posteromedial is inferior and paraseptal. The papillary muscles of the left ventricle are large, arise only from the left ventricular free wall, and cover the interior surface of the free wall to a major degree. Consequently, left ventriculotomy is difficult, except at the left ventricular apex. Because the papillary muscles of the left ventricle do not arise from the left ventricular septal surface, these papillary muscles may be described as "septophobic."

The **mitral valve** has a deep anterior leaflet, and a shallow posterior leaflet—very different from the

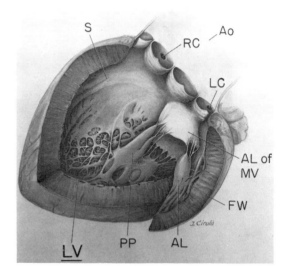

Figure 12. Interior of morphologically left ventricle (LV) (see Table 2). AL, anterolateral papillary muscle; AL of MV, anterior leaflet of mitral valve; Ao, ascending aorta; FW, free wall; LC, left coronary ostium; PP, posteromedial papillary muscle; RC right coronary ostium; S, septum. (From Van Praagh R, Vlad P: Dextrocardia, mesocardia, and levocardia. The segmental approach to diagnosis in congenital heart disease. In Keith JD, Rowe RD, Vlad P (eds): Heart Disease in Infancy and Childhood, 3rd ed. New York, Macmillan, 1978, pp. 638–695, with permission.)

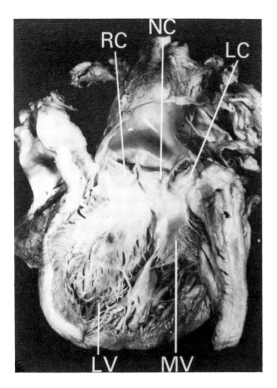

Figure 13. Photograph of interior of morphologically left ventricle (LV). LC, left coronary leaflet of aortic valve; MV, anterior leaflet of mitral valve; NC, noncoronary leaflet of aortic valve; RC, right coronary leaflet of aortic valve. (From Van Praagh R, et al: Tetralogy of Fallot: underdevelopment of the pulmonary infundibulum and its sequelae. Report of a case with cor triatriatum and pulmonary sequestration. Am J Cardiol 26:25–33, 1970, with permission.)

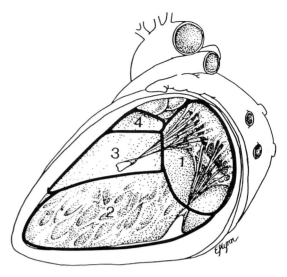

Figure 14. The four main anatomic and developmental components of the interventricular septum, left ventricular view. 1, septum of the atrioventricular canal; 2, trabeculated muscular ventricular sinus septum; 3, nontrabeculated muscular septum, corresponding to and continuous with the septal band or proximal conal septum from right ventricular view (Fig. 10); 4, parietal band or distal conal septum. (Reprinted with permission from the American College of Cardiology, Journal of the American College of Cardiology 14:1298–1299, 1989.)

tricuspid valve. The mitral valve is both an inflow and an outflow valve in the sense that the deep anterior leaflet is an important part of both the inflow and the outflow tracts of the left ventricle.

Normally there is little or no conal musculature beneath the noncoronary and the left coronary leaflets of the aortic valve (Figs. 12 and 13). This normal absence of conal free-wall musculature permits aortic-mitral fibrous continuity (Figs. 12 and 13). When the great arteries are normally related, the noncoronary–left coronary commissure of the aortic valve sits directly above the middle of the anterior mitral leaflet (Figs. 12 and 13). The noncoronary–right coronary commissure sits directly above the membranous septum, which in turn is located directly above the left bundle branch of the conduction system (Fig. 12). The conal septum runs beneath the right coronary leaflet of the aortic valve. The foregoing are highly important landmarks for transaortic therapeutic procedures (balloon dilatation or surgery).

The left ventricle may be described as a two-coronary ventricle, supplied by the **anterior descending** and the **circumflex** branches of the left coronary artery.

Typically, the **conduction system** of the left ventricle has two radiations (Fig. 12): the superior radiation to the superior (anterolateral) papillary muscle group, and the inferior radiation to the inferior (posteromedial) papillary muscle group.

The left ventricle also consists of **four anatomic components** (Fig. 14), which correspond to the four anatomic components that together make up the right ventricle (Fig. 10). Ventricular septal defects may involve each of these components, and also can occur between them.

Anatomic variations in the conus arteriosus are shown schematically in Figure 15. The conus can be: **subpulmonary** with normally related great arteries; **subaortic** with transposition of the great arteries; **bilateral** (subpulmonary and subaortic) typically with double-outlet right ventricle; or **bilaterally absent** (neither subpulmonary nor subaortic) with double-outlet left ventricle.

Comparison and Contrast of the Right and Left Ventricles

The anatomic features of the morphologically right and left ventricles are compared, contrasted, and summarized in Table 2. As with the atria (Table 1), so too with the ventricles (Table 2), virtually all of the anatomic details are distinctive and different. These anatomic features facilitate accurate morphologic diagnosis of the right and left ventricles, no matter where they may be located.

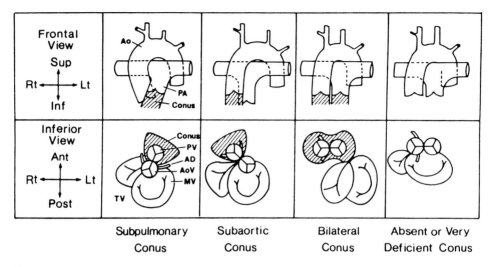

Figure 15. Anatomic types of subsemilunar infundibulum or conus arteriosus. AD, anterior descending coronary artery; Ant, anterior; AoV, aortic valve; Inf, inferior; Lt, left; MV, mitral valve; PA, main pulmonary artery; Post, posterior; PV, pulmonary valve; Rt, right; Sup, superior; TV, tricuspid valve. (Modified from Van Praagh R, Vlad P: Dextrocardia, mesocardia, and levocardia. The segmental approach to diagnosis in congenital heart disease. In Keith JD, Rowe RD, Vlad P (eds): Heart Disease in Infancy and Childhood, 3rd ed. New York, Macmillan, 1978, pp. 638–695.)

THE IMPORTANCE OF UNDERSTANDING NORMAL MORPHOLOGIC ANATOMY

An understanding of the normal morphologic anatomy of the right and left atria and of the right and left ventricles is not just a baseline or a frame of reference. Instead, an understanding of the morphologic anatomy of the four cardiac chambers is the indispensable key to the diagnosis of much of congenital heart disease: dextrocardia, mesocardia, isolated levocardia, ectopia cordis, superoinferior ventricles, crisscross atrioventricular relations, transposition of the great arteries, double-outlet right ventricle, single ventricle, etc. Accurate diagnosis of the aforementioned anomalies—and many more—is based on an understanding of normal morphologic anatomy.

REFERENCES

1. Van Praagh R: The segmental approach to diagnosis in congenital heart disease. In Bergsma D (ed): Birth Defects: Original Article Series 8:4–23, 1972.

2. Van Praagh R, Geva T, Kreutzer J: Ventricular septal defects: how shall we describe, name, and classify them? J Am Coll Cardiol 14:1298–1299, 1989.

3. Van Praagh R, Plett JA, Van Praagh S: Single ventricle: pathology, embryology, terminology, and classification. Herz 4:113–150, 1979.

4. Van Praagh R, Van Praagh S, Nebesar RA, et al: Tetralogy of Fallot: underdevelopment of the pulmonary infundibulum and its sequelae. Report of a case with cor triatriatum and pulmonary sequestration. Am J Cardiol 26:25–33, 1970.

5. Van Praagh R, Vlad P: Dextrocardia, mesocardia, and levocardia. The segmental approach to diagnosis in congenital heart disease. In Keith JD, Rowe RD, Vlad P (eds): Heart Disease in Infancy and Childhood, 3rd ed. New York, Macmillan, 1978, pp. 638–695.

6. Van Praagh S, Kreutzer J, Alday L, et al: Systemic and pulmonary venous connections in visceral heterotaxy, with emphasis on the diagnosis of the atrial situs: a study of 109 postmortem cases. In Clark EB, Takao A (eds): Developmental Cardiology, Morphogenesis and Function, Mt. Kisco, NY, Futura, 1990, pp. 671–727.

Chapter 4

SEGMENTAL APPROACH TO DIAGNOSIS

Richard Van Praagh, M.D.

The segmental approach[3,12,19,21] (sequential approach,[9,11] systematic approach[8]) to the diagnosis of congenital heart disease[2,3,6–15,19,21,24] is based upon an understanding of the morphologic and segmental anatomy of the heart. The **cardiac segments** are the anatomic and embryologic "building blocks" out of which all human hearts—normal and abnormal—are made.

CARDIAC SEGMENTS

The three main cardiac segments are (1) the viscera and atria, (2) the ventricular loop, and (3) the truncus arteriosus. Understanding of the three main cardiac segments is necessary for the diagnostic localization of (1) the atria, (2) the ventricles, and (3) the great arteries (Fig. 1).

The **two connecting or junctional cardiac segments** are (1) the atrioventricular canal and (2) the infundibulum or conus arteriosus. The atrioventricular canal normally consists of the atrioventricular valves and the atrioventricular septum. The distal or subsemilunar part of the conus arteriosus, or infundibulum, normally consists of a muscular cone or funnel beneath the pulmonary valve, separating the pulmonary valve from both atrioventricular valves (Fig. 1, row 1). Normally, there is aortic-mitral fibrous continuity, reflecting the normal absence of subaortic conal free wall myocardium.

Segmental Sets

How many types of human heart are there? Figure 1 provides a partial answer to this question. For each type of heart, the atria, the ventricles, and the great arteries may be regarded as the members of a set that are recorded in venoarterial sequence, or blood flow order: {atria, ventricles, great arteries}. Hence, in each segmental set, {1,2,3}, the atrial situs is #1, the ventricular situs (ventricular loop) is #2, and the great arterial situs is #3 (Fig. 1). **Situs** denotes the pattern of anatomic organization: solitus (usual or normal) or inversus (a mirror-image of solitus).

The types of visceroatrial situs are shown in Figure 1: solitus (S), as in {S,–,–}; or inversus (I), as in {I,–,–}; or ambiguus (A), as in {A,–,–} (not shown in Fig. 1). In situs ambiguus of the atria, the atrial situs is indicated by the connections of the suprahepatic segment of the inferior vena cava and the coronary sinus ostium. Hence, atrial situs ambiguus, probably basically situs solitus, may be recorded as {A(S),–,–}; and atrial situs ambiguus, probably basically situs inversus, can be rendered as {A(I),–,–} (see p. 597).

The types of ventricular situs are (Fig. 1): solitus or D-loop ventricles (D), as in {–,D,–}, the right ventricle being right-handed (Fig. 2) and the left ventricle being left-handed;[16,18] or inverted or L-loop (L), as in {–,L,–}, the right ventricle being left-handed (Fig. 3) and the left ventricle being right-handed.[16,18]

The types of great arterial situs are (Fig. 1): solitus (S), as in solitus normally related great arteries, as in {–,–,S} (row 1, column 1); and inversus (I), as in inverted normally related great arteries, as in {–,–,I} (row 1, column 3).

When the great arteries are abnormally related, the right-sided (dextro, or D) location of the aortic valve relative to the pulmonary valve is symbolized as D, as in {–,–,D}; and the left-sided (levo or L) location of the aortic valve relative to the pulmonary valve is symbolized as L, as in {–,–,L} (Fig. 1). D-malpositions of the great arteries are considered to be solitus or noninverted malpositions, the aortic valve normally being right-sided in situs solitus. L-malpositions of the great arteries are considered to be inverted or mirror-image malpositions because the aortic valve is left-sided relative to the pulmonary valve, as in situs inversus totalis (Fig. 1, row 1, column 3). In A-malpositions of the great arteries (not shown in Fig. 1), the right-left location of the aortic valve (directly anterior to the pulmonary valve) is equivocal (neither right nor left); hence, A-malpositions may be regarded as

TYPES OF HUMAN HEART:
Segmental Sets and Alignments

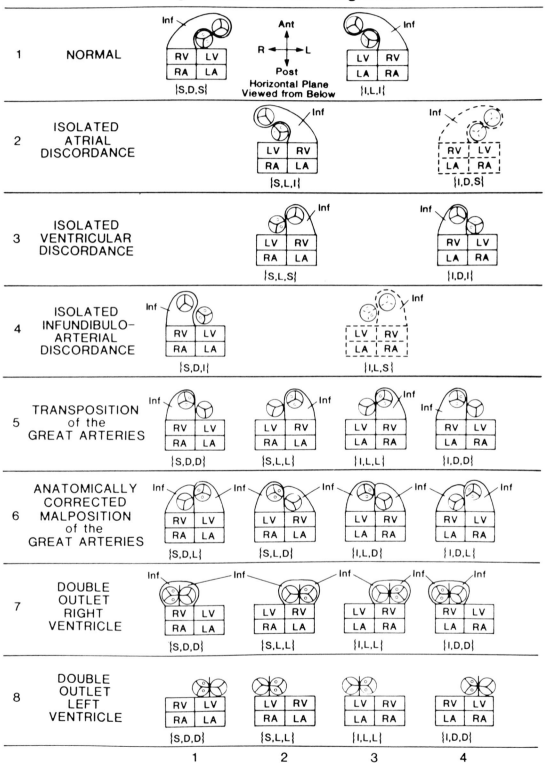

Figure 1. *See legend on opposite page.*

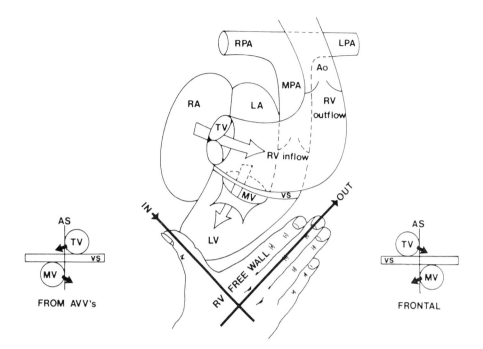

Figure 2. The D-loop, or solitus right ventricle, is right-handed. Figuratively speaking, the thumb of the right hand goes through the tricuspid valve (TV), indicating the RV inflow tract (IN). The fingers go into the right ventricular outflow tract (OUT). The palm of the right hand faces the right ventricular septal surface. The dorsum of the right hand is adjacent to the right ventricular free wall. Abbrevations are as in Figure 1, except: Ao, aorta; AS, atrial septum; AVV's, atrioventricular valves; LPA, left pulmonary artery; MPA, main pulmonary artery; MV, mitral valve; RPA, right pulmonary artery; and VS, ventricular septum. (From Van Praagh S, et al: Superoinferior ventricles, anatomic and angiocardiographic findings in 10 postmortem cases. In Van Praagh R, Takao A (eds): Etiology and Morphogenesis of Congenital Heart Disease. Mt. Kisco, NY, Futura, 1980, pp. 317–378, with permission.)

of uncertain situs (situs ambiguus of the great arteries).

Consequently, the segmental combinations shown in Figure 1 are **segmental situs sets.** In other words, these segmental combinations (Fig. 1) indicate the patterns of anatomic organization (situs) of each of the main cardiac segments {atria, ventricles, great arteries} of any type of congenital heart disease.

Segmental Alignments

Segmental alignments also are shown in Figure 1 as follows:

Atrioventricular alignments are **concordant** or appropriate when the morphologically right atrium is aligned with, and opens into, the morphologically right ventricle, and the morphologically left atrium is aligned with, and opens into, the morphologically left ventricle. Concordant atrioventricular alignments are shown in vertical columns 1 and 3.

Atrioventricular alignments are **discordant** or inappropriate when the morphologically right atrium is aligned with, and opens into, the morphologically left ventricle, and the morphologically left atrium is aligned with, and opens into, the mor-

---

Figure 1. Types of human heart: segmental sets and alignments. Heart diagrams are viewed from below, similar to a subxiphoid two-dimensional echocardiogram. Cardiotypes depicted in broken lines have not been documented as yet. Ant, anterior; Post, posterior; R, right; L, left; RA, morphologically right atrium; LA, morphologically left atrium; RV, morphologically right ventricle; LV, morphologically left ventricle; Inf, infundibulum. The aortic valve is indicated by the coronary ostia; the pulmonary valve is indicated by absence of the coronary ostia. Braces { } mean "the set of." The segmental sets are explained in the text. Rows 1–4 and 6 have ventriculoarterial (VA) concordance. Row 5, transposition of the great arteries, has VA discordance. Rows 7 and 8 have double-outlet RV and LV, respectively. Columns 1 and 3 have atrioventricular (AV) concordance, {S,D,–} and {I,L,–}, respectively. Columns 2 and 4 have AV discordance, {S,L,–} and {I,D,–}, respectively. (From Foran RB, et al: Isolated infundibuloarterial inversion {S,D,I}: a newly recognized form of congenital heart disease. Am Heart J 116:1337–1350, 1988, with permission.)

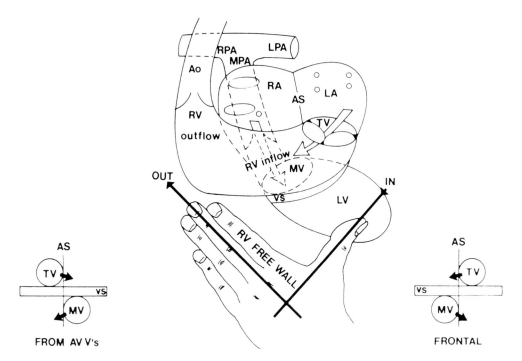

Figure 3. The L-loop or inverted right ventricle is left-handed. Figuratively speaking, the thumb of one's left hand goes through the tricuspid valve, indicating the right ventricular inflow tract (IN). The fingers of the left hand go into the right ventricular outflow tract (OUT). The palm of one's left hand faces the right ventricular septal surface and the dorsum of the left hand is adjacent to the right ventricular free wall. Abbreviations are as in previous illustrations. (From Van Praagh S, et al: Superoinferior ventricles, anatomic and angiocardiographic findings in 10 postmortem cases. In Van Praagh R, Takao A (eds): Etiology and Morphogenesis of Congenital Heart Disease. Mt. Kisco, NY, Futura, 1980, pp. 317–378, with permission.)

phologically right ventricle. Discordant atrioventricular alignments are shown in vertical columns 2 and 4.

Ventriculoarterial alignments are shown in the horizontal rows (Fig. 1) as follows:

The ventriculoarterial alignments are **concordant** or appropriate when the morphologically right ventricle is aligned with, and opens into, the pulmonary artery, and when the morphologically left ventricle is aligned with, and opens into, the aorta. Concordant ventriculoarterial alignments are of two types: (1) with normally related great arteries (rows 1 to 4, inclusive); and (2) with abnormally related great arteries, i.e., with anatomically corrected malposition of the great arteries (row 6).

The ventriculoarterial alignments are **abnormal** in rows 5 to 8, inclusive. The ventriculoarterial alignments are **discordant** in transposition of the great arteries (row 5): the morphologically right ventricle is aligned with, and opens into, the aorta, and the morphologically left ventricle is aligned with, and opens into, the pulmonary artery. Other types of abnormal ventriculoarterial alignment include **double-outlet right ventricle** (row 7) and **double-outlet left ventricle** (row 8).

Alignments Versus Connections

The distinction between segmental **alignments** and segmental **connections** should be understood. The atria do not connect directly with the ventricles muscle-to-muscle, except at the atrioventricular bundle of His, because of the interposition of the fibrous atrioventricular canal or junction. Hence, the atria and the ventricles are aligned in various ways (Fig. 1), even though they do not connect directly (muscle-to-muscle).

Similarly, the ventricles do not connect directly with the great arteries, tissue-to-tissue, because of the interposition of the infundibulum or conus arteriosus. Even though the ventricles do not connect directly with the great arteries, they are aligned in various ways (Fig. 1).

The main cardiac segments—the atria, ventricles, and great arteries (Fig. 1)—are **aligned** in various ways, even though they do not connect directly; like "bricks" in a wall, they are connected and separated by the "mortar." The **connecting** cardiac segments—the atrioventricular junction and the infundibulum (conus)—**connect** the main segments in various ways (Fig. 1); the connecting segments are the mortar. For example, the atria and the ventricles are **connected** by the fibrous atrio-ventricular junction; they are also **separated,** and normally are **electrically insulated,** from each other by the fibrous atrioventricular junction. If the atria and the ventricles **do** connect muscle-to-muscle, except at the His bundle, then this is an abnormality of electrophysiologic importance, as in the Wolff-Parkinson-White syndrome.

The fact that the atria really do not connect directly with the ventricles also is of great developmental importance. If the right atrium were connected directly with the right ventricle, and if the left atrium were connected directly with the left ventricle, a discordant ventricular L-loop in visceroatrial situs solitus, i.e., {S,L,–} as in column 2 (Fig. 1), probably would be developmentally impossible.

The same principles apply at the ventriculo-arterial junction. The fact that the right ventricle does not connect directly with the pulmonary artery, and the left ventricle with the aorta, appears to be an anatomic fact of great developmental importance. This explains why abnormal ventriculoarterial alignments are developmentally possible (Fig. 1): because the ventricles do not connect directly with the great arteries. The development of the conal connector between the ventricles (ventricular sinuses or pumping portions) and the great arteries appears to be of fundamental importance to the type of ventriculoarterial alignment that results (Fig. 1).

To summarize, the segmental alignments and connections are distinguished in the interests of anatomic and developmental accuracy. The distinction between alignments and connections is important because they are two different things. Different cardiac segments are involved. Segmental alignments and connections are both important.

The concepts of concordance and discordance apply well to segmental **alignments** (Fig. 1, columns 1 to 4), but **not** to **connections.** The difficulty with connections is that they are Janus-like structures: they "look" both proximally and distally at the same time. For example, the right-sided mitral valve in classical physiologically corrected transposition of the great arteries, i.e., transposition of the great arteries {S,L,L} (Fig. 1, row 5, column 2), connects the right-sided right atrium with the right-sided left ventricle. This right-sided mitral valve is concordant relative to the right-sided left ventricle, but discordant relative to the right-sided right atrium. The concordant/discordant concept applies unequivocally to alignments because alignments "look" in one direction only—distally (Fig. 1).

Associated Malformations

In addition to segmental situs sets and their **alignments** (Fig. 1), associated malformations of the main or connecting cardiac segments are also of great diagnostic importance. Associated malformations are omitted from Figure 1 for simplicity. Different segmental sets have distinctive and very different associated malformations: for example, discordant L-loop ventricles have very different associated malformations than do concordant D-loop ventricles.[23] Finally, the functional or **physiologic diagnosis** is every bit as important as is the aforementioned anatomic diagnosis. How does the segmental set and its alignments (Fig. 1), with or without associated malformations, function?

SPECIFIC EXAMPLES

Specific examples of this diagnostic approach, which has been used at The Children's Hospital in Boston for the past two decades, are summarized as follows (Fig. 1):

The Solitus Normal Heart

The solitus normal heart (row 1, column 1) is {S,D,S}, meaning the set of situs solitus of the viscera and atria (S), D-loop or solitus ventricles (D), and solitus normally related great arteries (S). Atrioventricular concordance, ventriculoarterial concordance, and a subpulmonary infundibulum with aortic-mitral direct continuity are present.

In this chapter, whenever the term "concordance" or "discordance" is used without other qualification, it always means **alignment** concordance or discordance, consistent with common usage. Parenthetically, there is another type of concordance or discordance that can be very important, namely **situs** concordance or discordance. One can have {S,D,S} with **straddling tricuspid valve,** or **double-inlet left ventricle.** In other words, when the atrioventricular alignments are concordant, as in the normal heart, nothing else need be said diagnostically. If something is not mentioned, one may assume that it is normal, or is as expected. However, when the atrioventricular alignments are abnormal, they must, of course, be specified, as above. In {S,D,S} with double-inlet left ventricle, there is atrioventricular **situs** concordance (**not** atrioventricular **alignment** concordance): the situs of the atrial segment and of the ventricular segment are both solitus.

The Inverted Normal Heart

The inverted normal heart (Fig. 1, row 1, column 3) is {I,L,I}—the set or combination of visceroatrial situs inversus (I), L-loop ventricles (L), and inverted normally related great arteries (I). There is a subpulmonary infundibulum with aortic-mitral fibrous continuity. Atrioventricular and ventriculoarterial concordance are present.

Ventricular Inversion with Inverted Normally Related Great Arteries in Visceroatrial Situs Solitus

Ventricular inversion with inverted normally related great arteries in visceroatrial situs solitus (Fig. 1, row 2, column 2) is {S,L,I}—the set of visceroatrial situs solitus (S), L-loop ventricles (L), and inverted normally related great arteries (I). The infundibulum is subpulmonary. As one would expect from the segmental situs set {S,L,I}, the atrioventricular alignments are discordant and the ventriculoarterial alignments are concordant. Since there is one discordant alignment, the circulations are physiologically uncorrected. In this rare segmental combination, an atrial inversion procedure (Senning or Mustard) results in an anatomic correction: postoperatively, the left ventricle is the systemic ventricle and the right ventricle is the pulmonary ventricle.

Because the aforementioned name of this anomaly is too long, attempts have been made to shorten it. **Isolated atrial noninversion** has been suggested because only the atria are in situs solitus, the ventricular and great arterial segments both being inverted. The difficulty with "isolated atrial noninversion" is that it is excessively cardiocentric: the noninversion of the atria may be isolated as far as the heart is concerned, but not as far as the body is concerned. Since all of the viscera also are in situs solitus, the atrial noninversion is hardly isolated. However, if understood as a **cardiac** diagnosis, "isolated atrial noninversion" is brief and not inaccurate. The briefest diagnosis is, of course, {S,L,I}.

Isolated Ventricular Inversion

Isolated ventricular inversion is {S,L,S} (Fig. 1, row 3, column 2), which means situs solitus of the viscera and atria (S), L-loop ventricles (L), and solitus normally related great arteries (S). As the segmental combination {S,L,S} suggests, there is atrioventricular discordance and ventriculoarterial concordance. Because there is one alignment discordance, i.e., one right-left switching error, the circulations are physiologically uncorrected. This is confirmed by the presence of atrioarterial alignment discordance: the right atrium and the aorta are ipsilateral, both right-sided; and the left atrium and the pulmonary artery are ipsilateral, both left-sided. As with all types of atrioventricular discordance with ventriculoarterial concordance, anatomic repair can be accomplished with an atrial inversion procedure.

Isolated Ventricular Noninversion

Isolated ventricular noninversion is {I,D,I} (Fig. 1, row 3, column 4)—the set of situs inversus of the viscera and the atria (I), D-loop ventricles (D), and inverted normally related great arteries (I). The infundibulum is subpulmonary, as one would expect with a form of normally related great arteries. As {I,D,I} suggests, there is atrioventricular discordance and ventriculoarterial concordance. Given one discordant alignment, the circulations are physiologically uncorrected. Note the atrioarterial discordance, the right atrium and the aorta being ipsilateral. Again, as in all anatomic types of atrioventricular discordance with ventriculoarterial concordance, an atrial inversion procedure results in an anatomic correction.

Isolated Infundibuloarterial Inversion

Isolated infundibuloarterial inversion is a newly discovered form of congenital heart disease with the segmental combination of {S,D,I} (Fig. 1, row 4, column 1):[4] situs solitus of the viscera and atria (S), D-loop ventricles (D), and inverted normally related great arteries (I). As {S,D,I} suggests, there is atrioventricular concordance and ventriculoarterial concordance. Consequently, one would expect to have no hemodynamic derangement. Usually, however, the inverted normal type of conotruncus is associated with a **tetralogy of Fallot** type of malformation. Pulmonary outflow tract obstruction (stenosis or atresia) with a large subaortic ventricular septal defect results in cyanotic congenital heart disease. Also characteristic of tetralogy of Fallot {S,D,I} are: dextrocardia, superoinferior ventricles, the appearance of crisscross atrioventricular relations, small right ventricular sinus (inflow tract), huge ventricular septal defect (confluent ventricular septal defect of atrioventricular canal type with conoventricular ventricular septal defect of the malalignment tetralogy type), and a tendency of the atrioventricular valves to straddle the ventricular septum. The right coronary artery runs across the obstructed pulmonary outflow tract, necessitating the use of an external conduit from the right ventricle to the pulmonary artery.

Transposition of the Great Arteries

Transposition of the great arteries (Fig. 1, row 5) is a specific type of malposition of the great arteries characterized by ventriculoarterial discordance. Only a few of the segmental combinations that occur with transposition of the great arteries are shown.[23]

1. **Transposition of the great arteries {S,D,D}** means transposition of the great arteries with the set of visceroatrial situs solitus (S), D-loop ventricles (D), and D-transposition of the great arteries (D). Typically, there is a subaortic infundibulum (conus), with pulmonary-mitral fibrous continuity. There is atrioventricular concordance with ventriculoarterial discordance. There being one segmental alignment discordance, the circulations are

physiologically uncorrected: note the atrioarterial alignment discordance, the right atrium and the aorta being ipsilateral (instead of contralateral as normally). This is the classical form of transposition of the great arteries.

In physiologically uncorrected transposition of the great arteries, the aortic valve can be directly anterior (antero or A) relative to the pulmonary valve, i.e., transposition of the great arteries {S,D,A} (not shown in Fig. 1). Or the aortic valve can be to the left (levo or L) relative to the pulmonary valve, i.e., transposition of the great arteries {S,D,L} (Fig. 2). Even though the aortic valve can lie to the left of the pulmonary valve, which may confusingly suggest physiologically corrected transposition of the great arteries, **segmental alignment analysis** clearly indicates that physiologically uncorrected transposition of the great arteries is present: there is only one discordance (right-left switching error) at the ventriculoarterial junction, not two. The vena caval return goes to the aorta (Fig. 2).

Transposition of the great arteries {S,D,D} (Fig. 1, row 5, column 1) is the classical form of transposition of the great arteries. In 1915, Abbott[1] called this anomaly **complete** transposition of the great arteries, as opposed to **partial** transposition of the great arteries, which is now called **double-outlet right ventricle.** As the term "transposition of the great arteries" is now used, all transpositions (row 5, Fig. 1) (physiologically uncorrected and corrected) are complete (as opposed to partial). However, Abbott's[1] usage of "complete" transposition of the great arteries to mean physiologically uncorrected transposition of the great arteries has stuck. Whenever "complete" transposition of the great arteries is used, it always means physiologically uncorrected transposition of the great arteries. Transposition of the great arteries {S,D,D} is often simply called **D-transposition of the great arteries,** for convenient brevity. Transposition of the great arteries {S,D,D} is **complete noninverted transposition of the great arteries.** "Complete" means that each great artery is placed completely across the ventricular septum, and so arises above the morphologically inappropriate ventricle. "Noninverted" means that the aortic valve is right-sided and the pulmonary valve is left-sided, as is normal in situs solitus: {S,D,S} (row 1, column 1).

2. **Transposition of the great arteries {S,L,L}** (Fig. 1, row 5, column 2) means transposition of the great arteries with the set of visceroatrial situs solitus (S), L-loop ventricles (L), and L-transposition of the great arteries (L). As {S,L,L} suggests, there is atrioventricular discordance. As transposition of the great arteries indicates, there is ventriculoarterial discordance. This is the classical form of **physiologically corrected transposition of the great arteries.** The two segmental discordances cancel each other. There is atrioarterial

alignment concordance, the left atrium and the aorta being ipsilateral. Transposition of the great arteries {S,L,L} is **complete inverted transposition of the great arteries.** "Complete" means that each great artery is placed completely across the ventricular septum, i.e., that "partial" transposition of the great arteries is not present. "Inverted" means that the semilunar valves are right-left reversed— a mirror-image of what is normal in situs solitus, i.e., {S,D,S} (Fig. 1, row 1, column 1). Because transposition of the great arteries {S,L,L} is by far the most common form of L-transposition, this anomaly is often briefly called **L-transposition of the great arteries.** However, {S,L,L} transposition of the great arteries is a little longer and is entirely specific, whereas "L-transposition of the great arteries" does not specify the atrial or ventricular situs, and consequently, is open to misinterpretation.

3. **Transposition of the great arteries {I,L,L}** (Fig. 1, row 5, column 3) denotes transposition of the great arteries with the segmental set of visceroatrial situs inversus (I), L-loop ventricles (L), and L-transposition (L). There is atrioventricular concordance with ventriculoarterial discordance, indicating a physiologically uncorrected circulation (one discordance), the right atrium and the aorta being ipsilateral. Transposition of the great arteries {I,L,L} exemplifies **physiologically uncorrected (complete) transposition of the great arteries in situs inversus.** Transposition of the great arteries {I,L,L} my be viewed as **noninverted transposition of the great arteries for situs inversus,** because the aortic valve usually is left-sided and the pulmonary valve is right-sided in situs inversus totalis, i.e., {I,L,I} (Fig. 1, row 1, column 3). Both in visceroatrial situs solitus and in visceroatrial situs inversus, **physiologically uncorrected transposition** typically is **noninverted transposition of the great arteries** (relative to the semilunar relationship that is usual for the situs, row 1).

4. **Transposition of the great arteries {I,D,D}** (Fig. 1, row 5, column 4) indicates transposition of the great arteries with the segmental combination (set) of visceroatrial situs inversus (I), D-loop ventricles (D), and D-transposition of the great arteries (D). There is atrioventricular discordance with ventriculoarterial discordance, indicating physiologically corrected transposition of the great arteries (two discordances). This is **physiologically corrected transposition of the great arteries in situs inversus.** Transposition of the great arteries {I,D,D} also may be viewed as **inverted transposition of the great arteries for situs inversus:** the semilunar interrelationship is right-left switched compared with the semilunar interrelationship that is usual in situs inversus totalis, i.e., {I,L,I} (row 1, column 3). Both in visceroatrial situs solitus and in visceroatrial situs inversus, **physiologically corrected transposition of the great arteries** typically

is **inverted transposition of the great arteries** (relative to the semilunar interrelationship that is usual for the situs, row 1).

Anatomically Corrected Malposition of the Great Arteries

Anatomically corrected malposition of the great arteries (Fig. 1, row 6) may be exemplified by the most common form, anatomically corrected malposition of the great arteries {S,D,L} (row 6, column 1), which means anatomically corrected malposition of the great arteries with the segmental set of visceroatrial situs solitus (S), D-loop ventricles (D), and L-malposition of the great arteries (L). As anatomically corrected malposition of the great arteries {S,D,L} suggests, there is atrioventricular concordance and ventriculoarterial concordance. A bilateral infundibulum (subaortic and subpulmonary) is more common than is a subaortic infundibulum with pulmonary-mitral fibrous continuity.

Although this form of anatomically corrected malposition of the great arteries has physiologically corrected circulations (the left atrium and aorta are ipsilateral), other forms such as **anatomically corrected malposition of the great arteries {S,L,D}** have physiologically uncorrected circulations, the right atrium and the aorta being ipsilateral (row 6, column 2).

Anatomically corrected malposition of the great arteries also occurs in visceroatrial situs inversus (row 6, columns 3 and 4): anatomically corrected malposition of the great arteries {I,L,D} with atrioventricular and ventriculoarterial concordance (physiologically corrected); and anatomically corrected malposition of the great arteries {I,D,L} with atrioventricular discordance and ventriculoarterial concordance (physiologically uncorrected).

In all forms of anatomically corrected malposition of the great arteries, the ventricles fold in one direction, and the conotruncus twists in the opposite direction (row 6). This may explain why anatomically corrected malposition of the great arteries is so rare.

The designation **anatomically corrected malposition**[5,20] means that the great arteries are malposed, but despite this fact, the great arteries nonetheless originate above the anatomically correct ventricles: the aorta above the morphologically left ventricle and the pulmonary artery above the morphologically right ventricle. Anatomically corrected malposition of the great arteries indicates that the ventriculoarterial concordance and normally related (and normally connected) great arteries are not synonymous. In anatomically corrected malposition of the great arteries, although the ventriculoarterial **alignments** are concordant, the ventriculoarterial **connections** are very abnormal—the conal connector being subaortic and subpulmonary, or subaortic only.

The meanings of the segmental symbols and of concordance and discordance should now be clear; hence, the other forms of anatomically corrected malposition of the great arteries need not be spelled out in detail.

Double-Outlet Right Ventricle

Double-outlet right ventricle (Fig. 1, row 7) means that both great arteries are entirely or predominantly above the morphologically right ventricle. A few of the segmental sets that occur[17] with double-outlet right ventricle are presented in row 7. For example, double-outlet right ventricle {S,D,D} means double-outlet right ventricle with the set of solitus atria (S), D-loop ventricles (D), and D-malposition of the great arteries (D). Atrioventricular concordance is typical. The ventriculoarterial alignments are, of course, those of double-outlet right ventricle. The segmental anatomy of the other forms of double-outlet right ventricle is self-evident (row 7).

Double-Outlet Left Ventricle

Double-outlet left ventricle (Fig. 1, row 8) means that both great arteries are entirely or predominantly above the left ventricle. Some of the segmental combinations that are now known to be associated with double-outlet left ventricle[22] are depicted in row 8 (Fig. 1). The most common is double-outlet left ventricle {S,D,D}, which means double-outlet left ventricle with the set of solitus atria (S), D-loop ventricles (D), and D-malposition of the great arteries (D). Typically, the atrioventricular alignments are concordant. By definition, the ventriculoarterial alignments are those of double-outlet left ventricle. Because the segmental anatomy of the other forms depicted should be understood by now, further description will be omitted in the interest of brevity.

SUMMARY

The foregoing is an introduction to the segmental anatomy of congenital heart disease. Diagnosis is based mainly on the following six criteria (Fig. 1): segmental situs, alignments, connections, spatial relations, associated malformations, and function.

The segmental approach to the diagnosis of congenital heart disease involves answering the following questions:

1. What type of visceroatrial situs is present?
2. What type of ventricular situs (ventricular loop) is present?
3. What anatomic type of infundibulum and great arteries (conotruncus) does the patient have?
4. What are the atrioventricular alignments?
5. What are the atrioventricular connections?

6. What are the ventriculoarterial alignments?
7. What are the ventriculoarterial connections?
8. Are there any associated malformations?
9. How does the segmental set, with or without associated malformations, function?

The segmental approach to diagnosis is concerned primarily with questions 1 to 8. The **anatomic diagnosis** (points 1 to 8) is highly relevant to the **physiologic diagnosis** (point 9), and both are important in surgical management.

REFERENCES

1. Abbott ME: Congenital cardiac disease. In Osler and McCrae's Modern Medicine, 2nd ed. Philadelphia, Lea & Febiger, 1915, Vol. 4, p. 323.
2. Ando M, Satomi G, Takao A: Atresia of tricuspid or mitral orifice: anatomic spectrum and morphogenetic hypothesis. In Van Praagh R, Takao A (eds): Etiology and Morphogenesis of Congenital Heart Disease. Mt. Kisco, NY, Futura Publishing Co., 1980, pp. 421–487.
3. Calcaterra G, Anderson RH, Lau KC, et al: Dextrocardia—value of segmental analysis in its categorization. Br Heart J 42:497–507, 1979.
4. Foran RB, Belcourt C, Nanton MA, et al: Isolated infundibuloarterial inversion {S,D,I}: a newly recognized form of congenital heart disease. Am Heart J 116:1337–1350, 1988.
5. Harris JS and Farber S: Transposition of the great cardiac vessels with special reference to the phylogenetic therapy of Spitzer. Arch Pathol 28:427, 1939.
6. Kirklin JW, Pacifico AD, Bargeron LM, et al: Cardiac repair in anatomically corrected malposition of the great arteries. Circulation 48:153–159, 1973.
7. Otero Coto E, Quero Jimenez M: Aproximacion segmentaria al diagnostico y clasificacion de las cardiopatias congenitas. Fundamentos y utilidad. Rev Esp Cardiol 30:557–566, 1977.
8. Rao PS: Systemic approach to differential diagnosis. Am Heart J 102:389–403, 1981.
9. Shinebourne EA, Macartney FJ, Anderson RH: Sequential chamber localization—logical approach to diagnosis in congenital heart disease. Br Heart J 38:327–339, 1976.
10. Stanger P, Rudolph AM, Edwards JE: Cardiac malpositions. An overview based on study of sixty-five necropsy specimens. Circulation 56:159–172, 1977.
11. Tynan MJ, Becker AE, Macartney FJ, et al: Nomenclature and classification of congenital heart disease. Br Heart J 41:544–553, 1979.
12. Van Praagh R: The segmental approach to diagnosis in congenital heart disease. The cardiovascular system. Birth Defects: Original Article Series 8:4–23, 1972.
13. Van Praagh R: Terminology of congenital heart disease. Glossary and commentary. Circulation 56:139–143, 1977.
14. Van Praagh R: Diagnosis of complex congenital heart disease: morphologic anatomic method and terminology. Cardiovasc Intervent Radiol 7:115, 1984.
15. Van Praagh R: The importance of segmental situs in the diagnosis of congenital heart disease. Semin Roentgenol 20:254–271, 1985.
16. Van Praagh R, David I, Gordon D, et al: Ventricular diagnosis and designation. In Godman MJ (ed): Pediatric Cardiology, 1980 World Congress. London, Churchill Livingstone, 1981, Vol 4, pp. 153–168.
17. Van Praagh S, Davidoff A, Chin A, et al: Double-outlet right ventricle: anatomic types and developmental implications based on a study of 101 autopsied cases. Coeur 13:389–440, 1982.
18. Van Praagh S, LaCorte M, Fellows KE, et al: Superoinferior ventricles, anatomic and angiocardiographic findings in 10 postmortem cases. In Van Praagh R, Takao A (eds): Etiology and Morphogenesis of Congenital Heart Disease. Mt. Kisco, NY, Futura Publishing Co., 1980, pp. 317–378.
19. Van Praagh R, Ongley PA, Swan HJC: Anatomic types of single or common ventricle in man. Morphologic and geometric aspects of sixty autopsied cases. Am J Cardiol 13:367–386, 1964.
20. Van Praagh R, Perez-Trevino C, Lopez-Cuellar M, et al: Transposition of the great arteries with posterior aorta, anterior pulmonary artery, subpulmonary conus and fibrous continuity between aortic and atrioventricular valves. Am J Cardiol 28:621–631, 1971.
21. Van Praagh R, Van Praagh S, Vlad P, et al: Anatomic types of congenital dextrocardia. Am J Cardiol 13:510–531, 1964.
22. Van Praagh R, Weinberg PM, Srebro J: Double-outlet left ventricle. In Adams FH, Emmanouilides GC, Riemenschneider TH (eds): Moss' Heart Disease in Infants, Children, and Adolescents, 4th ed. Baltimore, Williams & Wilkins, 1989, pp. 461–485.
23. Van Praagh R, Weinberg PM, Calder AL, et al: The transposition complexes: how many are there? In Davila JC (ed): Second Henry Ford Hospital International Symposium on Cardiac Surgery. New York, Appleton-Century-Crofts, 1977, pp. 207–213.
24. Van Praagh R, Weinberg PM, Foran RB, Van Praagh S: Malposition of the heart. In Moss AJ, Adams FH, Emmanouilides GC, Riemenschneider TH (eds): Heart Disease in Infants, Children and Adolescents, 4th ed. Baltimore, Williams & Wilkins, 1989, pp. 530–580.

Section III
Dysmorphology

Chapter 5

DYSMORPHOLOGY

Ronald V. Lacro, M.D.

In 1966, Smith proposed that the term *dysmorphology* be used to denote the study of abnormalities in morphogenesis, regardless of etiology, timing of origin, or severity.[78] This field has expanded dramatically over the last two decades, during which time the number of recognizable patterns of malformation has more than tripled. Furthermore, great strides have been made in our understanding of the developmental pathogenesis of certain structural defects, including those affecting the cardiovascular system. Progress has been made in the dysmorphology and genetics of pediatric heart disease, particularly in clinical diagnosis, management, and genetic counseling of families and patients with congenital heart disease, whether isolated or associated with one or more extracardiac malformations.

Frequently, cardiologists and cardiac surgeons are required to manage patients with multiple malformations involving multiple organ systems. As many as 4% of all infants have at least one major defect in structural development.[53] A significant proportion of these have congenital heart disease, for which the incidence in the general population is estimated to be between 0.4 and 1%[22] (see ch. 18). Furthermore, 25% of these patients have at least one extracardiac malformation.[29] Consultations between the cardiologist and a dysmorphologist, or clinical geneticist, play an integral part in the management of affected patients and their families.

APPROACH TO THE CHILD WITH STRUCTURAL DEFECTS

The two patients depicted in Figures 1 and 2 illustrate the importance of recognizing an overall diagnosis. The first patient (Fig. 1) has the Ellis-van Creveld syndrome and the second patient (Fig. 2) has the trisomy 18 syndrome, each with a characteristic pattern of multiple malformations associated with a distinctive pattern of cardiac anomalies. Although both children could well be referred to a cardiologist for management, the prognosis and risk of recurrence are quite different for the two disorders and should be taken into account when deciding on appropriate treatment and counseling. The Ellis-van Creveld syndrome (chondroectodermal dysplasia) is an autosomal recessive disorder manifested by growth deficiency of prenatal onset, short limbs, polydactyly, hypoplasia of the nails, and dental anomalies. Atrial septal defect or common atrium occurs in about half of these patients. Intelligence is normal. In contrast, babies with the trisomy 18 syndrome are feeble at birth and have a limited capacity for survival. Characteristic features include growth deficiency of prenatal onset, petite facial features (short palpebral fissures, small and malformed ears, and small nose, mouth, and jaw), a prominent occiput, clenched hands, and a short sternum. Thirty percent die within the first month and 50% die by two months of age. Of the 10% who survive the first year, all are severely retarded. Salient findings in a recent review of 41 postmortem cases of trisomy 18 included a ventricular septal defect in all cases, polyvalvular disease (redundant or thick myxomatous leaflets) in 93%, and striking absence of transposition of the great arteries and inversion at any level (visceral or cardiac).[83]

Figure 3 presents a rational clinical approach to the child with structural defects. The ultimate goal of this schema is a specific diagnosis so that accurate

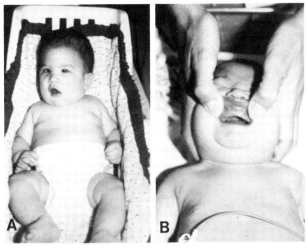
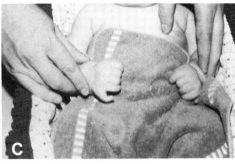

Figure 1. **A,** Ellis-van Creveld syndrome in a 6-month-old infant with a large atrial septal defect (common atrium). Note multiple frenulae between upper lip and alveolar ridge (**B**) and polydactyly (**C**).

prognosis can be made, the risk of recurrence can be determined, and an appropriate management plan may be formulated. When evaluating an infant or child with structural defects, it must first be determined whether the defect(s) is a problem with a prenatal or postnatal onset. Usually this distinction can be deduced from a careful history and physical examination. The term **prenatal onset** is used to designate structural abnormalities which are present at birth, whereas **postnatal onset** is used to designate structural abnormalities that are not present at birth, but rather develop postnatally.

Many structural defects are categorized as postnatal in onset even though the genetic alteration responsible for them was present prenatally. For example, children with genetically determined metabolic abnormalities that might be identified by amino acid screening are normal at birth, having appeared to thrive *in utero*. Neurologic problems frequently develop within the first few weeks of life, and rapid deterioration often follows. On the other hand, children with chromosomal abnormalities are abnormal at birth; however, the defects frequently remain static. Neurologic deterioration rarely occurs.

Once the distinction between prenatal and postnatal onset has been made, a rational differential diagnosis can be developed, since this determination narrows the diagnostic possibilities considerably. Figures 4 and 5 illustrate examples of prenatal and postnatal onset. When structural

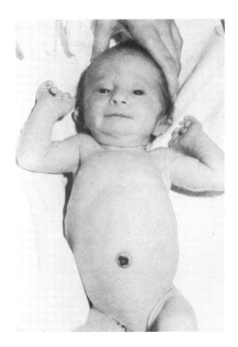

Figure 2. Trisomy 18 syndrome in a newborn infant with complex cardiac defects. Note petite facial features, clenched hands, and short sternum.

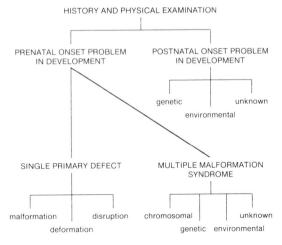

Figure 3. An approach to the child with structural defects.

malformations are present at the time of birth (prenatal onset), the diagnostic possibilities should include chromosomal abnormalities, genetically determined syndromes, and disorders due to prenatal exposure to a teratogen.

The child depicted in Figure 4 was born to a mother who used the acne medication, *cis*-retinoic acid (Accutane) during her pregnancy.[46] In these infants, malformations present at birth include craniofacial defects, especially anomalies of the ears and the Robin sequence, defects of the central nervous system (including hydrocephalus and microcephaly), thymic abnormalities, and a characteristic spectrum of conotruncal malformations (tetralogy of Fallot, double-outlet right ventricle, truncus arteriosus, supracristal ventricular septal defect, and type B interruption of the aortic arch). The retinoic acid embryopathy is an example of the effect of a teratogen on the developing embryo or fetus. In particular, it demonstrates how a specific teratogen can lead to a characteristic spectrum of cardiac lesions, presumably by acting via a common mechanism interfering with conotruncal development. Disorders caused by environmental agents take on special significance because prevention prior to conception may be feasible. In general, recognizing that a teratogenic agent was the cause

of the structural defect(s) means that the risk of recurrence is negligible if the mother avoids the use of that agent during subsequent pregnancies. Unfortunately, recent reports suggest that preconceptual use of a related compound, etretinate, which is stored in adipose tissue, may be associated with teratogenicity for indefinite periods of time after ingestion.[45] Other teratogens that are known to cause cardiac malformations include alcohol, anticonvulsants (hydantoins, trimethadione, valproic acid, carbamazepine), lithium, thalidomide, Coumadin, the rubella virus, maternal diabetes, and maternal phenylketonuria.[40,65,74,77]

Figure 5 depicts a patient with the Hurler syndrome (mucopolysaccharidosis I-H). The child was normal at birth, having appeared to thrive *in utero*. By 18 months of age, coarse facial features, cloudy corneas, poor growth, mental deficiency, and multiple skeletal anomalies became evident. Deposition of mucopolysaccharides in cardiac valve tissue and the intima of coronary vessels led to severe congestive heart failure due to marked mitral and aortic regurgitation. Postnatal onset of these structural defects should focus the diagnostic evaluation on the etiologic possibilities set forth in Figure 3, as they became manifest after birth. They include genetically determined inborn errors of metabolism, degenerative diseases of the central nervous system, and perinatal and postnatal environmental factors, such as anoxia, trauma, infection, and drugs.

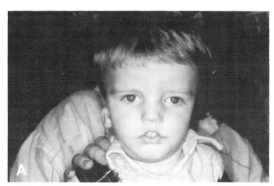

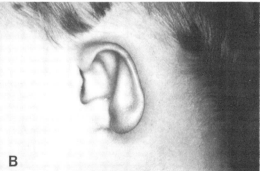

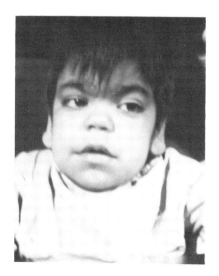

Figure 4. Retinoic acid embryopathy in a 2-year-old boy. **A,** Triangular facies, downslanting palpebral fissures, and widely spaced eyes. **B,** Malformed ears. Brain malformations (e.g., hydrocephalus) and conotruncal abnormalities are common.

Figure 5. Hurler syndrome. The facial features become progressively more coarse in this condition. Deposition of mucopolysaccharides in the valve tissue causes valvar insufficiency.

DEVELOPMENTAL PROBLEMS OF PRENATAL ONSET

Single Versus Multiple Malformations

Once a given problem has been determined to be of prenatal onset, a distinction should be made between those in which there is a single primary defect in development and those in which more than one system is involved, i.e., a multiple malformation syndrome (Fig. 3). Separation of prenatal onset problems into these two categories is useful because it permits some generalizations that can be helpful with respect to prognosis and to counseling about the risk of recurrence.

Conceptually, a single primary defect is a morphogenetic designation. In the majority of cases, the defect involves a single structure and the child is completely normal otherwise. The seven most common single primary defects in development include: cleft palate, cleft lip (with or without cleft palate), cardiac septal defects, pyloric stenosis, neural tube defects, congenital dislocation of the hip, and talipes equinovarus (clubfoot). For most single primary defects, the etiology is not known or is presumed to be heterogeneous.

In contrast to the anatomic concept of the single primary defect in development, the designation **multiple malformation syndrome** indicates that the observed structural defects all have the same known or presumed mode of etiology. The defects themselves usually include a number of anatomically unrelated errors in structural development. Multiple malformation syndromes are caused by chromosomal abnormalities, teratogens, and single gene defects inherited in mendelian patterns. Unfortunately, many multiple malformation syndromes currently have no identifiable cause.

The risk of recurrence depends entirely on an accurate diagnosis. For example, the risk for disorders due to a fresh gene mutation or to a teratogen with which the mother has no contact in subsequent pregnancies is 0%. However, the risk is 25% for disorders having an autosomal recessive mode of inheritance, 50% for autosomal dominant disorders in which one parent is affected, and 100% for the unusual case of a child with Down syndrome in which one parent is a balanced 21/21 translocation carrier.

From a practical standpoint, recognition that a child has a single primary defect of prenatal onset, such as an isolated atrial septal defect, suggests an approximate recurrence risk in the range of 2–4% for first-degree relatives (see below). However, recognition that a child has an atrial septal defect as one feature of a multiple malformation syndrome is not helpful with respect to counseling for risk of recurrence unless a specific overall diagnosis can be made. It should become obvious, then, that any child with a cardiac malformation or any other major malformation, for that matter, deserves a careful history and physical examination to rule out a broader pattern of malformation which will have an impact on the prognosis for that child and genetic counseling for that family.

Single Primary Defects. Single primary defects can be subcategorized according to the nature of the error in morphogenesis which produced the defect (Fig. 3). Thus, single primary defects involve **malformation, deformation,** or **disruption** of developing structures.[79]

Malformations. A malformation is a primary structural defect arising from a localized error in morphogenesis—a failure of normal development or a failure in formation. This definition implies an intrinsically abnormal developmental process within an organ, part of an organ, or larger region of the body leading to a structural morphologic defect. Most congenital cardiac defects fit this definition. The risk of recurrence for most isolated malformations is 2–4% for first-degree relatives with one affected family member, and higher if two or more family members are affected.[60]

Deformations. In contrast, deformations and disruptions are secondary events. A deformation (for example, congenital dislocation of the hip or clubfoot) is an alteration in the form, shape, or position of an intrinsically normal part caused by mechanical forces.[28] These forces may be extrinsic to the fetus as in intrauterine constraint, or intrinsic as with decreased mobility caused by a malformation of the central nervous system. The risk of recurrence depends on the cause of the abnormal forces. For example, if the mother has a uterine anomaly or fibroids, the risk could be high.

Some cardiac defects may result from deformation. The distribution of blood flow within the heart and great vessels is a determinant of chamber and vessel size and shape. Alteration in the relative volume of blood results in dramatic changes in the size of the cardiac chamber. For example, experimental obstruction of blood flow in the left side of the heart produces hypoplasia (deformation) of the left heart structures and a reciprocal increase in size (deformation) of the right heart structures.[35,80] A spectrum of defects related to altered fetal hemodynamics has been described.[9,44]

Disruptions. A disruption is a defect resulting from destruction of a previously normally formed part—extrinsic interference with an originally normal developmental process. With disruption, in contrast to malformation, the developmental potential of the involved organ was originally normal. Secondarily, an extrinsic factor interfered with development, which thereafter proceeded abnormally. By definition, a disruption cannot be inherited; however, inherited factors can predispose to and influence the development of a disruption. The two basic mechanisms known to produce disruption include amniotic bands and vascular infarction. As a general rule, the risk of recurrence for disruptions is negligible.

Even when the exact cause of a defect cannot be determined, its categorization as a malformation, deformation, or disruption will help to predict prognosis and risk of recurrence. Because development is intrinsically normal for most deformations and disruptions, the likelihood of congenital heart malformations occurring with such defects generally is low. In contrast, the incidence of cardiac malformations would be expected to be increased in association with other true malformations where the intrinsic developmental potential of the fetus is abnormal. This concept is illustrated by the fact that cardiac malformations frequently are associated with cases of omphalocele (**malformations**), but not with gastroschisis (vascular **disruptions** involving the omphalomesenteric artery).[37]

Multiple Defects. This category includes patients in whom a primary developmental anomaly of two or more systems has occurred, all of which are thought to have a common etiology; that is, a pattern of multiple anomalies thought to be pathogenetically related. As shown in Figure 3, multiple malformation syndromes can be categorized on the basis of their etiology: chromosomal, genetic, environmental, and unknown.

Chromosomal Abnormalities. The ability to perform chromosomal studies has led to the recognition of a large number of chromosomal multiple malformation syndromes that are usually caused by faulty chromosomal distribution at cell division. The most common disorder associated with a chromosomal abnormality, Down syndrome (trisomy 21), is also the most common recognizable multiple malformation syndrome. The characteristic stigmata of this disorder are present at birth, making a clinical diagnosis possible at that time.

The incidence of chromosomal aberrations at birth is about 1:200.[32] Recent studies utilizing chromosomal banding and high-resolution analysis have found that as many as 12.9% of all infants with congenital heart disease have chromosomal abnormalities, the vast majority of these having the trisomy 21 syndrome.[21] The "averaged" incidence of congenital heart disease among patients with unbalanced chromosome aberrations is probably about 20%. It is about 40% for autosomal chromosomal aberrations, including the Down syndrome, but only 2–3% for sex chromosome aberrations.[74] Overall, the incidences of the different types of congenital heart disease among liveborn children with chromosomal aberrations does not deviate strikingly from their overall incidences in all newborns. Ventricular septal defect, atrial septal defect, and patent ductus arteriosus are among the most frequent defects associated with many chromosomal aberrations. Transposition of the great arteries, truncus arteriosus, and endocardial

fibroelastosis seldom occur in children with chromosomal aberrations. However, for many individual chromosomal aberrations, there are marked deviations from the mean frequencies. For example, in the Down syndrome, endocardial cushion defects are overrepresented, whereas transposition of the great arteries has not been reported to the author's knowledge. In the cat eye syndrome, total anomalous pulmonary venous return occurs rather frequently. Most patients with the Turner syndrome and congenital heart disease have coarctation of the aorta; in boys with the karyotype 49,XXXXY and in 49,XXXXX girls, patent ductus arteriosus is overrepresented.

Heart and brain malformations are the most important life-limiting factors in chromosomal disorders; however, the group with congenital heart disease has a dramatically lower mean survival. In newborns with a chromosomal aberration and multiple abnormalities, including clinically significant congenital heart disease, the medical team needs to decide how far to proceed with diagnostic and therapeutic procedures. It is mandatory to have a rapid cytogenetic diagnosis, to be aware of other significant malformations (mainly involving the brain or kidneys), and to assess the probable clinical course and degree of mental handicap that could be expected. For example, if the child has a deletion of the long arm of chromosome 13, which often is associated with holoprosencephaly, it would be worthwhile to confirm or exclude severe forms of this malformation by neuroradiologic investigation. If holoprosencephaly is found, no extraordinary life-prolonging measures should be undertaken. The same is true for a number of autosomal chromosomal aberrations, including trisomy 18 and trisomy 13 (see p. 47), which are associated with poor survival and/or an unfavorable prognosis relative to mental development. On the other hand, if, in a patient with multiple malformations (including congenital heart disease), the cytogenetic examination reveals the cat eye chromosome, the prognosis for survival and mental development usually is relatively good. Thus, the withholding of therapeutic measures cannot be justified if there are no cerebral or severe renal malformations.

Disorders with Known Genetic Etiology. A single mutant gene (autosomal dominant or X-linked) or a pair of mutant genes (autosomal recessive) have been implicated as the cause of some recognizable multiple malformation syndromes of prenatal onset.[55] In most of these disorders correct diagnosis depends on clinical recognition, because in the vast majority of cases there is no confirmatory laboratory test. Family history indicating a similarly affected individual can be extremely helpful; however, in many patients with multiple malformation syndromes of genetic etiology, the occurrence is sporadic and represents a fresh gene mutation. In such situations all family members are normal, and diagnosis depends entirely on evaluation of the patient's phenotype.

Because variance in expression among patients with the same disorder is the rule in dominant conditions, the patient's phenotype, particularly if it represents a mild expression of the disorder, may not be conclusive. This can lead to serious problems in diagnosis and must also be taken into consideration when giving parents information regarding the risk of recurrence and the prognosis.

Disorders Caused by Teratogens. The role of teratogens in the etiology of congenital heart disease has been reviewed extensively.[8,65,74,77] Teratogens are chemical, physical, or biological agents capable of inducing congenital anomalies. Although the assignment of risk for any potential teratogen is difficult, as a group, these defects are the most amenable to preventive measures. It is difficult to predict the risk of congenital heart disease in a particular fetus exposed to a particular teratogen, but cardiac defects often have a serious impact on survival. Some teratogens produce distinct clinical syndromes or recognizable patterns of malformation, the most common being the fetal alcohol syndrome; other agents cause an increased incidence of single or multiple malformations without a specific syndromic pattern (for example, maternal ingestion of lithium or maternal diabetes). Table 1 summarizes the known or potential teratogens with respect to congenital heart disease.

DEVELOPMENTAL PROBLEMS OF POSTNATAL ONSET

With the exception of children with metabolic disorders such as the Hurler syndrome, the vast majority of patients with structural heart disease have developmental problems of **prenatal onset**. Children with developmental problems of **postnatal onset** are normal at birth, having appeared to thrive *in utero*. Neurologic problems frequently begin within the first week of life and deterioration often is rapid. Usually, a specific pattern of malformation does not occur; structural abnormalities are virtually always the result of neurologic deterioration. In disorders with a known metabolic aberration, other manifestations of the metabolic defect, such as cataracts, sparse hair, coarse facies, unusual skin pigmentation, and hepatosplenomegaly, are frequently present. As set forth in Figure 3, these disorders can be categorized on the basis of etiology.

Genetic. *Metabolic.* Most of these conditions are the result of a specific enzyme deficiency. Because of the possibility that early institution of dietary therapy may help to prevent mental retardation, these disorders are of particular interest. Also, these conditions are potentially amenable to

gene replacement therapy. Their incidence is extremely low, and most have an autosomal recessive mode of inheritance. Phenylketonuria (1:14,000 persons) is the most common and, in its untreated state, represents approximately 1% of institutionalized populations.

Central Nervous System Degenerative States. Probably, a metabolic defect will be found for most of these rare disorders. However, at present, although the clinical features and mode of inheritance have been delineated, the biochemical abnormality for many of them is not known. The most common of these disorders is Tay-Sachs disease, which is associated with hexosaminidase A deficiency.

Environmental. Trauma, infection, hypoxia, and metabolic derangements can result in severe neurologic impairment. Progressive joint immobility, abnormal positioning, and paralysis secondary to degeneration of the central nervous system are the most frequent causes of structural anomalies.

CARDIAC SYNDROMES

There are a great many malformation syndromes involving the cardiovascular system. The approach that has been described allows a systematic narrowing of diagnostic possibilities, such that one of the basic texts of dysmorphology can be consulted in a practical fashion.[5,25,26,39,55] Having reached a specific diagnosis, an accurate prognosis and risk of recurrence can be communicated to the family.

It is useful to view the multiple malformation syndromes with cardiovascular involvement as constituting a spectrum. On one end of the spectrum are multiple malformation syndromes, which are easy to diagnose and have a high incidence of cardiac malformations. Examples include Down and Turner syndromes. Because of the presence of multiple malformations, these patients should be seen early in the diagnostic process by a dysmorphologist, but they also require cardiac assessment and management. On the other end of the spectrum are multiple malformation syndromes, which are, in large part, defined by the cardiac defects associated with them (for example, the Holt-Oram syndrome). Frequently, these patients are evaluated by a cardiologist first because the cardiac defect is most prominent, but they require a dysmorphologist's evaluation because of associated extracardiac anomalies. The extracardiac malformations may be subtle, but nevertheless, awareness of them is essential for arriving at an accurate diagnosis. In the middle of the spectrum are disorders that engender close collaboration between cardiology and dysmorphology. Careful scrutiny of the pattern of cardiac and noncardiac anomalies often leads to a definitive systemic diagnosis. Ex-

Table 1. Abnormalities Caused by Teratogens

Recognizable Phenotypes (Syndromes)	Cardiac Abnormalities
Chemical teratogens	
Fetal alcohol syndrome	Ventricular septal defect, atrial septal defect, tetralogy of Fallot, coarctation of the aorta
Fetal hydantoin syndrome	Ventricular septal defect, tetralogy of Fallot, pulmonary stenosis, patent ductus arteriosus, atrial septal defect, coarctation of the aorta
Fetal trimethadione syndrome	Combined defects
Fetal valproate syndrome	Nonspecific
Fetal carbamazepine syndrome	Ventricular septal defect, tetralogy of Fallot
Retinoic acid embryopathy	Conotruncal malformations
Thalidomide embryopathy	Conotruncal malformations
Fetal warfarin syndrome	Patent ductus arteriosus, peripheral pulmonary stenosis
Biological teratogens	
Maternal PKU fetal effects	Tetralogy of Fallot, ventricular septal defect, coarctation of the aorta
Maternal lupus fetal effects	Complete heart block, cardiomyopathy, L-transposition of the great arteries
Fetal rubella syndrome	Patent ductus arteriosus, peripheral pulmonary stenosis, fibromuscular and intimal proliferation of medium and large arteries, ventricular septal defect, atrial septal defect
Non-Syndromic Increased Risk for Malformations	
Lithium	Ebstein's disease, tricuspid atresia, atrial septal defect
Maternal diabetes	Transposition of the great arteries, ventricular septal defect, coarctation of the aorta, hypertrophic cardiomyopathy

amples include Noonan, Williams, and Marfan syndromes.

Classification of Congenital Cardiac Malformations

Traditional nomenclature for classifying structural heart defects is based on presumed embryologic events or on their anatomic characteristics and location. Although helpful in naming complex cardiac defects, the traditional use of earlier classifications may have obscured important pathogenic relationships. More recently, congenital heart defects have been approached from the viewpoint of disordered mechanisms. Five developmental mechanisms (cell migration abnormalities, cardiac hemodynamics, cellular death, extracellular matrix abnormalities, and disordered targeted growth) are likely to play a role in causing cardiac malformations.[10] Although the specific cardiac defects involved are heterogeneous, they share the disordered mechanism. Evaluation of cases of congenital heart disease by mechanistic groups can help to clarify relationships among malformations, suggest underlying mechanisms, and elucidate familial patterns and risks of recurrence for relatives (Table 2).[6]

Genetic Counseling

Guidelines for genetic counseling for congenital heart defects were recently presented by Lin and Garver.[49] Requirements for optimal genetic counseling include (1) a thorough understanding of the anatomy, management, and outcome of the particular defect, (2) identification of other affected family members and careful pedigree analysis for prediction of familial risks, (3) identification of associated malformations or syndromes, and (4) options for prenatal diagnosis. Ideally, genetic counseling should be provided by both a dysmorphologist knowledgeable about cardiac defects and outcome and by a pediatric cardiologist with a keen awareness and interest in genetic issues.

As a general rule, congenital heart diseases are thought to have multifactorial origins with genetic and environmental influences; however, the familial occurrence of virtually all forms of congenital heart disease has been noted. Clinical and echocardiographic studies of first-degree relatives of patients with complete common atrioventricular canal and hypoplastic left heart syndrome have detected previously unsuspected congenital heart diseases that were clinically less significant than the proband's congenital heart disease but were part of the same mechanistic spectrum (e.g., atrioventricular type of septal defects and left-axis deviation for complete atrioventricular canal; left ventricular outflow obstruction for hypoplastic left heart syndrome).[7,14] Numerous instances of single gene (mendelian) inheritance of congenital heart

Table 2. Sibling Precurrence Rates for Congenital Heart Disease

Category of Disordered Cardiac Embryonic Mechanism	Siblings Affected/At Risk	Percent
Cell Migration Abnormality (Conotruncal)		
Truncus arteriosus	0/1	
Transposition of great arteries	0/24	
Double-outlet right ventricle	0/8	
Tetralogy of Fallot	0/22	
Type B interrupted aortic arch	0/1	
Ventricular septal defect (supracristal, malalignment)	0/2	
Flow Lesions		
Hypoplastic left heart syndrome	5/38	13.5
Coarctation	3/37	8.1
Aortic stenosis, valvar	0/12	
Bicuspid aortic valve	1/9	11.1
Patent ductus arteriosus	1/13	7.7
Secundum atrial septal defect	1/31	3.2
Pulmonic stenosis, valvar	3/33	9.1
Pulmonary atresia, intact ventricular septum	0/8	
Ventricular septal defect (membranous)	5/86	5.8
Cell Death		
Ebstein anomaly	0/10	
Ventricular septal defect (muscular)	0/9	
Extracellular Matrix		
Atrioventricular canal	0/10	
Ventricular septal defect (endocardial cushion type)	0	
Targeted Growth		
Anomalous pulmonary venous return, total	0/12	
Anomalous pulmonary venous return, partial	0/1	
Single atrium	0/1	
Other	1/37	2.8

Modified from Boughman JA, et al.,[6] with permission.

disease with autosomal recessive or dominant transmission have been reported.

Risk of Recurrence of Congenital Heart Disease in Siblings (Table 3). Initially, the empirical risk of recurrence to a family with one affected child was thought to be 1–3%, in accordance with a multifactorial model. Recent information from a large retrospective study suggests that familial **precurrence** rates (i.e., frequency of congenital heart disease in relatives of probands with isolated congenital heart disease) may be greater for specific groups of cardiac defects when they are classified according to the type of disordered mechanism (Table 2).[6] The sibling precurrence rates for all types of congenital heart disease were consistent with previously reported rates (1.8%); however, the rates for obstructive lesions of the left side of the heart (related to disordered cardiac hemodynamics) were significantly higher (fourfold to sixfold greater). Sibling precurrence rates for the hypoplastic left heart syndrome and coarctation of the aorta were 14 and 8%, respectively. In contrast, the sizable Second Natural History Study of Congenital Heart Defects found occurrence rates of congenital heart disease in siblings of subjects with ventricular septal defects, aortic stenosis, and pulmonary stenosis

to be 1.1, 1.6, and 1.1%, respectively.[16] The recurrence risk figures quoted in Table 3[60] represent combined data published between 1966 and 1985. Caution should be exercised in counseling families with left-sided obstructive lesions, given the more recent data presented by Boughman.[6] Further carefully designed epidemiologic studies are indicated.

Risk of Recurrence for Congenital Heart Disease Given One Affected Parent (Table 4). Initial reports indicated that the recurrence risk to offspring of parents with congenital heart disease was 2–4%, depending on the lesion, if one parent was affected. If both parents were affected or if there was one affected parent and a previously affected child, the risk was tripled. These data, consistent with a multifactorial model, were challenged seriously in a large prospective cohort study, which noted a 14.2% incidence of congenital heart disease in children born to women with congenital heart disease.[84] Similarly, another study found a recurrence risk of 8.8% in children born to parents with certain congenital heart disease.[71] A high recurrence risk (10–14%) in children of parents with complete atrioventricular canal has also been reported.[19] In contrast to these studies, the Second

Table 3. Recurrence Risks for Congenital Heart Defects in Siblings

	Percent at Risk	
Defect	1 Sibling Affected	2 Siblings Affected
Ventricular septal defect	3	10
Patent ductus arteriosus	3	10
Atrial septal defect	2.5	8
Tetralogy of Fallot	2.5	8
Pulmonary stenosis	2	6
Coarctation of aorta	2	6
Aortic stenosis	2	6
Transposition	1.5	5
Endocardial cushion defects	3	10
Fibroelastosis	4	12
Hypoplastic left heart	2	6
Tricuspid atresia	1	3
Ebstein anomaly	1	3
Truncus arteriosus	1	3
Pulmonary atresia	1	3

Based on combined data published during two decades from European and North American populations. (From Nora JJ, Nora AH: Update on counseling the family with a first-degree relative with a congenital heart defect. Am J Med Genet 29:137–142, 1988, with permission.)

Table 4. Suggested Percent Recurrence Risks for Congenital Heart Defects in Offspring Given One Affected Parent

Defect	Mother Affected	Father Affected
Aortic stenosis	13–18	3
Atrial septal defect	4–4.5	1.5
Atrioventricular canal	14	1
Coarctation of aorta	4	2
Patent ductus arteriosus	3.5–4	2.5
Pulmonary stenosis	4–6.5	2
Tetralogy of Fallot	2.5	1.5
Ventricular septal defect	6–10	2

From Nora JJ, Nora AH: Update on counseling the family with a first-degree relative with a congenital heart defect. Am J Med Genet 29:137–142, 1988, with permission.

Natural History Study of Congenital Heart Defects found much lower rates of congenital heart disease in children of subjects with ventricular septal defect, aortic stenosis, and pulmonary stenosis (2.92, 1.2, and 2.89%, respectively).[16] The recurrence risk figures quoted in Table 4 represent combined data published between 1966 and 1985. Risk projections should be based on the genetic and teratogenic history in the individual family and pregnancy.

Prenatal Diagnosis. In addition to the assessment and communication of risk of recurrence, genetic counseling should also provide information about prenatal diagnosis and referral to appropriate specialists. Fetal echocardiography,[63] beginning at 16 weeks' gestation, can be offered if either parent or a previous offspring has a congenital heart disease or if the mother has a risk factor predisposing the fetus to congenital heart disease (e.g., affected first-degree relative, teratogenic exposure, maternal diabetes). The parents should be counseled, ideally in conjunction with a pediatric cardiologist, regarding the specific cardiac anatomy, current medical or surgical options, and prognosis.

Fetal karyotype analysis is indicated when certain highly distinctive cardiac defects are detected prenatally, especially when associated with other extracardiac malformations, in order to determine the possibility of an associated chromosomal syndrome (e.g., common atrioventricular canal in the trisomy 21 syndrome, polyvalvular disease in the trisomy 18 syndrome, and interrupted aortic arch, type B, in the DiGeorge sequence).

During pregnancy, the mother should be monitored closely by a perinatologist and a cardiologist.

Delivery should occur near a tertiary neonatal unit that can provide immediate resuscitation and intensive care. Cardiology and dysmorphology evaluations should be performed after birth to confirm prenatal diagnoses and identify associated defects.

Heterogeneity: Pitfalls in Genetic Counseling. Previously, genetic counseling for isolated congenital heart disease (i.e., not associated with a malformation syndrome) was transmitted as generalized advice, with the use of an overall recurrence risk for first-degree relatives of 2–5%. Any given defect, however, has heterogeneous courses; therefore, risk projections should be based on the genetic and teratogenic history in an individual family or pregnancy.

Patent ductus arteriosus has a number of different known causes. Most common is that associated with prematurity. Birth at high altitudes increases the risk for patent ductus arteriosus. The fetal rubella syndrome, as well as a number of other multiple malformation syndromes, can cause patent ductus arteriosus. In some families, single gene (mendelian) transmission is implicated, whereas more commonly, multifactorial inheritance is involved.

Left-sided obstructive lesions may carry higher familial rates than previously reported. The risk of affected mothers having a child affected with a congenital heart defect may be in the range of 8–14%, although additional studies are needed to confirm this. Well-designed epidemiologic studies, replacing smaller, uncontrolled and anecdotal reports, are necessary to clarify the genetic aspects of congenital heart disease. The techniques of molecular genetics may be useful in the future for the study of familial congenital heart disease.

OTHER SYNDROMES WITH HEART DISEASE

Only the more common disorders frequently associated with cardiovascular defects will be described. Reference to general textbooks of dysmorphology and genetics is recommended.[5,25,26,39,55]

Chromosomal Aberrations

Trisomy 21 Syndrome (Down Syndrome). Although the classic description of Down syndrome was published in 1866,[15] cytogenetic confirmation of its trisomic etiology was not reported until 1959. Trisomy 21 is the most frequent chromosomal aberration affecting liveborn infants, with an incidence of 1 in 660 livebirths: 94% are due to nondisjunction, 3% to parental translocation, and 3% to mosaicism.[66] The clinical phenotype is so distinctive that cytogenetic analysis is done primarily to identify cases due to translocation or mosaicism.

The typical facies of an infant with trisomy 21 is shown in Figure 6. The skull shows microcephaly and brachycephaly, and the occiput is flattened. The face is also flattened with underdevelopment of the midface. The nasal bridge is low, and the nose is small. The palpebral fissures slant upward. Epicanthal folds, Brushfield spots, strabismus, and nystagmus are frequent findings. The ears are

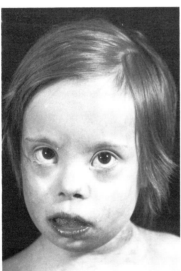

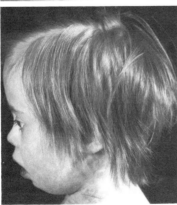

Figure 6. Trisomy 21 (Down) syndrome. Note the flat expressionless face, small nose, low nasal bridge, bilateral epicanthal folds, and protrusion of the tongue.

small. As part of the generalized hypotonia, the mouth is held open with the tongue thrust forward. The neck is short and webbed with loose skinfolds posteriorly. The stature is relatively small and the gait awkward. The joints are hyperextensible. The hands and fingers are short and broad; the fifth finger is particularly short and shows clinodactyly. Typically, there is a wide gap between the first and second toes. Mental retardation is present, but the children are quite sociable. A recent population-based epidemiologic study showed that 10.4% of 2102 infants with cardiovascular malformations had the trisomy 21 syndrome.[21] Cardiac malformations are found in at least 40% of patients with Down syndrome. There is a distinctive spectrum of cardiac defects with an overrepresentation of endocardial cushion defects compared with the general population. The most common lesions (in decreasing order of frequency) include common atrioventricular canal, ventricular septal defect, atrial septal defect, tetralogy of Fallot, and patent ductus arteriosus.[74] Left-sided obstructive lesions such as coarctation and valvar aortic stenosis are rare. Transposition of the great arteries has not been reported.

Most patients with Down syndrome who die during infancy do so within the first year of life, and congenital heart disease is the most important contributing factor. Recent studies have shown that 49.9% of patients with Down syndrome with congenital heart disease and 79.2% of patients with Down syndrome without congenital heart disease have a life expectancy of 30 years (Table 5). This compares with 92.2% for a cohort of patients with mental retardation not related to Down syndrome and 96.7% for normal controls.[4] Whether current medical and surgical therapy will affect life expectancy remains to be seen.

The risk for trisomy 21 increases with maternal age. The likelihood for recurrence of Down syndrome is 1%, except in cases of the rare translo-

Exhibit 1

Boston Children's Hospital Experience 1973–1987		
Down Syndrome with Congenital Heart Disease N = 666		
Cardiac Defect		No. of Patients
Endocardial cushion defects		328
Complete atrioventricular canal	262	
Ostium primum defect	51	
Other	15	
Ventricular septal defect		171
Tetralogy of Fallot		68
Patent ductus arteriosus		19
Atrial septal defect (secundum)		16
Double-outlet right ventricle		6
Coarctation of the aorta		5
Other		53

Table 5. Life Expectancy in Trisomy 21 Syndrome

Life Expectancy	With Congenital Heart Disease (%)	Without Congenital Heart Disease (%)
To age 1 year	76.3	90.7
To age 5 years	61.8	87.2
To age 10 years	57.1	84.9
To age 20 years	53.1	81.9
To age 30 years	49.9	79.2

The 30-year statistics compare to 96.7% for normals and 92.2% for a cohort with mental retardation without heart disease. (From Baird PA, Sadovnick AD: Life expectancy in Down syndrome. J Pediatr 110:849–854, 1987, with permission.)

cation carrier parent, when the risk will depend on the type of translocation and the sex of the parent that carries it.[39]

Trisomy 18 Syndrome. Trisomy 18 syndrome (Fig. 2) was first recognized as a specific entity in 1960 when the extra 18 chromosome was discovered in babies with a characteristic pattern of malformation.[17,64] Trisomy 18 is the second most frequent autosomal chromosomal aberration in man, with an incidence of 1 in 3500 newborns. Principal features found in virtually all affected individuals include clenched hands, a short sternum, a low arch pattern of the dermal ridges on the fingertips, and severe cardiac anomalies.

Cardiovascular defects are found in virtually all liveborn infants with trisomy 18. Recently the cardiac malformations in 41 karyotyped and autopsied cases of trisomy 18 were studied.[83] The salient findings included a ventricular septal defect in all cases, polyvalvular disease (malformations of more than one valve) in 93%, a subpulmonary infundibulum in 98%, and a striking absence of transposition of the great arteries and inversion at any level (cardiac or visceral), findings which appear to be characteristic of all trisomies. The ventricular septal defect was associated with anterosuperior conal septal malalignment in 61% of patients. The malformations of the atrioventricular and semilunar valves were characterized by redundant or thick myxomatous leaflets, long chordae tendineae, and hypoplastic or absent papillary muscles. Other findings included double-outlet right ventricle (10%), all with mitral atresia, and tetralogy of Fallot (15%).

Most infants with trisomy 18 syndrome have severe perinatal difficulties attributable to severe brain dysfunction as well as to severe cardiac malformations. The majority die within a week of birth, most commonly because of apneic spells. Cardiovascular failure and aspiration pneumonia are common. Occasionally, a patient has survived into the teens or to adult age, but all have been profoundly mentally retarded, completely dependent on care, and severely spastic. Because of the poor prognosis and fatal outcome of newborns with trisomy 18, no

life-prolonging and intensive therapeutic measures are justified.

Though no accurate empirical data are available, risk of recurrence is presumed to be less than 1%.

Trisomy 13 Syndrome. Trisomy 13 syndrome (Fig. 7) was not recognized generally until cytogenetic confirmation of its trisomic etiology was made by Patau.[64] The incidence is about 1 in 5000 live births. Principal features include cleft lip and palate; holoprosencephalic type of defects of the eye, nose, lip, and forebrain; polydactyly; and localized skin defects of the posterior portion of the scalp. Microphthalmia, colobomata of the iris, and retinal dysplasia are common. Apneic spells, seizures, and severe mental deficiency are hallmarks.

The incidence of cardiovascular malformations is about 80%. The most frequent malformations are as follows:[74] patent ductus arteriosus (63%), ventricular septal defect (48%), atrial septal defect (40%), abnormal valves (22%), coarctation of the aorta (10%), and dextrocardia (6%). About three-fourths of affected patients have complex defects.

Of infants with trisomy 13, 44% die within the first month and 69% by six months. Only 18% survive the first year. Although long-term survival has been observed occasionally, all survivors are profoundly retarded, completely dependent on care, and severely spastic. As in trisomy 18, infants with trisomy 13 syndrome have a dismally poor prognosis. Life-prolonging and intensive therapeutic measures are not justified. Although no accurate empirical data are available, the risk of recurrence is presumed to be less than 1%.

Turner Syndrome. This syndrome of short stat-

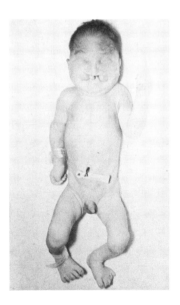

Figure 7. Trisomy 13 syndrome in a newborn infant with complex congenital heart disease. Note the bilateral cleft lip and palate and polydactyly.

ure, sexual infantilism, webbed neck, congenital lymphedema, and cubitus valgus was described by Turner[82] in 1938 (Fig. 8). Although common in the first trimester, the majority of XO conceptuses are spontaneously aborted. They constitute 25% of spontaneous abortions during the first trimester of pregnancy. The incidence of this chromosomal aberration among liveborn females is 1 in 5000. More than half the patients have a 45,X karyotype without evidence of mosaicism. The remainder show mosaicism and/or more complex rearrangements involving the X chromosome (ring, deletion, isochromosome Xq, isodicentric X, etc.).

On the average, intelligence is normal, but girls frequently display dysfunctional sensory-motor integration (gross and fine motor development).[72] Many phenotypic features, including the webbed neck, hypoplastic nails, and swelling of the dorsa of the hands and feet, are thought to be secondary to jugular lymphatic obstruction *in utero*.[39] There is suggestive evidence that the cardiac lesions may also be related to lymphatic obstruction.[44]

Between 20 and 40% of girls with Turner syndrome have significant heart defects, most commonly coarctation of the aorta (70%), often bicuspid aortic valve, and aortic stenosis, lesions normally not common in females. In a recent study of 35 patients with Turner syndrome who had no prior history of cardiovascular disease, echocardiography revealed a biscuspid aortic valve in 34% of patients, suggesting that the actual incidence of cardiac defects is higher than previously believed.[57]

Aortic dilatation, dissection, and rupture also have been reported with the Turner syndrome and have been related to changes described as cystic medial necrosis in the aorta. Several risk factors have been suggested, including coarctation, bicuspid aortic valve, and systemic hypertension (present in about 10% of patients with Turner syndrome). Two recent studies have found an unexpectedly high incidence of unrecognized aortic root dilatation (8.8–29%) among 85 patients with Turner syndrome who were prospectively evaluated by echocardiography.[2,50]

Disorders Caused by Teratogens

Fetal Alcohol Syndrome. One of the most frequent multiple malformation syndromes, with an estimated frequency greater than 1:1000 liveborn infants, the fetal alcohol syndrome is also one of the most frequent single causes of mental retardation (Fig. 9).[42,47] About half of all patients with the full fetal alcohol syndrome have congenital heart disease.[52,73] By far the most common defect is ventricular septal defect, followed by atrial septal defect and tetralogy of Fallot. Less commonly reported malformations include atrioventricular canal, hypoplasia or absence of one pulmonary artery, subaortic stenosis, and other complex lesions.

The most serious consequence of prenatal alcohol exposure is its effects on brain development and function. Spontaneous abortion and perinatal mortality are high. Affected individuals tend to be irritable young infants, hyperactive children and adolescents, but more sociable adults. The amount of alcohol consumption, severity of maternal alcoholism, and extent and severity of the pattern of malformation seem to be the most predictive of the ultimate prognosis.

Fetal Anticonvulsant Syndromes. Distinct patterns of malformation have been identified for several anticonvulsant agents: **fetal hydantoin syndrome,**[33,34] **fetal trimethadione syndrome,**[20,24,86]

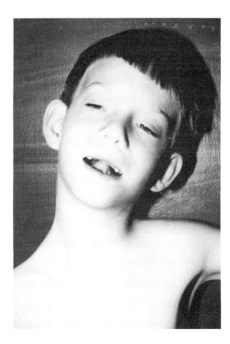

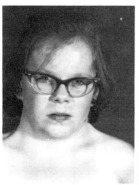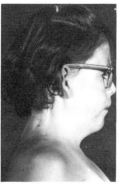

Figure 8. Turner syndrome in a young woman with coarctation of the aorta. Note the webbed neck, broad chest, prominent ears, and multiple pigmented nevi.

Figure 9. Fetal alcohol syndrome. Typical facies in a child with severe manifestations of prenatal alcohol exposure. Note the short, downslanting, palpebral fissures, short upturned nose, long smooth philtrum, and thin upper lip.

fetal valproate syndrome,[3,13,38,65] and **fetal carba-mazepine effects.**[40]

The approximate risk for the fetal hydantoin syndrome in exposed infants is 10%, with an additional 33% showing some effects of the disorder. The incidence of congenital heart disease in infants exposed prenatally to hydantoins is not clear; however, the most frequently reported defects include ventricular septal defect, tetralogy of Fallot, valvar pulmonary stenosis, atrial septal defect, patent ductus arteriosus, and coarctation of the aorta. The degree of mental retardation has the greatest impact on prognosis.

More than two-thirds of prenatally exposed infants show abnormalities consistent with the fetal trimethadione syndrome. Cardiac malformations (most often combined defects) occur in about 50% of affected patients and are the most important life-limiting defects.

Prenatal exposure to valproic acid has been associated with a relative risk for cardiac defects of 3.7–4.3%.[65]

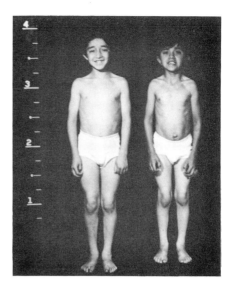

Figure 10. Noonan syndrome. These brothers have short stature, webbed neck due to prominence of the trapezius muscle, cryptorchidism, and dysplastic pulmonary valve stenosis.

Single Gene Defects

Noonan Syndrome. Although sporadic reports of probable cases of Noonan syndrome appeared in 1883 and 1928, it was not until 1963 that Noonan and Ehmke[59] provided further delineation of the clinical phenotype of this disorder and documented its association with dysplastic pulmonary stenosis.[56] Principal features include short stature of prenatal onset, seen in about half of affected individuals; mental retardation (usually mild), seen in about 25% of cases; characteristic facial appearance; a short, webbed neck with low posterior hairline; a shield chest deformity with pectus carinatum superiorly and pectus excavatum inferiorly; cubitus valgus; and cryptorchidism among males (Fig. 10).[56] There is a variable but specific and predictably changing phenotype dependent on chronological age (Fig. 10).[1]

At least 50% of patients with Noonan syndrome have congenital heart disease, although there may be ascertainment bias toward cardiac defects among the cases published in the literature. At least 75% of those with congenital heart disease have valvar pulmonary stenosis secondary to a dysplastic pulmonary valve with thickened valve leaflets. Particularly unusual is the high incidence of a leftward or superior frontal QRS vector, even in the face of severe right ventricular hypertrophy, presumably due to a conduction abnormality. Other congenital heart diseases reported include atrial septal defect (30%) (usually associated with pulmonary stenosis), patent ductus arteriosus (10%) and ventricular septal defect (10%). Rare lesions include tetralogy of Fallot, coarctation of the aorta, subaortic stenosis, Ebstein's malformation, and complex defects. A cardiomyopathy associated with asymmetric septal hypertrophy is rare, but may develop at any age, and appears to be independent of the presence or severity of pulmonary stenosis.

Aside from the cardiac defects, there is no unusual propensity to illnesses. Mental deficiency is seldom severe, and social performance is usually better than would be predicted based on the intelligence quotient (IQ). Particularly in milder cases, affected individuals lead an active, normal life.

Holt-Oram Syndrome. This syndrome of upper limb and cardiovascular malformations was first described in 1960 by Holt and Oram,[36] who noted the association of radial anomalies with atrial septal defect (Fig. 11). It is an autosomal dominant disorder with variable expression, but complete or nearly complete penetrance. An affected individual may have only hand, only heart, or both, anomalies. All gradations of skeletal defects involving the upper limb and shoulder girdle, ranging from mild hypoplasia of the thumb to phocomelia, can occur, even within a single pedigree.[51] All patients with involvement of the upper limbs have defects of the thumb. There is no correlation between the severity of the defect of the limb and the cardiac defect.

Congenital heart defects are seen in at least half of affected individuals, although there may be an ascertainment bias toward cardiac malformations. Atrial septal defect is the most frequent lesion. Together with ventricular septal defect, it accounts for most of the congenital heart disease.

Prognosis is dependent on the degree of skeletal deformity and the nature of the congenital heart

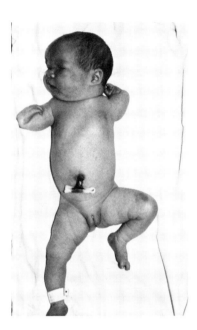

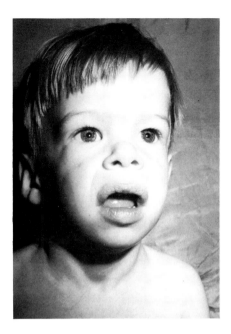

Figure 11.   Holt-Oram syndrome in a newborn infant with an atrial septal defect. Note the bilateral deficiency of the upper limbs.

Figure 12.   Williams syndrome in a 2-year-old boy with supravalvar aortic stenosis. Note the typical facies including a stellate pattern of the iris, short anteverted nose, long philtrum, prominent lips, and open mouth.

disease. There are no associated visceral anomalies. Intelligence is normal.

Ellis-van Creveld Syndrome *(Chondroectodermal Dysplasia).* Ellis and van Creveld described this autosomal recessive disorder in 1940 (Fig. 1). Principal features include a short stature of prenatal onset (short limbs), ectodermal dysplasia manifested by hypoplastic nails and dental anomalies (neonatal teeth, partial anodontia, small teeth, and/or delayed eruption), postaxial polydactyly, narrow thorax, and cardiac defects. About 50% of the patients have congenital heart disease, which is the major cause for the high infant mortality. Atrial septal defect or common atrium occurs in about half of patients. Other less frequent defects include patent ductus arteriosus, persistent left superior vena cava, hypoplastic left heart, coarctation of the aorta, total anomalous pulmonary venous return, and transposition of the great arteries. About half of the patients die in infancy, almost all from cardiovascular failure. Most survivors have normal intelligence. Eventual stature is in the range of 43–60 inches. Dental problems are frequent.

Syndromes of Unknown Etiology

Williams Syndrome. In 1961, Williams and colleagues described this condition in four unrelated children with mental retardation, an unusual facies, and supravalvar aortic stenosis (Fig. 12).[85] Hypercalcemia has been an infrequent finding, particularly beyond the neonatal period. Cardiovascular anomalies, including supravalvar aortic

stenosis, have been variable, but features such as the unusual facies and behavior, and the growth and mental deficiency are more consistent relative to diagnosis.[41,58]

About half of the patients have cardiovascular defects. Supravalvar aortic stenosis is the most frequent single defect. Other aortic abnormalities are also common, including valvar aortic stenosis, hypoplasia of the aorta, and coarctation. Peripheral pulmonary artery stenosis, stenosis of peripheral systemic arteries (for example, the renal arteries) (see Fig. 16, ch. 34), and hypoplasia of one coronary artery have been described also. Ventricular septal defect, atrial septal defect, mitral and tricuspid anomalies, and complex lesions are less often encountered. Management is particularly difficult when there is bilateral outflow obstruction. Histologically, the arterial narrowings are associated with disorganization of the media and intimal hypertrophy, often accompanied by focal necrosis, round cell infiltration, and calcification.[61,76]

Psychomotor retardation occurs in most patients, but the overall IQ varies widely from the normal range to severe mental retardation. Systemic hypertension has been reported in 7 of 42 children (17%) and 8 of 17 adults (47%) with Williams syndrome[58] (see ch. 21).

The etiology is not known. Isolated supravalvar aortic stenosis with autosomal dominant inheritance and Williams syndrome probably represent clinically distinct entities.[75]

Connective Tissue Disorders

Marfan Syndrome. Originally described by Marfan in 1896, this disorder is the most common and best characterized of the connective tissue disorders with significant cardiovascular manifestations (Fig. 13).[54] Marfan syndrome is an autosomal dominant condition with a wide variability of expression of skeletal, ocular, and cardiovascular malformations.[69] The basic defect in connective tissue has yet to be identified.

At least one-third of affected individuals have normal cardiovascular findings on clinical examination, but nearly all patients have cardiovascular involvement, such as aortic dilatation, mitral valve prolapse, or dilatation of the sinuses of Valsalva, which is detectable by echocardiography. Aortic disease predominates, particularly early in the course. Mitral valve dysfunction generally occurs later.

Patients with mitral valve prolapse and mild dilatation of the aortic root should have electrocardiographic and echocardiographic examinations on a yearly basis. As the aorta dilates and regurgitation appears, or in the presence of significant mitral regurgitation, these examinations should be performed more frequently. Because the mitral valvar cusps are abnormal, even in the clinical absence of prolapse or regurgitation, antibiotic prophylaxis against infective endocarditis is recommended for all patients.

Aortic dissection and dilatation are thought to be related to the shearing force of ventricular ejection. Wall tension is increased because of the increase in the radius of the lumen of the vessel and the decreased thickness of its wall. Physical activity should be restricted: there should be no participation in contact sports, activities that require maximal exertion, or isometric exercise. Beta-adrenergic blockade has been shown to delay or prevent the development of aortic regurgitation or dissection. Propranolol 3 or 4 times a day at a dosage that increases the pre-injection period/left ventricular ejection time by 30% has been recommended.[68] Atenolol may have some advantages over propranolol because of its cardiac selectivity, longer half-life, and fewer side effects.

Pregnant women with Marfan syndrome face two risks: a 50% risk of passing the disorder to the fetus, and a risk for aortic dissection or rupture during or shortly after pregnancy. The latter is particularly high if there is preexisting aortic disease. However, if the aortic root is less than 4.0 cm in diameter and cardiopulmonary function is not compromised, pregnancy is less perilous than previously suspected.[69]

Replacement of the ascending aorta with a composite graft is recommended for the following indications: aortic regurgitation with evidence of left ventricular dysfunction, acute or chronic aortic dissection, and an aortic diameter greater than 6.0 cm, with or without aortic regurgitation.[27] Patients with severe mitral regurgitation require replacement of the mitral valve.

The mean age of survival has been reported to be 43 years for males and 46 years for females; however, the long-term benefits of more recently introduced beta-adrenergic blockade and composite grafts on longevity are still unknown. Noncardiac management issues include screening and treatment of scoliosis, which tends to worsen during periods of rapid growth, and management of ophthalmologic problems. Although affected individuals are of normal intelligence, neuropsychologic impairment, including learning disabilities and attention deficit, was noted in 42% of children and teenagers in one study.[69]

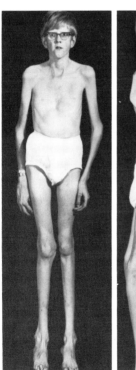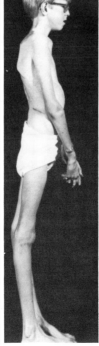

Figure 13. Marfan syndrome in a teenager with aortic root dilatation, myopia with retinal detachment, pectus excavatum, and the typical body habitus. (From Nadas AS, Fyler DC: Pediatric Cardiology, Philadelphia, W.B. Saunders Co., 1972, with permission.)

Branchial Arch Disorders

DiGeorge Sequence. A sequence is a pattern of multiple anomalies derived from a single known or presumed prior anomaly or mechanical factor. The pattern of malformation emphasized by DiGeorge is theorized to arise from a primary defect in the development of the third and fourth pharyngeal pouches and the fourth branchial arch, and should be classified as a sequence rather than a syndrome. This pattern of malformation variably includes developmental defects of the thymus (hypoplasia to aplasia, associated with defects in cellular immunity), parathyroids (hypoplasia to aplasia, associated with hypocalcemia and seizures), and great vessels (aortic arch anomalies and conotruncal malformations). The facial dysmorphism may not be particularly striking, but includes hypertelorism, downslanting palpebral fissures, and ear anomalies. The majority of patients have cardiovascular malformations, most frequently, interruption of the aortic arch, type B (1/3). About half of all cases of type B interrupted arch have the DiGeorge sequence.[11] Other frequent malformations include aberrant right subclavian artery, right aortic arch, and conotruncal malformations, including truncus arteriosus and tetralogy of Fallot.[11,23]

When one of the typical cardiovascular malformations is encountered, particularly type B interrupted aortic arch, an evaluation for the DiGeorge sequence, including testing for calcium homeostasis, parathyroid function, and cellular immunity (lymphocyte studies) is indicated. Chromosomal analysis should be performed to identify possible familial cases. All blood products should be irradiated prior to transfusion to reduce the risk for graft versus host reaction. The presence or absence of a thymus should be documented at the time of surgery.

The etiology of the DiGeorge sequence is unknown. Although usually it occurs sporadically in otherwise normal families, the pattern is etiologically heterogeneous. The sequence can occur as one feature of a broader pattern of malformation (for example, as part of the fetal alcohol syndrome, CHARGE association, or retinoic acid embryopathy). A minority of cases have been associated with a chromosomal deletion of segment 22q11, and these may be familial.[12,43]

Most patients with the full expression of the DiGeorge sequence die. Congenital heart disease is the most common cause of death, followed by infections and seizures due to hypocalcemia. Mild to severe degrees of mental retardation have been reported. Because of an increased index of suspicion for this condition in infants with arch anomalies and conotruncal malformations, increasing numbers of infants with a "partial" DiGeorge phenotype have been encountered at The Children's Hospital in Boston. These patients seem to do better than those described in the literature who have the full expression of the disorder. Spontaneous recovery from the immune deficiency has been noted among survivors with thymic hypoplasia. Improved surgical results for the cardiovascular defects combined with prospective identification and management of seizures and infections should improve overall survival.

Facioauriculovertebral Spectrum. This spectrum includes Goldenhar syndrome, first and second branchial arch syndrome, oculoauricular vertebral dysplasia, and hemifacial microsomia. The principal defects in this nonrandom association of anomalies represent problems in development of the first and second branchial arches, sometimes accompanied by vertebral and ocular anomalies.[30,67] The separate designations of the first and second branchial arch syndrome, oculo-auriculo-vertebral dysplasia, hemifacial microsomia, and Goldenhar syndrome are thought to represent gradations in severity of a similar error in morphogenesis, rather than distinct "syndromes." Cardinal features include external ear anomalies, epibulbar dermoids and lid colobomas, facial hypoplasia and asymmetry, vertebral defects, and cardiac malformations (Fig. 14).

About half of the patients have congenital heart disease, which presents the most serious handicap for patients with this condition. Tetralogy of Fallot and ventricular septal defect are the most frequent defects, followed by patent ductus arteriosus and coarctation of the aorta. Other anomalies of the

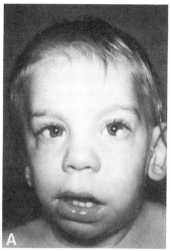
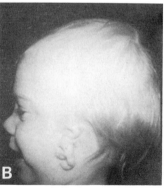

Figure 14. Facioauriculovertebral spectrum. **A,** Facial asymmetry and epibulbar dermoid of the eye. **B,** Severe external ear malformation.

great vessels are common also, especially right-sided aortic arch and abnormal position of the subclavian arteries.

Most patients have normal intelligence. Mental retardation occurs more frequently with microphthalmia. Management centers primarily around cosmetic surgery, evaluation and treatment of hearing disorders, and treatment of cardiovascular defects.

The etiology is not known and is probably heterogeneous. It usually occurs sporadically, although familial cases have been reported. Vascular disruption may play a role in pathogenesis.

ASSOCIATIONS

An association is a nonrandom occurrence of multiple anomalies not known to be a developmental field defect, sequence, or syndrome. The definition refers solely to statistically (not pathogenetically or causally) related anomalies. A given association, such as the VATER association, can occur in isolation or as part of a broader pattern of malformation, such as in trisomy 18 syndrome or infants of diabetic mothers. The two most common associations that include congenital heart diseases are the VATER and CHARGE associations.

VATER Association. The VATER association refers to the nonrandom occurrence of defects, including vertebral defects, anal atresia, tracheoesophageal fistula with esophageal atresia, and radial and renal dysplasia.[70,81] The spectrum has been extended to include cardiac defects, single umbilical artery, and growth deficiency of prenatal onset. Although ventricular septal defects are most common, a wide variety of cardiac lesions has been seen. The etiology of this pattern of malformation is not known. Generally, it has occurred sporadically in an otherwise normal family. Identification of VATER association defects in a particular patient does not, in itself, imply a diagnosis. Rather, the presence of one or more VATER-associated malformations should alert the clinician to the presence of other VATER defects.

CHARGE Association. The CHARGE association is a nonrandom association of congenital anomalies including coloboma, heart disease, atresia choanae, retarded growth and development and/or central nervous system anomalies, genital anomalies and/or hypogonadism, and ear anomalies and/or deafness.[31,62] Other medically significant associated malformations include renal anomalies, tracheoesophageal fistula, facial palsy, micrognathia, cleft lip, cleft palate, omphalocele, and the DiGeorge sequence. Heart defects have been described in 50–70% of the patients. Of those with congenital heart disease, 42% had conotruncal anomalies (tetralogy of Fallot, double-outlet right ventricle, truncus arteriosus) and 36% had aortic

arch anomalies (vascular ring, aberrant subclavian artery, interrupted aortic arch).[48] Other defects include patent ductus arteriosus, atrioventricular canal, ventricular septal defect and atrial septal defect. Most patients have some degree of mental deficiency and/or defects of the central nervous system. In some instances, the severity of the malformations has led to death in the perinatal period. The etiology of the CHARGE association is not known, but it usually occurs sporadically.

REFERENCES

1. Allanson JE, Hall JG, Hughes HE, et al: Noonan syndrome: The changing phenotype. Am J Med Genet 21:507–514, 1985.
2. Allen DB, Hendricks SA, Levy JM: Aortic dilation in Turner syndrome. J Pediatr 109:302–305, 1986.
3. Ardinger HH, Atkin JF, Blackston RD, et al: Verification of the fetal valproate syndrome phenotype. Am J Med Genet 29:171–185, 1988.
4. Baird PA, Sadovnick AD: Life expectancy in Down syndrome. J Pediatr 110:849–854, 1987.
5. Bergsma DS: Birth Defects Atlas and Compendium, 2nd ed. Baltimore, Williams & Wilkins, 1979.
6. Boughman JA, Berg KA, Astemborski JA, et al: Familial risks of congenital heart defect assessed in a population-based epidemiologic study. Am J Med Genet 26:839–847, 1987.
7. Brenner JI, Berg KA, Schneider DS, et al: Cardiac malformations in relatives of infants with hypoplastic left-heart syndrome. Am J Dis Child 143:1492–1494, 1989.
8. Briggs GG, Freeman RK, Yaffe SJ: Drugs in pregnancy and lactation. Baltimore, Williams & Wilkins, 1986.
9. Clark EB: Cardiac embryology, its relevance to congenital heart disease. Am J Dis Child 140:41–44, 1986.
10. Clark EB: Mechanisms in the pathogenesis of congenital cardiac malformations. In Pierpont MEM, Moller JH (eds): The Genetics of Cardiovascular Disease. Boston, Martinus Nijhoff, 1986, ch. 1.
11. Conley ME, Beckwith JB, Mancer KFK, et al: The spectrum of the DiGeorge syndrome. J Pediatr 94:883–890, 1979.
12. De la Chapelle A, Herva R, Koivisto M, et al: A deletion in chromosome 22 can cause DiGeorge syndrome. Hum Genet 57:253–256, 1981.
13. DiLiberti JH, Farndon PA, Dennis NR, et al: The fetal valproate syndrome. Am J Med Genet 19:473–481, 1984.
14. Disegni E, Pierpont ME, Bass JL, et al: Two-dimensional echocardiographic identification of endocardial cushion defect in families. Am J Cardiol 55:1649–1652, 1985.
15. Down JLH: Observations on an ethnic classification of idiots. Clinical Lecture Reports, London Hospital 3:259, 1866.
16. Driscoll DJ, Michels V, Gersony WM, et al: Occurrence of congenital heart defects in offspring of patients with ventricular septal defect, aortic stenosis, or pulmonary stenosis: Results of the Second Natural History Study of Congenital Heart Defects (abstract). J Am Coll Cardiol 13:136A, 1989.
17. Edwards JH, Harnden DG, Cameron AH, et al: A new trisomic syndrome. Lancet 1:787–790, 1960.
18. Ellis RWB, van Creveld S: A syndrome characterized by ectodermal dysplasia, polydactyly, chondro-dysplasia

and congenital morbus cordis. Report of three cases. Arch Dis Child 15:65–84, 1940.

19. Emanuel R, Somerville J, Inns A, et al: Evidence of congenital heart disease in the offspring of parents with atrioventricular defect. Br Heart J 49:144–147, 1983.

20. Feldman GL, Weaver DD, Lovrien EW: The fetal trimethadione syndrome. Am J Dis Child 131:1389–1392, 1977.

21. Ferencz C, Neill CA, Boughman JA, et al: Congenital cardiovascular malformations associated with chromosome abnormalities: an epidemiologic study. J Pediatr 114:79–86, 1989.

22. Ferencz C, Rubin JD, McCarter RJ, et al: Congenital heart disease prevalence at live birth—the Baltimore-Washington Infant Study. Am J Epidemiol 121:31–36, 1985.

23. Freedom RM, Rosen FS, Nadas AS: Congenital cardiovascular disease and anomalies of the third and fourth pharyngeal pouch. Circulation 46:165–172, 1972.

24. German J, Lowal A, Ehlers KH: Trimethadione and human teratogenesis. Teratology 3:349–361, 1970.

25. Goodman RM, Gorlin RJ: Atlas of the Face in Genetic Disorders, 2nd ed. St. Louis, C.V. Mosby Co., 1979.

26. Gorlin RJ, Cohen MM, Levin LS: Syndromes of the Head and Neck, 3rd ed. Oxford, Oxford University Press, 1989.

27. Gott VL, Pyeritz RE, Magovern G, et al: Surgical treatment of aneurysms of the ascending aorta in Marfan syndrome. Results of composite-graft repair in 50 patients with Marfan syndrome. N Engl J Med 314:1070–1074, 1986.

28. Graham JM: Smith's Recognizable Patterns of Human Deformation, 2nd ed. Philadelphia, W.B. Saunders Co., 1988.

29. Greenwood RD, Rosenthal A, Parisi L, et al: Extracardiac abnormalities in infants with congenital heart disease. Pediatrics 55:485–492, 1975.

30. Greenwood RD, Rosenthal A, Sommer A, et al: Cardiovascular malformations in oculo-auriculo-vertebral dysplasia (Goldenhar syndrome). J Pediatr 85:818–821, 1974.

31. Hall BD: Choanal atresia and associated anomalies. J Pediatr 95:395–398, 1979.

32. Hamerton JL, Canning N, Ray M, et al: A cytogenetic survey of 14,069 newborn infants. I. Incidence of chromosomal abnormalities. Clin Genet 8:223–243, 1975.

33. Hanson JW, Smith DW: The fetal hydantoin syndrome. J Pediatr 87:285–290, 1975.

34. Hanson JW, Myrianthopoulos C, Harvey MAS, et al: Risks to the offspring of women treated with hydantoin anticonvulsant, with emphasis on the fetal hydantoin syndrome. J Pediatr 89:662–668, 1976.

35. Harh JY, Paul MH, Gallen WJ, et al: Experimental production of hypoplastic left heart syndrome in the chick embryo. Am J Cardiol 31:51–56, 1973.

36. Holt M, Oram S: Familial heart disease with skeletal malformations. Br Heart J 22:236, 1960.

37. Hoyme HE, Higginbottom MC, Jones KL: The vascular pathogenesis of gastroschisis: intrauterine interruption of the omphalomesenteric artery. J Pediatr 98:228–231, 1981.

38. Jager-Roman E, Deichl A, Jakob S, et al: Fetal growth, major malformations, and minor anomalies in infants born to women receiving valproic acid. J Pediatr 108:997–1004, 1986.

39. Jones KL: Smith's Recognizable Patterns of Human Malformation, 4th ed. Philadelphia, W.B. Saunders Co., 1988.

40. Jones KL, Lacro RV, Johnson KA, et al: Pattern of malformations in the children of women treated with car-

bamazepine during pregnancy. N Engl J Med 320:1661–1666, 1989.

41. Jones KL, Smith DW: The Williams' elfin facies syndrome. A new perspective. J Pediatr 86:718–723, 1975.

42. Jones KL, Smith DW, Ulleland CN, et al: Pattern of malformation in offspring of chronic alcoholic mothers. Lancet 1:1267–1271, 1973.

43. Kelley RI, Zackai EH, Emanuel BS, et al: The association of the DiGeorge anomalad with partial monosomy of chromosome 22. J Pediatr 101:197–200, 1982.

44. Lacro RV, Jones KL, Benirschke K: Pathogenesis of coarctation of the aorta in the Turner syndrome: a pathologic study of fetuses with nuchal cystic hygromas, hydrops fetalis, and female genitalia. Pediatrics 81:445–451, 1988.

45. Lammer E: Etretinate and pregnancy (letter). Lancet 1:109, 1989.

46. Lammer EJ, Chen DT, Hoar RM, et al: Retinoic acid embryopathy. N Engl J Med 313:837–841, 1985.

47. Lemoine P, Harrousseau H, Borteyro JP, et al: Les enfants de parents alcooliques. Ouest Med 21:476–482, 1968.

48. Lin AE, Chin AJ, Devine W, et al: The pattern of cardiovascular malformation in the CHARGE association. Am J Dis Child 141:1010–1013, 1987.

49. Lin AE, Garver KL: Genetic counseling for congenital heart defects. J Pediatr 113:1105–1109, 1988.

50. Lin AE, Lippe BM, Geffner ME, et al: Aortic dilation, dissection, and rupture in patients with Turner syndrome. J Pediatr 109:820–826, 1986.

51. Lin AE, Perloff JK: Upper limb malformations associated with congenital heart disease. Am J Cardiol 55:1576–1583, 1985.

52. Loser H, Majewski F: Type and frequency of cardiac defects in embryofetal alcohol syndrome. Report of 16 cases. Br Heart J 39:1374–1379, 1977.

53. Marden PM, Smith DW, McDonald MJ: Congenital anomalies in the newborn infant including minor variants. J Pediatr 64:357–371, 1964.

54. Marfan AB: Un cas de déformation congénitale des quatre membres plus prononcée aux extrémities charactérisée par l'allongement des os avec un certain degré d'amincissement. Bull Mem Soc Med Hop (Paris) 13:220, 1896.

55. McKusick VA: Mendelian Inheritance in Man: Catalogs of Autosomal Dominant, Autosomal Recessive, and X-linked Phenotypes, 8th ed. Baltimore, The Johns Hopkins University Press, 1988.

56. Mendez HM, Opitz JM: Noonan syndrome: a review. Am J Med Genet 21:493–506, 1985.

57. Miller MJ, Geffner ME, Lippe BM, et al: Echocardiography reveals a high incidence of bicuspid aortic valve in Turner syndrome. J Pediatr 102:47–50, 1983.

58. Morris CA, Demsey SA, Leonard CO, et al: Natural history of Williams' syndrome: Physical characteristics. J Pediatr 113:318–326, 1988.

59. Noonan JA, Ehmke DA: Associated noncardiac malformations in children with congenital heart disease (abstract). J Pediatr 63:469–470, 1963.

60. Nora JJ, Nora AH: Update on counseling the family with a first-degree relative with a congenital heart defect. Am J Med Genet 29:137–142, 1988.

61. O'Connor WN, Davis JB Jr, Geissler R, et al: Supravalvular aortic stenosis. Clinical and pathologic observations in six patients. Arch Pathol Lab Med 109:179–185, 1985.

62. Pagon RA, Graham JM, Zonana J, et al: Coloboma, congenital heart disease and choanal atresia with multiple anomalies: CHARGE association. J Pediatr 99:223–227, 1981.

63. Parness IA, Yeager SB, Sanders SP, et al: Echocardiographic diagnosis of fetal heart defects in midtrimester. Arch Dis Child 63:1137–1145, 1988.

64. Patau K, Smith DW, Therman E, et al: Multiple con-

genital anomaly caused by an extra autosome. Lancet 1:790–793, 1960.

65. Pexieder T: Teratogens. In Pierpont MEM, Moller JH (eds): The Genetics of Cardiovascular Disease. Boston, Martinus Nijhoff, 1986, Ch. 3.

66. Pierpont MEM, Gorlin RJ, Moller JH: Chromosomal abnormalities. In Pierpont MEM, Moller JH (eds): The Genetics of Cardiovascular Disease. Boston, Martinus Nijhoff, 1986, Ch. 5.

67. Pierpont MEM, Moller JH, Gorlin RJ, et al: Congenital cardiac, pulmonary, and vascular malformations in oculoauriculovertebral dysplasia. Pediatr Cardiol 2:297–302, 1982.

68. Pyeritz RE: Propranolol retards aortic root dilatation in the Marfan syndrome (abstract). Circulation 68(Suppl III):365, 1983.

69. Pyeritz RE: Heritable disorders of connective tissue. In Pierpont MEM, Moller JH (eds): The Genetics of Cardiovascular Disease. Boston, Martinus Nijhoff, 1986, Ch. 13.

70. Quan L, Smith DW: The VATER association: Vertebral defects, Anal atresia, T-E fistula with esophageal atresia, Radial and Renal dysplasia: a spectrum of associated defects. J Pediatr 82:104–107, 1973.

71. Rose V, Gold RJ, Lindsay G, et al: A possible increase in the incidence of congenital heart defects among the offspring of affected parents. J Am Coll Cardiol 6:376–382, 1985.

72. Salbenblatt JA, Meyers DC, Bender BG, et al: Gross and fine motor development in 45,X and 47,XXX girls. Pediatrics 84:678–682, 1989.

73. Sandor GGS, Smith DF, MacLeod PM: Cardiac malformations in the fetal alcohol syndrome. J Pediatr 98:771–773, 1981.

74. Schinzel AA: Cardiovascular defects associated with chromosomal aberrations and malformation syndromes. In Steinberg AG, Bearn AG, Motulsky AG, et al (eds): Progress in Medical Genetics. Genetics of Cardiovascular Disease. Philadelphia, W.B. Saunders Co., 1983, vol. 5, pp. 303–379.

75. Schmidt MA, Ensing GJ, Michels VV, et al: Autosomal dominant supravalvular aortic stenosis: large three-generation family. Am J Med Genet 32:384–389, 1989.

76. Schmidt RE, Gilbert EF, Amend TC, et al: Generalized arterial fibromuscular dysplasia and myocardial infarction in familial supravalvular aortic stenosis syndrome. J Pediatr 74:576–584, 1969.

77. Shepard TH: Catalog of Teratogenic Agents, 6th ed. Baltimore, The Johns Hopkins University Press, 1989.

78. Smith DW: Dysmorphology (teratology). J Pediatr 69:1150–1169, 1966.

79. Spranger J, Benirschke K, Hall JG, et al: Errors of morphogenesis: concepts and terms. Recommendations of an international working group. J Pediatr 100:160–165, 1982.

80. Sweeney LJ: Morphometric analysis of an experimental model of left heart hypoplasia in the chick (thesis). Omaha, NE, University of Nebraska Medical Center, 1981.

81. Temtamy SA, Miller JD: Extending the scope of the VATER association: Definition of a VATER syndrome. J Pediatr 85:345–349, 1974.

82. Turner HH: A syndrome of infantilism, congenital webbed neck, and cubitus valgus. Endocrinology 23:566–574, 1938.

83. Van Praagh S, Truman T, Firpo A, et al: Cardiac malformations in trisomy 18: a study of 41 postmortem cases. J Am Coll Cardiol 13:1586–1597, 1989.

84. Whittemore R, Hobbins JC, Engle MA: Pregnancy and its outcome in women with and without surgical treatment of congenital heart disease. Am J Cardiol 50:641–651, 1982.

85. Williams JCP, Barratt-Boyes BG, Lowe JB: Supravalvular aortic stenosis. Circulation 24:1311–1318, 1961.

86. Zackai E, Mellman MJ, Neiderer B, et al: The fetal trimethadione syndrome. J Pediatr 87:280–284, 1975.

Section IV
Normal Circulatory Physiology

Chapter 6

FETAL AND TRANSITIONAL CIRCULATION

Michael D. Freed, M.D.

FETAL CIRCULATION

Most of our modern understanding of the circulation before birth comes from more than 40 years of research on fetal lambs.[1,5,13,14,17,18]

The fetal circulation is arranged in parallel, rather than in series, the right ventricle delivering the majority of its output to the placenta for oxygenation, and the left ventricle delivering the majority of its output to the heart, brain, and upper part of the body (Fig. 1).[16] However, there is mixing of the streams at the atrial and great vessel level which diverts blood from the immature lungs to the placenta for oxygen exchange. This parallel circulation permits fetal survival despite a wide variety of complex cardiac lesions.

Normally, blood returning from the placenta via the umbilical venous return splits in the liver; some of it goes into the hepatic veins and the portal system of the liver, while the remainder (slightly over half) passes through the ductus venosus into the inferior vena cava near its junction with the right atrium. In the right atrium the blood from the inferior vena cava is divided into two streams by the crista dividens. About 40% of the blood returning from the inferior vena cava (27% of the combined ventricular output) passes across the foramen ovale into the left atrium where it joins with the pulmonary venous return from the lung, passing through the mitral valve into the left ventricle. This blood is then pumped out the ascending aorta where it supplies the coronary, carotid, and subclavian arteries, with approximately a third of this stream (10% of combined ventricular output) passing across the aortic arch into the descending aorta.

The majority of blood returning from the inferior vena cava joins the superior vena caval drainage and coronary sinus return before passing through the tricuspid valve into the right ventricle and pulmonary artery. Because the fluid-filled lungs and constricted pulmonary arterioles offer a high resistance to flow, most of the blood, almost 90%, passes not to the lungs, but through the open ductus arteriosus into the low-resistance descending aorta and placenta.

The oxygen content of the blood in the fetus is considerably lower than that in the neonate or child, because of the lower efficiency of the placenta compared with the lung as an organ for oxygen exchange (Fig. 2). Blood returning from the placenta via the umbilical veins has the highest pO_2 (32–35 torr; oxygen saturation, 70%). The blood that passes into the left ventricle has already mixed with the less saturated vena caval and pulmonary venous return, lowering the pO_2 to 26–28 torr (oxygen saturation about 65%) before its distribution to the ascending aorta and upper half of the body.

The umbilical venous return destined for the right ventricle mixes with the superior vena caval return (pO_2, 12–14 torr; oxygen saturation, 40%), reducing the oxygen content of blood passing into the right ventricle, main pulmonary artery, and descending aorta to about 20–22 torr (oxygen saturation, 50–55%). Thus, blood with the highest oxygen content is diverted to the coronary arteries and brain, and that with the lowest oxygen content is diverted to the placenta, increasing the efficiency of oxygen pickup. An additional fetal adaptation to oxygen transport at low oxygen saturations is the presence of high levels of fetal hemoglobin with its high affinity for oxygen and its low p50 (partial pressure of oxygen at the point where 50% of the

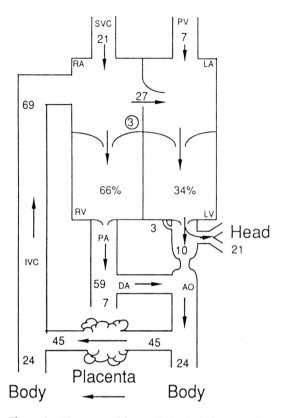

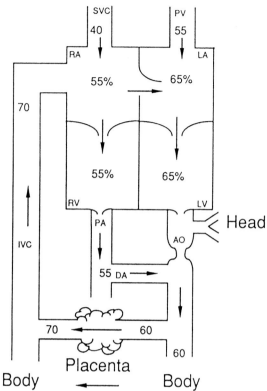

Figure 1. The course of the circulation in the late gestation fetal lamb. The numbers represent the percentage of combined ventricular output. Some of the return from the inferior vena cava (IVC) is diverted by the crista dividens in the right atrium (RA) through the foramen ovale into the left atrium (LA), where it meets the pulmonary venous return (PV) and passes into the left ventricle (LV) and is pumped into the ascending aorta. Most of the ascending aortic flow goes to the coronary, subclavian, and carotid arteries, with only 10% of combined ventricular output passing through the aortic arch (indicated by the narrowed point in the aorta) into the descending aorta (AO). The remainder of the inferior vena cava flow mixes with return from the superior vena cava (SVC) and coronary veins (3%) and passes into the right atrium and right ventricle (RV) and is pumped into the pulmonary artery (PA). Because of the high pulmonary resistance, only 7% percent passes through the lungs (PV), with the rest going into the ductus arteriosus (DA) and then to the descending aorta (AO), to the placenta and lower half of the body. (Modified from Rudolph AM: Congenital Diseases of the Heart. Chicago, Year Book Publishers, 1974, pp. 1–48.)

Figure 2. The numbers indicate the percent of oxygen saturation in the late gestation lamb. The oxygen saturation is the highest in the inferior vena cava, representing flow that is primarily from the placenta. The saturation of the blood in the heart is slightly higher on the left side than on the right side. The abbreviations in this diagram are the same as in Figure 1. (Modified from Rudolph AM: Congenital Diseases of the Heart. Chicago, Year Book Publishers, 1974, pp. 1–48.)

hemoglobin is oxidized) of approximately 18 or 19 torr. This leftward shift of the oxygen association curve facilitates oxygen uptake at the relatively low pO_2 levels of the placental vasculature.

The wide communication between the atria allows for equalization of pressures in the atria (Fig. 3); similarly, the patency of the ductus arteriosus results in equalization of pressures in the aorta and pulmonary artery. Because atrial and great vessel pressures are equal, in the absence of pulmonic or aortic stenosis, the ventricular pressures are equal

also, with a systolic pressure of approximately 70 mm, using amniotic pressure as zero.

It has been shown that the fetus has a limited ability to adjust cardiac output. The primary determinants of cardiac output are heart rate, filling pressure (preload), resistance against which the ventricles eject (afterload), and myocardial contractility. It has been known that there are spontaneous changes in heart rate associated with electrocortical activity as well as with the sleep state and fetal activity. Using continuous measurements of left and right ventricular output, utilizing electromagnetic flow probes, Rudolph and Heymann have shown that spontaneous increases in heart rate are associated with increasing ventricular output, whereas decreases in heart rate result in a considerable fall of both right and left ventricular output.[19] By electrically pacing the right atrium above the resting level of 160–180, the left ventricular output eventually increases to about 15% above resting levels. Decreasing the heart rate by 50% by vagal stimulation caused a fall in output of approximately 30%.

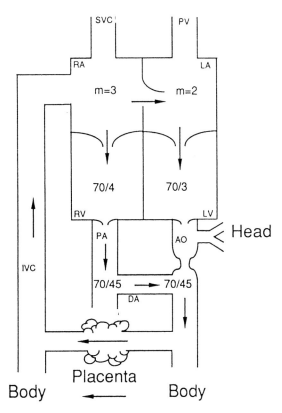

Figure 3. The numbers indicate the pressures observed in late gestation lambs. Because large communications between the atrium and great vessels are present, the pressures on both sides of the heart are virtually identical. The abbreviations are the same as in Figure 1. (Modified from Rudolph AM: Congenital Diseases of the Heart. Chicago, Year Book Publishers, 1974, pp. 1–48.)

Contrary to the significant effects of increasing or decreasing heart rate on fetal cardiac output, increasing preload (even to levels as high as a right atrial pressure of 20 mm Hg) produces only very small increases in ventricular output,[11] suggesting that the fetal ventricle normally functions near the top of its function curve and has little reserve to increase cardiac output. Increasing the work of the heart by increasing afterload (by inflating a balloon in the fetal descending aorta or by methoxamine)[10] produces a dramatic fall in right ventricular output, suggesting that the fetal heart is very sensitive to increases in afterload.

Morphometric studies on the fetal myocardium have demonstrated a significant decrease in myofibrillar content per tissue volume, suggesting that the fetal myocardium has much less contractile tissue than the adult. The active tension produced in excised strips of fetal myocardium was less than that produced by adult myocardium,[8] possibly because of the myofibrillar content, a reduced content of sarcoplasmic reticulum and/or the T-tubule system[12] (see ch. 1).

All of the above data suggest that the fetal my-

ocardium is structurally and functionally immature compared with that of the older child or adult. The fetal heart appears to work at the peak of its ventricular function curve, with increases in preload causing little or no change in cardiac output, and increases in afterload resulting in a marked depression. The limited ability of the fetal heart to respond to stress seems to be mediated primarily through increasing the heart rate.

The structure, hemodynamics, and myocardial function of the fetal circulation have significant consequences in the neonate with congenital heart disease:

1. The parallel circulation, with connections at the atrial and great vessel level, allows a wide variety of cardiac malformations to provide adequate transport of blood to the placenta to pick up oxygen and deliver it to the tissues.

2. The right ventricle performs approximately two-thirds of the cardiac work before birth. This is reflected in the size and thickness of the right ventricle before and after birth and may explain why left-sided defects are poorly tolerated after birth, compared with right-sided lesions.

3. Because the normal flow across the aortic isthmus is small (10% of ventricular output), the aortic isthmus is especially vulnerable to small changes in intracardiac flow from various congenital defects. This may account for the relatively high incidence of narrowing (coarctation of the aorta) or atresia (interrupted aortic arch) in this region.

4. Because the pulmonary flow *in utero* is very small compared with that immediately after birth, anomalies preventing normal pulmonary return (total anomalous pulmonary return, mitral stenosis, etc.) may be masked *in utero* when pulmonary venous return is so low anyway.

5. The low levels of circulating oxygen before birth (pO$_2$, 26–28 torr in the ascending aorta and 20–22 torr in the descending aorta) may account for the relative level of comfort of infants with cyanotic heart disease who may be quite active and comfortable, and may feed well with an arterial pO$_2$ of 20–25, a level that would lead to cerebral and cardiac anoxia, acidosis, and death within a few minutes for the older child or adult.

6. The limited ability of the fetal myocardium to respond to stress makes the hemodynamic consequences of congenital heart disease after birth that much more difficult to tolerate.

7. Birth is a time of stress for the left ventricle. Because of the switch from parallel to serial circulation, there is an increased amount of blood to pump. The ductus arteriosus may, at least briefly, shunt left to right. The work of respiration must be assumed. Of greater importance is the loss of the incubator effect of the uterus; the body metabolism and the circulation must adapt to maintaining body temperature. The possible role of the thyroid in these events has been noted.[2]

TRANSITIONAL CIRCULATION

Within a few moments of birth, profound changes must occur as the newborn rapidly switches from the placenta to the lung as the organ of respiration.[5,15] Failure of any one of a complex series of pulmonary or cardiac events that take place within minutes of birth leads to generalized hypoxemia and brain damage or death.

Soon after the onset of spontaneous respiration, the placenta is removed from the circulation, either by clamping the umbilical cord or, more naturally, by constriction of the umbilical arteries. This suddenly increases the systemic resistance as the lower-resistance placenta is excluded from the circulation. At approximately the same time the onset of spontaneous respiration expands the lungs and brings oxygen to the pulmonary alveoli. Reduction in the pulmonary vascular resistance results both from simple physical expansion of the vessels and from the chemo-reflex vasodilatation of the pulmonary arterioles caused by the high level of oxygen in the alveolar gas.

This sudden increase in systemic vascular resistance and drop in pulmonary vascular resistance causes a reversal of the flow through the ductus arteriosus and an increase in pulmonary flow. Before birth the relative pulmonary and systemic resistances cause 90% of the blood to go through the ductus arteriosus into the descending aorta; by a few minutes after birth 90% goes to the pulmonary arteries, with the pulmonary blood flow increasing from 35 ml/kg/min to 160–200 ml/kg/min.

The rapid drop in systemic venous return to the inferior vena cava as the umbilical venous flow is cut off, as well as the increase in pulmonary venous return as the pulmonary blood flow increases, causes the left atrial pressure to rise and the right atrial pressure to fall. When left atrial pressure exceeds right atrial pressure, the flap valve of the foramen ovale closes against the edge of the crista dividens, eliminating left-to-right or right-to-left shunting (Fig. 3).

There have been questions in the past regarding how much these marked circulatory changes are influenced by the mechanical changes in the lung parenchyma due to the onset of ventilation, how much by the vasodilatory effects of oxygen, and how much by the increase in systemic vascular resistance, with constriction of the umbilical vessels removing the low-resistance placenta from the circulation. Recently, Tietel,[20] using monitored fetal sheep near term, found that ventilation alone caused dramatic changes in the central flow patterns, attributable to a large decrease in pulmonary vascular resistance and an associated increase in pulmonary blood flow. Ventilation alone increased the pulmonary venous return from 8% of combined ventricular output to 31%, whereas right ventricular output (which had formerly ejected 90% to the

ductus arteriosus) was reduced to less than 50%. Oxygenation further changed the flow patterns so that more than 90% of the flow from the main pulmonary artery went to the lungs rather than through the ductus arteriosus. Umbilical cord occlusion had few additional effects.

Usually, the ductus arteriosus remains patent for several hours or days after birth. Initially, the pulmonary vascular resistance exceeds systemic vascular resistance so that there is a small right-to-left (pulmonary artery-to-aorta) shunt with some systemic desaturation to the lower half of the body. Anything that increases the pulmonary vascular resistance, such as acidosis, hypoxemia, polycythemia, or lung disease, may exacerbate or prolong the normal transient right-to-left shunt. Within a few hours of birth, however, in the normal child, the pulmonary vascular resistance has fallen lower than systemic vascular resistance, resulting in a small "physiologic" left-to-right (aorta-to-pulmonary artery) shunt. Normally, within 10–15 hours of birth, the ductus arteriosus has closed, although permanent structural closure may not take place for another 2–3 weeks.

The mechanism of closure of the ductus arteriosus is not completely understood. It has been clear for some time that oxygen plays a role.

Coceani and Olley[4] have shown that prostaglandins of the E series are responsible for maintaining patency of the ductus arteriosus during fetal life. It has been possible to keep the ductus open for days, weeks, or months, or even longer in infants with congenital heart disease, by infusion of exogenous prostaglandins E,[7] and it has been possible to close the ductus arteriosus in about 80% of preterm infants weighing less than 1750 gm with indomethacin, a nonselective prostaglandin synthetase inhibitor.[9]

Clyman and coworkers[3] observed a decrease in the ability of the ductus arteriosus to dilate and contract within a few hours of postnatal ductal constriction, before the loss of an anatomically patent lumen, in both human newborns and full-term lambs. They postulated that this change reflects early ischemic damage to the inner muscle wall. Fay and Cook[6] proposed that irreversibility reflects a mechanical restraint imposed by cellular necrosis, with a loss of intact endothelium leading to constriction from opposing walls until an anatomic lumen is eliminated. The etiology of the necrosis is unknown but it has been postulated that it is caused by interruption of luminal blood flow.

Although some hypoxemia is present soon after birth, because of right-to-left shunting through the ductus arteriosus over the first few hours of life, with continued vasodilatation and improved ventilation/perfusion ratios, the normal arterial pO_2 gradually increases from 50 torr at 10 minutes to 62 at 1 hour and 75–83 between 3 hours and 2 days of age. With continued vasodilatation the pulmonary pressure gradually falls to about 30 torr within approximately 48 hours. Although further falls in the pulmonary vascular resistance continue for several weeks, the transition to adult circulation is virtually completed within the first few days of life.

REFERENCES

1. Barcroft J: Researches of Pre-natal Life. Springfield, IL, Charles C Thomas, 1947.
2. Breall JA, Rudolph AM, Heymann MA: Role of thyroid hormone in postnatal circulatory and metabolic adjustments. J Clin Invest 73:1418–1424, 1984.
3. Clyman RI, Mauray F, Roman C, et al: Factors determining the loss of ductus arteriosus responsiveness to prostaglandin E. Circulation 68:433–436, 1983.
4. Coceani F, Olley PM: The response of the ductus arteriosus to prostaglandins. J Physiol Pharmacol 51:220–225, 1973.
5. Dawes GS: Foetal and Neonatal Physiology: A Comparative Study of the Changes at Birth. Chicago, Year Book Medical Publishers, 1968, pp 90–101, 160–187.
6. Fay FS, Cooke PH: Guinea pig ductus arteriosus. II Irreversible closure after birth. Am J Physiol 222:841–849, 1972.
7. Freed MD, Heymann MA, Lewis AB, et al: Prostaglandin E in infants with ductus arteriosus dependent congenital heart disease. Circulation 64:899–905, 1981.
8. Friedman WF: The intrinsic properties of the developing heart. In Friedman WF, Lesch M, Sonnenblick EH (eds): Neonatal Heart Disease. New York, Grune and Stratton, 1973, pp. 21–49.
9. Gersony WM, Peckham GJ, Ellison RC, et al: Effects of indomethacin in premature infants with patent ductus arteriosus: results of a national collaborative study. J Pediatr 102:895–906, 1983.
10. Gilbert RD: Effects of afterload and baroreceptors on cardiac function in fetal sheep. J Dev Physiol 4:299–309, 1982.
11. Heymann MA, Rudolph AM: Effects of increasing preload on right ventricular output in fetal lambs in-utero (abstract). Circulation 48(Suppl):37, 1973.
12. Hoerter J, Mazet F, Vassort G: Perinatal growth of the rabbit cardiac cell: possible implications for the mechanism of relaxation. J Mol Cell Cardiol 13:725–740, 1982.
13. Lind J, Wegelius C: Human fetal circulation: changes in the cardiovascular system at birth and disturbances in the post-natal closure of the foramen ovale and ductus arteriosus. Cold Spring Harbor Symposium. Quant Biol 19:109–125, 1954.
14. Lind J, Stern L, Wegelius C: Human Foetal Neonatal Circulation. Springfield, IL, Charles C Thomas, 1964.
15. Rudolph AM: The changes in the circulation after birth: their importance in congenital heart disease. Circulation 41:343–359, 1970.
16. Rudolph AM: Congenital Diseases of the Heart. Chicago, Year Book Publishers, 1974, pp. 1–48.
17. Rudolph AM, Heymann MA: The circulation of the fetus in utero. Circ Res 21:163–184, 1967.
18. Rudolph AM, Heymann MA: Circulatory changes with growth in the fetal lamb. Circ Res 26:289–299, 1970.
19. Rudolph AM, Heymann MA: Cardiac output in the fetal lamb: the effects of spontaneous and induced changes of heart rate on right and left ventricular output. J Obstet Gynecol 124:183–192, 1976.
20. Teitel DF, Iwamoto HS, Rudolph AM: Effects of birth related events on central flow patterns. Pediatr Res 22:557–566, 1987.

Section V

Problems Caused by Heart Disease

Chapter 7

CONGESTIVE HEART FAILURE

Michael D. Freed, M.D.

Congestive heart failure is defined as the pathologic condition in which the heart is unable to pump sufficient blood to meet the metabolic demands of the body. In broad terms there are two causes of heart failure: (1) the imposition of an excessive work load, usually a volume or pressure overload secondary to congenital or acquired heart disease, in the presence of a normal myocardium, or (2) a normal workload faced by a myocardium that has been damaged by, for example, inflammatory disease. In the perinatal period and infancy, heart failure is more commonly caused by a structural defect, whereas in the older child either structural or myocardial disease may be found.

Congestive heart failure results in a variety of signs and symptoms due to the failure of the body's adaptive mechanisms. This chapter reviews the more common causes of congestive heart failure and describes the clinical manifestations and current approaches to management.[1,3-6]

CAUSES OF CONGESTIVE HEART FAILURE

In the Fetus

With the advent of echocardiography, congestive heart failure has been increasingly recognized in the fetus as hydrops. Whereas previously the most common cause was anemia secondary to hemolysis from Rh disease, fetal/maternal transfusion, or hypoplastic anemia, more recently heart failure has been found to be associated with cardiac arrhythmias (Table 1). Other causes of *in utero* congestive heart failure include massive semilunar or atrioventricular valve insufficiency (sometimes seen in fetuses with complete atrioventricular canal or Ebstein's disease), large systemic arteriovenous

Table 1. Causes of Heart Failure *In Utero*

Anemia
  Hemolytic secondary to RH sensitization
  Fetal maternal transfusion
  Hypoplastic anemia
Arrhythmias
  Supraventricular tachycardia
  Atrial flutter
  Atrial fibrillation
  Ventricular tachycardia
  Complete heart block
Volume Overload
  Atrioventricular valve regurgitation in AV canal
  Tricuspid regurgitation in Ebstein's disease
  Arteriovenous fistula
Myocarditis

fistula, premature closure of the foramen ovale, or inflammatory disease of the myocardium.

Neonatal Period

Myocardial dysfunction in the neonatal period is relatively rare and almost invariably associated with other perinatal problems such as asphyxia, sepsis, hypoglycemia, or other organ system damage. Undoubtedly, this is because a normal circulatory system is necessary *in utero* after the embryo is three to four cells thick; significant abnormalities that prevent adequate tissue perfusion in fetal life result in first trimester spontaneous abortions.

Structural problems, silent *in utero* while the circulatory system was arranged in parallel with high pulmonary resistance, may cause hemodynamic embarrassment as the ductus arteriosus closes and the pulmonary vascular resistance drops (Table 2). Neonates with increased pressure work

63

Table 2.   Causes of Congestive Heart
Failure in Neonates

Myocardial Dysfunction
  Asphyxia
  Sepsis
  Hypoglycemia
  Myocarditis
Pressure Overload
  Aortic stenosis
  Coarctation of the aorta
  Hypoplastic left heart syndrome
Volume Overload
  Great vessel level shunts
    patent ductus arteriosus
    truncus arteriosus
    aortopulmonary window
  Ventricular level shunts
    ventricular septal defect
    single ventricle without pulmonic stenosis
    atrioventricular canal
  Arteriovenous fistula
Tachyarrhythmias
  Supraventricular tachycardia
  Atrial flutter
  Atrial fibrillation
Bradyarrhythmias
  Congenital complete heart block

on the left side of the heart, usually secondary to aortic stenosis or coarctation of the aorta, become sick in the first week or two of life. Those with right-sided lesions that cause pressure overload usually do not present with congestive heart failure, because the patent foramen ovale allows the right side to decompress by right-to-left shunting, leading to cyanosis rather than the usual symptoms of congestive failure.

Because the pulmonary vascular resistance is high in the first few weeks of life, children with communications between the left and right side of the heart do not commonly develop heart failure in the first week or two. By the third or fourth week, however, the pulmonary vascular resistance has dropped sufficiently so that a significant left-to-right shunt at the ventricular or great-vessel level can result in enough pulmonary blood flow to cause ventricular dilatation and congestive failure. Heart failure from a large left-to-right shunt may result from shunting at the great-vessel level (patent ductus arteriosus, aortopulmonary window or truncus arteriosus), or at the ventricular level (ventricular septal defect, single ventricle, complete atrioventricular canal). Systemic arteriovenous fistulas (usually of the head or liver) produce a volume overload lesion independent of pulmonary vascular resistance and are usually noticed earlier in the perinatal period (see p. 707).

Abnormal variations in heart rate may also lead to congestive heart failure, either when the heart rate is too fast (paroxysmal supraventricular tachycardia, atrial flutter, or atrial fibrillation), or when it is too slow (congenital complete heart block).

Occasionally, hematologic abnormalities can cause circulatory failure; severe anemia can lead to high output failure, and marked polycythemia can cause a hyperviscosity syndrome.

Infancy

During infancy heart failure is usually caused by structural problems, although abnormalities in the heart muscle are seen occasionally. By four weeks of age the pulmonary vascular resistance has usually dropped significantly, and connections between the systemic and pulmonary circulations, if sufficiently large, often lead to congestive heart failure (Table 3). Volume overload lesions with left-to-right shunting at the great-vessel level (patent ductus arteriosus, truncus arteriosus, or aortopulmonary window) become symptomatic at this age. Failure may also be seen in a child with a large ventricular septal defect as an isolated lesion or with more complicated heart disease, such as transposition of the great arteries or tricuspid atresia. Usually atrial level shunts do not cause congestive heart failure, but total anomalous pulmonary venous return often does.

Heart muscle abnormalities that are seen in infancy include endocardial fibroelastosis, Pompe's type of glycogen storage disease, inflammatory myocarditis, coronary calcinosis, or occasionally anomalous origin of the left coronary artery from the pulmonary artery with myocardial ischemia. Metabolic cardiomyopathies, especially systemic carnitine deficiency, may be seen occasionally. Other less common causes of congestive heart failure during infancy include renal failure, systemic hypertension, hypothyroidism, Kawasaki's disease, and, occasionally, overwhelming sepsis.

Table 3.   Causes of Congestive Heart
Failure in Infants

Volume Overload
  Great vessel level shunts
    patent ductus arteriosus
    truncus arteriosus
    aortopulmonary window
  Ventricular level shunts
    isolated ventricular septal defect
    VSD with transposition
    VSD with tricuspid atresia
    single ventricle
  Atrial level shunts
    total anomalous pulmonary venous return
Heart Muscle Abnormalities
  Endocardial fibroelastosis
  Glycogen storage disease (Pompe's)
  Myocarditis, viral, Kawasaki
Secondary Heart Failure
  Renal disease
  Hypertension
  Hypothyroidism
  Sepsis

Childhood

By early and mid childhood most of the congenital defects have been repaired or palliated. However, congestive heart failure may be seen with increasing atrioventricular valve regurgitation in children with complete atrioventricular canal or as a result of palliative procedures such as large systemic-to-pulmonary artery shunts (Table 4). Acquired heart disease, such as rheumatic fever, viral myocarditis, or bacterial endocarditis, may cause failure in the child or adolescent. Noncardiac lesions leading to heart failure include acute hypertension (usually secondary to glomerulonephritis), thyrotoxicosis, cancer therapy toxicity (including radiation or doxorubicin [Adriamycin]), sickle cell anemia, or cor pulmonale secondary to cystic fibrosis.

CLINICAL MANIFESTATIONS

The signs and symptoms of heart failure are due to low cardiac output, the systemic adaptation to the low output state and/or systemic venous or pulmonary venous congestion. Although the underlying physiology may be similar, the clinical manifestations of congestive heart failure in infancy and in childhood differ.

Infancy

Feeding difficulties are the most prominent symptoms in infants with failure. While a normal infant feeds vigorously, often completing a feeding within 15 or 20 minutes, the infant with congestive heart failure has more difficulty. Nursing is prolonged and associated with significant tachypnea and increased perspiration. Some infants struggle for 5 or 10 minutes and fall asleep, only to waken an hour or so later voraciously hungry again. Others seem to tire and fall asleep after taking in only 1 or 2 oz. Presumably the feeding difficulties result from the combined effort of sucking and maintaining a rapid respiratory rate, as well as from the limited cardiac reserve. The total caloric intake, under these circumstances, may be reduced to under 75 kcal/kg/day, which is not sufficient to sustain growth.

Table 4. Causes of Heart Failure in Childhood

Palliated congenital heart disease
Atrioventricular valve regurgitation
Rheumatic fever
Viral myocarditis
Bacterial endocarditis
Secondary Causes
Hypertension secondary to glomerulonephritis
Thyrotoxicosis
Doxorubicin (Adriamycin) cardiomypathy
Sickle cell anemia
Cor pulmonale secondary to cystic fibrosis

Parents often note **excessive perspiration** (especially while feeding) that is out of proportion to the ambient temperature or clothing. This is caused by increased autonomic nervous system activity in an attempt to improve myocardial performance.

On physical examination the children are almost invariably **tachycardic,** with resting heart rates of more than 160 beats per minute in the neonate, and more than 120 in the older infant. Tachycardia is also the result of increased circulating catecholamines that augment cardiac output by increasing myocardial contractility and heart rate.

Tachypnea (a resting respiratory rate greater than 60 in the neonate or greater than 40 in the older infant) usually is present and is associated with increased stiffness of the lung secondary to increased interstitial fluid from either elevated pulmonary venous pressure (pulmonary edema) or high flow left-to-right shunts. As heart failure becomes more severe, ventilatory function may become more compromised and flaring of the alae nasi, intercostal retractions, and grunting may be seen. Distention of the neck veins is not commonly appreciated in neonates, but may be seen in some older infants. The elevated systemic venous pressure does result in enlargement of the liver, but peripheral edema is not common in infants and is associated with only very severe heart failure. Cool extremities, weakly palpable pulses, and a low arterial blood pressure with narrow pulse pressure may be seen as manifestations of low cardiac output. Mottling of the extremities and slow capillary refill are signs of more severe vascular compromise.

Occasionally, examination of the chest shows **mild wheezing** that may be confused with bronchiolitis or pneumonia and may be exacerbated from compression of the airways by distended pulmonary vessels. Rales are not common unless there is coexisting pneumonia, a not infrequent association.

The findings at cardiac examination are variable depending upon the etiology of the heart failure. An infant with primary disease of the heart muscle usually has a quiet precordium; one with heart failure from volume overload usually has a very active precordium; one with pressure overload may have a systolic thrill. Frequently, a gallop rhythm is present but it is difficult to appreciate with the rapid heart rates.

The chest x-ray almost always demonstrates **cardiomegaly;** its absence must seriously challenge the diagnosis. Notable exceptions include left atrial obstructive lesions such as cor triatriatum and total anomalous pulmonary venous return with obstruction. Excessive pulmonary blood flow is present in those with heart failure secondary to a large left-to-right shunt, and a diffuse haziness secondary to pulmonary venous congestion is found in most of the remainder. Redistribution of pulmonary blood flow to the upper lobes is not common in infants who spend most of their time supine. Increased lung volumes with hyperexpansion and flattened diaphragms are common, and an enlarged left atrium may cause collapse of the left lower lobe.

The electrocardiogram is rarely useful in the diagnosis, but is almost invariably abnormal, with the specific abnormality dependent upon the lesion causing the heart failure.

The echocardiogram, on the other hand, is very useful in assessing left ventricular function. The left ventricular shortening fraction, left-sided systolic time intervals, and the rate of circumferential fiber shortening as a function of the end-systolic wall stress have been used to evaluate muscle function. The echocardiogram can also rule out pericardial effusion. With volume-overload lesions the myocardial performance may be normal; the signs and symptoms of congestive heart failure in these cases are caused by the enormous volume load of the heart in the presence of normal or even enhanced myocardial function.

Childhood

The signs and symptoms of congestive heart failure in the older child more closely resemble those in the adult. **Breathlessness** is a common sign of left ventricular decompensation in the child. This is usually manifested by exertional dyspnea and exaggeration of the usual response of breathlessness on severe exercise. At first the decreased ability may be within the range of normal variation, but eventually, as heart failure progresses, the child may find difficulty with the demands of everyday life, including walking up steps at school. A chronic hacking cough, secondary to congestion of the bronchial mucosa, may also be present in some children. As left atrial pressure increases, the child may develop orthopnea, requiring elevation of the head on several pillows at night. Fatigue and weakness are relatively late manifestations.

On physical examination, children with mild or moderate heart failure appear to be in no distress, but those with severe heart failure may be dyspneic at rest. If the onset of heart failure has been relatively abrupt, the child may appear anxious but well developed and well nourished; those in whom a more chronic process has occurred usually do not appear anxious but may be malnourished and wasted.

Like infants, children with congestive heart failure are usually **tachycardic** because of increased sympathetic activity and **tachypneic** because of increased lung water. The low output may cause peripheral vasoconstriction, resulting in coolness, pallor and cyanosis of the digits, with poor capillary refill.

Increased systemic venous pressure may be de-tected by distention of the neck veins with venous pulsations visible above the clavicle while the patient is sitting. The liver may be enlarged on percussion or palpation, and if the enlargement is relatively acute, there may be tenderness owing to stretching of the liver capsule.

Children may also develop **peripheral edema.** At first the signs may be subtle, but when there has been a 10% increase in weight, the face, especially the eyelids, begins to appear puffy and edema develops in dependent parts of the body. Longstanding edema can result in reddening and induration of the skin, usually over the shins and ankles. Exudation of fluid into body cavities may be discovered as ascites and, occasionally, hydrothorax.

On cardiac examination there is almost invariably **cardiomegaly.** The cardiac impulse may be quiet when there is primarily cardiac muscle disease (e.g., myocarditis or cardiomyopathy), but it is usually hyperactive when congestive failure is due to volume overload from a left-to-right shunt or atrioventricular valve regurgitation. A third heart sound occurring in mid diastole may be a normal finding in children but it is frequently associated with increased ventricular stiffness in those with heart disease. **Pulsus alternans,** characterized by a regular rhythm with alternating strong and weak pulsations, can be felt occasionally; however, it is more easily appreciated while measuring the systemic blood pressure or monitoring the arterial pressure. Pulsus alternans has been thought to be caused by an alteration in left ventricular volume, owing to incomplete recovery of the myocardium on alternate beats. **Pulsus paradoxus** (a fall in blood pressure on inspiration and a rise on expiration), secondary to marked swings of intrapulmonary pressures which affect ventricular filling (as in pericardial tamponade), is seen occasionally in older children.

In children, the chest x-ray almost invariably shows cardiac enlargement. The normal pulmonary arterial flow pattern (that is, increased flow to the lung bases compared with the apices) is reversed. When the capillary pressures exceed 20–25 mm Hg, interstitial pulmonary edema may be seen, causing a cloudiness throughout the lung field, especially in a "butterfly pattern" around the hili. This may result in Kerley's lines, sharp linear densities in the interlobar septa.

In chronic congestive heart failure, proteinuria and high specific gravity of the urine are common findings, and there may be an increase in the blood urea nitrogen and creatinine levels, secondary to reduced renal blood flow. The level of sodium in the urine is usually less than 10 mEq/L. Serum electrolyte values are usually normal prior to treatment but hyponatremia, secondary to increased water retention, may be seen in cases of severe, longstanding heart failure. Congestive hepatomegaly and cardiac cirrhosis may lead to abnormalities in liver enzymes and/or elevation of bilirubin in rare instances.

TREATMENT

The successful treatment of congestive heart failure in the child is predicated on an understanding of the nature and physiologic consequences of the specific cardiac defect leading to the failure, and of the treatment modalities available. For those with structural disease and an associated or aggravating condition that may be the precipitating cause of the heart failure (fever, dysrhythmias or anemia), prompt recognition and treatment may result in dramatic improvement. If there is a specific anatomic lesion amenable to palliative or corrective surgery, pharmacologic or other attempts at ameliorating the signs and symptoms of heart failure may be superfluous; mechanical problems frequently require mechanical solutions. If, however, surgery is unavailable or inappropriate, a variety of general and pharmacologic measures are available to improve the patient's clinical status.

Because the causes of congestive heart failure in the child are so varied, it is difficult to generalize regarding treatment. Nevertheless, some general principles hold. Pharmacologically, the treatment is a three-tiered approach to improve the pumping performance of the heart, control the excessive salt and water retention, and reduce the workload. The approach to improving pumping performance usually relies, at first, on the administration of digitalis. If heart failure is not controlled by digitalis alone, the excessive salt and water retention is usually treated with diuretics (preload reduction). If these two measures are not effective, a reduction in the workload of the heart with systemic vasodilators (afterload reduction) is usually tried. If these approaches are not effective, further attempts at improving pumping performance of the heart with other sympathomimetic agents or other positive inotropic agents may be tried. If none of these measures is effective, cardiac transplantation may be required.

General Measures

While **reduced physical activity** is a mainstay of the treatment of heart failure in adults, this issue is more problematic in children. Competitive, strenuous, or isometric exercises ought to be discouraged, but it is difficult to ensure compliance in children when they are out of sight of the physician or parents. With severe heart failure, however, physical activity should be severely restricted. While a period of bed rest during the day is desirable, it must be remembered that having a child quietly sitting fingerpainting may be consid-

erably more "restful" than having him or her screaming uncontrollably in bed.

Before the availability of potent diuretic agents, **restriction of dietary sodium** played an important role in the management of heart failure. While very salty foods (pretzels, popcorn, potato chips, and some candies) ought to be avoided and the salt shaker eliminated from the dinner table, it does not seem necessary to restrict salt intake excessively. Low-salt foods are almost invariably unpalatable; it seems better to maintain an adequate diet, increasing the dose of diuretics as needed. In infants the use of a very low sodium diet is probably unnecessary for the same reason. Because the retention of fluid is primarily dependent upon total body sodium content, it would seem unnecessary, and in some cases ill advised, to restrict free water except in far-advanced congestive heart failure, when dilutional hyponatremia occurs.

The use of **oxygen** may be very helpful for those with pulmonary edema, especially when there is underlying right-to-left shunting with chronic hypoxemia. However, oxygen does not seem to have a role in the treatment of chronic congestive heart failure.

Digitalis

For more than 200 years digitalis has been a mainstay for the treatment of congestive heart failure. While its utility in those with primarily "muscle failure" is unarguable, there have been some questions recently concerning its utility in children with large left-to-right shunts (especially in the premature baby with a ductus arteriosus), where heart failure results from a volume overload to the heart without evidence of depressed myocardial function.

Digitalis refers to a group of related steroid compounds that exert a positive inotropic effect and have certain electrophysiologic effects. Although a wide variety of different, closely related compounds have been used in the past in pediatric cardiology, digoxin is the preparation used almost exclusively because of its excellent bioavailability, its absorption, and the relatively rapid excretion rate that allows for adjustment to meet individual demands.

The principal effect of the digitalis glycosides is to increase the force and the velocity of cardiac muscle contraction. This "inotropic" effect is present in cardiac but not skeletal muscle and is dependent upon the concentration of a number of ions, including potassium, sodium, calcium, and magnesium; it seems to be unrelated to the catecholamine response. Recently, a consensus has been reached, suggesting that the inotropic effects result from digitalis binding to, and thereby inhibiting, sodium-potassium (Na-K) adenosine triphosphatase, the enzyme that maintains high intracellular concentrations of sodium in myocardial cells. This poisoning of the sodium pump alters the excitation-contraction coupling, making more calcium available to the contractile elements, resulting in increased force of contraction. For children with myocardial failure, this inotropic effect increases cardiac output, resulting in a reduction or elimination of symptoms.

Because the Na-K adenosine triphosphatase pump is the mechanism needed to maintain an 80–90 millivolt transmembrane resting potential in cardiac cells, it is not surprising that digitalis affects electrophysiologic properties in the heart, in addition to its inotropic effects. Clinically, the most important effect is an increase in the effective refractory period of the conduction system, which tends to slow the ventricular response to atrial fibrillation or atrial flutter. In addition, digitalis increases the sensitivity of the arterial baroreceptor reflex, resulting in an increase in vagal and a decrease in sympathetic efferent activity, thereby reducing the resting heart rate.

Pharmacokinetics

Digoxin may be given orally or intravenously (see Appendix, p. 760). The absorption from the gastrointestinal tract is rapid, with peak plasma levels and the onset of action occurring within 15–30 minutes. About 75% of the dose is absorbed in the gastrointestinal tract, with the remainder excreted in the feces unchanged. The half-life is about 37 hours in the full-term infant, 57 hours in the premature infant, and somewhere in between for the older child.

The dosage of digoxin is determined by individual titration. The premature infant, somewhat more sensitive to digoxin, is usually digitalized with 20 μg/kg of body weight. Full-term neonates with better renal function are given 30–40 μg/kg. For infants, 1 month to 2 years of age, the dose is usually 30–50 μg/kg, and for older children 20–30 μg/kg is usually sufficient. The total digitalizing dose, a loading dose, is usually given over 12–24 hours, but may be given over 6–12 hours in semiemergency situations. In the usual case we give half the digitalizing dose followed by another quarter approximately 12 hours later and the final quarter approximately 6 hours after that. The daily maintenance dose, used to replace renal losses, is approximately one-fourth the total digitalizing dose, usually divided into two doses, approximately 12 hours apart. When intravenous digitalization is preferred, approximately 80% of the above dosages are used, because absorption is complete.

Decreased renal function reduces the dose of digoxin required. In adults, the percentage of digoxin loss per day equals 14 plus creatinine clearance (ml/min) divided by 5. This probably applies to infants, children, and adolescents as well. To calculate an approximate value for the daily dose, one should multiply the percentage lost each day by the total digitalizing dose.

Several points have been emphasized in the past by other authors but deserve repetition.

1. **Digitalization remains an individualized procedure.** There are wide variations in individual response and the dose must be adjusted according to the patient's needs and response. This is especially true when dealing with inflammatory diseases of the myocardium, in which enhanced sensitivity to the drug is common. One should probably start with approximately half the usual digitalizing dose in these patients.

2. **The dose calculation should be done in duplicate,** at a minimum, by a physician and a nurse, and preferably checked again. Digoxin comes as an oral preparation containing 50 μg/ml, tablets of 0.125 mg, 0.25 mg and 0.5 mg, and as a parenteral solution of 0.1 mg/ml and 0.25 mg/ml. Explicit instructions must be given with the dosage in milligrams and milliliters to the person administering the digoxin. Although it may seem unnecessary to emphasize these details, the toxic-therapeutic range is narrow and the author has personally seen significant errors occur every few years, sometimes with tragic results.

3. When young children are discharged, **parents need to be shown how to use the calibrated dropper and to be told the signs of digitalis toxicity,** including nausea, vomiting, and loss of appetite. At home the digoxin should be kept in a locked cabinet away from other siblings. If the child vomits within 5 or 10 minutes of getting the dose, we usually recommend readministering it; if vomiting occurs after that period, we recommend waiting until the next dose 12 hours later.

Enhanced Sensitivity and Drug Interactions. Enhanced sensitivity to digitalis preparations may also be seen with electrolyte disturbances, including hypokalemia, hypomagnesemia, hypercalcemia, or hyponatremia. Thyroid disease affects digitalis pharmacokinetics, with the half-life being prolonged in children who have hypothyroidism,[2] and accelerated in those with hyperthyroidism; appropriate adjustments in the dosage may be necessary. Certain drugs may interact with digitalis through different mechanisms. Neomycin and some of the nonabsorbable antacids lower the absorption. Quinidine seems to reduce the renal and nonrenal elimination of digoxin, resulting in an average twofold increase in serum digoxin concentration. When adding this drug to someone on a maintenance dose of digoxin, the digoxin dose should be decreased.

Serum Digoxin Concentration. Since the advent of an accurate radioimmunoassay for measuring digoxin concentration, attempts have been made to correlate efficacy of the inotropic effect and toxicity with serum concentrations. It has been shown that in adults positive inotropic effects may be demonstrated at low serum levels and there is evidence, also in adults, that further inotropic benefit may not occur with serum levels greater than 1.0–2.0 ng/ml. In adults without evidence of toxicity, the mean serum or plasma digoxin concentrations averages about 1.4 ng/ml. Serum digoxin levels have been shown to be higher in infants (in a range of 2.8 ± 1.9 ng/ml) without obvious evidence of toxicity. In fact, at the usual recommended dosages, more than half the infants achieve levels greater than 2 ng/ml, which would be considered evidence of toxicity in adults. Toxic symptoms usually occur with digoxin levels in the range of 4–5 ng/ml in infants and 3 ng/ml in children up to 3 years old. Because the therapeutic effects of more than 2 ng/ml appear to be limited (at least in children), one should probably err on the side of lower serum digoxin levels than are currently being used.

Measurement of the serum digoxin level is difficult and the accuracy in some laboratories has been questioned. The absorption and distribution of digoxin take some time, and if the serum digoxin levels are drawn less than 6 hours after administration, falsely elevated levels may be obtained that do not represent muscle-bound digoxin levels.

Digitalis Intoxication. Fortunately, the incidence of digoxin toxicity in infants and children is considerably less than it is for adults. Nevertheless, the potential exists for life-threatening arrhythmias, and vigilance and a high index of suspicion are necessary. Although gastrointestinal symptoms such as anorexia, nausea, and vomiting are common presenting symptoms of digitalis toxicity in adults, they are less commonly recognized in children. Whether this is a physiologic difference or merely a difference in communication skills remains to be clarified. The most common evidence of cardiac toxicity in infants and children is arrhythmia. Although supraventricular tachycardia, ectopic atrial tachycardia, and ventricular dysrhythmias are frequent in the adult, it appears that bradyrhythmias are a more common toxic manifestation in children and, fortunately, ventricular tachycardia and ventricular ectopy are relatively rare.

For minor digoxin toxicity, stopping the drug and waiting the one or two half-lives necessary for the drug level to drop into the therapeutic range, followed by a downward modification of a chronic dosage, are usually sufficient. Constant electrocardiographic monitoring is useful for awhile in order to be certain that more malignant arrhythmias do not occur.

For more significant arrhythmias, hospital admission for treatment is usually necessary. For those with mild sinus bradycardia, atropine may be all that is necessary. If the drop in heart rate leads to hemodynamic embarrassment, and especially if higher grade atrioventricular block is present, a pacemaker is usually required. The ectopic tachycardias, whether they are atrial or ventricular, may respond to phenytoin (Dilantin) or lidocaine. Usually, potassium is recommended when hypokalemia is present, but it must be used carefully in those with severe digitalis intoxication, because inhibition of the Na-K adenosine triphosphatase may lead to inability of the sodium pump to transport potassium into the cell, causing severe elevations of the serum potassium level. Propranolol, quinidine, and procainamide have been used with some success in those with severe dysrhythmias. Direct current countershock is generally not advisable in the presence of digoxin intoxication because of the severe arrhythmias that can be elicited. However, it must be used in life-threatening arrhythmias when all other methods have failed.

For children who have ingested a potentially lethal dose, usually by accident or suicidal intent, the use of cardiac glycoside–specific antibodies and their "FAB" fragments may be lifesaving by reversing the cardiac glycoside–induced inhibition of the myocardial Na-K adenosine triphosphatase. When used, the electrocardiographic manifestations of toxicity usually disappear within a half hour.

Diuretics

The low-output state associated with congestive heart failure results in increased sodium reabsorption in the kidneys. This increased sodium leads to volume expansion, which in turn may lead to pulmonary edema if accumulated in the lungs, or to peripheral edema, or ascites, if sequestered in the systemic circulation. Diuretics are drugs that increase the urinary excretion of salt and water. They act indirectly by increasing renal blood flow or, more commonly, by directly inhibiting solute and water absorption, thereby increasing urine volume. Diuretics may have an effect in the proximal tubule (carbonic anhydrase inhibitors such as acetazolamide), the loop of Henle (furosemide, ethacrynic acid, bumetanide, and the organic mercurials), or in the distal convoluted tubule (thiazides, spironolactone, triamterene, and amiloride).

The most commonly used diuretic in pediatrics is **furosemide,** and to a lesser extent, **ethacrynic acid** and **bumetanide.** By blocking the luminal transport in the loop of Henle, reabsorption of sodium and chloride is prevented and up to 25% of the filtered sodium can be excreted, bringing water out with it. Furosemide is usually given as 1 mg/kg/dose, but may be given in larger doses in refractory cases (see Appendix, p. 760). If given intravenously, the response is usually prompt and impressive when there is an adequate cardiac output. The oral dosage is usually 2–5 mg/kg/day in two or three divided doses.

In cases in which such a prompt and vigorous diuresis is not necessary, we at Children's Hospital in Boston have usually used one of the thiazide diuretics, usually chlorothiazide (Diuril). The usual dosage is 20–50 mg/kg/day in two divided doses. Because the most common complication of diuretic therapy is potassium depletion, we have made extensive use of **spironolactone,** an aldosterone antagonist. Spironolactone acts by inhibiting sodium absorption and potassium secretion indirectly by binding to the receptors of aldosterone, displacing the hormone and preventing its effect. Although not a terribly effective diuretic in its own right, it is usually given in conjunction with one of the more potent diuretics (furosemide, ethacrynic acid, or one of the thiazide diuretics) to prevent potassium loss. The dose is 1–2 mg/day in one dose, and the half-life is measured in days. Triamterine and amiloride also inhibit the distal reabsorption of sodium and secretion of potassium, but work by a different mechanism and are effective even in the absence of aldosterone.

The **carbonic anhydrase inhibitors (acetazolamide)** act on the proximal tubule by interfering with hydrogen ion secretion, which is coupled to sodium reabsorption. This inability to secrete hydrogen ions prevents reabsorption of bicarbonate, which in turn decreases the movement of sodium and chloride. Acetazolamide is a relatively weak diuretic, however, and is not used routinely, although it may be effective in children who develop a normokalemic-hypochloremic alkalosis as a consequence of treatment with furosemide and spironolactone.

Complications of Diuretic Therapy. The diuretic agents presently available, especially furosemide and ethacrynic acid, are potent and may result in **volume depletion.** If elevated preload is necessary for compensation, this lowered intravascular volume may exacerbate the low-output state. This results in an increasing level of urea nitrogen in the blood, with a relatively preserved creatinine level. Reducing the dosage of the diuretics, switching to a less potent agent, or administering the dose on alternate days rather than daily is usually sufficient to increase blood volume.

The second most common complication of diuretics is **hypokalemia.** Most of the potent diuretics enhance potassium secretion. Initially potassium moves from the extracellular stores into intravascular space, but eventually the whole body is depleted of potassium and the serum potassium level falls. This can be especially dangerous for children receiving digoxin, because toxicity is increased in the presence of low serum potassium. The treatment is to reduce the level of diuresis, institute potassium chloride supplements, or administer a potassium-sparing diuretic such as spironolactone or triamterene.

A third complication of diuretic therapy is **hyponatremia.** If water intake is increased, hyponatremia may result. Furosemide, ethacrynic

acid, and the thiazides can cause a larger loss of solute than water, resulting in relatively concentrated urine. The treatment is usually to restrict water intake, reduce or interrupt the diuretic therapy, and, if possible, improve cardiac function. Dilutional hyponatremia is a serious complication; it may be difficult to diagnose and has a poor prognosis.

Metabolic alkalosis secondary to chloride depletion is seen occasionally with the potent loop diuretics, and, along with volume contraction, stimulates aldosterone production. Oral potassium chloride supplements may be effective, but if the alkalosis persists ammonium chloride may be necessary.

In some older children on diuretic therapy, **hyperuricemia** is an occasional problem. Most patients tolerate the hyperuricemia well and no specific therapy is necessary, although if gout occurs, treatment with allopurinol may be necessary.

One of the most serious complications is **ototoxicity,** which may be caused by furosemide or ethacrynic acid and is usually dose related. This occurs most commonly in patients with renal insufficiency and is usually, but not invariably, reversible.

Vasodilator Therapy

It has been known for some time that alterations in the resistance and the capacitance of the peripheral vascular bed can alter the performance of the heart. For example, by imposing an increased afterload on the heart from an anatomic lesion such as coarctation, or from suddenly increasing the peripheral vascular resistance, the workload facing the heart will be increased and, if cardiac reserve is minimal, the cardiac output will be reduced. By dilating systemic arterioles and reducing the afterload, cardiac output may be augmented in the reverse fashion.

Cardiac performance is also dependent on preload. Increasing the ventricular end-diastolic pressure and volume, and thereby atrial pressures, increases cardiac output by the Starling effect for any given level of contractility or afterload. However, this increased preload can result in pulmonary or systemic venous congestion. Frequently, by using venodilators, one can reduce the systemic venous or pulmonary venous pressures enough to relieve symptoms without markedly reducing cardiac output. From a theoretical standpoint, a pure venodilator would be desirable in patients whose symptoms are related to systemic or pulmonary venous congestion with preserved or nearly preserved cardiac output, whereas an afterload reducing agent would be preferable in patients with increased peripheral vascular resistance. However, most available agents affect both preload and afterload, and are thus best suited for patients with rather advanced congestive heart failure in whom systemic vascular resistance and atrial filling pressures are increased and in whom the agents can improve cardiac output and reduce signs and symptoms of systemic and pulmonary venous congestion.

Specific Agents. Nitroprusside, a short-acting agent that must be given intravenously, acts on both preload and afterload by relaxing vascular smooth muscle in the arteries and veins. The usual dose is approximately 5 μg/kg/min, but it may be increased substantially if hypotension does not occur (see Appendix, p. 760).

The most common toxic effect is **hypotension,** an exaggeration of the therapeutic effect, which can be reversed by stopping the medicine for 10 or 15 minutes. If hypotension is severe, the administration of fluid and/or a concomitant vasoconstrictor such as phenylephrine or epinephrine may be necessary. The metabolism of nitroprusside releases hydrocyanic acid, which, in the presence of thiosulfate, is converted to thiocyanate. The thiocyanate is excreted by the kidney and when renal function is impaired, the use of nitroprusside has led to thiocyanate toxicity. This causes, primarily, central nervous symptoms, especially convulsions, psychosis, muscle twitching, and abdominal pain. Patients with renal impairment who receive high doses of nitroprusside should have serum levels determined; the dose should be tapered or discontinued at serum levels higher than 6 mg/dl.

Hydralazine, an orally effective vasodilator that acts on smooth muscle, has been shown to have beneficial effects in studies of patients with large left-to-right shunts, cardiomyopathies, and postoperative hypertension after coarctation repair. The side effects include headache, nausea, vomiting, drug-induced fever, rash, and the more serious lupus-like syndrome, usually reversible, seen occasionally in people who are slow acetylators.

Because the renin-angiotensin system is activated in many patients with congestive heart failure, leading to vasoconstriction and elevated afterload, angiotensin-converting enzyme inhibitors such as captopril, and more recently, enalapril, have been used. These drugs are balanced **vasodilators** with actions on both the arterial and venous beds, and have been shown experimentally to cause a marked reduction in systemic vascular resistance and in right and left atrial pressures. These agents have been used with some success in children with large left-to-right shunts and in hypertensive patients following repair of coarctation of the aorta. They should be used carefully in patients receiving potassium supplements or potassium-sparing diuretics.

Prazosin, an oral alpha-adrenergic receptor blocking agent, is a balanced vasodilator equally effective in both arteries and veins and produces effects similar to those seen with nitroprusside. It is absorbed rapidly with maximum effectiveness within an hour and maintains hemodynamic effects for approximately 6 hours. Side effects include polyarthralgias, transient headache, urinary incontinence, rashes, and dry mouth. Occasionally, in adults, the first dose has been reported to cause transient faintness, dizziness, palpitations and, rarely, syncope.

Other Inotropic Agents

Sympathomimetic amines, catecholamines, and other sympathomimetics may improve low cardiac output by interacting with the beta receptors, leading to increased contractility and heart rate. Drugs that have been used to stimulate beta-1 cardiac receptors include isoproterenol, dopamine, dobutamine, and epinephrine.

Isoproterenol. Isoproterenol has pure beta-1 and beta-2 activity and augments contractility, increases heart rate, and causes vasodilatation. Its principal disadvantages are that it causes significant tachycardia, which may interfere with coronary perfusion and increase the beta-2 activity that causes vasodilatation, predominantly of vessels in the skeletal muscle rather than the renal or mesenteric vascular beds; this leads to hypotension. These disadvantages have limited its clinical use.

Dopamine. Dopamine is the immediate precursor of norepinephrine and is a potent beta-1 agonist, releasing norepinephrine at the sympathetic nerve terminals. At low doses it causes vasodilation primarily of the renal, mesenteric, cerebral, and coronary beds. At higher doses (greater than 20 μg/kg/min) it is a vasoconstrictor. The chronotropic effects are significantly less than those of isoproterenol. It has been found to be effective in low-output states that occur after cardiac surgery or after myocardial failure.

Dobutamine. Dobutamine acts primarily as a beta-1 agonist that improves contractility with little change in heart rate. However, unlike dopamine, at usual doses dobutamine does not increase renal blood flow and actually causes a redistribution of cardiac output in favor of coronary and skeletal muscle beds rather than mesenteric beds. In children it has been shown to increase cardiac output by increasing stroke volume rather than heart rate, resulting in a slight fall in systemic vascular resistance. The increase in cardiac output, however, is more than the fall in systemic resistance, resulting in an increase of blood pressure.

Epinephrine. Epinephrine has both alpha-peripheral and beta-1 cardiac activity. Occasionally it is used after cardiac surgery, where its very potent inotropic stimulation makes it useful in the low-output state with severe vasoconstriction that sometimes follows surgery. A major drawback, the marked increase in heart rate frequently seen, limits its usefulness.

The presently available sympathomimetic amines must be given intravenously with continuous, careful monitoring of arterial pressure, and thus are useful only for those in the perioperative period or with the life-threatening low-output state frequently associated with cardiogenic shock. Several oral agents have undergone research testing but none is presently available for use in children.

Amrinone. Amrinone is the first of a new class of drugs, dissimilar to both catecholamines and digitalis, with positive inotropic and vasodilator activity that works through a mechanism separate from the cardiac glycosides or sympathomimetic amines. Recent evidence suggests that it works through inhibition of phosphodiesterase activity, thereby resulting in significantly higher levels of intracellular cyclic adenosine monophosphate.

Several studies have documented increased cardiac output with an improved left ventricular ejection fraction and lower atrial pressures. These responses usually lead to an increased cardiac output both at rest and at exercise without major alteration in heart rate or blood pressure. Amrinone has serious side effects, however, including thrombo-cytopenia, fever, and hepatomegaly. As with the sympathomimetic amines, it is available in an intravenous preparation and thus has limited utility in those with chronic congestive heart failure.

REFERENCES

1. Artman M, Graham TP: Congestive heart failure in infancy: recognition and management. Am Heart J 103:1040–1055, 1982.
2. Croxson MS, Ibbertson HK: Serum digoxin in patients with thyroid disease. Br Med J 3:566–568, 1975.
3. Friedman WF, George BL: Treatment of congestive heart failure by altering loading conditions of the heart. J Pediatr 106:697–706, 1985.
4. Hougen TJ: Use of digoxin in the young. In Smith TW (ed): Digitalis Glycosides. New York, Grune and Stratton, 1986, pp. 169–207.
5. Smith TW, Braunwald E: The management of heart failure. In Braunwald E (ed): Heart Disease: A Textbook of Cardiovascular Medicine, 3rd ed. Philadelphia, W.B. Saunders Co., 1988.
6. Talner NS: Heart failure. In Adams FH, Emmanouilides GC, Riemenschneider TA (eds). Moss' Heart Disease in Infants, Children and Adolescents, 4th ed. Baltimore, Williams & Wilkins, 1989, pp. 660–675.

Chapter 8

HYPOXEMIA

Alexander S. Nadas, M.D.

Congestive heart failure and hypoxemia are the two principal handicaps that may result from congenital heart disease. Heart failure, as discussed in chapter 7, is a clinical syndrome (a combination of signs and symptoms) based on certain physiologic phenomena (increased end-diastolic ventricular pressure and inadequate cardiac output to meet the metabolic needs). By contrast, hypoxemia is a biochemical phenomenon (arterial oxygen saturation lower than 90% in room air) that is associated with a number of clinical signs and symptoms. It may be reasonable to state right at the outset that hypoxemia may be due to respiratory causes or to a right-to-left shunt (i.e., the mixture of venous into arterial blood) within or without the heart. The simplest way to differentiate between respiratory and shunt (cardiac) cyanosis is by determining the arterial pO_2 (through an arterial puncture or pulse oximetry) at room air after 100% oxygen has been inhaled for 10 minutes. The resting, room-air, arterial pO_2 is normally between 90 and 100 torr ($\pm$ 5%). In patients with hypoxemia, arterial pO_2 may vary anywhere from 10–80 torr. If the hypoxemia is respiratory in nature, inhalation of 100% oxygen will raise it to between 400 and 500 torr. By contrast, in shunt cyanosis the pO_2 seldom, if ever, rises above 150 torr.

For practical purposes an oxygen test is not necessary to differentiate between cardiac and respiratory cyanosis. When watching the patient quietly, in the office or at the bedside, the increased respiratory effort of respiratory hypoxemia is usually quite obvious. Plain chest films will also quickly reveal pulmonary pathology and show depressed diaphragms. In rare cases in which the distinction is not clear, the oxygen test is helpful.

CLINICAL CORRELATES OF HYPOXEMIA

Having defined the chemical substrate of hypoxemia and discussed the two principal causes, one should list, briefly, the clinical correlates of hypoxemia.

Cyanosis

Cyanosis is the bluish color of the skin, best noted at the fingernails, toenails, and the mucous membranes of the lips and conjunctivae. More than 60 years ago Lundsgaard and Van Slyke[3] determined that the abnormal color becomes perceptible when 5 gm of reduced hemoglobin is present in the capillaries (instead of the normal 2.25 gm), corresponding to approximately 70% saturation with a normal hemoglobin level. The experienced observer can usually detect saturation of 80–85%, corresponding, under average circumstances (hemoglobin 15 gm), to 3 gm of reduced hemoglobin.

Cyanosis may be present even if the arterial saturation is normal. This occurs most commonly if the cardiac output is reduced and the arteriovenous difference widens from the usual 40% to as much as 60% or more, giving rise to an increased amount of reduced hemoglobin at a capillary level. The amount of reduced hemoglobin required for this phenomenon is the same as it is for shunt cyanosis; only the mechanism by which it is created is different. Low-output cyanosis is acrocyanosis: it is most notable (even exclusively so) at the tip of the fingers or the tip of the nose, but not so much at the mucous membranes. Patients with acrocyanosis usually have cool extremities and small pulse volume. Clinical conditions resulting in low-output cyanosis include, among others, critical mitral stenosis and pulmonary vascular obstructive disease.

Another instance of visible cyanosis, not associated with arterial unsaturation, is due to polycythemia. In the pediatric age group this is most common in the newborn period when the hematocrit and hemoglobin are normally very high. The normal arteriovenous difference of approximately 40% can easily give rise to more than 3 gm of reduced hemoglobin in the capillaries of these babies. All pediatricians—even obstetricians—are familiar with the plethoric cyanosis of newborns which sometimes may be hard to differentiate from hypoxemia.

The reciprocal of the above phenomenon, the

absence of cyanosis in the face of true hypoxemia due to low hematocrit or hemoglobin level, should also be discussed here. For instance, in the case of anemia, with a hemoglobin of 10 gm and an average arteriovenous difference of 40%, the amount of reduced hemoglobin in the capillaries may not be more than 2 gm; thus, no cyanosis may be detected, although the percent arterial saturation is 80%.

Therefore, when discussing cyanosis three factors should be considered: (1) arterial oxygen saturation, (2) oxygen capacity (hemoglobin), and (3) arteriovenous oxygen difference. Cyanosis will be noted if the arterial oxygen saturation is low, if the oxygen capacity is high, or if the arteriovenous difference is increased.

Clubbing

A common and striking concomitant of hypoxemia is clubbing or hypertrophic osteoarthropathy (see Fig. 1, ch. 11). In its fully developed form, this consists of a widening and thickening of the ends of the fingers and toes accompanied by convex (hourglass) fingernails. Earlier forms of clubbing consist of shininess and tenseness of the skin over the terminal phalanges, obliterating the wrinkles usually present in this part of the skin. This incipient clubbing is usually accompanied by fiery red fingers, a characteristic of early, slight, arterial unsaturation. Full-blown clubbing in severely cyanotic children may be seen as early as 2 or 3 weeks of age. Ordinarily, however, it does not make its appearance until a child is a year or two old. For some reason, it appears earliest and most pronounced on the thumbs. Physiologic and histologic studies indicate that clubbed fingers have an increased number of capillaries and increased blood flow through a myriad of arteriovenous aneurysms.[5] This is accompanied by an increase of connective tissue in the terminal phalanges.

In children, clubbing almost always indicates congenital heart disease of the cyanotic variety, although occasionally cirrhosis of the liver, infective endocarditis, lung abscess, malabsorption syndromes, or even a familial hereditary condition may be responsible for it.

Polycythemia

Polycythemia, with increased hemoglobin content, is another consequence of arterial unsaturation. That a low arterial oxygen content acts as a stimulus to bone marrow (via release of erythropoietin from the kidneys) has been amply demonstrated, not only in patients with congenital malformation of the heart but also in people living at high altitudes with low atmospheric tension.[1] The increased oxygen-carrying capacity and oxygen delivery achieved by this means constitute a useful compensatory mechanism until the polycythemia

reaches hematocrit levels of 80% or more. At these levels, however, the benefits derived from the increase in available oxygen are probably outweighed by the disadvantages of the high viscosity and, actually, capacity increased beyond a "reasonable level" (70–75% hematocrit) may result in decreased oxygen delivery. The therapeutic implications of these considerations will be discussed later.

Children whose hematocrit level rises during adolescence may become symptomatic. Initially, the symptoms are vague, such as: feeling logy, being tired, having a full sensation in the head, and having headaches. Later the symptoms are no longer vague; the patient simply cannot do what was possible before. Symptoms begin to appear when the hematocrit reaches levels in excess of 70%. It is important that the hematocrit be measured by the centrifuging technique, because the density methods in common use give erroneous readings for these high levels. On examination, murmurs, readily audible before, may no longer be heard, the viscosity having a significant influence on the turbulence required to produce an audible murmur. Symptoms are relieved by reducing the hematocrit. This is best accomplished by a pheresis machine that receives blood from one arm, centrifuges it, and returns the patient's plasma to the opposite arm. The hematocrit is continuously monitored and is reduced by 10%; a greater reduction would reduce oxygen-carrying capacity to an uncomfortable degree. Between 35 and 45 such red cell phereses are performed annually for patients with congenital heart disease at The Boston Children's Hospital.[2] The same result can be attained by removing blood and replacing it with an equal volume of plasma or albumin. It is important to maintain the blood volume or the arterial pressure may fall and, in the presence of a ventricular defect, this would result in increased right-to-left shunting and decreased pulmonary blood flow.[6] Phlebotomy, for these reasons, is contraindicated.

Squatting

Squatting, described by Taussig,[7] is a characteristic posture assumed after exertion by patients with certain types of cyanotic congenital heart disease, specifically tetralogy of Fallot and, less commonly, pulmonary stenosis with an open foramen ovale (Fig. 1). It first makes its appearance at 1 or 2 years of age, or when the child starts walking. Usually, though not invariably, social pressure abolishes it at 8–10 years of age. Detailed studies at The Children's Hospital in Boston and elsewhere[4] indicate that oxygen saturation, diminished by effort, can be raised to normal more rapidly in a squatting than in a standing position (Fig. 2). Probably, this beneficial effect is caused by exclusion of the highly unsaturated lower extremity

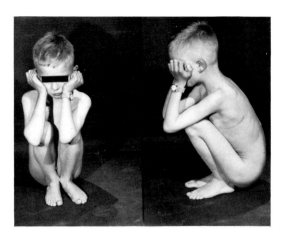

Figure 1. Child squatting. (From Nadas AS, Fyler DC: Pediatric Cardiology. Philadelphia, W.B. Saunders Co., 1973, with permission.)

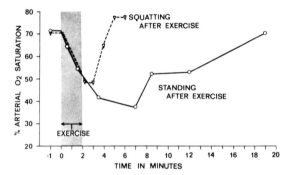

Figure 2. Effect of squatting on exercise-induced arterial oxygen unsaturation in a patient with cyanotic heart disease. (From Nadas AS, Fyler DC: Pediatric Cardiology. Philadelphia, W.B. Saunders Co., 1973, with permission.)

blood from the circulation, augmenting the peripheral resistance and thus diminishing the degree of right-to-left shunt. That initial increased systemic venous return also occurs in squatting is demonstrated by the fact that immediately after assumption of this characteristic posture, a brief drop in oxygen saturation occurs, corresponding to the "dumping" of highly unsaturated blood from the inferior vena cava into the common pool. This, then, is followed by the increase in peripheral saturation owing to the shutting out of venous return from the legs and the increase in systemic resistance.

Hypoxic Spells (Cyanotic Spells)

These are *the* most traumatic consequences of hypoxemia. Ordinarily, they consist of irritability, uncontrollable crying, tachypnea, deepening of cyanosis, disappearance of an ejection murmur, metabolic acidosis, and even loss of consciousness. These spells may affect babies with only mild cy-

anosis at rest or with no cyanosis at all. They are sudden, episodic phenomena that may occur for no obvious reason at all, usually early in the morning. Precipitating causes include bowel movements, crying with hunger, or medical interventions (finger pricks for hemograms or cardiac catheterization, etc.). This experience is frightening, not only for inexperienced parents but also for physicians and nurses.

As a rule, the vicious circle of crying, leading to hypoxemia, leading to more crying, can be interrupted by placing the baby on the shoulder with knees pressed against the abdomen, and soothing the infant by quietly patting the back. If the attack is not terminated within minutes, surely within half an hour, morphine should be administered subcutaneously, and oxygen may be administered by face mask to increase the dissolved oxygen in the plasma. Administration of beta blockers, presumably to release the infundibular spasm underlying the increase in the right-to-left shunt, is the next step in our armamentarium. If all else fails and the infant is unconsolable, general anesthesia has been administered, and even emergency shunt operations have been performed in years past. Surely, in the 1990s, the presence of hypoxic spells is an indication for early corrective surgery. In the author's view, pharmacologic prevention (beta blockers) of these episodes is too unreliable, and corrective surgery is safe and effective enough to make it the treatment of choice.

For some reason the spells do not occur in the newborn period; usually their onset is at 3–4 months of age. Careful questioning of new mothers with presumably "pink" infants who have tetralogy of Fallot may elicit a story of morning irritability, attacks of "teething," or momentary "loss of contact." All of these symptoms should raise the suspicion that, indeed, these may be cyanotic spells that might require surgical intervention. These spells may lead to cerebrovascular accidents and even death. Less traumatically, they may lead to decreased intelligence quotients or to more subtle neurologic impairment or learning disability. At The Children's Hospital in Boston the present policy is that even one major hypoxic spell is too much and should lead to early surgery.

Exercise Intolerance

This is a less traumatic but equally serious consequence of hypoxemia. The physiologic principle is that the common ejectile chamber, consisting of the right and left ventricle, connected by a large ventricular defect, faces an overriding aorta and an obstructed pulmonary infundibulum in patients with tetralogy of Fallot. Exercise (and this may not be more than sucking on a bottle) results in increased demand, which is met by a drop in systemic resistance, and a fixed, and maybe even

Exhibit 1

Boston Children's Hospital Experience 1973–1987 Cardiac Patients with Scoliosis*	
Diagnosis	% of Diagnostic Group with Scoliosis
Ventricular septal defect	0.66
Pulmonary valve abnormality	1.06
Tetralogy of Fallot	3.57
Aortic valve abnormality	0.94
Atrial septal defect	0.79
Patent ductus arteriosus	0.35
Coarctation of the aorta	1.59
D-transposition of the great arteries	0.79
Endocardial cushion defect	0.56
Myocardial disease	1.08
Malposition	1.79
Mitral valve abnormality	3.04
Hypoplastic left ventricle	0.00
Pulmonary atresia with ventricular septal defect	1.56
Double-outlet right ventricle	0.89
Single ventricle	6.25
Tricuspid valve abnormality	1.99
Tricuspid atresia	0.00
Truncus arteriosus	2.88
OVERALL	1.14

*There were 175 patients who developed scoliosis. Scoliosis was more common among cyanotic patients, especially among patients with tetralogy of Fallot, single ventricle, truncus arteriosus, malpositions, and tricuspid atresia. Because there were more patients with tetralogy of Fallot, more patients with scoliosis had this diagnosis than any other. Among the acyanotic patients, those with coarctation of the aorta or mitral valve disease were most likely to have scoliosis.

Exhibit 2

Boston Children's Hospital Experience 1973–1987 Birth Dates of Patients with Scoliosis*	
Date of Birth	Number of Patients
1950–54	30
1955–59	46
1960–64	33
1965–69	25
1970–74	14
1975–79	6
1980–84	2
1985–89	0

*There were 19 patients born before 1973 who had no birth date recorded. Most of the patients with scoliosis were born before 1975; indeed, the majority were born before 1965. This suggests that present methods for the correction of cyanotic defects prevent scoliosis. However, this conclusion must be taken with caution because scoliosis does not become manifest until the child is 10 years old and, therefore, must have been born more than 10 years earlier to have developed the problem.

increased, pulmonary resistance caused by circulating catechols. This results in a decrease in arterial saturation, dyspnea, hyperpnea and, possibly, even metabolic acidosis. It is interesting to note that older children do not really know how limited their exercise tolerance is, because they have never experienced a "normal" exercise tolerance. Occasionally, a high-school student or young adult states that his exercise tolerance is "normal" when, in fact, he or she is severely limited. Not until after successful surgery, curative or palliative, do these patients realize how limited they were. With cardiac surgery early in infancy, these stories of heroism and stoicism are less and less common.

Brain Abscess

In a patient with hypoxemia, symptoms of the central nervous system (headache, focal neurologic signs, convulsions, or loss of consciousness) should raise the immediate suspicion of brain abscess, because this is the one etiology explaining these symptoms and signs that is clearly treatable. Vascular lesions of the central nervous system, the alternative possibility, may be manageable but not curable (see p. 79, ch. 9).

Cerebrovascular Accidents

Cerebrovascular accidents not associated with brain abscess, and ranging from transient motor deficit to full-blown hemiplegia, are usually attributable to vascular lesions such as emboli or thrombi, but most commonly they are due to hypoxic damage occurring as a consequence of hypoxic spells. With more aggressive, early surgical correction, these have become rarities in this country within the past decade (see p. 78, ch. 9).

Scoliosis

Scoliosis is a complication among surviving cyanotic patients (Exhibits 1 and 2).

REFERENCES

1. Hurtado A: Aspectos fisiologicos y patologicos de la altura. Lima, Ed. Rimac, 1943.
2. Kevy S: Personal communication.
3. Lundsgaard C, Van Slyke DD: Cyanosis. Medicine 2:1–76, 1923.
4. Lurie PR: Postural effects in tetralogy of Fallot. Am J Med 15:297–306, 1955.
5. Mendlowitz M: Clubbing and hypertrophic osteoarthropathy. Medicine 21:269–306, 1942.
6. Rosenthal A, Button LN, Nathan DG et al: Blood volume changes in cyanotic congenital heart disease. Am J Cardiology 27:162–167, 1971.
7. Taussig HB: Congenital malformations of the heart. Cambridge, The Commonwealth Fund, Harvard University Press, 1960, Vols. I and II, pp. 1–1019.

Chapter 9

CENTRAL NERVOUS SYSTEM SEQUELAE OF CONGENITAL HEART DISEASE

Jane W. Newburger, M.D., M.P.H.

Recent dramatic improvements in surgical mortality of congenital heart lesions have been accompanied by the recognition that survivors frequently suffer neurologic sequelae. The prevalence of injury to the central nervous system ranges from 5–56%, the latter in children with D-transposition of the great arteries.[4,41] Often, brain injury is related to complications of cardiovascular surgery or diagnostic procedures, but neurologic outcome may also be influenced by preexisting brain abnormalities, severe chronic hypoxemia, congestive heart failure, episodes of arrhythmia or cardiac arrest, thromboembolic events unrelated to surgery, nutritional status, and infection of the central nervous system (i.e., brain abscess or meningitis).

CARDIOVASCULAR SURGERY

Cardiopulmonary Bypass

The association between central nervous system disorders and extracorporeal circulation has been recognized for some time. In retrospective studies, the incidence of focal neurologic complications after conventional cardiopulmonary bypass has ranged from 1.3–9%.[1,57] Prospective evaluation by neurologists after the use of extracorporeal circulation in adults has shown much higher rates of neurologic morbidity (23–53%).[53,58] Usually neurologic events resulting from cardiopulmonary bypass are attributed to either thromboembolic problems or diminished perfusion leading to ischemic insults.

Deep Hypothermia. In repairing complex congenital heart lesions in infancy, deep hypothermia is used together with either (1) total circulatory arrest ("circulatory arrest"), or (2) continuous low-flow cardiopulmonary bypass ("low-flow bypass"). Animal experiments and clinical experience have shown apparent safety of hypothermia as low as 15–20°C.[33] The protective effect of hypothermia during cerebral ischemia is derived, in part, from

a reduction in metabolic activity, reflected in reduced oxygen consumption. Additional mechanisms of hypothermic cerebral protection during ischemia include preservation of intracellular stores of high-energy phosphates and of high intracellular pH, as well as protection against reperfusion injury (including the "no-reflow" phenomenon), calcium influx, and free radical damage.[32] An understanding of the mechanism of cerebral protection during hypothermia has led to improved adjunctive methods, such as the use of the alpha-stat strategy to preserve high intracellular pH,[45] administration of agents that further suppress cerebral metabolism (e.g., barbiturates), and regulation of blood sugar and hematocrit.

Total Circulatory Arrest. Since its introduction in the early 1960s, circulatory arrest has been used widely in open heart surgery for infants.[34,66] A great advantage of this technique is the absence of perfusion cannulas and of blood from the operative field. The use of circulatory arrest for open heart surgery assumes that there is a "safe" duration of total circulatory arrest which is inversely related to body temperature.[33] The organ with the shortest "safe" circulatory arrest time is the brain.

Evidence for transient cerebral injury during circulatory arrest comes from laboratory and clinical investigations. Experimental studies on brain structure and function after use of circulatory arrest have suggested that, at a core temperature of 15–20°C, a 30-minute total arrest time is "safe" with respect to central nervous system damage.[25,62] Conflicting results have been reported with circulatory arrest times between 45 and 60 minutes.[24,38,62] Electrophysiologic studies using electroencephalograms and somatosensory, cortical-evoked potentials have clearly shown that at least transient cerebral dysfunction does occur after these prolonged periods of circulatory arrest.[16,67] The "reappearance latency" and "latency to continuous electroencephalographic activity" have been related to duration of circulatory arrest.

Functional disturbances following circulatory arrest include transient choreoathetosis, which occurs at an incidence reported between 1 and 19% on the second to sixth postoperative day.[10,11,60] Although usually transient, severe choreoathetosis may result in permanent abnormalities of movement. Transient seizures occur in 4–10% of infants in the immediate postoperative period after circulatory arrest.[11,14,19] Subclinical changes in brain morphology without concomitant abnormalities in neurologic examination have also been reported after circulatory arrest.[40] Finally, the serum level of creatinine kinase, brain isoenzyme (CK-BB), has been reported to be significantly higher among children who had surgery using circulatory arrest than among those with closed procedures (i.e., without extracorporeal circulation or circulatory arrest).[48] The length of circulatory arrest had a marked influence on the peak concentration of CK-BB, presumably reflecting the severity of cerebral ischemic insult.

Despite a relatively large number of studies on development after circulatory arrest, the developmental impact of this technique remains uncertain. Studies on cognitive, behavioral, and linguistic development of children who underwent circulatory arrest have shown evidence of deficits in these areas, sometimes related to duration of circulatory arrest.[52,65,68] Patients who underwent cardiac surgery with the use of circulatory arrest in infancy had scores on the McCarthy scale which were significantly worse than those of their siblings; these differences were positively associated with duration of circulatory arrest.[65] Other reports have shown no significant differences in those who had circulatory arrest when compared with controls.[6,14,18,47,59] Children with similar heart surgery who were operated upon under moderate hypothermia with continuous cardiopulmonary bypass had scores comparable to those of their siblings.

Low-flow Cardiopulmonary Bypass. Low-flow bypass at less than 0.5 L/min/m² of body surface has been shown to support a cerebral oxygen consumption appropriate for temperature in clinical and experimental studies.[26,27] Furthermore, latency and amplitude of somatosensory cortical-evoked potentials are maintained in normal ranges for temperature at perfusion rates as low as 0.50 L/min/m² for the duration of hypothermia (21–25°C), but disappear at lower rates of flow and with circulatory arrest.[46] However, at flow rates of 0.5 L/min/m² in animal studies, cerebral metabolic reserves were reduced, as indicated by a significant decrease in cerebral ATP levels.

CARDIAC CATHETERIZATION

The cooperative study on cardiac catheterization monitored complications arising from cardiac catheterization between 1963 and 1965 in 12,367 children and adults.[7] Unfortunately, this study included very few small infants, the patients who are most at risk for injury of the central nervous system. Still, recognized complications of the central nervous system were reported in approximately 0.2% of patients. Convulsions, headaches, and impairment of consciousness were reported as late as several hours after catheterization and were usually associated with contrast injection. In 13 patients, focal neurologic injury was presumed to be secondary to embolic events resulting from the use of catheters in the left side of the heart.

The risk of stroke may be particularly high in infants with D-transposition of the great arteries treated at catheterization with balloon atrial septostomy;[63,64] perhaps this is secondary to venous thrombosis occurring in femoral veins through which large-bore septostomy catheters are placed in these patients with profound right-to-left shunts (see Fig. 15, ch. 35).

CEREBROVASCULAR ACCIDENTS

Among young children, and especially among cyanotic infants, cerebral infarction caused by emboli, thrombosis in situ, or venous thrombosis has been described.[61] Many of these events occur in temporal relation to cardiac surgery, left-sided cardiac catheterization, or catheterization of cyanotic infants. However, occasionally emboli may arise from thrombosis in the heart chambers or the systemic venous circulation. It has been proposed that relative anemia,[17,37] secondary to cyanosis, leads to increased blood viscosity, increased coagulability and, thereby, venous thrombosis.[61]

CHRONIC HYPOXEMIA

Among children with cyanotic congenital heart disease, Cottrill[17] noted that the most common lesion was cerebral venous thrombosis. Of 25 cases studied at autopsy, arterial thrombi were involved in only 3, whereas in 18 there were antemortem cerebral venous clots, predominantly in the superior sagittal sinus. The majority of children were under one year of age and had either tetralogy of Fallot or transposition of the great arteries. All but one patient had an abnormally low mean corpuscular hemoglobin concentration, despite polycythemia. The authors postulated that abnormal red cell indices in relative anemia may lead to increased blood viscosity. An association of cerebrovascular accidents in young children with anemia has also been reported by Martelle[37] and by Phornphutkul.[44]

Children with cyanotic congenital heart disease have lower intelligence quotients and poorer perceptual and gross motor function than children with acyanotic heart disease or well children (Fig. 1).[35,36,44] The longer the infant is allowed to remain cyanotic, the greater the potential for measurable

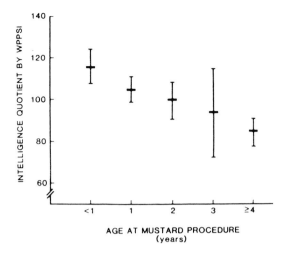

Figure 1. The relation of intelligence quotient, measured by the Wechsler Preschool and Primary Scale of Intelligence (WPPSI) at age five years, to the age at which Mustard's procedure was performed. These data demonstrate a decreasing mean intelligence quotient the longer the children are exposed to reduced amounts of arterial oxygen. (From Newburger JW, et al: Cognitive function and duration of hypoxemia in children with transposition of the great arteries. N Engl J Med 310:1495–1499, 1984, with permission.)

deficit at a later age.[41,54] Several hypotheses may be advanced to explain this finding. It may be related to a general effect of arterial hypoxemia on central nervous system function and development. For example, chronic hypoxemia, interacting with such other factors as hemoglobin level and cardiac output, may limit brain oxygenation, causing cumulative interference with normal brain maturation and function. Both chronic and acute hypoxemia affect the frequency at which flicker is perceived.[5,43,56] In children with chronic hypoxemia that is secondary to cyanotic congenital heart disease, there is a direct relation between the severity of cyanosis, as measured by the level of arterial oxygen saturation, and critical flicker frequency.[2]

Human neuropathologic studies support the hypothesis of a time-dependent effect of chronic hypoxemia on the brain.[55] White-matter gliosis has been reported in children and adults with congenital heart disease. Infants with congenital heart disease who die before the age of four months have a 39% prevalence of abnormalities in parietal white matter[51] (approximately twice the prevalence in infants who die of other causes). Among children with congenital heart disease who die after the age of one year, similar white matter abnormalities were found in 72%, representing a significant increase in cumulative risk with age. In addition to the increase in prevalence, the distribution of white-matter abnormalities changed with age as well. White-matter gliosis in the anterior temporal lobe was not encountered in infants under the age of two months, but it was present in the brains of 75% of

children with congenital heart disease who were more than one year old.

Perceptual motor function seems to be more profoundly impaired than other cognitive functions in children with cyanotic (and acyanotic) heart disease. The effect of early hypoxemia and hemodynamic disturbances on perceptual motor function may be explained by greater vulnerability of the related areas of the developing nervous system during the first year of life.[30]

Yakolev and Lecours,[69] studying patterns of myelination, delineated differences in the ages at which maturation occurs in various regions and fiber systems in the central nervous system. Fiber systems mediating optic, propriokinesthetic, and some motor functions myelinate rapidly during the first year of life, whereas the commissural and association systems of the cerebral hemispheres mature predominantly after the age of one year. However, the relation of the stage of development (and hence, the metabolism) of neurologic tissue to vulnerability to hypoxemia and hemodynamic stresses is conjectural.

HEMORRHAGE

Intracranial hemorrhage in the form of subarachnoid, subdural, or intraventricular hemorrhage is encountered in newborns who are very ill for a variety of reasons. It is not surprising, therefore, that these have been reported occasionally in very ill infants with congenital heart disease.[64,69]

CENTRAL NERVOUS SYSTEM INFECTION

Brain abscess is one of the most serious complications of cyanotic congenital heart disease, with a reported incidence in this population of 2%.[15] Conversely, cyanotic congenital heart disease is associated with 5–10% of all cases of brain abscess.[15,22,42] This predisposition of patients with cyanotic heart disease to brain abscess is thought to relate to the fact that bacteria in venous blood may not pass through the normally effective phagocytic filtering action of the pulmonary capillary bed. In addition, the polycythemia and consequent hyperviscosity associated with chronic hypoxemia are thought to reduce capillary blood flow in the brain, leading to microinfarction and reduced tissue oxygenation, complicated later by bacterial colonization.[23] Bacterial endocarditis is associated with brain abscess only rarely; it occurred in only 4 of 148 cases of brain abscess in two series.[39,50] The most common bacteria isolated in brain abscess are streptococci, often microaerophilic species.[23] Brain abscess is exceedingly rare in patients less than two years of age, presumably because they do not yet have periodontal disease.

While the more cyanotic the patient, the more likely a brain abscess will develop,[15] patients with minimal or intermittent cyanosis are encountered with this problem. The classic triad of symptoms of brain abscess (that is, fever, headaches, and focal neurologic deficit) is present in a minority of patients.[23] Headache is the most common symptom, occurring in approximately 70% of patients.[8,22,49,50] The majority of patients also have a change in mental status.[22,31,50] Fever and focal findings each are present in approximately 50% of patients.[3,22,28,29,31,49,50] Symptoms and signs of brain abscess are necessarily dependent on intracranial location. The often subtle symptoms of brain abscess, together with its high morbidity and mortality, mandate a rapid evaluation for this diagnosis in any patient with cyanotic heart disease and possible or definite neurologic findings.

The diagnosis of brain abscess is made using computed tomography (CT) with contrast enhancement.[9] Examination of peripheral blood is not often helpful; indeed, in 40% of patients with brain abscess the white blood cell count is normal.[12,22,50] In patients with brain abscess, lumbar puncture sometimes leads to clinical deterioration or death.[31,49,50] Thus, patients with cyanotic heart disease, fever, and focal neurologic findings should undergo a CT scan before lumbar puncture is performed. If meningitis is strongly suspected, one should obtain blood cultures and begin antibiotic therapy before the CT scan; lumbar puncture should be performed promptly if the CT scan is negative.[23]

Few published reports address optimal antibiotic therapy of brain abscess. A combination of intravenous penicillin and chloramphenicol or metronidazole are frequently administered.[23] The choice of antibiotics must be guided by consideration of in-vitro activity against the etiologic agent(s), as well as antibiotic penetration into the abscess; most patients with brain abscess require surgical management, although the timing and type of surgical procedure vary depending on the "stage" of the abscess.[13,20,21] Attempts to drain an area of cerebritis before there is liquefaction may be counterproductive. Management must be directed by the neurosurgeon, in close consultation with specialists in infectious disease and cardiology, as clinical deterioration can occur precipitously.[3,22,28,29,31,49,50]

The mortality from brain abscess depends on the location of the lesion, the presence of multiple or multiloculated lesions, rupture of the abscess into a ventricle, the etiologic agent, and the choice of antibiotics. The overall mortality of brain abscess in recent series is approximately 15–20%.[22,23,29] A seizure disorder requiring long-term anticonvulsant medication follows brain abscess in 35% of cases.[22,29]

Meningitis has been reported to be more common among infants with cyanotic heart disease than among those with acyanotic heart disease or well children.[58,59]

FUTURE

The neurologic outcome for children with congenital heart disease represents one of the most important issues in pediatric cardiology today. Survival as a goal has largely been achieved. Future studies are needed to assess the prevalence and determinants of brain injury, so that central nervous system sequelae of congenital heart disease may be reduced.

REFERENCES

1. Aberg T, Kihlgren M: Cerebral protection during open-heart surgery. Thorax 32:525–533, 1977.
2. Aisenberg RB, Rosenthal A, Wolff PH, et al: Hypoxemia and critical flicker frequency in congenital heart disease. Am J Dis Child 128:335–358, 1974.
3. Beller AJ, Sahar A, Praiss I: Brain abscess. Review of 89 cases over 30 years. J Neurol Neurosurg Psychiatry 36:757–768, 1973.
4. Berthrong M, Sabiston DC, Jr: Cerebral lesion in congenital heart disease: a review of autopsies on 162 cases. Bull Johns Hopkins Hosp 89:384–401, 1951.
5. Birren JE, Fisher MB, Vollmer E, et al: Effects of anoxia on performance at several simulated altitudes. J Exp Psychol 36:35–49, 1946.
6. Blackwood M, Haka-Ikse K, Steward D: Developmental outcome in children undergoing surgery with profound hypothermia. Anesthesiology 65:437–440, 1986.
7. Branwald E, Swan HJC: Cooperative Study of Catheterization. American Heart Association Monograph No. 20. Circulation 37(Suppl):III-1–III-103, 1968.
8. Brewer NS, MacCarty CS, Wellman WE: Brain abscess: a review of recent experience. Ann Intern Med 82:571–576, 1975.
9. Britt RH, Enzmann DR: Clinical stages of human brain abscesses on serial CT scans after contrast infusion. Computerized tomographic, neuropathological, and clinical correlations. J Neurosurg 59:972–989, 1983.
10. Brunberg JA, Doty DB, Reilly EL: Choreoathetosis in infants following cardiac surgery with deep hypothermic and circulatory arrest. J Pediatr 84:232–238, 1974.
11. Brunberg JA, Reilly EL, Doty DB: Central nervous system consequences in infants of cardiac surgery using deep hypothermia and circulatory arrest. Circulation 49:62–68, 1974.
12. Carey ME: Brain abscesses. Contemp Neurosurg 3:1, 1982.
13. Carey ME, Chou SN, French LA: Experience with brain abscesses. J Neurosurg 36:1–9, 1972.
14. Clarkson PM, MacArthur BA, Barratt-Boyes BG: Developmental progress following cardiac surgery in infants using profound hypothermia and circulatory arrest. Circulation 62:855–861, 1980.
15. Cohen MM: The central nervous system in congenital heart disease. Neurology 10:452–456, 1970.
16. Coles JG, Taylor MJ, Pearce JM: Cerebral monitoring of somatosensory evoked potentials during profoundly hypothermic circulatory arrest. Circulation 70:96–102, 1984.
17. Cottrill CM, Kaplan S: Cerebral vascular accidents in cyanotic congenital heart disease. Am J Dis Child 125:484–487, 1973.
18. Dickinson D, Sambrooks J: Intellectual performance in children after circulatory arrest with profound hypothermia in infancy. Arch Dis Child 54:1–6, 1979.
19. Ehyai A, Fenichel GM, Bender HW: Incidence and

prognosis of seizures in infants after cardiac surgery with profound hypothermia and circulatory arrest. JAMA 252:3165–3167, 1984.

20. Enzmann D, Britt RH, Placone R: Staging of human brain abscess by computed tomography. Radiology 146:703–708, 1983.

21. Epstein F, Whelan M: Cerebritis masquerading as brain abscess: case report. Neurosurgery 10:757–759, 1982.

22. Fischbein CA, Rosenthal A, Fischer EG: Risk factors for brain abscess in patients with congenital heart disease. Am J Cardiol 34:97–102, 1974.

23. Fischer EG, McLennan JE, Suzuki Y: Cerebral abscess in children. Am J Dis Child 135:746–749, 1981.

24. Fisk GC, Wright JS, Hicks RG: The influence of duration of circulatory arrest at 20°C on cerebral changes. Anaesth Intens Care 4:126–134, 1976.

25. Folkerth TL, Angell WW, Fosburg RG, et al: Effect of deep hypothermia, limited cardiopulmonary bypass, and total arrest on growing puppies. In Recent Advances in Studies on Cardiac Structure. Baltimore, University Park Press, 1975, pp. 411–421.

26. Fox LS, Blackstone EH, Kirklin JW: Relatinship of whole body oxygen consumption to perfusion flow rate during hypothermic cardiopulmonary bypass. J Thorac Cardiovasc Surg 83:239–248, 1982.

27. Fox LS, Blackstone EH, Kirklin JW: Relationship of brain blood flow and oxygen consumption to perfusion flow rate during profoundly hypothermic cardiopulmonary bypass. J Thorac Cardiovasc Surg 87:658–664, 1984.

28. Garfield J: Management of supratentorial intracranial abscess: a review of 200 cases. Br Med J 2:7–11, 1969.

29. Garvey G: Current concepts of bacterial infections of the central nervous system. Bacterial meningitis and bacterial brain abscess. J Neurosurg 59:735–744, 1983.

30. Gilles F, Leviton A, Jammes J: Age-dependent changes in white matter in congenital heart disease (abstract). J Neuropathol Exp Neurol 32:179, 1973.

31. Heinneman HS, Braude AI: Anaerobic infection of the brain. Observations on eighteen consecutive cases of brain abscess. Am J Med 35:682–697, 1963.

32. Hickey PR, Anderson NP: Deep hypothermic circulatory arrest: a review of pathophysiology and clinical experience as a basis for anesthetic management. J Cardiothoracic Anesth 1:137–155, 1987.

33. Kirklin JW, Barratt-Boyes BG (eds.): Cardiac Surgery. New York, John Wiley and Sons, 1986, pp. 30–74.

34. Kirklin JW, Dawson B, Devloo RA, et al: Open intracardiac operations: Use of circulatory arrest during hypothermia induced by blood cooling. Ann Surg 154:769–776, 1961.

35. Linde LM, Rasof B, Dunn OJ: Mental development in congenital heart disease. J Pediatr 71:198–203, 1967.

36. Linde LM, Rasof B, Dunn OJ: Longitudinal studies of intellectual and behavioral development in children with congenital heart disease. Acta Paediatr Scand 59:169–176, 1970.

37. Martelle RR: Cardiovascular accidents with tetralogy of Fallot. Am J Dis Child 101:206–215, 1961.

38. Molina JE, Einzig S, Mastri AR: Brain damage in profound hypothermia; perfusion versus circulatory arrest. J Thorac Cardiovasc Surg 87:596–604, 1984.

39. Morgan H, Wood M, Murphey F: Experience with 88 consecutive cases of brain abscess. J Neurosurg 38:698–704, 1973.

40. Muraoka R, Yokota M, Aoshima M: Subclinical changes in brain morphology following cardiac operations as reflected by computed tomographic scans of the brain. J Thorac Cardiovasc Surg 81:364–369, 1981.

41. Newburger JW, Silbert AR, Buckley LP, et al: Cognitive function and duration of hypoxemia in children with transposition of the great arteries. N Engl J Med 310:1495–1499, 1984.

42. Nielsen H, Gyldensted C, Harmsen A: Cerebral abscess. Aetiology and pathogenesis, symptoms, diagnosis and treatment. Acta Neurol Scand 65:609–622, 1982.

43. O'Dougherty M, Wright FS, Garmezy N, et al: Later competence and adaptation in infants who survive severe heart defects. Child Dev 54:1129–1142, 1983.

44. Phornphutkul C, Rosenthal A, Nadas AS, et al: Cerebrovascular accidents in infants and children with cyanotic congenital heart disease. Am J Cardiol 32:329–334, 1973.

45. Rahn H, Reeves RB, Howell BJ: Hydrogen ion regulation, temperature and evolution. Am Rev Resp Dis 112:165–172, 1975.

46. Rebeyka IM, Coles JG, Wilson GJ: The effect of low-flow cardiopulmonary bypass on cerebral function: An experimental and clinical study. Ann Thorac Surg 43:391–396, 1987.

47. Richter JA: Profound hypothermia and circulatory arrest: Studies on intraoperative metabolic changes and later postoperative development after correction of congenital heart disease. In deLange S, Hennis PJ, Kettler D, et al (eds): Cardiac Anesthesia: Problems, Innovations. Boston, Nijhoff, 1986, pp. 121–142.

48. Rossi R, Ekroth R, Lincoln C: Detection of cerebral injury after total circulatory arrest and profound hypothermia by estimation of specific creatinine kinase isoenzyme levels using monoclonal antibody techniques. Am J Cardiol 58:1236–1241, 1986.

49. Samson DS, Clark K: A current review of brain abscess. Am J Med 54:201–210, 1973.

50. Scheld MW, Winn RH: Brain abscess. In Mandell GL, Douglas RG, Bennett JE, (eds): Principles and Practice of Infectious Diseases. New York, John Wiley and Sons, 1985, pp. 585–591.

51. Schilz W: Uber den Einfluss chronischen Sauerstoffmangels auf das menschliche Gehirn (Aug Grund des Hirnbefundes eines Achtzehnjahrigen mit Morbus caeruleus bei angeborenem Herzfehler). Z Gesamte Neurol Psychiatr 171:426–450, 1941.

52. Settergren G, Ohqvist Gun Lundberg S: Cerebral blood flow and cerebral metabolism in children following cardiac surgery with deep hypothermia and circulatory arrest. Clinical course and follow-up of psychomotor development. Scand J Thorac Cardiovasc Surg 16:209–215, 1982.

53. Shaw PJ, Bates D, Cartlidge NEF: Neurologic and neuropsychological morbidity following major heart surgery: comparison of coronary artery bypass and peripheral vascular surgery. Stroke 18:700–707, 1987.

54. Silbert A, Wolff PH, Mayer B, et al: Cyanotic heart disease and psychological development. Pediatrics 43:192–200, 1969.

55. Simonson E, Brozek J: Flicker fusion frequency: background and applications. Physiol Rev 32:349–378, 1972.

56. Simonsen E, Winchell P: Effect of high carbon dioxide and of low oxygen concentration on fusion frequency of flicker. J Appl Physiol 3:637–641, 1951.

57. Sotaniemi KA: Neuropsychologic outcome after openheart surgery. Arch Neurol 38:2–8, 1981.

58. Sotaniemi KA: Cerebral outcome after extracorporeal circulation. Comparison between prospective and retrospective evaluations. Arch Neurol 40:75–77, 1983.

59. Stevenson J, Stone E, Dillard D, et al: Intellectual development of children subjected to prolonged circulatory arrest during hypothermic open heart surgery in infancy. Circulation 49(Suppl II):54–59, 1974.

60. Stewart RW, Blackstone EH, Kirklin JW: Neurological dysfuction after cardiac surgery. In Parenzan L, Crupi G, Graham G (eds): Congenital Heart Disease in the First Three Months of Life. Medical and Surgical Aspects. Bologna, Italy, Patron Editore, 1981, p. 431.

61. Terplan KL: Patterns of brain damage in infants and children with congenital heart disease. Am J Dis Child 125:175–185, 1973.

62. Treasure T, Naftel DC, Conger KA, et al: The effect of hypothermic circulatory arrest time on cerebral function, morphology, and biochemistry. An experimental study. J Thorac Cardiovasc Surg 86:761–770, 1983.

63. Tynan M: Survival of infants with transposition of the great arteries after balloon septostomy. Lancet 1:621–623, 1971.

64. Venables AW: Balloon septostomy in complete transposition of the great arteries in infancy. Br Heart J 32:61–65, 1970.

65. Wells F, Coghill S, Caplan H, et al: Duration of circulatory arrest does influence the psychological development of children after cardiac operation in early life. J Thorac Cardiovasc Surg 86:823–831, 1983.

66. Weiss M, Piwnica A, Lenfant C, et al: Deep hypothermia with total circulatory arrest. Trans Am Soc Artif Intern Organs 6:227–239, 1960.

67. Weiss M, Weiss J, Nicolas F, et al: A study of the electroencephalograms during surgery with deep hypothermia and circulatory arrest. J Thorac Cardiovasc Surg 70:316–329, 1975.

68. Wright J, Hicks R, Newman D: Deep hypothermic arrest: Observations on later development in children. J Thorac Cardiovasc Surg 77:466–469, 1979.

69. Yakovlev PI, Lecours AR: The myelogenetic cycles of regional maturation of the brain. In Minkowski A (ed): Regional Development of the Brain in Early Life. Oxford, Blackwell, 1967, pp. 3–70.

Chapter 10

PULMONARY HYPERTENSION

Thomas J. Kulik, M.D.

There are multiple facets to pulmonary physiology, but of most concern to the pediatric cardiologist are the factors that influence resistance to blood flow through the lung. The pulmonary vascular bed is normally a low resistance circuit, but it is prone to develop increased resistance to blood flow, which can result in serious disability. As a consequence, "the lesser" circulation: (1) is a major factor in the natural history of many cardiac lesions, (2) determines the type of operative procedure feasible for many patients with cardiac lesions, and (3) influences the morbidity and mortality of cardiac operations (Fig. 1). In addition, the pediatric cardiologist may be asked to evaluate and treat patients with pulmonary hypertension not related to congenital heart lesions.

Unfortunately, our understanding of the factors that determine pulmonary vascular resistance is rudimentary, and consequently our ability to influence pulmonary resistance in the clinical situation is limited.

NORMAL PULMONARY VASCULAR DEVELOPMENT

There are detailed reviews of the development and structure of normal airways,[18] as well as of the pulmonary[78] and bronchial vasculature.[31] It is worth emphasizing here that the lung's circulation undergoes important physiologic and anatomic changes in the first few hours, weeks, and months of life. *In utero*, the pulmonary arteries are relatively thick-walled, and pulmonary vascular resistance is very high. *At birth*, there is an immediate and large reduction in pulmonary vascular resistance, because of the combined effects of mechanical expansion of the lung, relief of alveolar hypoxia, and, probably, the release of humoral substances such as bradykinin and dilator prostaglandins.[58,155] Pulmonary vascular resistance continues to decrease until the adult level is reached between 1 and 3 weeks of age.[39,152,154] Dilatation of pulmonary arteries at birth is reflected in the virtually immediate decrease in wall thickness (ratio of wall thickness to external diameter) of pulmonary arteries less than 200 microns in diameter. Larger pulmonary arteries show a slower regression of wall thickness, but reach the adult level in the first several months.[78] Failure of the normally high fetal pulmonary vascular resistance to regress normally appears to be an essential element of at least one form of pulmonary hypertension (see p. 93), and it may be important in other clinical settings. A delayed fall in pulmonary vascular resistance commonly occurs with large intracardiac communications (such as ventricular septal defect), and may account for the fact that the onset of heart failure from left-to-right shunting lesions usually occurs well after pulmonary vascular resistance has normally fallen to low levels.[154]

Postnatally, the pulmonary vascular bed also undergoes considerable growth. Although the branching pattern of the larger pulmonary arteries and veins is established with the airway branching pattern at 16 weeks of gestation, the number of small pulmonary vessels increases proportionate to the number of alveoli. This increase in small pulmonary vessels is very large, since at birth there are approximately 20 million "primitive saccules" (precursors to alveoli), whereas by about 8 years of age there are 300 million alveoli.[78] Factors that cause pathologic changes in the pulmonary vascular bed in the child (e.g., congenital heart lesions) affect existing vessels and may interfere with this normal growth of the vascular bed (see p. 87). Hence, early intervention in patients with heart lesions is required to eliminate stimuli that interfere with normal pulmonary vascular development during the critical first 18 months or so, when such rapid growth takes place.

PULMONARY VASCULAR RESISTANCE

Measurement

The relationship between pressure and flow in the pulmonary circulation is complex.[42] One may

83

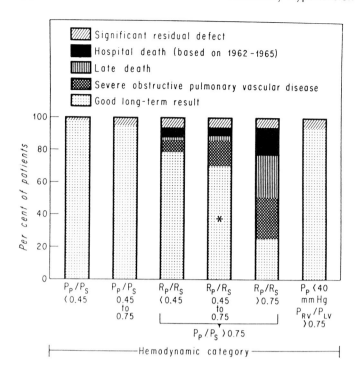

Figure 1. Results of repair of ventricular septal defect at the Mayo Clinic, from 1962 through 1965, in patients older than six months of age. Although these patients were operated on when intracardiac surgery was relatively new, short- and long-term results were excellent in patients with low preoperative pulmonary vascular resistance. As preoperative pulmonary vascular resistance increased, so did the risk of an unsatisfactory outcome. P_p, pulmonary arterial systolic pressure; P_s, systemic arterial systolic pressure; P_{RV}, right ventricular systolic pressure; P_{LV}, left ventricular systolic pressure; R_p, pulmonary vascular resistance; R_s, systemic vascular resistance. (From Cartmill TB, et al: Results of repair of ventricular septal defect. J Thorac Cardiovasc Surg 52:486–501, 1966, with permission.)

think of resistance to blood flow as a function of the number, luminal area, and length of pulmonary vessels (Poiseuille),[10] but even from this highly simplified viewpoint things are knotty. The number and luminal diameter of patent pulmonary "resistance" vessels depend not only on the architecture of the pulmonary vascular bed,[138,139] but also on pulmonary blood flow, left atrial pressure, pulmonary vascular smooth muscle tone, and "critical closing pressure."[98,116] In addition, because blood flow is pulsatile, the total energy expended by the right ventricle cannot be calculated using only mean pressure and flow.[120] Nevertheless, the clinician must start somewhere, and the resistance to blood flow through the lungs is generally reckoned in a way analogous to that used to calculate resistance in an electrical circuit:

$$R_p = P_{pa}/Q_p$$

where R_p = pulmonary vascular resistance, sometimes referred to as "total pulmonary vascular resistance;" P_{pa} = mean pulmonary artery pressure; and Q_p = pulmonary blood flow. Because using absolute pulmonary blood flow fails to take into account body size, in pediatrics, pulmonary flow is often divided by the body surface area to yield the pulmonary flow index. The pressure necessary for blood to flow in the pulmonary circuit depends on both resistance within the lung and left atrial pressure, and both of these factors are accounted for in this equation. To determine the resistance to flow that resides within the lung itself, mean left atrial pressure (LAP) is subtracted from mean

pulmonary artery pressure and pulmonary arteriolar resistance (R_p) is calculated:

$$R_p \text{ (mm Hg/L/min/m}^2) = P_{pa} \text{ (mm Hg)} - P_{la} \text{ (mm Hg)} / Q_p \text{ (L/min/m}^2)$$

where P_{la} = mean left atrial pressure. Resistance in mm Hg/L/min/m² ("Wood units," after Earl Wood) is sometimes multiplied by 80 in order to convert the value to dynes-sec-cm⁻⁵.

When the measurement of pulmonary flow is impractical, the ratio of pulmonary to systemic resistance (R_p:R_s) can be calculated using only pressure and blood oxygen saturation data:

$$R_p{:}R_s = (P_{pa} - P_{la}) ([AO] - [MV]) / (P_{ao} - P_{ra}) ([PV] - [PA])$$

where P_{ao} = mean aortic pressure; P_{ra} = mean right atrial pressure; [AO] = aortic blood oxygen content; [MV] = mixed venous blood content; [PV] pulmonary venous blood oxygen content; and [PA] = pulmonary arterial blood oxygen content. This expression is often taken as an estimate of pulmonary vascular resistance, especially in patients with intracardiac shunting (normal R_p:R_s is <.23),[97] the implicit assumption being that systemic vascular resistance is essentially normal.

Normal Values

Immediately following birth pulmonary artery pressure approximates that of the aorta, but it falls rapidly and is usually half of the systemic pressure or less within the first 1–2 days;[39] it reaches adult levels within the first 1–3 weeks of life.[39,152,154] Normal mean pulmonary arterial pressure (zero pressure taken at mid-chest level) after the first few weeks of life is 10–20 mm Hg.[97,156] Total pulmonary vascular resistance (indexed) in essentially normal children was found by Lock and associates[112] in 1978 to be 269 ± 19 dynes-sec-cm^{-5}. This is similar to that reported for young adults.[62]

Pathophysiology of Increased Pulmonary Vascular Resistance

Patients with increased pulmonary vascular resistance (especially when secondary to congenital heart lesions) are often said to have "pulmonary vascular disease" or "pulmonary vascular obstructive disease." This term generally implies pathologic structural changes in small pulmonary vessels. Actually, increased pulmonary vascular resistance may result not only from structural changes in the pulmonary vascular bed (decreased luminal area of pulmonary arteries and veins or diminished number of pulmonary vessels), but also from active constriction of pulmonary vessels.[6,23,142,144] Because it is difficult or impossible to eliminate all active tone from pulmonary vessels *in vivo*, one can never be certain precisely how an elevated pulmonary vascular resistance is partitioned between structural changes and vasoconstriction.

Pathologic Changes in Pulmonary Vascular Structure. Heath and Edwards described the progressive changes in pulmonary vascular structure that occur with pulmonary hypertension secondary to congenital septal defects.[67,73] **Grade 1** changes, which are the mildest, consist of medial hypertrophy and the extension of smooth muscle into normally nonmuscular arteries. These are the initial findings observed with congenital lesions which are associated with increased pulmonary arterial pressure (e.g., large ventricular septal defect). When there is increased pulmonary flow associated with normal pressure (e.g., atrial septal defect), intimal proliferation is usually the earliest pathologic change, this is followed by medial hypertrophy only after elevation of pulmonary arterial pressure.[67] **Grade 2** changes show more medial hypertrophy and cellular intimal proliferation. **Grade 3** changes include fibrosis of the intima, sometimes with early generalized vascular dilatation. Intimal fibrosis first occurs in pre-acinar arteries (arteries accompanying airways proximal to terminal bronchioles). These areas of intimal obstruction may cause the distal pulmonary artery to have normal or even decreased wall thickness; this "predilatation phase" appears to precede the development of Grade 4 changes.[70] The arteries in **Grade 4** show thinning of the media and generalized dilatation, as well as local areas of dilatation ("dilatation lesions"). Dilatation lesions are of three types, known

as "plexiform" lesions, "angiomatoid" lesions, and "vein-like" branches of hypertrophied (usually occluded) muscular pulmonary arteries.[165] In Grade 4 plexiform lesions are present, but the other types are found in **Grade 5**, where medial fibrosis also occurs. **Grade 6** indicates the presence of necrotizing arteritis (Fig. 2).

Because plexiform lesions may be found in pulmonary vascular obstruction due to increased pulmonary arterial pressure and flow, it is sometimes referred to as "plexiform arteriopathy"; similar histologic findings are present in primary pulmonary hypertension (see p. 90). On the other hand, plexiform lesions do not occur in other forms of pulmonary hypertension (e.g., that secondary to hypoxia); hence, the progression of histologic changes outlined above does not apply to pulmonary hypertension of all etiologies. Nevertheless, at least some of these histologic abnormalities (e.g., medial hypertrophy) are found in pulmonary hypertension of other causes.[180]

Analysis of the pulmonary vascular bed after the injection of a barium-gelatin mixture in postmortem specimens shows better quantified changes in medial thickness and distal extension of medial muscle, and has demonstrated a decreased number of small pulmonary arteries in the hypertensive lung.[69,141,144,180] These morphometric studies describe pathologic structural changes in terms of three grades:[71,139,141] **Grade A** signifies the appearance of muscle more peripherally than normal, with or without medial hypertrophy of normally muscular vessels; **Grade B** signifies distal extension of muscle plus medial wall thickness 1.5–2 times normal (B mild), or more than two times normal (B severe); **Grade C** denotes Grade B plus a decreased density of peripheral arteries relative to alveoli. **Grade C "mild"** indicates a less than 50% decrease in density of peripheral arteries, with **Grade C "severe"** being a reduction of more than 50%. These morphometric findings appear to correlate reasonably well with pulmonary pressures and resistances.[139]

The mechanism(s) responsible for pathologic vascular changes is not known. Insights gained from the study of systemic vascular pathology, and in particular atherogenesis, may be pertinent,[46,71,80] as the pathogenesis of systemic and pulmonary vascular lesions appear to share at least some features: in both, intimal proliferation appears to be due to collections of smooth muscle or smooth muscle-like cells.[74,161,165] Increased intraluminal pressure appears to be a stimulus for medial hypertrophy in at least some forms of pulmonary and systemic hypertension.[80,162,185] Endothelial cell damage may play a role in the genesis of systemic atherogenesis,[24,57] and it has been speculated that shear stress, secondary to increased pulmonary flow, may damage endothelium and thus cause vascular remodeling in the lung.[143] Although there is little evi-

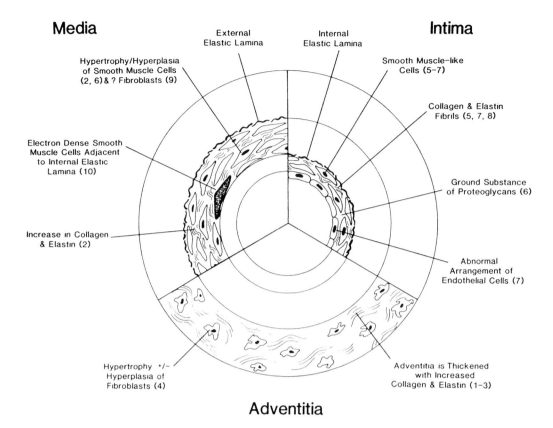

Media

External Elastic Lamina

Internal Elastic Lamina

Intima

Hypertrophy/Hyperplasia of Smooth Muscle Cells (2, 6) & ? Fibroblasts (9)

Smooth Muscle–like Cells (5–7)

Collagen & Elastin Fibrils (5, 7, 8)

Electron Dense Smooth Muscle Cells Adjacent to Internal Elastic Lamina (10)

Ground Substance of Proteoglycans (6)

Increase in Collagen & Elastin (2)

Abnormal Arrangement of Endothelial Cells (7)

Hypertrophy +/– Hyperplasia of Fibroblasts (4)

Adventitia is Thickened with Increased Collagen & Elastin (1–3)

Adventitia

Figure 2.   Some of the histologic features of pathologically remodeled pulmonary arteries are summarized in this diagram of a cross-section of a small pulmonary artery. Some or all of the histologic abormalities depicted can be secondary to a congenital heart defect, but they also can occur with pulmonary hypertension of other etiologies. Depending on the severity of the pathologic remodeling, not all of these features will be present. Numbers indicate references for each part of the diagram: (1) Heath D, Edwards J: The pathology of hypertensive pulmonary vascular disease. Circulation 18:533–547, 1958. (2) Meyrick B, Reid L: Ultrastructural findings in lung biopsy material from children with congenital heart defects. Am J Pathol 101:527–532, 1980. (3) Mecham RP, Whitehouse LA, Wrenn DS, et al: Smooth muscle-mediated connective tissue remodeling in pulmonary hypertension. Science 237:423–437, 1987. (4) Meyrick B, Reid L: Hypoxia-induced structural changes in the media and adventitia of the rat hilar pulmonary artery and their regression. Am J Pathol 100:151–178, 1980. (5) Smith P, Heath D: Electron microscopy of the plexiform lesion. Thorax 34:177–186, 1979. (6) Heath D, Smith P: Electron microscopy of hypertensive pulmonary vascular disease. Br J Dis Chest 77:1–13, 1983. (7) Rabinovitch M, Bothwell T, Hayakawa BN, et al: Pulmonary artery endothelial abnormalities in patients with congenital heart defects and pulmonary hypertension. Lab Invest 55:632–653, 1986. (8) Harris P, Heath D: The Human Pulmonary Circulation, 2nd ed. New York, Churchill Livingstone, 1977, p. 248. (9) Sobin SS, Tremer HM, Hardy JD, et al: Changes in arteriole in acute and chronic hypoxic pulmonary hypertension and recovery in rat. J Appl Physiol 55:1445–1455, 1983. (10) Heath D, Smith P, Gosney J: Ultrastructure of early plexogenic pulmonary arteriopathy. Histopathology 12:41–52, 1988.

dence for significant pulmonary endothelial cell denudation with congenital heart lesions,[118] increased pulmonary arterial pressure and flow are associated with changes in endothelial cell morphology and ultrastructure (Fig. 3).[137] Current interest focuses on the control of the smooth muscle phenotype, function, and growth,[11,161] endothelial cell modulation of vascular growth,[24] and the role of growth factors in promoting normal and pathologic vascular growth.[161] Regulation of connective tissue production by smooth muscle and other cells is another area of active investigation.[93,96,167,168]

Active Vasoconstriction. Some patients with increased pulmonary vascular resistance secondary to congenital heart disease,[23] pulmonary parenchymal disease,[92] or primary pulmonary hypertension[6,142] respond to pharmacologic vasodilators with a decrease in pulmonary vascular resistance, indicating the presence of active vasoconstriction. Many endogenous agents and stimuli are pulmonary vasoconstrictors, including neural stimulation,[83] catecholamines,[5] angiotensin II,[9] serotonin,[103] histamine,[113] prostaglandins and thromboxane A_2,[75,87] leukotrienes,[75,100] alveolar hypoxia,[176] and possibly mechanical stress or strain.[102] Except for patients with pulmonary parenchymal disease and alveolar hypoxia,[41] it has not been possible to establish a clear link between a given agent

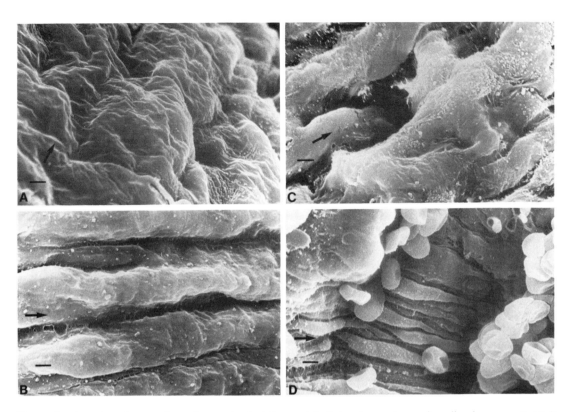

Figure 3. Scanning electron photomicrographs depicting endothelial surface patterns of small pulmonary arteries in patients with congenital heart defects. Pulmonary arteries with increased blood flow but normal pressure, which were normal or nearly normal on light microscopy, showed either a "crinkled" appearance when dilated (**A**), or narrow, corduroy-like ridges when constricted (**B**). With increased pulmonary pressure and flow, and severe medial hypertrophy and cellular intimal hyperplasia, endothelial surfaces were comprised of thick, deep, intertwined ridges with increased density of surface microvilli (**C**). With increased pressure and flow, and more severe histologic changes (Heath-Edwards grades 3 and 4), the endothelial surface showed high convoluted ridges which alternated with relatively flat areas; the endothelial cells were uneven in size and twisted (**D**). (From Rabinovitch M, et al: Pulmonary artery endothelial abnormalities in patients with congenital heart defects and pulmonary hypertension. Lab Invest 55:632–653, 1986, with permission.)

and clinically observed pulmonary hypertension. The relationship between vasoconstriction and structural changes in pulmonary vessels is also unclear. It is possible that active vasoconstriction, by increasing pulmonary arterial pressure, stimulates pathologic remodeling of the pulmonary circulation through mechanical stimulation of pulmonary vessels. Also, agents that contract smooth muscle may directly cause hyperplasia or hypertrophy of smooth muscle,[15,51] although these effects are incompletely characterized thus far.

PULMONARY HYPERTENSION IN THE CLINICAL SETTING

Pulmonary Hypertension with Congenital Cardiac Lesions

The development of increased pulmonary vascular resistance may complicate a variety of congenital heart lesions. Alterations in pulmonary arterial pressure and flow appear to be the chief, but not the only, stimuli for pulmonary vascular obstruction associated with congenital heart defects. Increased pressure appears to be a considerably more potent stimulus for pulmonary vascular obstruction than increased flow, as even considerably increased pulmonary flow usually does not result in pulmonary vascular obstruction, and even when it does the pathologic changes occur at a later age than those associated with increased pressure.

Hemodynamic Settings. *Increased Pulmonary Arterial Pressure.* Cardiac lesions associated with increased pulmonary venous pressure but normal or even decreased pulmonary flow (such as mitral stenosis, cor triatriatum, or obstructed pulmonary venous return) may cause increased pulmonary arteriolar resistance and pathologic pulmonary vascular changes.[27,67,129] Medial hypertrophy and intimal fibrosis are observed in both arteries and veins, although dilatation lesions are rarely, if ever, present.[67,180] Adult patients with mitral stenosis, and even severely increased pulmonary arteriolar resistance, usually show a large reduction in pulmonary arteriolar resistance (although not necessarily to normal levels) following relief of even long-standing left atrial hypertension.[29,193] Relatively little information is available for pediatric patients, although it appears that the same is true for infants and children.[27,66] This is unlike the situation observed with pulmonary hypertension secondary to left-to-right shunting lesions, where markedly increased pulmonary vascular resistance often fails to resolve after cardiac repair, especially in patients more than two years of age (see p. 89).

Increased Pulmonary Arterial Flow. Small increases in pulmonary flow without elevation in pressure (as occur with the small atrial septal defect, small ventricular septal defect, or small patent ductus arteriosus) pose little risk for the pulmonary circulation.[186] On the other hand, a large increase in pulmonary flow, even with initially normal pressure (e.g., with a large atrial septal defect), will cause pulmonary vascular obstruction in some patients (albeit a small minority). With most lesions that cause excessive flow, the pulmonary arterial oxygen saturation is also increased, but the latter is not the sole cause of pulmonary vascular obstruction with increased flow, as pathologic changes are often found in the normally perfused lung of patients with congenital unilateral absence of the opposite pulmonary artery.[135] The risk of developing pulmonary vascular obstruction with an atrial septal defect is small but significant (approximately 10%),[188] although structural changes usually (but not always)[192] occur considerably later (the third decade and beyond)[14] than they do with lesions causing increased flow *and* pressure. On the other hand, patients with D-transposition of the great vessels (and intact ventricular septum) usually have increased pulmonary blood flow with normal pulmonary arterial pressure after the early neonatal period,[4,90] but have a relatively high risk of developing pulmonary vascular obstruction in the first year of life.[26,104] The reason(s) for this propensity to develop early vascular changes is unclear.[80]

Increased Pulmonary Arterial Pressure and Flow. In cardiac lesions with a large communication between the systemic ventricle and the pulmonary circulation, there is increased pulmonary arterial pressure and flow (the latter as long as pulmonary vascular resistance is less than systemic resistance). Examples include, but are not limited to: large ventricular septal defects, large patent ductus arteriosus, double-outlet right ventricle or single ventricle without pulmonary stenosis, truncus arteriosus, and excessively large systemic-to-pulmonary shunts that may occur following surgery.

The risk of development, and rate of progression of vascular changes, appear to depend on pulmonary arterial pressure and flow, the type of heart lesion, the propensity of the individual to develop pulmonary vascular obstruction, and perhaps to other factors as well. The Joint Study on the Natural History of Congenital Heart Defects[186] found that patients with a ventricular septal defect who had pulmonary arterial pressure less than 50 mm Hg had only about a 2% risk of suffering an increase in pressure over the duration of the study (4–8 years), whereas about a third of the patients with greater pulmonary arterial pressure had an increase. While this does not suggest that anatomic vascular changes were lacking in patients with pressure less than 50 mm Hg, it does indicate that the rate of progression of vascular disease may be related in part to pulmonary pressure.

The type of heart lesion is important. For example, with isolated ventricular septal defect, pathologic vascular changes greater than Heath and Edwards Grade 1 are very infrequent in the first year of life,[72,178] whereas with D-transposition of the great vessels associated with ventricular septal defect or patent ductus arteriosus,[40,127] or truncus arteriosus,[85] more advanced vascular changes are common in infancy. Several factors may be responsible for the relatively rapid development and progression of pulmonary vascular obstruction with certain types of congenital heart lesions: increased hematocrit (and therefore blood viscosity), systemic cyanosis, formation of microthrombi in the pulmonary vessels, increased left atrial pressure, and bronchopulmonary collaterals may be significant.[80] The rapidity with which irreversible vascular changes develop importantly influences the timing of surgery, as discussed on p. 89.

Decreased Pulmonary Arterial Flow. Pulmonary or subpulmonary stenosis with right-to-left shunting (in the absence of large systemic-to-pulmonary collateral vessels) leads to deceased pulmonary pressure and flow. Histologic studies of small pulmonary arteries in tetralogy of Fallot differ. Although the number of small arteries appears to be increased,[77] the media has been found to be of normal, increased, or decreased thickness.[77,86,180] Mild, eccentric intimal proliferation and fibrosis, and organized and recanalized microvascular thrombi are also observed.[86,180] The extremely low incidence of pulmonary hypertension following repair of tetralogy of Fallot (save for those with large vessel abnormalities or surgically-created shunts)[94] suggests that regardless of histologic findings, subnormal flow *per se* does not generally prevent development of an adequate pulmonary microvascular bed.

Therapy. The ideal, and essentially the only, effective therapy for pulmonary vascular obstruction associated with congenital heart defects is actually prevention, meaning timely repair of the defect. In some situations in which complete repair is not feasible (e.g., an infant with single ventricle without pulmonary stenosis), pulmonary artery banding is usually effective in preventing significant pathologic vascular changes,[128,183] provided that pulmonary arterial pressure is sufficiently reduced. At the Children's Hospital in Boston, such banding operations are generally performed in the first month of life. In the case of infants with cyanosis from inadequate pulmonary blood flow, the choice of systemic-to-pulmonary arterial shunt is important, especially since many such patients will subsequently be considered for a Fontan repair. Systemic-to-pulmonary shunts of the Waterston and Potts variety often result in excessive pulmonary arterial pressure and, thus, pulmonary vascular obstruction. Blalock-Taussig and so-called modified Blalock-Taussig shunts are much less likely to cause excessive pulmonary arterial pressure and, therefore, are not frequently associated with pulmonary vascular obstruction.

What constitutes "timely" repair or palliation depends on the type of cardiac lesion and the hemodynamics of the individual patient. Because pulmonary vascular structural changes usually develop relatively late in uncomplicated atrial septal defect (either ostium primum or secundum), repair is often deferred until the child is four or five years of age. On the other hand, patients with isolated ventricular septal defect and significantly elevated pulmonary vascular resistance who are operated on after two years of age often do not have normal pulmonary arterial pressure postoperatively, and may even suffer an increase in pulmonary vascular resistance with time.[36,45,63] Because the risk of significant residual vascular disease following closure of a ventricular septal defect is small in patients operated on within the first two years of life,[36,164] repair is undertaken in most centers within that period. However, occasionally a patient will develop advanced vascular lesions before two years of age, and one report suggests that the likelihood of normal pulmonary arterial pressure following repair may be somewhat greater in patients operated on within the first nine months of life than in those undergoing surgery between 9 and 24 months of age.[141] As a result, at The Boston Children's Hospital and in some other centers, the current practice is not to delay operation beyond the first year of life for large ventricular septal defect or complete atrioventricular canal.[70,191] In patients with evidence of increased pulmonary vascular resistance (e.g., complete atrioventricular canal defect without evidence of heart failure in the first few months), catheterization and operation are undertaken even earlier. Because advanced vascular lesions may appear in the first six months in patients with D-transposition of the great vessels and ventricular septal defect or patent ductus arteriosus, at The Boston Children's Hospital, operation for this lesion is generally undertaken within the first three months of life. Similarly, other lesions prone to the early development of pulmonary vascular obstruction, such as truncus arteriosus or large ventricular septal defect with coarctation, are generally operated on within the first three to six months of life.

Repair of Congenital Heart Defects with High Pulmonary Vascular Resistance. Few patients less than one year of age have severely elevated pulmonary vascular resistance ($R_p:R_s > .75$). Generally, given the remarkable capacity of the young pulmonary vascular bed to normalize following relief of hypertension,[36,141] such infants are offered surgical repair when technically feasible, as long as pulmonary vascular resistance is not suprasystemic. On the other hand, repair of malformations in older patients with severely elevated pulmonary vascular resistance carries a considerable surgical mortality, and, in patients operated on after two years of age, a high risk of a progressive increase in pulmonary vascular resistance despite repair.[25,36,45] Because a progressive rise in pulmonary vascular resistance may actually be better tolerated with an intracardiac communication (to allow for decompression of the right ventricle), surgical repair in such patients may actually shorten their life span.[79] In an effort to separate those who will suffer increased pulmonary vascular resistance following repair from those whose pulmonary vascular resistance may remain stable or fall following closure, vasodilators (100% oxygen, tolazoline, isoproterenol, and other agents) have been employed preoperatively. The notion is that patients with "reactive" pulmonary vascular beds (i.e., those who decrease their pulmonary vascular resistance with vasodilators) are more likely to respond favorably to surgical closure than are those with a "fixed" elevation in pulmonary vascular resistance.[19] Although data from patients studied at high altitude (5000 feet) indicate that response to tolazoline may be a reasonable predictor of postoperative outcome with ventricular septal defect,[177] there are few data to suggest that studies conducted at sea level, using either pharmacologic agents or 100% inspired oxygen, are useful.[111]

Lung biopsy (usually as an adjunct to hemodynamic data) has also been advocated as a means of determining suitability for surgical repair.[138] Indeed, it has been shown that a preoperative biopsy (analyzed by Heath and Edwards and morphometric criteria) may be predictive of persistent pulmonary hypertension in patients older than two years of age following repair of interventricular communications.[141] However, there is relatively little published follow-up data correlating preoperative biopsy and hemodynamic findings with eventual outcome, and it is not clear whether biopsy can separate patients who will have persistent but tolerable levels of residual pulmonary hypertension from those who will have a progressive rise in pulmonary vascular resistance. In addition, there is considerable overlap among patients with severe pathologic vascular changes who do well following repair and those who suffer severe postoperative hypertension, making biopsy of dubious utility in deciding suitability for operation.[50,70]

Eisenmenger Syndrome. As used by Paul Wood and most authors subsequently, this term refers to patients with congenital heart defects who have a systemic level of pulmonary arterial pressure and high pulmonary vascular resistance (> 800 dsc⁻⁵), with right-to-left or bidirectional shunting.[187] At least for older patients who reside at sea level,[19] it implies that the heart lesion is inoperable, although, as was noted above, young patients (in the first year or two of life) with subsystemic pulmonary vascular resistance may still be candidates for repair. In fact, the fully developed clinical picture (including cyanosis, clubbing, and polycythemia) is seldom seen before the second decade of life, although the onset of cyanosis often occurs in the first few years.[187,192] Patients with the Eisenmenger syndrome may suffer dyspnea, syncope, congestive heart failure, hemoptysis, bacterial endocarditis, or sudden death, as well as complications of cyanosis, such as stroke and cerebral abscess.[187] The duration of survival varies considerably, with some patients succumbing in early childhood, while most remain stable for many years and live into the fourth decade.[187,192] Conventional therapy is nonspecific: anticongestive therapy for congestive heart failure, red cell pheresis to reduce the hematocrit when indicated, and vigorous treatment of pulmonary and other infections. Heart-lung transplantation has been undertaken in relatively few of these patients,[145] but with good short-term results.

"Primary" Pulmonary Hypertension

Pulmonary hypertension not associated with congenital heart malformations, pulmonary parenchymal disease, left atrial hypertension, hypoventilation, or other known causes of pulmonary hypertension, are encountered rarely in adults,[47,68,148] and even less frequently in infants and children.[172] Which patients should be included in this category is not entirely clear. Newborns with increased pulmonary vascular resistance and right-to-left shunting are usually considered to have "persistent pulmonary hypertension of the newborn,"[35,107,163] whereas older infants and children are said to have "primary" or "unexplained" pulmonary hypertension.[46] There is overlap between these two groups, as evidenced by reports of patients who, as newborns, had symptoms suggestive of pulmonary hypertension and who developed increased evidence of pulmonary hypertension over the ensuing several weeks.[22,106,173] Some children with primary pulmonary hypertension have persistence of the fetal pattern of elastic lamellae in the main pulmonary artery, suggesting the presence of elevated pulmonary pressure since birth.[172,181] The vascular structural abnormalities

observed in primary pulmonary hypertension of the newborn (medial hypertrophy and distal extension of smooth muscle) are similar to those observed in children with primary pulmonary hypertension.[48,181] However, increased pulmonary vascular resistance in the first few days of life is distinguished from that in the older patient by its short course (culminating in either resolution or death within a few days),[106] and the frequent association of neonatal pulmonary hypertension with perinatal stress.[35] This section deals specifically with patients who are first seen by the physician after the first month of life. Primary pulmonary hypertension of the newborn is discussed on p. 93.

Pathologic Findings. If one excludes recurrent thromboembolic and pulmonary veno-occlusive disease (both are rare in infants and children;[181] see discussion below), histologic findings in primary pulmonary hypertension are identical to those of congenital cardiac malformations with systemic-to-pulmonary communications.[68] To some extent, the pathologic changes may be age-related. The Wagenvoorts[181] found that patients less than one year of age who died with primary pulmonary hypertension had considerable medial hypertrophy but few intimal changes; intimal fibrosis was significant only after children reached one to six years of age, and was even more marked from 6–12 years of age. On the other hand, Thilenius and coworkers reported severe intimal fibrosis and/or necrotizing arteritis in patients as young as eight months of age.[172]

Clinical Manifestations. Primary pulmonary hypertension is not consistently associated with other diseases, although it is occasionally familial.[82,148,172] A positive antinuclear antibody test or Raynaud's phenomenon, suggesting an underlying collagen-vascular cause, is found in a significant number of patients, largely adults.[148,184] **Symptoms** include dyspnea, easy fatigue, syncope (sometimes described as seizures), chest pain, dry cough, and vomiting.[148,172]

Physical examination may reveal slight cyanosis. Often there is a right ventricular heave and, sometimes, a palpable second heart sound. The second heart sound is single or narrowly split and the pulmonic component is accentuated. Many patients have a soft systolic ejection murmur along the upper left sternal border. An early high-frequency diastolic murmur at the upper left sternal border, due to pulmonic regurgitation, is often present. Patients may show signs of right ventricular failure, such as an increased jugular "a" wave (although this is often difficult to appreciate in young patients), hepatomegaly, or ascites.

The **electrocardiogram** typically shows right-axis deviation and right ventricular hypertrophy. Depressed S-T segments and T waves, suggesting "strain," may also be present in the anterior, and even lateral, chest leads.

The **chest x-ray** may show cardiac enlargement, a prominent main pulmonary artery segment, and the appearance of decreased vasculature in the peripheral lung fields (Fig. 4). **Echocardiography** shows evidence of right ventricular hypertension (see ch. 13) and is particularly useful in excluding other anatomic lesions that may cause pulmonary hypertension (mitral stenosis, cor triatriatum, pulmonary vein stenosis).

Cardiac Catheterization. Cardiac catheterization reveals elevated pulmonary arterial pressure but normal pulmonary capillary wedge or left atrial pressures. Right atrial pressure is frequently elevated. There may be mild systemic arterial desaturation secondary to intra-atrial or intrapulmonary shunting.[91,148] Cardiac output is normal or decreased. Contrast injection into the main pulmonary artery carries the risk of decompensation in these patients,[91] but the author and others have found selective injection into the left and right pulmonary arteries to be of low risk.[148] At The Boston Children's Hospital the current practice is to perform bilateral pulmonary wedge angiograms, as they yield data regarding pulmonary vascular structure,[140] are helpful in identifying the presence of macroscopic peripheral pulmonary emboli, and, on levophase, nicely outline the pulmonary veins.

Natural History. Walcott and colleagues reported 23 cases of primary pulmonary hypertension in adults. All but two of their patients were more

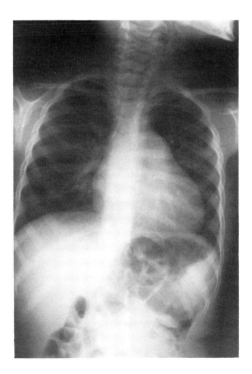

Figure 4. Chest x-ray of a three-year-old girl with primary pulmonary hypertension. Note the very prominent main pulmonary segment.

than 15 years of age: seven survived less than two years from the onset of symptoms, 13 survived less than three years, and only three lived for more than 10 years.[184] Fuster and associates[47] reported that only about 40% of their patients (mostly adults) with primary pulmonary hypertension were alive three years after diagnosis. The natural history appears to be even more unfavorable in young children, as approximately 75% die within one year after the onset of symptoms (Fig. 5).[172]

Therapy. There is no consistently efficacious therapy for primary pulmonary hypertension. The medications currently most favored for treatment include hydralazine, diazoxide, nifedipine, and diltiazem,[60,142,146] although alpha-adrenergic blocking agents are employed occasionally.[6] Unfortunately, all of these drugs relax systemic as well as pulmonary vascular smooth muscle, and in many patients have little effect on the pulmonary circulation. As a consequence, therapy for primary pulmonary hypertension has been only inconsistently effective, with only about a third of adults deriving benefit from chronic vasodilators.[60,142] Children may be more likely to show a favorable response to therapy: Barst found that five of nine patients, ages 9 months to 23 years, showed a significant decrease in pulmonary arterial pressure with nifedipine (n = 4), or phenoxybenzamine (n = 1), and younger patients were more likely to respond than older ones (Fig. 6).[6] Because the medications employed are inconsistently efficacious and have potentially serious side effects, such as systemic hypotension and depression of ventricular function,[133] and because relatively high doses may be required,[60,146] therapy should be initiated and followed in conjunction with cardiac catheterization for measuring pulmonary, systemic, right atrial, and pulmonary capillary wedge pressures and cardiac output.[60,142]

Though still an investigational drug, and available only in intravenous form, prostaglandin I_2 (prostacyclin) has been employed in a few centers, primarily as a means of assessing the reactivity of the pulmonary vascular bed.[60,142] Experience suggests that this agent may be used to ascertain the likelihood that the lung will favorably respond to orally active vasodilators, as patients whose pulmonary vascular resistance does not decrease with prostacyclin are not likely to experience a decrease with other drugs.[6,142] Long-term (months) infusion of prostacyclin has also been employed in symptomatic adults who are awaiting heart-lung transplantation.[76,145]

Thrombi are often found in small pulmonary vessels in adults with primary pulmonary hypertension[47,181] and one retrospective study found that patients with primary pulmonary hypertension treated with oral anticoagulants of the warfarin class lived somewhat longer than those not treated.[47] These observations have led some to ad-

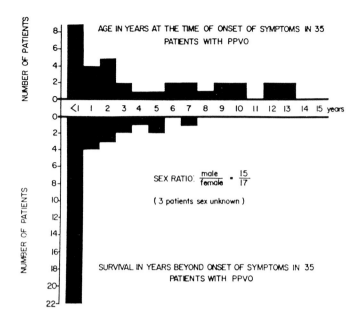

Figure 5. Age at the time of onset of symptoms, and survival beyond that point, for 35 children with primary pulmonary hypertension. Seventy-five percent of all children survived less than one year after the onset of symptoms. (Reproduced by permission of Pediatrics 36:75–87, 1965.[172])

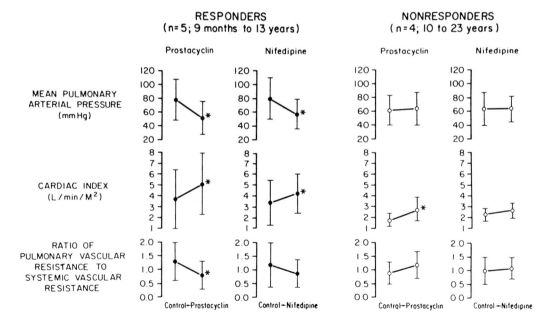

Figure 6. Nine patients with primary pulmonary hypertension underwent acute testing with prostacyclin (9–38 ng/kg/min) and nifedipine (0.5–2.0 mg/kg). Those who responded to prostacyclin had a 20% or greater decrease in mean pulmonary arterial pressure, a rise in cardiac index, and no change or a decrease in the pulmonary-to-systemic vascular resistance ratio. Patients who responded to prostacyclin also showed similar hemodynamic improvement with nifedipine. Those who responded (mean age, five years) were considerably younger than those who did not (mean age, 17.3 years). (From Barst RJ: Pharmacologically induced pulmonary vasodilation in children and young adults with primary pulmonary hypertension. Chest 89:497–503, 1986, with permission.)

vocate the use of anticoagulants,[47,149] but it is unclear whether the benefits outweigh the risks of such therapy.

Atrial septostomy, using a Park blade septostomy catheter, has been used to increase systemic blood flow (by allowing for a right-to-left atrial shunt) in patients with refractory right ventricular failure[130] or multiple syncopal episodes.[101] Although this procedure has provided relief of symptoms over the short term in some patients,[101,130] it is not without potential hazard.[147]

Persistent Pulmonary Hypertension of the Newborn

The term "persistence of the fetal circulation" was first used to describe two newborn infants without roentgenographic lung disease who had cyanosis secondary to right-to-left atrial and ductal shunting.[53] It referred to the persistently elevated pulmonary vascular resistance that normally falls precipitously at birth. Subsequently, other terms have been applied to this condition (perhaps the most descriptive being "primary pulmonary hypertension of the newborn"). Pulmonary hypertension with right-to-left shunting across the ductus arteriosus and/or foramen ovale has been observed in multiple settings: with meconium aspiration, pneumonia,[170] primary pulmonary hypoplasia,[171] congenital diaphragmatic hernia,[17] ventricular dysfunction,[21,151] cerebral arteriovenous malformation,[28] various metabolic abnormalities,[52] and after perinatal asphyxia.[35]

Pathophysiology. Although catheter studies have shown that babies with characteristics of primary pulmonary hypertension of the newborn usually have pulmonary arterial pressure at or above systemic pressure,[34,35,107,134,163] in some infants increased pulmonary vascular resistance is not the major cause of cyanosis. Riemenschneider and coworkers[151] described infants with cyanosis, heart failure, and normal newborn pulmonary arterial pressure, but systemic hypotension; when systemic pressure was increased using epinephrine, right-to-left ductal shunting was decreased or abolished. Right ventricular myocardial dysfunction with tricuspid insufficiency may also cause right-to-left atrial shunting, with normal pulmonary arterial pressure.[21] Decreased right ventricular compliance not associated with pulmonary hypertension may also result in a right-to-left intracardiac shunt. Twenty neonates with the diagnosis of primary pulmonary hypertension of the newborn (descending aortic $pO_2 < 60$ torr, with $FiO_2 = 1.0$ and $pCO_2 < 30$ torr, plus right-to-left shunting at the ductal and/or atrial level by echocardiography) were catheterized at The Children's Hospital in Boston.[44] At catheterization, five of the babies had pulmonary arterial systolic pressure less than 0.8 of the systemic, with three having right-to-left

shunting at the atrial level only. Although the pulmonary arterial pressure may have been higher at an earlier time in these five babies, it does appear that in a minority of infants with primary pulmonary hypertension of the newborn atrial shunting is due to decreased right ventricular compliance, with elevated pulmonary vascular resistance not being a major factor. It is important to distinguish, if possible, between cyanotic patients who have pulmonary hypertension and those who do not, as therapy for pulmonary hypertension carries the risk of serious complications (see p. 94).

The mechanism(s) responsible for the increased pulmonary vascular resistance is not known. Babies who have died within the first few days of life from primary pulmonary hypertension of the newborn typically have a normal number of small pulmonary arteries and veins, but have medial hypertrophy and distal extension of smooth muscle. Focal areas of microvascular thrombi and proliferation of the adventitia are also observed. Because these abnormalities are observed within the first 24 postnatal hours, it is suggestive that the original stimulus for increased pulmonary vascular resistance must have happened *in utero*.[48] Hypoxia, especially in combination with acidosis, is a powerful pulmonary vasoconstrictor in the fetus and newborn,[155] and the immature lung may respond to hypoxia with vasoconstriction that persists even after the hypoxic stimulus is removed.[1] These observations, and the fact that perinatal asphyxia is often associated with primary pulmonary hypertension of the newborn,[35] suggest that hypoxia may be an important stimulus for increased pulmonary vascular resistance in the newborn. Underdevelopment of the pulmonary vasculature (e.g., with congenital diaphragmatic hernia and other structural abnormalities[48]), is probably significant in some patients, although even in such babies there is a large component of active vasoconstriction as well.[38,170] Bacterial and other toxins[54,64] and endogenously elaborated vasoconstrictors may also be important,[65] although as yet they are uncharacterized.

Clinical Manifestations. The history, physical findings, and laboratory data consistent with primary pulmonary hypertension of the newborn have been well summarized.[43] Briefly, these newborns are seen because of respiratory distress and cyanosis. Although differential cyanosis may be present (because of right-to-left ductal shunting), right-to-left atrial shunting may result in desaturation of the ascending aorta, and there may be no difference between right radial arterial and descending aortic oxygen saturations. Often, cyanotic congenital heart disease can be ruled out on the basis of physical findings, the chest x-ray, the presence of differential cyanosis, and the response of arterial pO_2 to hyperoxia and hyperventilation,[43] but in some cases echocardiography is necessary. Besides ruling out structural heart disease, echocardiography may be useful in demonstrating ventricular function and the presence and level of intracardiac shunting.

Therapy. Mechanical hyperventilation, to achieve hypocarbia and alkalosis, appears to be the most consistently efficacious therapy. Alkalosis is a pulmonary vasodilator,[160] and respiratory alkalosis has been demonstrated to decrease the pulmonary-to-systemic pressure ratio and to increase descending aortic oxygen tension in babies with primary pulmonary hypertension of the newborn.[34] In fact, the salutary effect of hyperventilation has led to its widespread use,[43] although not all investigators agree on the need for, or desirability of, using this therapy in primary pulmonary hypertension of the newborn.[190] Certainly, the high mean airway pressures used to achieve hypocarbia (as well as the high FiO_2 usually employed) can lead to pulmonary parenchymal damage, necessitating careful evaluation of the need for hyperventilation.[43] High levels of inspired oxygen are virtually always used, and are often necessary to maintain adequate arterial oxygen saturation.[43]

Pharmacologic therapy for primary pulmonary hypertension of the newborn has been hindered by the lack of a selective pulmonary dilator. Numerous drugs have been employed in an attempt to decrease pulmonary vascular resistance in this setting, without consistent success.[33,89,99,166] Tolazoline (Priscolene) is the most often used, but it is inconsistently effective in increasing arterial oxygen saturation.[43,99] Ionotropic support, using dopamine and other agents,[32] often appears useful, especially because these infants often have low cardiac output and/or systemic hypotension.[44]

The extracorporeal membrane oxygenator has been used to provide adequate oxygenation and augmentation of cardiac output in patients who fail conventional therapy.[7] Although this therapy is relatively labor-intensive and requires the services of specially trained personnel, the results (as yet, short-term) from many centers are good, and use of this mode of therapy has grown considerably over the last five years.[114]

Pulmonary Hypertension Associated with Alveolar Hypoxemia

Pulmonary hypertension may result from disorders of pulmonary structure or function whose primary effect is to cause alveolar hypoxemia. The pulmonary hypertension resulting from these disorders leads to cor pulmonale (right ventricular enlargement from disorders which affect the structure or function of the lung).[41] Cystic fibrosis,[125] bronchopulmonary dysplasia,[12,132] and upper airway obstruction[109] are the most frequent of these disorders encountered in pediatrics, although there are others, including parenchymal lung disease, chest wall deformity, hypoventilation mediated through the central nervous system, and disorders caused by residence at high altitude.[123]

Because, in this setting, pulmonary hypertension is often reversible with the administration of oxygen or relief of hypoventilation, it can be concluded that alveolar hypoxia is the primary cause of elevated pulmonary vascular resistance.[41] On the other hand, not all patients with pulmonary disease or hypoventilation show a decrease in pulmonary vascular resistance with inspired oxygen sufficient to fully saturate arterial blood,[13,55,56] suggesting that other factors may also act to increase pulmonary vascular resistance. In patients with parenchymal lung disease, the pulmonary vascular bed may be reduced in cross-sectional area because of a decreased number of pulmonary vessels[157] or medial hypertrophy and intimal fibrosis.[174] Increased blood viscosity, secondary to increased hematocrit, may also contribute to elevated pulmonary hypertension.[79]

Clinical Manifestations. Patients with pulmonary hypertension secondary to alveolar hypoxia may have physical and laboratory findings similar to those described for primary pulmonary hypertension (see p. 90). Echocardiography is often useful in excluding cardiac malformations that may cause pulmonary hypertension, in estimating right ventricular pressure, and in evaluating left ventricular function, which may be diminished in some patients with cor pulmonale.[8] Radionuclide angiography is useful in determining the right and left ventricular ejection fractions. Patients with frank right ventricular failure may exhibit the usual signs and symptoms associated with right ventricular decompensation. Signs, symptoms, and laboratory evidence of pulmonary arterial hypertension and right ventricular failure may be lacking, or difficult to differentiate from pulmonary disease, in patients with cystic fibrosis or hyperinflated lungs secondary to other diseases.[41,169] In such patients, fluid retention, with increasing hepatomegaly and peripheral edema, may be a better indicator of right ventricular decompensation than are auscultatory findings, heart size, or the electrocardiogram.

Therapy. Relief or diminution of alveolar hypoxemia is clearly the most effective therapy, when possible. Diuresis reduces symptoms, and digitalis is often employed, although its efficacy in right ventricular failure is a matter of dispute, and patients with pulmonary disease appear to be more susceptible than others to digitalis toxicity.[59,115]

Vasodilators such as nifedipine and hydralazine have been employed in patients with bronchopulmonary dysplasia[16,20,56] and cystic fibrosis,[49,119] and in adults with chronic obstructive lung disease.[92,153] The short-term results of such vasodilator therapy have been mixed; it appears that only some patients respond to such vasodilator therapy with a reduction in pulmonary arterial pressure and pulmonary vascular resistance, and an increase in cardiac output.[49,56,119,153] There is little information regarding the long-term effects of vasodilator therapy in these patients, and the effect on patient survival is unknown.[133] As with the use of vasodilators for primary pulmonary hypertension, initiation and follow-up of vasodilator therapy should be carried out in conjunction with careful monitoring of the relevant hemodynamic variables.

Other Causes of Pulmonary Hypertension

Chronic Thromboembolism. Chronic, recurrent pulmonary thromboemboli are rare in children[189] but can occur secondary to ventriculoatrial shunts (for hydrocephalus) and other indwelling vascular catheters[117,189] or to deep venous thrombosis.[149,150] Chronic pulmonary hypertension can result from restriction of the pulmonary vascular bed. It is usually impossible to differentiate pulmonary hypertension secondary to recurrent thromboemboli from primary pulmonary hypertension on clinical grounds, but radionuclide ventilation-perfusion lung scans have been found to be a sensitive and specific way of demonstrating chronic thromboembolic disease.[30,149] Surgical thrombectomy, anticoagulants, caval plication, and intravascular filters have been employed as therapy.[149]

Pulmonary Veno-occlusive Disease. This is a rare, apparently usually acquired, disease that primarily affects children and young adults. Its clinical presentation is usually similar to that of primary pulmonary hypertension but, unlike the latter, the chest x-ray usually shows pulmonary edema. The hemodynamic findings are similar to those of primary pulmonary hypertension, and the pulmonary capillary wedge pressure is usually normal or only modestly elevated. Histologic examination of the lungs shows obliteration of veins and venules by fibrous tissue and thrombosis. Nodal areas of edema, hemorrhage, interstitial inflammation, and fibrosis are also seen.[179] There is no known therapy for this disorder, other than heart-lung transplantation, and that is associated with a poor prognosis.

Collagen Vascular Disease. Pulmonary hypertension frequently occurs in association with systemic sclerosis and the CREST syndrome variant.[136,158,159] The hypertension can be severe, and may result in death.[159] Although some degree of restrictive lung disease is often present in these patients, the severity of parenchymal disease is poorly correlated with the severity of pulmonary hypertension,[158] suggesting that the former is not the primary cause of the latter. Intimal proliferation and, to a lesser extent, medial hypertrophy of small and medium-sized pulmonary arteries are observed.[159] Pulmonary hypertension has also been reported, although much less frequently, with rheumatoid arthritis,[84] systemic lupus erythematosus,[3,126] and mixed connective tissue disease.[81]

Drugs. *Aminorex.* Ingestion of the appetite suppressant, aminorex,[61] has been associated with pulmonary hypertension in adults.

Cyclooxygenase Inhibitors. These constrict the ductus arteriosus and cause medial hypertrophy of pulmonary arterioles in the fetal lamb, suggesting that ingestion of such drugs during pregnancy might result in pulmonary hypertension in the newborn.[108] A study of 14 *human* fetuses of 26.5 to 31 weeks' gestation showed that half of them developed echocardiographic findings consistent with ductal constriction after maternal indomethacin treatment.[122] There are also several reports of babies with primary pulmonary hypertension of the newborn whose mothers had ingested salicylates, indomethacin, or naproxen during pregnancy.[175] On the other hand, a large experience with cyclooxygenase inhibitors used as tocolytics suggests that such therapy is *not* causally linked with pulmonary hypertension in the newborn,[75] leaving the question of the possible link between cyclooxygenase inhibitors and pulmonary hypertension in the newborn unresolved.

Oral Contraceptives. There are anecdotal reports of oral contraceptives being associated with rapid progression of pulmonary hypertension in patients with cardiac shunting lesions[131] and in women without an obvious predisposing cause for pulmonary vascular disease.[95] There has been no evidence of thromboemboli to account for the pulmonary hypertension in these patients, suggesting that oral contraceptives may act to cause intimal and medial changes in pulmonary vessels.[95] However, there are relatively few reported cases of pulmonary hypertension with these drugs, especially given their widespread use. Large retrospective[47] and prospective[148] studies of patients with primary pulmonary hypertension have failed to demonstrate a relationship between use of oral contraceptives and primary pulmonary hypertension. Whether oral contraceptives are causally linked with pulmonary vascular obstruction is, therefore, unclear.

Additional Causes of Pulmonary Hypertension. Sickle cell anemia,[124] portal hypertension,[37,110] sarcoidosis,[121] carcinoma,[2,88] several forms of systemic arteritis,[105] and parasites[182] can also cause pulmonary hypertension.

REFERENCES

1. Abman SH, Accurso FJ, Wilkening RB, et al: Persistent fetal pulmonary hypertension after acute hypoxia. Am J Physiol 253:H941–H948, 1987.
2. Altemus LR, Lee RE: Carcinomatosis of the lung with pulmonary hypertension. Arch Intern Med 119:32–38, 1967.
3. Aszkenasy OM, Clarke TJ, Hickling P, et al: Systemic lupus erythematosus, pulmonary hypertension, and left recurrent laryngeal nerve palsy. Ann Rheum Dis 46:246–247, 1987.

4. Aziz KU, Paul MH, Rowe RD: Bronchopulmonary circulation in d-transposition of the great arteries: possible role in genesis of accelerated pulmonary vascular disease. Am J Cardiol 39:432–438, 1977.

5. Barer GR: The physiology of the pulmonary circulation and methods of study. Pharmacol Ther 2:247–273, 1976.

6. Barst RJ: Pharmacologically induced pulmonary vasodilation in children and young adults with primary pulmonary hypertension. Chest 89:497–503, 1986.

7. Bartlett RH, Roloff DW, Cirnell RG, et al: Extracorporeal circulation in neonatal respiratory failure: a prospective randomized study. Pediatrics 76:479–487, 1985.

8. Baum GL, Schwartz A, Llamas R, et al: Left ventricular function in chronic obstructive lung disease. N Engl J Med 285:361–365, 1971.

9. Baum MD, Kot PA: Response of pulmonary vascular segments to angiotensin and norepinephrine. J Thorac Cardiovasc Surg 63:322–328, 1972.

10. Bayliss LE: The rheology of blood. In Hamilton WF (ed): The Handbook of Physiology, Section 2. Circulation. Washington, D.C., American Physiological Society, 1962, Vol. 1, pp. 137–150.

11. Benitz WE, Lessler DS, Coulson JD, et al: Heparin inhibits proliferation of fetal vascular smooth muscle cells in the absence of platelet-derived growth factor. J Cell Physiol 127:1–7, 1986.

12. Berman W, Katz R, Yabek SM, et al: Long-term follow-up of bronchopulmonary dysplasia. J Pediatr 109:45–50, 1986.

13. Berman W, Yabek SM, Dillon T, et al: Evaluation of infants with bronchopulmonary dysplasia using cardiac catheterization. Pediatrics 70:708–712, 1982.

14. Besterman E: Atrial septal defect with pulmonary hypertension. Br Heart J 23:587–598, 1961.

15. Blaes N, Boissel J-P: Growth-stimulating effect of catecholamines on rat aortic smooth muscle cells in culture. J Cell Physiol 116:167–172, 1983.

16. Blanchard DW, Brown TM, Coates AL: Pharmacotherapy in bronchopulmonary dysplasia. Clin Perinatol 14:881–910, 1987.

17. Bloss RS, Turmen T, Beardmore HE, et al: Tolazoline therapy for persistent pulmonary hypertension after congenital diaphragmatic hernia repair. J Pediatr 97:984–988, 1980.

18. Boyden EA: Development and growth of the airways. In Hodson WA (ed): Lung Biology in Health and Disease. New York, Marcel Dekker, 1977, Vol. 6, pp. 3–35.

19. Brammell HL, Vogel JHK, Pryor R, et al: The Eisenmenger syndrome. Am J Cardiol 28:679–692, 1971.

20. Brownlee JR, Beekman RH, Rosenthal A: Acute hemodynamic effects of nifedipine in infants with bronchopulmonary dysplasia and pulmonary hypertension. Pediatr Res 24:186–190, 1988.

21. Bucciarelli RL, Nelson RM, Egan EA, et al: Transient tricuspid insufficiency of the newborn: a form of myocardial dysfunction in stressed newborns. Pediatrics 59:330–337, 1977.

22. Burnell RH, Joseph MC, Lees MH: Progressive pulmonary hypertension in newborn infants. Am J Dis Child 123:167–170, 1972.

23. Bush A, Busst C, Booth K, et al: Does prostacyclin enhance the selective vasodilator effect of oxygen in children with congenital heart disease? Circulation 74:135–144, 1986.

24. Campbell JH, Campbell GR: Endothelial cell influences on vascular smooth muscle phenotype. Ann Rev Physiol 48:295–306, 1986.

25. Cartmill TB, DuShane JW, McGoon DC, et al: Results of repair of ventricular septal defect. J Thorac Cardiovasc Surg 52:486–501, 1966.

26. Clarkson PM, Neutze JM, Wardill JC, et al: The pulmonary vascular bed in patients with complete transposition of the great arteries. Circulation 53:539–543, 1976.

27. Collins-Nakai RL, Rosenthal A, Castaneda AR, et al: Congenital mitral stenosis: a review of 20 years' experience. Circulation 56:1039–1047, 1977.

28. Cumming GR: Circulation in infants with intracranial arteriovenous fistula and cardiac failure. Am J Cardiol 45:1019–1024, 1980.

29. Dalen JE, Matloff JM, Evans GL, et al: Early reduction of pulmonary vascular resistance after mitral-valve replacement. N Engl J Med 277:387–394, 1967.

30. D'Alonzo G, Bower J, Dantzker DR: Differentiation of patients with primary and thromboembolic pulmonary hypertension. Chest 85:457–461, 1984.

31. Deffebach ME, Charan NB, Lakshminarayan S, et al: The bronchial circulation. Am Rev Respir Dis 135:463–481, 1987.

32. Drummond WH: Use of cardiotonic therapy in the management of infants with PPHN. Clin Perinatol 11:715–728, 1984.

33. Drummond WH, Lock JE: Neonatal "pulmonary vasodilator" drugs. Dev Pharmacol Ther 7:1–20, 1984.

34. Drummond WH, Gregory GA, Heymann MA, et al: The independent effects of hyperventilation, tolazoline, and dopamine on infants with persistent pulmonary hypertension. J Pediatr 98:603–611, 1981.

35. Drummond WH, Peckham GJ, Fox WW: The clinical profile of the newborn with persistent pulmonary hypertension. Clin Pediatr 16:335–341, 1977.

36. DuShane JW, Krongrad E, Ritter DG, et al: The fate of raised pulmonary vascular resistance after surgery in ventricular septal defect. In Rowe RD, Kidd BSL (eds): The Child with Congenital Heart Disease After Surgery. Mount Kisco, NY, Futura Publishing Co., 1976, pp. 299–312.

37. Edwards BS, Weir EK, Edwards WD, et al: Coexistent pulmonary and portal hypertension: morphologic and clinical features. J Am Coll Cardiol 10:1233–1238, 1987.

38. Ein SH, Barker G, Shandling B, et al: The pharmacologic treatment of newborn diaphragmatic hernia—a 2 year evaluation. J Pediatr Surg 15:384–394, 1980.

39. Emmanouilides GC, Moss AJ, Duffie ER, et al: Pulmonary arterial pressure changes in human newborn infants from birth to 3 days of age. J Pediatr 65:327–333, 1964.

40. Ferencz C: Transposition of the great arteries. Circulation 33:232–241, 1966.

41. Fishman AP: Chronic cor pulmonale. Am Rev Respir Dis 114:775–794, 1976.

42. Fishman AP: Pulmonary circulation. In Geiger SR (ed): Handbook of Physiology, Section 3, The Respiratory System, Vol. I: Circulation and Nonrespiratory Functions. Bethesda, American Physiological Society, 1985, pp. 93–165.

43. Fox WW, Duara S: Persistent pulmonary hypertension in the neonate: diagnosis and management. J Pediatr 103:505–514, 1983.

44. Freed MD, Murphy J, Epstein M, et al: Cardiac catheterization in severely hypoxemic neonates without structural heart disease. In press.

45. Friedli B, Kidd BSL, Mustard WT, et al: Ventricular septal defect with increased pulmonary vascular resistance. Am J Cardiol 33:403–409, 1974.

46. Friedman WF: Proceedings of National Heart, Lung,

and Blood Institute Pediatric Cardiology Workshop: pulmonary hypertension. Pediatr Res 20:811–824, 1986.

47. Fuster V, Steel PM, Edwards WD, et al: Primary pulmonary hypertension: natural history and the importance of thrombosis. Circulation 70:580–587, 1984.

48. Geggel RL, Reid LM: The structural basis of persistent pulmonary hypertension of newborn. Clin Perinatol 2:525–549, 1984.

49. Geggel RL, Dozor AJ, Fyler DC, et al: Effect of vasodilators at rest and during exercise in young adults with cystic fibrosis and chronic cor pulmonale. Am Rev Respir Dis 131:531–536, 1985.

50. Geggel RL, Fried R, Helgason G, et al: Role of lung biopsy in patients undergoing a modified Fontan procedure (abstract). Circulation 76:IV–554, 1987.

51. Geisterfer AAT, Peach MJ, Owens GK: Angiotensin II induces hypertrophy, not hyperplasia, of cultured rat aortic smooth muscle cells. Circ Res 62:749–756, 1988.

52. Gersony WM: Persistence of the fetal circulation: a commentary. J Pediatr 82:1103–1106, 1973.

53. Gersony WM, Due GV, Sinclair JC: "PFC" syndrome (persistence of the fetal circulation) (abstract). Circulation 40(Suppl III):11, 1969.

54. Gibson RL, Truog RE, Redding GJ: Hypoxic pulmonary vasoconstriction during and after infusion of group B streptococcus in neonatal piglets: vascular pressure-flow analysis. Am Rev Respir Dis 137:774–778, 1988.

55. Goldring RM, Fishman AP, Turino GM, et al: Pulmonary hypertension and cor pulmonale in cystic fibrosis of the pancreas. J Pediatr 65:501–524, 1964.

56. Goodman G, Perkin RM, Anas NG, et al: Pulmonary hypertension in infants with bronchopulmonary dysplasia. J Pediatr 112:67–72, 1988.

57. Gordon D, Schwartz SM: Replication of arterial smooth muscle cells in hypertension and atherosclerosis. Am J Cardiol 59:44A–48A, 1987.

58. Gordon JB, Tod ML, Wetzel RC, et al: Age-dependent effects of indomethacin on hypoxic vasoconstriction in neonatal lamb lungs. Pediatr Res 23:580–584, 1988.

59. Green LH, Smith TW: The use of digitalis in patients with pulmonary disease. Ann Intern Med 87:459–465, 1977.

60. Groves BM, Turkevich D, Donnellan K, et al: Current approach to therapy of primary pulmonary hypertension. Chest 93(Suppl III):175S–178S, 1988.

61. Gurtner HP: "Plexogenic pulmonary arteriopathy" and the appetite depressant drug aminorex: post or propter. Bull Eur Physiopathol Respir 15:897–923, 1979.

62. Gurtner HP, Walser P, Fassler B: Normal values for pulmonary hemodynamics at rest and during exercise in man. Prog Respir Res 9:295–315, 1975.

63. Halladie-Smith KA, Wilson RSE, Hart A, et al: Functional status of patients with large ventricular septal defect and pulmonary vascular disease 6 to 16 years after surgical closure of their defect in childhood. Br Heart J 39:1093–1101, 1977.

64. Hammerman C, Komar K, Abd-Khudair H: Hypoxic vs. septic pulmonary hypertension. Am J Dis Child 142:319–325, 1988.

65. Hammerman C, Lass N, Strates E, et al: Prostanoids in neonates with persistent pulmonary hypertension. J Pediatr 110:470–472, 1987.

66. Hammon JW, Bender HW, Graham TP, et al: Total anomalous pulmonary venous connection in infancy. J Thorac Cardiovasc Surg 80:544–551, 1980.

67. Harris P, Heath D: The Human Pulmonary Circulation, 2nd ed. New York, Churchill Livingstone, 1977, pp. 259, 344–364.

68. Haworth SG: Primary pulmonary hypertension. Br Heart J 49:517–521, 1983.

69. Haworth SG: Pulmonary vascular disease in different types of congenital heart disease. Implication for interpretation of lung biopsy findings in early childhood. Br Heart J 52:557–571, 1984.

70. Haworth SG: Pulmonary vascular disease in ventricular septal defect: structural and functional correlations in lung biopsies from 85 patients, with outcome of intracardiac repair. J Pathol 152:157–168, 1987.

71. Haworth SG, Hislop A: Pulmonary vascular development: normal values of peripheral vascular structure. Am J Cardiol 52:578–583, 1983.

72. Haworth SG, Sauer U, Buhlmeyer K, et al: Development of the pulmonary circulation in ventricular septal defect: a quantitative structural study. Am J Cardiol 40:781–788, 1977.

73. Heath D, Edwards J: The pathology of hypertensive pulmonary vascular disease. Circulation 18:533–547, 1958.

74. Heath D, Smith P, Gosney J, et al: The pathology of the early and late stages of primary pulmonary hypertension. Br Heart J 58:204–213, 1987.

75. Heymann MA: Prostaglandins and leukotrienes in the perinatal period. Clin Perinatol 14:857–880, 1987.

76. Higenbottam T: The place of prostacyclin in the clinical management of primary pulmonary hypertension. Am Rev Respir Dis 136:782–785, 1987.

77. Hislop A, Reid L: Structural changes in the pulmonary arteries and veins in tetralogy of Fallot. Br Heart J 35:1178–1183, 1973.

78. Hislop A, Reid L: Growth and development of the respiratory system, anatomical development. In Davis JA, Dobbing J (eds): Scientific Foundation of Pediatrics. London, Heinemann Medical Publications, 1981, pp. 390–431.

79. Hoffman JIE, Heyman MA: Pulmonary arterial hypertension secondary to congenital heart disease. In Weir EK, Reeves JT (eds): Pulmonary Hypertension. Mt. Kisco, NY, Futura Publishing Co., 1984, pp. 73–114.

80. Hoffman JIE, Rudolph AM, Heymann MA: Pulmonary vascular disease with congenital heart lesions: pathologic features and causes. Circulation 64:873–877, 1982.

81. Hosoda Y, Suzuki Y, Takano M, et al: Mixed connective tissue disease with pulmonary hypertension: a clinical and pathological study. J Rheumatol 14:826–830, 1987.

82. Husson GS, Wyatt TC: Primary pulmonary obliterative vascular disease in infants and young children. Pediatrics 23:493–506, 1959.

83. Hyman AL, Dempsey CW, Fontana C, et al: Pulmonary vascular responses to forebrain stimulation in the cat. Circ Res 63:493–501, 1988.

84. Jordan JD, Snyder CH: Rheumatoid disease of the lung and cor pulmonale. Am J Dis Child 108:174–180, 1964.

85. Juaneda E, Haworth SG: Pulmonary vascular disease in children with truncus arteriosus. Am J Cardiol 54:1314–1320, 1984.

86. Juaneda E, Haworth SG: Pulmonary vascular structure in patients dying after a Fontan procedure. Br Heart J 52:575–580, 1984.

87. Kadowitz PJ, Lippton HL, McNamara DB, et al: Action and metabolism of prostaglandins in the pulmonary circulation. In Oates JA (ed): Prostaglandins and the Cardiovascular System. New York, Raven Press, 1982, pp. 333–356.

88. Kane RD, Hawkins HK, Miller JA, et al: Microscopic pulmonary tumor emboli associated with dyspnea. Cancer 36:1473–1482, 1975.

89. Kappa P, Koivisto M, Ylikorkala O, et al: Prostacyclin in the treatment of neonatal pulmonary hypertension. J Pediatr 107:951–953, 1985.

90. Keane JF, Ellison C, Rudd M, et al: Pulmonary blood flow and left ventricular volumes in transposition of the great arteries and intact ventricular septum. Br Heart J 35:521–526, 1973.

91. Keane JF, Fyler DC, Nadas AS: Hazards of cardiac catheterization in children with primary pulmonary vascular obstruction. Am Heart J 96:556–558, 1978.

92. Kennedy TP, Michael JR, Huang C-K, et al: Nifedipine inhibits hypoxic pulmonary vasoconstriction during rest and exercise in patients with chronic obstructive pulmonary disease. Am Rev Respir Dis 129:544–551, 1984.

93. Kerr JS, Ruppert CL, Tozzi CA, et al: Reduction of chronic hypoxic pulmonary hypertension in the rat by an inhibitor of collagen production. Am Rev Respir Dis 135:300–306, 1987.

94. Kinsley RH, McGoon DC, Danielson GK, et al: Pulmonary arterial hypertension after repair of tetralogy of Fallot. J Thorac Cardiovasc Surg 67:110–120, 1974.

95. Kleiger RE, Boxer M, Ingham RE, et al: Pulmonary hypertension in patients using oral contraceptives. Chest 69:143–147, 1976.

96. Kollros PR, Bates SR, Mathews MB, et al: Cyclic AMP inhibits increased collagen production by cyclically stretched smooth muscle cells. Lab Invest 56:410–417, 1987.

97. Krovetz LJ, McLoughlin TG, Mitchell MB, et al: Hemodynamic findings in normal children. Pediatr Res 1:122–130, 1967.

98. Kulik TJ, Lock JE: The assessment of pulmonary vascular tone: a review of experimental methodologies. Pediatr Pharmacol 4:73–83, 1984.

99. Kulik TJ, Lock JE: Pulmonary vasodilator therapy in persistent pulmonary hypertension of the newborn. Clin Perinatol 11:693–701, 1984.

100. Kulik TJ, Lock JE: Leukotrienes and the immature pulmonary circulation. Am Rev Respir Dis 136:220–222, 1987.

101. Kulik TJ, Lock JE: Unpublished data.

102. Kulik TJ, Evans JN, Gamble WJ: Stretch-induced contraction in pulmonary arteries. Am J Physiol 255:H1391–H1398, 1988.

103. Kulik TJ, Johnson DE, Elde RP, et al: Pulmonary and systemic vascular effects of serotonin in conscious newborn lambs. Dev Pharmacol Ther 11:135–141, 1988.

104. Lakier JB, Stanger P, Heymann MA, et al: Early onset of pulmonary vascular obstruction in patients with aortopulmonary transposition and intact ventricular septum. Circulation 51:875–880, 1975.

105. Lande A, Bard R: Takaysu's arteritis: an unrecognized cause of pulmonary hypertension. Angiology 27:114–121, 1976.

106. Levin DL, Cates L, Newfeld EA, et al: Persistence of the fetal cardiopulmonary circulatory pathway: survival of an infant after a prolonged course. Pediatrics 56:58–64, 1975.

107. Levin DL, Heymann MA, Kitterman JA, et al: Persistent pulmonary hypertension of the newborn infant. J Pediatr 89:626–630, 1976.

108. Levin DL, Mills LJ, Weinberg AG: Hemodynamic, pulmonary vascular, and myocardial abnormalities secondary to pharmacologic constriction of the fetal ductus arteriosus. Circulation 60:360–364, 1979.

109. Levin DL, Muster AJ, Pachman LM, et al: Cor pulmonale secondary to upper airway obstruction. Chest 68:166–171, 1975.

110. Levine OR, Harris RC, Blanc WA, et al: Progressive pulmonary hypertension in children with portal hypertension. J Pediatr 83:964–972, 1973.

111. Lock JE, Einzig S, Bass JL, et al: The pulmonary vascular response to oxygen and its influence on operative results in children with ventricular septal defect. Pediatr Cardiol 3:41–46, 1982.

112. Lock JE, Einzig S, Moller JH: Hemodynamic responses to exercise in normal children. Am J Cardiol 41:1278–1284, 1978.

113. Lock JE, Hamilton F, Luide H, et al: Direct pulmonary vascular responses in the conscious newborn lamb. J Appl Physiol 48:188–196, 1980.

114. Marx G: Prediction of nonsurvival in critically ill infants with respiratory failure. Am J Dis Child 142:261–262, 1988.

115. Mathur PN, Powles AC, Pugsley SO, et al: Effect of digoxin on right ventricular function in severe chronic airflow obstruction. Ann Intern Med 95:283–288, 1981.

116. McGregor M, Sniderman A: On pulmonary vascular resistance: the need for more precise definition. Am J Cardiol 55:217–221, 1985.

117. McMahon DP, Aterman K: Pulmonary hypertension due to multiple emboli. J Pediatr 92:841–845, 1978.

118. Meyrick B, Reid L: Ultrastructural findings in lung biopsy material from children with congenital heart defects. Am J Pathol 101:527–532, 1980.

119. Michael JR, Kennedy TP, Fitzpatrick S, et al: Nifedipine inhibits hypoxic pulmonary vasoconstriction during rest and exercise in patients with cystic fibrosis and cor pulmonale. Am Rev Respir Dis 130:516–519, 1984.

120. Milnor WR: Pulsatile blood flow. N Engl J Med 287:27–34, 1972.

121. Moffat RE, Sobonya RE, Chang CHJ: Childhood sarcoidosis with fatal cor pulmonale. Pediatr Radiol 7:180–182, 1978.

122. Moise KJ, Huhta JC, Sharif DS, et al: Indomethacin in the treatment of premature labor. N Engl J Med 319:327–331, 1988.

123. Morgan AD: Cor pulmonale in children: review and etiological classification. Am Heart J 73:550–562, 1966.

124. Moser KM, Shea JG: The relationship between pulmonary infarction, cor pulmonale, and the sickle states. Am J Med 22:561–579, 1957.

125. Moss AJ: The cardiovascular system in cystic fibrosis. Pediatrics 70:728–741, 1982.

126. Nair SS, Askari AD, Popelka CG, et al: Pulmonary hypertension and systemic lupus erythematosus. Arch Intern Med 140:109–111, 1980.

127. Newfeld EA, Paul MH, Muster AJ, et al: Pulmonary vascular disease in complete transposition of the great vessels. Am J Cardiol 34:75–82, 1974.

128. Newfeld EA, Sher M, Paul MH, et al: Pulmonary vascular disease in complete atrioventricular canal defect. Am J Cardiol 39:721–726, 1977.

129. Newfeld EA, Wilson A, Paul MH, et al: Pulmonary vascular disease in total anomalous pulmonary venous drainage. Circulation 61:103–109, 1980.

130. Nihill M: Personal communication.

131. Oakley C, Somerville J: Oral contraceptives and progressive pulmonary vascular disease. Lancet 1:890, 1968.

132. O'Brodovich HM, Mellins RB: State of the art: bronchopulmonary dysplasia. Am Rev Respir Dis 132:694–709, 1985.

133. Packer M: Therapeutic application of calcium-channel antagonists for pulmonary hypertension. Am J Cardiol 55:196B–201B, 1985.

134. Peckham GJ, Fox WW: Physiologic factors affecting pulmonary artery pressure in infants with persistent

pulmonary hypertension. J Pediatr 93:1005–1010, 1978.

135. Pool PE, Vogel JHK, Blount SG: Congenital unilateral absence of a pulmonary artery. Am J Cardiol 10:706–732, 1962.

136. Pressly TA, Winkler A, Alpert MA, et al: Value and limitations of calcium channel blockade in the therapy of pulmonary hypertension associated with CREST—case reports. Angiology 39:385–389, 1988.

137. Rabinovitch M, Bothwell T, Hayakawa BN, et al: Pulmonary artery endothelial abnormalities in patients with congenital heart defects and pulmonary hypertension. Lab Invest 55:632–653, 1986.

138. Rabinovitch M, Castaneda AR, Reid L: Lung biopsy with frozen section as a diagnostic aid in patients with congenital heart defects. Am J Cardiol 47:77–84, 1981.

139. Rabinovitch M, Haworth SG, Castaneda AR, et al: Lung biopsy in congenital heart disease: a morphometric approach to pulmonary vascular disease. Circulation 58:1107–1122, 1978.

140. Rabinovitch M, Keane JF, Fellows KE, et al: Quantitative analysis of the pulmonary wedge angiogram in congenital heart defects. Circulation 63:152–164, 1981.

141. Rabinovitch M, Keane JF, Norwood WI, et al: Vascular structure in lung tissue obtained at biopsy correlated with pulmonary hemodynamic findings after repair of congenital heart defects. Circulation 69:655–667, 1984.

142. Reeves JT, Groves BM, Turkevich D: The case for treatment of selective patients with primary pulmonary hypertension. Am Rev Respir Dis 134:342–346, 1986.

143. Reeves JT, Herget J: Experimental models of pulmonary hypertension. In Weir EK, Reeves JT (eds): Pulmonary Hypertension. Mt. Kisco, NY, Futura Publishing Co., 1984, pp. 73–114.

144. Reid LM: The pulmonary circulation: remodeling in growth and disease. Am Rev Respir Dis 119:531–546, 1979.

145. Reitz B: Heart-lung transplantation. Chest 93:450–451, 1988.

146. Rich S, Brundage BH: High-dose calcium channel-blocking therapy for primary pulmonary hypertension: evidence for long-term reduction in pulmonary arterial pressure and regression of right ventricular hypertrophy. Circulation 76:135–141, 1987.

147. Rich S, Lam W: Atrial septostomy as palliative therapy for refractory primary pulmonary hypertension. Am J Cardiol 51:1560–1561, 1983.

148. Rich S, Dantzker DR, Ayres SM, et al: Primary pulmonary hypertension. Ann Intern Med 107:216–223, 1987.

149. Rich S, Levitsky S, Brundage BH: Pulmonary hypertension from chronic pulmonary thromboembolism. Ann Intern Med 108:425–434, 1988.

150. Riedel M, Stanek V, Widimsky J, et al: Longterm follow-up of patients with pulmonary thromboembolism. Chest 81:151–158, 1982.

151. Riemenschneider TA, Nielsen HC, Ruttenberg HD, et al: Disturbances of the transitional circulation: spectrum of pulmonary hypertension and myocardial dysfunction. J Pediatr 89:622–625, 1976.

152. Rowe RD, James LS: The normal pulmonary arterial pressure during the first year of life. J Pediatr 51:1–4, 1957.

153. Rubin LJ, Peter RH: Hemodynamics at rest and during exercise after oral hydralazine in patients with cor pulmonale. Am J Cardiol 47:116–122, 1981.

154. Rudolph AM: The foetal circulation, circulatory adjustments after birth and the influence of congenital heart lesions on pulmonary hemodynamics. In Watson H (ed): Pediatric Cardiology. St. Louis, C.V. Mosby Co., 1968, p. 52.

155. Rudolph AM: Fetal and neonatal pulmonary circulation. Ann Rev Physiol 41:383–395, 1979.

156. Rudolph AM, Cayler GG: Cardiac catheterization in infants and children. Pediatr Clin North Am 5:907–943, 1958.

157. Ryland D, Reid L: The pulmonary circulation in cystic fibrosis. Thorax 30:285–292, 1975.

158. Sackner MA, Akgun N, Kimbel P, et al: The pathophysiology of scleroderma involving the heart and respiratory system. Ann Intern Med 60:611–630, 1964.

159. Salerni R, Rodnan GP, Leon DF, et al: Pulmonary hypertension in the CREST syndrome variant of progressive systemic sclerosis. Ann Intern Med 86:394–399, 1977.

160. Schreiber MD, Heymann MA, Soifer SJ: Increased arterial pH, not decreased $PaCO_2$ attenuates hypoxia-induced pulmonary vasoconstriction in newborn lambs. Pediatr Res 20:113–117, 1986.

161. Schwartz SM, Campbell GR, Campbell JH: Replication of smooth muscle cells in vascular disease. Circ Res 58:427–444, 1986.

162. Seidel CL, Schildmeyer LA: Vascular smooth muscle adaptation to increased load. Ann Rev Physiol 49:489–499, 1987.

163. Siassi B, Goldberg S, Emmanouilides GC, et al: Persistent pulmonary vascular obstruction in newborn infants. J Pediatr 78:610–615, 1971.

164. Sigmann JM, Perry BL, Behrendt DM, et al: Ventricular septal defect: results after repair in infancy. Am J Cardiol 39:66–71, 1977.

165. Smith P, Heath D: Electron microscopy of the plexiform lesion. Thorax 34:177–186, 1979.

166. Soifer SJ, Clyman RI, Heymann MA: Effects of prostaglandin D_2 on pulmonary arterial pressure and oxygenation in newborn infants with persistent pulmonary hypertension. J Pediatr 112:774–777, 1988.

167. Stenmark KR, Orton EC, Reeves JT, et al: Vascular remodeling in neonatal pulmonary hypertension: Role of the smooth muscle cell. Chest 93(Suppl III):127s–133s, 1988.

168. Stepp MA, Kindy MS, Franzblau C, et al: Complex regulation of collagen gene expression in cultured bovine aortic smooth muscle cells. J Biol Chem 261:6542–6547, 1986.

169. Stern RC, Borkat G, Hirschfeld SS, et al: Heart failure in cystic fibrosis. Am J Dis Child 134:267–272, 1980.

170. Stevenson DK, Kasting DS, Darnall RA, et al: Refractory hypoxemia associated with neonatal pulmonary disease: the use and limitation of tolazoline. J Pediatr 95:595–599, 1979.

171. Swischuck LE, Richardson CJ, Nichols MM, et al: Primary pulmonary hypoplasia in the neonate. J Pediatr 95:573–577, 1979.

172. Thilenius OG, Nadas AS, Jockin H: Primary pulmonary vascular obstruction in children. Pediatrics 36:75–87, 1965.

173. Teisberg P, Hognestad J: Primary pulmonary hypertension in infancy. Acta Paediatr Scand 62:69–72, 1973.

174. Tomashefski JF, Opperman HC, Vawter GF, et al: Bronchopulmonary dysplasia: a morphometric study with emphasis on the pulmonary vasculature. Pediatr Pathol 2:469–487, 1984.

175. Turner GR, Levin D: Prostaglandin synthesis inhibition in persistent pulmonary hypertension of the newborn. Clin Perinatol 11:581–589, 1984.

176. Voelkel NF: Mechanisms of hypoxic pulmonary vasoconstriction. Am Rev Respir Dis 133:1186–1195, 1986.

177. Vogel JHK, Grover RF, Jamieson GG, et al: Long-

term physiologic observations in patients with ventricular septal defects and increased pulmonary vascular resistance. Adv Cardiol 11:108–122, 1974.

178. Wagenvoort CA: The pulmonary arteries in infants with ventricular septal defect. Med Thorac 19:354–366, 1962.

179. Wagenvoort CA: Pulmonary veno-occlusive disease. Chest 69:82–86, 1976.

180. Wagenvoort CA: Lung biopsies and pulmonary vascular disease. In Weir EK, Reeves JT (eds): Pulmonary Hypertension. Mt. Kisco, NY, Futura Publishing Co., 1984, pp. 73–114.

181. Wagenvoort CA, Wagenvoort N: Primary pulmonary hypertension. Circulation 42:1163–1184, 1970.

182. Wagenvoort CA, Heath D, Edwards JE: The Pathology of the Pulmonary Vasculature. Springfield, IL, Charles C Thomas, 1964, pp. 314–318.

183. Wagenvoort CA, Wagenvoort N, Draulans-Noe Y: Reversibility of plexogenic pulmonary arteriopathy following banding of the pulmonary artery. J Thorac Cardiovasc Surg 87:876–886, 1984.

184. Walcott G, Burchell HB, Brown AL: Primary pulmonary hypertension. Am J Med 49:70–79, 1970.

185. Webb RC, Bohr DF: Recent advances in the pathogenesis of hypertension: consideration of structural, functional, and metabolic vascular abnormalities resulting in elevated arterial resistance. Am Heart J 102:251–264, 1981.

186. Weidman WH, Blount SG, DuShane JW, et al: Clinical course in ventricular septal defect. Circulation 56(Suppl. I):I-56–I-69, 1977.

187. Wood P: The Eisenmenger syndrome: or pulmonary hypertension with reversed central shunt. Br Med J 2:701–709; 755–762, 1958.

188. Wood P: Diseases of the Heart and Circulation, 3rd ed. Philadelphia, J.B. Lippincott Co., 1968, p. 429.

189. Woodruff WW, Merten DF, Wasner ML, et al: Chronic pulmonary embolism in children. Radiology 159:511–514, 1986.

190. Wung J-T, James LS, Kilchevsky E, et al: Management of infants with severe respiratory failure and persistence of the fetal circulation, without hyperventilation. Pediatrics 76:488–494, 1985.

191. Yeager SB, Freed MD, Keane JF, et al: Primary surgical closure of ventricular septal defect in the first year of life. J Am Coll Cardiol 3:1269–1276, 1984.

192. Young D, Mark H: Fate of the patient with the Eisenmenger syndrome. Am J Cardiol 28:658–669, 1971.

193. Zener JC, Hancock EW, Shumway NE, et al: Regression of extreme pulmonary hypertension after mitral valve surgery. Am J Cardiol 30:820–826, 1972.

Section VI
Tools of Diagnosis

Chapter 11

HISTORY, PHYSICAL EXAMINATION, AND LABORATORY TESTS

Donald C. Fyler, M.D., and Alexander S. Nadas, M.D.

HISTORY

When a child is referred because of a suspected cardiac problem, most commonly because of a murmur, a complete pediatric history is taken. The possibilities of associated anomalies (10–20% of patients with congenital heart disease) or acquired diseases are almost unlimited. Any noncardiac questions discovered are evaluated in the context of the cardiac abnormality.

The circumstances surrounding history taking are important. It is almost mandatory, even at the bedside, that the doctor sit down. The physician must convey an unhurried, compassionate concern. If this is the initial examination of a child referred because of heart disease, it may be the start of a continuing relationship which, later on, may involve serious decisions about the health of the child. The stronger the relationship between the parents and the physician, the easier it will be to manage the later problems requiring emotional strength. The cardiologist must understand the parents, their circumstances, their strengths, weaknesses, and concerns.

Pediatric history taking ranges from the purely veterinarian approach for infants to a typical medical encounter with an adult and all stages in between. Every attempt should be made to obtain information from the patient, with the parents serving as confirmatory observers. Most of the history can be obtained from the child by age 10 to 12; for patients age 15 or 16, the parents (one or the other or both) might, under some circumstances, be better kept out of the room, at least part of the time. Often the parents are out of the room during the physical examination, at which time further historical data are sometimes forthcoming.

Parents who, in their concern for the child, dominate the discussion can at times be annoying, even disruptive. It should be remembered that the consulting physician has undertaken the responsibility to provide the best for the child, surmounting all obstacles, including occasionally, the parents. The tendency for some parents to dominate their offspring well into adulthood is common, especially when there is a medical problem. The author has in mind a 35-year-old "child" with cyanotic heart disease who, with his septuagenarian father, has visited every few months for the past 30 years.

Specifically, the cardiac history should consider the following general issues:

1. **Birth.** The details of the birth are recorded in detail. Was the infant cyanotic? How well did the baby do in the first days of life? Was oxygen needed? If oxygen was used, did it help?

2. **Growth.** Growth failure because of heart disease is sufficiently common that detailed plotting of the growth curve is mandatory. It is of interest how well the child grows relative to siblings and how well the child grows relative to the size of the parents. Are the height and weight disproportionate? What are the actual percentiles?

3. **Exercise Tolerance.** Most of the history is concerned with evaluating the child's physical abilities. Can the baby take usual feeding in an appropriate amount of time or does he tire, become short of breath, or need to rest while feeding? How

101

much exercise produces fatigue? Does it cause shortness of breath? How does the child function relative to contemporaries? The child's lifestyle provides clues to physical ability. What is the child's involvement and capacity in sports? How far can he walk, at his own pace, on a nice day?

Is the exercise limitation a function of shortness of breath or is it caused by fatigue? What are the limitations of the exercise assessment? Does the child (perhaps like his parents) lead a sedentary life without limitation on a cardiac basis? Or does the child keep up with contemporaries at great personal discomfort? Is it possible that he has never known what it is like to have normal exercise tolerance and believes his capability is normal?

4. **Palpitations.** Some time after the age of two children begin to report episodes of tachycardia and occasional irregularity. Why one of two children of the same age, with the same kind of ectopy, at the same heart rate, notices the aberrant rhythm and the other does not, cannot be explained. Conventional wisdom suggests that a child who has had ectopy for some years does not notice it as much as someone who has recently begun to experience a problem. In older children an attempt should be made to distinguish rate from irregularity.

5. **Chest Pain.** Chest pain is a common reason for referral to a pediatric cardiologist. The circumstances surrounding the pain should be considered in some detail. If it is related to exercise, what time of day does it occur? Does it happen while watching television? Is it noticed while going to sleep? What relieves the pain? How long does it last? Where is it located? The child who reports pain in his "heart" prompts further discussion of his environmental circumstances. What is the source of the idea that the pain in his chest comes from his heart? Do the parents regularly ask whether the child has pain in his heart, or does grandma have angina, or is this simply a learned idea from television or overheard discussions of heart attacks? Children are not born with the idea that chest pain comes from the heart.

6. **Cyanosis.** Among patients who are cyanotic the tendency to squat suggests labile blood oxygen saturation. Even more important are episodes resembling cyanotic spells (see p. 75). It is our belief that a single cyanotic spell in a patient with potentially operable heart disease requires a surgical procedure. Detailed and careful documentation of a spell are required before recommending surgical repair.

7. **Syncope.** Any episode suggesting syncope or near syncope should be reviewed in detail: What were the events immediately preceding the episode? How long did it last? Were there any injuries? Were there convulsive movements? How often has it happened? Were there premonitory symptoms? A typical fainting episode may be a well-defined historical event, but near-syncope (a dizzy spell) requires detailed discussion to make certain that the symptom may have a cardiac origin.

8. **Prior Observations.** Because virtually all of our patients are referred by another physician, the data accumulated elsewhere are reviewed as part of the historical information.

PHYSICAL EXAMINATION

The physical examination of the child suspected of having heart disease should follow along well-established pediatric lines. It is valuable to have a routine sequence that will reduce omissions to a minimum. The uncomfortable parts of the examination should be reserved until last. Toddlers are often best examined on the mother's lap, the auscultation being completed first while the infant remains distractable. In a hospital setting it is highly recommended simply to watch a baby lying quietly, without touching.

General Examination

Does the child appear ill, or is he happy and playful? Is he in distress of any sort, and if so, what kind? What is the state of the peripheral circulation? Are the pulses weak or are they absent? Is the child pale or blue? The temperature of the extremities should be noted and an opinion of circulatory competence formulated.

Respiration

Is there tachypnea? The respiratory rate, possible subcostal retractions, and flaring alae nasi should be observed with the patient quiet. The infant's response to his respiratory problems should be noted; does he seem distressed and anxious or is he "happily tachypneic"? Rapid, shallow respiration in excess of 50–60 breaths per minute in an otherwise happy newborn infant, if observed repeatedly, is abnormal and implies elevated pulmonary venous pressure until proved otherwise. This pattern is particularly common in infants with excessive pulmonary blood flow. The anxious infant with rapid, deep respirations, associated with cough and distress may have pneumonia.

Growth

Is the child's growth appropriate for his age? How does this assessment compare to the measured weight and height in terms of percentiles? The developmental chart should be updated. Generally cardiac disease dating from birth affects the weight before the height, resulting in a scrawny infant. Those with more severe problems show delays in both weight and weight. In general, obstructive lesions without congestive failure, such as coarctation, aortic stenosis, or pulmonary stenosis, are associated with normal growth. In patients with cyanotic lesions, such as tetralogy of Fallot, there may be generalized growth retardation, whereas in those who have lesions associated with congestive heart failure, such as left-to-right shunts (septal defects), weight is more affected than height. Complete cessation of growth, even weight loss, is seen in patients with severe congestive heart failure. Growth charts are a vital and indispensable tool in the assessment of infants with heart disease.

Extracardiac Anomalies

The possibility of associated congenital anomalies should be considered. Is there a syndrome such as Down, Turner, Noonan, Marfan, Williams, or Holt-Oram? (See pp. 45–53.) The overall incidence of extracardiac anomalies among children with congenital heart disease is high[1,2] (in the order of 20% of all patients). There is considerable variation: with some cardiac defects (e.g., truncus arteriosus) there is an incidence of extracardiac anomalies as high as 50%, whereas in others the incidence of associated anomalies seems lower than in the general population (e.g., transposition of the great arteries). Some extracardiac anomalies tend to be associated with a particular cardiac disease (e.g., Down syndrome with atrioventricularis communis) (see ch. 36).

Scoliosis

Scoliosis is common among adolescent children with cyanotic congenital heart disease, the severity being roughly proportionate to the severity of arterial unsaturation.[7] Examination of the spine with this possibility in mind is a required part of the examination of children with congenital heart disease.

Cyanosis

No general description of a child suspected of having congenital heart disease should fail to mention whether there is evidence of cyanosis. If it is present, its depth and distribution are always pertinent. Sometimes patients with minimal arterial unsaturation are not frankly cyanotic; their cheeks and lips have a peculiar high color, however, with a slight bluish tinge. Noticing this, the experienced observer will estimate the arterial oxygen saturation to be in the 85–90% range. Often this color is misleading, however, and even the trained clinician may mistake the flush of a healthy child entering a warm room for borderline cyanosis. The particular combination of cyanosis and pallor in patients with cyanotic heart disease and relative anemia used to be known as "Picasso blue" in our clinic.

Cyanosis of the fingernails, toenails, and mucous membranes strongly suggests congenital heart disease and is commonly accompanied by **clubbing.**

Clinically, clubbing has at least two components: one is the rounding of the fingernails, especially the thumbnails; the other is a thickening and shininess of the terminal phalanges with disappearance of the normal creases (Fig. 1).

Patients with congenital heart disease often have **red fingers and toes.** We have learned to recognize this phenomenon as a precursor of cyanosis and clubbing; it is fairly characteristic of those whose arterial oxygen saturation is permanently or paroxysmally low normal or slightly abnormal (± 90%).

Edema

Puffiness of the eyelids and roundness of the face are common manifestations of right-sided congestive failure in small children, whereas pitting edema of the extremities is rare.

Arterial Pulses

Observation of the radial, carotid, and femoral pulses should be a matter of routine. Specific simultaneous comparison of the strength and timing of femoral and right radial pulses is mandatory in evaluating the possibility of coarctation of the aorta. Feeling the femoral pulses is an indispensable part of physical examination. Strong radial pulses with weak or absent femoral pulses is the hallmark of coarctation of the aorta.

Bounding peripheral pulsations suggest systemic hypertension or lesions associated with an aortic runoff, either back into the left ventricle (aortic regurgitation), into the pulmonary artery (patent ductus arteriosus), or even exclusively into the peripheral vascular bed (thyrotoxicosis, anemia). Prominent carotid pulsations may be seen in patients with hypertrophic subaortic stenosis. Lesser degrees of carotid hyperactivity may simply be the result of excitement.

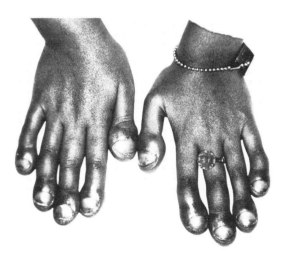

Figure 1. Clubbed fingers.

One important clue to be obtained from carotid pulses in patients with aortic stenosis should be mentioned. The patient with critical aortic valve obstruction usually does not have strong carotid pulsations, a fact related to the small pulse pressure and the slow upstroke time in these patients. In contrast, in functional, muscular, subaortic stenosis, the initial part of the central aortic and carotid tracing has a rapid upstroke. Consequently, these patients may present a picture of critical aortic stenosis with bounding carotid pulses.

Respiratory variations in pulse pressure of more than 10 mm Hg (**pulsus paradoxus**) (Fig. 2) may indicate pericardial tamponade, although on rare occasions severe respiratory distress (asthma, emphysema, or pleural fluid) may give rise to pulsus paradoxus of 20–25 mm Hg.

Arterial Pressure

Determination of blood pressure in the arm is an integral part of the examination. It is important to measure the systolic blood pressure in the arms as well as in the legs in all patients in whom congenital heart disease is suspected; thus, coarctation of the aorta will not be missed by clinical examination. The auscultatory method, using a mercury sphygmomanometer, is an easy and well-accepted procedure for adults and older children (see ch. 21). The results can be interpreted without much hesitation. In infants, however, especially in the younger age groups, the problem is far from simple. To begin with, the patient usually does not cooperate. Second, limbs of different sizes require different cuff sizes. Finally, the results have to be interpreted according to the age of the patient.

To ensure optimal cooperation, it is worthwhile, if possible, to explain the procedure to the child beforehand. Often an older child may be distracted by watching the up-and-down movements of the mercury. Infants may have to be pacified with a bottle while the blood pressure is being taken. Finally, in some instances, sedation with chloral hydrate may be necessary to ensure some degree of cooperation when the observation is considered vital.

The **size of the cuff** is important; as a rough guide, the cuff should cover two thirds or more of the upper arm or leg. A cuff that is too small gives falsely high readings. One does not get into trouble by using too large a cuff. For accurate results the pediatrician should have available the following cuff sizes: 5 cm, 7 cm, 12 cm, and 18 cm widths. The bag should be completely deflated and applied evenly, snugly, without bulging, around the upper arm or leg, and should completely encircle the limb.

Once a cuff of proper size has been applied to the patient, it may be well to obtain a quick reading of the systolic pressure by palpation. The cuff should be inflated to a point well above the disappearance of the radial pulse, then slowly released (2–3 mm Hg per beat) until the radial pulse reappears. This point clearly corresponds to the systolic pressure determined by direct measurement.

Once the systolic pressure has been determined by palpation, the systolic and diastolic pressures should be estimated by the auscultatory method. Reference to standard tables and graphs for normal data is required (see ch. 21).

In the most difficult situations (e.g., an apprehensive infant in whom coarctation is suspected), the authors prefer the use of a Doppler sensing device as the best-tolerated approach. It may be necessary to sedate the patient in order to measure blood pressure, often in association with sedation for other frightening tests such as echocardiography.

The systolic pressure in the legs is usually significantly higher than in the arms because of a summation effect of the forward pulse wave with the rebound wave (Fig. 3).[9] A reversal of this re-

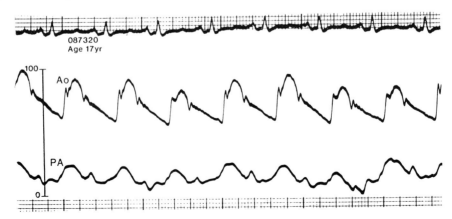

Figure 2.　Pulsus paradoxus in a patient with constrictive pericarditis. Simultaneous systemic arterial and pulmonary arterial pressures and electrocardiogram. The variations in arterial pressures are a direct function of respiration and exceed the expected variation under normal circumstances.

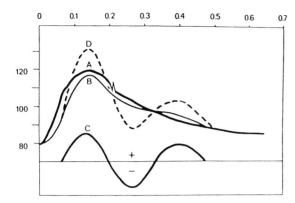

Figure 3. Diagram illustrating the principles of damping and wave summation in the arterial system. **A,** Aortic pulse. **B,** Changes in contour and amplitude due to damping. **C,** Nature of rebound wave. **D,** Summation of curves B and C (ordinate pressure in mm Hg; abscissa lines in 0.1 second). (From Wiggers CJ: Circulatory Dynamics: Physiologic Studies. New York, Grune & Stratton, 1952, with permission.)

lationship is pathologic and implies the presence of an aortic block in patients more than one year of age. Normal systemic blood pressure gradually rises over the lifetime of children (see ch. 21).

Pulse Pressure

The pulse pressure may be calculated by subtracting the diastolic from the systolic pressure. A widened pulse pressure, detectable by the bounding, water-hammer pulse, is commonly seen in (1) fever, anemia, thyrotoxicosis, and after vigorous exercise, (2) aortic runoffs (aortic regurgitation, patent ductus arteriosus, aortopulmonary window, and arteriovenous fistulas), and (3) complete heart block. Conversely, narrow pulse pressures may be observed in (1) low cardiac output, (2) mitral or aortic stenosis, and (3) pericardial tamponade or constrictive pericarditis.

Two peculiarities of the pulse may best be detected while determining blood pressure. **Pulsus paradoxus,** characteristic of the accumulation of an appreciable amount of fluid in the pericardial sac, consists of a decrease of systolic pressure and narrowing of the pulse pressure on deep inspiration (Fig. 2). **Pulsus alternans,** a sign of left ventricular failure, consists of a drop in systolic pressure in alternate beats. Both pulsus paradoxus and pulsus alternans are more reliably documented while observing the blood pressure rather than by palpating the pulse itself.

Venous Pressure

With practice, in children who cooperate, especially the older ones, simple inspection furnishes valuable information about venous pressure. Perhaps the simplest and most reliable method is inspection of the jugular vein of the patient when he is sitting upright. In a child as tall as the usual 6-year-old, venous distention or pulsation should not be visible above the clavicle unless the venous pressure is elevated. Not all patients have readily visible external jugular veins. Internal jugular pulsations usually can be seen with the patient lying flat; if still present when the patient is in a sitting or upright position, they are abnormal. More than one pulse per heart beat in an undulatory pattern, particularly in the absence of palpable neck pulsations, usually can be interpreted as venous pulsations inconsistent with an arterial pulse. A crude estimation of venous pressure is furnished by measuring the height of the jugular venous column, vertically, above the level of the right atrium, in a sitting patient. If the patient is recumbent at a 45° angle, the height of the jugular venous column should not rise above an imaginary straight line across the manubrium of the sternum (Fig. 4).[4] It follows that when the patient is lying flat, venous pulsations are always present unless the superior cava is not connected to the right atrium (e.g., the Glenn operation)

When there is doubt, a needle inserted into an accessible vein and connected to a transducer (available in modern intensive care units) will provide not only an accurate measure of pressure (zero = level of right atrium) but will show pulsatile waveforms.

Chest Deformity

Left chest deformity is a feature of congenital heart disease. This results largely from increased cardiac size and activity during the time that the chest wall is being formed. It is seen commonly in patients with large left-to-right shunts. Vigorous pulsations of a significantly enlarged right or left ventricle which last for several months lead to visible left-sided chest prominence, particularly in young patients, who have an elastic rib cage.

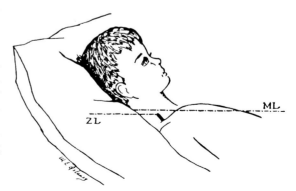

Figure 4. Clinical estimation of venous pressure. With the patient lying down at approximately 45°, the pressure (ZL) in the right atrium does not rise above the manubrium (ML). (From Lewis T: Diseases of the Heart Described for Practitioners and Students, 2nd ed. New York, Macmillan, 1937.)

Cardiac Impulse

Observations and palpation of the cardiac impulse may be revealing. Visible pulsations, sometimes rocking the entire chest, are characteristic of certain patients with congenital heart disease involving large volume change (patent ductus arteriosus, large ventricular septal defect, and ventricular defect with aortic regurgitation), or of children with severe mitral regurgitation. On the other hand, a relatively quiet beat may be seen in the presence of marked cardiac enlargement in patients with Ebstein's deformity, cardiomyopathy and, of course, pericardial effusion. It is hard to imagine a patient suffering from severe mitral regurgitation without having a prominent cardiac impulse. Similarly, the diagnosis of a small patent ductus arteriosus associated with a grossly hyperactive cardiac impulse is suspicious.

A good estimation of the hypertrophy of the right or left ventricle can be achieved by noting the point of maximal impulse of the heart beat. If this is at the xiphoid process or the lower left sternal border, with visible up-and-down pulsations, the chances are that the right ventricle is dominant. Conversely, if the cardiac impulse is maximal at the apex, probably the left ventricle is enlarged. A cardiac impulse palpable at both the xiphoid and the apex strongly suggests combined hypertrophy. The nature of the cardiac impulse may be tapping and quick, suggesting movement of large volumes, or heaving and slow, suggesting increased pressures.

Heart Size

The location of the cardiac apex with the child in the sitting position correlates with the cardiac apex on the upright chest x-ray and provides a reasonable estimation of heart size. Percussion of the entire cardiac silhouette is tiresome, time-consuming, and barely justifiable in this age of easy availability of radiograms and echocardiograms. At best, this procedure can give the physician only an approximate idea of the size of the heart; at worst, it may be completely misleading.

Thrills

The presence of thrills and their timing, intensity, and localization should be noted. Because the vast majority of thrills are systolic, the notion that *all* thrills are systolic should be guarded against. The old clinical axiom that apical thrills are almost invariably diastolic is worth remembering.

Auscultation

The most cost-effective tool for cardiac diagnosis is the stethoscope. Systematic evaluation of heart sounds and murmurs is inexpensive, often diagnostic, readily repeated, and can be learned by almost everyone. For some cardiac lesions (e.g.,

aortic regurgitation), it is a most sensitive tool. It is an efficient means of discovering new cases and accounts for most of the referrals to a cardiology unit each year. This is the one cardiac diagnostic tool remaining to the pediatrician. The "experts" have expropriated most of the other tools and charge handsomely for them.

After inspection and palpation have furnished information about the size of the heart and the intensity and localization of its pulsations, the examiner should concentrate on auscultation. To obtain maximal benefit from this most valuable part of the physical examination, the proper instrument must be used. The tiny, disposable "pediatric stethoscope" is almost totally useless for reliable auscultation of the heart. Equally useless in the examination of infants are the huge adult stethoscopes, especially the ones with only a diaphragm chest-piece; these instruments, when placed on the tiny chest of a baby, cover practically the entire cardiac silhouette. A third kind of stethoscope should be used only when necessary—someone else's stethoscope. The pernicious practice of picking up any stethoscope in a hospital ward is to be deplored. A stethoscope is a personal instrument. Best results can be achieved only by the continuous use of the same ear- and chest-pieces. Not everyone's aural canals are the same size and shape. The ear-pieces have to fit the canals snugly without discomfort to assure optimal auscultation.[6]

What type of stethoscope should be carried for the examination of infants or children with heart disease? It should be a so-called binaural stethoscope with a combined bell and diaphragm chest-piece. The length of the thick-walled rubber tubing should be the shortest comfortable length (not more than 18″) with a bore of $\frac{1}{8}$″.[6] Its efficiency will depend on its length from chest-piece to ear-piece, its total enclosed volume, its internal diameter, and the physical characteristics of the tubing, but perhaps most important, over and above who is between the ear-pieces, is the integrity of the acoustic seal from skin surface to auditory canal. Any leak, anywhere, not only will admit outside noises, but will interfere with appropriate sound transmission. By and large, stethoscopes with small internal volume, a small end-piece, and good skin-contact give more faithful reproduction, although everybody has experienced situations in which a faint aortic diastolic murmur is revealed only by an end-piece with a large diaphragm. In general, low-frequency sounds are heard best with a bell-shaped end-piece, whereas high-frequency murmurs are best heard with a diaphragm.

Sadly, the techniques for recording and analysis of external physiologic tracings, including phonocardiography, have fallen into disuse (Fig. 5). It can be assumed that as the new field of echocardiography exhausts its enormous potential for new development, return to externally measured phys-

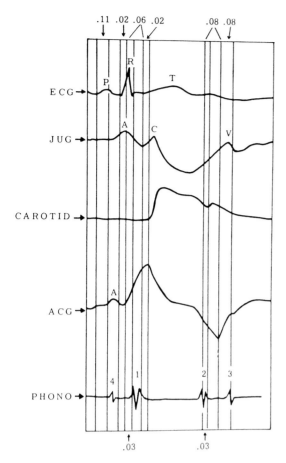

Figure 5. Correlation of the electrocardiogram and various external reference tracings. (From Tavel ME: Clinical Phonocardiography and External Pulse Recording. 2nd ed. Chicago, Year Book Medical Publishers, Inc., 1976, with permission.)

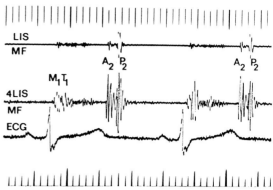

Figure 6. Components of the first and second heart sounds. Because this patient has complete right bundle branch block, the right and left ventricles contract asynchronously and both first and second heart sounds are split.

iologic parameters will take place, perhaps in conjunction with echocardiograms. Fortunately, there is abundant phonocardiographic experience to document the physiologic basis for auscultation. See Leatham or Tavel for classic texts.[3,8]

First Heart Sound. The first heart sound is largely produced by a combination of mitral and tricuspid valve closures. This sound marks the beginning of systole (Fig. 6), and is coincident with the q wave on the electrocardiogram. The fourth heart sound contributes to increased intensity of the first heart sound if the PR interval is short. Alternatively, the first heart sound tends to be of decreased intensity if the PR interval is long. For this reason, the first heart sound commonly varies in intensity when there is complete heart block (Fig. 7). Generally, fourth sounds are dull, low-frequency, indistinct, soft thuds that precede the first sound; they are best heard with the bell. Early systolic clicks may be easily confused with the first sound. A click is a short, snappy, high-frequency, clicking noise (Fig. 8) that follows the first sound

and is best heard with a diaphragm. First sounds are loud in patients with atrial septal defects (Fig. 9), whereas delayed, loud first sounds are heard in patients with mitral stenosis (Fig. 10). The time lapse between the q wave of the electrocardiogram and the first heart sound is proportionate to the severity of the mitral stenosis and can be readily recorded on a phonocardiogram. The longer the Q1-S1 interval, the more severe the mitral stenosis.[8]

Second Heart Sound. In most instances the second heart sound (Fig. 11) is audibly split (at least 0.03 sec) into two components, originating from closure of the aortic and the pulmonary valves. Because of the differences in spread of electrical activity of the ventricles and differences between pressure in the aorta and pulmonary artery, pulmonary valve closure normally is heard after aortic valve closure. Respiration produces different effects on the pulmonary and systemic circulations, inspiration being associated with greater inflow of systemic venous blood into the thorax. The result is variation in splitting of the second heart sound, depending on whether the right ventricle has received more or less blood because of the coincident phase of respiration. The degree of splitting increases with inspiration and decreases, usually to the point of no audible split, on expiration. If no split is observed on inspiration, an explanation is needed. Is there perhaps only one semilunar valve (e.g., pulmonary valve atresia)? Is there pulmonary artery hypertension at systemic levels, or do the ventricles eject simultaneously because of a large ventricular septal defect or single ventricle (Fig. 12)?

With open communication between the atria via an atrial septal defect, the effect of respiration on the splitting of the second heart sound is diminished. Further, the atrial left-to-right shunt greatly increases the right ventricular stroke volume, accentuating the split. Thus, a widely-split second heart sound (> 0.05 sec) that does not audibly vary

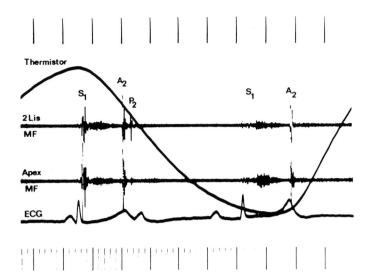

Figure 7. Note that when the PR interval on the electrocardiogram is short the first heart sound (S1) is loud and when the PR interval is long the first heart sound is much less intense. This tracing emphasizes the contribution of the fourth heart sound to the intensity of the first.

with respiration is almost diagnostic of an atrial septal defect (Fig. 13).

The second heart sound may be widely split because of complete right bundle branch block (Fig. 6) or because of pulmonary stenosis. With obstruction of either semilunar valve, the appropriate ventricle may necessarily be delayed in emptying and the second heart sound may be widely split in the case of pulmonary stenosis or less than normally split in patients with aortic stenosis. It is rarely paradoxically split—the aortic closure following the pulmonary closure sound and the split closing with inspiration.

Children less than five years old can rarely control respiration on demand; hence, observing the effects of inspiration and expiration in young children requires some other approach. A useful technique is to listen while the child is lying down and, while continuing to listen, to sit the child upright. The first several beats while sitting will show variation in splitting; if not, the split may be fixed.

The intensities of the aortic and pulmonary closure sound are dependent on the aortic and pulmonary arterial pressure, as well as on the distance from the valve to the chest wall. Consequently, only rarely may systemic or pulmonary hypertension be diagnosed confidently by auscultation. When there is a thin chest and pulmonary hyper-

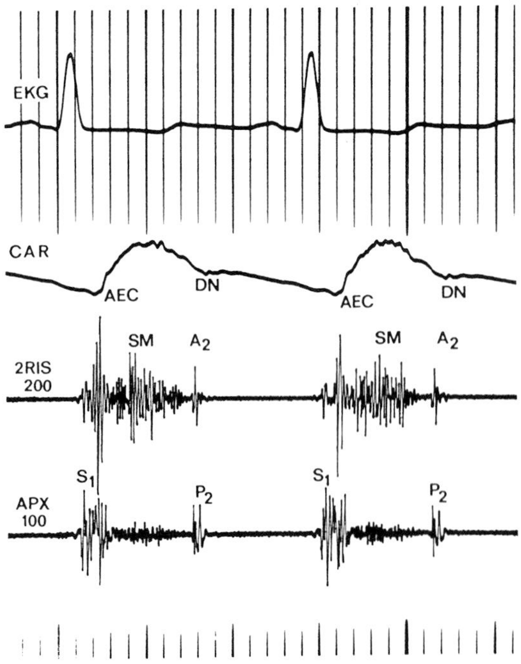

Figure 8. Note the click (AEC) following the second heart sound in this patient with aortic stenosis.

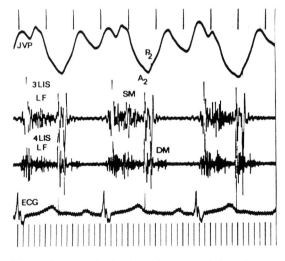

Figure 9. Note the loud first heart sound, best demonstrated at 3LIS, the diamond-shaped systolic murmur, the widely split second heart sound, and the diastolic rumbling murmur best seen at the lower left sternal border.

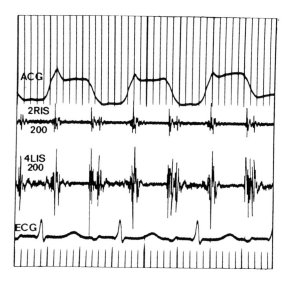

Figure 10. Note the loud and delayed first heart sound in this patient with mitral stenosis.

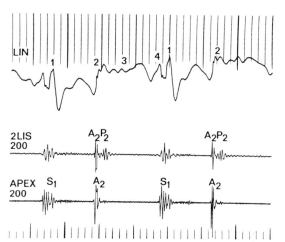

Figure 11. Note the splitting of the second heart sound at the second left intercostal space.

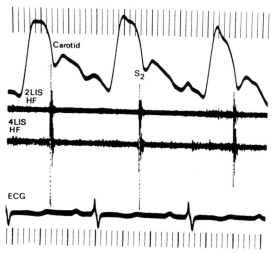

Figure 12. Note the very loud, single, second heart sound, audible at both the upper and lower left sternal borders. This patient has pulmonary hypertensive vascular disease with a ventricular septal defect.

tension, the second heart sound may palpable. Similarly, the second heart sound may be loud when the great vessels are transposed because of the proximity of the aortic valve to the chest wall. When there is low pulmonary artery pressure and low pulmonary flow, the pulmonary component of the second heart sound may be so faint that only aortic closure is audible.

Opening Snap. The opening snap of the mitral valve usually is considered part of the second heart sound. Ordinarily, this sound is not audible, but it may be shown on a phonocardiographic tracing recorded at the apex. When there is mitral stenosis, the opening snap may be accentuated and is often heard at the lower sternal border or apex about 0.08 sec (0.04–0.12) after the second heart sound (Fig. 14).

Third Heart Sound. The third heart sound is heard during diastole in the first period of rapid inflow into the ventricle. In adults an audible third sound signifies cardiac pathology, whereas many normal, thin children have a readily audible third heart sound. The sound, being of low frequency, is best heard with the bell of the stethoscope and in the presence of tachycardia, produces a **gallop rhythm** (Fig. 15). Third heart sounds, in the context of a gallop, are heard in patients with congestive heart failure, particularly those with myocardial disease. With any abnormality accompanied by excessive blood flow across an atrioventricular valve, such as a left-to-right shunt, there is also likely to be an audible third heart sound. If the shunt is large, the third heart sound may be the beginning of a diastolic rumble. As a practical clinical matter, if the third heart sound seems to have more than slight duration, a diastolic rumble should be suspected.

Fourth Heart Sound. A remote, brief thud heard immediately before the first heart sound is usually the fourth heart sound (Fig. 16), and is rarely a normal finding at any age. This sound is associated with atrial contraction, with excessive flow across the atrioventricular valves, and with atrial hypertension (e.g., congestive heart failure). Because fourth heart sounds result from atrial contraction, they are not audible in rhythm abnormalities such as atrial fibrillation or junctional tachycardia.

Clicks. Brief, high-frequency, early systolic clicks are heard in patients with semilunar valvar lesions (pulmonary stenosis, aortic stenosis or bicuspid aortic valve), in those with dilated great arteries, and in those with pulmonary hypertension. If there is no audible click, the diagnosis of

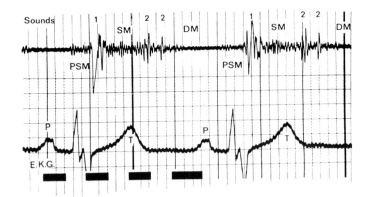

Figure 13. Atrial septal defect. Note the widely split second heart sound, which does not vary with respiration. There is an associated minimal systolic murmur and a minimal presystolic murmur.

valvar pulmonary or aortic stenosis is in doubt. The timing of the click in pulmonary stenosis gives some clue as to the severity of the obstruction; the earlier the click, the more severe the valvar pulmonary stenosis. However, the same relation does not hold for valvar aortic stenosis (Fig. 8).

The presence of a variable **midsystolic click** is characteristic of mitral valve prolapse. Clicks are usually high-frequency sounds, best heard with a diaphragm, and often heard best with the patient standing up or doing the Valsalva manuever. A midsystolic click is **not diagnostic** of mitral valve prolapse; often no organic basis can be found.

Systolic Murmurs. The majority of murmurs occur in systole (Fig. 17). They are associated with passage of blood through a limited orifice (e.g., stenotic semilunar valves, regurgitant atrioventricular valve, ventricular septal defects, or mild obstructions within the pulmonary arteries or the aorta, as in coarctation of the aorta). In general, the intensity of the murmur is proportionate to the pressure loss across the orifice and to the amount of blood involved.

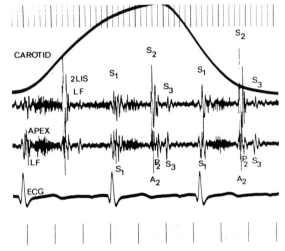

Figure 15. Gallop rhythm consisting of the first sound, second sound and loud third heart sound (S3).

A very loud murmur (grade 5) may produce a thrill (palpable vibrations of the chest wall). The lower the frequency of the murmur, the more likely a thrill will be palpable. For this reason, the murmur of aortic stenosis is often associated with a thrill, whereas the murmur of mitral regurgitation rarely is.

Much has been made of the characteristics of systolic murmurs. Murmurs with maximal intensity in mid systole are described as **ejection murmurs** (diamond-shaped) (Fig. 17), and those with the same intensity throughout systole are **regurgitant murmurs** (pan systolic, plateau type) (Fig. 18). In general, diamond-shaped murmurs are associated with larger pressure gradients (as in aortic stenosis) and plateau murmurs with little or no pressure gradient (as in mitral regurgitation). While these descriptions are correct, their practical value is limited, particularly for small children.

The location of maximal intensity of a systolic murmur may be of diagnostic help. A murmur localized to the left infrascapular area suggests coarctation of the aorta; a murmur at the right lower

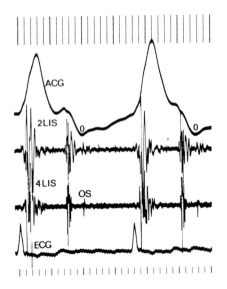

Figure 14. Opening snap (OS) in a patient with mitral stenosis.

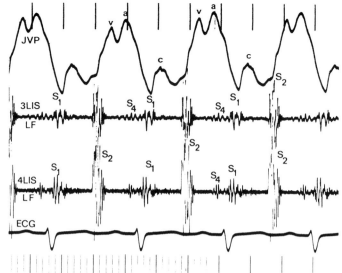

Figure 16. Loud atrial or fourth sound noted at the third and fourth left intercostal spaces.

sternum, increasing with inspiration, indicates tricuspid valve incompetence, and an apical murmur radiating toward the axilla, mitral regurgitation.

Murmurs emanating from normal hearts (functional, innocent murmurs) are discussed in chapter 19.

Diastolic Murmurs. The early diastolic murmur of aortic regurgitation has a high-frequency, blowing quality (Fig. 19). Because of the logarithmic nature of human hearing, the murmur of minimal

aortic regurgitation is detectable almost before aortic regurgitation can be discerned by other means. The murmur is best heard along the left sternal border, with the patient in the sitting position, in expiration, and leaning forward; the diaphragm is used to exclude lower frequency sounds. The murmur of pulmonary regurgitation in patients with normal pulmonary arterial pressure is of low frequency and is heard best in the pulmonary area or the lower left sternal border. Confusion between

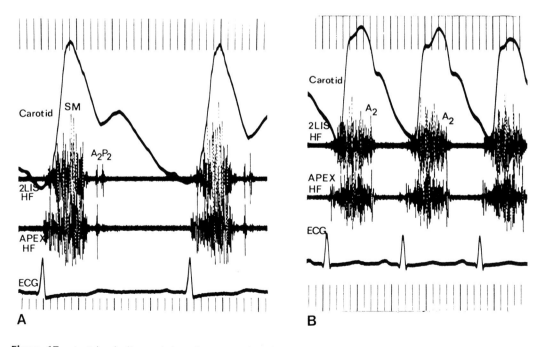

Figure 17. **A,** A loud, diamond-shaped murmur of aortic stenosis. **B,** A loud, diamond-shaped murmur of pulmonary stenosis. Note that the murmur of pulmonary stenosis extends through to the second component of the second heart sound (pulmonary closure), whereas the aortic murmur ends before aortic closure.

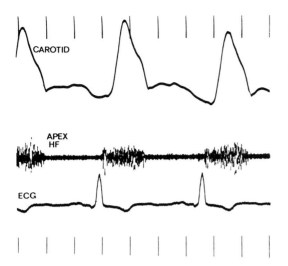

Figure 18. A plateau-shaped, high-frequency murmur of mitral regurgitation. Note that the murmur extends from the first to the second heart sounds.

the murmurs of aortic and pulmonary regurgitation may arise in patients with high pulmonary arterial pressure in whom the long, loud, early diastolic murmur may sound like that of aortic regurgitation. The low-frequency murmur of pulmonary regurgitation is most often heard after pulmonary outflow surgery, whereas aortic regurgitation is most often a natural phenomenon. Furthermore, a wide pulse pressure may help to identify the presence of aortic regurgitation.

While early diastolic blowing murmurs have the highest frequencies encountered in clinical auscultation, mid and late diastolic rumbles have the lowest—so low as to be occasionally palpable but inaudible. Rumbles are mostly heard at the lower sternal border and apex, and occur at the time of maximal diastolic inflow into either of the ventricles. These murmurs are best heard with the bell held lightly against the chest. Excess inflow through a normal atrioventricular valve, as in left-to-right shunts (Fig. 20), or pathologic narrowing of the inflow orifice, can result in a diastolic rumble. The timing of diastolic rumbles in children is almost invariably at the first period of rapid inflow, immediately following the third heart sound. A severely obstructed mitral valve may produce a rumble extending into presystole, with accentuation during the second period of rapid inflow during atrial contraction.

Continuous Murmurs. A murmur extending from systole into diastole, through the second heart sound (without a hiatus) and sometimes even throughout the entire cardiac cycle, is described as continuous (Fig. 21). Generally it results from communication between two blood vessels with a continuous, although possibly variable, pressure difference. Connections between arteries and veins, between the systemic arterial and pulmo-

nary circulation, or between systemic arteries and cardiac chambers can result in continuous murmurs. The classic example is patent ductus arteriosus, heard best at the second left interspace. Other common causes include: excessive bronchial collateral circulation (often heard over the back), coronary arteriovenous fistula (often at the third or fourth interspace to the right or left of the sternum), and systemic arteriovenous fistula (anywhere over the body). The intensity of the murmurs is an indication of the pressure difference between the two structures as well as the amount of blood being shunted. Consequently, some murmurs are loudest during systole and diminish in diastole as the pressure differences become smaller. In children with patent ductus arteriosus and pulmonary hypertension, the differences in pressure during diastole may be sufficiently small that the murmur becomes inaudible in early or mid diastole. It follows that the point of maximal intensity of the murmur is at about the second heart sound, giving a crescendo-decrescendo quality. This is useful in recognizing patients who have systolic murmurs by reason of valvar stenosis or ventricular defects associated with pulmonary or aortic regurgitation. In this case (to-and-fro murmur) the systolic component may appear to extend into diastole, but careful auscultation will reveal that the peak intensity of the systolic murmur is before the second heart sound. Because maximal flow occurs during diastole in a coronary arterial fistula, this variety of continuous murmur has its peak intensity in diastole.

Perhaps the most common continuous murmur encountered in everyday practice is the venous hum, a continuous but inconsistent, high-frequency murmur that varies with position and is heard maximally just beneath the clavicle or in the neck (Fig. 22) (see ch. 19).

Squeaks and Honks. Rarely, peculiar squeaking or honking noises are encountered. Often these are related to the cardiac cycle, although not necessarily. These sounds vary from time to time in intensity and presence, and in the absence of other findings have little significance.

Lungs

The lungs, like the heart, should be examined by inspection, percussion, and auscultation of the chest. Inspection gives invaluable information about respiratory rate and the visible effort of breathing. The sensation of shortness of breath or dyspnea can sometimes be deduced in small infants; on the other hand, more often, tachypnea is not associated with recognizable distress. Dyspnea or tachypnea is frequently the clue to excessive pulmonary blood flow or an elevated capillary wedge pressure. Auscultation not only reveals the wheezes or rales characteristic of infection or con-

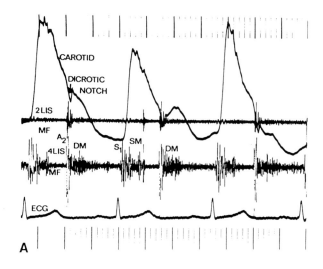

Figure 19. The murmurs of **(A)** aortic regurgitation and **(B)** pulmonary regurgitation are high-frequency, decrescendo murmurs immediately following the respective valve closures.

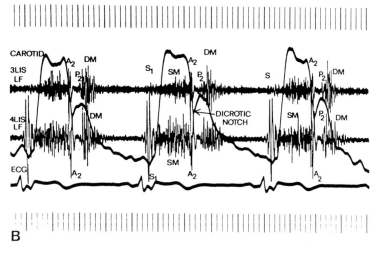

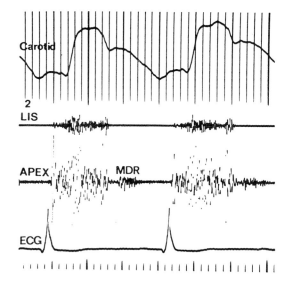

Figure 20. Note the low-frequency, mid-diastolic rumble at the apex in this patient with ventricular septal defect.

gestion, but also give basic information as to whether too little, sufficient, or too much air is being exchanged. An old pediatric technique that gives helpful information about tidal volume consists of holding the stethoscope in front of the baby's mouth.

Liver

One evidence of elevated central venous pressure is the presence of hepatomegaly. A liver edge that is more than 3 cm below the right costal margin is abnormal. Apparent hepatomegaly often results from respiratory distress and thereby a lower diaphragm. Furthermore, most normal infants have a palpable but not enlarged liver. Hepatomegaly as a sign of congestive heart failure has been overemphasized; tachypnea is a much more important and reliable indicator of congestive failure in pediatric cardiology. Still, daily observation as to the size of the liver is one of the guides in the estimation of progress in controlling congestive failure in infants.

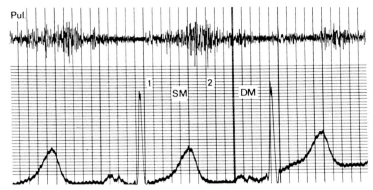

Figure 21. Continuous murmur of patent ductus arteriosus. Note the presence of the murmur in all phases of the cardiac cycle. The murmur is loudest at the second heart sound.

Generally, if there is abnormal hepatomegaly in an older child, the neck veins will also be visible when the child is in the sitting position. A pulsatile liver may easily be felt in patients who have tricuspid regurgitation or critical pulmonic stenosis with an intact ventricular septum (see Fig. 4, p. 309).

Spleen

Although many young children normally have a palpable spleen, definite splenomegaly is one of the cornerstones in the diagnosis of bacterial endocarditis. By contrast, an enlarged spleen is seldom caused by congestive failure. Abdominal situs inversus, with or without thoracic situs inversus, may suggest associated congenital heart disease.

ROUTINE LABORATORY TESTS

Routine laboratory tests performed on all children, including those with cardiac disease, will not be described here in detail. However, their par-

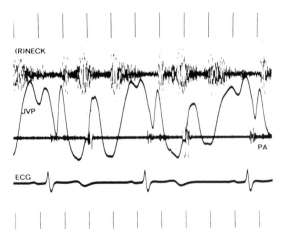

Figure 22. Venous hum in the right side of the neck. Note the continuous high-frequency sounds. These murmurs are commonly heard over the upper chest, particularly when the patient is sitting.

ticular applicability to children with heart disease should be mentioned briefly.

Urinalysis

Patients with congestive failure, as well as those with longstanding arterial unsaturation, may have albuminuria, a urine of high specific gravity, and mild hematuria. Hematuria is also found in patients with bacterial endocarditis.

Complete Blood Cell Count

Leukocytosis of moderate degree may be present in congestive failure, bacterial endocarditis, and acute rheumatic fever, with or without failure. Thrombocytopenia is common in adolescents with severe cyanosis.

Hematocrit

In following any patient with congenital heart disease, it is important to observe the hematocrit. Among those who are cyanotic the hematocrit is largely reflective of the prevailing arterial oxygen content in the blood during the course of the day. The hemoglobin level may serve the same purpose. Cyanotic children with low hematocrit may be in particular difficulty. They may exhibit hypoxic spells more readily than if the oxygen-carrying capacity were normal. While it is important that such children receive iron therapy, it is equally important that the course of response to iron therapy be monitored carefully, because the hematocrit may be driven quickly to undesirably high levels, causing high blood viscosity.

The modern method of measuring hematocrit (densitometry) gives somewhat erroneous results in the high ranges. The more precise centrifugation measurement is used for decisions about red cell pheresis.

Transcutaneous Oxygen

In following children with cyanosis, it is useful to have some idea of arterial oxygen saturation. Often, comparative measurements at rest and on exercise are useful. Transcutaneous pO_2, although somewhat unstable and not perfect, gives a reasonable estimate of the percentage of oxygen saturation. Monitoring the percentage of oxygen saturation by transcutaneous techniques is helpful for following cyanotic neonates being maintained on prostaglandin E1.

Blood Gases

Arterial pH, pO_2, and pCO_2 determinations obtained from umbilical catheter samples are indispensable in the management of newborns with cardiorespiratory distress. No baby should be catheterized without the monitoring of blood gases, and the postoperative care of patients who have undergone cardiopulmonary bypass is inadequate unless careful attention is paid to these measurements.

In some situations, particularly in cyanotic newborns, measurements of blood gases may be especially useful. The discovery of acidosis or retained carbon dioxide requires an explanation.

Comparison of right arm or right temporal arterial blood gases with those obtained from the umbilical artery is a useful test. If there is notable difference in the partial pressure of oxygen in these two areas, it can be concluded that there is a right-to-left shunt through a patent ductus arteriosus.

Having the patient breathe 100% oxygen for 10 minutes while measuring arterial pO_2 can be revealing. Any cyanotic child who can raise his pO_2 to levels higher than 200 torr probably has a primary pulmonary problem (including pulmonary edema) that accounts for the low arterial oxygen saturation. Individuals who cannot raise their pO_2 higher than 100 torr while breathing 100% oxygen for 10 minutes probably have congenital heart disease with a right-to-left shunt, particularly if there is no obvious lung disease apparent on a chest x-ray.

Blood Chemistries

It is useful to measure a variety of electrolyte, coagulation, and metabolic products in managing patients with cardiac problems. The blood levels of virtually all cardioactive drugs can be measured as needed.

Blood Cultures

A positive blood culture is an integral, although not indispensable, part of diagnosis of bacterial endocarditis (see ch. 26).

CHEST X-RAY

A chest radiograph provides an impression of the overall cardiac size and an estimation of the pulmonary blood flow. If it were for these features alone, echocardiograms would be more revealing without the necessity for exposure to X-radiation. The major value of the chest radiograph is as a screen for ancillary observations such as: abnormal vessels, right aortic arch, scimitar syndrome, aberrant pulmonary vessels, abnormal position of bronchi, vascular rings, or associated pulmonary abnormalities (e.g., pneumonia, atelectasis, or emphysema).

RADIOISOTOPE SCANS

Radioisotopes provide information not otherwise readily available in some children with heart disease. The techniques vary. Either the initial bolus of radioisotope is followed through the intrathoracic circulation (first pass) or the patient is observed after the radioisotope has been distributed throughout the circulation (equilibrium).

A first-pass scan is a crude angiogram; gross anatomic abnormalities can be identified. Radionuclear perfusion scans to determine relative blood flow to different parts of the lung are valuable in patients with congenitally or iatrogenically distorted pulmonary arteries. The decay in pulmonary radiation counts in patients with suspected left-to-right shunts is proportionate to the size of the shunt. Shunts with pulmonary blood flow 1.5 times larger than the systemic flow can be confidently identified by this technique.[5]

The relative blood flow to the right versus the left lung can be estimated from the relative number of counts of radioactivity over each lung after injection of the isotope. This technique is particularly useful in assessing the possibility of success preoperatively for patients who might be candidates for a Fontan operation but who might have major blood flow to only one lung. It is also useful in assessing pulmonary blood flow preoperatively and postoperatively in patients with tetralogy of Fallot and pulmonary atresia, with some blood supply to the lungs via collateral vessels or by operative shunts.

When there is concern about localized myocardial ischemia or even infarction, thallium scans with the patient at rest and during exercise may help to demarcate the area and therefore the extent of injury. With increasing interest in arterial switching operations for transposition of the great arteries and the consequent necessity to manipulate coronaries, thallium scans have become a useful tool in determining success.

EXERCISE TESTING

As a matter of practice, most cardiac observations are made with the patient in a resting, relaxed state. Further observations during graded physical exercise add information about the patient's cardiovascular reserve (see ch. 16).

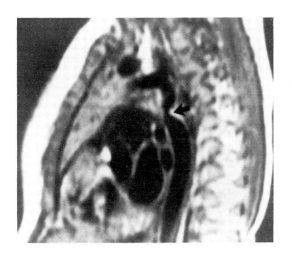

Figure 23.   Note the well-demonstrated coarctation of the aorta.

MAGNETIC RESONANCE IMAGING

Magnetic resonance imaging (Fig. 23) has yet to realize its potential in imaging vascular structures. The necessity to stop the motion of the beating heart presents a problem that may be managed by gating.

COMPUTERIZED TOMOGRAPHY

The problems of motion pose a problem for the routine use of computerized tomography in pediatric cardiology.

REFERENCES

1. Fyler DC, Buckley LP, Hellenbrand WE, et al: Report of the New England Regional Infant Cardiac Program. Pediatrics 65(Suppl):376:460, 1980.
2. Greenwood RD, Rosenthal LA, Parisi L, et al: Extracardiac abnormalities in infants with congenital heart disease. Pediatrics 55:485–492, 1975.
3. Leatham A: Auscultation of the Heart and Phonocardiography. New York, Churchill Livingstone, 1975.
4. Lewis T: Diseases of the Heart Described for Practitioners and Students, 2nd ed. New York, Macmillan, 1937.
5. Maltz DL, Treves S: Quantitative radionuclide angiocardiography: determination of $Q_p:Q_s$ in children. Circulation 47:1049–1056, 1973.
6. Rappaport MB, Sprague HB: Physiologic and physical laws that govern auscultation, and their clinical application. Am Heart J 21:257–318, 1941.
7. Roth A, Rosenthal A, Hall JE, et al: Scoliosis in congenital heart disease. Clin Orthop Rel Res 93:95–102, 1973.
8. Tavel ME: Clinical Phonocardiography and External Pulse Recording. 2nd ed. Chicago, Year Book Medical Publishers, Inc., 1976.
9. Wiggers CJ: Circulatory Dynamics: Physiologic Studies. New York, Grune & Stratton, 1952.

Chapter 12

ELECTROCARDIOGRAPHY AND INTRODUCTION TO ELECTROPHYSIOLOGIC TECHNIQUES

Edward P. Walsh, M.D.

Of the benefits which graphic methods have conferred upon practical medicine, it is my desire to speak but briefly. These records have placed the entire question of irregular or disordered mechanism of the human heart upon a rational basis . . . , they have influenced prognosis . . . , they have potentially abolished the promiscuous administration of certain cardiac poisons, and have clearly shown the line which therapy should follow.

Thomas Lewis, 1924[12]

Electrocardiography, accurate physical examination, and radiology form the tripod on which rests the clinical diagnosis in pediatric cardiology. Omission of, unfamiliarity with or misinterpretation of any of these three tools spells disaster.

Alexander S. Nadas, 1957[14]

The graphic registration of cardiac electrical activity continues to be an invaluable tool in pediatric cardiology. The optimism of Sir Thomas Lewis and the cautions of Doctor Nadas remain valid even today. However, the study of electrophysiologic phenomenon is no longer limited to recordings from the body surface alone. To better appreciate the strengths and limitations of the electrocardiogram, it is helpful first to review some basic principles of cellular depolarization and alternate recording techniques.

BASIC ELECTROPHYSIOLOGY

Cellular Action Potential

The electrocardiogram is several steps removed from electrical activity at the cellular level, but the two are intimately related. Cellular events must be recorded using microelectrodes equipped with tips that are small enough to pierce individual cell membranes. When an electrode invades a normal cardiac cell, it encounters a field of net negative charge relative to the outside environment. This is the **diastolic potential** or **resting potential** of the cell, which is maintained by the selective permeability of the membrane to extracellular ions, as well as the operation of the $Na^+ - K^+$ pump. If the cell interior becomes slightly depolarized (i.e., less negatively charged), it may reach a critical value referred to as the **threshold potential**. At this point, a dramatic change in membrane permeability will allow a sudden flood of positive ions to enter the cell, and an **action potential** develops.

Two distinct types of cardiac action potentials have been observed. The most common, known as the "fast-response" or "sodium channel" type, occurs in cells of atrial muscle, ventricular muscle, His-Purkinje cells, and probably in accessory atrioventricular conduction tissue (such as the Kent bundle in the Wolff-Parkinson-White syndrome). These cells generally register a resting potential at around -90 mV, and rely upon sodium ions as the positive charge carrier for their initial rapid phase 0 depolarization (Fig. 1).

A second variety of action potential occurs predominantly in cells of the sinus node and the AV node; it is referred to as the "slow response" or

Fast–Response or Sodium–Channel Action Potential

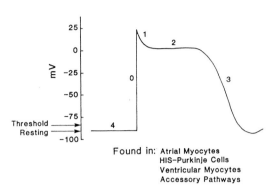

Figure 1. Diagrammatic action potential of a "fast response" cardiac cell. Depolarization during phase 0 is caused by rapid sodium influx.

Slow–Response or Calcium–Channel Action Potential

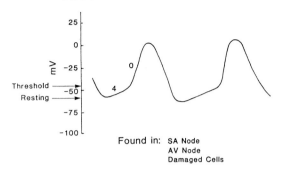

Found in: SA Node
AV Node
Damaged Cells

Figure 2. Diagrammatic action potential of a "slow response" cardiac cell. Depolarization during phase 0 is due to calcium and sodium influx. Note gradual spontaneous depolarization during phase 4 which imparts the property of automaticity to such cells.

"calcium channel" type. It is distinguished by a very blunt contour for the initial phase 0 upstroke, and utilizes calcium (along with some sodium) to provide the inward ionic current for depolarization (Fig. 2). An important feature of many slow response cells is the property of **automaticity**. Upward drift of the diastolic potential during phase 4 enables the cell to reach threshold of its own accord and thereby act as a natural pacemaker for the heart (Fig. 3). Likewise, some fast response cells may be capable of spontaneous automaticity but at much slower rates.

Cell-to-Cell Conduction

When a cardiac cell depolarizes, it usually stimulates neighboring tissue in such a way that the activation sequence is transmitted from cell to cell throughout the heart. For this process to repeat smoothly, cells must have sufficient time to recover between stimuli. If the initiating impulse is **pre-**

mature, the cells may not be prepared, or may be only partially prepared, for reactivation. The time needed to recover from a prior stimulus is known as the **refractory period** and usually lasts until cells have nearly completed their repolarization process (late phase 3 or early phase 4). During the **absolute refractory period** a cell does not respond in any way to a new impulse, regardless of the strength of the stimulus. During the **relative refractory period** a cell may respond occasionally, but only if the premature stimulus is sufficiently strong. During the early phase of the relative refractory period, a cell sometimes responds to a premature stimulus with an incomplete and low-amplitude action potential that is too weak to propagate any further to cells downstream. This is designated the **effective refractory period** (ERP). The distinction between absolute and effective refractoriness is subtle but important, because the ERP may be measured in the intact heart with clinical electrophysiologic techniques. For practical purposes, the **effective**

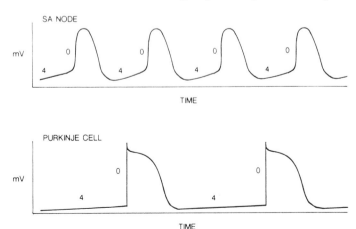

Figure 3. Comparison of the rate for spontaneous automaticity of a slow response cell (e.g., sinus node) with that of a fast response cell (e.g., Purkinje cell); differences are due to the slope of phase 4 depolarization.

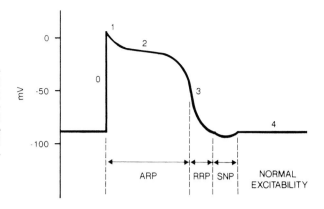

Figure 4. Diagrammatic fast response action potential showing the time course of refractoriness and excitability. During the absolute refractory period (ARP), the cell cannot be reexcited regardless of stimulus strength. During the relative refractory period (RRP), only large amplitude stimuli can reexcite the cell. Some cells may display a supernormal period (SNP) at the end of phase 3, which permits excitability with low-amplitude stimuli.

and **absolute** refractory periods can be considered similar (Fig. 4).

Conduction Through the Intact Heart

A normal heart beat begins with the spontaneous depolarization of a cell in the sinus node, located at the junction of the superior vena cava and right atrium, in the area of the sulcus terminalis. This event then activates adjacent atrial muscle cells so that a wave of depolarization spreads out from high in the right atrium like ripples in a pond. The wave front reaches the lower part of the right atrium after about 30 msec and finishes at the lateral part of the left atrium after approximately 80 msec. The electrical activity from sinus node depolarization is too small to be recorded from the body surface, but atrial muscle cell depolarization is clearly registered as the P wave on the electrocardiogram. The P wave corresponds to phase 0 of the action potentials from individual atrial myocytes and reflects the leading edge of the depolarization wave front as it travels from cell to cell. Once all atrial cells have undergone their initial rapid depolarization and entered the phase 2 plateau, the P wave is complete. Phase 3 repolarization of atrial cells causes a very small deflection on the surface electrocardiogram, referred to as the T_A wave. This wave form is rarely seen because it is usually obscured by the QRS complex, but under special conditions (such as heart block) the atrial repolarization wave may be appreciated (Fig. 5).

As the atrial activation wave front passes through

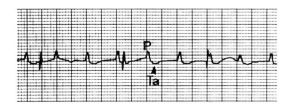

Figure 5. The Ta wave of atrial repolarization clearly seen in a patient with complete heart block and atrial enlargement.

the lower right atrium, depolarization of the AV node is initiated. This node is a complete interface consisting predominantly of slow-response cells, located in an anatomic region referred to as the triangle of Koch (Fig. 6). Conduction velocity within the AV node is relatively slow, and it varies according to the timing of atrial impulses. Premature beats or accelerated atrial rhythms exaggerate nodal delay in a gradual and progressive manner, which ultimately can produce the sterotypic sequence of conduction block known as Wenckebach periodicity (Fig. 7). This pattern (often described as **decremental conduction**) is rather specific to slow-response cells.

Unfortunately, electrical activity within the AV node is not directly registered on the surface electrocardiogram. One must rely on upstream events (P wave) and downstream events (ventricular activation) as indirect measures of the process. On the surface electrocardiogram, the P-R interval provides an estimation of AV node conduction, but there is much more to this interval than AV node activity alone. To be precise, the P-R interval includes conduction times: (1) from high to low in the right atrium, (2) in the AV node proper, and (3) in the His-Purkinje system. To dissect the P-R interval into these individual components, a multielectrode intracardiac catheter is positioned just across the tricuspid valve to straddle an area near the bundle of His. This recording reveals: (1) localized low-right atrial activation, (2) a small deflection from the common bundle of His, and (3) localized right ventricular activation. An index of true AV node conduction time is obtained by measuring the interval between low right atrial depolarization and the initial depolarization of the bundle of His, the so-called **A-H interval** (Fig. 8).

Beyond the AV node, the excitation process enters the common bundle of His, which crosses the A-V junction on the right ventricular side, just beneath the membranous septum (Fig. 6). Cells of the His-Purkinje system have fast response action potentials and, generally, rapid conduction velocity. The propagated impulse traverses the common bundle of His, splits into right and left bundle

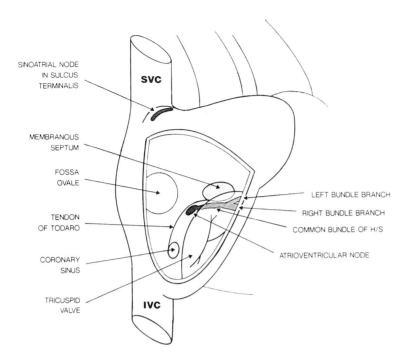

Figure 6. Schematic view of the interior of the right atrium emphasizing the landmarks of the normal conduction system. The AV node lies within the "triangle of Koch." The apex of this triangle lies at the membranous septum, with its long sides marked by the tendon of Todaro and the rim of the tricuspid valve; its base is at the coronary sinus.

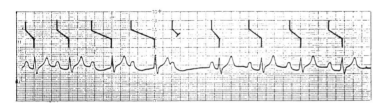

Figure 7. Lead II rhythm strip and laddergram demonstrating AV nodal Wenckebach phenomenon.

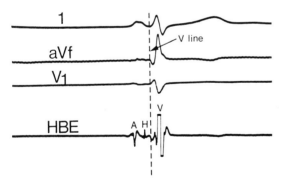

Figure 8. Simultaneous surface ECG leads and the His bundle electrogram (HBE). The A-H interval is measured from the beginning of the "A" deflection to the beginning of the "H" deflection. The H-V interval is measured from the beginning of the "H" deflection to the "V line," which marks the earliest ventricular activation in any lead.

branches, and finally exits from the tips of the terminal Purkinje fibers to begin activation of ventricular myocytes, all in about 40 msec. On the intracardiac His recording, the time from the initial His deflection to the beginning of ventricular activation (**H-V interval**) is an accurate measure of His-Purkinje conduction time (Fig. 8).

Conduction along the His-Purkinje network occurs as the cells are depolarizing (i.e., during phase 0). Their repolarization begins long after the excitation wave front has passed on to lower portions of the heart. Indeed, final repolarization of His-Purkinje cells tends to be one of the last electrical events during a cardiac cycle and is thought to be responsible for the small terminal U wave on the surface electrocardiogram.

As the excitation wave front leaves the His-Purkinje system, phase 0 of ventricular myocyte depolarization begins. The His-Purkinje system is highly arborized in its terminal portion, and these multiple exit sites promote depolarization of several different ventricular regions at one time, a process that is further complicated by the heart's three-dimensional geometry. To better visualize ventricular activation, it is useful to divide events into small time components and examine the order of regional depolarization. A simplification of the sequence is shown in Figure 9, beginning with left-to-right septal activation, followed by activation of the left and right apex, the endocardium of the right and left ventricular free walls, the free wall epicardium, the base of the left ventricle and, finally, the right ventricular outflow tract. The ad-

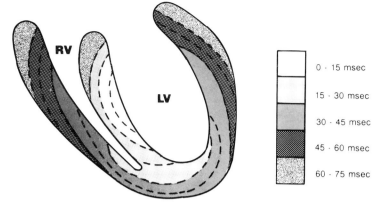

Figure 9. Simplification of ventricular activation sequence showing a rough approximation of the time course for regional depolarization.

	0 - 15 msec
	15 - 30 msec
	30 - 45 msec
	45 - 60 msec
	60 - 75 msec

vancing wave front in each region generates a signal that can be recorded from the body surface as the QRS complex.

The QRS is complete once all ventricular cells have depolarized (usually within 90 msec). The S-T segment is registered while the cells remain at the phase 2 plateau. At the onset of phase 3 repolarization, inscription of the T wave begins. Repolarization is less homogeneous than depolarization; hence, there is a rather protracted duration for the T wave. Additionally, the repolarization sequence is just the opposite of depolarization and appears to follow the reverse direction of epicardium toward endocardium.

When all ventricular myocytes are back to phase 4, the T wave is complete. After the late Purkinje cell repolarization and registration of the U wave, the heart has completed its electrical cycle and all cells remain at phase 4 until a single cell once again generates a new action potential to reinitiate the process.

Graphic Recording of Cardiac Electrical Activity

It should be apparent from the preceding discussion that the signal registered on the surface electrocardiogram occurs during abrupt changes in cellular conditions: the P wave and QRS complex mark the acute transition from resting potential to the fully depolarized state, with the T_A, T, and U waves marking repolarization back to the base line. Indeed, when all cells in a given cardiac chamber are either fully depolarized (phases 1 and 2) or fully repolarized (phase 4), no signal is recorded from the body surface even though intracellular conditions differ dramatically. Thus, what is measured with an electrocardiogram is not individual cellular voltages, but rather the current that arises at the boundary between depolarized and repolarized cells as activation or deactivation wave fronts move through a cardiac chamber. This boundary acts as a dipole, which generates current because of the presence of opposing charges in front and behind.

Movement relative to the electrode produces the electrocardiographic signal (Fig. 10). During depolarization the leading edge of the activation wave front is charged positive and the trailing edge negative. Movement toward a recording electrode results in an upward deflection on the electrocardiogram, and movement away results in a downward deflection. Repolarization wave fronts have a negative leading edge and generate signals of opposite direction. In addition to direction, electrocardiographic signals can be further qualified by amplitude, which is largely proportional to the muscle mass transmitting the wave front. Thus, these electrical events can be described as vectors.

The simplest example of body surface recording is the cycle of atrial activation, recorded in Figure 11 by three hypothetical leads on the left arm, right arm, and leg. The normal atrial depolarization wave front advances from high in the right atrium, resulting in a mean vector that inscribes positive P waves in the left arm and leg leads, with a negative deflection in the right arm lead. Repolarization follows in the same path after a short isoelectric period, generating a T_A wave of opposite polarity.

The ventricular cycle results in a more complex series of vectors (Fig. 12). The process begins with septal activation, which generates a small negative deflection (Q wave) in the left arm lead and a small positive deflection in the leg lead. The right arm, being nearly at right angles to this vector, records little activity at this point. With left apex depolarization, the vector abruptly shifts leftward and inferior, beginning the inscription of an R wave in the left arm, further increasing the positive amplitude of the leg recording, with a negative deflection now appearing in the right arm lead. As events proceed to the ventricular free walls, there is competition between the simultaneous vectors of left- and right-sided depolarization. In a normal heart, the left ventricle wins out by virtue of its larger muscle mass, and the resultant "net" vector continues leftward. Final depolarization of the left base and right outflow tract generates superior and

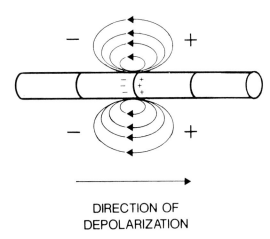

DIRECTION OF
DEPOLARIZATION

Figure 10. The dipole created by advancing depolarization along a series of cardiac cells generates fields of extracellular current.

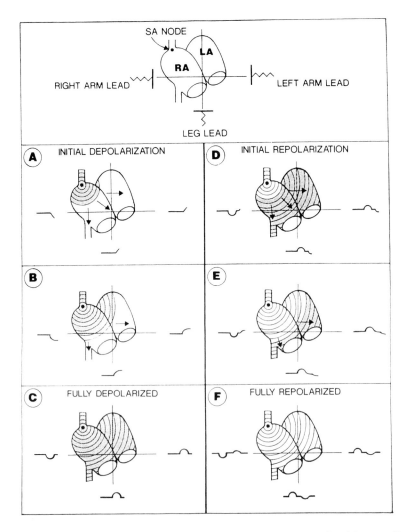

Figure 11. Genesis of the P wave and Ta wave. **A,** Onset of the P wave. **C,** Completed P wave. **D,** Onset of Ta. **F,** Completion of P-Ta.

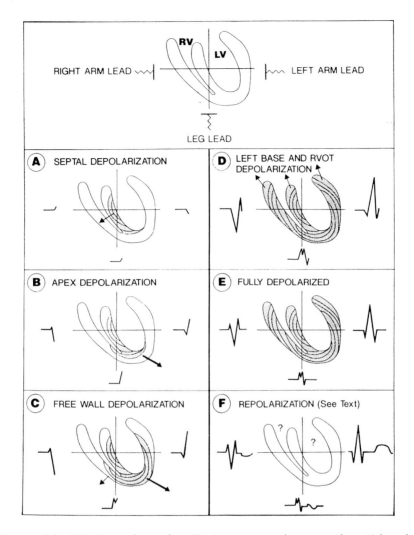

Figure 12. Genesis of the QRS. Ventricular repolarization is a more complex process than atrial repolarization (see p. 119). **A–E,** The spread of ventricular depolarization (QRS). **F,** Repolarization (T wave).

rightward vectors, causing inscription of a negative S wave in the left arm and leg leads, with a positive deflection in the right arm lead.

An alternate method for graphic display of ventricular depolarization is the technique of vectorcardiography. This system utilizes specially positioned body surface leads and arranges the data in a format that involves the principle of vector addition. The QRS is divided into small time segments and the "net instantaneous" vector during each time frame is calculated and plotted as shown in Figure 13. The vectorcardiogram is slightly more quantitative than the standard QRS, but measures essentially an identical body surface phenomenon.

The repolarization process of the ventricle is even more complex. Unlike the atrium, the vectors of repolarization do not exactly retrace the same steps as depolarization, because ventricular myocytes generally repolarize in an epicardial to endocardial direction. For this reason, the direction

of the T wave is similar to that of the QRS, and not reversed as is the case with atrial tissue or simple experimental models of isolated cardiac muscle fibers (Fig. 14).

The principles of cardiac excitation and recording are summarized in Figure 15. The interested reader is referred to several excellent reviews[7,8,15,20] for further details of these topics.

THE SURFACE ELECTROCARDIOGRAM

This section reviews the basics of interpreting the body surface electrocardiogram as they apply to pediatric heart disease. Although the topic has occupied entire textbooks,[7,15] this discussion is necessarily limited to those highlights that could be of most use to the novice. Although it must be admitted today that detailed cardiac anatomy and physiology are best determined by echocardiog-

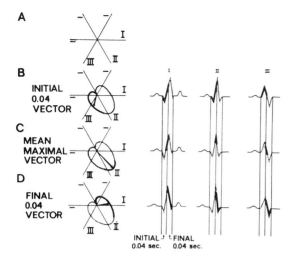

Figure 13. Relationship of the surface electrocardiogram to the frontal plane vectorcardiogram. The QRS loop can be described by its rotation (clockwise or counterclockwise) and its maximum spatial vector [i.e., the vector with the largest amplitude (arrow) at any point in the loop].

raphy or catheterization, the electrocardiogram is not (and never will be) obsolete. It remains the quickest, safest, and least expensive cardiac diagnostic tool and is quite sensitive in registering arrhythmias, conduction defects, and many varieties of cardiac chamber enlargement. With proper interpretation, the electrocardiogram also offers an accurate reflection of cardiac position or myocardial injury.

Lead Systems and Recording Technique

The standard electrocardiogram evolved from a three-lead system, introduced by Einthoven, to a 15-lead tracing in current use for pediatric recording. The two major lead groupings include the limb or "frontal plane" leads and the precordial or "horizontal plane" leads. The limb leads can be further divided into Einthoven's standard bipolar system (I, II, and III) and an "augmented" variation of Wilson's unipolar lead system (aV_R, aV_L, and aV_F). Einthoven's leads record potentials between electrode pairs: left arm (positive) to right arm (negative) = lead I; left leg (positive) to right arm (negative) = lead II; and left leg (positive) to left arm (negative) = lead III. Wilson's leads record from a single limb in reference to a zero potential central terminal: right arm (positive) = aV_R; left arm (positive) = aV_L; and left leg (positive) = aV_F. A wave front moving toward the positive terminal of one of these leads registers a positive deflection on the electrocardiogram. These leads form a compass around the frontal plane, which is divided into 360°, with lead positions and degree coordinates as shown in Figure 16.

The precordial leads (V_{4R} through V_7) view the electrical activity in the horizontal plane. They are all unipolar (positive) and are referenced to a zero potential central terminal, but without augmentation. Electrode placement is slightly modified in pediatric studies to obtain lead positions far out on the right side of the chest and laterally on the left side of the chest (Fig. 17).

Routine recordings are made with a chart paper

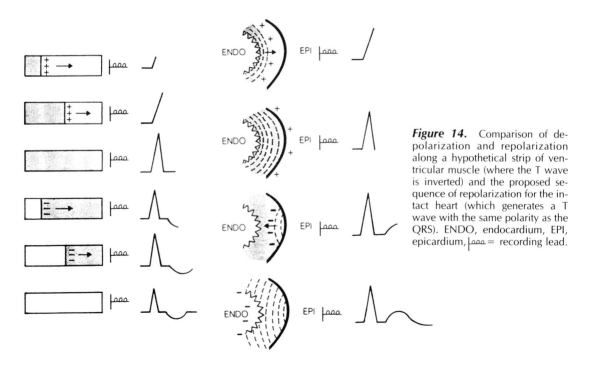

Figure 14. Comparison of depolarization and repolarization along a hypothetical strip of ventricular muscle (where the T wave is inverted) and the proposed sequence of repolarization for the intact heart (which generates a T wave with the same polarity as the QRS). ENDO, endocardium, EPI, epicardium, ∫₀₀₀ = recording lead.

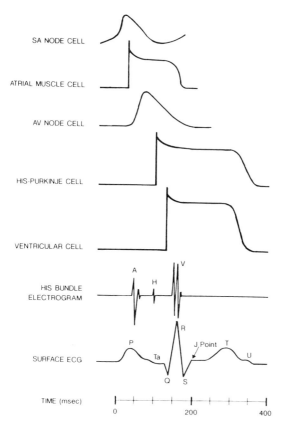

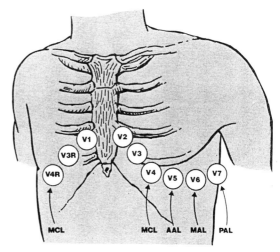

Figure 17. Location of the precordial leads for pediatric ECG recording. MCL, midclavicular line; AAL, anterior axillary line; MAL, midaxillary line; PAL, posterior axillary line.

Figure 15. Comparative time course of cellular action potentials, intracardiac electrograms from the bundle of His, and the surface ECG.

speed of 25 mm/sec and standardized with an amplitude response of 1 mV/cm. The amplitude calibration mark must be clearly documented and recorder sensitivity should be reduced on one-half or one-fourth standard if a QRS overshoots the width of the paper.

The Normal Electrocardiogram

The normal values referred to in this discussion have been drawn from our experience at The Children's Hospital in Boston and the publications of Davignon,[4] Garson,[7] and Fisch.[6] Data are abstracted for easy reference in Table 1. The electrocardiogram should be read in a systematic fashion, beginning with measurements of axes and intervals, and followed by wave-form analysis, all of which must be synthesized into a final impression based on history and physical examination.

Axes

The electrical axis refers to the predominant direction (or "mean" vector) of a wave form in the frontal plane. By identifying the limb lead with the largest positive deflection for the wave form in question, and remembering the coordinates for this lead on the frontal compass face, one can assign a value in "degrees" for the mean axis. The easiest example involves the P wave. Because normal atrial activation begins near the sinus node and spreads through the atrium high-to-low and right-to-left, the wave front of depolarization flows toward the southeast quadrant of the frontal plane. Lead II (+60°) best records this area and usually registers the largest positive P wave. A lead from the northwest quadrant (aV$_R$) simultaneously registers a deep negative P wave. Leads that record at nearly right angles to the P wave vector (aV$_L$

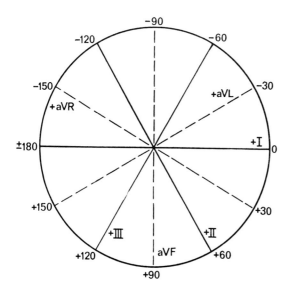

Figure 16. Degree coordinates and positive pole of the limb ECG leads in the frontal plane.

Table 1. Normal Range and Mean Values for Selected ECG Measurements in Children*

	0–7 days	1 wk–1 mo	1 mo–6 mos	6 mos–1 yr	1 yr–5 yrs	5–10 yrs	10–15 yrs	>15 yrs
Heart rate/min	90–160 (125)	100–175 (140)	110–180 (145)	100–180 (130)	70–160 (110)	65–140 (100)	60–130 (90)	60–100 (80)
P–R (sec) lead II		.08–.15 (.10)			.08–.15 (.12)		.09–.18 (.14)	.10–.20 (.16)
QRS duration (sec)		.03–.07 (.05)			.04–.08 (.06)		.04–.09 (.07)	.06–.09 (.08)
Maximum QTc (sec)†	.45 max				.44 max			.43 max
QRS axis (degrees)	70–180 (120)	45–160 (100)	10–120 (80)		5–110 (60)			
QRS V$_1$ Q (mm)	0	0	0	0	0	0	0	0
QRS V$_1$ R (mm)	5–25 (15)	3–22 (10)	3–20 (10)	2–20 (9)	2–18 (8)	1–15 (5)	1–12 (5)	1–6 (2)
QRS V$_1$ S (mm)	0–22 (7)	0–16 (5)	0–15 (5)	1–20 (6)	1–20 (10)	3–21 (12)	3–22 (11)	3–13 (8)
QRS V$_5$ Q (mm)	0–1 (.5)	0–3 (.5)	0–3 (.5)	0–3 (.5)	0–5 (1)	0–5 (1)	0–3 (.5)	0–2 (.5)
QRS V$_5$ R (mm)	2–20 (10)	3–25 (12)	5–30 (17)	10–30 (20)	10–35 (23)	13–38 (25)	10–35 (20)	7–21 (13)
QRS V$_5$ S (mm)	2–19 (10)	2–16 (8)	1–16 (8)	1–14 (6)	1–13 (5)	1–11 (4)	1–10 (3)	0–5 (2)
QRS V$_6$ Q (mm)	0–2 (.5)	0–2 (.5)	0–2 (.5)	0–3 (.5)	0–4 (1)	0–4 (1)	0–3 (1)	0–2 (.5)
QRS V$_6$ R (mm)	1–12 (5)	1–17 (7)	3–20 (10)	5–22 (12)	6–22 (14)	8–25 (16)	8–24 (15)	5–18 (10)
QRS V$_6$ S (mm)	0–9 (3)	0–9 (3)	0–9 (3)	0–7 (3)	0–6 (2)	0–4 (2)	0–4 (1)	0–2 (1)
T wave V$_1$ (mm)	0–4 days = −3 to +4(0); 4–7 days = −4 to 2(−1)		−6 to −1 (−3)		−6 to +2 (−2)		−4 to +3 (−1)	−2 to +2 (+1)

Adapted from Davignon,[4] Garson,[7] and Fisch.[6]

*Values reported as 2%–98% (mean), except for QTc (given as max value only) and >15 yr data, which reports range as ±1SD.

†Q–Tc = Q–T/√R–R.

and III) are equiphasic or isoelectric, with relatively low amplitude. The P-wave axis for a normal heart in sinus rhythm should be between 0° and +90° regardless of the patient's age. An abnormal axis can be seen in ectopic atrial rhythms or atrial malpositions.

The mean QRS axis is calculated in a similar fashion by identifying the limb lead with the largest positive R wave and assigning the corresponding degree value. In contrast to the P-wave axis, the normal QRS axis has wide age-dependent variation. In newborns, in whom the right ventricle is relatively hypertrophied by virtue of its intrauterine work load, the axis is directed rightward, usually about 120°. As the left ventricle becomes relatively more dominant within the first 6 months of life, the axis gradually shifts toward +60° and should remain between about 0° and +90° thereafter. An abnormal QRS axis can be seen with ventricular hypertrophy, malpositions, intraventricular conduction disturbances, and infarction.

The T-wave axis is usually "concordant" with the QRS. There may be some discrepancy in the early months of life, but by the time the child is 6 months old, the frontal plane QRS and T axes should not differ by more than 60°. An abnormal T-wave axis can be seen in marked hypertrophy with ventricular "strain," ischemia, myopathy, and some intraventricular conduction disturbances.

Rhythm and Rate

Cardiac excitation arising from the sinus node generates a P wave with a normal axis at a rate within the limits for age (Table 1). Rate determination is usually a straightforward exercise (Fig. 18). **Respirophasic sinus arrhythmia** (at times pronounced) is a normal finding in healthy children, as is the observation of a **shifting atrial pacemaker,** where a subsidiary P wave (different axis than sinus rhythm) takes over during episodic slowing of the sinus node.

The P Wave

The contour and magnitude of the P wave are an indirect measure of atrial size. The normal P wave should have a smooth dome shape in lead II, and should never be taller than 0.3 mV or wider than 0.12 sec in duration. Occasionally, there may be a small notch in the P wave of lead II, but this is acceptable if amplitude and duration fall within the normal range.

The T_A Wave

The shallow wave of atrial repolarization is rarely seen on the normal electrocardiogram because of its low amplitude and superimposition of the QRS complex. It may be seen occasionally in patients with heart block when the QRS is late or dissociated. The normal T_A wave is directed opposite from the P wave and is usually less than 0.1 mV in depth. Atrial enlargement or inflammation distort the T_A wave.

The P-R Interval

The P-R interval is measured from the beginning of the P wave to the initial deflection of ventricular activation (it is more precisely a "P-Q" interval) and, as noted earlier, comprises several electrical events, AV node conduction accounting for the major portion. The normal P-R interval is less than 0.16 sec in young children or 0.18 sec in adolescents and adults. A prolonged P-R interval can be due to enhanced vagal tone, cardiac medications (digoxin and antiarrhythmic agents), or disease involving either the AV node or the His-Purkinje system. A shortened P-R interval (less than 0.08 sec) may be observed in anterograde preexcitation (Wolff-Parkinson-White syndrome), "enhanced" AV node conduction, and some congenital anatomic defects.

The QRS Complex

Registration of the QRS begins when cardiac excitation leaves the His-Purkinje system and the ventricular myocytes begin to depolarize. The complex is evaluated for its morphology, amplitude, and duration.

QRS morphology is dictated by the sequence of regional ventricular activation and the balance (right versus left) of ventricular muscle mass, as previously discussed. The normal heart leaves a characteristic "signature" in each lead of the electrocardiogram, which may change because of distortions of activation sequence or hypertrophy. Beyond infancy, the normal pattern is one of a small Q wave, followed by a large R and a small S wave in left-sided leads (I, II, or aV_L, V_3–V_6), while right-sided leads (aV_R, III, V_{4R}–V_2) typically register a small R followed by a deep S wave.

QRS amplitude is a more quantitative measure of ventricular mass and compliments QRS morphology when evaluating a trace for hypertrophy. Normal values are established for R-wave amplitude, as well as for Q- and S-wave amplitudes, for each individual lead. Measurements in the pre-

MAJOR DIVISION = 0.20 secs
MINOR DIVISION = 0.04 secs

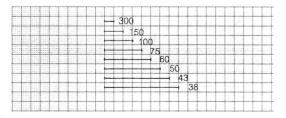

Figure 18. At chart paper speed of 25 mm/sec, each major division = 0.20 sec, and each minor division = 0.04 sec. Heart rate in beats per minute can be determined from the number of large divisions between the QRSs.

cordial leads are particularly sensitive indicators of an abnormality. Normal amplitudes vary widely with patient age, and tables of normal data should be on hand during review of all pediatric cardiograms.

The duration of the QRS complex is related to the speed of conduction within the His-Purkinje system, as well as from myocyte to myocyte within the ventricles. Duration increases slightly with age. In normal infants the QRS width should be less than 0.08 sec and in those older than 6 months, less than 0.10 sec. Prolongation of the QRS may be seen with a block of His-Purkinje conduction pathways (bundle branch blocks), slow myocyte conduction (due to muscle injury, drugs or electrolyte disturbances), or severe ventricular hypertrophy.

The S-T Segment

Ventricular muscle cells are in the plateau phase of their action potential (phase 2) during the S-T segment. Because no electrical wave fronts are advancing or retreating through the heart, the body surface recording is normally isoelectric. The **J point** at the termination of the S wave marks the beginning of the S-T segment and should not deviate more than 1 mm from the base line.

Deviations in S-T level may be caused by ischemia, inflammation, severe hypertrophy, and some medications. One normal variant is the **early repolarization** pattern, seen occasionally in healthy adolescent patients, where the J point can be elevated 2–4 mm. Usually, this elevation is observed in the lateral (V_4–V_6) and inferior (II, III, aV_F) leads and is accompanied by strikingly tall T waves (Fig. 19). The diagnosis of benign early repolarization should not be made if the elevation is more than 4 mm and/or the T-wave is of low amplitude.

The T Wave

The T wave corresponds to phase 3 repolarization of ventricular myocytes. The normal T-wave amplitude is variable and is not routinely quantitated. On the other hand, the direction of the T wave deserves careful attention. As mentioned,

generally the T wave should follow the same net direction as the QRS, so that the frontal axes are similar within ±60°. Discordance of the axis in the limb leads usually suggests pathology, but there are some important age-dependent exceptions in the precordial leads. Normally, in children from birth to 4–7 days of age, the T wave is upright in all precordial leads. After this, the T wave becomes negative over the right chest (V_{4R}–V_1), while remaining positive in the left chest leads. This pattern persists until adolescence, when the T waves tend to resume an upright direction in all chest leads. This sequence is critical to remember during analysis of electrocardiograms in children; an upright T wave in the right precordial leads between the age of 7 days and early adolescence can suggest right ventricular hypertrophy.

The Q-T Interval

The Q-T interval is a crude reflection of the duration of action potential for ventricular myocytes. It is measured from the onset of the QRS to T-wave termination. Because the normal Q-T interval varies with heart rate (longer at slow rates, shorter at fast rates), the measurement is adjusted with the formula: Q-T (second)/(square root R-R) (second). This rate-corrected interval (QT_c) should be less than 0.45 sec in infants, 0.44 sec in children, and 0.43 sec in adults.

A prolonged Q-T_c interval can be of dramatic clinical significance. The hereditary syndromes in which there are long Q-T intervals are potentially fatal disorders and early detection on an electrocardiogram is crucial. The Q-T_c is also affected by many antiarrhythmic drugs, and some electrolyte imbalances.

The U Wave

The U wave is thought to reflect the relatively late repolarization of His-Purkinje cells and is not always visible on the cardiogram of normal patients. Generally, it is of low amplitude (less than one-fourth the height of the T wave) and has the same polarity as its T wave. When the U wave is

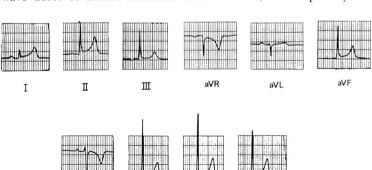

I   II   III   aVR   aVL   aVF

V_1 V_4 V_5 V_6

Figure 19. A dramatic example of early repolarization in a healthy athletic 15-year-old boy.

abnormally prominent (more than half the height of the T wave), it probably should be included in the measurement of the Q-T interval. Occasionally, the U wave may be pronounced, secondary to hypokalemia, antiarrhythmic drugs, and some cases of long Q-T syndrome.

Clinical Correlation

After wave forms and intervals have been analyzed, the proper next step is to consider how the data apply to the clinical history and physical examination. The electrocardiogram should never be interpreted in isolation and there should always be specific questions to answer when the test is ordered (regarding rhythm, hypertrophy, myocardial injury, etc.). Additionally, one should constantly bear in mind that a child can have serious heart disease with a normal-appearing electrocardiogram, particularly in the first few days of life!

The Abnormal Electrocardiogram

Cardiac Malpositions

Chamber orientation is reflected on the electrocardiogram by the axis and the morphology of the P wave and the QRS complex. Atrial situs is determined with considerable accuracy by deciding which side of the atrium contains the sino-atrial (SA) node. In situs solitus, the SA node fires high in the right atrium, and the resultant atrial depolarization wave front generates a P-wave axis of about $+60$, whereas in situs inversus the activation eminates from high in the left atrium so that the P axis is at $+120°$ (Fig. 20). Variable patterns may be seen in the "heterotaxy" syndromes. For example, patients with asplenia ("bilateral right-sidedness") may, in fact, have bilateral sinus nodes, and the P-wave axis may alternate between $+60°$

and $+120°$. In polysplenia ("bilateral left-sidedness") there may not be a true sinus node, and such patients usually rely on a subsidiary atrial pacemaker focus which can have a variable location.

Ventricular orientation is best estimated from the precordial leads. Normal **levocardia** has a characteristic pattern of relatively low (or predominately negative) voltage in the right chest leads (V_{4R} to V_2) with positive forces of higher amplitude in the mid and left chest leads. In **dextrocardia** (Figs. 20 and 21), the pattern is classically reversed (unfortunately, marked right ventricular hypertrophy in levocardia can mimic this appearance, making it a less than perfect diagnostic observation). Further insight into ventricular anatomy may be gained by determining the embryologic ventricular "looping." The normal **D-looped** orientation has an anatomic right ventricle and tricuspid valve located on the right side of the heart. In an **L-looped** anomaly, the ventricular relationship is inverted; hence the septal activation wave front must travel right-to-left. This changes the QRS morphology to one of initial Q waves in right-sided limb and/or precordial leads, with small initial R waves on the left side (Fig. 21).

Atrial Enlargement

The surface electrocardiogram is a fair indicator of atrial enlargement. Because the right atrium is the first to depolarize, indicators of right-sided enlargement are found in the early portions of the P wave. The diagnostic criterion for isolated **right atrial enlargement** is the presence in lead II of a peaked, narrow P wave greater than 0.30 mV in amplitude in lead II. This is often accompanied by either a tall P wave or a biphasic P wave with an early deep negative deflection in lead V_1 (Fig. 22).

Left atrial enlargement is reflected in the terminal portion of the P wave. The classic findings

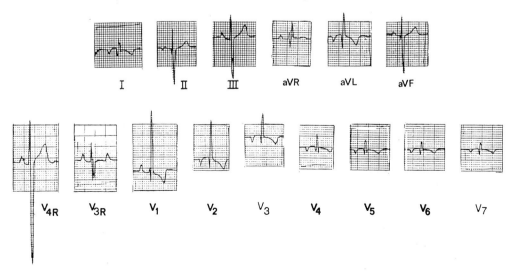

Figure 20. Electrocardiogram from a 6-year-old patient with documented situs inversus and a P wave axis of $+150°$. Dextrocardia is also present.

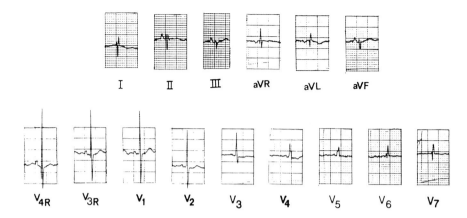

Figure 21. The ECG in a patient with L-looped ventricles (note the RSR pattern in V_4–V_7, and the QRS pattern in V_{4R} and V_{3R}) and dextrocardia (note prominent voltage in the right chest leads).

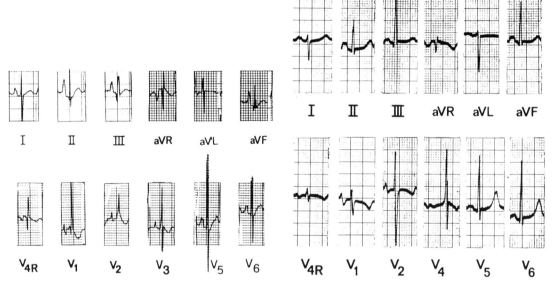

Figure 22. Electrocardiogram showing right atrial enlargement.

Figure 23. Electrocardiogram showing left atrial enlargement.

include a broad, notched P wave in lead II (duration greater than 0.10–0.12 sec), or a deep, slurred terminal portion of a biphasic P wave in V_1 (Fig. 23).

A combination of the above amplitude and duration criteria is indicative of **biatrial enlargement** (Fig. 24).

Ventricular Hypertrophy

Identification of ventricular hypertrophy from the surface electrocardiogram is far from perfect. Although criteria are generally accurate for right ventricular hypertrophy (RVH), the diagnosis of left-sided hypertrophy (LVH) is sometimes difficult until the process is far advanced.

Right Ventricular Hypertrophy. Screening for

RVH is particularly important in pediatric patients because the more common congenital defects impose an increased work load on this chamber. Fortunately, the criteria that have evolved are fairly sensitive.

R-Wave Amplitude in V_1 Higher than the 98th Percentile for Age. This finding is very specific outside of the newborn period. The height of the R wave in this lead correlates well with right ventricular systolic pressure and is sufficiently quantitative to allow prediction of right ventricular pressure for isolated pulmonary valve stenosis using the formula: R wave height (in millimeters) × 5 = peak systolic pressure (mm Hg).

Abnormal T-Wave Direction in V_1. As previously mentioned, the T-wave direction in lead V_1

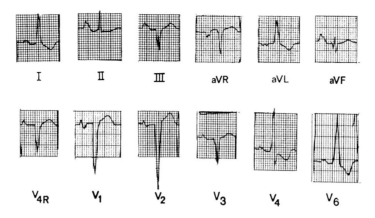

Figure 24. Electrocardiogram showing biatrial enlargement.

changes with time: it is upright in newborns, negative beyond the age of 7 days, and positive again in adolescents and adults. A persistently upright T wave after the seventh day of life is a sensitive indicator of elevated right ventricular pressure, and when combined with R wave amplitude, even greater precision is possible.[7] Mild degrees of RVH may show a normal R-wave amplitude but an upright T wave in V_1. Moderate RVH is characterized by abnormal height of the R wave in conjunction with the upright T wave. In marked RVH, the R wave remains excessive, but the T wave may now be deeply inverted in what is referred to as a "strain" pattern (Fig. 25).

S-Wave Depth in V_6 Lower than the 98th Percentile for Age. This measurement is useful in patients with increased right ventricular pressure secondary to chronic lung disease. Respiratory diseases such as cystic fibrosis can lower the voltage pattern recorded from the right chest because of

heart rotation and hyperexpansion of the lungs. Despite low anterior forces, RVH can still be diagnosed when the lateral S wave is deep. This pattern of RVH, when associated with right atrial enlargement in a patient with severe pulmonary disease, is characteristic of "cor pulmonale" (Fig. 26).

Right Axis Deviation. Isolated right axis deviation is not specific for RVH and may be observed in conduction disturbances such as left posterior hemiblock. When present in conjunction with other RVH criteria, it lends additional support for the diagnosis.

QR Pattern in V_1. This criterion is likewise not absolute for RVH, but is supportive evidence when associated with a tall R wave in the right chest leads. A QR pattern may also be seen with L-looped ventricles and anterior infarction.

RSR' Pattern in V_1. It is important to understand the significance and limitations of this finding in the pediatric population. Increased right ventricular volume loads, imposed by common lesions such as an atrial septal defect, may create a pattern of V_1 of a small initial R wave, followed by an S wave, terminating with a tall R' wave (Fig. 27). RVH should be diagnosed only when the secondary R' wave is large in amplitude. Some normal children may have a similar pattern with a lower-amplitude R' wave. Often it is useful to examine the distribution of the RSR' pattern in multiple pre-

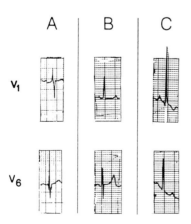

Figure 25. ECG patterns with varying degrees of right ventricular pressure load hypertrophy. **A,** *Mild RVH* in a 9-month-old suggested by an upright T wave in V_1, but without excess R-wave voltage. **B,** *Moderate RVH* in a 4-year-old with an upright T wave and excess R-wave voltage in V_1. **C,** *Marked RVH* in a 7-year-old showing a very tall R wave with an inverted T wave ("strain" pattern) in V_1.

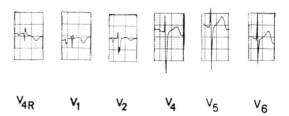

Figure 26. The pattern of RVH seen in chronic lung disease (cystic fibrosis in this case), characterized by deep, lateral S waves and by normal voltages in the right chest.

A   B

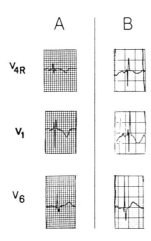

V_{4R}

V_1

V_6

Figure 27. The RSR' pattern in lead V_1: **A,** Normal patient without heart disease. **B,** Patient with increased RV volume load due to large atrial septal defect. Note the tall R' wave in the abnormal trace.

cordial leads; for large right ventricular volume loads the RSR' may extend from V_{4R} all the way across to V_3 or V_4, whereas the pattern does not usually extend beyond V_1 in normal children. An RSR' pattern may also be caused by incomplete right bundle branch block.

Abnormal R/S Ratio in V_1 or V_6. Normal values for R/S ratios are well established and these data can be drawn upon when the decision regarding RVH is questionable. However, it is rare to see abnormal ratios as an isolated finding, and one should hesitate to make a firm diagnosis of RVH on the basis of this criterion alone.

Left Ventricular Hypertrophy. It is difficult to predict LVH accurately from the electrocardiogram. The diagnosis is best entertained when multiple criteria are fulfilled.

R-Wave Amplitude in V_5–V_6 Higher than the 98th Percentile for Age. The "voltage criteria" for LVH are not very exact. Hypertrophy may be present with normal left precordial forces, and in some normal children (particularly athletic teenagers) the R-wave amplitude may exceed the 98th percentile. Attempts have been made to improve diagnostic accuracy by examining the reciprocal S-wave depth in lead V_1 as an indicator of LVH (using isolated S-wave measurement or a combination of S in V_1 plus R in V_6), but there remain limitations to voltage data alone.

Lateral T-Wave Inversion: The "Strain Pattern." In the Natural History Study of congenital aortic stenosis,[17] T-wave abnormalities were identified as the most specific indications of LVH. Left ventricular strain presents a pattern of inverted T waves in the inferior limb leads (II, III, aV_F) and left precordial leads (V_5 and V_6), sometimes associated with depression of the S-T segment. There may or may not be concomitant voltage indications of LVH

(Fig. 28). Although the presence of these T-wave changes usually suggests advanced degrees of hypertrophy, the presence of ischemia or myocardial inflammation must be excluded before this criterion can be applied with certainty.

Left Axis Deviation. An abnormal leftward axis is supportive evidence for LVH. The utility of this criterion is best appreciated in the neonate, where the QRS axis is normally directed rightward. The presence of a "mature" axis in the 0° to +90° range, or a "superior" axis in the 0° to −90° range in early infancy suggests a definite cardiac abnormality (although not necessarily LVH). Left axis deviation may also be due to conduction disturbances such as left anterior hemiblock.

Abnormal Lateral Q Wave. The Q wave in leads V_5 and V_6 (septal depolarization) may be distorted if the left ventricle is very dilated or markedly thick, because of rotation of septal position and increased competition from vectors of left apex and left free-wall depolarization. As a broad generalization, a dilated, "volume loaded" left ventricle tends to have an abnormally deep Q wave at the lateral leads in such lesions as aortic regurgitation, patent ductus, or ventricular septal defect (Fig. 29). Concentric hypertrophy from a "pressure load" (e.g., aortic stenosis) is more likely to be associated with a small or absent Q wave (Fig. 30).

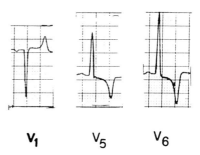

V_1   V_5   V_6

Figure 28. LVH with "strain" pattern in a patient with aortic stenosis. The T-wave inversion is dramatic even though the R-wave voltage does not exceed normal limits.

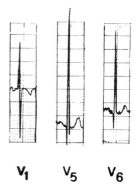

V_1   V_5   V_6

Figure 29. The typical ECG pattern for LVH due to a large volume load, with deep Q waves in V_5 and V_6 in an infant with a large ventricular septal defect.

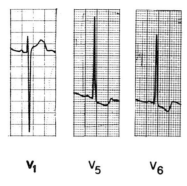

Figure 30. The typical ECG pattern for LVH due to increased pressure, with minimal Q waves in V_5 and V_6, from a patient with aortic stenosis.

Left Ventricular Hypertrophy Scoring Systems. Frustration with the inaccurate diagnosis of LVH has led to the development of more quantitative schemes where points are assigned for the magnitude of excessive voltages, the presence of T-wave changes, left axis deviation, the coexistence of left atrial enlargement, etc. Such scoring systems may improve diagnostic accuracy slightly, but are only as good as each individual measurement and are somewhat difficult to memorize. The "maximum spatial vector to the left" of the vectorcardiogram also has limited value. For the present, it must be realized that electrocardiographic techniques are inaccurate for detection of LVH in about 50% of cases.

Bilateral Ventricular Hypertrophy (BVH) and Single Ventricle Hypertrophy (SVH). When two normal ventricles are present, the diagnosis of BVH can be made if voltage criteria are met in both the right and left precordial leads (Fig. 31). In practice, this is not commonly observed because the depolarization vectors from the right and left sides compete and may cancel each other out, to a large extent, on the body surface. An alternate criterion is abnormal total amplitude for the R plus the S wave in the midprecordial lead V_4 (the "Katz-Wachtel" criterion). When the additive forces exceed the 98th percentile, BVH is suggested. The Katz-Wachtel criterion should not be applied in the absence of supporting evidence of ventricular enlargement in the other chest leads. Some normal newborns, especially premature infants, have impressive midprecordial voltages but show normal forces in the rightward and lateral leads.

There are no firm criteria to apply for hypertrophy of a single ventricle in complex congenital anomalies. What is most surprising is that, occasionally, an electrocardiogram in such conditions may look fairly normal, at least in the newborn. However, voltage criteria for single ventricles generally exceed those for either RVH or LVH in some precordial lead. The exact QRS morphology is variable, depending on the presence and location of the ventricular septum, which anatomic ventricle is indeed present, and on the rotation of the abnormal heart in the thorax. One may be able to predict which ventricle is absent by noting which side of the precordium has deficient positive voltage (Fig. 32). Absent ventricle (or hypoplastic ventricle) may also be suspected if the "septal" Q wave is absent in every precordial lead, including V_7.

Intraventricular Conduction Abnormalities

From the common bundle of His, intraventricular conduction fibers divide into the right and left bundle branches. The left bundle actually fans out alone the entire left ventricular septal surface, but may be considered to split into two major divisions: the left anterior and left posterior fascicles. Partial or complete block at any one of these sites creates delay in regional ventricular activation and a characteristic change in QRS pattern. Likewise, the presence of "accessory" conduction pathways distorts regional activation.

Incomplete Right Bundle Branch Block. An RSR′ pattern in the right precordial leads with normal QRS duration may indicate an incomplete conduction disturbance in the right bundle branch. However, an identical pattern may be seen in healthy normal individuals or in patients with right ventricular volume overload, as previously discussed. Probably, the diagnosis of incomplete block should be reserved for situations in which the QRS duration is only slightly prolonged, and then it should be used only if a left-to-right shunt at the atrial level has been excluded.

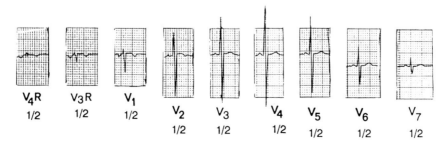

Figure 31. Biventricular hypertrophy suggested by midprecordial voltages above the 98th percentile. The combined R + S waves in lead V_4 are 95 mm (trace is shown at half of standard size).

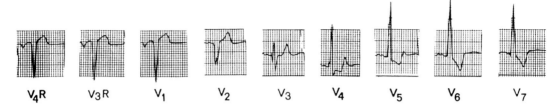

| V_4R | V_3R | V_1 | V_2 | V_3 | V_4 | V_5 | V_6 | V_7 |

Figure 32. Absent RV forces (no R wave in right chest leads) in a patient with tricuspid atresia.

Complete Right Bundle Branch Block. When transmission is interrupted along the right bundle branch, the septum and left ventricle can activate normally, but the right ventricle must depend upon slower cell-to-cell activation spreading left-to-right. The resultant QRS complex has prolonged duration (greater than 0.10 sec for infants, greater than 0.12 sec for older patients) and a characteristic morphology that reflects the late, slow-activation wave front spreading toward the right heart. The initial portion of the QRS is generated by the usual septal and initial left ventricular depolarization and, thus, is quite similar to normal (small R wave in V_1, QR in V_6). The subsequent slow wave front traveling toward the right heart inscribes a tall, slurred R′ wave in V_1 and an equally sluggish S wave in V_6 (Fig. 33). A pattern of complete right bundle branch block is a frequent observation following surgical repair of ventricular septal defects and tetralogy of Fallot. Of interest, the classic electrocardiographic picture of complete right bundle branch block can be seen with interruption of either the "peripheral" portions of the right His-Purkinje network, or of the "central" right bundle branch itself. Although the surface electrocardiographic patterns are indistinguishable, by using an intracardiac electrode catheter, normal conduction times to the right ventricular apex can be measured in the former condition, whereas apex activation is delayed with a central injury.

The ability to diagnose ventricular hypertrophy on the electrocardiogram is lost in complete bundle branch block. Attempts to correlate right ventricular pressure with the height of the R′ wave in V_1, or the extent of RSR′ distribution across the precordium, have met with limited success. Additionally, bundle branch block results in diffuse changes in the level of the S-T segment and the shape of the T wave, so that the usual electrocardiographic markers of ischemia or strain are lost.

Left Anterior Hemiblock. Conduction block in the left anterior fascicle produces a shift in QRS axis to the range of $-60°$, without prolongation of QRS duration. Whereas the anterior-superior and posterior-inferior portions of the normal left ventricle are usually depolarized simultaneously by their respective fascicles, block in the anterior limb changes the sequence. The inferior regions activate normally, but the depolarization wave front must then spread upward, producing a superiorly directed vector in the frontal plane (Fig. 34). Isolated block in the anterior fascicle is rare in children, but may occur with myocardial inflammation, ischemia, and surgical or catheter trauma.

Certain congenital cardiac anomalies, notably endocardial cushion defects and tricuspid atresia, have electrocardiographic patterns with a leftward superior QRS axis that mimic left anterior hemiblock. The abnormal axis is not due to true conduction defects in these cases, but instead results

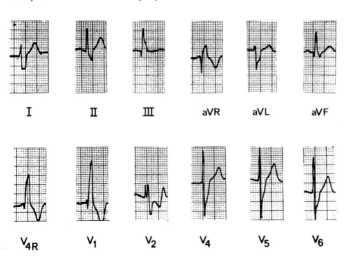

| I | II | III | aVR | aVL | aVF |

| V_4R | V_1 | V_2 | V_4 | V_5 | V_6 |

Figure 33. Electrocardiographic pattern of complete right bundle branch block.

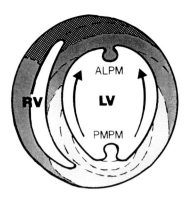

Figure 34. Axis shift in left anterior hemiblock. Depolarization of the LV spreads from inferior to superior, generating a superior axis. ALPM, anterolateral papillary muscle; PMPM, posteromedial papillary muscle.

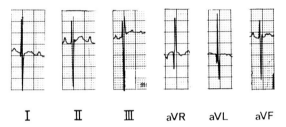

I   II   III   aVR   aVL   aVF

Figure 35. Superior QRS axis (− 90°) in a patient with AV canal defect.

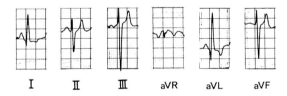

I   II   III   aVR   aVL   aVF

Figure 36. Superior axis (− 60°) in a patient with tricuspid atresia.

from the abnormal anatomic location of the conduction fibers in cushion defects (Fig. 35) or the unusual left ventricular shape and orientation in tricuspid atresia (Fig. 36).

Left Posterior Hemiblock. The QRS duration remains normal, but the axis is shifted right and inferior to about + 120° when the posterior fascicle is interrupted. The activation pattern in the left ventricle is just the reverse of anterior hemiblock (Fig. 37). Because right axis deviation is seen in normal infants and older children with variable degrees of right ventricular hypertrophy, the diagnosis of posterior hemiblock should be reserved for instances when an abrupt and dramatic axis shift has occurred between serial electrocardiograms.

Complete Left Bundle Branch Block. When the main left bundle branch is interrupted, ventricular activation begins solely via the right bundle. The septum must now depolarize right to left, and the left ventricle must rely on late transmission of the

activation wave front which is directed leftward and posterior. The QRS is prolonged, slurred, and directed away from the right chest leads (mostly negative in V_1) and toward the lateral precordial leads (positive in V_5–V_7) (Fig. 38). As with complete right bundle branch block, ventricular hypertrophy and ischemic changes cannot be interpreted from electrocardiograms. Very advanced degrees of concentric left ventricular hypertrophy can produce an electrocardiographic pattern identical to that of complete left bundle branch block, and the two conditions may be impossible to distinguish by body surface recording.

Bifascicular Block. The combination of complete right bundle branch block and left anterior hemiblock may occur after surgical correction of complex congenital heart defects. For example, following repair of tetralogy of Fallot, bifascicular block of this type is present in 10% of patients. The electrocardiographic pattern is essentially a combination of the findings for the two individual conduction defects. Recall that in right bundle branch

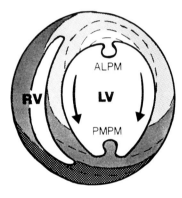

Figure 37. Axis shift in left posterior hemiblock. Depolarization of the LV spreads from superior to inferior. ALPM, anterolateral papillary muscle; PMPM, posteromedial papillary muscle.

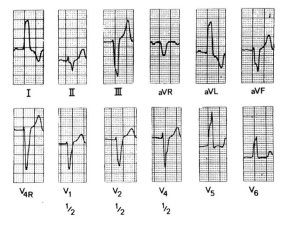

I   II   III   aVR   aVL   aVF

V_{4R} V_1 V_2 V_4 V_5 V_6
                $\frac{1}{2}$ $\frac{1}{2}$ $\frac{1}{2}$

Figure 38. Electrocardiographic pattern of complete left bundle branch block.

block, the initial portion of the QRS reflects the normal pattern of septal and left ventricular activation. If a new shift in the superior axis is detected for this early portion of the QRS, in conjunction with the terminal slurring characteristic of complete right bundle branch block, the coexistence of left anterior hemiblock should be considered (Fig. 39).

Combined right bundle and left posterior fascicular block is less common in the pediatric age group and is difficult to diagnose from the electrocardiogram. The initial portion of the QRS, representing septal and left ventricular activation, is shifted rightward in this case. Because children undergoing cardiac surgery often have preexistent right axis deviation from right ventricular hypertrophy, it may be impossible to appreciate this particular conduction change in the postoperative period.

Preexcitation. Preexcitation implies that a portion of ventricular tissue is being activated ahead of schedule relative to normal His-Purkinje conduction. In the **Wolff-Parkinson-White (WPW) syndrome** this early activation occurs over an accessory connection between atrial and ventricular muscle located along the right or left atrioventricular groove (so-called bundle of Kent). As an atrial depolarization wave front approaches the ventricles, it may advance over both the accessory pathway and the normal AV node. AV-node conduction is relatively slow, but the abnormal pathway allows almost immediate depolarization of a focal ventricular segment. The focus of early activation generates a "delta wave" on the electrocardiogram (Fig. 40) with a short P-R (actually a P-delta) interval. Because some portion of ventricular activation still occurs over the normal His pathways, there is fusion between the preexcitation and the normal depolarization sequence.

The electrocardiographic patterns in the WPW syndrome are variable, depending on the location of the accessory pathway and its conduction characteristics. Generally, left-sided accessory pathways tend to produce positive delta waves in the right limb and precordial leads, since the early activation vector is traveling left-to-right. For the most part, the right ventricle is activated by the normal conduction pathways, but only after a small delay imposed by the AV node, thus generating an overall QRS morphology reminiscent of right bundle branch block. This general pattern for a left-sided pathway is sometimes referred to as "type A" WPW syndrome (Fig. 41). Right-sided pathways, by comparison, are usually associated with positive delta waves in the left-sided leads (Fig. 42) and a QRS pattern more closely resembling left bundle branch block ("type B" WPW syndrome). Knowledge of accessory pathway location is of considerable relevance: as many as 50% of children with right-sided tracts have a structural heart lesion (usually Ebstein's anomaly) in addition to the electrical abnormality.[5]

A less common form of preexcitation is associated with the presence of a **Mahaim fiber.** This pathway arises from the AV node or proximal His-Purkinje system and usually inserts in right ventricular muscle. Since excitation must pass through the AV node before reaching this fiber, the P-R interval remains normal on the electrocardiogram. However, activation through the Mahaim pathway preexcites a portion of the right ventricle and generates a delta wave pattern similar to that in type B WPW syndrome (Fig. 43). Mahaim fibers are rare and may require intracardiac electrophysio-

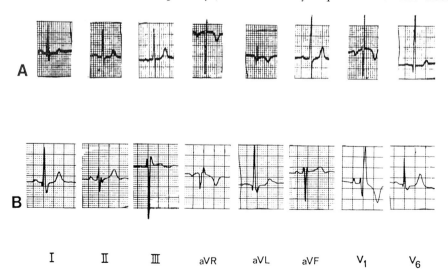

I   II   III   aVR   aVL   aVF   V₁   V₆

Figure 39. Preoperative (**A**) and postoperative (**B**) ECG recordings from a patient with tetralogy of Fallot, showing right bundle branch block and a superior shift in the axis for initial LV depolarization consistent with left anterior hemiblock.

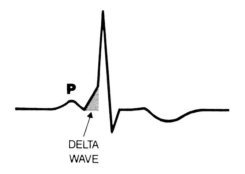

Figure 40. Short P-R interval and the delta wave of ventricular preexcitation.

logic study to confirm their presence or distinguish them from the WPW syndrome.

In both WPW and Mahaim preexcitation, the ability to use the electrocardiogram for evaluation of hypertrophy and changes in the S-T segment and T wave is completely lost (similar to bundle branch block).

A final type of preexcitation involves a conduction pathway running from low in the atrium to the common bundle of His. This arrangement permits conduction to bypass the AV node. When normal nodal delay is lost, the P-R interval is short, but because the ventricles activate over normal His-Purkinje branches, the QRS remains normal (Fig. 44). It is not clear whether this pattern results from a true accessory pathway (so-called "James" fiber) or just represents "enhanced" conduction in the AV node itself. The combination of a short P-R interval and recurrent SVT is often referred to as **Lown-Ganong-Levine syndrome**.

Pathologic Changes in the S-T Segment and T Wave

No other aspect of the interpretation of an electrocardiogram is so dependent on good clinical history as the evaluation of abnormalities of the S-T segment and T wave. Unfortunately, pathologic changes are often nonspecific. Elevation or depression of the J point and changes in the T wave can be seen in most any condition involving injury to myocytes or in certain electrolyte disturbances.

Pericarditis and Pericardial Effusion. Pericardial inflammation produces a sequence of changes in the S-T segment and T wave which evolve as the disorder progresses. The earliest finding is elevation of the S-T segment with preservation of normal T-wave amplitude and direction. Later the S-T segment returns to the baseline, but the T wave becomes flattened and, ultimately, inverted. As opposed to the focal changes in the S-T segment and T wave which are seen in ischemic syndromes, the electrocardiographic findings in pericarditis are diffuse and usually involve all leads except, perhaps, aV_R and the right precordium. Additionally, pericarditis affects both atrial and ventricular surfaces, such that noticeable depression of the T_A wave may sometimes be observed.

Occasionally, the presence of a large effusion in the pericardial space can result in diminished ventricular voltages and a pattern of QRS-amplitude variation known as electrical alternans (Fig. 45).

Myocarditis. The electrocardiographic findings in myocarditis are variable, but usually involve diminished ventricular voltages and T-wave inversion during the acute illness. Atrioventricular and intraventricular conduction disturbances, along with ventricular arrhythmias, are common (Fig. 46).

Hypertrophic Cardiomyopathy. The changes in the S-T segment and T wave seen in hypertrophic cardiomyopathy are similar to the left ventricular "strain" pattern that occurs with advanced hypertrophy from any cause. The lateral T waves are inverted and the J point may be depressed. Voltage criteria for LVH are usually present (Fig. 47). About 30% of patients also have prominent Q waves in the lateral and inferior leads and may display left axis deviation. A small number of patients have been found to have true preexcitation from accessory atrioventricular pathways (WPW syndrome). The P-R interval may be short in hy-

Figure 41. Electrocardiogram showing Wolff-Parkinson-White syndrome in a patient with a left posterolateral accessory pathway. The precordial pattern is akin to right bundle branch block (so-called Type A pattern).

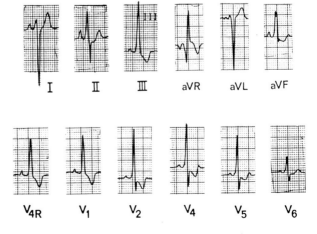

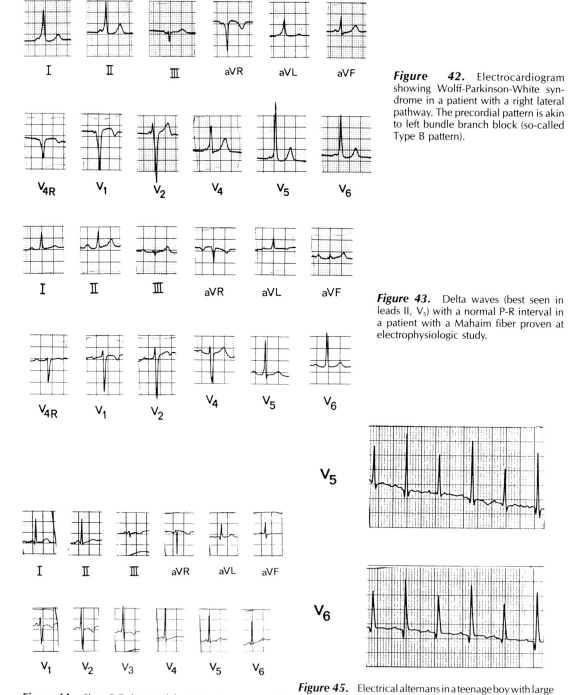

Figure 42. Electrocardiogram showing Wolff-Parkinson-White syndrome in a patient with a right lateral pathway. The precordial pattern is akin to left bundle branch block (so-called Type B pattern).

Figure 43. Delta waves (best seen in leads II, V_5) with a normal P-R interval in a patient with a Mahaim fiber proven at electrophysiologic study.

Figure 44. Short P-R, but no delta wave, in a 3-year-old with recurrent supraventricular tachycardia.

Figure 45. Electrical alternans in a teenage boy with large pericardial effusion. Note also the nonspecific flattening of the T wave in V_5 and V_6.

pertrophic myopathy even when such pathways are absent.

Dilated Cardiomyopathy. There are no specific electrocardiographic findings to aid in the diagnosis of the dilated myopathies, although the electrocardiogram is rarely normal in such cases. Because the etiology is so variable, the electrocardiogram can include most any of the patterns seen with inflammatory disease or hypertrophy, although S-T depression (rather than elevation) is most common.

Ischemia. Myocardial ischemia is a rare problem in pediatric practice, but it may occur with congenital anomalies or inflammation of the coronary arteries. Hypoxic insult results in an evolution of electrocardiographic findings which tend to parallel cellular events. During the initial **ischemic**

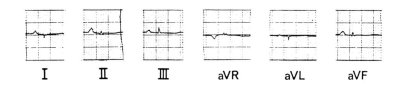

Figure 46. Dramatically low QRS voltage in a patient with dilated myopathy from myocarditis.

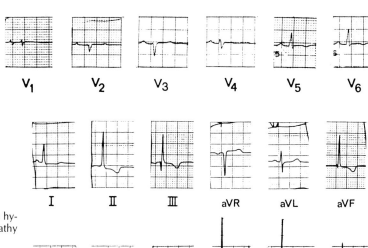

Figure 47. ECG from a patient with hypertrophic obstructive cardiomyopathy showing LVH and "strain."

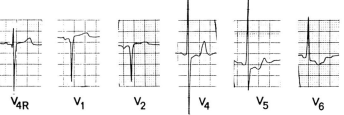

phase, the most dramatic changes occur in the T wave, which becomes tall and peaked in those leads which record near the affected myocardial segment; these changes are usually accompanied by some deviation of the S-T segment (Fig. 48). If the pathologic process is promptly reversed, these changes can resolve. However, if the insult persists, the **injury phase** commences and may be seen on the electrocardiogram as a more dramatic shift in the S-T segment. The S-T deviation may be upward or downward, depending on whether the injured cells are epicardial or endocardial (Fig. 49). During the injury phase, correction of the underlying cause may still result in reversion to a normal electrocardiogram. When the injury persists, cell death (infarction) follows, reflected on the electro-

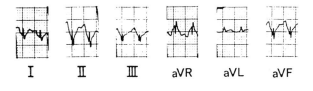

Figure 48. ECG showing acute ischemia with lateral (V₄–V₆) and inferior (aV_F) elevation of the S-T segment.

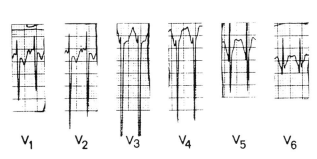

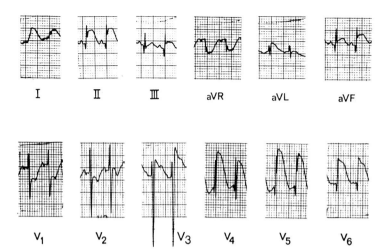

I   II   III   aVR   aVL   aVF

V_1 V_2 V_3 V_4 V_5 V_6

Figure 49. ECG from the same patient as in Figure 48 several hours later, showing marked changes in the S-T segment caused by myocardial injury.

cardiogram as a diminution of R-wave voltage and the appearance of Q waves in those leads facing the infarcted segment (Fig. 50).

The most common cause of myocardial ischemia in pediatric practice involves **anomalous origin of the left coronary from the pulmonary artery**. At initial presentation, variable degrees of injury or infarction are apparent, typically involving ventricular muscle in the area of distribution of the left anterior descending artery (i.e., anterior and septal areas). The electrocardiographic findings in severely afflicted infants include deep Q waves in leftward and lateral leads (I, aV_L, V_3–V_6) and loss of the mid-precordial R wave (V_3–V_5), with a normal QRS axis (Fig. 51). Children who present beyond infancy are more likely to have left axis deviation, smaller Q waves in the leftward and lateral leads, and increased voltages suggestive of LVH (Fig. 52).

Kawasaki's disease is another potential cause of coronary insufficiency in children (see ch. 23). Early in the disease the electrocardiogram may indicate myocardial inflammation (e.g., low QRS voltages, nonspecific T-wave changes). The late se-

quelae of coronary aneurysms can predispose to acute obstruction of coronary flow and the evolution of injury and infarction, as previously described.

Electrolyte Abnormality. Significant changes may occur on the surface electrocardiogram with certain electrolyte disturbances, notably potassium, calcium, and magnesium imbalance. For **hyperkalemia,** the electrocardiographic findings are quite specific for more than mild abnormalities. Moderate elevation of serum potassium concentration (greater than 6.0 mEq/L) causes tall, peaked T waves, along with some widening of the QRS complex (Fig. 53). Marked elevation (more than 8.0 mEq/L) causes profound widening of the P wave and QRS complex, resulting in a pattern for sinus rhythm that resembles a sine wave or mimics wide ventricular tachycardia (Fig. 54). Elevations beyond this point are likely to cause degeneration to ventricular fibrillation or asystole. **Hypokalemia** (less than 3.0 mEq/L) results in a low-amplitude, flattened T wave, with the appearance of prominent U waves.

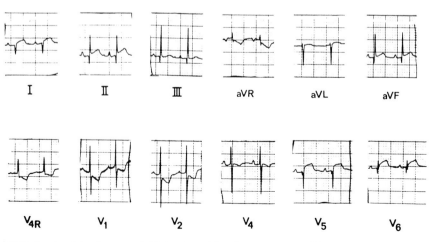

I   II   III   aVR   aVL   aVF

V_{4R} V_1 V_2 V_4 V_5 V_6

Figure 50. ECG showing lateral myocardial infarction with a deep Q wave and loss of the R wave in lead V_5.

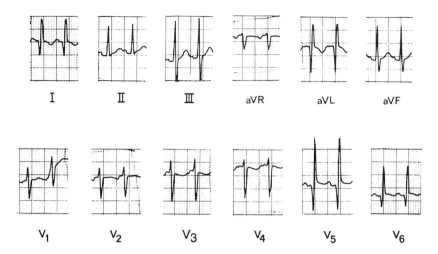

Figure 51. ECG from infant with origin of the left coronary artery from the pulmonary artery who arrived at the hospital in shock. Note the deep, wide Q waves in V_5 and V_6, and the small R wave in V_4.

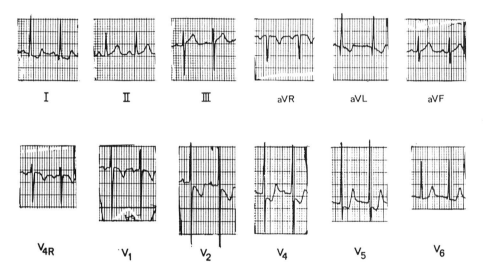

Figure 52. ECG from an asymptomatic 12-year-old with the origin of the left coronary artery from the pulmonary artery. Except for mild left axis deviation, borderline LVH, and nonspecific changes in the S-T segment, the trace is deceptively unimpressive.

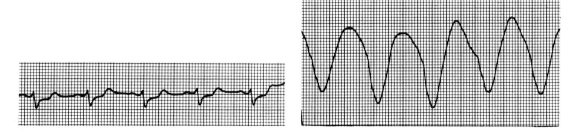

Figure 53. Electrocardiographic pattern of moderate hyperkalemia ($K^+ = 7.0$). Note the widening of the QRS.

Figure 54. Electrocardiographic pattern of marked hyperkalemia ($K^+ = 8.9$) showing a "sine-wave" pattern.

Calcium and **magnesium** predominantly influence speed of cellular repolarization. Low levels of either ion prolong the Q-T interval (Fig. 55), whereas high serum levels may shorten the Q-T.

Pathognomonic Electrocardiographic Patterns. Table 2 lists those cardiac conditions and/or syndromes where the electrocardiographic findings are sufficiently specific to allow rapid diagnosis. These disorders are discussed individually elsewhere in this text, but are abstracted here for quick reference.

RHYTHM MONITORING ("HOLTER") AND "EVENT" RECORDING

Unless one is fortunate enough to have an electrocardiograph hooked up during a clinical arrhythmia, alternate techniques for long-term recording must be employed. Until recently, the only tool for this purpose was the tape recording system developed by Holter—the **Holter monitor**.[9] These devices are small, battery-driven, cassette tape recorders that register the cardiogram from adhesive electrodes placed on the chest (Fig. 56). Two simultaneous channels, which are synchronized to a 24-hour time tract, are usually recorded. (One resembles a right precordial lead and the other resembles a left precordial lead.) The patient or family maintains a diary to correlate activity or symptoms with rhythm status. The 24-hour tape is played back later on a high-speed analysis system

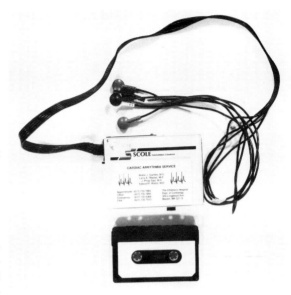

Figure 56.   Standard 2-channel Holter monitor recorder.

at about 60 × or 120 × real time. A skilled technician, often aided by computerized arrhythmia-detection templates in the analyzer, can then pick out events of interest and print hard copy of those rhythm strips that require review (Fig. 57). Most analysis systems also calculate heart rate trends (minimum, maximum and mean) and quantitate supraventricular or ventricular ectopy.

The Holter monitor is a wonderful tool, but is useful only if arrhythmias occur at a frequency greater than once in 24 hours. Some patients may go days or weeks between events, and it is often impractical to use the Holter technique in this setting. To overcome this deficiency, "**event**" **recorders** have been developed. The basic device is a small portable recorder (Fig. 58) with adhesive electrodes or flat metal contact plates which are positioned on the chest. When the device is activated, a single-channel electrocardiogram will be recorded for 1 minute or so and stored in memory. Later the recording is played back as an oscillating audio signal, which is decoded into an electrocardiogram wave-form. One major advantage of this technology is the fact that the audio signals can be sent long distance over a standard telephone to a receiving station at the hospital, thus saving the patient travel time while also hastening detection of potentially serious rhythm disorders.

Event recorders demand that a patient or family is capable of recognizing symptoms from the arrhythmia, so that timely activation of the device is possible. Proper use requires careful rehearsal and family cooperation, particularly with young children. Event recording is extremely useful for the diagnosis of episodic palpitations of undetermined etiology or for evaluation of vague symptoms (e.g., mild dizziness or chest pain) where arrhythmia is part of the differential diagnosis.

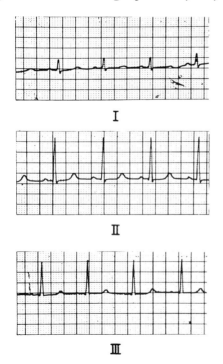

I

II

III

Figure 55.   Prolongation of the Q-T interval in a patient with hypocalcemia.

Table 2. Syndromes and Diseases of Childhood with Distinctive ECG Findings

Anatomic Heart Disease

Atrioventricular Canal Defects	Superior QRS axis (-30 to -120), RVH
Tricuspid Atresia	Superior QRS axis (-30 to -120), decr. right volts (V_4R-V_1), LVH, BAE, $\pm$ short P–R
Holt-Oram Syndrome (ASD)	AVB, RVH
Ventricular Inversion (L-Loop)	RSR left leads (V_5, V_6, aV_L); QR in right leads (V_1, aV_R); AVB, CHB
Situs Inversus/Dextrocardia	P axis $+120$, incr. right volts (V_4R-V_1), decr. left volts (V_3-V_7)
Origin LCA from PA	Deep left Q waves (I, aV_L, V_3-V_6), decr. mid volts (V_3-V_5), $\pm$ LAD, $\pm$ LVH
Hypertrophic Cardiomyopathy	LVH with "strain," deep Q waves (V_4-V_6, I, II, III, aV_F), $\pm$ LAD, $\pm$ short P–R, SVT, VT

Congenital Conduction Disorders

Wolff-Parkinson-White Syndrome	Short P-R, delta wave, SVT
Mahaim Fiber	Normal P-R, delta wave, SVT
Lown-Ganong-Levine Syndrome	Short P-R, no delta wave, SVT
Romano-Ward Syndrome	Long QT_c, VT (autosomal dominant normal hearing)
Jervell-Lange-Nielsen Syndrome	Long QT_c, VT (autosomal recessive congenital deafness)

Systemic Disorders

Maternal Lupus (fetal exposure)	CHB
Refsum's Syndrome	IVCD, AVB, CHB
Pompe's Disease	Short P-R, increased volts, $\pm$ deep Q waves
Friedreich's Ataxia	Sinus tachycardia, LVH, SVT, VT
Becker's Muscular Dystrophy	IVCD, AVB, SVT
Duchenne's Muscular Dystrophy	RVH, deep Q wave (I, aV_L), SVT, VT
Myotonic Dystrophy	Sinus bradycardia, IVCD, SVT
Kerns-Sayre Syndrome	IVCD, AVB, CHB
Hypothyroidism	Sinus bradycardia, AVB, absent S-T segment ("mosque sign")
Hyperkalemia	Peaked T wave, wide QRS, "sine-wave" pattern, VT
Hypokalemia	Low-amplitude T wave, increased U wave
Hypocalcemia/Magnesemia	Long QT_c
Chagas Disease	IVCD, AVB, CHB
Lyme Disease	IVCD, AVB, CHB

ASD, atrial septal defect
AVB, 1° and/or 2° atrioventricular block
BAE, biatrial enlargement
CHB, complete heart block
IVCD, intraventricular conduction delay/bundle branch or fascicular block
LCA, left coronary artery

LVH, left ventricular hypertrophy
PA, pulmonary artery
RVH, right ventricular hypertrophy
SVT, supraventricular tachycardia
VT, ventricular tachycardia
LAD, left axis deviation

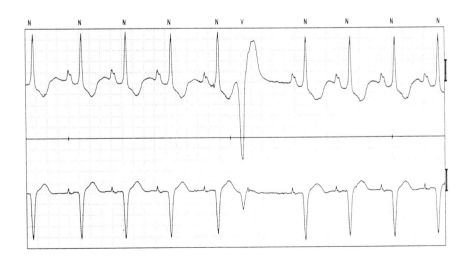

Figure 57. Example of printout from a Holter scanning device showing a ventricular premature beat. N, normal complex; V, ventricular premature beat.

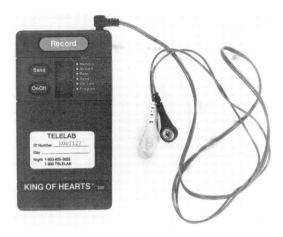

Figure 58. An event recorder with a "memory loop" that locks in the preceding 30 sec of rhythm and a subsequent 30 sec when the device is activated.

EXERCISE TESTING AND AUTONOMIC STUDIES

The manipulation of autonomic tone often provides information regarding rhythm status that is not always available on a resting electrocardiogram. Enhancement of sympathetic drive during dynamic exercise permits analysis, not only of exercise capacity and hemodynamic response to stress, but also of sinus node function, intracardiac conduction, and arrhythmias.

The most widely employed exercise technique involves the Bruce Protocol on an adjustable treadmill, where the belt speed and slope are increased at 3-minute intervals, during which heart rate, blood pressure, and surface electrocardiograms are recorded (see ch. 16). Normal values for exercise tolerance, peak sinus rate, and blood pressure responses are well established for sex and age.

Exercise testing can be utilized as a rough indicator of sinus node integrity by comparing the maximal achieved heart rate to the expected normal for age. Some reports suggest a blunted heart rate response to exercise may be observed in patients with the "sick sinus syndrome." The conduction characteristics of the AV node during sinus tachycardia can also be used to evaluate low-to-moderate grades of AV blocks. For patients with known complete heart block, the chronotropic response of their junctional escape rhythm, or the appearance of ventricular ectopy during exercise, may assist in determining the need for pacemaker insertion.[18]

By far the most common arrhythmic issue addressed with exercise testing is **ventricular ectopy.** Children who demonstrate ectopy on an electrocardiogram or on Holter monitoring are usually subjected to maximal exercise testing as part of their evaluation. The testing serves two purposes.

First, it is sometimes helpful to determine whether ectopy is suppressed or aggravated by exercise. In asymptomatic patients with single premature beats, ectopy which is suppressed by exercise is thought to have a benign prognosis,[10] although there may be some exceptions to this rule. On the other hand, an increased frequency of premature contractions at **peak exercise,** or the new appearance of couplets or ventricular tachycardia at **any stage of testing,** may suggest pathology (Fig. 59). The second purpose for this testing is to establish a baseline arrhythmia density, against which follow-up studies can be compared while the patient is on antiarrhythmic drugs.

Generally, supraventricular arrhythmias do not lend themselves to evaluation by stress testing, with the notable exception of the preexcitation syndromes. In patients with the WPW syndrome, exercise testing often yields important clues regarding the conduction characteristics of the accessory pathway, and in some cases it may precipitate reentry tachycardia. Patients who demonstrate clear delta waves and short P-R intervals at rest (i.e., are preexcited in the anterograde direction) can be exercised to accelerate their atrial rate. A rate may eventually be reached where the capacity of the accessory path to conduct anterograde is exceeded, so that all forward conduction must travel over the AV node, at which point the QRS complex and the P-R interval normalize (Fig. 60). The rate at which anterograde preexcitation is blocked correlates fairly well with the more accurate measurements of effective refractory periods for the accessory pathway obtained at electrophysiologic study. Many accessory pathways are capable of conducting at rates greater than the maximum achieved heart rate.

Exercise testing serves to increase sympathetic tone while minimizing the effect of vagal tone. More exacting manipulation of autonomic influence has recently become available with the development of "autonomic testing" laboratories. The applications for these are rapidly expanding, but presently include analysis of sinus node dysfunction, atrioventricular conduction disturbances, or recurrent syncope. The usual equipment includes a "tilt-table," which can quickly move a patient from a supine to a 60° upright position, along with equipment for constant electrocardiographic monitoring and measurement of respiratory rate and blood pressure. Orthostatic changes in all vital signs are recorded in baseline condition and then are repeated during an infusion of isoproterenol. The study can also be repeated after "total autonomic blockade" with atropine (to eliminate vagal influence) and a short-acting beta blocker (to eliminate catecholamine influences). Autonomic testing may help identify neurally mediated mechanisms as the etiology for syncope[1] or episodic arrhythmias (e.g., abrupt sinus bradycardia or transient AV block). Treatment can be tailored more exactly to the underlying cause in such cases.

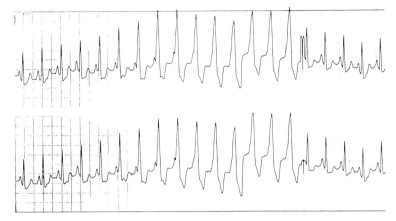

Figure 59. ECG recording from an exercise test showing slow ventricular tachycardia which developed during recovery from exercise.

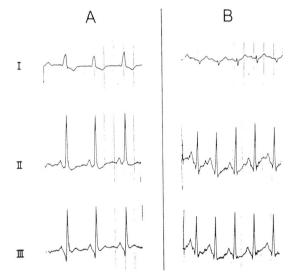

Figure 60. **A,** Exercise testing in a patient with Wolff-Parkinson-White syndrome showing a delta wave and a short P-R in early exercise, but (**B**) disappearance of the preexcitation at sinus rates of more than 160 BPM at 9 minutes of exercise. This suggested long, anterograde refractoriness of the pathway which was later confirmed at electrophysiologic study.

SIGNAL AVERAGING OF THE SURFACE CARDIOGRAM

Signal averaging produces a high-resolution, high-amplitude electrocardiogram from which one can view subtle electrical events which are too small in amplitude to be seen on the standard surface recording. This is usually accomplished by recording several hundred consecutive wave forms and superimposing them one on top of the other in the computer memory of a recording device, thereby producing a composite or "average" signal for the multiple beats. Random electrical noise that is not part of the composite wave form is then subtracted. Because this sample is so "clean," the average wave form can be greatly amplified,

thereby permitting a glimpse of small cardiac signals that go undetected on the standard electrocardiogram.

This technique may be used to display two varieties of low-amplitude electrical data. The first is depolarization within the His-Purkinje system. Recall that the P-R interval includes transmission through both the AV node and the bundle of His, and that measurements of the A-H and H-V intervals usually require placement of an intracardiac catheter. With signal averaging, a small signal corresponding to the His deflection can often be seen during the highly amplified P-R interval; this allows fairly reliable measurement of the His-Purkinje conduction time (Fig. 61).

The second item that may be examined with this technique is "late potentials" from damaged ventricular muscle. Late potentials are thought to arise from areas of slow cell-to-cell conduction and may be markers of potential reentry sites. During normal ventricular depolarization healthy cells depolarize quickly and inscribe the sharp QRS complex, but areas of slow conduction may continue to generate small amplitude signals that outlast the QRS duration. On the averaged and amplified electrocardiogram these small late potentials may be observed in the early portions of the S-T segment (Fig. 62). The significance of late potentials is still under investigation, but they may help identify patients at risk for reentry ventricular tachycardia.[3]

TRANSESOPHAGEAL RECORDING AND PACING

The proximity of the mid portion of the esophagus to the left atrium allows for placement of a recording and/or pacing electrode very near to atrial tissue. A properly positioned esophageal lead records a sharp, high-amplitude atrial electrogram (representing local left atrial depolarization) that is far superior to a surface electrocardiogram for identifying atrial activity during complex arrhythmias when the P wave and QRS complex may be su-

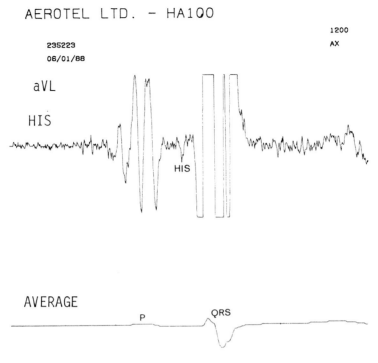

Figure 61. Signal-averaged ECG showing a sharp deflection corresponding to probable depolarization of the His bundle.

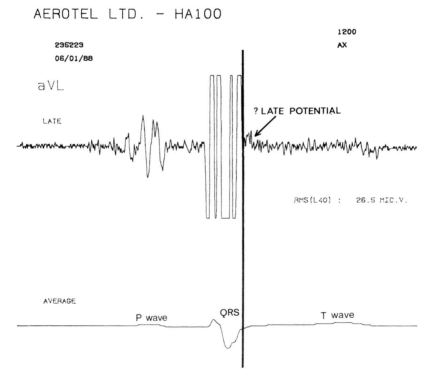

Figure 62. Signal-averaged ECG showing low-amplitude activity at the end of the QRS that may represent late potentials from abnormal cells.

perimposed. One may also pace the atrium through such a lead to correct arrhythmias or to gather electrophysiologic data.[2]

Equipment and Technique

Two types of electrodes are commercially available for transesophageal studies (Fig. 63). One variety is a small bipolar "pill" electrode that can be encased in a gelatin capsule or buried in a spoonful of ice cream and is generally acceptable for older children and adolescents to swallow. For infants and children unable to tolerate the pill electrode, a flexible bipolar pacing wire can be inserted by mouth or through the nares. Proper lead positioning is crucial, not only to obtain a good quality electrogram, but also to achieve the lowest possible threshold for successful pacing. The position may be checked by moving the lead up and down the esophagus, looking for the largest atrial electrogram (Fig. 64), but it is usually sufficient to rely on published data[2] for insertion depth based on the patient's height for ideal lead placement.

Any equipment capable of recording electrophysiologic signals can be used to display the electrogram from an esophageal lead, although optimal data are obtained with multichannel equipment that can register the esophageal trace simultaneously with at least one surface electrocardiographic lead (Fig. 65). If adjustable frequency filters are available on the recorder the ideal esophageal trace is obtained by sampling between 10 and 250 Hz.

Transesophageal pacing requires a substantially higher pacemaker output than that used for an electrode in direct contact with atrial tissue. Whereas intracardiac pacing is routinely done at a pulse width of about 2.0 msec, the capacity for wider pulses of up to 10.0 msec is needed for an esophageal lead. The expanded pulse width allows use of relatively low-amplitude settings (usually 8–15 mA) to minimize patient discomfort. Except in rare instances, ventricular pacing is not possible with an esophageal electrode.

Applications

An esophageal electrogram is helpful for recording atrial activity during complex arrhythmias when the mechanism is unclear on a surface electrocardiogram. A classic example is atrial flutter with 2:1 conduction to the ventricles. In this case, because every other flutter wave is buried by a QRS on the surface electrocardiogram, the diagnosis may be surprisingly difficult. The esophageal electrogram can clearly demonstrate the hidden flutter wave (Fig. 66). During some other forms of supraventricular tachycardia, esophageal recording may be used to clarify the timing of P waves, which may be indistinct on the surface electrocardiogram (Fig. 67).

Atrial pacing via the esophageal lead can be used for temporary correction of sinus bradycardia, but it is more frequently employed for rapid overdrive pacing of the atrium to interrupt reentry supra-

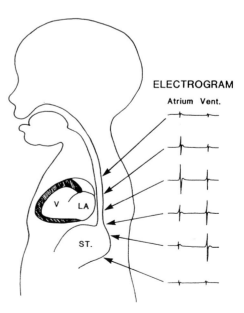

Figure 64. The anatomic relationship of the infant esophagus to cardiac chambers. The ideal electrogram at mid-esophagus has an atrial spike which is equal to, or larger than, the ventricular signal. V, ventricle; LA, left atrium; ST, stomach.

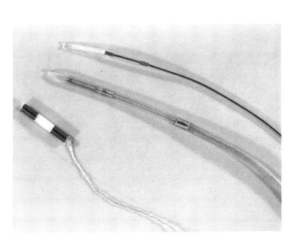

Figure 63. Electrodes for transesophageal pacing and recording: a "pill" electrode and two types of flexible bipolar catheters.

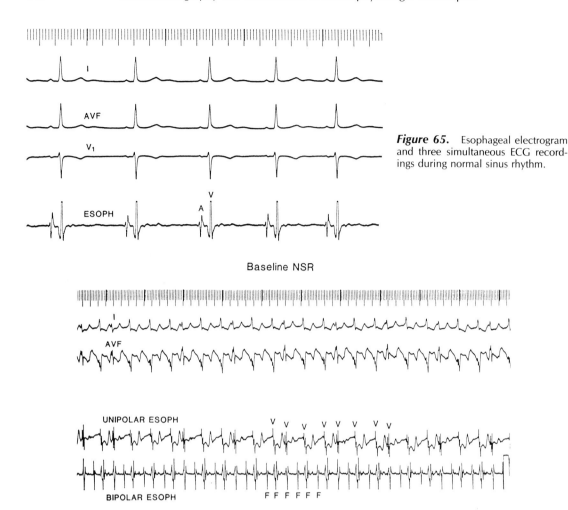

Figure 65. Esophageal electrogram and three simultaneous ECG recordings during normal sinus rhythm.

Baseline NSR

Atrial Flutter with 3:2 Conduction

Figure 66. Two surface ECG leads (I and aV$_F$) recorded simultaneously with esophageal electrograms in a patient with atrial flutter and alternating 2:1 and 3:2 conduction. Note how the bipolar esophageal signal clarifies atrial activity. A unipolar esophageal recording will highlight only ventricular activity.

ventricular tachycardia. The overdrive technique is extremely successful in converting reentry circuits within the AV node or those involving an accessory pathway (Fig. 68), and it may be successful in as many as 80% of cases involving atrial flutter (Fig. 69). Overdrive pacing is not applicable to atrial fibrillation or automatic focus tachycardias.

In addition to terminating supraventricular arrhythmias, esophageal pacing can also be used to initiate reentry tachycardias in susceptible individuals. These stimulation studies are done in a controlled setting by introducing progressively premature paced beats into sinus rhythm until a precise time sequence is found that will initiate the reentry circuit (Fig. 70). The mode of tachycardia initiation helps to determine the mechanism for the arrhythmia and aids in selection of treatment. Later, follow-up studies can be done while the patient is taking antiarrhythmic medications to test drug efficacy.

INTRACARDIAC ELECTROPHYSIOLOGIC (EP) TESTING

Practical recording of intracardiac electrograms in man was first described in 1969,[16] and the method of pacing (programmed stimulation) to induce clinical arrhythmias and study conduction characteristics is less than 20 years old. Despite this short history, electrophysiologic studies have expanded our understanding of clinical arrhythmias by a quantum leap and have helped pave the way for newer treatment modalities such as surgery for arrhythmias and catheter ablation for refractory rhythm disorders.

Equipment and Technique

Studies are performed using specialized catheters (ranging in size from 3 to 7 French) equipped with variable arrays of electrodes at the distal tip

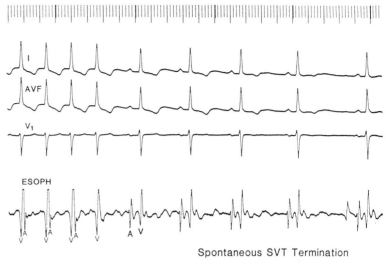

Figure 67. Esophageal and surface cardiograms during supraventricular tachycardia and at the moment of spontaneous conversion to sinus rhythm. The esophageal record confirms that the P wave was buried in the QRS during SVT, a finding that supports AV-node reentry as the probable tachycardia mechanism.

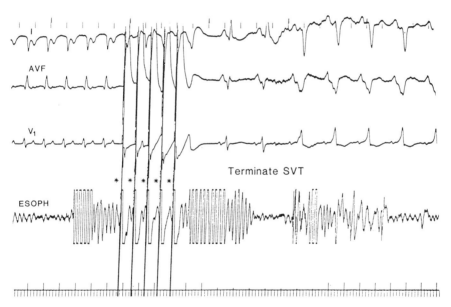

Figure 68. Termination of supraventricular tachycardia with 5 beats of esophageal burst pacing in a patient with the WPW syndrome. Note that the preexcitation returns after the second sinus beat.

(Fig. 71), through which one can pace and/or record from various cardiac sites. Procedures are done in a catheterization laboratory using standard percutaneous techniques for vascular access. The number and types of catheters employed depend on the specific goals of the study, ranging from a single atrial catheter for assessment of sinus node function to four or five separate catheters for precise mapping of arrhythmias. The standard pacing and/or recording sites are shown in Figure 72 and include the high right atrium, the bundle of His, the coronary sinus, and the right ventricular apex.

High Right Atrium (HRA)

The HRA site is located at the superior vena cava–right atrial junction, in close proximity to the sino-atrial node. This site records local atrial depolarization and is used for routine atrial pacing to assess SA node function and atrioventricular conduction, or to study supraventricular tachycardia (SVT).

His Bundle Electrogram (HBE)

The HBE is obtained by positioning the catheter just across the tricuspid valve at its posterior and superior rim, near the area of the common bundle of His. Because the catheter straddles the valve, it records both low, right atrial depolarization, and right ventricular inflow depolarization, along with a distinct His deflection. The HBE dissects atrioventricular conduction into AV-node and His-Purkinje components. It is a crucial recording site for

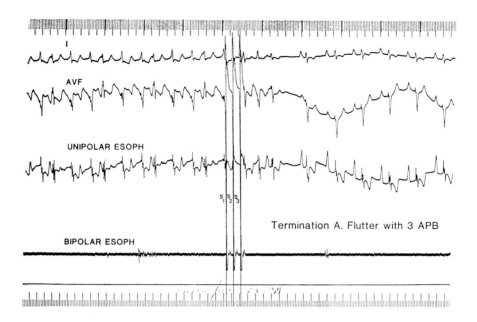

Figure 69. Termination of atrial flutter with three premature beats (APB) delivered by transesophageal pacing.

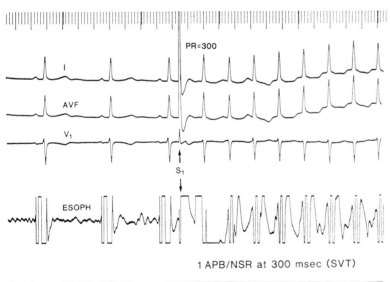

Figure 70. Induction of supraventricular tachycardia with a single premature beat delivered by transesophageal pacing. APB, atrial premature beat; NSR, normal sinus rhythm.

analysis of atrioventricular conduction disturbances and for evaluation of SVT.

Coronary Sinus (CS)

A catheter in the coronary sinus records both atrial and ventricular signals from the left heart. Usually, catheters must be positioned from the superior vena cava, using a subclavian or arm approach. The CS catheter is mandatory for evaluation of SVT, particularly if an accessory pathway is involved.

Right Ventricular Apex (RVA)

The RVA provides a stable site for ventricular pacing and recording. It is used for evaluation of complex SVT, as well as for the study of ventricular arrhythmias. Additional ventricular pacing sites (such as the right ventricular outflow area, or left ventricular apex) may be included for ventricular stimulation in some cases.

The electrograms are displayed on a multichannel recorder, along with simultaneous surface electrocardiogram leads (most often I, aV_F, and V_1). Recording paper speeds of 100 mm/sec are routinely employed; this permits time resolution of ±5 msec for most data. The equipment is backed up by a magnetic tape recording and often includes a freeze-screen oscilloscope for quick reference. Pacing is performed with a device capable of vari-

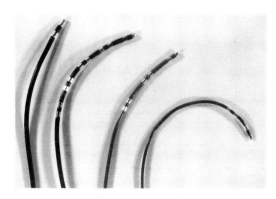

Figure 71. Example of electrode catheters for intracardiac electrophysiologic study. Shown here are 4 Fr quadrapolar, 5 Fr hexapolar, 6 Fr decapolar, and 7 Fr "large tip" bipolar.

able-rate pacing, as well as the delivery of a premature beat(s) at finely adjustable intervals. Defibrillation equipment must be readily available for emergency use.

Applications

Electrophysiologic studies involve three general categories of data: (1) baseline rhythm, (2) pacing maneuvers to evaluate functional characteristics, and (3) programmed stimulation with premature beats to initiate tachycardias. A comprehensive study for SVT or ventricular arrhythmia involves an orderly collection of all these items as outlined below.

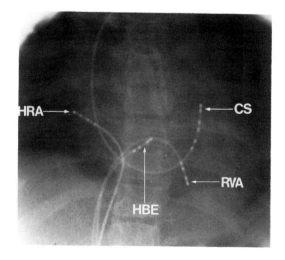

Figure 72. Standard catheter positions for electrophysiologic study. Note that the CS catheter is usually positioned via the superior vena cava. HRA, high right atrium; HBE, His bundle electrogram; CS, coronary sinus; RVA, right ventricular apex.

Baseline Recording

Resting rhythm may be examined to determine conduction times and activation sequence throughout the heart (Fig. 73). Signals are not routinely observed from sinus node depolarization; however, local atrial depolarization can be recorded from the HRA, HBE, and CS electrodes. In normal sinus rhythm the HRA electrode is the first to register electrical activity by virtue of its close proximity to the SA node, followed by the electrode in the low right atrium (HBE catheter) 20–25 msec later, and finally, the "distal" CS electrode after about 60 msec. Ectopic foci or other forms of SVT shift the atrial sequence in favor of the site of origin of the abnormal rhythm.

Conduction time within the AV node may be determined by measuring the A-H interval of the HBE recording. The normal A-H interval varies between 40 and 100 msec in children. A prolonged A-H interval can be observed in patients taking certain antiarrhythmic drugs, those with high vagal tone, and in patients with disease of the AV node. It is shortened under conditions of high circulating catecholamines and in patients with "enhanced" AV-node conduction or the Lown-Ganong-Levine syndrome.

The H-V interval, representing conduction time in the His-Purkinje system, is also recorded by the HBE electrode, and is between 35 and 55 msec in normal children. Prolonged resting H-V intervals usually suggest His-Purkinje pathology. A short H-V may be observed in the preexcitation syndrome, including the WPW syndrome and nodoventricular (Mahaim) fibers.

Final baseline measurements involve regional ventricular activation times. Data points from the standard catheter position include the apex of the right ventricle (from the RVA catheter), the inflow area of the right ventricle (from the HBE catheter) and the left ventricular base (from the CS catheter). Measurements are indexed against a "V-line," which is marked at the earliest evidence of ventricular activation in any lead (including the surface QRS). Normally, the RVA displays the earliest signals among these recording sites, approximately 10–35 msec after onset of the QRS. Block in the central right bundle branch can cause delayed RVA activation (>50 msec). In the WPW syndrome, preexcitation via a right-sided accessory pathway may promote early activation of the right ventricular inflow area, or conversely, a left-sided pathway may cause the left ventricular base to activate ahead of schedule.

Functional Characteristics of the SA Node

Unfortunately, electrophysiologic techniques are not perfect indicators of SA-node integrity.

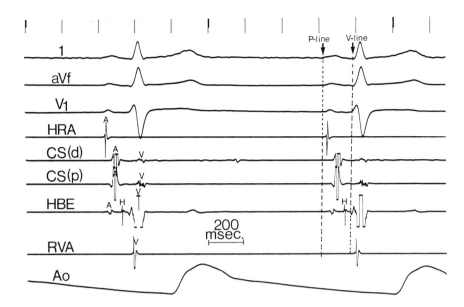

Figure 73. Baseline signals during normal sinus rhythm, including three surface ECG leads, along with multiple intra-cardiac recordings. Atrial activation is indexed against a "P-line" and shows the earliest activation in HRA near the sinus node. Ventricular activation is indexed against the "V-line," and normally shows the earliest activity in RVA. HRA, the high right atrium; CSd, distal coronary sinus; CSp, proximal coronary sinus; HBE, His bundle electrogram; RVA, right ventricular apex; and Ao, arterial blood pressure.

When testing is grossly abnormal the data are useful, but false-negative results are not uncommon. Thus, these techniques must be used in conjunction with clinical history and noninvasive monitoring when evaluating the sinus node.

Two pacing maneuvers have evolved to evaluate SA node status. The first, **sinus node recovery time** (**SNRT**), involves pacing the HRA for 30–60 sec at rates above normal baseline rhythm. When pacing is abruptly terminated there is usually a very brief pause before the resumption of sinus beats in a normal individual, but if the pause is protracted, sinus node dysfunction is suggested. The recovery time is usually "corrected" by subtracting the rest-

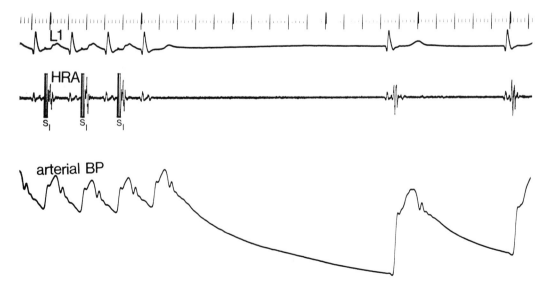

Figure 74. An example of depressed sinus node recovery. After 60 sec of pacing (S1) in the HRA at a rate of 150/min, pacing is abruptly terminated. There is a pause of nearly 3.0 sec before a junctional escape beat restores the rhythm. HRA, high right atrium.

ing cycle length (i.e., the time in milliseconds between two normal sinus beats, designated A1–A1) from the recovery cycle length (i.e., the time from the last beat of pacing until the first spontaneous sinus beat, designated A2–A3) to yield a "corrected sinus node recovery time" or CSNRT. Normal values for CSNRT should be less than 275 msec for children.[19] These same data may also be reported as a percentage [%SNRT = (A2–A3)/(A1–A1) × 100] where values less than 166% are considered normal. When there is advanced disease of the SA node, the abnormal SNRT is usually not subtle and involves a "painful pause" at the cessation of pacing (Fig. 74).

The SA node may also be evaluated by determining the **sino-atrial conduction time (SACT)**. The SACT essentially measures how fast impulses are conducted into and out of the SA node, and it is prolonged in disease involving nodal cells or the surrounding atrial tissue. Single-paced beats are delivered at the HRA at progressively premature intervals until a reproducible noncompensatory pause or "reset zone" is encountered. This pause is made up of three components (Fig. 75): (1) the time it takes the premature beat to penetrate back into the node, (2) the normal resting cycle length of SA node depolarization (A1–A1), and (3) the time it takes for SA node depolarization to exit back out to atrial tissue. The total SACT = ("reset" A_2–A_2) − ("resting" A_1–A_1) and should normally be less than 200 msec.[11]

Functional Characteristics of the AV Node

The simplest technique for evaluation of atrioventricular conduction involves short bursts of pacing in the HRA while observing the ventricular response. The pacing cycle length is decreased in 10-msec increments until a rate is encountered at which the Wenckebach phenomenon occurs. For normal children this is usually not observed until the pacing cycle length is less than about 350 msec (i.e., rate faster than 171/minute).

More precise evaluation of the AV node is performed with the introduction of single premature beats at the HRA, delivered at an interval that is progressively shortened in 10-msec increments (Fig. 76). As the stimulus is moved earlier, a gradual and progressive increase in the A-H interval is seen, related to the normal decremental conduction properties of the slow-response cells in the AV node. Eventually, a stimulus can be delivered early enough to block at the AV node. This registers on the HBE electrogram as an atrial signal without a His or ventricular deflection. The premature interval at which this conduction fails to occur is defined as the effective refractory period (ERP) for the node and normally ranges from 200–270 msec in children. As the stimulus timing is further shortened, a point will be reached where the atrial tissue no longer depolarizes. This is the atrial muscle ERP and is encountered between 150 and 200 msec in normal children.

Functional Characteristics of His-Purkinje Conduction

Function of the His-Purkinje system may likewise be evaluated with the single extrastimulus technique. Normally, the H-V interval tends to remain constant and the QRS complex tends to remain narrow during premature atrial stimula-

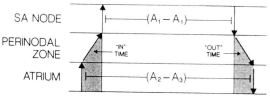

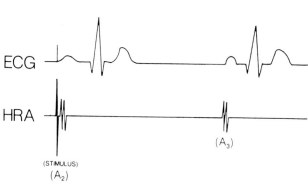

Figure 75. Calculation of total sino-atrial conduction time (SACT). HRA, high right atrium.

TOTAL SACT = (RESET TIME) − (RESTING SINUS RATE)

= $(A_2 − A_3) − (A_1 − A_1)$

= "IN TIME" + "OUT TIME"

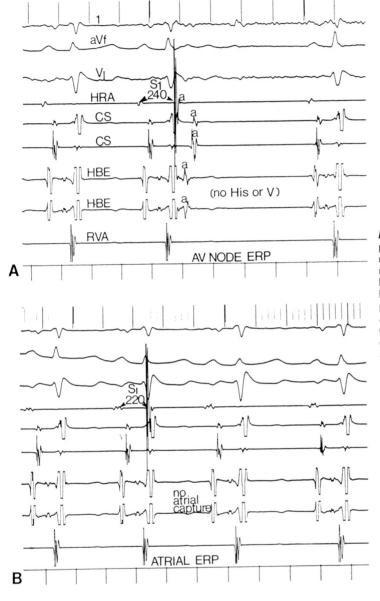

Figure 76. The effective refractory periods of the AV node (**A**) and atrial muscle (**B**). In sequence A, the premature beat captures the atrium but blocks at the AV node such that no His bundle signal is seen. A slightly earlier premature beat fails to capture the atrium entirely. HRA, high right atrium; CS, coronary sinus; HBE, His bundle electrogram; RVA, right ventricular apex.

tion. Some patients may develop QRS aberration (due to rate-related bundle branch block) in response to early beats, but this is usually a benign finding. More significant is the observation of block in the common bundle of His with an early stimulus, which registers on the HBE as an atrial spike followed by a His deflection but without conduction to the ventricles. When the ERP of the common bundle of His is encountered ahead of the AV node ERP, primary His-Purkinje disease may be suggested.

Functional Characteristics of Ventricular Tissue

The ERP can also be measured for ventricular muscle, using the single extra stimulus technique.

This information is most useful during the study of ventricular arrhythmias, when one must compare baseline conditions to the alteration in ERP related to antiarrhythmic drugs. The longest premature interval at which a stimulus fails to capture the ventricle is defined as the ventricular muscle ERP, and it normally occurs at 200–260 msec. The administration of antiarrhythmic agents often prolongs the ERP.

Evaluation of Supraventricular Tachycardia (SVT)

Many patients with SVT can be well managed without electrophysiologic study. However, if the arrhythmia has been refractory to first-line management or is associated with serious symptoms,

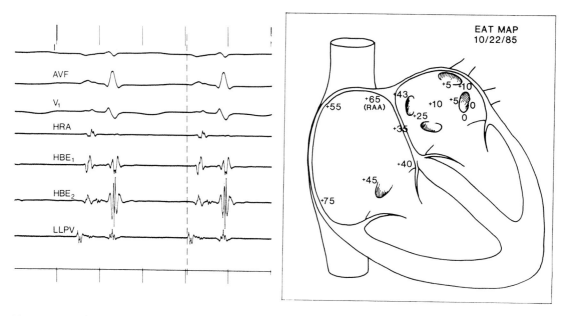

Figure 77.   An example of atrial activation sequence-mapping in a patient with ectopic atrial tachycardia. The earliest atrial activity was found with mapping near the left, lower pulmonary vein (LLPV); HBE, His bundle electrogram; HRA, high right atrium.

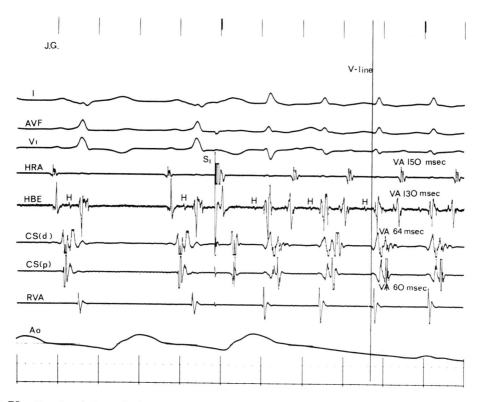

Figure 78.   Mapping during orthodromic reentry tachycardia in a patient with the WPW syndrome. Tachycardia is induced with a single premature beat (S1) that conducts to the ventricle over the AV node and returns to the atrium over the accessory pathway. The shortest VA time (i.e., the earliest retrograde atrial signal) is seen in the proximal coronary sinus, corresponding to a left-sided accessory pathway. HRA, high right atrium; HBE, His bundle electrogram; CS(d), distal coronary sinus; CS(p), proximal coronary sinus; RVA, right ventricular apex; Ao, arterial blood pressure.

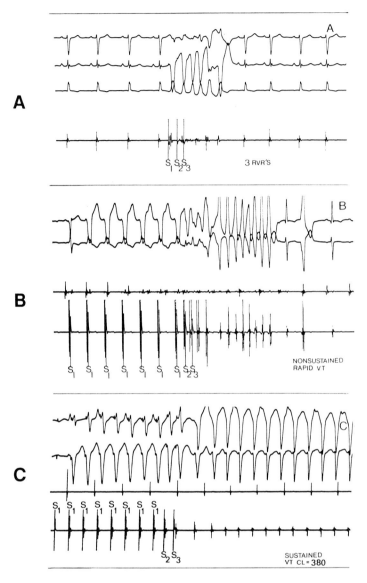

Figure 79. Examples of possible responses to ventricular programmed stimulation; A, repetitive ventricular responses (RVRs); B, nonsustained ventricular tachycardia; and C, sustained ventricular tachycardia.

intracardiac study is indicated to determine the mechanism of the arrhythmia, to evaluate drug responses, and to map the location of foci or pathways that could potentially be ablated with surgical or catheter techniques.

Such studies require catheters at the four standard recording sites. Resting rhythm is first examined for the atrial activation sequence and any evidence for preexcitation (e.g., short A-H or H-V interval). A routine evaluation of the functional status of the entire conducting system is then performed as described previously. During these maneuvers, or with more aggressive stimulation, SVT may be induced.

There is a long list of mechanisms for pediatric SVT (see ch. 27) but, as a starting point, one may divide them into the broad categories of "automatic focus" versus "reentry circuits." The automatic va-

riety tend to occur spontaneously or in response to increased catecholamine levels, but generally are not induced or terminated with pacing techniques. Reentry, by far the more common mechanism in the pediatric population, appears in response to approximately-timed premature beats and can usually be interrupted with standard overdrive pacing techniques.

Mapping of an arrhythmia location begins by determining whether the AV node and/or ventricle are critical components of the disorder. Those SVTs that arise from the area of the SA node or atrial muscle (so-called "primary-atrial" SVT) usually display some intermittent block at the AV node which does not modify the atrial SVT rate. By comparison, tachycardias with a fixed 1:1 atrioventricular relationship (so-called "AV reciprocating" SVT) terminate promptly whenever this ratio is disturbed.

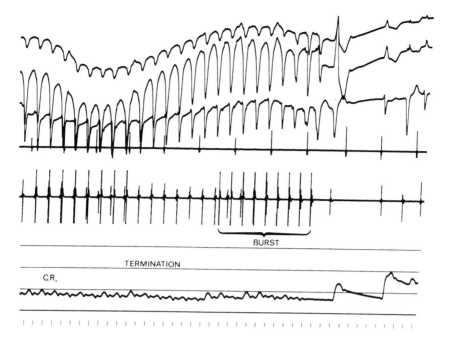

Figure 80. Termination of sustained monomorphic ventricular tachycardia with burst pacing.

The latter pattern is typical for SVT due to reentry within the AV node or via an accessory pathway (e.g., the WPW syndrome).

Finer tuning of the arrhythmia location is possible by examining the atrial activation sequence during SVT (Fig. 77). Precise mapping of both automatic foci and reentry pathways is possible with careful attention to the location of the earliest atrial signals (Fig. 78).

Determining SVT mechanisms is of more than just academic interest. Rational choices of antiarrhythmic drug therapy demand knowledge of the types of cardiac cells responsible for an automatic focus or reentry circuit. For example, reentry within the AV node operates through slow-response cells which are highly dependent on calcium channel activity. A drug such as verapamil can modify these channels and represents an intelligent choice for first-line therapy. On the other hand, atrial flutter (atrial muscle reentry) is more likely to respond to a drug that modifies sodium channels, such as quinidine. Determination of the mechanism, in conjunction with careful mapping, also allows consideration of surgical or catheter ablation as an alternative to long-term drug use.

Evaluation of Ventricular Arrhythmias

Studies of ventricular stimulation are performed with three major goals in mind. First, some arrhythmias that appear to be ventricular tachycardia (VT) on a surface electrocardiogram are, in fact, atypical supraventricular arrhythmias. Because the prognosis and treatment differ so significantly, electrophysiologic testing is indicated to establish

the exact mechanism. Second, programmed stimulation can be performed in an attempt to induce reentry VT, and the ease of induction may be used as an index of a patient's risk for spontaneous arrhythmia. Finally, the patient can be retested after drug loading to evaluate therapeutic response,[13] or if drugs prove inadequate, the VT focus can be mapped with a view to surgical or catheter ablation.

A complete VT study begins with baseline recording from at least three sites—HRA, HBE, and RVA—followed by atrial stimulation to evaluate functional characteristics of the conducting system and to rule out atypical SVT as the cause of the clinical arrhythmia. A ventricular stimulation protocol is then carried out in an attempt to induce VT. Protocols vary, and it must be remembered that a point can be reached where the stimulation becomes so provocative that an induced arrhythmia is nonspecific and bears little resemblance to the clinical tachycardia. Additionally, some forms of VT may involve a mechanism other than classic reentry, and normal stimulation techniques may be unsuccessful in reproducing the disorder. In general, studies usually include some minor modifications of the following protocol:

1. Stimulation begins at the right ventricular apex with introduction of the stimuli, delivered at progressively premature intervals (shortened in 10-msec increments) until the ventricular muscle is refractory:

  A. Single premature beats (S1) in sinus rhythm

  B. Double premature beats (S1, S2) in sinus rhythm

  C. Single premature beats following 8 beats of

ventricular pacing (S1 × 8, S2), using three different cycle lengths for S1 (usually 600, 500, and 400 msec)

   D. Double premature beats following 8 beats of pacing (S1 × 8, S2, S3) at three S1 cycle lengths

   E. Triple premature beats in sinus rhythm (S1, S2, S3)

   F. Triple premature beats following 8 beats of pacing (S1 × 8, S2, S3, S4) at one or more S1 cycle lengths

2. Stimulation at a second site, usually the right ventricular outflow tract, with an identical sequence.

3. Optional additions to the protocol:

   A. The standard sequence at a third ventricular site such as the left ventricular apex

   B. Stimulation with four premature beats after an 8-beat drive train (S1 × 8, S2, S3, S4, S5)

   C. Burst ventricular pacing at rapid rates

   D. Stimulation during an infusion of isoproterenol

The possible responses to ventricular stimulation are shown in Figure 79. Whenever sustained arrhythmias are induced, the team must react quickly to terminate the condition. For sustained VT, this can most often be accomplished with rapid overdrive pacing of the ventricles (Fig. 80), but very rapid VT or ventricular fibrillation needs to be terminated with standard DC shock. Obviously, such studies require an experienced laboratory team to ensure patient safety. If a significant ventricular arrhythmia is induced at the initial study, it is possible to test drug efficacy by repeating the protocol after intravenous or oral drug loading. This process may require several return trips to the electrophysiology lab until an optimal treatment regimen is found.

REFERENCES

1. Almquist A, Goldenberg IF, Milstein S, et al: Provocation of bradycardia and hypotension by isoproterenol and upright posture in patients with unexplained syncope. N Engl J Med 320:346–351, 1989.
2. Benson DW, Dunnigan A, Benditt DG, et al: Transesophageal cardiac pacing: history, application, technique. Clin Prog Pacing Electrophysiol 2:360–372, 1984.
3. Breithardt G, Borggrefe M: Recent advances in the identification of patients at risk of ventricular tachyarrhythmias: role of ventricular late potentials. Circulation 75:1091–1096, 1987.
4. Davignon A, Rautaharju PM, Boisselle E, et al: Normal ECG standards for infants and children. Pediatr Cardiol 1:123–131, 1979.
5. Deal BJ, Keane JF, Gillette PC, et al: Wolff-Parkinson-White syndrome and supraventricular tachycardia during infancy: management and follow-up. J Am Coll Cardiol 5:130–135, 1985.
6. Fisch C: Electrocardiography and vectorcardiography. In Braunwald E (ed): Heart Disease. Philadelphia, W.B. Saunders, 1984, p. 200.
7. Garson A: Recording the sequence of cardiac activity. In The Electrocardiogram in Infants and Children. Philadelphia, Lea & Febiger, 1983, pp. 19, 99.
8. Gilmore RF, Zipes DP: Cellular basis for cardiac arrhythmias. Cardiol Clin 1:3–11, 1983.
9. Holter NJ: New method for heart studies. Science 134:1214–1220, 1961.
10. Jacobsen JR, Garson A, Gillette PC, et al: Premature ventricular contractions in normal children. J Pediatr 92:36–38, 1978.
11. Kugler JD, Gillette PC, Mullins CE, et al: Sinoatrial conduction in children: an index of sinoatrial node function. Circulation 59:1266–1276, 1979.
12. Lewis T: The Mechanism and Graphic Registration of the Heart Beat. London, Shaw and Sons et al., 1925, preface, p. vi.
13. Mason JW, Winkle RA: Electrode catheter arrhythmia induction in the selection and assessment of antiarrhythmic drug therapy for recurrent ventricular tachycardia. Circulation 58:971–985, 1978.
14. Nadas AS: Electrocardiography. In Pediatric Cardiology. Philadelphia, W.B. Saunders, 1957, p. 42.
15. Plonsey R: The biophysical basis for electrocardiography. In Liebman J, Plonsey R, Gillette RC (eds): Pediatric Electrocardiography. Baltimore, Williams & Wilkins, 1982, p. 1.
16. Scherlag BJ, Lau SH, Helfant RA, et al: Catheter technique for recording His bundle activity in man. Circulation 39:13–18, 1969.
17. Wagner JR, Weidman WH, Ellison RC, et al: Indirect assessment of severity of aortic stenosis. Circulation 56(Suppl I):21–24, 1977.
18. Winkler RB, Freed MD, Nadas AS: Exercise induced ventricular ectopy in children and young adults with complete heart block. Am Heart J 99:87–92, 1980.
19. Yabek SM, Jarmakani JM, Roberts NK: Sinus node function in children: factors influencing its evaluation. Circulation 53:28–32, 1976.
20. Zipes DP: Genesis of cardiac arrhythmias: electrophysiological considerations. In Braunwald E (ed): Heart Disease. Philadelphia, W.B. Saunders Co., 1984, p. 605.

Chapter 13

ECHOCARDIOGRAPHY

Stephen P. Sanders, M.D.

The current status of cardiovascular ultrasound as the primary diagnostic modality for structural heart defects is the product of some 35 years of development. Edler and Hertz first described the use of reflected ultrasound for imaging the heart in 1954.[22] At that time the images were crude, displaying only the walls of the left ventricle and the mitral valve leaflets. Initially, the principal use of echocardiography was to detect mitral stenosis by measuring the rate of closure of the mitral leaflets (E to F slope).[21] By the mid-1960s the uses of echocardiography had expanded to include detection of pericardial effusion and dilated cardiomyopathy, despite little improvement in image quality.[24]

Interest in echocardiography grew rapidly over the next decade. Technologic advances in transducer design and image processing led to improved image quality. The discovery of contrast echocardiography[32] allowed investigators to identify structures seen on the echocardiogram. Techniques for positioning and directing the transducer were developed that allowed several heart structures to be displayed on a single recording (Fig. 1). By the late 1970s attempts had been made to use M-mode echocardiography, alone or with contrast, to diagnose many congenital heart defects. However, the limited view of the heart afforded by M-mode echocardiography proved to be insufficient for reliable diagnosis of most defects.

The development of two-dimensional echocardiography transformed the field.[33,45] For the first time tomographic images of the beating heart were available to the clinician (Fig. 2). The size, location, orientation, and pattern of motion of nearly any cardiac structure could be determined precisely. Virtually every congenital defect or acquired abnormality could be rapidly demonstrated by two-dimensional imaging. By the mid-1980s, two-dimensional echocardiography had become the primary diagnostic tool in pediatric cardiology.

Concurrent with the development of ultrasonic imaging techniques, methods were devised for investigating blood flow, using the Doppler principle. Doppler analysis of reflected sound waves was first used to detect obstruction of peripheral arteries and veins.[50,88] Other investigators directed the Doppler beam at the heart to study patterns of blood flow within the heart and great vessels.[5] Doppler flow analysis combined with two-dimensional imaging allowed sampling of flow velocity and direction at selected sites within the heart and great vessels.[43] Doppler color flow mapping, the newest combined Doppler-imaging modality, overlaid information about the direction and velocity of blood flow in color on the gray scale, two-dimensional image.[13,60,61] Doppler echocardiography has proved to be extremely valuable for the detection and estimation of severity of valvar dysfunction and for the detection of shunt lesions.

For a variety of reasons, cardiovascular ultrasound is especially suited to infants and small children. First, the path that the sound energy may traverse is short, allowing use of high-frequency sound energy without sacrificing the strength of the returning signal. The quality of the image depends largely on the frequency of the sound energy used, with higher frequencies producing better images. Second, more and better echocardiographic "windows" are available in infants and children. For example, the subxiphoid views allow comprehensive imaging of the heart and associated structures in infants and small children, but are much less useful in older children and adults. Third, the kinds of questions that generally arise in pediatric cardiology relate to gross anatomic details. Cardiovascular ultrasound is uniquely suited to answer the vast majority of such questions. In fact, for an increasing number of cardiac defects, ultrasound provides all the information needed to undertake surgical intervention. Consequently, it is essential for the pediatric cardiologist to be well versed in the uses and limitations of all aspects of cardiovascular ultrasound.

159

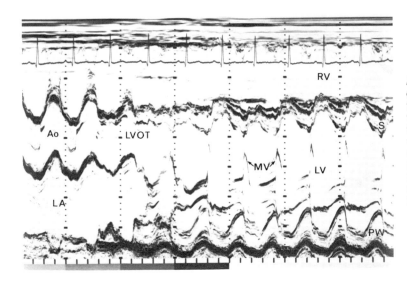

Figure 1. A current M-mode echocardiogram illustrating a scan from the aortic root to the body of the left ventricle. By sweeping the transducer in an arc, the entire left ventricle from body to outflow tract can be imaged. Ao = aorta; LA = left atrium; LV = left ventricle; LVOT = left ventricular outflow tract; MV = mitral valve leaflets; RV = right ventricle.

PHYSICAL PRINCIPLES OF CARDIOVASCULAR ULTRASOUND

A detailed discussion of the physics of sound can be found elsewhere[23] and is beyond the scope of this text. However, a few basic concepts are essential.

Sound

Sound waves, unlike electromagnetic waves, are mechanical and require a physical medium in which to propagate. The speed and efficiency with which a medium transmits sound energy depend on the stiffness and density of the medium. Stiffer substances, such as solids, transmit sound energy more rapidly than do less stiff materials, such as liquids or gases. Sound energy is reflected at an interface between two media of different trans- mission properties. The greater the difference in acoustic transmission properties between the two media, the more sound energy is reflected and the less energy crosses the interface into the second medium. Such naturally occurring, large tissue in- terfaces (e.g., between blood and endocardium or endocardium and myocardium) in the heart and other organs form the basis for ultrasonic imaging. On the other hand, an interface between tissues having very different acoustic transmission char- acteristics, such as gas-filled bowel or lung and soft tissue, or bone and soft tissue, results in reflection of virtually all the incident sound energy. Struc- tures beneath the highly reflective interface cannot be imaged because no sound energy reaches them. Consequently, echocardiographic "windows" must be selected to provide access to the heart and ves- sels without intervening lung or bone.

If the surface that reflects sound energy (e.g., a red blood cell) is moving with respect to the sound source (the transducer), the frequency of the re- flected sound energy is changed, as described by the Doppler equation. The change in frequency is proportional to the velocity of the reflector. The direction of the frequency change (increase or de- crease in frequency) indicates the direction of mo- tion of the reflector. This is the basis for Doppler echocardiography and will be discussed in more detail later.

Imaging

Ultrasonic imaging devices consist of a pulse generator, a timer, a transducer and an image pro- cessor and display screen. Electrical pulses are sent from the pulse generator to the transducer. In re- sponse to electrical stimulation, the transducer emits a short burst of sound energy at a charac- teristic frequency. After each pulse the transducer acts as a receiver, waiting for reflected sound en-

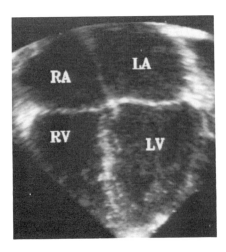

Figure 2. A two-dimensional echocardiogram in apical four-chamber view. LA = left atrium; LV = left ventricle; RA = right atrium; RV = right ventricle.

ergy to return from tissue interfaces. Reflected sound energy that returns to the transducer is converted back into an electrical impulse that is sent to the image processor. As each pulse of sound energy is transmitted, the timer is started. When sound energy returns to the transducer, the timer is consulted to determine the time required for the sound energy to travel to the target and back. Then the distance from the transducer to the target is calculated using the known speed of propagation of sound in soft tissue (1530 m/sec). A dot is placed on the image display at a position corresponding to the calculated location of the target. This process is rapidly repeated to build up an image. The typical pulse rate, or rate at which pulses of sound energy are emitted by the transducer, is 1000 Hz, or 1000 times per second. Because the transducer generates very brief pulses of sound energy (1 μsec in duration), most of the time is spent listening for returning signals.

M-Mode Echocardiography. M-mode echocardiography provides an "icepick" view of the heart. A thin beam of sound energy is directed into the heart, and only structures that lie along the line of sight of this beam are displayed. The temporal and spatial resolution of M-mode echocardiography is extremely high, making it particularly useful for measuring linear dimensions and rate of change of dimension (e.g., transverse dimension of a heart chamber or the thickness of the wall of a chamber). M-mode echocardiography is now used mostly for evaluation of ventricular size and function. Because of the limited view of the heart afforded by M-mode echocardiography, this modality has no place in the diagnosis of structural heart defects.

Two-Dimensional Echocardiography. Two-dimensional echocardiography provides a cross-sectional, or tomographic, view of the heart. The two-dimensional image is constructed by sweeping the sound beam through an arc. This can be accomplished either by rocking the transducer or electronically steering the sound beam. The image can be thought of as many M-mode lines radiating outward from the apex of the arc.

Two-dimensional echocardiography is exceptionally useful for diagnosis of structural heart defects. The tomographic images demonstrate structures and relationships within the image plane. By sweeping the transducer across the heart in many planes, the experienced examiner can mentally construct a three-dimensional image of the heart. The entire heart and associated structures can be visualized in detail, yielding a wealth of anatomic information. In addition, 2-D echocardiography is proving to be useful in a quantitative sense. Although linear measurements are not as precise and time resolution is lower than with M-mode echocardiography, two-dimensional imaging allows planar areas to be measured for volume calculations. Cross-sectional images allow linear measurements

to be made even at angles to the direction of propagation of the sound waves. However, the accuracy of such measurements is less than that for measurements made parallel to the direction of propagation of the sound waves.

Generally, the resolving power of imaging devices is thought of as having two components, axial resolution and lateral resolution. Axial resolution is the ability to discriminate between two closely spaced objects along the axis of the sound beam. The principal determinant of axial resolution is the length or duration of the pulse of sound energy emitted by the transducer. The shorter the pulse length, the better is the axial resolution. The pulse length, in turn, is a function of the frequency or wave length of the sound energy and the damping characteristics of the transducer. Today, most transducers are critically damped, emitting as few cycles of sound energy with each pulse as possible. Therefore, the major variable determinant of axial resolution is sound frequency or wave length. As the frequency of sound energy increases the wave length decreases, leading to improved axial resolution.

Lateral resolution is the ability to discriminate between two closely spaced objects perpendicular to the sound beam and it is largely determined by the width of the sound beam. The width can be altered by mechanically or electronically focusing the sound beam. In mechanical systems, the beam is narrow, and lateral resolution is favorable near the focal point. The beam diverges rapidly outside the focal zone, resulting in poor lateral resolution in the near and far fields. The rate of divergence depends on the frequency of the sound energy (with higher frequencies diverging less rapidly) and the distance between the transducer and the focal point. Modern electronic imaging systems can change the focal point dynamically, extending the focal zone to encompass the entire depth of field.

Doppler Analysis

Physics. As noted previously, motion of the reflector relative to the transducer results in a shift in the frequency of the reflected sound waves proportional to the velocity of the reflector, as described by the Doppler equation:

$$f_d = \frac{v \times f_o \times \cos \theta}{2c}$$

where f_d = Doppler frequency shift, v = reflector velocity, f_o = frequency of the incident sound energy, θ = angle between the direction of motion of the reflector and the direction of propagation of the sound waves, and c = speed of sound propagation in tissue.

Because one is generally interested in determining the velocity of the reflector (usually red blood cells), it is helpful to rearrange the Doppler equation, solving for velocity:

$$v = f_d \times \frac{2c}{f_o} \times \frac{1}{\cos \theta}$$

The variables that must be known in order to calculate the velocity of the reflector are the Doppler frequency shift (f_d), the transmitted frequency (f_o), and the angle between the direction of propagation of the sound waves and the direction of motion of the reflector (θ).

Consider a small boat at anchor on a lake. If a large stone is dropped into the water some distance from the boat, waves propagate on the surface of the water toward the boat much as sound waves do in tissue. As long as the boat remains stationary, the frequency of the waves reflected by the bow of the boat is the same as the frequency of the waves incident on the bow of the boat (Fig. 3A). In the special case in which velocity of the reflector is zero, the Doppler shift, or the change in frequency of the reflected waves, is also zero. If the boat begins to move toward the source of the waves, however, the bow strikes the crest of each wave a little sooner than it would have if the boat were stationary (Fig. 3B). Consequently, the distance between crests of the reflected waves is shorter and the frequency is higher than for the incident waves. This difference in frequency between the incident and reflected waves is the Doppler frequency shift. Similarly, if the boat began to move away from the source of the waves, the stern of the boat would strike the crest of each successive wave a little later than if the boat were stationary (Fig. 3C). The distance between crests of the reflected waves would be greater and the frequency lower than for the incident waves. In either case, the faster the boat moves, the more it changes the frequency of the reflected waves. The Doppler frequency shift is directly proportional to the velocity of the reflector, and the direction of the shift (increase or decrease in frequency) is determined by the direction of motion of the reflector, with motion toward the sound source increasing frequency and motion away from the sound source lowering frequency.

The angle between the direction of propagation of the sound waves and the direction of motion of the reflector also affects the Doppler frequency shift. Consider a case in which the source of the waves on the lake is directly upwind from the boat, so that it must be approached on a tack (Fig. 3D). Now the boat is moving at some angle θ with respect to the direction of propagation of the waves. The component of the velocity vector of the boat that projects in the direction of motion of the waves is inversely proportional to the angle. Only this component of the velocity vector acts to alter the frequency of the reflected waves. If the boat is moving perpendicularly to the direction of propagation of the waves, there is no Doppler frequency shift at all because the component of the velocity vector in the direction of propagation of the waves is zero. The relation between the angle θ and the Doppler frequency shift is described by the cosine function of the angle. The larger the angle θ, the less is the Doppler frequency shift for any given reflector velocity. For practical purposes angles less than 15–20° can be ignored, because the cosine function is 0.94 or greater.

The Doppler frequency shift for any given reflector velocity also varies directly with the frequency of the transmitted sound energy. Returning to the boat analogy, the distance traveled by the boat and the consequent change in wave length become relatively larger as the base wave length decreases. Thus, the Doppler frequency shift is not only a function of the velocity of the reflector, but also of the frequency of the incident sound energy.

Doppler instruments are of two basic types, continuous-wave or pulsed-wave.

Continuous-wave Doppler. These devices have two transducers, one that continuously transmits sound energy and one that continuously acts as a receiver. The transducers are oriented so that sound energy from the transmitter is reflected back to the receiver. Any reflectors that lie along the line of sight of the transducer system contribute to the recorded Doppler frequency shift. If multiple reflectors lie along the path of the Doppler beam, it is impossible to determine which part of the overall frequency shift results from any one reflector. Hence, continuous-wave Doppler has no spatial resolution. On the other hand, because the field of interest is being sampled continuously, the maximum Doppler shift or target velocity that can be unambiguously recorded is essentially unlimited. Consequently, continuous-wave Doppler is useful for recording high-velocity signals associated with stenotic lesions, atrioventricular valve regurgitation, and some shunt lesions, but not for localizing the source of the signal.

Pulsed Doppler. This method uses the same principle as M-mode echocardiography to achieve spatial resolution. Instead of a pair of transducers continuously sending and receiving sound energy, pulsed Doppler uses a single transducer that emits brief pulses of sound energy. As in echocardiography, the transducer is free to act as a receiver between pulses. If the transducer is active as a receiver for a very short time, only the reflected sound energy from a discrete locus in the field of view is analyzed for a Doppler frequency shift. Because the speed of propagation of sound energy in soft tissue is known, it is possible to calculate

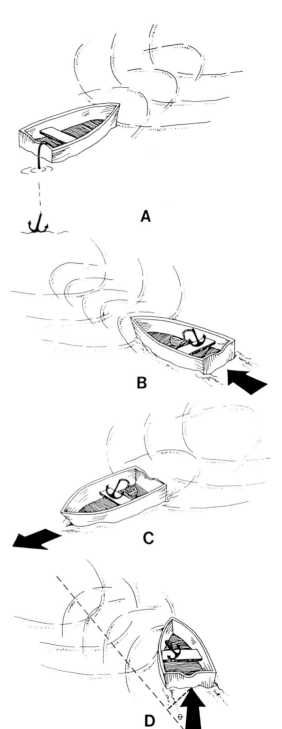

Figure 3. An illustration of the Doppler principle: **A,** The frequency and wave length (distance between wave crests) of the waves reflected by the boat at anchor are the same as for the incident waves, because the boat is not moving with respect to the source of the waves. **B,** If the boat is moving toward the source of the waves, the frequency of the reflected waves is greater and the wave length shorter than for the incident waves. Because the boat is moving into the waves, the bow reaches each successive wave front a little sooner than if it were stationary. The faster the boat moves the sooner it reaches the next wave front. The increase in frequency is proportional to the velocity of the reflector. **C,** Conversely, if the boat moves away from the source of the waves, each wave front reaches the stern of the boat a little later than if the boat were at rest. In this case the frequency of the reflected waves is lower and the wave length longer than for the incident waves. Again, the faster the boat moves, the larger will be the difference in frequency between the incident and reflected waves. **D,** If the boat moves at some angle θ with respect to the direction of propagation of the waves, only that portion of the velocity vector of the boat which projects along the direction of propagation of the waves acts to alter the frequency of the waves. This is described by the cosine function of the angle between the direction of motion of the boat and the direction of propagation of the waves. The larger the angle, the smaller the cosine function, and the less the Doppler frequency shift.

the appropriate interval during which the receiver must be active in order selectively to capture the sound energy from the target of interest. The active interval for the receiver, or time gate, can be moved to sample the Doppler shift produced by any target in the field.

Of course, there is a price to be paid for introducing spatial resolution. Because the sampling rate is finite, there is a maximum velocity or Doppler shift that can be recorded unambiguously, as defined by the sampling theorem.[14] If the sampling rate is too low, aliasing, or invalid representation of the Doppler shift, occurs. A familiar example of aliasing occurs in old movies when the wheels of the stagecoach begin to spin. At first the direction and rate of motion of the wheels is correct. As the stage accelerates, however, the wheels suddenly appear to be spinning backward. This occurs because the rate of motion of the wheels exceeds the maximum velocity that can be properly recorded by the movie camera. To avoid aliasing, the sampling rate should be as high as possible. However, the maximum distance from the transducer that can be sampled is inversely related to the sampling rate because of the finite time required for the sound energy to travel to the sampling site and back. These competing constraints on the sampling rate are an inherent limitation of pulsed Doppler that can be overcome only in part.

Doppler Color Flow Mapping. This is an extension of pulsed Doppler.[13,60,61,86] Instead of flow being sampled at a single site in the field, returning signals from multiple sites along each image line are analyzed for Doppler shift. Then the direction and velocity of the flow at many sites along each image line are mapped in color on top of the gray-scale, two-dimensional image. The benefits of Doppler color flow mapping derive from its ability to display flow over large areas. Visualization of blood flow helps in identification of normal structures such as pulmonary veins (Fig. 4). Abnormal patterns of flow, such as jets through regurgitant valves (Fig. 5) or septal defects (Fig. 6), are much more quickly and easily recognized than they are with pulsed Doppler. Continuous or nearly continuous flow, as seen with a patent ductus arteriosus (Fig. 7) or a coronary artery fistula (Fig. 8) is readily apparent with Doppler color flow mapping. A major limitation of Doppler flow mapping is the low aliasing threshold (Fig. 9).

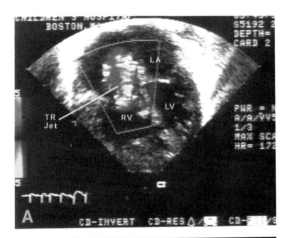

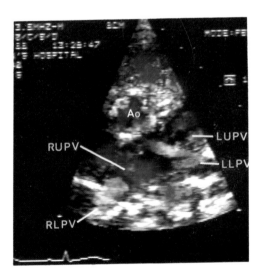

Figure 4. Suprasternal notch views illustrating the use of color Doppler in identifying pulmonary veins. All four pulmonary veins are seen entering the left atrium. Ao = aorta; LLPV = left lower pulmonary vein; LUPV = left upper pulmonary vein; RLPV = right lower pulmonary vein; RUPV = right upper pulmonary vein.

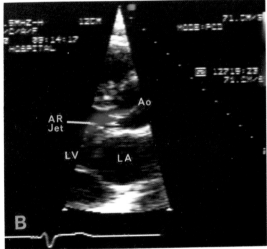

Figure 5. A, Apical four-chamber view demonstrating a jet of tricuspid regurgitation. **B,** Parasternal long-axis view showing mild aortic regurgitation. Ao = aorta; AR = aortic regurgitation; LA = left atrium; LV = left ventricle; RV = right ventricle; TR = tricuspid regurgitation.

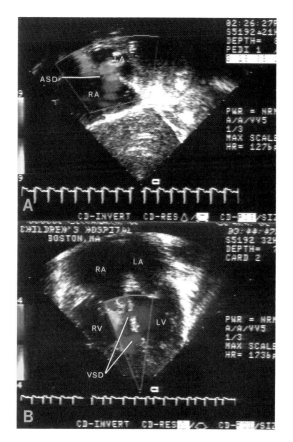

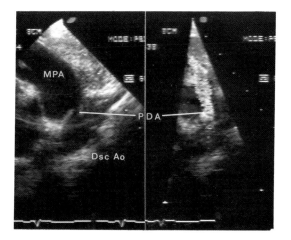

Figure 6. **A,** A secundum atrial septal defect with left-to-right flow in a subxiphoid parasagittal plane view. **B,** Multiple, muscular ventricular septal defects demonstrated in this apical four-chamber view. ASD = atrial septal defect; LA = left atrium; LV = left ventricle; RA = right atrium; RV = right ventricle; VSD = ventricular septal defect.

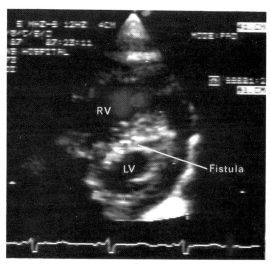

Figure 8. Coronary artery fistulas in the setting of complex congenital defects can be appreciated using color Doppler but would be extremely difficult to detect by imaging alone or with other types of Doppler. In this patient with hypoplastic left heart syndrome and transposition of the great arteries, a fistula connects the hypoplastic left ventricle with the left anterior descending coronary artery. LV = left ventricle; RV = right ventricle.

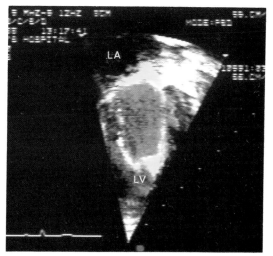

Figure 7. High, left sternal border view showing flow from aorta to pulmonary artery through a ductus arteriosus. Continuous nature of the flow can be appreciated in real time. The gray scale image (left panel) is shown for orientation. Dsc Ao = descending thoracic aorta; MPA = main pulmonary artery; PDA = patent ductus arteriosus.

Figure 9. Normal mitral infow in a child. The inflow signal has a blue center that is caused by the low aliasing threshold of color Doppler. LA = left atrium; LV = left ventricle.

EXAMINATION TECHNIQUE

For cardiovascular ultrasound to be used to full advantage, the examination must be carried out with the proper equipment, under optimal conditions, by qualified personnel, using the correct views to answer the questions posed, and must be interpreted by physicians with a thorough understanding of cardiac anatomy and physiology who are *fully apprised of the clinical setting.*

Equipment

The equipment needs of an echocardiography laboratory depend upon the mission of the laboratory. If the only purpose of the laboratory is to screen for heart defects in children, a device with suitable imaging characteristics and Doppler is all that is needed. At least two transducers, a 5-mHz near-focus and a 3- or 3.5-mHz medium-focus transducer, are needed to cover the size range. Pulsed and continuous-wave Doppler should be available. A video tape recorder helps the examiner to learn from experience. Unless the tapes are archived there is no way to review previous examinations.

An echocardiography laboratory for the sophisticated medical and surgical treatment of infants and children with heart defects has additional requirements. If small premature infants will be examined, a 7.5-mHz transducer may be desirable. Doppler color flow mapping is extremely useful for delineating the complex anatomy and physiology often encountered. A video tape recorder is essential, both for the education of the examiner and for comparison of serial examinations. In a busy laboratory additional video players and high resolution monitors are needed for review of current and previous examinations in real-time, slow-motion, and stop-frame modes. A strip chart recorder is necessary for recording M-mode echocardiograms and Doppler. Measurements made from hard copy are more reliable and reproducible than measurements made from a video monitor. Using a page printer to generate a hard copy of the frozen video screen is not adequate, because the resolution of the video screen is much lower than that of a strip chart recorder. At least two physiology channels, one for an indirect pulse tracing or pressure tracing and one for a phonocardiogram, are needed on the echocardiographic machine for analysis of ventricular loading conditions and contractility (see ch. 15). In addition, an automatic device for blood pressure measurement is useful for calibrating the indirect tracing and for interpreting some Doppler-derived pressure estimates.

A device for quantitative analysis of echocardiograms and Doppler recordings is desirable. Electronic calipers capable of making linear and area measurements from the video screen permit cal-culation of the ventricular volume and ejection fraction. A desktop computer and digitizing tablet allow more sophisticated analysis of M-mode echocardiograms, and Doppler recordings than can be performed with calipers. Digitizing M-mode echocardiograms reduces the observer bias in dimension measurements and allows calculation of indices of diastolic function, such as rate of chamber enlargement and rate of wall thinning. Digitizing Doppler recordings facilitates the calculation of peak and mean pressure gradients and pressure half-time.

Examination Room

The room must be large enough to accommodate comfortably the patient, one or two examiners, and at least one parent. A parent standing by, or holding a hand, goes a long way toward calming an apprehensive child. The examining table should be as comfortable as possible since examinations may require an hour or more. The table should be mobile, with lockable wheels, because it may be useful to have access to both sides of the patient. A cutout in the left side of the mattress facilitates obtaining apical views in older children and adults. Adequate storage space for linen, gowns, strip chart paper, and other items saves steps on the part of the examiner. A sink in the room facilitates hand washing and cleanup. The lights should have a dimmer switch, or a small lamp should be available to optimize viewing of the video screen. The room temperature should be 70–72°F, warm enough for the patient to be comfortable but cool enough to prevent damage to the equipment. Carpeting reduces the noise level and makes the room more comfortable.

Preparation of the Patient

For older children and adults a brief explanation of the procedure is generally sufficient. Assurance that the test is painless and involves no hazardous radiation usually allays the fears of both the patient and the parents. A pamphlet describing the echocardiogram, which the referring physician can give to the patient and parents, is an efficient means of transmitting this information. Babies from about 3 months to 3 years old are rarely able to cooperate adequately. In this age range it is almost always necessary to sedate the patient. It has been found that chloral hydrate, in a dose range of 50–100 mg per kg of body weight, up to a total dose of 1 gm, is both safe and effective. The dose must be adjusted for the age and health of the patient. In healthy patients more than 6 or 8 months of age, a dose of 90–100 mg/kg is used, scaling the dose down for younger patients or patients with severe cyanosis or congestive heart failure. The drug seems to be more efficient if the patient has fasted for 2 or 3 hours prior to administration. A small number of patients, especially those at the higher end of the age range, become agitated and difficult to control before falling asleep. This adverse effect may last for 15 or 20 minutes and is generally followed by sleep. The parents should be reassured and the child protected from self-harm during this period.

Echocardiographic Views

Four standard transducer locations or echocardiographic views serve as starting points or frames of reference for the echocardiographic examination.[64,82,85,91] **Although these views should be obtained in virtually every patient, and represent the minimum acceptable examination, the examiner should not feel constrained to use only the standard views. Improvisation and variations on standard themes are to be encouraged if additional information is desired.** When using unconventional views, it is well to record a description of the transducer location and orientation on the audio channel for future reference.

Subxiphoid Views. The subxiphoid space provides an excellent window for examining the heart and vessels in infants and small children. Using this view the heart and proximal great arteries can be imaged as a unit, which facilitates understanding the relationships between structures. The examination is begun with the transducer in the subxiphoid space, pointing directly posteriorly, and the scan plane oriented from left to right (Fig. 10). The resulting transverse view of the trunk at the level of the diaphragm shows the relationship between the inferior vena cava, the descending aorta, and the spine, and is used to determine viscero-atrial situs (Fig. 11A). Next, the transducer is

slowly angled superiorly and anteriorly. This sweep, sequentially, displays the inferior cavo-atrial junction, the right and left atria with the interatrial septum, the left ventricular inflow tract, a long-axis view of the left ventricle with the outflow tract (Fig. 11B), and, finally, a coronal plane view of the right ventricle with its outflow tract. By the end of the sweep the image plane is nearly parallel to the frontal or coronal plane of the trunk. Next, the transducer is rotated clockwise 90° so that the scan plane is parallel to the sagittal plane of the trunk (Fig. 12). By angling slightly to the patient's right, the junction of both cavae with the right atrium can be seen (Fig. 13A). Slowly sweeping the transducer to the patient's left reveals the atria and atrial septum, the atrioventricular valves in cross-section, the right ventricular sinus and infundibulum in a parasagittal plane (Fig. 13B), and, finally, the mid and apical portions of the left ventricle.

The examination in infants and small children is begun with the subxiphoid views because these views provide an excellent overview of the anatomy. With this general information as background, the echocardiographer can then systematically investigate the details of cardiac anatomy using other views.

Apical Views. To obtain apical views, the apex impulse of the heart is palpated and the tip of the transducer is placed over it, with the scan plane oriented from left shoulder to right hip (Fig. 14). Usually the patient must be rolled into a left decubitus position for optimal images. In this position the heart is tipped toward the chest wall, displacing any intervening lung. The four-chamber projection displays the four chambers of the heart and the atrioventricular valves (Fig. 2). Often, the pul-

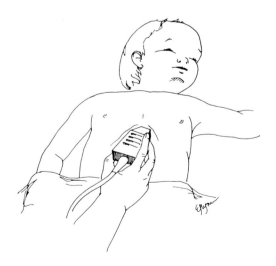

Figure 10. Orientation of the transducer for the subxiphoid transverse or long-axis scan.

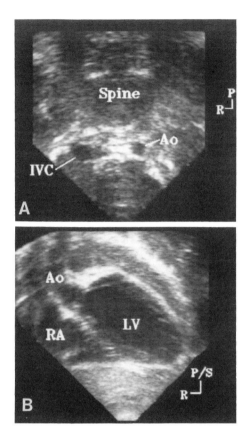

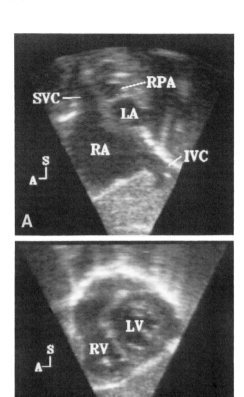

Figure 11. **A,** Subxiphoid transverse view of the abdomen showing the spine, inferior vena cava, and the descending aorta in cross-section. **B,** Continuing the scan demonstrates the left ventricle in long axis with the outflow tract. Ao = aorta; IVC = inferior vena cava; LV = left ventricle; P = posterior; R = right; RA = right atrium; S = superior.

Figure 13. **A,** A right parasagittal plane through the junctions of the inferior and superior vena cavae with the right atrium. **B,** Short-axis cut through the right ventricular outflow tract. A = anterior; IVC = inferior vena cava; LA = left atrium; LV = left ventricle; RA = right atrium; RPA = right pulmonary artery; RV = right ventricle; S = superior; SVC = superior vena cava.

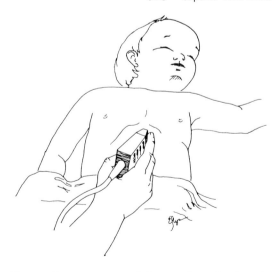

Figure 12. Orientation of the transducer for the subxiphoid parasagittal or short-axis scan.

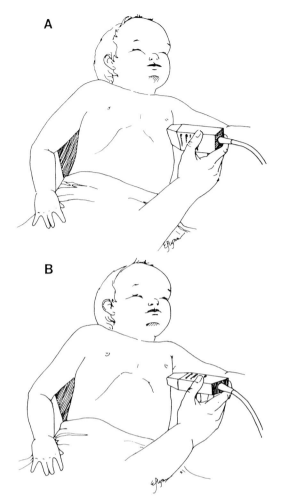

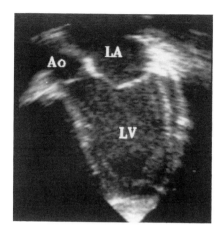

Figure 15. Apical two-chamber or long-axis view obtained by rotating the transducer 75–90° from the four-chamber view. Ao = aorta; LA = left atrium; LV = left ventricle.

Figure 14. Orientation of the transducer for (**A**) the apical long-axis view and (**B**) apical four-chamber view.

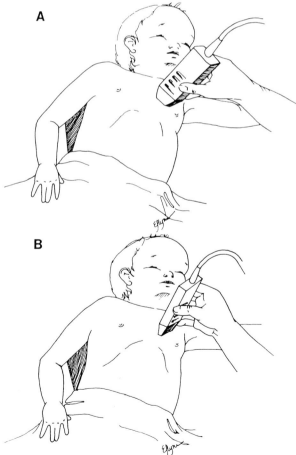

monary veins are seen well in this view. By angling posteriorly, the posterior aspect of the heart, including the coronary sinus, is displayed. By angling anteriorly from the four-chamber plane, the left ventricular outflow tract can be seen. Rotation of the transducer about 75–90° clockwise produces a two-chamber, or apical long-axis, view of the left ventricle (Fig. 15). This is the best view for examining the left ventricular outflow tract, especially when looking for subvalvar obstruction.[20]

Parasternal Views. Probably the most familiar echocardiographic view is the parasternal long-axis view of the left ventricle, obtained with the transducer directed posteriorly in the third or fourth left intercostal space and the image plane oriented from the right shoulder to the left hip (Fig. 16). As for the apical views, it is usually necessary to turn the patient into a left decubitus position for optimal images. This view displays the left ventricular inflow and outflow tracts, the aortic valve, and the proximal ascending aorta (Fig. 17). By an-

Figure 16. Orientation of the transducer for (**A**) the parasternal long-axis view and (**B**) the parasternal short-axis view.

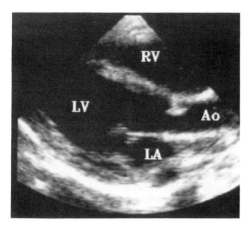

Figure 17. Standard parasternal long-axis view of the left ventricle showing the mitral valve, left ventricular inflow and outflow and the aortic valve. Ao = aorta; LA = left atrium; LV = left ventricle; RV = right ventricle.

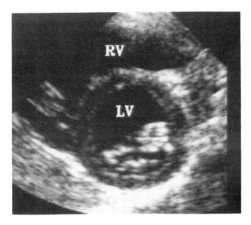

Figure 18. Parasternal short-axis view showing the left ventricle in cross section. LV = left ventricle; RV = right ventricle.

gling the transducer inferiorly and rightward across the ventricular septum, the tricuspid valve and right ventricular inflow tract are displayed. By angling to the left and superiorly from the parasternal long-axis view, the right ventricular outflow tract can be traced through the pulmonary valve to the main pulmonary artery. Clockwise rotation of the transducer about 90° from the parasternal long-axis view yields a parasternal short-axis, or transverse, view (Fig. 18). By sweeping toward the base of the heart, the aortic valve can be seen in cross-section and the right ventricular outflow tract and pulmonary valve can be seen in long axis. Scanning toward the apex of the heart reveals the mitral valve and left ventricle in cross-section. Sliding the transducer superiorly one or two interspaces while maintaining approximately the same orientation of the scan plane makes it possible to see the bifurcation of the pulmonary artery and the proximal

branches of the pulmonary arteries. Similar long- and short-axis views obtained from the right sternal border are useful for displaying the interatrial septum (Fig. 19).

Suprasternal Notch Views. Proper positioning of the patient is essential for obtaining optimal images from the suprasternal notch (Fig. 20). A sheet or towel rolled into a flattened cylinder and placed beneath the shoulders (not the neck) produces the proper amount of extension of the neck. Too much extension tightens the skin over the notch, limiting access, whereas too little extension leaves the chin in the way of the transducer. It may be necessary to turn the head to one side or the other to facilitate the examination. Usually this view is left for last, because it requires major repositioning of the patient and may be frightening for apprehensive children. Often in small infants the same information may be obtained from the left infraclavicular space.

The examination is begun with the transducer aimed inferiorly and posteriorly, at about 45° to the frontal plane, with the image plane oriented from

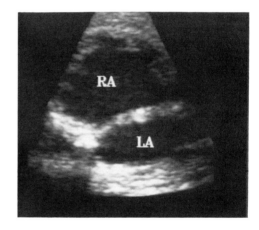

Figure 19. Right sternal border view displaying the interatrial septum. LA = left atrium; RA = right atrium.

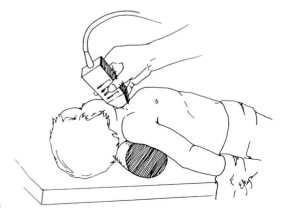

Figure 20. Proper position of the patient and orientation of the transducer for suprasternal notch views.

left to right. This view displays an oblique section of the ascending aorta and the right pulmonary artery in long axis behind it. By angling posteriorly, the pulmonary veins and left atrium are displayed. By sweeping anteriorly, the superior vena cava can be tracked to the innominate vein, and the left innominate vein can be seen in the long-axis view. Counterclockwise rotation of the transducer about 30°, with leftward angulation, makes it possible to see the left pulmonary artery in long axis. Further counterclockwise rotation, with rightward angulation, reveals the aortic arch with the origins of the brachiocephalic vessels (Fig. 21).

Integration of Doppler Examination and Imaging

Doppler echocardiography is used in concert with 2-D echocardiography. The way in which these modalities are integrated may vary at the discretion of the examiner. Doppler examination while imaging obviates the need to repeat each view to perform the Doppler examination. Nonetheless, it is often necessary to repeat parts of the Doppler examination with a lower frequency transducer because either the velocity of flow was too high to be recorded unambiguously with the higher frequency transducer, or the signal strength with the higher frequency transducer was insufficient for reliable interpretation. Also, if a very high-velocity jet is encountered, continuous-wave Doppler, or pulsed Doppler at a high sampling rate, will be necessary to record the peak velocity of the jet. If measuring the velocity of the jet for estimation of pressure drop is one of the primary objectives of the examination, it is wise to take the time to use continuous-wave Doppler sooner rather than later.

Flow through the **atrioventricular valves** is eval-

uated using both the apical four-chamber view and the parasternal long-axis view. Doppler color flow mapping is most efficient for detecting regurgitation, but the same information is available using pulsed Doppler. Pulsed or continuous-wave Doppler is used to record the flow velocity on the ventricular side of the valve, seeking evidence of stenosis. If a stenotic jet is identified, imaging the jet with color Doppler facilitates aligning the pulsed or continuous-wave Doppler beam with the jet.

Similarly, flow is evaluated on both sides of the **semilunar valves,** using apical and parasternal long-axis views for the aortic valve and parasternal short- and long-axis views for the pulmonary valve. Again, Doppler color flow mapping is probably more sensitive than pulsed Doppler for detecting regurgitation. Pulsed or continuous-wave Doppler is then used to record the maximum flow velocity through the valve in order to detect stenosis.

The flow from the **pulmonary veins** can be imaged using subxiphoid, apical, or suprasternal notch views. Imaging flow from the pulmonary veins, using Doppler color flow mapping, facilitates identification of these structures and helps in detecting stenosis of individual veins (Fig. 4). The integrity of the **interatrial septum** is best evaluated by scanning the septum with Doppler color flow mapping in subxiphoid or right sternal border views. Although there are reports describing the use of pulsed Doppler to detect atrial septal defects,[54] at The Children's Hospital in Boston we have found it unreliable, largely because of the difficulty in distinguishing normal superior or inferior vena cava flow from flow across an atrial septal defect. Similarly, the **interventricular septum** should be scanned with Doppler color flow mapping in parasternal, apical, and subxiphoid views, looking for ventricular septal defects. Pulsed Doppler can be used for this purpose but the process is time-consuming and less sensitive than Doppler color flow mapping. Flow in the **pulmonary arteries** and **aortic arch** is best evaluated from a high left sternal border view using Doppler color flow mapping. This approach is most sensitive for detection of the flow in the pulmonary arteries associated with a patent ductus arteriosus (Fig. 7) and the narrowing of the flow stream in the proximal descending aorta associated with coarctation of the aorta. Although similar information can be obtained using pulsed Doppler, more time and effort are required and it appears to be less sensitive than Doppler color flow mapping. Finally, pulsed Doppler is used to record the pattern of flow in the **descending aorta** at the diaphragm (Fig. 22). This is a sensitive screening technique for coarctation of the aorta[74,80] and provides an estimation of the severity of run-off lesions from the proximal aorta, such as aortic regurgitation,[92] patent ductus arteriosus, and arteriovenous fistula.

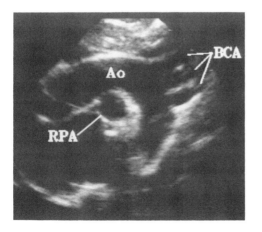

Figure 21. Counterclockwise rotation, nearly into a parasagittal plane, displays the aortic arch and brachiocephalic vessels. Ao = aorta; BCA = brachiocephalic arteries; RPA = right pulmonary artery.

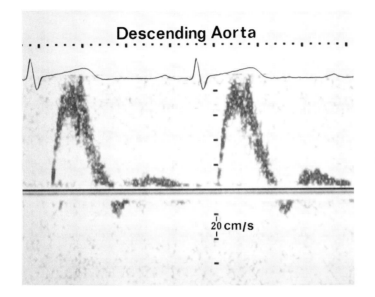

Figure 22. Normal flow pattern in the descending aorta at the diaphragm.

Who Should Perform the Examination?

The qualifications and experience of the examiner, like the equipment, depend on the mission of the laboratory. In general, an experienced technologist can screen for straightforward heart defects in older children without the examination being directly supervised by a cardiologist. In any case, the recorded examination must be reviewed and interpreted by a cardiologist. On the other hand, the examination of an infant or small child with potentially complex heart disease must be performed, or directly supervised, by a pediatric cardiologist with special expertise in echocardiography. It is essential that the person responsible for the examination be thoroughly familiar with the anatomic possibilities and their physiologic implications. Further, because many infants and young children require sedation for the examination, the cardiologist must ensure that all essential information is obtained before the patient awakens.

At Boston Children's Hospital a cardiologist-echocardiographer is always present in the laboratory to supervise and assist with examinations as needed. While technologists and fellows perform large portions of the examinations, the staff cardiologist directs the progress of each examination and often actively participates in obtaining difficult views or sorting out confusing information. The results of the cardiac ultrasound examination are most reliable when an experienced cardiologist performs a physical examination in conjunction with the ultrasound examination. If the physical findings are not adequately explained by the ultrasound examination, the latter should be repeated, in part or in whole, until the discrepancy is eliminated. This point is especially applicable in patients with semilunar valve stenosis when the physical examination suggests a more severe lesion than was detected by Doppler. More than likely the direction of the stenotic jet is unusual and not readily accessible from the usual transducer locations. In such cases other transducer positions should be tried or the direction of the jet evaluated using Doppler color flow mapping. Similarly, the presence of a murmur suggestive of a ventricular septal defect when none was detected on the initial scan should prompt another more careful search for the defect. The point of maximal intensity of a well-localized murmur is the best place to start the search.

INTERPRETATION

Obtaining adequate images is only half the battle. The examination must be interpreted and the results communicated to the referring physician.

Anatomic Analysis

Although most of the information available through ultrasound is apparent at the time the examination is being performed, it is essential that the tapes be reviewed using a device capable of display in slow motion and stop-frame as well as in real-time mode. This allows the cardiologist to be more certain about anatomic details that may be difficult to appreciate in real time, especially at heart rates typical for infants and children. While reviewing each examination requires a substantial time investment, the enhanced accuracy is worth the effort.

A complex structure such as the heart is analyzed best by breaking it down into its components, studying each one separately, and synthesizing the resultant information to generate a comprehensive set of diagnoses.[70–72] The most useful framework for this purpose is the segmental approach to cardiac anatomy proposed by Van Praagh and colleagues (see ch. 4). According to this concept the heart is composed of five segments, three main segments and two connecting segments. The three main segments are the atria, the ventricles, and the great arteries; the atrioventricular canal connects the atria with the ventricles and the infundibulum connects the great arteries with the ventricles. One could examine the heart sequentially, segment by segment. However, this would require skipping around from view to view, repositioning the patient and possibly disturbing the flow of the examination. Preferably, all the views needed for a complete examination are obtained in a relatively fixed order and segmental analysis is applied during the review. Of course, the examiner must go over a mental checklist segment by segment while the examination is being performed to be sure all the data are gathered.

Veno-atrial Segment. First the viscero-atrial situs is determined using a subxiphoid transverse view of the trunk.[41] In situs solitus the descending aorta is posterior and to the left of the spine, whereas the inferior vena cava is anterior and to the right of the spine (Fig. 11A). Tracking the inferior vena cava cranially shows its junction with the right-sided right atrium. The opposite is true in situs inversus (see ch. 37). Systemic venous connections are seen best using subxiphoid and suprasternal notch views. Subxiphoid transverse and parasagittal plane views are best for seeing the connection of the inferior vena cava and hepatic veins to the right atrium, and the suprasternal transverse view is best for the superior vena cava and innominate veins. The coronary sinus can be seen using subxiphoid, apical four-chamber, or parasternal long-axis views. The pulmonary venous connections to the left atrium are normally seen using subxiphoid, apical, and suprasternal notch views.

The atria can be seen from most views, but the subxiphoid and apical (Fig. 2) views are best for determining morphology and estimating size. The morphologically right atrium receives the inferior vena cava and/or hepatic veins, and the coronary sinus, if present; it has septum secundum on its septal surface. In contrast, the morphologically left atrium has septum primum on its septal surface. In infants and small children the interatrial septum is most reliably imaged from subxiphoid views, especially in the parasagittal plane. In older patients the apical and right sternal border (Fig. 19) views afford the best display of the interatrial septum,[93] keeping in mind that false dropout of the mid portion of the septum is common in the apical four-chamber view because the sound beam is parallel to the thin fossa ovalis. Finally, the atrial appendages can be seen in either a subxiphoid or para-

sternal short-axis view through the atrioventricular junction.

Atrioventricular Canal. The septum of the atrioventricular canal, including the portion of the interatrial septum nearest the atrioventricular valves and the membranous and atrioventricular canal portions of the interventricular septum, is best seen in the subxiphoid and apical (Fig. 2) views. The entire septum must be scanned from its most posterior aspect to the aortic root. The atrioventricular valves should be examined in several views because they are complex structures. The annular diameters can be measured in parasternal, apical or subxiphoid views.[44] Because the valve annuli are not circular, measurements should be made in two orthogonal planes. The mitral valve typically has two leaflets, a larger lateral leaflet and a smaller medial leaflet. The chordae from both leaflets attach to two major sets of free-wall papillary muscles, the anterolateral and posteromedial groups. The base of each papillary muscle divides into several heads that are arranged in a horseshoe around the appropriate commissure of the mitral valve. Leaflet motion of the mitral valve is optimally appreciated in parasternal long- and short-axis and apical four- and two-chamber views. The tricuspid valve classically has three leaflets, but may have two or four. The tricuspid valve has multiple papillary muscles in the right ventricle, originating from the septum, the moderator band and the free wall. Leaflet motion of the tricuspid valve is seen best in a parasternal long-axis view, angled to the right, and in the apical four-chamber view. The papillary muscle attachments of both valves are optimally seen using the subxiphoid parasagittal or short-axis view and the parasternal short-axis view.

Ventricles. The right and left ventricles have characteristic morphologic features that permit identification of each ventricle no matter what its position in space.[26,35,90] The echocardiographic features typical of a left ventricle include (1) an ellipsoidal shape (Fig. 11B), (2) an atrioventricular valve with only free-wall papillary muscle attachments and a more basal septal insertion of the annulus (Fig. 2), (3) a smooth septal surface, (4) an outflow tract between the atrioventricular valve and the septum, and (5) a finely trabecular apical septum and free wall. The characteristic echocardiographic features of the right ventricle include (1) a triangular or trapezoidal shape, (2) an atrioventricular valve with septal and free-wall papillary muscle attachments (Fig. 13B) and a more apical septal insertion of the annulus (Fig. 2), (3) no outflow tract between the atrioventricular valve and the septum, (4) a moderator band crossing the ventricle from the septum to the free wall, and (5) a coarsely trabecular septum and free wall. The loop or situs of the ventricles is determined by first identifying both ventricles and then examining the internal organization of each. The D-loop or solitus right ventricle is organized so that when one looks at the septal surface, the inflow of the ventricle is to the right and the outflow is to the left. Just the opposite is true for the L-loop or inversus right ventricle. By contrast, in the D-loop or solitus left ventricle, the inflow is to the left and the outflow to the right. Again the opposite is true for the L-loop or inversus left ventricle. A practical and easy test is to compare the location of the atrioventricular valve annuli. The tricuspid valve annulus is to the right of the mitral annulus in D-loop ventricles, whereas the tricuspid annulus is to the left in L-loop ventricles.

The interventricular septum is comprised of several regions or parts (Fig. 23). The atrioventricular canal portion of the septum is posterior and inferior to the membranous septum and abuts the tricuspid valve annulus. This segment may be difficult to image because of overlying tricuspid valve tissue; it is best seen using subxiphoid, apical four-chamber, and parasternal short-axis views. The membranous septum is usually seen from subxiphoid short-axis, parasternal short-axis and apical four- or two-chamber views. The muscular septum is usually divided into a mid portion, an apical portion and an anterior portion that is anterior to the septal band. The coarse trabeculations on the right ventricular side of the septum make detection of defects in this region especially difficult by imaging alone. The subxiphoid parasagittal plane or short-axis,[9] parasternal short-axis and apical four-chamber views should be used to examine this part of the septum. The area of the septum being examined is determined from the orientation of the transducer and the relation to the septomoderator band. The infundibular septum lies between the semilunar roots, divides the outflow tracts of the ventricles, and joins the "Y" of the septal band. This segment can be seen using subxiphoid short-axis or parasternal short-axis views. In a parasternal short-axis plane, just apical to the aortic valve, the membranous septum is at about 8 to 11 o'clock, whereas the infundibular septum is between 12 and 2 o'clock.

The outflow tract of the left ventricle is seen best using the parasternal long-axis (Fig. 17) and the apical two-chamber views (Fig. 15). The latter view is more sensitive for detecting membranous subvalvar stenosis.[20]

Infundibulum. The right ventricular outflow tract or infundibulum is seen best in infants and young children using subxiphoid coronal plane and parasagittal plane or short-axis views. In older patients a parasternal short-axis view is most satisfactory. In the solitus normal heart the infundibulum is oriented from right and inferior to left and superior, and it crosses the left ventricular outflow tract as it connects the pulmonary valve and artery with the right ventricle. The orientation of the infundibulum is exactly the opposite in the inversus normal heart. Any other orientation of the infundibulum is strong evidence for an abnormal ventriculoarterial connection and/or alignment.

Great Arteries. Normally, both semilunar valves have three leaflets and three commissures. The leaflets and commissures of the aortic valve are easily demonstrated using a parasternal short-axis view. The parasternal long-axis view demonstrates leaflet separation and allows reliable measurement of the diameter of the annulus (Fig. 17). The pulmonary valve is rarely in position to be imaged in cross-section, so the number of leaflets and commissures cannot be determined in most cases. The parasternal short-axis view displays the pulmonary valve showing leaflet separation. The diameter of the annulus can also be measured in this view.

The identity of each great artery is determined by its morphology.[40,73] The pulmonary artery is directed posteriorly and bifurcates a short distance above the valve. In contrast, the aorta runs anteriorly, forms an arch, and gives rise to two or more brachiocephalic arteries. The course and branching pattern of the great arteries can be seen from several views, including the subxiphoid, parasternal, and suprasternal views.

Ventriculoarterial Alignments. These are determined by identifying both ventricles and both great arteries and visually assessing which is related to which.[10,73] At The Children's Hospital in Boston, we find the subxiphoid and parasternal views most suitable because the ventricles and great arteries can be imaged simultaneously. The relative posi-

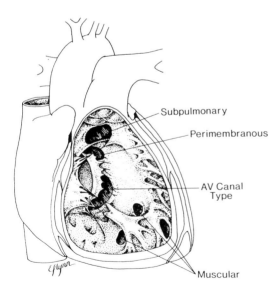

Figure 23. The locations and names of various types of ventricular septal defects. Note that the septo-moderator band is the landmark used to distinguish the types of muscular ventricular septal defects. Apical muscular defects are apical to the septal insertion of the moderator band. Anterior muscular defects are anterior to the septal band. (From Sanders SP: Echocardiography 1:333–391, 1984, with permission.)

tions of the great arteries (semilunar roots) are best determined from a parasternal short-axis view rotated clockwise so that the scan plane is oriented from right to left. In solitus normally related great arteries, the aorta is posterior and rightward, whereas the pulmonary artery is leftward and anterior. The right-left orientation is reversed, with no change in the anterior-posterior position, in inversus normally related great arteries. Any other arrangement is highly suggestive of a malposition of the great arteries.

The bifurcation of the pulmonary artery can be seen using a parasternal short-axis view, from either the standard position or one to two interspaces higher. The branches of the pulmonary artery are seen best from the suprasternal notch. The aortic arch is seen best from the suprasternal notch or the left infraclavicular space (Fig. 21). The location of the aortic arch (left or right) is determined from the branching pattern and the orientation of the transducer when imaging the arch in long axis. In a normal left arch the first branch is directed toward the right and bifurcates into the right common carotid and subclavian arteries, while the left common carotid and subclavian arteries arise separately as the second and third branches, respectively (Fig. 21). Further, the arch is directed toward the left as determined by the orientation of the transducer when imaging the arch. A right aortic arch is directed to the right and gives rise to a left innominate artery as the first branch, with the right common carotid and subclavian arteries as the second and third branches, respectively. Usually, the aortic isthmus is not seen well from the suprasternal notch view. Instead, placing the transducer in the left infraclavicular or first intercostal space, with the scan plane parallel to the sagittal plane of the trunk, is the best way to display the isthmus (Fig. 24).[40]

Quantitative Analysis

In addition to the delineation of cardiac anatomy, cardiovascular ultrasound permits noninvasive measurement of ventricular size and function, cardiac output, and the severity of valve dysfunction.

Ventricular Volume, Mass, and Ejection Fraction. Several techniques have been described for estimating the volume and muscle mass of the left ventricle.[83] Estimation of right ventricular volume and mass is more difficult and less reliable because the shape of the right ventricle lends itself much less to geometrical modeling.[95] The Simpson's rule algorithm appears to be the most accurate method for both ventricles.

Doppler Analysis. Several useful measurements can be made from the Doppler recordings. Measurements made from hard copy of the Doppler recordings are more reproducible than measure-

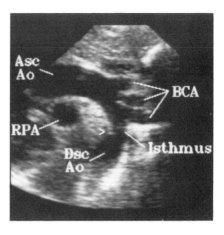

Figure 24. Left infraclavicular view with the scan plane in a parasagittal plane of the trunk, used to image the aortic isthmus. Asc Ao = ascending aorta; BCA = brachiocephalic arteries; Dsc Ao = descending thoracic aorta; RPA = right pulmonary artery.

ments made from the video screen. The peak velocity of flow across an orifice can be measured from the Doppler recording using calipers or a computer with a digitizing board. The peak velocity of flow is used to calculate the peak instantaneous pressure drop across the orifice, using the simplified Bernoulli equation:[67]

$$\Delta p = 4 \times v^2$$

where Δp is pressure drop and v is velocity of flow. Severity of semilunar valve stenosis is often expressed as the peak instantaneous pressure drop across the valve (Fig. 25).

Other uses for this technique include (1) estimation of the pressure difference between right and left ventricles in the presence of a ventricular septal defect,[55] (2) estimation of the pressure difference between the aorta and pulmonary artery in patients with a ductus arteriosus or other aortopulmonary communication,[56] (3) estimation of right ventricular systolic pressure using the peak velocity in a regurgitant jet through the tricuspid valve,[100] and (4) evaluation of the efficacy of a pulmonary artery band.[28]

Mean velocity of flow or mean pressure drop is more difficult to calculate, generally requiring a computer and digitizing board. The mean pressure drop is especially useful for evaluating stenosis of an atrioventricular valve. Values for the peak, mean, and end-diastolic pressure drop are all calculated and reported.

The pressure half-time, or the time required for the pressure difference across an orifice to decrease by half, has also been shown to be useful for evaluating stenosis of an atrioventricular valve[36] and aortic regurgitation.[57] Again, a computer and dig-

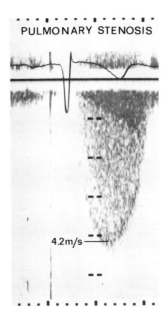

Figure 25. Transvalvar continuous-wave Doppler recording in a patient with valvar pulmonary stenosis. The peak velocity is 4.2 m/sec. The peak pressure drop is calculated as 4 times the square of the peak velocity (in m/sec). The same technique can be used to calculate the pressure drop across any discrete orifice.

itizing board facilitate measuring the half-time, although nomograms have been constructed to estimate atrioventricular valve area directly from the Doppler tracing. The half-time is especially useful in patients with a large variation in heart rate (e.g., mitral stenosis with atrial fibrillation) where mean or end-diastolic gradients may vary widely.[36] In aortic regurgitation the pressure half-time indicates how rapidly the aortic and left ventricular diastolic pressures tend to equilibrate. The more rapidly they equilibrate, the more severe is the regurgitation. In adults half-times greater than 1 sec indicate mild regurgitation; between 0.5 and 1 sec, moderate; and less than 0.5 sec, severe regurgitation.[57] Similar ranges are not available in children.

The time to peak velocity or acceleration time, the peak acceleration, and the mean acceleration have been investigated as indicators of pulmonary artery pressure.[46,49] Although the acceleration time, especially if adjusted for the ejection time, is a fair predictor of pulmonary artery pressure, the reliability of this index is not sufficient for clinical use. Peak and mean acceleration, although correlated with the pulmonary artery pressure, have a low predictive value. All three indices appear to be sensitive to pulmonary flow as well as pressure and may cause confusion when dealing with a patient who has a left-to-right shunt.[79]

The Doppler recording can be used to calculate both right and left ventricular systolic time inter-

vals.[37,38] The pre-ejection period is measured from the Q wave of the electrocardiogram to the onset of flow on the Doppler tracing. The ejection time extends from the onset of flow to the apex of the retrograde flow peak at the end of ejection.

Systemic and pulmonary blood flows can also be measured using Doppler examination.[30,42,65,75,77] Both blind continuous-wave Doppler from the suprasternal notch or right sternal border[66] and pulsed Doppler directed from the apex or subxiphoid space[75] can be used for estimation of systemic blood flow. At The Children's Hospital in Boston we have used only pulsed Doppler from the left sternal border to measure pulmonary blood flow.[75] In any case, the diameter of the vessel in which flow is to be estimated must be measured. Generally, a parasternal long-axis view is most satisfactory for the aorta, and a parasternal short- or long-axis view for the pulmonary artery. The diameter of the annulus is measured in early to mid systole at the base of the valve leaflets. If pulsed Doppler is used, the sample volume should be placed in, or slightly above, the valve annulus. The envelope of the continuous-wave Doppler tracing represents the highest velocity in the ascending aorta, which is assumed to originate from the valve annulus, because under usual circumstances, that is the narrowest part. Stroke volume is calculated as the product of the cross-sectional area of the vessel, calculated from the measured diameter, and the area under the Doppler time-velocity curve. Systemic or pulmonary flow is then calculated as the product of stroke volume and heart rate. Although methods have been described for estimating flow using the atrioventricular valve Doppler recordings,[25,96] at Boston Children's Hospital we have not found them to be reliable.

CLINICAL APPLICATIONS

Applications of cardiovascular ultrasound in pediatric cardiology fall into one of a few general categories which include (1) structural heart defects, (2) valvar heart disease, (3) ventricular function, and (4) miscellaneous.

Structural Heart Defects

As noted previously, 2-D echocardiography coupled with Doppler cardiography is extremely accurate and reliable for diagnosing or excluding structural heart defects. These modalities, used in concert, are especially useful for screening sick neonates in whom heart defects are suspected. Significant heart defects can be excluded reliably in infants with neonatal lung disease, persistent pulmonary hypertension, or infection. In the vast majority of infants with heart defects, a precise anatomic and physiologic diagnosis can be made by cardiovascular ultrasound. Infants with patent ductus arteriosus, total anomalous pulmonary venous connection,[51] interrupted aortic arch, or coarctation are repaired without catheterization. Palliative procedures are also performed without cardiac catheterization in infants with hypoplastic left heart syndrome[6] and tetralogy of Fallot with pulmonary atresia.[68] In older children coarctation, primum[52] and secundum atrial septal defect,[27] patent ductus arteriosus, and some ventricular septal defects are repaired without catheterization.

On the other hand, cardiovascular ultrasound has definite limitations. First, **there must be adequate windows to the heart and great vessels.** Midline abdominal defects and chest deformities may seriously impair cardiac imaging by limiting access to the heart. Following heart surgery, bandages and chest tubes may prevent adequate cardiac imaging. As patients get older and larger, some windows, such as the subxiphoid space or suprasternal notch, become less useful. Calcification of intercostal cartilage impairs the parasternal windows. Patients with chronic lung disease and overexpanded lungs may also have poor parasternal or apical windows. After cardiac surgery access to the heart may become limited, especially if the thymus is removed or part of the lung becomes entrapped between the heart and the anterior chest wall. In general, less satisfactory images are obtained in older and larger patients. Transesophageal echocardiography is especially useful in older patients with poor transthoracic windows.

Second, **some structures are not accessible to ultrasound because of location.** The branches of the pulmonary arteries in or near the parenchyma of the lung cannot be imaged by cardiovascular ultrasound. All of the incident sound energy is reflected at the air-tissue interfaces in the overlying lung and none reaches the intraparenchymal branch of the pulmonary artery. Individual pulmonary veins may be difficult to image, especially in older patients, because they are the most posterior cardiac structures. In fact, isolated partially anomalous pulmonary venous connection in the older child or young adult is one of the very few lesions that remains difficult or impossible to diagnose using ultrasound. In a small number of children the proximal descending aorta, including the aortic isthmus, is inaccessible because of overlying lung or airway. Similarly, the bifurcation of the left main coronary artery and the proximal left anterior descending coronary artery may be covered by the left lung, which prevents it from being imaged in a few infants and children ($< 10\%$). This is especially important in patients with tetralogy of Fallot or transposition of the great arteries. The more distal parts of the anterior descending and circumflex coronary arteries can rarely be imaged adequately.

Third, **some defects are beyond the resolution of current ultrasound systems.** Small, or even moderate, muscular ventricular septal defects may be difficult or impossible to distinguish from intertrabecular spaces by imaging alone. Multiple small fenestrations of septum primum in the atrial septum may also be impossible to distinguish from false dropout by echocardiography alone. However, Doppler cardiography, especially Doppler color flow mapping, has proved very sensitive for detecting flow through such small defects in both the atrial and ventricular septa.[69] Although insufficient data are available for a confident evaluation, early experience indicates that Doppler color flow mapping can detect additional small ventricular septal defect, even in the presence of another large defect and systemic right ventricular pressure.

Valvar Heart Disease

Both the morphology and function of the heart valves may be optimally evaluated and followed using 2-D echocardiography and Doppler cardiography. The structure of congenitally deformed valves (including isolated cleft,[84] double orifice[94] or abnormal papillary attachments[17] of atrioventricular valves, and commissural fusion of semilunar valves[15]) can be determined reliably. Rheumatic mitral valve disease is also reported to have characteristic features,[99] including thickening of the leaflets with fusion of commissures and chordae; however, at The Children's Hospital in Boston, our experience with rheumatic heart disease is too limited to comment further. Although valve morphology is often important, Doppler assessment of valve function is usually of more clinical relevance.

Atrioventricular Valve Regurgitation. Atrioventricular valve regurgitation can be evaluated by estimating the area of the atrium over which the disturbed flow from the regurgitant jet is detected.[11,59,97] The greater the area of disturbed flow, the more severe is the regurgitation. This method requires careful mapping of the atrium with pulsed Doppler and should be performed in two planes. Doppler color flow mapping greatly simplifies this task and is probably as reliable as pulsed Doppler.[58] Another parameter worth noting is the diameter of the regurgitant jet at the level of the valve.[12] This provides an estimate of the size of the gap in the closure line of the valve and correlates with the severity of the regurgitation. The velocity of flow in the regurgitant jet is not predictive of the severity of regurgitation, but rather of the difference in pressure between the atrium and ventricle. Although Doppler evaluation of atrioventricular valve regurgitation generally correlates well with angiographic assessment, there are potential pitfalls. Using pulsed Doppler alone, it is easy to miss or underestimate the size of regurgitant jets that are directed along the wall of the atrium. Two or more small jets may be misinterpreted as a single large jet, leading to overestimation of severity.

Careful use of Doppler color flow mapping largely eliminates these potential sources of error. The size of the patient is also a determinant of the quality of the Doppler examination; the signal-to-noise ratio progressively deteriorates with increasing patient size, resulting in low sensitivity in large patients. In such cases regurgitant jets may be missed or the size of the jet underestimated.

Atrioventricular Valve Stenosis. Numerous methods have been devised for estimating the severity of atrioventricular valve stenosis. In rheumatic mitral stenosis the diameter or area of the opening in the valve can be measured directly.[53] This is less practical in congenital mitral stenosis, because there may not be a discrete primary orifice to measure. Rather, the secondary orifice of the valve, the interchordal spaces, may be the major means of egress. In a congenitally hypoplastic valve where the subvalvar apparatus appears normally formed, the diameter of the annulus is an excellent indicator of the severity of stenosis. Pulsed Doppler is useful for detecting high-velocity diastolic flow through the valve, and may be able to record the peak velocity in mild or moderate obstruction. Continuous-wave Doppler is much more reliable for recording the diastolic flow signal from the valve. The peak, mean, and end-diastolic pressure drop across the valve can be calculated easily from this tracing, yielding an excellent index of the severity of stenosis. If the heart rate is slow enough to separate the rapid filling wave from the atriosystolic filling wave, the pressure half-time can be determined from the slope of the downward limb of the rapid filling wave. The pressure half-time is less sensitive to changes in heart rate than is the pressure gradient and it is highly predictive of the functional valve area.[36] Doppler color flow mapping may be useful for detecting the disturbed flow pattern associated with atrioventricular valve stenosis. The direction of the stenotic jet can also be determined using Doppler color flow mapping, thus facilitating alignment of the pulsed or continuous-wave Doppler beam with the jet. Also the size of the functional or flow orifice through the valve can be determined by measuring the diameter of the flow stream as imaged by color Doppler.

There are several potential sources of error in estimating the severity of atrioventricular valve stenosis. First, the area or diameter of a stenotic valve will be overestimated if the measurement is not made at the tips of the leaflets. Because the proximal parts of the valve leaflets dome, measurement of the cross-sectional area even a small distance higher on the valve may cause serious underestimation of the severity of stenosis. There may be stenosis at more than one level of the valve, making measurement of an area at one part of the valve of little value in predicting the overall severity of obstruction. For example, a supravalvar stenosing ring is often present with a parachute mitral valve or typical congenital mitral stenosis.

The jet through the stenotic valve may be eccentric and directed at an acute angle with respect to the plane of the valve annulus. In such cases the Doppler beam may not be aligned with the flow jet, resulting in a falsely low measurement of velocity. This is particularly a problem in mitral stenosis associated with a small left ventricle, because the mitral jet is often directed posteriorly, but the only apical transducer window is anterior, at the right ventricular apex. Doppler color flow mapping aids in recognizing the orientation of the flow jet.

Low flow across a stenotic valve results in little or no pressure gradient. Low cardiac output may hamper accurate evaluation of a stenotic valve if the cardiac output is not measured. Similarly, it may be very difficult to evaluate the severity of atrioventricular valve stenosis in the presence of an atrial septal defect. Blood may be shunted preferentially across the atrial septal defect with little passing through the stenotic valve. Consequently little or no pressure gradient will be recorded.

Semilunar Valve Regurgitation. Semilunar valve regurgitation is more difficult to evaluate by Doppler examination. Although the length and area covered by the regurgitant jet have been used as indicators of severity,[18] at The Children's Hospital in Boston we have not found this particularly useful. Mapping the regurgitant jet of aortic regurgitation is complicated by the concomitant, and often superimposed, mitral inflow signal. Others have reported, and our experience would indicate, that the diameter of the regurgitant jet at the valve is an excellent indicator of severity.[63] As mentioned previously, the pressure half-time of the regurgitant jet is also a good index of severity in adults[57] but has not been proved in children. The pattern of flow in the descending aorta at the diaphragm (retrograde diastolic flow) is also a fair indicator of severity of aortic regurgitation.[92] Putative indicators of the severity of pulmonary regurgitation have not been evaluated because of the lack of a standard for comparison.

Mapping the regurgitant jet in the ventricle is not only difficult but also error-prone. Jets that hug the septum may be missed or underestimated, whereas those that intermix with the mitral inflow signal may be overestimated. Even the velocity of the flow signal may not be helpful in distinguishing between the regurgitant flow and normal mitral inflow, because the velocity of the regurgitant jet decreases substantially as the jet approaches the apex of the ventricle. The pressure half-time of the regurgitant jet has not been evaluated at the higher heart rates seen in children. Although the half-time should be insensitive to heart rate, this has not been verified. The flow pattern in the descending aorta may lead to underestimation of the severity of aortic regurgitation in the presence of a dilated aortic root. Apparently the high capacity root buffers the effect of regurgitation on flow more distal in the aorta.

Semilunar Valve Stenosis. Cardiovascular ultrasound has proved to be reliable for evaluating semilunar valve stenosis. The peak pressure difference across both the pulmonary and aortic valves can be accurately measured using the modified Bernoulli equation.[16,87] In many cases this correlates well with the peak-to-peak pressure difference measured at cardiac catheterization. The difference between the peak instantaneous pressure and the peak-to-peak pressure difference appears to increase with milder stenosis and in patients with substantial semilunar regurgitation. Studies in which measurements were made by Doppler examination simultaneously with catheter measurements have demonstrated a close correlation between the two techniques.[19,76] However, Doppler measurements made the day before catheterization in the same patients differed significantly from the simultaneous Doppler and catheter measurements, indicating that the day-to-day variation in pressure gradients may be large.[19] Apparent discrepancies between Doppler and catheter measurements may be largely due to biologic variation.

The major potential source of error in the Doppler assessment of semilunar stenosis is a large angle between the flow jet and the Doppler beam, which can be overcome by recording the Doppler signal from several different transducer positions. For the aortic valve, the apex, right sternal border and suprasternal notch are used, and for the pulmonary valve, the high and low left sternal border and the subxiphoid space. Also Doppler color flow mapping may be of value in determining the direction of the jet. Low cardiac output may result in underestimation of the severity of aortic stenosis, as noted for atrioventricular valves.

Prosthetic Valves. Cardiovascular ultrasound is also an excellent method for following patients with prosthetic valves. The valve should be imaged from several transducer positions, looking for excessive motion of the sewing ring, occluder or leaflet motion, and masses associated with the valve. Normally the sewing ring should move in concert with, and to about the same extent, as the surrounding cardiac tissue. Excessive or discordant motion suggests dehiscence. The motion of the occluder device of mechanical prosthetic valves is observed

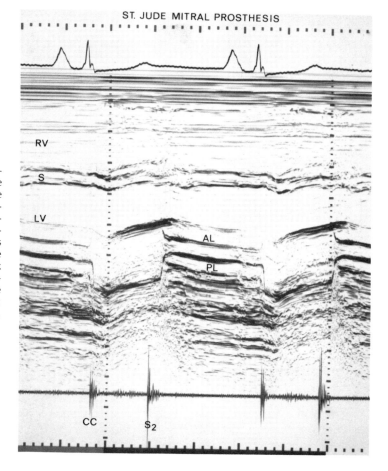

Figure 26. M-mode echocardiogram of a St. Jude prosthesis in the mitral position. Note the motion of the 2 "leaflets" of this mechanical prosthesis. The opening and closing motions are rapid and the interval between A2 and the valve opening is constant. AL = anterior "leaflet" of the prosthetic valve; CC = closing click of the prosthetic valve; LV = left ventricle; PL = posterior "leaflet" of the prosthetic valve; RV = right ventricle; S = septum; S_2 = second heart sound.

best using M-mode echocardiography (Fig. 26). The timing of the opening and closing of the valve should be measured for several cycles. At a constant heart rate, variation of more than a few percent in the time to opening, or the duration of opening, of the valve is highly suggestive of dysfunction. Delay in opening is most often due to ingrowth of pannus or the development of a clot around the seating ring of the valve (Fig. 27). M-mode echocardiography is also useful for recording the motion of the leaflets of bioprosthetic valves. Coarse vibration of a valve leaflet has been associated with rupture of the leaflet.[1] Diminished excursion of the leaflets may indicate calcification.

Pulsed or continuous-wave Doppler examination is used to evaluate prosthetic valve functions as was described for native valves. Most mechanical prosthetic valves in the atrioventricular valve position have a substantial early diastolic pressure drop across the valve, even when functioning normally. However, the pressure gradient should decay rapidly, so that by end-diastole the gradient is less than 7–8 mm Hg. Again, Doppler flow mapping is useful for determining the orientation of the flow jet through the valve and for evaluating regurgitation. Periprosthetic regurgitation can be localized and distinguished from transvalvar regurgitation by scanning parallel to the valve ring with Doppler color flow mapping. Because the sound energy may not penetrate metallic or plastic valve material, views must be selected that display the upstream chamber without traversing the valve. For example, the parasternal long-axis view is excellent for detecting prosthetic mitral regurgitation, because the left atrium can be imaged without the sound beam crossing the prosthetic valve.

Ventricular Function

Now that infants and children survive with severe heart defects, pediatric cardiologists are becoming concerned with the functional status of survivors. Ventricular function is a major determinant of the quality of life of these children and young adults. Cardiovascular ultrasound is an ideal technique for serially evaluating ventricular function. The technique does not influence ventricular function and can be repeated as often as needed without discomfort or risk. Numerous parameters of both systolic and diastolic function can be measured with cardiovascular ultrasound. In addition, the loading conditions of the left ventricle can be assessed. Knowledge of both the functional state and the loading conditions of the ventricle allows inference about the contractile state of the muscle. At present about 25–30% of the echocardiograms

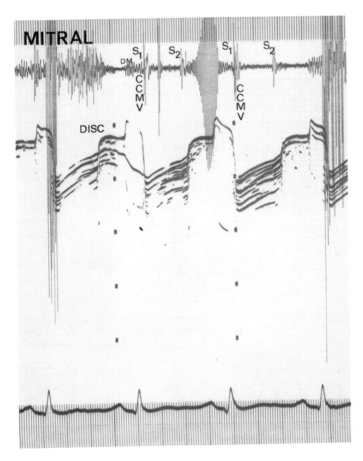

Figure 27. M-mode echocardiogram of Bjork-Shiley prosthesis in the mitral position. Note the step-wise opening motion of the valve. Opening is not complete until atrial systole. In this case the occluder motion was obstructed by pannus ingrowth around the sewing ring. CCMV = closing click of the prosthetic valve; Disc = occluder of the prosthetic valve; DM = diastolic murmur; S_1 = first heart sound; S_2 = second heart sound.

performed at The Children's Hospital in Boston are specifically for assessment of ventricular function. For a complete discussion of specific techniques, see chapter 15.

Miscellaneous Indications for Cardiac Ultrasound Examination

Pericardial Effusion. A common reason for obtaining an echocardiogram, especially in the postoperative patient, is the suspicion of a pericardial effusion. Two-dimensional imaging from multiple transducer locations is essential in evaluating such patients (Fig. 28). Although a large effusion can generally be seen from any position, small or loculated fluid collections can be missed on a casual examination or on an M-mode examination alone. The location of the fluid should be described and the thickness of the layer of fluid measured in two or three standard locations. If the fluid collection is large and requires drainage, it is helpful to determine a safe route of approach to the pericardium. The preferred route is from the subxiphoid space. Imaging from this location shows the amount of fluid between the heart and the pericardium. Also, adhesions between the pericardium and the heart wall can be seen. If a clear path to the fluid cannot be identified, other approaches must be investigated. The left parasternal or apical windows are other potential points of attack.

Masses. Cardiac masses are of two types: intracavitary thrombi and/or vegetations and tumors. Intracardiac thrombi may occur in the presence of an indwelling catheter, ventricular dysfunction, an atrial arrhythmia, or a prosthetic valve. Usually, the thrombus is attached to the heart or indwelling device, but, rarely, it may be floating free in the cavity. Typically irregular in outline, thrombus is more reflective than myocardium and is of uneven density (Fig. 29). A vegetation is distinguishable

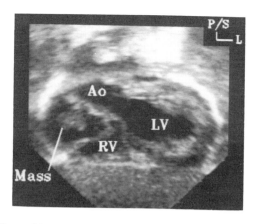

Figure 29. A thrombus (Mass) in the right atrium of an infant who had previously had an indwelling central venous catheter for alimentation. Ao = aorta; L = left; LV = left ventricle; P = posterior; RV = right ventricle; S = superior.

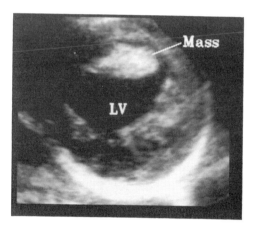

Figure 30. A rhabdomyoma (Mass) in the left ventricular (LV) free wall of this child with tuberous sclerosis.

from thrombus only by location and association. Signs and symptoms of infective endocarditis are usually present, and vegetations are almost always located on valve leaflets or other sites of turbulence in the heart and vessels. Although cardiovascular ultrasound is capable of detecting thrombus or vegetation, the sensitivity is low in adults[81,89] and unknown in children. The ability to distinguish between thrombus and vegetation is poor, being based on the soft criteria described above. A negative examination does not exclude the presence of thrombus or vegetation.

Solid tumors of the heart, including rhabdomyomas, teratomas, and, rarely, myxomas and fibromas, can be detected with high sensitivity using cardiovascular ultrasound (Fig. 30).[29] However, the histologic type of the tumor cannot be determined reliably. The physiologic consequences of the tumor(s) can be determined using Doppler cardiography.

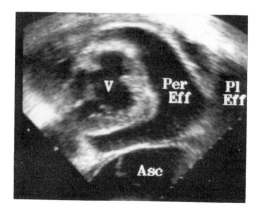

Figure 28. A large pericardial effusion (Per Eff) following a Fontan operation. Note also the ascites (Asc) below the diaphragm and the left pleural effusion (Pl Eff).

Catheter Placement. Vascular catheters or pacing leads can be localized easily and accurately using multiple plane imaging. The position of umbilical arterial and venous catheters can be checked using this technique. An umbilical venous catheter readily crosses into the left atrium through a patent foramen ovale. Imaging the catheter passing through the foramen or a contrast injection demonstrates the position of the catheter. Balloon atrial septostomy is commonly performed with echocardiographic guidance.[3]

The exact location of the tip of an electrode catheter is often important when mapping the source of a ventricular arrhythmia. Using cardiovascular ultrasound, the tip can be localized with respect to familiar intracardiac structures. This is particularly important if surgical or catheter ablation is being considered.

Special Applications

Two relatively new applications of cardiovascular ultrasound include fetal echocardiography and intraoperative echocardiography.

Fetal Echocardiography. Prenatal screening for congenital heart defects is now possible even in the previable fetus. Most major heart defects can be reliably diagnosed by 18–20 weeks of gestation.[2,4,7,48,62] The indications for prenatal echocardiography include a previous child with a heart defect, a parent with a heart defect, maternal diabetes, a known chromosomal anomaly, or multiple noncardiac anomalies. The examination is approached much the same as it is in the newborn infant, except that the examiner has little control over the position of the fetus, and, thus, over the views obtained (Figs. 31 and 32). However, if the segmental approach is employed, even complex defects can be diagnosed accurately.[62] Defects that remain difficult or impossible to detect *in utero* include atrial septal defect, patent ductus arteriosus, ventricular septal defect, coarctation, and some valve abnormalities.[7,62] Usually, it is impossible to distinguish between normal patency of the foramen ovale and an atrial septal defect. Patency

of the ductus arteriosus is, of course, normal prior to birth. Even moderate-sized ventricular septal defects may be below the resolution of the imaging equipment. An examination later in gestation (35 weeks) may improve the detection rate of ventricular septal defects.[7] Coarctation of the aorta may not be apparent until after closure of the ductus arteriosus, or may not be detected *in utero* because of limited resolution. However, a disparity in ventricular size (right ventricle larger than the left ventricle) is a sensitive, although not specific, marker for coarctation.[8]

The ability to detect heart defects in the previable fetus avails the parents of the option to terminate the pregnancy. On the other hand, plans can be made to expedite the neonatal management of the fetus known to have a heart defect.[39] Most commonly, anxious parents can be assured that the fetus has no detectable heart defect. This is especially important to parents who previously have lost a child with a heart defect.

The other major use of fetal echocardiography is for the management of arrhythmias in the fetus.[47,98] Atrial premature beats, either conducted or blocked, are the most common rhythm disturbance detected *in utero*. These are almost always benign, and only if frequent or associated with short bursts of tachycardia do they require specific follow-up. Supraventricular tachycardia and atrial flutter are the two most common serious arrhythmias encountered in the fetus. Either may cause congestive heart failure manifested by hydrops fetalis. Both require close follow-up and, often, pharmacologic therapy via the placenta. The diagnosis is made using two-dimensionally directed M-mode echocardiography or Doppler examination to demonstrate a rapid, regular atrial rate with corresponding ventricular activity at the same rate or with some degree of atrioventricular block. Atrial tachycardia should be suspected in any hydropic fetus for which no other cause is found. Even intermittent tachycardia, which can be missed on a brief ultrasound examination, can cause hydrops. In such cases arrangements should be made for frequent sampling of the fetal heart rate over a

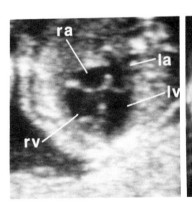 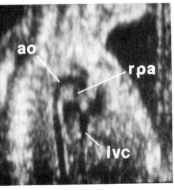

Figure 31. (**left**). Two-dimensional echocardiogram in a 21-week fetus showing a four-chamber view. la = left atrium; lv = left ventricle; ra = right atrium; rv = right ventricle.

Figure 32. (**right**). Sagittal plane view in a 22-week fetus showing the aortic arch. ao = aorta; ivc = inferior vena cava; rpa = right pulmonary artery.

period of several hours, or until tachycardia is detected.

Ventricular tachyarrhythmias are rare in the fetus. Isolated ventricular beats may be distinguished from premature beats of atrial origin by noting the sequence of activation of the atria and ventricles on the M-mode strip.

Complete heart block is the most common prolonged bradyarrhythmia detected in utero. The diagnosis is made using 2-D or M-mode echocardiography to demonstrate independent contraction of the atria and ventricles. Complete heart block usually occurs in the setting of maternal lupus erythematosus[78] or with some structural heart defects such as complete common atrioventricular canal or corrected transposition.[47] It is important to distinguish complete heart block from the bradycardia accompanying fetal distress, in order to avoid unnecessary cesarean section.

Intraoperative Echocardiography. Direct application of the transducer onto the exposed heart at surgery provides exceptional images of intracardiac anatomy.[31,34] This technology has proved valuable for sorting out complex anatomy at the operating table and for detecting residual structural problems. In addition, ventricular function can be assessed in the period immediately following cardiopulmonary bypass. More common uses have included assessment of the severity of atrioventricular valve regurgitation after valvoplasty, localization of residual ventricular septal defects, evaluation of the subaortic region after resection of subaortic stenosis, and evaluation of regional left ventricular function following suspected coronary artery injury. Because of the relatively low cardiac output in the immediate post-bypass period, measured gradients are often lower than gradients measured later, after output has returned to normal.

It is fair to say that the potential of intraoperative imaging and Doppler examination is only now being explored. Early efforts indicate that this technique will prove to be useful in surgical management of children with heart defects.

REFERENCES

1. Alam M, Madrazo AC, Magilligan DJ, et al: M-mode and two-dimensional echocardiographic features of porcine valve dysfunction. Am J Cardiol 43:502–509, 1979.
2. Allan LD, Crawford DC, Anderson RH, et al: Echocardiographic and anatomical correlations in fetal congenital heart disease. Br Heart J 52:542–548, 1984.
3. Allan LD, Leanage R, Wainwright R, et al: Balloon atrial septostomy under two-dimensional echocardiographic control. Br Heart J 47:41–43, 1982.
4. Allan LD, Tynan M, Campbell S, et al: Identification of congenital cardiac malformations by echocardiography in midtrimester fetus. Br Heart J 46:358–362, 1981.
5. Baker DW, Rubenstein SA, Lorch GS: Pulsed Doppler echocardiography: principles and applications. Am J Med 63:69–80, 1977.
6. Bash SE, Vick GW, Gutgesel HP: Hypoplastic left heart syndrome: is echocardiography accurate enough to guide surgical palliation? J Am Coll Cardiol 7:610–616, 1986.
7. Benacerraf BR, Pober BR, Sanders SP: Accuracy of fetal echocardiography. Radiology 165:847–849, 1987.
8. Benacerraf BR, Saltzman DH, Sanders SP: Sonographic sign for the prenatal diagnosis of coarctation of the aorta. Radiology 165:847–849, 1987.
9. Bierman FZ, Fellows K, Williams RG: Prospective identification of ventricular septal defects in infancy using two-dimensional echocardiography. Circulation 62:807–817, 1980.
10. Bierman FZ, Williams RG: Prospective diagnosis of d-transposition of the great arteries in neonates by subxiphoid two-dimensional echocardiography. Circulation 60:1469–1502, 1979.
11. Blanchard D, Diebold B, Guermonprez JL: Noninvasive quantification of tricuspid regurgitation by Doppler echocardiography (abstract). Circulation 64:IV–256, 1981.
12. Bolger A, Eigler N, Pfaff JM, et al: Computer analysis of color Doppler images of flow jets in a phantom model (abstract). J Am Coll Cardiol 7:59A, 1986.
13. Bommer WJ: Basic principles of flow imaging. Echocardiography 2:501–509, 1985.
14. Bracewell R: The Fourier Transform and Its Applications. New York, McGraw-Hill, 1965, p. 189.
15. Brandenburg RO, Tajik AJ, Edwards WD, et al: Accuracy of 2-dimensional diagnosis of congenitally bicuspid aortic valve: echocardiographic-anatomic correlation in 115 patients. Am J Cardiol 51:1469–1473, 1983.
16. Callahan MJ, Tajik AJ, Su Fan Q, et al: Validation of instantaneous pressure gradients measured by continuous-wave Doppler in experimentally induced aortic stenosis. Am J Cardiol 56:989–993, 1985.
17. Chin AJ, Bierman FZ, Sanders SP, et al: Subxiphoid 2-dimensional echocardiographic identification of left ventricular papillary muscle anomalies in complete common atrioventricular canal. Am J Cardiol 51:1695–1699, 1983.
18. Ciobanu M, Abbasi AS, Allen M, et al: Pulsed Doppler echocardiography in the diagnosis and estimation of severity of aortic insufficiency. Am J Cardiol 49:339–343, 1982.
19. Currie PJ, Seward JB, Reeder GS, et al: Continuous-wave Doppler echocardiographic assessment of severity of calcific aortic stenosis: a simultaneous Doppler-catheter correlative study in 100 adult patients. Circulation 71:1162–1169, 1985.
20. Disessa TG, Hagan AD, Isabel-Jones JB, et al: Two-dimensional echocardiographic evaluation of discrete subaortic stenosis from the apical long-axis view. Am Heart J 101:774–782, 1981.
21. Edler I, Gustafson A: Ultrasonic cardiogram in mitral stenosis. Acta Med Scand 159:85–90, 1957.
22. Edler I, Hertz CH: Use of ultrasonic reflectoscope for continuous recording of movements of heart walls. Kungl Fysiogr Sallsk Lund Forhandl 24:5–9, 1954.
23. Feigenbaum H: Echocardiography, 4th ed. Philadelphia, Lea & Febiger, 1985, pp. 1–50.
24. Feigenbaum H, Zaky A, Waldhausen JA: Use of ultrasound in the diagnosis of pericardial effusion. Ann Intern Med 65:443–452, 1966.

25. Fisher DC, Sahn DJ, Friedman MJ, et al: The mitral valve orifice method for noninvasive two-dimensional echo Doppler determination of cardiac output. Circulation 67:872–877, 1983.

26. Foale R, Stefanini L, Rickards A, et al: Left and right ventricular morphology in complex congenital heart disease defined by two-dimensional echocardiography. Am J Cardiol 49:93–99, 1982.

27. Freed MD, Nadas AS, Norwood WI, et al: Is routine preoperative cardiac catheterization necessary before repair of secundum and sinus venosus atrial septal defects? J Am Coll Cardiol 4:333–336, 1984.

28. Fyfe DA, Currie PJ, Seward JB, et al: Continuous-wave Doppler determination of the pressure gradient across pulmonary artery bands: hemodynamic correlation in 20 patients. Mayo Clin Proc 59:744–750, 1984.

29. Fyke FE, Seward JB, Edwards WD, et al: Primary cardiac tumors: experience with 30 consecutive patients since the introduction of two-dimensional echocardiography. J Am Coll Cardiol 5:1465–1473, 1985.

30. Gardin JM, Dabestani A, Matin K, et al: Reproducibility of Doppler aortic blood flow velocity measurements: studies on intra-observer, interobserver and day-to-day variability in normal subjects. Am J Cardiol 54:1092–1098, 1984.

31. Goldman ME, Mindich BP: Intraoperative two-dimensional echocardiography: new application of an old technique. J Am Coll Cardiol 7:374–382, 1986.

32. Gramiak R, Shah PM, Kramer DH: Ultrasound cardiography: contrast studies in anatomy and function. Radiology 92:939–948, 1969.

33. Griffith JM, Henry WI: A sector scanner for real time two-dimensional echocardiography. Circulation 49:1147–1152, 1974.

34. Gussenhoven EJ, van Herwerden LA, Roelandt J, et al: Intraoperative two-dimensional echocardiography in congenital heart disease. J Am Coll Cardiol 9:565–572, 1987.

35. Hagler DJ, Tajik AJ, Seward JB, et al: Atrioventricular and ventriculoarterial discordance (corrected transposition of the great arteries): Wide-angle two-dimensional echocardiographic assessment of ventricular morphology. Mayo Clin Proc 56:591–600, 1981.

36. Hatle L, Bjorn A, Tromsdal A: Noninvasive assessment of atrioventricular pressure half-time by Doppler ultrasound. Circulation 60:1096–1104, 1979.

37. Hegrenaes L: Left ventricular systolic time intervals: a comparison between conventional carotid pulse wave method and the Doppler ultrasound method. Eur Heart J 4:313–319, 1983.

38. Hsieh KS, Sanders SP, Colan SD, et al: Right ventricular systolic time intervals: comparison of echocardiographic and Doppler-derived values. Am Heart J 112:103–107, 1986.

39. Huhta JC, Carpenter RJ Jr, Moise KJ Jr, et al: Prenatal diagnosis and postnatal management of critical aortic stenosis. Circulation 75:573–576, 1987.

40. Huhta JC, Gutgesell HP, Latson LA, et al: Two-dimensional echocardiographic assessment of the aorta in infants and children with congenital heart disease. Circulation 70:417–424, 1984.

41. Huhta JC, Smallhorn JF, Macartney FJ: Two-dimensional echocardiographic diagnosis of situs. Br Heart J 48:97–108, 1982.

42. Huntsman LL, Stewart DK, Barnes SR, et al: Noninvasive Doppler determination of cardiac output in man. Circulation 67:593–602, 1983.

43. Johnson SL, Baker DW, Lute RA, et al: Doppler echocardiography: the localization of cardiac murmurs. Circulation 48:810–822, 1973.

44. King DH, O'Brien-Smith E, Huhta JC, et al: Mitral and tricuspid valve annulus diameter in normal children determined by two-dimensional echocardiography. Am J Cardiol 55:787–789, 1985.

45. Kisslo J, VonRamm OT, Thurstone F: Cardiac imaging using a phased array ultrasound system. II. Clinical technique and applications. Circulation 53:262–267, 1976.

46. Kitabatake A, Inoue M, Asao M, et al: Noninvasive evaluation of pulmonary hypertension by a pulsed Doppler technique. Circulation 68:302–309, 1983.

47. Kleinman CS, Donnerstein RL, Jaffe C, et al: Fetal echocardiography. A tool for evaluation of in utero cardiac arrhythmias and monitoring of in utero therapy: analysis of 71 patients. Am J Cardiol 51:237–243, 1983.

48. Kleinman CS, Hobbins JC, Jaffe CC, et al: Echocardiographic studies in the human fetus: prenatal diagnosis of congenital heart disease and cardiac dysrhythmias. Pediatrics 65:1059–1067, 1980.

49. Kosturakis D, Goldberg SJ, Allen HD, et al: Doppler echocardiographic prediction of pulmonary arterial hypertension in congenital heart disease. Am J Cardiol 53:1110–1115, 1984.

50. Lavenson GS, Rich NM, Baugh JH: Value of ultrasonic flow detection in the management of peripheral vascular diseases. Am J Surg 120:522–526, 1970.

51. Lincoln CR, Rigby ML, Mercanti C, et al: Surgical risk factors in total anomalous pulmonary venous connection. Am J Cardiol 61:608–611, 1988.

52. Lipschultz SE, Sanders SP, Mayer JE, et al: Are routine preoperative cardiac catheterization and angiography necessary before repair of ostium primum atrial septal defect? J Am Coll Cardiol 11:373–378, 1988.

53. Martin RP, Rakowski H, Kleiman JH, et al: Reliability and reproducibility of two-dimensional echocardiographic measurements of the stenotic mitral valve orifice area. Am J Cardiol 43:560–568, 1979.

54. Marx GR, Allen HD, Goldberg SJ: Transatrial septal velocity measurement by Doppler echocardiography in atrial septal defect—correlation with QP:QS ratio. Am J Cardiol 55:1162—1167, 1985.

55. Marx GR, Allen HD, Goldberg SJ: Doppler echocardiographic estimation of systolic pulmonary artery pressure in pediatric patients with interventricular communications. J Am Coll Cardiol 6:1132–1137, 1985.

56. Marx GR, Allen HD, Goldberg SJ: Doppler echocardiographic estimation of systolic pulmonary artery pressure in pediatric patients with aortico-pulmonary shunts. J Am Coll Cardiol 7:880–885, 1986.

57. Masuyama T, Kodama K, Kitabatake A, et al: Noninvasive evaluation of aortic regurgitation by continuous-wave Doppler echocardiography. Circulation 73:460–466, 1986.

58. Miyatake K, Izumi S, Okamoto M, et al: Semiquantitative grading of severity of mitral regurgitation by real-time two-dimensional Doppler flow imaging technique. J Am Coll Cardiol 7:82–88, 1986.

59. Miyatake K, Okamoto M, Kinoshita N, et al: Evaluation of tricuspid regurgitation by pulsed Doppler and two-dimensional echocardiography. Circulation 66:777–783, 1982.

60. Omoto R (ed): Color Atlas of Real-Time Two-Dimensional Doppler Echocardiography. Philadelphia, Lea & Febiger, 1984.

61. Omoto R, Kasai C: Basic principles of Doppler color flow imaging. Echocardiography 3:463–473, 1986.

62. Parness IA, Yeager SB, Sanders SP, et al: Echocardiographic diagnosis of fetal heart defects in mid trimester. Arch Dis Child 63:1137–1145, 1988.

63. Perry GJ, Helmcke F, Nanda N, et al: Evaluation of aortic insufficiency by Doppler color flow mapping. J Am Coll Cardiol 9:952–959, 1987.

64. Popp RL, Fowles R, Coltart J, et al: Cardiac anatomy viewed systematically with two-dimensional echocardiography. Chest 75:579–585, 1979.

65. Rein AJJT, Colan SD, Parness IP, et al: Regional and global left ventricular function in infants with anomalous origin of the left coronary artery from the pulmonary trunk: preoperative and postoperative assessment. Circulation 75:115–123, 1987.

66. Rein AJJT, Hsieh KS, Elixson M, et al: Cardiac output estimates in the pediatric intensive care unit using a continuous-wave Doppler computer: validation and limitations of the technique. Am Heart J 112:97–103, 1986.

67. Requarth JA, Goldberg SJ, Vasko SD, et al: In vitro verification of Doppler prediction of transvalve pressure gradient and orifice area in stenosis. Am J Cardiol 53:1369–1373, 1984.

68. Rice MJ, Seward JB, Hagler DJ, et al: Impact of 2-dimensional echocardiography on the management of distressed newborns in whom cardiac disease is suspected. Am J Cardiol 51:288–292, 1983.

69. Ritter SB, Rothe WA, Kawai D: Identification of ventricular septal defects by Doppler color flow mapping. A study in enhanced sensitivity (abstract). Clin Res 36:311A, 1988.

70. Sanders SP: Echocardiography and related techniques in the diagnosis of congenital heart defects. I. Veins, atria and interatrial septum. Echocardiography 1:185–217, 1984.

71. Sanders SP: Echocardiography and related techniques in the diagnosis of congenital heart defects. II. Atrioventricular valves and ventricles. Echocardiography 1:333–391, 1984.

72. Sanders SP: Echocardiography and related techniques in the diagnosis of congenital heart defects. Part III: Conotruncus and great arteries. Echocardiography 1:443–493, 1984.

73. Sanders SP, Bierman FZ, Williams RG: Conotruncal malformations: diagnosis in infancy using subxiphoid two-dimensional echocardiography. Am J Cardiol 50:1361–1367, 1982.

74. Sanders SP, MacPherson D, Yeager SB: Temporal flow velocity profile in the descending aorta in coarctation. J Am Coll Cardiol 7:603–609, 1986.

75. Sanders SP, Yeager S, Williams RG: Measurement of systemic and pulmonary blood flow and Qp/Qs ratio using Doppler and two-dimensional echocardiography. Am J Cardiol 51:952–956, 1983.

76. Scholler GF, Colan SD, Sanders SP, et al: Noninvasive estimation of the left ventricular pressure waveform throughout ejection in young patients with aortic stenosis. J Am Coll Cardiol 12:492–497, 1988.

77. Schuster AH, Nanda NC: Doppler echocardiography. I. Doppler cardiac output measurements: perspective and comparison with other methods of cardiac output determination. Echocardiography 1:45–54, 1984.

78. Scott JS, Maddison PJ, Taylor PV, et al: Connective-tissue disease, antibodies to ribonucleoprotein, and congenital heart block. N Engl J Med 309:209–212, 1983.

79. Serwer GA, Cougle AG, Eckerd JM, et al: Factors affecting use of the Doppler-determined time from flow onset to maximal pulmonary artery velocity for measurement of pulmonary artery pressure in children. Am J Cardiol 58:352–356, 1986.

80. Shaddy RE, Snider AR, Silverman NH: Pulsed Doppler findings in patients with coarctation of the aorta. Circulation 73:82–88, 1986.

81. Shrestha NK, Moreno FFL, Narciso FV: Two-dimensional echocardiographic diagnosis of left atrial thrombus in rheumatic heart disease. Circulation 67:341–347, 1983.

82. Silverman NH, Schiller NB: Apex echocardiography. A two-dimensional technique for evaluating congenital heart disease. Circulation 57:503–511, 1978.

83. Silverman NH, Ports TA, Snider AR, et al: Determination of left ventricular volume in children: echocardiographic and angiographic comparisons. Circulation 62:548–557, 1980.

84. Smallhorn JF, DeLeval M, Stark J, et al: Isolated anterior mitral cleft. Two-dimensional echocardiographic assessment and differentiation from "clefts" associated with atrioventricular septal defects. Br Heart J 48:109–116, 1982.

85. Snider AR, Silverman NH: Suprasternal notch echocardiography: a two-dimensional technique for evaluating congenital heart disease. Circulation 63:165–173, 1981.

86. Snider AR, Stevenson JG, French JW, et al: Comparison of high pulse repetition frequency and continuous wave Doppler echocardiography for velocity measurement and gradient prediction in children with valvular and congenital heart disease. J Am Coll Cardiol 7:873–879, 1986.

87. Stevenson JG, Kawabori I: Noninvasive determination of pressure gradients in children: two methods employing pulsed Doppler echocardiography. J Am Coll Cardiol 3:179–192, 1984.

88. Strandness DE, McCutcheon EP, Rushmer RF: Application of transcutaneous Doppler flow meter in evaluation of occlusive arterial disease. Surg Gynecol Obstet 122:1039–1045, 1966.

89. Strom J, Becker R, Davis R: Echocardiographic and surgical correlation in bacterial endocarditis. Circulation 62(Suppl I):164–167, 1980.

90. Sutherland GR, Smallhorn JF, Anderson RH, et al: Atrioventricular discordance: cross-sectional echocardiographic-morphologic correlative study. Br Heart J 50:8–20, 1983.

91. Tajik AJ, Seward JB, Hagler DJ, et al: Two-dimensional real-time ultrasonic imaging of the heart and great vessels. Mayo Clin Proc 53:271–303, 1978.

92. Takenaka K, Dabestani A, Gardin JM, et al: A simple Doppler echocardiographic method for estimating severity of aortic regurgitation. Am J Cardiol 57:1340–1343, 1986.

93. Tei C, Tanaka H, Kashima T, et al: Real-time cross-sectional echocardiographic evaluation of the interatrial septum by right atrium-interatrial septum-left atrium direction of ultrasound beam. Circulation 60:539–546, 1979.

94. Trowitzsch E, Bano-Rodrigo A, Burger BM, et al: Two-dimensional echocardiographic findings in double orifice mitral valve. J Am Coll Cardiol 6:383–387, 1985.

95. Trowitzsch E, Colan SD, Sanders SP: Two-dimensional echocardiographic estimation of right ventricular area change and ejection fraction in infants with systemic right ventricle (transposition of the great arteries or hypoplastic left heart syndrome). Am J Cardiol 55:1153–1157, 1985.

96. Valdes-Cruz LM, Horowitz S, Mesel E, et al: A pulsed Doppler echocardiographic method for calculating pulmonary and systemic blood flow in atrial level shunts: validation studies in animals and initial human experience. Circulation 69:80–86, 1984.

97. Veyrat C, Ameur A, Bas S, et al: Pulsed Doppler echocardiographic indices for assessing mitral regurgitation. Br Heart J 51:130–138, 1984.

98. Walsh EP, Keane JF, Sanders SP: Fetal cardiac dysrhythmias: detection and management. In Milunsky A, Friedman EA, Gluck L (eds): Advances in Perinatology. New York, Plenum Medical Book Co., 1985, Vol. 4, pp. 63–94.

99. Wann LS, Feigenbaum H, Weyman AE, et al: Cross-sectional echocardiographic detection of rheumatic mitral regurgitation. Am J Cardiol 41:1258–1263, 1978.

100. Yock PG, Popp RL: Noninvasive estimation of right ventricular systolic pressure by Doppler ultrasound in patients with tricuspid regurgitation. Circulation 70:657–662, 1984.

Chapter 14

CARDIAC CATHETERIZATION

James E. Lock, M.D., John F. Keane, M.D.,
Valerie S. Mandell, M.D., and Stanton B. Perry, M.D.

Stephen Hales' measurement of equine arterial pressure,[39] Werner Forssmann's celebrated auto-cannulation,[29] and Andre Cournand's assessment of pulmonary arterial pressures in human disease[16] mark the known beginnings of cardiac catheterization. The first cardiac catheterization in a case of congenital heart disease was reported in 1946.[13] Until that time, the notion that an atrial septal defect resulted in a left-to-right shunt was surmised from the anatomic findings of a large right heart. This hypothesis was supported by the case of a 32-year-old woman with an atrial septal defect who has a superior vena caval oxygen content of 10.4 ml per 100 cc, an inferior vena caval content of 9.5 ml per 100 cc, and a right atrial oxygen content of 12.1 ml per 100 cc.

The first therapeutic cardiac catheterization procedures in congenital heart disease were described in the remarkable reports from the Institute for Cardiology from Mexico City where Rubio-Alvarez and his colleagues used their own blade-equipped catheter (Fig. 1).[99,100] Using this device in a 32-year-old woman, they reduced the systolic pulmonary valve gradient from 90 to 30 mm Hg. Despite such successes, transcatheter therapy remained dormant until the development of the lifesaving balloon septostomy technique for transposition of the great arteries by Rashkind and Miller.[91]

Since these pioneering studies, the capabilities of cardiac catheterization in children have increased enormously. All parts of the normal and abnormal circulation are routinely cannulated. Many forms of heart disease that previously required operative management are now corrected with transcatheter techniques (some on an outpatient basis) and some diseases that previously were inoperable can now be effectively managed at cardiac catheterization.[66]

INDICATIONS FOR CARDIAC CATHETERIZATION

Because of its capability for showing excellent anatomic detail and the possibility for repeated examinations, echocardiography has largely supplanted angiography as the prime source for examining cardiac anatomy.[31] Angiography is still needed when there are poor echocardiographic windows and when there is intervening bone or air-filled lung (e.g., scoliosis or abnormalities of the peripheral pulmonary arteries). Echocardiograms are especially useful for infants; it is difficult to get comparable visualization in fully grown patients.

When it comes to physiologic measurements, the estimates based on indirect echocardiographic observations are statistically valid but less precise than those obtained at cardiac catheterization. At the same time the ability to get repeated observations easily makes the echocardiogram the prime tool in following physiologic abnormalities (e.g., pressure gradients or myocardial function). Still, when a decision to undertake surgery is being debated, cardiac catheterization frequently is required.

In the past few years, catheterization has become safer and more precise. New, smaller catheters, more flexible shafts, flow-directed balloons, less toxic contrast agents, improved anatomic understanding provided by the precatheterization noninvasive evaluation, and imaging systems that offer superior resolution with less radiation have all contributed to this improved safety.

In general, cardiac catheterization is used (1) when precise physiologic measurements are needed (e.g., in estimating the severity of aortic stenosis or studying the feasibility of a Fontan procedure); (2) when the anatomic features are poorly visualized by echocardiography (e.g., peripheral pulmonary structures or poor windows); (3) when electrophysiologic studies are needed; or (4) when therapeutic catheterization is planned.

Given the enormous variability of congenital heart disease, skill at echocardiographic diagnosis, surgical approaches, and experience at interventional techniques, a listing of the indications for cardiac catheterization that would apply to each

187

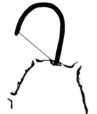 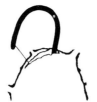 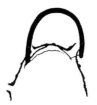

Figure 1. Diagram of the first interventional catheter used by Rubio-Alvarez in 1953 to successfully open a stenotic pulmonary valve.

cardiac institution simply is not possible. Table 1 summarizes the indications used at Boston Children's Hospital at the present time on a lesion by lesion basis. Further discussion of indications will be presented in the chapters on individual lesions.

RISKS OF CATHETERIZATION

The number of complications of catheterization have decreased over the years. However, they still occur, particularly in sick neonates and infants with complex lesions and unstable cardiovascular status. Major complications are noted in about 30% of infants classified as high risk, 14% in the medium-risk group and 4% of those in the low-risk category.[15] In addition, the incidence of complications requiring treatment was 12% in infants less than 4 months old, compared with 1.5% in the older infants.

Deaths. When deaths occurring within 24 hours

Table 1. Indications for Cardiac Catheterizations

Diagnosis	Catheterization Usually Indicated?	Potential or Real Indication for Catheterization
Ventricular septal defect, preop.	Yes	Multiple ventricular septal defects, pulmonary arterial resistance
Pulmonary stenosis	Yes	Balloon valvotomy
Tetralogy of Fallot, preop. shunt	No	Central pulmonary artery, arch anatomy
Tetralogy of Fallot, preop. repair	Yes	Pulmonary artery anatomy, multiple ventricular septal defects, coronary arteries, etc.
Aortic stenosis, preop.	Yes	Balloon valvotomy
Aortic stenosis, postop.	Yes	Restenosis, left vetricular function, balloon valvotomy
Atrial septal defect secundum	Yes	Transcatheter closure
Patent ductus arteriosus	Yes	Transcatheter closure
Coarctation	No	Balloon angioplasty
Transposition of the great arteries	Yes	Balloon septostomy, left ventricle and pulmonary artery pressure, coronary anatomy
Atrial septal defect primum	No	Associated defects, mitral regurgitation
Complete atrioventricular canal	No	Multiple ventricular septal defects, atrioventricular valve regurgitation
Hypoplastic left ventricle, preop.	No	Right ventricular function, arch anatomy
Hypoplastic left ventricle, postop.	Yes	Arch obstruction, atrial septal defect obstruction, pulmonary artery distortion, tricuspid valve incompetence
Tetralogy of Fallot, pulmonary atresia	Yes	Collateral size, distribution of pulmonary arteries, coronary arteries
Single ventricle, preop. shunt	No	Central pulmonary artery, arch anatomy
Single ventricle, postop. band, shunt	Yes	Pulmonary artery pressure, anatomy
Single ventricle, preop. band, Stansel	Yes	Aortic outflow obstructions
Truncus arteriosus	Yes	Truncal valve, pulmonary artery anatomy
Total anomalous pulmonary venous return	No	Mixed venous drainage, small left ventricle
Pulmonary atresia, intact septum	Yes	Right ventricle size, pressure, coronary fistulas and stenosis
Recurrent aortic gradient	Yes	Balloon angioplasty
Venous baffle obstruction	Yes	Balloon angioplasty
Pulmonary arteriovenous malformation	Yes	Transcatheter closure
Left superior vena cava-to-left atrium	Yes	Transcatheter closure
Cardiac transplantation	Yes	Cardiac biopsy
Pericardial tamponade	Yes	Placement of drain

of cardiac catheterization, including those after cardiac surgery, were analyzed, mortality was higher in neonates than in older children.[110] The average rate has been reported at 16.0% in the first week of life, 9.7% in infants less than 1 month old and 4.5% in those less than 1 year of age, the overall mortality for all ages being 2.0%. In another study mortality was 3.8% within 24 hours and 8.3% within 48 hours of cardiac catheterization in the first year of life.[15] When lesions, such as hypoplastic left heart, and surgical deaths were excluded, no deaths directly attributable to catheterization occurred during the first 24 hours, and the mortality within 48 hours was 0.3%.

The 1980–1988 overall mortality rate within 48 hours of catheterization in 6101 studies at The Boston Children's Hospital was 1.7%, ranging from 10.2% in the first week of life to 0.5% in patients more than 1 year of age (Exhibit 1). Rarely, death has occurred in patients with primary pulmonary hypertension[49] and in those with severe diffuse peripheral pulmonary stenosis. Since the advent of interventional procedures, the authors have encountered fatalities (approximately 1% of all interventional procedures) primarily in patients with severe peripheral pulmonary stenosis and in infants with critical aortic stenosis.

Arterial and Venous Complications. Virtually all catheterizations at The Boston Children's Hospital are now carried out percutaneously via the femoral vessels. With this approach, arterial occlusion is extremely rare beyond infancy. In the first six months of life, using a 4F pigtail catheter for retrograde arterial catheterizations, temporary or permanent pulse loss occurred in 10% of the babies.[48] Pulse loss occurred less frequently if a smaller (3F) pigtail catheter was used.[47] The use of heparin,[30] and, more recently, streptokinase[113] has been effective in achieving recovery of pulses in most of these infants.

Thrombosis of the inferior vena cava or iliac vein in the first six months of life is a recognized problem of uncertain magnitude. In the authors' early experience, vena caval occlusion was identified in 16% of babies following a percutaneous study, compared with 1.2% using the cutdown approach.[50] No definite risk factors other than the technique used were identified although other investigators have implicated the use of balloon septostomy catheters.[10,74] Following the addition of sheath aspiration and routine heparinization in all cases, the incidence of vena caval occlusion after percutaneous studies in infants has decreased to 7%. At subsequent catheterization, the iliac vein has been patent in 59% and occluded in 15%, whereas patency of the iliac vein was uncertain in the other 26%.

Arrhythmias. Catheter-related atrial or ventricular premature beats are frequent and of no significance. Sustained atrial tachycardias occur occasionally and are generally easily terminated by catheter-induced atrial or ventricular extrasystoles, by overdrive atrial pacing, or by electrical cardioversion if necessary. Ventricular tachycardia or fibrillation is rare, usually occurring in critically ill infants and responding to countershock and appropriate medical management. Atrioventricular conduction disturbances occur but are almost invariably transient in nature, although the authors have encountered one instance of catheter-induced complete block requiring permanent pacing in the last 5000 cases (a patient with tetralogy of Fallot).

Myocardial Stain and/or Perforation. Since the advent of pigtail and balloon catheters, these complications of angiography are now rarely seen. More common are vascular stains that may occur with selective contrast injections into aortopulmonary collaterals. These vessels may carry considerable flow, have a very unpredictable course, and frequently are cannulated with endhole catheters. Rapid hand injections may stain the vascular wall; although pain-producing, they are well tolerated.

Hypoxia and Acidosis. These complications have been observed in infants with tetralogy of Fallot, when the catheter has traversed the right ventricular outflow tract and a **cyanotic spell** has been induced. For this reason the authors avoid this maneuver.

Apnea. Apnea is a known and troublesome side effect of the use of prostaglandin palliation. The

Exhibit 1

	Boston Children's Hospital Experience 1980–1988				
	6101 Catheterizations **Percent Mortality Within 48 Hours**				
	Ages				
Patients	0–6 days	7–28 days	29 days–1 year	>1 year	All Ages
All	10.2	4.4	1.1	0.5	1.7
Nonsurgical	6.3	1.5	0.2	0.27	0.85
Nonsurgical, excluding hypoplastic left heart, persistent fetal circulation, malignancies, conjoined twins	2.7	1.1	0.2	0.08	0.41

apnea may occur during catheterization. Because virtually all infants who need prostaglandins also need an early operation, such babies are routinely intubated prior to catheterization and subsequent surgery.

Air Emboli. Air emboli are associated with angiography. Usually, the bubbles are small and can be prevented by inserting a transparent section of tubing between the catheter and the injector. At The Boston Children's Hospital there have been two instances of large air emboli associated with an open sheath in an umbilical vein, fortunately, without permanent sequelae; hence, only sheaths with a diaphragm are used when entering the umbilical vein.

Other Complications. Transient neurological deficits are rare and are presumably embolic in origin. **Transient hematuria** is seen occasionally and has been reported to be related to contrast agents. **Transient fevers** are not uncommon during the first few hours following catheterization and are generally of uncertain etiology. **Endocarditis** is extremely rare, but in recent years the authors have seen 2 instances following prolonged interventional procedures in newborns who were not on antibiotic therapy.

HEMODYNAMIC EVALUATION

A complete description of the methods used to evaluate physiologic variables in congenital heart disease is beyond the scope of this book and has been discussed elsewhere.[66,101] What follows is an overview designed to help the reader to gain understanding of the techniques being used.

Pressure Measurements

Recording systems consist of a fluid-filled catheter, a pressure transducer, an amplifier and a recorder (printer). The fluid-filled catheter allows transmission of the pressure wave from the heart to the transducer. The transducer converts the energy of pressure to an electrical impulse through mechanical displacement of a movable diaphragm. The electrical impulse that is generated is proportional to the displacement of the diaphragm and, therefore, to the pressure. The electrical signal generated is small and must be amplified and then converted to an analog of the pressure wave in the recorder. Each component from the catheter to the recorder can contribute to error in measurement.

The demands on a recording system vary with heart rate. At a heart rate of 60 a system capable of recording 10 Hertz is adequate, but at a heart rate of 180, a rate not unknown in infants, a system capable of recording 30 cycles per second is required.

The response of the system depends, in part, on damping (i.e., anything that dissipates energy and reduces the amplitude of oscillations in the diaphragm). Underdamping (which causes an artificial increase in pressure fluctuation) generally is not a problem when using clinically relevant catheters. Overdamping (artificial reduction in pressure fluctuation) is much more common. Thus, damping increases as the catheter diameter decreases and its length and compliance increase. Overdamping due to a small diameter of the catheter is especially relevant when catheterizing pediatric patients. Damping is also increased by the presence of air, blood, and clots in the system or loose connections (e.g., between the catheter and transducer).

In addition to inaccuracies introduced by the system, there are other sources of error. By convention, the pressure at the level of the heart is set to 0 mm Hg by opening the transducer to air at the level of the heart and adjusting the recorder to read zero. It is assumed that the heart is at mid chest for this setting. Using a mercury manometer, the transducer is then calibrated over a range of pressures appropriate for the procedure, usually 200 mm Hg. Failure to adjust the height of the transducer and calibrate the equipment properly leads to inaccurate pressure recordings. The stability or drift of a system is defined by its tendency, once calibrated, to change over time. Although the drift of commonly used systems is minimal, it is prudent to check the calibration during a catheterization. Commonly, pressure recordings during cardiac catheterization are subject to motion artifacts caused by catheter movement within the heart; the amplitude of these artifacts can be decreased by maneuvers that increase damping of the system.

Pressure recorders allow pressures to be displayed or recorded at different attenuations; that is, the scale of the pressure tracing can be changed.

Pressures are displayed or recorded as phasic or mean pressures. A phasic recording shows the instantaneous fluctuations in pressure and is important for determining systolic and diastolic pressures and the presence of normal and abnormal waves. Modern pressure recorders automatically determine and display the mean, time-averaged pressure by electronic damping. The mean pressure of atria and arteries are routinely recorded and used, for example, to calculate vascular resistance.

In choosing a catheter to record pressure, several factors need to be considered. As discussed earlier, ideally, one would choose the stiffest, largest, and shortest catheter. Obviously, the selection is determined to a large extent by the size of the patient and the vessel to be entered. In addition, the number and position of holes are an important consideration. Endhole catheters are required to record pulmonary capillary or venous wedge pressures and are optimal for localizing gradients. Occlusion of the end hole by the wall of the heart is not uncommon but easily recognized. Also, endhole catheters, especially balloon-tipped catheters, can become entrapped (for example, in the atrial appendage, ventricular apex, or trabeculae), leading to falsely elevated pressure. Because the tracing often has a normal contour, entrapment is difficult to recognize. The use of catheters with multiple side holes eliminates the problem of entrapment. However, they cannot be used for wedge pressures and are not optimal for localizing gradients. For example, if some of the side holes are proximal (high pressure) and some distal (low pressure) to a coarctation, the pressure recorded will be some combination of the two sites. Double-lumen catheters, one with a single end hole and the second with a single side hole, can be useful for recording gradients. For example, in a patient with pulmonary stenosis, the end hole is positioned in the pulmonary artery and the side hole in the right ventricle. Each lumen is connected to a separate transducer and simultaneous pulmonary artery and right ventricular pressures can be recorded.

Right Atrial Pressure. The normal right atrial pressure consists of the a, c, and v waves and x and y descents (Figs. 2 and 3). The a wave is associated with atrial contraction at the end of diastole. It is usually the dominant wave in the right atrium. The c wave is associated with displacement of the tricuspid valve toward the right atrium in early systole and is generally seen as a small notch on the descending side of the a wave. The v wave peaks during late systole and is related to continued atrial filling against the closed tricuspid valve. The x descent records the fall in pressure following the a and c waves and is due to a decrease in pericardial pressure and movement of the tricuspid valve away from the right atrium during ventricular ejection. The y descent shows the decrease in pressure following the v wave and is due to opening of the tricuspid valve at the beginning of diastole.

Flow in the venae cavae is greatest during the x and y descents and ventricular filling is greatest during early diastole, with only about 30% of filling associated with atrial contraction. Pressure and flow also vary with respiration. Right atrial pressure is highest at the end of expiration and drops during inspiration, because of variation in intrathoracic pressure. Because of the low pressure, right atrial and ventricular filling are increased during inspiration. By convention, right atrial pressure is measured at the end of expiration.

Normally, the mean right atrial pressure is 3 mm Hg. The a wave is the dominant wave, commonly 2–3 mm Hg higher than the v wave. As it appears to have little clinical significance and commonly is not seen, the c wave is not measured routinely. Abnormalities of right atrial pressure include changes in mean pressure and changes in the normal pattern and relationships among the **waves** and **troughs.** Increases in right atrial mean pressure are associated with right ventricular dysfunction (decreased compliance) and outflow obstruction (tricuspid stenosis or atresia associated with a restrictive interatrial communication). In tricuspid regurgitation, the v wave may be dominant.

Superior and Inferior Vena Caval Pressure. Pressures in the superior and inferior vena cava are not recorded routinely, but they have contours similar to the right atrial pressure tracing. However, they should be measured in any patient suspected of having caval obstruction. The classic example of this is the patient who has undergone atrial inversion for transposition of the great arteries (Mustard or Senning procedure).

Left Atrial Pressure. The a, c, and v waves and x and y descents are also seen in the left atrial pressure tracing. In contrast to right atrial pressure, the v wave is dominant in the normal left atrium. The mean left atrial pressure is normally 8 mm Hg. Elevations in left atrial pressure occur in patients with left ventricular dysfunction and in those with outflow obstruction (mitral stenosis or atresia with a restrictive interatrial communication). The v wave is increased in mitral regurgitation and decreased in total anomalous pulmonary venous return.

Pulmonary Artery "Wedge" Pressure. The pulmonary artery wedge pressure is measured by advancing an endhole catheter, with or without a balloon, into a branch of the pulmonary artery until the vessel is occluded by the catheter or, more commonly, by inflating the balloon. The pressure recorded through the end hole reflects distal pressure, that is, the left atrial pressure. It is important to be sure the catheter is indeed wedged. The wedge pressure is routinely recorded simultaneously with the left ventricular end-diastolic pressure and normally there is no gradient. Differences

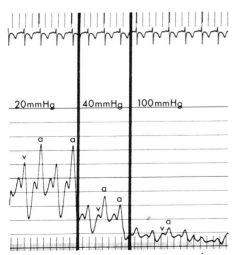

Figure 2. Right atrial tracing at three different attenuations. In addition to phasic intracardiac changes, the pressure falls during inspiration.

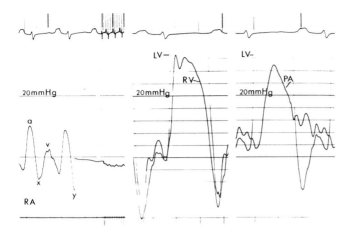

Figure 3. Normal pressure tracings. RA = right atrial pressure tracing; RV = right ventricular pressure tracing; PA = Pulmonary artery tracing; LV = left ventricular tracing, which is only partially seen. Note the similarity of the right ventricular and pulmonary artery systolic trace and the similarity of the right and left ventricular diastolic pressure tracings.

in pressure suggest disease, improperly calibrated transducers, or a defective wedge pressure. The latter occurs both when the catheter is "overwedged" or only partially wedged. The wedge pressure should look like a left atrial tracing, demonstrate respiratory variation, and be lower than the pulmonary artery pressure. The "wedge" position of the catheter can be confirmed by checking the oxygen saturation; the blood should be fully saturated in normal patients. The "wedged" position can also be demonstrated by injecting a small amount of contrast by hand, which will not wash out if the catheter is properly wedged.

Because of the intervening capillaries and pulmonary veins, the "wedge" pressure is delayed and damped, compared with direct measurement of the left atrial pressure. When important left atrial gradients are suspected, they should be measured directly.

Pulmonary Vein Pressure. Normal pressure tracings of pulmonary veins are similar to left atrial tracings. Abnormal elevation of pulmonary vein pressure in the presence of a normal left atrial valve suggests stenosis of the pulmonary veins. However, this diagnosis can be difficult. For example, if only one or two of the veins are stenotic, flow within the lungs is redistributed and no gradient can be measured across the stenotic veins.

Pulmonary Vein "Wedge" Pressure. If a catheter is wedged in a pulmonary vein, with or without a balloon, the pressure measured may reflect pulmonary artery pressure. This technique is conceptually similar to that used to measure pulmonary arterial wedge pressure. Achieving proper wedge position involves similar attention to detail. Although not employed routinely, obtaining pulmonary vein wedge pressure is the only way to estimate pulmonary artery pressure when the pulmonary arteries cannot be entered directly (e.g., patients with pulmonary atresia without shunts or with shunts that cannot be crossed). Although the wedge pressure estimate tends to be lower than actual pulmonary artery pressure, it is relatively

accurate in patients with low or normal pulmonary artery pressure.

Right Ventricular Pressure. Normal ventricular pressures are easily distinguishable from atrial and arterial pressures. The right ventricular pressure wave consists of a rapid upstroke during isovolumic contraction, a systolic plateau, and a fall to near zero during isovolumic relaxation. There is, then, a gradual increase in pressure during diastole with a late diastolic increase associated with the a wave of atrial contraction (Fig. 3). The peak systolic and end-diastolic pressures, which vary with respiration, are measured routinely. "End-diastole" is identified as the point where the right atrial and ventricular tracings cross at the end of diastole or at the junction of the a wave and the rapid upstroke in the ventricular tracing. The former is the most accurate, but because simultaneous right atrial and right ventricular pressures are not routinely recorded, the latter is the more commonly utilized. The normal right ventricular systolic pressure is less than 30 mm Hg and the end-diastolic pressure, 5 mm Hg.

Abnormal elevation of right ventricular systolic pressure occurs in outflow obstruction (e.g., pulmonary valve stenosis, pulmonary artery bands, or stenosis of the pulmonary artery branches), pulmonary artery hypertension, or lesions such as ventricular septal defects. In double-chambered right ventricle, anomalous muscle bundles obstruct the outflow portion of the right ventricle and create a proximal high-pressure chamber and a distal low-pressure chamber (Fig. 4).

Left Ventricular Pressure. The left ventricular pressure contour is similar to that of the right ventricle except the upstroke is usually more rapid, the systolic plateau flatter, and the a wave more prominent (Fig. 5). End-diastolic pressure varies with respiration and is measured in the same way as for the right ventricle.

Normally the left ventricular systolic pressure is equal to the aortic systolic pressure, which increases with age. The end-diastolic pressure is nor-

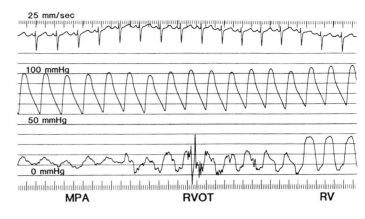

Figure 4. Pressure pullback in a patient with double-chambered right ventricle. Upper tracing = electrocardiogram. Middle tracing = arterial pressure. Lower tracing obtained from the catheter as it was withdrawn from the pulmonary artery to the right ventricle. Note that the pressure gradient occurs within the ventricle. MPA = main pulmonary artery; RV = right ventricle. Stenosis below the pulmonary valve will produce a characteristic pressure tracing in the right ventricular outflow tract (RVOT), with a further gradient into the body of the right ventricle.

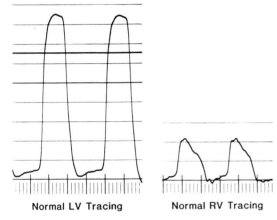

Figure 5. Normal right and left ventricular pressure tracing. A normal left ventricular pressure tracing has a flattened systolic pressure phase and very rapid upslopes and downslopes.

mally less than 12 mm Hg and is slightly higher than the left atrial mean pressure.

Pulmonary Artery Pressure. Normally, the systolic pressure in the pulmonary artery is equal to that in the right ventricle, but the diastolic pressure is higher because of closure of the pulmonary valve. Respiratory variation is common and, by convention, pressures are measured at the end of expiration. Normal mean pulmonary artery pressure is less than 20 mm Hg.

Aortic Pressure. The normal central aortic pressure wave consists of a systolic rise and a plateau, with a dicrotic notch on the downstroke. Normally, the systolic pressure in the ascending aorta is equal to the left ventricular systolic pressure. Closure of the aortic valve causes the diastolic pressure to remain well above the ventricular diastolic pressure. The aortic pressure and contours of the tracing vary, depending on where the pressure is measured. As the catheter is moved more peripherally (e.g., in the descending aorta or iliac arteries), the systolic pressure increases and the diastolic pressure decreases owing to amplification of the pulse ("standing wave"). Thus, for example, when mea-

suring gradients across the aortic valve, it is improper to compare left ventricular systolic pressure directly with femoral artery systolic pressure.

Aside from systemic hypertension or hypotension, abnormalities in aortic pressure usually are related to the presence of gradients (e.g., supravalvar aortic stenosis or coarctation of the aorta) or abnormalities in pulse pressure (systolic minus diastolic pressure). Lesions associated with increased run-off (e.g., aortic regurgitation, shunts, patent ductus arteriosus, aortopulmonary collaterals, systemic arteriovenous malformations and decreased systemic resistance) are associated with increased pulse pressure.

Gradients. A pressure gradient is the difference in pressure between two sites in the cardiovascular system and can be measured as a **mean gradient,** a **peak gradient** or an **instantaneous gradient.** The severity of stenotic lesions commonly is described in terms of pressure gradients, although, in fact, the gradient depends on the cross-sectional area of the obstruction and the flow across it. Thus, a severe narrowing may be associated with only a minimal gradient if the flow across the lesion is low.

Several techniques can be used for measuring gradients. Most commonly a catheter is withdrawn across the obstruction while the pressure is being continuously recorded. Although this provides nearly simultaneous pressure recordings and allows easy measurement of peak and mean gradients, determination of instantaneous gradients requires that the two tracings be superimposed.

When assessing gradients, it is important to measure, or at least estimate, flow across the lesion at the same time the gradient is measured. For example, when assessing aortic valve stenosis, one should measure cardiac output. However, some lesions are so complex that accurate assessment of severity, using gradients and flows becomes nearly impossible. For example, with stenosis of multiple branches of the pulmonary artery, it is not possible to assess flow across each lesion. In such situations, assessment of obstruction must rely on imaging techniques.

Oxygen Content and Saturation

The oxygen content, or saturation of the blood from the various chambers of the heart, the veins, and the arteries, is used to detect and quantify shunts and, when combined with oxygen consumption, to determine cardiac output. **Oxygen saturation** is the percent of hemoglobin which is present as oxyhemoglobin and it can be measured using reflectance oximetry. **Oxygen content** is defined as the total amount of oxygen present in the blood, both as oxyhemoglobin and that dissolved in the plasma. Formerly, it was measured directly, using the method of Van Slyke, but now oxygen sensing cells are used. Oxygen content may be calculated from oxygen saturation:

$$O_2 \text{ Content} = (O_2 \text{ Sat} \times 1.36 \times 10.)$$

The O_2 Sat is the percent of oxygenated hemoglobin. The value of 1.36 is the amount of O_2 a gram of hemoglobin will carry when fully saturated. The 10 is used to convert 100 ml to liters. The contribution of dissolved O_2 is small and commonly ignored except in saturations when the pO_2 is very high, such as when 100% oxygen is being administered to the patient.

Oxygen contents (O_2 con) and oxygen consumption (VO_2) are used to calculate blood flow using the equations:

$$\text{Pulmonary blood flow} = \frac{VO_2 \text{ (ml/min)}}{PV\ O_2 \text{ con} - PA\ O_2 \text{ con}}$$

$$\text{Systemic blood flow} = \frac{VO_2 \text{ (ml/min)}}{SA\ O_2 \text{ con} - MV\ O_2 \text{ con}}$$

where PV is pulmonary vein, PA is pulmonary artery, SA is systemic artery, and MV is mixed (systemic) venous.

If complete mixing of inferior vena caval, superior vena caval, and coronary sinus blood occurred the right atrium, the right atrial, right ventricular, and pulmonary arterial oxygen saturations would equal the mixed venous oxygen content. In fact, studies have shown that variability in oxygen content is greatest in the right atrium[32] and least in the pulmonary artery, owing to incomplete mixing in the right atrium. Thus, in the absence of shunts, the pulmonary arterial saturation is used as the mixed venous oxygen saturation. In the presence of left-to-right shunts (see below), mixed venous oxygen contents must be obtained proximal to the site of the shunt.

In the absence of pulmonary disease and right-to-left shunts, mixing in the left side of the heart is not a significant problem because there is little variation in oxygen content in the various pulmonary veins. In the presence of right-to-left shunts, the oxygen content must be measured proximal to the site of the shunt to calculate pulmonary blood flow.

Shunts. Both extracardiac and intracardiac defects allow shunting of blood between the pulmonary (right-sided) and systemic (left-sided) circulations. Shunts may be left-to-right, right-to-left or bidirectional. Shunts can be localized using angiography or Doppler echocardiography and a variety of indicators, including oxygen saturation, radionucleotides, and indocyanine green dye. This section will focus on detection and quantification of shunts using oxygen content or saturations.

Left-to-Right Shunts. In a left-to-right shunt, the flow of blood from the left side of the heart to the right leads to an increase in oxygen saturation in the right side of the heart. To detect this increase, a series of samples is drawn from each chamber of the right side of the heart. To be considered significant, the increase in saturation between chambers must exceed the normal variation for that chamber.[32] Thus, the saturation in the right atrium normally varies between 5% and 6%, and a rise would be significant only if the right atrial saturation exceeded the superior vena caval saturation by at least 6%.

Right-to-Left Shunt. With a right-to-left shunt there is a decrease in oxygen saturation in the left side of the heart. Unlike evidence for a left-to-right shunt, virtually any fall in oxygen saturation which can be repeated is diagnostic. For practical purposes, any decrease from normal arterial saturation is considered as evidence of a right-to-left shunt in a child with heart disease until proved otherwise.

CALCULATIONS IN CARDIAC CATHETERIZATION

Shunts

A left-to-right shunt (Q_{L-R}) increases pulmonary blood flow (Q_p) compared with systemic blood flow (Q_s) and the shunt can be quantified by the equation:

$$Q_{L-R} = Q_p - Q_s$$

Usually, in children, the superior vena caval (SVC) oxygen content is taken as the mixed venous oxygen content. In discussing shunts it is common to refer to the pulmonary-to-systemic flow ratio (Q_p/Q_s).

$$\frac{\dfrac{\text{Oxygen consumption}}{PV\ O_2\% - PA\ O_2\%}}{\dfrac{\text{Oxygen consumption}}{SA\ O_2\% - MV\ O_2\%}} = Q_p/Q_s = \frac{SA\ O_2 - MV\ O_2}{PV\ O_2 - PA\ O_2}$$

Thus, the Q_p/Q_s can be determined without measuring or assuming an oxygen consumption, using either oxygen saturations or contents.

In addition to pulmonary and systemic flows, the concept of effective flow (Q_{EFF}) is useful in calculating shunts. The effective pulmonary blood flow is the volume of unoxygenated blood flowing to the lungs (i.e., the amount of blood that picks up oxygen on passing through the lungs). For example, with a pure left-to-right shunt, effective pulmonary blood flow would equal the total pulmonary blood flow (Q_p) minus the shunt flow (Q_{L-R}) which equals systemic blood flow (Q_s).

In bidirectional shunts, the left-to-right shunt is calculated as $Q_p - Q_{EFF}$, and the right-to-left shunt is calculated as $Q_s - Q_{EFF}$.

Several comments should be made about quantifying shunts. First, it is important to obtain the saturations as nearly simultaneously as possible to ensure that measured variation is not due to changes in hemodynamic status. For this reason oximetry series are always performed at least twice. If the values of the two series are different or if they suggest a shunt of borderline significance, more series are performed or another indicator is used. In deciding exactly which protocol to use for oximetry runs and in choosing saturations for calculations, it should be kept in mind that shunts are quantified to get a general idea of their size. Thus, it is important to know that the Q_p/Q_s is 2 rather than 4, but to suppose that one can distinguish Q_p/Q_s ratios of 2 versus 2.2 or 1.8 is to ignore the variations inherent in the measurements. The error is especially obvious when measuring large shunts. Assume the superior vena cava saturation is 80, the pulmonary artery saturation 95, and the systemic artery saturation 100. The Q_p/Q_s is $(100 - 80)/(100 - 95)$ or 4. If the oximetry run is repeated and the superior vena cava saturation is 78, the pulmonary artery saturation 95, and systemic artery saturation 99, the Q_p/Q_s ratio is $(99 - 78)/(99 - 96)$ or 7. Large shunts are reported as equal to or greater than 4, rather than giving the exact number calculated.

In certain lesions it may be possible to obtain adequately mixed samples to perform the calculations of shunt size. For example, with a patent ductus arteriosus the saturation in the left pulmonary artery is commonly higher than that in the right, and it is not possible to obtain mixed pulmonary arterial saturations. Averaging the values assumes that flow to both lungs is equal. With total anomalous pulmonary venous connections it may be impossible to obtain mixed venous saturations.

Finally, some patients have more than one defect associated with left-to-right shunts. Thus, a patient may have an atrial septal defect, a ventricular septal defect, and a patent ductus arteriosus. Analyzing saturations from oximetry runs in a stepwise fashion, one might attempt to calculate the magnitude of the left-to-right shunt associated with each lesion. This assumes complete mixing at each level, which is unlikely to occur. It also assumes that the increase at each level is due to only the lesion at that level. This may not be the case if, for example, the ventricular septal defect is associated with a left ventricular-to-right atrial shunt or there is tricuspid regurgitation. Finally, even if the calculations can be made, their clinical relevance is not clear.

Calculations for right-to-left shunts are fundamentally similar to calculations for left-to-right shunts. A right-to-left shunt (Q_{R-L}) leads to a decrease in left-sided saturations at or distal to the site of the shunt and to increased systemic blood flow (Q_s) compared with pulmonary blood flow. It can be calculated as:

$$Q_{R-L} = Q_s - Q_p$$

$$Q_p/Q_s = \frac{SA\ O_2 - MV\ O_2}{PV\ O_2 - PA\ O_2}$$

In addition to right-to-left shunts, left-sided oxygen unsaturation can be caused by pulmonary venous unsaturation in a patient with lung disease. There are a number of options for determining the cause of left-sided unsaturation. If the left atrium and pulmonary veins can be entered, the pulmonary venous saturation should be measured in as many pulmonary veins as possible. If the measurements are low, lung disease is suggested and administering 100% oxygen to the patient usually increases the pulmonary venous saturation. If the intrapulmonary shunt is due to a pulmonary arteriovenous malformation, the low saturation will not be corrected. Alternatively, if there is an atrial septal defect, an attempt should be made to occlude the defect with a balloon and measure the left atrial or systemic arterial saturation, which will normalize if the desaturation is due to a right-to-left shunt through the defect.

Cardiac Output

Cardiac output refers to the amount of blood pumped into the systemic circulation by the heart and is expressed as liters per minute. When corrected for body surface area (liter/minute/meter²), cardiac output is referred to as the "cardiac index." In patients with no shunts, pulmonary, systemic, and effective blood flows are equal (the minimal contribution of the bronchial circulation is ignored), and under stable conditions the term "cardiac output" can be used without confusion. However, in the presence of shunts, pulmonary, systemic, and effective blood flows may be unequal. In these patients, the more specific terms, "pulmonary," "systemic," and "effective" blood flows are used.

Measurements of cardiac output, resistances, and valve area are a routine part of most cardiac catheterizations. Indicator-dilution measurements are most commonly used to measure cardiac output. In general, if one knows the amount of indicator (I) added to or subtracted from a flowing fluid and the concentration of the indicator before (upstream) (C_b) and after (downstream) (C_a) its addition, one can calculate the volume of fluid (V) from the equation.

$$V = \frac{I}{C_a - C_b}$$

Assuming constant flow during the period of measurement, flow (Q) can be calculated by the introduction of a time term (t) into the equation:

$$Q = \frac{I}{(C_a - C_b)\, t}$$

Using these concepts, numerous indicators have been used to measure cardiac output. The most common methods currently used are thermodilution, in which the indicator is cold, and the Fick method, in which the indicator is oxygen. The use of indocyanine green dye, although common in the past, has largely been replaced by thermodilution.

Thermodilution Cardiac Output. The cardiac output is calculated as:

$$CO = \frac{V \times D_i \times S_i \times (T_b - T_i)}{dT \times t \times D_b \times S_b \times 1000/60}$$

where CO = cardiac output, V = volume injected minus dead space, D_i = density of injectate, S_i = specific heat of injectate, T_b = temperature of blood, T_i = temperature of injectate, dT = average temperature change, t = duration of temperature change (sec), D_b = density of blood, S_b = specific heat of blood, and 1000/60 = 1000 ml per 60 sec.

Using this technique, the indicator is cold saline. Most commonly the saline is injected in the right atrium, and a thermistor in the pulmonary artery senses the temperature. The measured flow is equal to pulmonary blood flow and, in the absence of shunts, to the systemic blood flow. The thermodilution catheters that are used have two lumens with a thermistor at the distal end. Various sizes are available so that when the thermistor is in the pulmonary artery, the proximal port, which is in the right atrium, can be used for injection.

The curve showing the change in temperature with time at the thermistor and the calculations of output are made by dedicated computers.

The term "dT × t" in the denominator is the area under the curve, and cardiac output is inversely proportional to this area. The temperature at the thermistor is determined by the temperature of the blood, the temperature of the injectate, and the flow. However, the injectate is also warmed by contact with the catheter and the vessel walls. The extent of this warming is related primarily to duration of contact. Thus, with low cardiac outputs, the transit time between the site of injection and the thermistor is increased, warming is increased, and the cardiac output will be overestimated. For this reason, thermodilution outputs are least accurate when cardiac output is low.

Although not routinely performed, thermodilution techniques can be used to measure flows in specific vessels or organs by positioning the thermistor and making injections at appropriate sites. For example, blood flow to the right lung in a patient with a Glenn anastomosis can be measured by injecting the superior vena cava with the thermistor in the right pulmonary artery. This technique assumes complete mixing of the thermal bolus.

Fick Method. Using the Fick method, the indicator is oxygen and cardiac output or flow (Q) is calculated from oxygen consumption/minute (VO_2) divided by the difference in oxygen content between arterial (C_a) and venous (C_v) blood.

$$Q = \frac{VO_2\ (L/min)}{(C_a - C_v)}$$

Under stable conditions in the absence of left-to-right or right-to-left shunts, the pulmonary blood flow is equal to the systemic blood flow. That is, the amounts of blood pumped by the right and left ventricles are equal. Pulmonary blood flow (Q_p) is:

$$Q_p\ (L/min) = \frac{VO_2\ (L/min)}{PV\ O_2\ con - PA\ O_2\ con}$$

where PV O_2 con and PA O_2 con are the pulmonary venous and the pulmonary arterial oxygen contents. Similarly the systemic blood flow (Q_s) is:

$$Q_s\ (L/min) = \frac{VO_2\ (L/min)}{SA\ O_2\ con - MV\ O_2\ con}$$

where SA O_2 con and MV O_2 con are the systemic arterial and mixed venous oxygen contents.

Several devices are available for measuring oxygen consumption. Often, the entire volume of air expired by a patient is collected. The volume of the expired gas is determined, as well as the relative volumes of oxygen, nitrogen, and/or carbon dioxide. Comparing the concentrations of gases in inspired (room air) and expired air and knowing the volume of inspired and expired air allow calculation of the oxygen consumption.

The second method does not involve collecting expired air, but is performed using a device consisting of a hood and a pump to withdraw air from the hood to an oxygen sensing device. The principle is that air is withdrawn from the hood at a fixed rate (V_m) so that the fractional content of O_2 at the oxygen sensor remains constant at 0.199. (An example of this device is the MRM-2 oxygen consumption monitor, Waters Instruments, Inc.)

Vascular Resistance

Calculations of vascular resistance (R) are made by relating the mean pressure change (delta P) across a circuit to the flow (Q) across the circuit, using the equation:

$$R = \frac{delta\ P}{Q}$$

Thus, systemic vascular (SVR) and pulmonary vascular (PVR) resistances are calculated:

$$SVR = \frac{Ao - RA}{Q_s} \qquad PVR = \frac{PA - LA}{Q_s}$$

where Ao is the mean aortic pressure, RA is the mean right atrial pressure, PA is the mean pulmonary artery pressure, and LA is the mean left atrial pressure. The pulmonary capillary wedge pressure is commonly substituted for the left atrial pressure. The pressures are in mm Hg and the flows in liters/minute and, thus, resistance is expressed as mm Hg/l/min (or Wood units). These can also be referred to as R units (dynes-sec-cm^{-5}) by multiplying Wood units by 80. Resistance is commonly normalized for body surface area (BSA) using one of the following equations:

$$R\ index = \frac{delta\ P}{Q/BSA} \ or\ R\ index = R \times BSA$$

Valve Areas

The most commonly used formula for calculating valve areas is based on the work of Gorlin and Gorlin in 1951,[38] using two basic equations. The

first is $A = F/VC_c$, where A is the valve area, F is the flow rate, V is the velocity of flow, and C_c is the coefficient of orifice contraction. The second, which relates velocity to pressure gradient, is $V = C_v\ 2gh$, where C_v is the coefficient of velocity, g is acceleration due to gravity (980 cm/sec/sec), and h is the pressure gradient. Combining these equations yields:

$$Valve\ area = \frac{F}{(C)\ (44.3)\ h}$$

where C is a constant. Flow across a valve is not constant but occurs during diastole at the mitral and tricuspid valves, and in systole at the aortic and pulmonary valves. The final formula takes this into account by including the diastolic filling period (DFP, sec/beat) or the systolic ejection period (SEP, sec/beat) and the heart rate (HR, beats/sec).

$$A = \frac{CO/(DFP\ or\ SEP)\ HR}{44.3\ (C)\ \sqrt{delta\ P}}$$

where A is the area in cm^2, CO is the cardiac output in cm^3/min, and delta P is the mean pressure gradient. The beginning and end of the diastolic filling period are the points where the atrial and ventricular pressure tracings intersect, and the systolic ejection period is defined by the intersection of ventricular and arterial tracings at the beginning and end of systole. When determined in this way, the constant, C, is 0.85 for the mitral valve and 1 for the aortic, pulmonary, and tricuspid valves.

As can be seen from the equation, for any given valve area, decreasing the flow across the valve decreases the gradient and increasing the flow increases the gradient. Thus, a patient with a stenotic valve could have a relatively low transvalvar gradient if the cardiac output were low. Therefore, it is logical to classify severity of valvar stenoses in terms of valve area. However, traditionally, cardiologists have not done this but have defined severity in terms of transvalvar gradients. Because most children with stenosis of pulmonary or aortic valves have normal cardiac outputs, the flow term in the equation tends to be a constant and severity varies directly with the gradient.

ANGIOGRAPHIC EVALUATION[20,34,58,80]

Image Production

Basic equipment for image production includes the generator, the x-ray tube, and image intensifier mounted opposite each other on a fixed stand or

C-arm, and a high quality television camera (Fig. 6). A digital recording and processing system, although not essential, can be helpful. For pediatric studies, simultaneous biplane cineangiography is virtually mandatory to provide sufficient anatomic information with minimal contrast material.

The x-ray generator supplies and controls three variables: kilovoltage (kv) (which determines the energy spectrum of the x-rays), milliamperes (ma) (the tube current which determines the number of x-ray photons produced), and milliseconds (msec) (the length of exposure or pulse width in cineangiography). Inside the x-ray tube a thin tungsten filament, the cathode, boils off electrons at a rate controlled by the current applied. When a high voltage current is applied, electrons accelerate across the tube and strike the rotating anode, causing x-ray photons to be emitted.

During standard fluoroscopy, x-rays are produced at a constant, but relatively low, level. Some newer systems improve resolution by providing more radiation, but delivering it in short pulses instead of in a continuous manner. During cineangiography, the x-ray output is always pulsed; radiation is delivered at a much higher level, but only during that fraction of time that the camera shutter is open. The length of each pulse, or "pulse width," determines the exposure for each individual frame. Pulse widths should be kept short to prevent blurring, but need to be long enough to provide a sufficient number of photons so that the image will not be too grainy. The pulse width in cineangiography should not exceed 4–6 msec.[34]

The image intensifier is the large canister mounted above or to the side of the patient. Its broad circular face, closest to the patient's body, contains the "input phosphor," a screen of cesium iodide crystals which produces visible light when struck by x-ray photons. The distribution of light produced by the phosphor corresponds to the spatial information formed by the attenuation of the x-rays by the patient's heart or by contrast agents used in angiocardiography. Light produced by the phosphor is detected by an immediately adjacent photocathode that generates low-energy electrons; these electrons are accelerated, and then focused by electronic lenses to produce a bright but minified image on the 1-inch "output phosphor" at the other end of the image intensifier (Fig. 7). The intensification of the image is produced both by minification (that is, by concentrating the light into a smaller, thus brighter, area), and by electronic gain, thereby using the lowest possible x-ray dose. The total gain in brightness achieved by modern image intensifiers is 2000–6000 fold.[20]

The effective input phosphor varies from 4–14 inches. Because the output phosphor is the same size regardless of the input phosphor, the image obtained at the face of a 6-inch input field will be magnified relative to the image obtained at the face

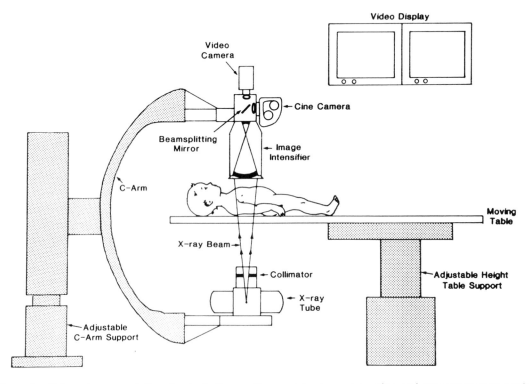

Figure 6. Schematic representation of a single C-arm with x-ray tube, image intensifier, and cine camera over moving table top.

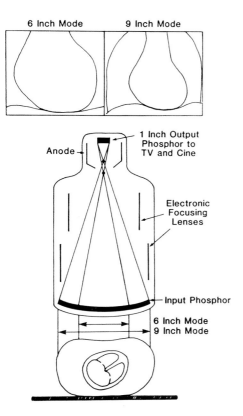

Figure 7. Drawing of dual-mode image intensifier illustrating the principles involved in magnification modes.

of a 9-inch input field size. Thus, a 9-inch image intensifier may be electronically switched to input the image from a 6-inch field and the image will be magnified. A small input phosphor field size is important for infant angiocardiography to provide adequate magnification and spatial resolution.

Image Recording

The light from the image produced by the output phosphor is split during cineangiography: 10% goes to the television monitor and 90% to the cine film. Continuous fluoroscopy is performed at a very low tube current (3–6 mA); when the cine pedal is depressed, the current is boosted about 10-fold. The 10% that is still directed to the TV camera allows the operator to monitor the actual injection and simultaneously record the injection on a high quality video tape or disc. An additional television monitor for each plane can provide a freeze-frame image of the injection.

Cineangiographic Film and Processing

Cineangiographic film for medical imaging may vary according to speed and contrast. A faster film requires less light and, therefore, less radiation for the same relative film density. Because this desirable quality is achieved by using larger silver gran-

ules activated by fewer x-ray photons, it produces a grainier image. Although a high contrast film sounds ideal, medium contrast films provide the wider gray scale necessary to image a wide range of structures from ventricular chambers to pulmonary collaterals and coronary arteries. It is important that the film, the iris settings on the camera, and developing conditions be compatible for the production of an optimal image.

Often, cineangiographic film processing is an underrated part of the imaging chain. Processing variables include temperature, film speed, chemical supply, and drying temperature. Regular quality control is essential; thus, two strips of film, one of a test pattern exposed to cineangiography under standard exposure factors, and one exposed to a light sensitometer alone, should be developed daily. A variation in the readings of the cineangiographic test strip with no change in the reading of the light exposed strip suggests a problem in the imaging chain. Conversely, a problem in the processing system affects both strips. Cineangiographic recording of a resolution phantom in all modes should be performed also, so that line pairs per mm can be measured and recorded and any degradation in resolution detected early.[34]

Digital Processing

Modern images of all types, including those obtained at cardiac angiography, are viewed and processed by television. The visual image is converted to digital information (pixels) that can be computerized and thereby usefully manipulated, often in unexpected ways. Contrast enhancement, digital subtraction, and computed tomography provide advantages in selected situations. As television systems, fiberoptic transmission of signals, and storage capacity for digital information improve and increase, major changes in handling of cardiovascular images are anticipated. The technical details are beyond the scope of this book.[12,14,26,43,59,80]

Radiation Exposure and Protection

Radiation units include the Roentgen (R), a unit of radiation exposure; the rad, a unit of absorbed dose; and the rem, a unit of dose equivalent (rads multiplied by a quality factor to measure biologic effect). For practical purposes, these three units can be thought of as equal.

Fluoroscopic patient exposure is expressed as skin dose and is usually about 0.5–1.0 R/mA per minute of fluoroscopic time. For cineangiography, the skin dose is about 20–30 mcR per frame.[58] Thus, it is apparent that the total dose to the patient, and the total scatter dose to personnel is determined by the length of fluoroscopic time (usually recorded in minutes) and by the length of cineangiographic time and the frame rate. Of course, total exposure is doubled for biplane usage. By comparison, 1 second of cineangiography at 60 frames per second is equivalent to 10–20 seconds of fluoroscopy.[80] Usually, in a diagnostic study, the major exposure to both patient and operator occurs during cineangiography rather than fluoroscopy. If interventional cases are considered, lengthy fluoroscopic time contributes significantly to the dose to the patient and personnel.

Cooperative studies have reported patient exposure rates for a complete adult cardiac catheterization of 20–47 R.[8,57,79,94] To put this dose range into perspective, it can be compared with doses for other x-ray studies on adults: chest x-ray, 95–150 mR; intravenous pyelogram, 3–4 R; barium enema, 2–5 R. Naturally occurring background radiation is about 50–500 mR per year.[33,40]

Personnel exposure is largely due to scattered x-ray photons, the x-ray dose being inversely related to the square of the distance from the x-ray source. Lead aprons, preferably wraparound, are necessary; thyroid shields and lead glasses are recommended, but ordinary glass eyeglasses are quite effective also in reducing scatter to the lens.[94,95]

In a review of radiation exposures from different laboratories, Reuter reported the dosage to the operator from a single catheterization procedure to be in the following range:[94] 4.6–154 mR to the hand of the angiographer, 3.5–33 mR to the thyroid, and 6.4–30 mR to the eye. The National Council on Radiation Protection and Measurement (NCRP) and the International Commission on Radiological Protection have set up guidelines for permissible yearly exposure. NCRP recommends a limit of radiation per year of 5 rems to the whole body, 75 rems to the hands, 15 rems to the thyroid, and 5 rems to the limbs.[105]

Good habits for fluoroscopy should be taught and practiced consistently. The image intensifier should be as close as possible to the patient's chest; the operator should always collimate carefully, making sure that the edges of the shutters are visible on the television monitor. Fluoroscopic time should be reserved for catheter manipulations and test injections; biplane fluoroscopy should be used only when absolutely necessary.

Contrast Agents

Contrast agents used in cardiac angiography are water-soluble, complex organic compounds, sharing in common the basic building block of three iodine atoms bound to a benzene ring. Modern contrast agents can be divided into either high-osmolality or low-osmolality agents. Both types of contrast, using an equivalent concentration of iodine, produce angiographic images which are of equal radiographic contrast. Low-osmolality agents cause less patient discomfort, and perhaps are safer, but cost considerably more.

Chemistry. Ionic agents are salts of the tri-io-dinated benzene derivatives of diatrozoic or iothalamic acid (the anions), which are bound to either sodium or methylglucamine (the cations) (Fig. 8). When in solution, the number of particles is immediately doubled; this results in a solution that is extremely hypertonic, with osmolality six to seven times that of blood. The hypertonicity of these agents not only causes the pain and warmth which the patient feels, but is responsible in part for a number of other adverse physiologic responses.[11]

Recently, two new classes of low-osmolality contrast agents (nonionic and dimeric) have been introduced. Nonionic contrast is formulated by replacing the carboxyl group of the benzene ring with a nonionizing side chain, so that the compound does not dissociate in solution; thus, its osmolality is half as great as an ionic compound (Fig. 8). Nonionic agents include iohexol and iopamidol.[1,111]

The other approach to reducing osmolality is to link two tri-iodinated benzoic acids together to form a dimer (Fig. 8). This is prepared as a salt of sodium or meglumine, which then dissociates in solution into two particles as conventional ionic agents do. Because each anionic particle contains six rather than three iodine atoms (as in conventional contrast), fewer particles are needed for a given iodine concentration, and the osmolality is reduced by one-half.[21,111] Table 2 compares various contrast agents and their physical properties.

Physiology. When high-osmolality contrast agents are injected, there is a rapid shift of fluid from interstitial and intracellular spaces into the intravascular space, causing volume expansion, a slight drop in hematocrit, and a change in electrolyte concentration.[28,35,45] With normal renal excre-

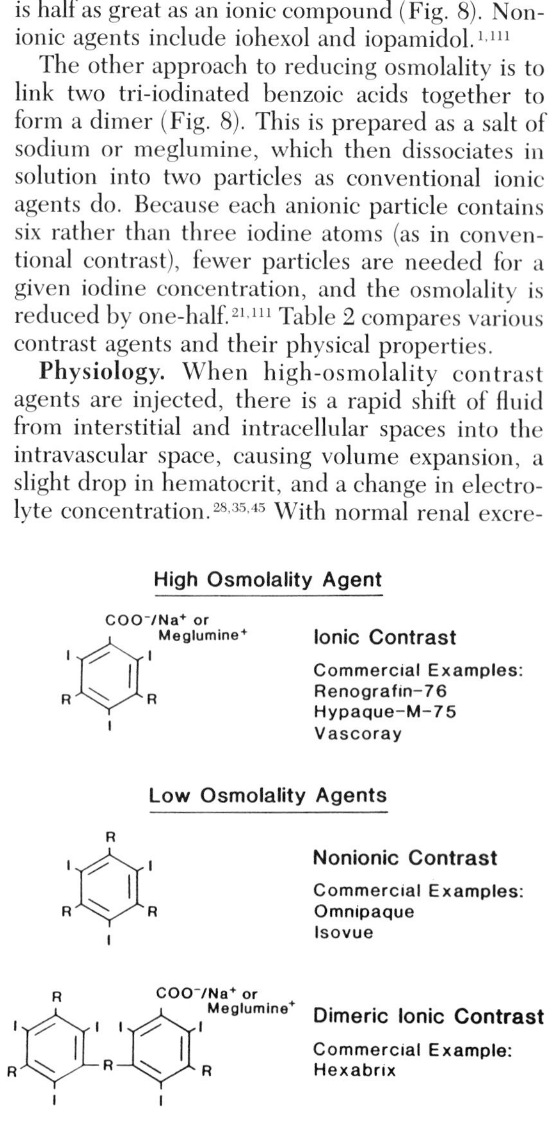

Figure 8. Chemical composition of various contrast agents.

Table 2. Comparison of the Physical Properties of Various Contrast Agents

Generic Name	Brand Name	Iodine mg/ml	Osmolality mOsm/kg	Viscosity at 37° (centipoise)
Ionic Agents				
Diatrozoate Sodium 10% Meglumine 66%	Renografin 76 Squibb	370	1689	9.1
Diatrozoate Sodium 8% Meglumine 52%	Renografin 60 Squibb	288	1511	3.9
Diatrozoate Sodium 35% Meglumine 34.3%	Renovist Squibb	370	1983	6.0
Diatrozoate Sodium 50% Meglumine 25%	Hypaque M-75% Winthrop	385	2108	8.3
Diatrozoate Sodium 10% Meglumine 66%	Angiovist-370 Berlex	370	1380	9.0
Iothalamate Sodium 26% Meglumine 52%	Vascoray Mallinckrodt	400	2150	9.0
Dimeric Agents				
Ioxaglate Sodium 19.6% Meglumine 39.3%	Hexabrix Mallinckrodt	320	600	7.5
Nonionic Agents				
Iohexol	Omnipaque Winthrop-Breon	300	709	6.8
Iopamidol	Isovue Squibb	300	616	4.7

tion, values can be expected to return to baseline within a few minutes, but newborns, fragile infants, and any patient with severely compromised cardiac function will be adversely affected.[103] Because this volume shift is an effect of contrast hypertonicity, it is much less severe when low-osmolality agents are used.[18,19]

Injection of high-osmolality contrast into the pulmonary vascular bed causes a rise in pulmonary artery pressure owing to a combination of vasospasm[1,22] and elevation of left atrial pressure.[28] The release of histamine from mast cells and basophils, platelet dysfunction, and sludging of distorted red cells may play a role also.

Reflex tachycardia occurs in response to contrast-induced hypotension, and with increased intravascular volume, there is a transient increase in cardiac output, along with a rise in ventricular diastolic pressure.[41] In the already compromised patient, this depressant effect, combined with volume expansion secondary to injection of the contrast, may precipitate pulmonary edema. Low-osmolality agents may produce less systemic hypotension, less tachycardia, and less ventricular dysfunction.[5,75,93] Finally, high-osmolality contrast decreases the threshold for ventricular fibrillation.[116]

Other toxic effects of high-osmolar contrast agents include decreased red cell pliability and increased viscosity, osmotic diuresis, proteinuria, hematuria, and, occasionally, renal failure.

Adverse Reactions. Arterial injection of a high-osmolality agent produces a hot flash or significant pain; when injected into a pulmonary artery or vein coughing is produced. These problems do not occur with low-osmolality agents.

Life-threatening reactions, including bronchospasm, laryngeal edema, and vascular collapse, have been reported in from 1/3000 to 1/14,000 patients, but fortunately most patients can be resuscitated, the reported mortality being 1/10,000 to 1/40,000.[3,4] These reactions probably have some allergic basis, as patients with any history of allergy have a two to three times greater incidence of reaction than does the nonallergic population.[3,106] However, one reaction does not foretell a second, with or without pretreatment, although from 15–60% of patients with a previous history of a severe contrast reaction have another severe reaction when catheterization is repeated.[106,107] Recent evidence indicates that an increased production of bradykinin may play a significant role in contrast reaction in patients with a history of allergy.[56] Preliminary reports suggest that severe reactions may be less frequent with low-osmolality agents than with high-osmolality contrast.[56]

Choice of Contrast Agents. For the reasons just discussed, at The Boston Children's Hospital, we use low-osmolality agents in newborns, unstable infants, children in whom the contrast load is anticipated to be high, those in heart failure, and those in whom peripheral injections would be painful otherwise.

Angiocardiography

The first step in any form of selective angiography is vascular access to the necessary chamber with an appropriate catheter. Usually, femoral vessels are used for percutaneous vascular access in nearly all forms of congenital heart disease, with the umbilical, subclavian, jugular, and upper limb vessels available for special circumstances. In general, angiograms are performed with sidehole catheters adequate to deliver a large volume of contrast rapidly; the volume and speed are determined by multiple factors, including chamber size and flow. A more complete discussion of angiographic techniques in general, and special procedures such as balloon occlusion angiography, wedge angiography, and coronary angiography in children is available elsewhere.[65,72]

Modern biplane C-arm equipment has facilitated the acquisition of the axial views, introduced in the late 1970s, which are necessary for accurate delineation of various parts of the cardiac anatomy.[9,25,27,109] Because in most cases today the basic diagnosis has been established by echocardiography prior to arrival in the catheterization laboratory, each angiographic view can be chosen to answer a specific anatomic question.

Axial angiography was developed to profile specific parts of the heart along the x-ray beam. For example, the ventricular septum runs neither in the sagittal nor the coronal plane, but obliquely, in such a way that a left anterior oblique view shows the ventricular septum better than a simple lateral view does. Further, the septum is a curved structure. The long axis of the heart is between horizontal and vertical. The bifurcation of the pulmonary artery is horizontal and the aortic arch runs obliquely from front to back. Axial views were developed to take account of these anatomic facts and provide specific information about each chamber or vessel. However, simple frontal and lateral views are still useful, or even preferred, for demonstration of certain anatomic areas or when the abnormalities are so deranged that a preliminary view is desired.

The most common and useful views are (1) posterior-anterior, (2) lateral, (3) long axial oblique, and (4) hepatoclavicular.[9,25] A long axial oblique view is obtained by placing the intensifier at 70° left anterior oblique with a 20° cranial angulation. Usually this is combined with the orthogonal right anterior oblique view (Fig. 9A). In left ventriculography, the long axial oblique projection provides good visualization of the mid and apical muscular septum, the membranous septum, and the subaortic area (Fig. 9B). This enables the viewer to see the motion of the anterior leaflet of the mitral valve, and the ventricular wall motion in the septal, apical, and posterior aspects, as well as mitral regurgitation and left ventricular-to-right atrial shunts. The aortic valve, the coronary arteries, and the arch and great vessels are well displayed. The right anterior oblique, orthogonal view provides information about anterior muscular septal and subpulmonary defects (Fig. 9C), both of which are difficult to pinpoint on other views. In tetralogy of Fallot, the infundibulum, pulmonary valve, and right pulmonary artery are nicely demonstrated.

The hepatoclavicular view was so named to describe the direction of the x-ray beam from the liver below to the clavicle above. Technically, it is a shallower (40°) long axial oblique view with steeper (40°) cranial angulation compared with the usual long axial oblique (Fig. 10A). This view specifically focuses on the posterior aspect of the ventricular septum, in the region of the atrioventricular canal. In this projection, one can actually visualize a common atrioventricular valve, rather than infer its presence by an angiographic sign such as the "gooseneck" (Fig. 10B). This view is also called the four-chambered view because both atria and both ventricles can be seen in each of four quadrants of the image, so that valvular regurgitation, defects from the left ventricle to the right atrium and left or right overriding or atresia of the atrioventricular valves can be recognized (Fig. 10C).

The frontal view with 40° cranial angulation (Fig. 11A, B) is particularly useful for displaying the pulmonary artery bifurcation. The complementary orthogonal lateral view of the right ventricle (Fig. 11C) displays the pulmonary infundibulum and valve as well as the main and left pulmonary artery in profile. In tetralogy, septal malalignment is particularly well illustrated, as the conal septum is profiled in its excessively anterior position (Fig. 11C).

The most common angiographic views and the diagnoses and injected chambers in which they are most helpful are displayed in Table 3.

INTERVENTIONAL CATHETERIZATION

In recent years the introduction of interventional techniques in the management of patients with congenital heart disease has revolutionized pediatric cardiac care (Exhibit 2). Some techniques have become accepted as standard therapy; others are under development. In this whirlwind of change, it is hard to imagine what the future holds.

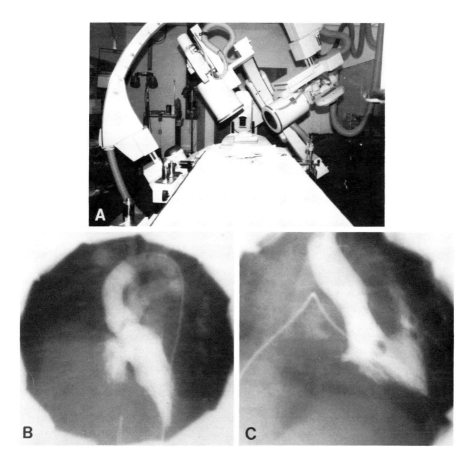

Figure 9. **A,** View of biplane equipment positioned for long axial oblique and right anterior oblique views. **B,** Left ventriculogram taken in the long axial oblique view illustrating a perimembranous ventricular septal defect. **C,** Left ventriculogram taken in the right anterior oblique view illustrating an anterior muscular ventricular septal defect.

Myocardial Biopsy

Endomyocardial biopsy is being performed in pediatric patients with increasing frequency because of studies demonstrating its relative safety, the development of smaller bioptomes, and the increasing number of cardiac transplants in pediatric patients. Despite this, indications for this procedure remain debatable. The most clear-cut indication is for the detection of immunologic rejection of a transplanted heart. In other patients, endomyocardial biopsy can be used to diagnose a long list of diseases affecting the myocardium, including metabolic and storage diseases, although both of these are rare and usually can be diagnosed by other means. Furthermore, generally, they are not treatable.[88] Thus, for most patients with cardiomyopathies the findings on biopsy are nonspecific and rarely influence therapy. On the other hand, biopsy may provide useful information for determining prognosis, for genetic counseling and for evaluation prior to transplantation. Finally, serial biopsies may be useful in the treatment of myocarditis.

Technique. The techniques for right and left ventricular biopsies have been described elsewhere in detail.[71,98] One of two basic techniques can be used. The first involves using a preformed, long sheath that is advanced to the ventricle to be biopsied (Fig. 12). The curves formed depend on the site of vascular access and on which ventricle is being biopsied. The bioptome is advanced through this sheath directly to the ventricle. The long-sheath technique is used routinely for the left ventricle and is used for the right ventricle when access is from the femoral vein. In the second technique, a standard short sheath with a back-stop valve is used. The bioptome is then preformed so that it can be manipulated and advanced to the ventricle without the aid of a long sheath. This technique is used routinely when the right ventricle is biopsied from the internal jugular or subclavian veins.

Right ventricular biopsies are taken from the interventricular septum near the apex to minimize complications such as perforation and damage to the tricuspid valve. The left ventricle can be ap-

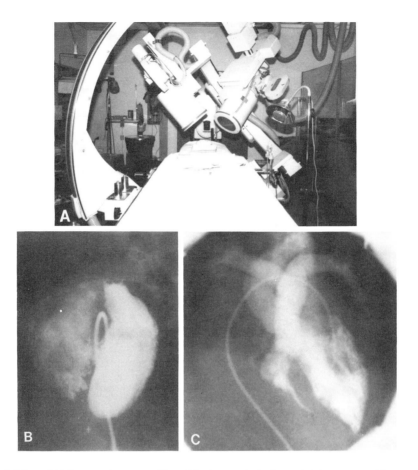

Figure 10. **A,** View of biplane equipment positioned for hepatoclavicular and right anterior oblique views. Note that the obliquity is less steep and has more cranial angulation than that used in Figure 9 for the long axial oblique view. **B,** Left ventriculogram taken in the hepatoclavicular view illustrating a common atrioventricular canal defect. **C,** Left ventriculogram taken in the hepatoclavicular view illustrating anatomy in a patient with tricuspid atresia.

proached retrograde, across the aortic valve, from the femoral artery or anterograde, across the atrial septum, from the femoral veins, using either a patent foramen ovale or a transseptal puncture. The bioptome is directed to the interventricular septum near the apex.

A 5.5-French bioptome (Cordis) with a 6-French sheath is used for older children and a 5-French bioptome (Fehling [Inrad] or Cook) with a 5-French sheath for children weighing less than 15 kg (Exhibit 2).

Balloon Valvotomy

Valvar Pulmonary Stenosis

Following the initial report of Kan and associates in 1982,[46] using a noncompliant balloon to treat valvar pulmonary stenosis, use of this therapy quickly became widespread. Except for dysplastic valves, it is effective and safe, providing relief of obstruction at least equivalent to the surgical approach.[54,89,96,97] In addition, it is now evident that this technique is also effective in neonates[119] and among those with residual postoperative valvar obstruction. Even with right ventricular pressure at the systemic level, pulmonary stenosis is well tolerated for some years, and because large catheters are needed for effective relief, elective use of this technique is delayed until patients are two years of age. Exceptions are made for neonates with critical obstruction.

Older Patients. _Technique._ Following routine catheterization of the right and left sides of the heart, the pulmonary valve annulus is measured from a lateral right ventriculogram. A balloon diameter as much as 140% of the size of the annulus is chosen and positioned over a guide wire (preferably advanced to the left lower lobe) across the stenotic valve. It is inflated wih dilute contrast until the waist is abolished (Fig. 13), and then rapidly deflated. Occasionally, among older patients, two balloons are necessary,[118] both of which may be introduced via the same femoral vein. The hemodynamic parameters are then reassessed, care be-

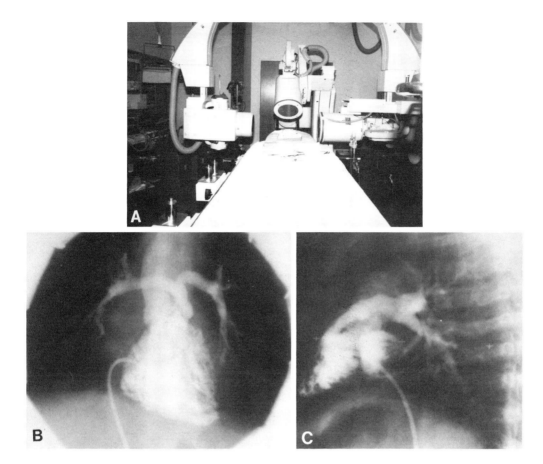

Figure 11. **A,** View of biplane equipment positioned for a frontal view with cranial angulation and a lateral view. **B,** Right ventriculogram in a frontal projection with cranial angulation demonstrating the pulmonary artery befurcation in a patient with tetralogy of Fallot. **C,** Right ventriculogram in the lateral projection demonstrating anterior malalignment of the conal septum with resulting infundibular narrowing and a ventricular septal defect in a patient with tetralogy of Fallot.

ing taken to measure any residual gradients at valvar as well as infundibular levels, after which a right ventricular cineangiogram is made.

Results. Among 27 of the patients so treated at The Boston Children's Hospital, the initial mean gradient of 65.0 ± 19.0 mm Hg was reduced to 15.9 ± 7.6 mm Hg, the residual gradient being less than 25 mm in 93% (Fig. 14). Significant residual infundibular gradients were identified in seven patients, the largest of which (60 mm Hg) had virtually disappeared at a follow-up catheterization. No significant complications occurred. A murmur of pulmonary regurgitation appeared in 19%. In another nine patients with residual postoperative obstruction, the mean gradient of 59.7 ± 29 mm Hg was reduced to 19.1 ± 7.5 mm Hg, with a regurgitant murmur being present in two.[89]

Neonates with Critical Obstruction. Technique. Virtually all these babies are cyanotic because of right to left atrial shunting and many are intubated and receiving prostaglandin E. Following right and left heart catheterization, the size of the annulus

is measured from a right lateral ventricular cineangiogram. The valve is then traversed, sometimes with difficulty, with a 5F balloon endhole catheter or a modified 3–4F multipurpose thinwalled, right-angled endhole catheter. A small (0.018″ or 0.025″) exchange guide wire is then passed via a patent ductus arteriosus to the descending aorta or, preferably, to a lower lobe pulmonary artery. A low profile 5- or 6-mm balloon, 2 cm in length, is used first to dilate the valve (Fig. 15), followed by a larger balloon (140% the annulus size). Hemodynamic parameters are remeasured, after which a right ventricular cineangiogram is made.

Results. Among the first six babies so treated at The Children's Hospital in Boston, the valve was crossed and dilated in five.[119] The final balloon diameters ranged from 6–10 mm, being 95–133% of the annular diameter. In one, a larger balloon was not used because of difficulty in accessing the vein. The right ventricular pressure, initially suprasystemic in all (mean, 122.8 ± 6.8 mm Hg), decreased

Table 3. Views Used to Demonstrate the Anatomy of Congenital Heart Lesions

LONG AXIAL OBLIQUE 70° LAO, 20° Cranial	HEPATOCLAVICULAR FOUR-CHAMBER VIEW 40° LAO, 40° Cranial	RAO OR ORTHOGONAL VIEW TO LONG AXIAL OBLIQUE OR HEPATOCLAVICULAR	FRONTAL AND LATERAL
Left Ventriculogram	*Left Ventriculogram*	*Left Ventriculogram*	*Pulmonary Arteriogram*
VSD–midmuscular apical membranous	VSD–post muscular common AV canal type	VSD–subpulmonary anterior muscular	TAPVR–venous return
Tetralogy–malalignment VSD multiple VSDs	Tricuspid Atresia–size of VSD size of RV outflow	Tetralogy–pulmonary infundibulum	*Innominate View*
D-TGA–Subpulmonary area and VSD	Straddling Tricuspid Valve	Mitral valve–mitral insufficiency mitral prolapse	Persistent LSVC
DORV–VSD location and size	Single Ventricle	LV function–anterior wall motion	*Right Ventriculogram*
Sub AS–LV outflow and mitral valve	*Right Ventriculogram*	apical wall motion	Pulmonary stenosis
LV function–septal wall posterior wall	Tetralogy–PA bifurcation proximal LPA	inferior wall motion	Pulmonary atresia–intact septum
Aortogram	*Aortogram*	*Aortogram*	*Inferior Vena Cava or Superior Vena Cava*
PDA	*Pulmonary Arteriogram*	Coronary arteries	TGA–post Senning or Mustard
Tetralogy–coronary arteries	Tetralogy–PA bifurcation (postop.) proximal LPA	*Pulmonary Arteriogram*	*Ventriculogram*
AS–aortic valve morphology aortic insufficiency	*Aortogram*	Right pulmonary artery	Complex ventricular anatomy
Arch abnormalities–hypoplasia coarctation	Similar to long axial oblique	FRONTAL VIEW WITH CRANIAL ANGULATION 40° Cranial	Heterotaxy syndromes
	FRONTAL VIEW WITH CAUDAL ANGULATION 30–40° caudal	*Right Ventriculogram*	*Pulmonary View Injection*
	Aortogram (balloon occlusion)	Tetralogy–PA bifurcation	Pulmonary atresia–to find true PA (wedge injection)
	Coronary Arteries in Transposition	*Pulmonary Arteriogram*	Anomalous venous drainage
		Tetralogy–postop. bifurcation	

AS = aortic stenosis
DORV = double-outlet right ventricle
D-TGA = D-transposition of the great arteries
LAO = long axial oblique
LPA = left pulmonary artery

LSVC = left superior vena cava
LV = left ventricle
PA = pulmonary artery
PDA = patent ductus arteriosus
RAO = right axial oblique

RV = right ventricle
TAPVR = total anomalous pulmonary venous return
TGA = transposition of the great arteries
VSD = ventricular septal defect

Exhibit 2

Procedure (n = number of patients)	Years						Number of Procedures
	1984	1985	1986	1987	1988	1989	
Myocardial biopsy* n = 104	4	9	24	47	78	112	274
Peripheral pulmonary stenosis n = 187	5	24	29	47	78	61	244
Pulmonary valvoplasty n = 192	12	26	40	38	43	44	203
Coil vessel occlusion n = 130	3	14	28	43	45	69	202
Aortic valvoplasty n = 174	2	22	44	36	44	46	194
Rashkind procedure n = 160	12	20	17	38	46	49	182
Patent ductus closure n = 123	0	8	11	19	26	59	123
Coarctation of aorta dilation n = 102	8	20	26	26	16	18	114
Atrial septal defect closure n = 71	0	1	2	3	9	67	82
Systemic vein dilation or occlusion n = 16	1	0	5	5	3	7	21
Ventricular septal defect closure n = 18	0	0	0	2	4	12	18
Mitral valvoplasty n = 12	0	1	2	2	4	3	12
Other procedure n = 109	2	3	19	20	28	47	119

Boston Children's Hospital Experience
1980–1990
**Interventional Cardiac Catheterization
Number of Procedures***

*As of March 1990, 300 procedures have been performed in 110 patients. The right ventricle alone was biopsied in 256 cases, the right and left ventricles in 42 cases, and the left ventricle alone in 2 cases. The patients ranged in age from 2 days to 22 years and in size from 2.5 to 96 kg. There were 39 procedures in patients less than 1 year of age (2.5 to 7.7 kg), 86 procedures in patients aged 1 to 5 years (7 to 20 kg), 31 procedures in patients aged 5 to 10 years (15 to 28 kg), and 144 procedures in patients more than 10 years of age (23 to 96 kg). An average of 4 pieces were taken at each procedure.

Of the 300 procedures, 198 were performed in 16 patients who had undergone cardiac transplantation. Venous access was from an internal jugular in 128, a femoral vein in 52, and a subclavian vein in 16. The internal jugular has been used routinely in patients as small as 10 kg.

There were 102 procedures in 96 patients who did not have transplants. Indications for biopsy in this group included dilated cardiomyopathy in 46, arrhythmia in 24, myocarditis in 16, and hypertrophic cardiomyopathy in 11. In only 2 of the 42 patients undergoing biopsy of both ventricles did the histology differ between ventricles. Both patients had endocardial fibroelastosis.

Complications included transient atrial arrhythmias in 3, transient third-degree block in 2, and transient right bundle branch block in 2. There was 1 asymptomatic perforation associated with a small pericardial effusion in an infant weighing 4 kg. There was 1 case of asymptomatic air embolism during biopsy of the left ventricle. There was loss of a femoral artery pulse which returned following administration of streptokinase. During serial biopsy in two transplant patients approximately 1 year of age, 1 femoral vein and 1 right subclavian vein were found to be occluded. Subsequently all patients for biopsy have been routinely heparinized.

to systemic level or less (mean, 58.8 ± 6.7 mm Hg), and residual gradients ranged from 7–35 mm Hg. At recatheterization the residual gradient was 6 mm Hg in one infant, was considered mild, at most, in three others, and was severe in the baby in whom the smaller balloon was used.

Complications. Complications consisted of occlusion of the iliac vein in one and persistent right bundle branch block in another. Since this initial experience, one baby has had endocarditis (safely treated with antibiotics), which was probably related to a successful valvotomy.

Valvar Aortic Stenosis

Soon after the report of balloon valvotomy for congenital pulmonary stenosis, use of this technique in the management of aortic stenosis was described. It became clear that, in comparison, the procedure was more difficult and dangerous, particularly in infants, and that gradient reduction was

LONG SHEATH CARDIAC BIOPSY

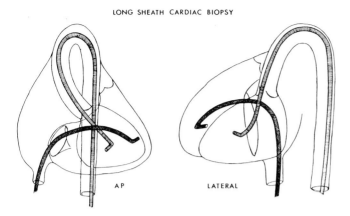

Figure 12. The long sheath technique for cardiac biopsy (developed by Dr. Paul Lurie) allows relatively precise placement of the bioptome on both the left (light catheter) and right side of the ventricular septum.

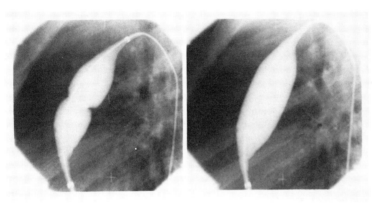

Figure 13. Pulmonary valve dilation using the static balloon technique of Dr. Jean Kan. A waist appears in the 18-mm balloon at 2 atmospheres of pressure and disappears at 4 atmospheres.

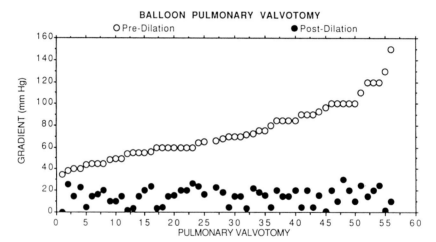

Figure 14. Peak systolic ejection gradient before (Pre) and immediately following (Post) dilatation in childen with typical valvar pulmonary stenosis.

less effective.[17,42,55,76,77,102,112,117] From experimental data in lambs,[42] it is evident that balloon sizes greater than the valve annulus, particularly greater than 120%, result in significant valvar and perivalvar damage.

At the present time, balloon valvotomy is undertaken in children and adolescents with peak systolic ejection gradients greater than 50–60 mm Hg without significant (mild at most) aortic regurgitation and is undertaken in infants with critical obstruction regardless of the gradient value.

Older Patients. *Technique.* Following routine right and left heart catheterization, including aortography, a pigtail catheter is placed in the contralateral femoral artery for subsequent pressure measurement and angiography. The valve annulus is measured from a left ventricular angiogram taken in the long axial oblique view (Fig. 16). A balloon,

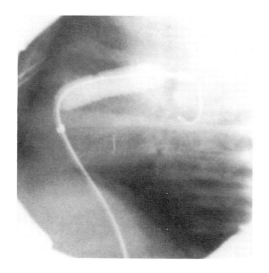

Figure 15. The first balloon being inflated in neonate with a critically stenotic pulmonary valve. The right ventricular outflow is shorter, more curved, and there is less room for an inflated balloon.

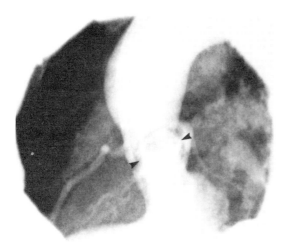

Figure 16. Measurement of an annulus size is taken from the valve hinge points.

4–6 cm long and with a diameter less than 90% of the annulus, is advanced over an exchange wire, the distal end having been looped in the ventricle. The balloon is positioned across the valve and inflated rapidly to abolish the usually subtle waist, and deflated immediately, the inflation-deflation cycle being 15 seconds or less. A team member auscults for regurgitation and the residual gradient is measured using the other arterial catheter. If the gradient has been reduced by 50% or more, the dilating catheter is removed; hemodynamic parameters, including cardiac output, are measured and aortography is repeated. If gradient reduction is minor, dilatation is repeated with the next largest balloon. In some older patients it may be necessary to use two balloons and an Amplatz extra-stiff Cook

guide wire. Stiff-shafted balloon catheters are helpful in maintaining stable balloon position across the valve. All patients are monitored overnight.

Neonates with Critical Obstruction. *Technique.* These babies are particularly fragile, are prone to ventricular fibrillation, and often have low gradients across the valve because of diminished cardiac output. The size of the left ventricular cavity is less than normal in some. The usually patent foramen ovale allows monitoring of the left ventricular pressure throughout. While the initial hemodynamic and angiographic evaluation may be carried out quickly in many via the umbilical vessels, prolonged use of the umbilical artery for the dilating procedure can be hazardous. Thus, if the initial approach through the umbilical artery is not easy, a femoral artery is used. A 3F pigtail is passed to the left ventricle using an .0018″ wire. An exchange wire is then placed and the valve is dilated with a balloon 4–6 mm in diameter and 2 cm long (90% of the annulus size). Hemodynamic measurements and angiography are carried out as for older patients.

Results. Among 80 procedures in 75 patients,[108] the mean gradient was reduced from 76 ± 26 mm Hg to 33 ± 20 mm Hg, representing overall a 55 ± 22% gradient reduction (Fig. 17). Gradient reductions among 15 who had had prior surgical valvotomy and among 12 neonates were similar, being 51 ± 9% and 52 ± 27% respectively. Among 16 who underwent follow-up catheterization, the gradient reduction persisted in the majority, the single major increase occurring in an infant (90 mm gradient) dilated as a neonate. This latter gradient decreased to 30 mm after a second dilatation.

Complications. *Deaths.* There were three deaths in the series, all in neonates. Severe aortic regurgitation was induced in two of these, one of whom had a small left ventricle (66% of normal). The remaining infant succumbed to septicemia after a prolonged unsuccessful attempt to dilate the valve via the umbilical artery.

Aortic Regurgitation. Aortic regurgitation was present in 49% prior to the procedure and was evident in 71% immediately afterward. The increase in aortic regurgitation was grade 1 in 61% of the 31 patients in whom aortic regurgitation appeared or increased. In four patients it increased to grade 4; two of these later underwent valve replacement and the other two, both infants, died. There was an 11% risk of more than a grade 1 increase when the balloon/valve annulus ratio was less than 100% and a 26% risk with a ratio of more than 100%.

Severe Mitral Regurgitation. Mitral regurgitation was evident at the conclusion of the procedure in two children, both of whom required surgical intervention consisting of successful plication of tears in the anterior mitral leaflet. At the time of surgery it was noted that both aortic valves had

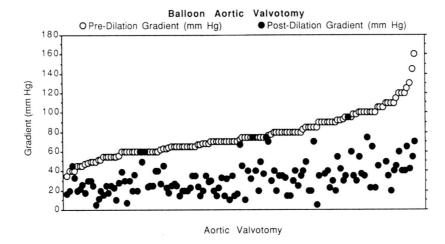

Figure 17. Peak systolic ejection gradient before (pre-dilation median, 70 mm Hg) and immediately following (post-dilation median, 31 mm Hg) dilatation in first consecutive 132 patients with valvar aortic stenosis.

been adequately and appropriately opened by the balloon valvotomy.

Ventricular Fibrillation. Ventricular fibrillation occurred in two infants and one older child and was converted electrically. Left bundle branch block occurred in 14 patients and was transient in all but one, aged 9 months.

Arterial Pulse Loss. Arterial pulse loss immediately following the procedure occurred in 24 patients (30%). Sixty percent of these were infants and 15% were older. In one infant who weighed 4 kg, the external iliac artery was ruptured during attempts to introduce a 7F sheath; this required surgical ligation, which was accomplished without complication. Following the administration of heparin, with or without streptokinase therapy, pulses returned in two-thirds of the patients. A femoral artery was found to be severely stenotic in a 5-year-old boy at follow-up catheterization.

Subaortic Stenosis

To date, our limited experience with attempts to dilate discrete or diffuse varieties of this lesion has not resulted in lasting relief of the gradient, although early success in some discrete forms has been reported.[23,53]

Mitral Valvar Stenosis

Balloon valvotomy for mitral stenosis was first reported in 1984.[44] Subsequent reports, with some modifications in technique, suggest this is a safe, and at least initially effective, method of treating severe rheumatic stenosis,[2,7,67,78] although perhaps it is less effective for congenital obstruction.[52]

Technique. Following standard right and left catheterization and left ventriculography to exclude significant mitral regurgitation, an 8-mm balloon may be needed to dilate the atrial septum to allow later passage of one or two larger dilating catheters. One or two preformed guide wires are

placed in the left ventricular cavity. An 18- to 25-mm balloon is then passed over the guide wire to straddle the valve in younger patients, or two balloons (each usually 20 mm) in adults. Inflation is carried out rapidly to abolish the waist and the balloon(s) are quickly deflated and removed (Fig. 18). Hemodynamic measurements, including left ventriculography, are then repeated.

Results. In our experience with 11 patients at The Boston Children's Hospital, including one who had had a prior surgical valvotomy and another with Scheie's syndrome, the predilation mean gradient of 18.9 ± 5.6 mm Hg was reduced to 8.2 ± 4.8 mm Hg and the mean indexed valve area increased from 0.8 ± 0.3 cm^2 to 1.4 ± 0.4 cm^2. Only one patient developed mitral regurgitation, this being mild. A transient small effusion due to perforation by a ventricular wire occurred in another and a small atrial shunt was the only other complication. Among six patients who were recatheterized, restenosis has occurred in two, but to a lesser degree than the original value.

Prosthetic Valve Stenosis

Attempts to dilate stenotic porcine valves, either within right heart conduits or in the tricuspid position, have not been very successful.[60]

Our experience at The Boston Children's Hospital consists of attempts in 11 patients ranging in age from 3–22 years, 9 of whom had porcine valves in conduits and two, in the tricuspid position.[54] The gradient was reduced by 33–58% in 3 of the former and by 54% in 1 of the latter, being unchanged in the others. While unsuccessful in many, it will allow postponement of conduit or valve replacement in some patients.

Balloon Angioplasty

Pulmonary Arteries

Surgical enlargement of narrowed central pulmonary arteries is essential to the management of

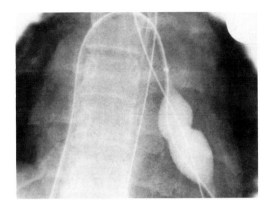

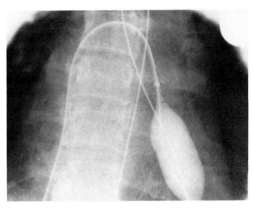

Figure 18. From the first successful transseptal dilatation of a mitral valve in a child. The initial balloons were short (3 cm) to avoid damage to the atrial septum and left ventricular apex, a precaution that proved unnecessary. Top shows the waist; bottom, the waist has disappeared.

many patients with tetralogy of Fallot and similar lesions; usually it is successful, restenosis is not common, and patch enlargement may be carried out into the pulmonary artery branches for a short distance with success. However, more distal obstructions and long-segment stenoses (so-called hypoplastic pulmonary arteries) have proved refrac-

tory to standard operative management. Balloon angioplasty offers an alternative approach.

Initial studies in lambs indicated that dilatation of narrowed pulmonary artery branches was feasible and produced long-lasting success.[69,97] Preliminary clinical studies[64,96] have demonstrated that most forms of pulmonary arterial narrowings in children can be dilated also. The procedure is not without risk; hemodynamic instability and vascular rupture have resulted in significant morbidity and occasional mortality.

Stenosis of pulmonary artery branches is the most common postoperative abnormality found at catheterization in patients with tetralogy of Fallot (Fig. 19). Balloon angioplasty for rehabilitation of diminutive pulmonary arteries in patients with tetralogy of Fallot or atresia is now the most common interventional procedure performed during catheterization at The Boston Children's Hospital.

Technique. Precatheterization evaluation of these patients should include not only estimates of the severity of right ventricular outflow obstruction (murmur intensity, right ventricular hypertrophy on the electrocardiogram, septal position, and regurgitant jets by echocardiography), but also an estimate of the flow distribution to the two lungs. In any child with bilateral disease, the lung that receives the least flow will have the greatest degree of obstruction. For obvious reasons, the worst lesion is always dilated first.

The need for pulmonary arterial dilatation is assessed by routine right and left heart catheterization. Candidates should have one or more of the following abnormalities attributable, at least in part, to the arterial narrowings: (1) cyanosis, (2) signs or symptoms of right heart failure, (3) near-systemic right ventricular pressures, or (4) less than 20% of the cardiac output directed to one lung. Pulmonary arterial anatomy is determined from selective biplane right and left pulmonary arteriograms; care is taken to outline distal as well as proximal arterial anatomy. The worst, most distal lesion is dilated first; distal lesions are the most difficult to reach but can be occluded without major

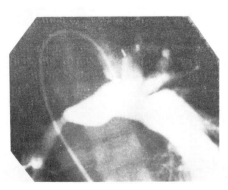

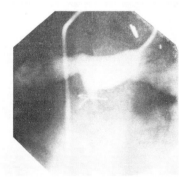

Figure 19. Successful experimental dilatation of a right pulmonary artery via a left Blalock-Taussig shunt.

hemodynamic instability. An appropriate catheter is advanced into the largest vessel distal to the obstruction (usually the lower lobe artery), taking care to avoid small branches. The guiding wire should be as stiff and as large as possible.

With the position of the wire established, a balloon about 4 times the size of the narrowed vessel is selected if a small patient is being dilated or about 3–3.5 times for an adolescent or adult. The most distal lesion is dilated first, using inflation pressures as high as the balloon will tolerate, until the waist disappears. If no waist is seen, larger balloons or better balloon positions are needed. Care is taken never to cross a recently dilated arterial site; angiograms and pressure measurements may be repeated without losing distal wire position if Y-adaptors are used. Generally, multiple narrowings along the same artery are dilated at one sitting (in the so-called "hypoplastic" artery). Only recently have both right and left pulmonary arteries been dilated in the same catheterization. Postdilatation angiograms delineate success or failure, identify postdilatation tears and aneurysms, and outline any residual lesions (Figs. 20 and 21).

Results. At The Children's Hospital in Boston, 218 vessels have been dilated in 135 patients. The results are highly dependent on the type of patient, the nature of the lesion, and the patient's age. In general, we consider a dilatation to be successful if the diameter of the pulmonary artery is enlarged by at least 50%. By this criterion about 55–60% of the dilatations are successful.

Perhaps the most useful role of pulmonary arterial angioplasty has been as part of the rehabilitation of diminutive pulmonary arteries. After establishment of right ventricular-to-pulmonary

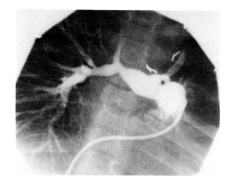

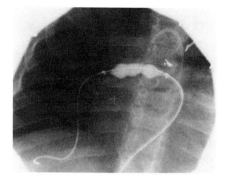

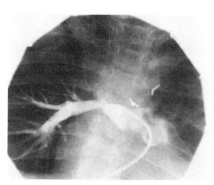

Figure 21. Dilation of two obstructions in the right pulmonary artery. The distal right lower lobe is enlarged, but the proximal, shunt-related lesion is unchanged.

arterial continuity with small (8–10 mm) homografts during early childhood, balloon dilatation is used to relieve the distal stenoses that invariably remain. Transcatheter closure of remaining collaterals and surgical relief of remaining obstructions, along with closure of any ventricular septal defect, complete the process and permit successful repair in many (if not most) of these patients (Fig. 22).

Complications. The overall mortality for this procedure has been 4 of 218: two of the deaths were due to pulmonary arterial rupture in the immediate postoperative period in children who remained in shock after a Fontan operation. In these children, dilatation was known to be very risky: surgical dissection may remove part of the adven-

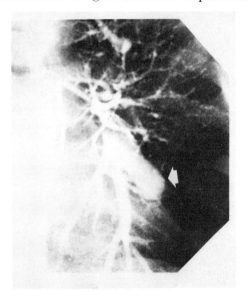

Figure 20. Postdilation aneurysm in a left pulmonary artery. Increased exerience and improved technique have made this an avoidable complication.

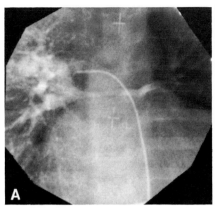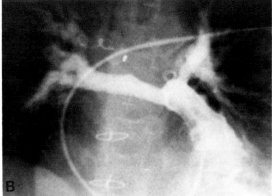

Figure 22. **A,** Patient with tetralogy of Fallot with pulmonary atresia and excess collaterals. Note the tiny right and left pulmonary arteries which were opacified by injection into a right collateral vessel. **B,** Same patient after coil occlusion of collaterals, surgical opening of the outflow tract, and balloon dilatation of the pulmonary arteries.

titia, a structure necessary to prevent vascular rupture in experimental dilatation.

Aside from arterial rupture in early postoperative patients, two deaths were due to hemodynamic instability. One infant had pulmonary arterial pressures of 170 mm Hg; just advancing the 7F angioplasty balloon into the main pulmonary artery produced cardiac arrest and the patient could not be resuscitated. A second child with truncus arteriosus and interrupted arch had had a prior pulmonary arterial band; successful left pulmonary artery dilatation produced a distal left pulmonary artery pressure of 110/70 and marked, and ultimately fatal, hemodynamic instability of uncertain etiology.

Morbidity has included hemoptysis (in five patients), unilateral pulmonary edema,[6] and aneurysms.

Unrepaired Coarctation of the Aorta

An unrepaired aortic coarctation can be dilated with a high frequency of initial gradient relief and minimal short-term complications. In general, however, benefit is less than complete (and indeed less than that obtained at surgery). Successful procedures succeed by tearing the vascular intima and part or all of the media.[61,68] This process may result in the development of aneurysms both in experimental animals and in children.[73] Thus, the role of balloon dilatation in the management of the child or infant with an uncomplicated, unrepaired aortic coarctation remains unclear at this time. There is no doubt, however, that balloon dilation can be a useful procedure in the infant or child who may be at very high risk for standard surgical management.

Technique. With few exceptions, vascular access is obtained percutaneously via the femoral arteries. Biplane angiography outlines the severity and dimensions of the coarctation and the diameter of

the aorta above and below the obstruction. Initially, balloons about 2.5–3 times the diameter of the narrowing are used. Frequently, larger balloons are required when no improvement is seen on the initial postdilatation angiogram (in more than 50% of the cases). To avoid injuring "normal" aorta, long balloons (more than 3 cm) and balloons more than 50% larger than the unaffected aorta are avoided.

Results. At The Boston Children's Hospital, initial results in dilating unrepaired neonatal coarctations demonstrated a recurrence rate approaching 100% in the first 6 months after dilatation.[61] More recent reports have noted some long-lasting gradient relief,[55,81] but nonetheless the recurrence rate persists. The absence of angiographically visible tears in the vessels following dilatation of neonatal coarctations, and the "soft" nature of the lesions (a waist is rarely seen in the balloon) suggests that dilatation may stretch ductal tissue, which subsequently contracts again.

In older patients, restenosis is not common. Dilatation has been carried out in four patients with coarctations who had severe mitral stenosis, recent intracranial hemorrhages, severe left ventricular dysfunction,[77] or other relative contraindications to surgery. The systolic gradients fell about 50% and each patient's clinical condition was improved. However, the result was less satisfactory than that usually seen following surgery.

Complications. In the small experience at The Boston Children's Hospital, complications are rare.

Postoperative Coarctation of the Aorta

Unlike unrepaired aortic coarctation, postoperative aortic obstruction can be a formidable surgical challenge: mortality rates are higher, morbidity can be considerable, and gradient relief frequently is incomplete. Balloon angioplasty has been a very useful tool in the management of arch obstructions that remain after repair of aortic coarctations, interrupted aortic arches, and the hypoplastic left heart syndrome.[104] Indeed, balloon dilatation has become the procedure of choice for most such patients.

Technique. The procedure is similar to that outlined for unrepaired aortic coarctation. Initially, balloon size is chosen to be 2.5–3 times the size of the obstruction, but the final balloon size frequently is larger (on average, nearly 4 times the narrowest diameter). As with unrepaired coarctations and dilatations of the pulmonary artery branches, the use of a Y-adaptor (to allow frequent measurement of gradients and angiographic diameters) is helpful in deciding when a large enough balloon has been used.

Results. At The Boston Children's Hospital we have attempted to dilate 25 patients with obstructions following end-to-end repair of coarctation, 34 patients with obstructions following other forms of coarctation repair, 10 patients with narrowings after repair of interrupted aortic arch, and six patients with obstructions after palliation for the hypoplastic left heart syndrome. Gradient reduction (50% or more) was achieved in more than 80% of patients,[104] and has been largely independent of the lesion (Fig. 23). Failure to reduce the gradient has occurred in long-segment stenosis (Fig. 24), whereas discrete lesions appear to be dilatable regardless of underlying anatomy or the patient's age.

Complications. One death occurred in the first 52 patients: a 3-month-old child with a postoperative coarctation and severe congestive heart failure had retroperitoneal bleeding which, in retrospect, began 4–6 hours after a successful dilatation procedure. Reliable venous access and blood for transfusion were not immediately available when hemodynamic instability became clear, and the patient expired. In retrospect, it seems likely that a branch of the iliac artery was severed during dilatation, become occluded during manual tampon-ade at the end of the procedure, and reopened later. Of five infants who had severely obstructed arches after first stage palliation for hypoplastic left heart syndrome, three developed severe hemodynamic instability at the time of antegrade balloon dilatation. All were successfully dilated and then resuscitated.

Other complications have included temporary and permanent loss of the femoral pulse. Although there has been no long-term serious morbidity, in two infants who had obstruction following repair of subclavian flap coarctation, obstruction recurred within 3 months after dilatation. Two children with multiple severe obstructions after repair of an interrupted aortic arch underwent successful dilatation with excellent clinical results; on follow-up they had small-to-moderate aneurysms of the arch (Fig. 25). In each the condition appears to be nonprogressive, and neither has required operative intervention.

Obstructed Venous Baffles

Until recently the mainstay of surgical corrections for transposition of the great arteries, the atrial inversion operations (Mustard, Senning) are complicated occasionally by obstructions in the superior or (rarely) inferior limb of the systemic venous baffle. Generally, these obstructions are at the level of the old atrial septum, a structure that can be dilated successfully.[62] Although the late results of the procedure are not yet known, balloon angioplasty has become an attractive alternative to surgical revision of the baffle.

Technique. These lesions are extremely compliant and generally require very large balloons or even two balloons. Successful dilatations occur when the obstruction is at, or near, the old atrial septum; thus, predilatation definition of the anatomy is important. Initially, balloons about 5 times the diameter of the narrowing are inflated to low pressures (1–2 atmospheres). Larger and larger

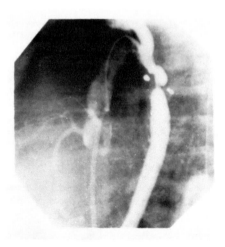 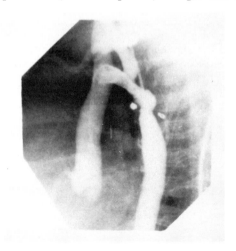

Figure 23. Successful dilatation of a recurrent coarctation following subclavian flap repair.

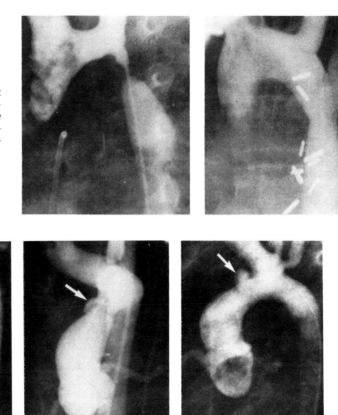

Figure 24. Examples of recurrent coarctations that proved to be undilatable. Patient on left had a long, severe obstruction; patient on right had significant gradient despite subtle anatomic obstruction.

| Pre Dilation | Immediately Post Dilation | 1 Yr. Post Dilation |

Figure 25. Balloon dilatation of arch obstruction which persisted after repair of interrupted aortic arch. Late aneurysm seen 1 year later.

balloons are used until the waist is seen at low pressures and disappears at high pressures. Balloons as much as 10 times larger than the narrowed segment may be needed. Indeed, the need for such large balloons in this lesion resulted in the early use of the double-balloon technique in children. After successful dilatation, pressure measurements and angiography are repeated (Fig. 26).

Results. Small baffle gradients are common and generally well tolerated, however, any discrete lesions producing gradients of more than 5 mm Hg are dilated. Twelve lesions in two centers (Boston Children's Hospital, Texas Children's Hospital) have been dilated, with an average reduction in gradient of 65% and at least some reduction in 8 of the 10 cases. Unsuccessful dilatations have occurred when the baffle obstruction has not been localized to the atrial septal rim. Postdilatation restenosis has occurred in at least one patient, whereas the others have remained largely asymptomatic. Late follow-up (more than 2 years) is not available.

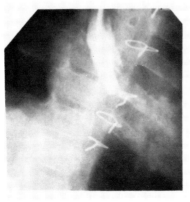
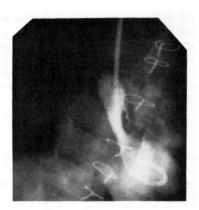

Figure 26. Successful dilatation of an obstructed venous baffle following the atrial inversion procedure.

Complications. This procedure has been safe, without mortality or significant morbidity, in this small group of patients. Specifically, there have been no baffle leaks and no late embolic events.

Pulmonary Venous Obstructions

Congenital narrowings of pulmonary veins, or stenoses, that occur after surgical repair of a number of lesions remain among the most vexing problems in congenital heart disease. Generally progressive and frequently fatal, they have not been successfully managed with standard surgical therapy. They were among the first congenital lesions to be approached with balloon catheters.[24] Despite initial success, restenosis and progressive further stenosis has occurred in every dilated patient, including 10 patients in The Boston Children's Hospital series.[62] As a result, further dilations in this group of patients have been suspended until vascular stents become available, an approach that may reduce the incidence and severity of restenosis.

Technique. Venous access must be obtained from the femoral veins and the atrial septum crossed either via the foramen ovale or using a Brockenbrough procedure. Most pulmonary venous stenoses (especially in isolated lesions) are relatively soft lesions; no waist is seen, although postdilatation angiograms frequently show improvement. On occasion, multiple lesions have been dilated using larger and larger balloons (as large as 8 times the narrowing) in an effort to reduce the incidence of restenosis.

Results. With the exception of an occasional case of pulmonary venous stenosis associated with complex congenital heart lesions, dilatation has produced short-term improvement, with restenosis evident within 2 months.

Complications. Patients with suprasystemic right ventricular pressures due to stenosed pulmonary veins are unstable; such patients need to be intubated, ventilated, and treated as critically ill during any dilatation procedure. Temporary occlusion of a pulmonary vein may increase right heart pressures and was associated with pulmonary hemorrhage in one patient. Although there has been no procedure-induced mortality, the consistent lack of success makes this morbidity appear unwarranted.

Balloon and Blade Atrial Septostomy

Balloon atrial septostomy, introduced by Rashkind and Miller in 1966 remains the standard method of creating an atrial septal defect in the newborn.[91] Although intracardiac complications occurred occasionally during the early years, with the advent of biplane fluoroscopy these have virtually disappeared. As experience accumulated, limitations became evident; the duration of septal patency was temporary in many infants and septostomy was ineffective in the majority when carried out in infants more than 1 month of age. Nonetheless, balloon septostomy remains the procedure of choice in the newborn, being particularly useful in the baby with D-transposition in whom an arterial switch procedure can be carried out within days if the ventricular septum is intact or within a few months if a ventricular septal defect is present.

Currently, if creation of an atrial defect is required in infants and young children older than 1 month, the Park blade[82,83] is used first and followed by a balloon septostomy. Rarely, the defect may be created using large dilating balloons.

Technique. In recent years the Miller TM septostomy (American Edwards Laboratories), introduced through a 7F sheath with a diaphragm, has been used exclusively. Entry is through an umbilical or percutaneous femoral venous site. Usually, the balloon is inflated with a 4 ml of dilute contrast in the left atrium, provided that the cavity is large enough to accept this inflated size (smaller amounts are necessary in most infants with hypoplastic left heart syndrome). The balloon is then rapidly jerked across the septum; this is repeated at least once. The defect is then measured and hemodynamic parameters are noted.

In patients older than 1 month, the Park blade is first introduced into the left atrium either directly across an existing communication or via a transseptally placed long sheath. With the former route, it is mandatory to ensure first, by echocardiography or left atrial angiography in the hepatoclavicular view, that the defect is not in the septum primum, to avoid cutting the atrioventricular valves. The blade is partially opened in the left atrium, repositioned to ensure that the arms are free, and then rotated until the tip is **anteroleftward.** Firm constant pressure pulls the blade into the right atrium. Following the blade septostomy, a balloon septostomy is carried out, the size of the defect is determined, and hemodynamic parameters are remeasured. At the conclusion, particularly in those in whom a modified Fontan procedure is anticipated, the transatrial mean gradient should be, at most, 3 mm Hg.

Results. In recent years, balloon septostomy has been adequate and without intracardiac complications in the majority of newborns, particularly those with D-transposition. However, in three patients with stenosis or atresia of the left atrioventricular valve, in whom balloon septostomy was the only procedure performed, surgical septectomy was required within 2 days to 5 months.[85]

Among some 30 patients who had blade septostomies followed by balloon dilatation, some of whom had had previous surgical septectomies, there have been no intracardiac complications; both of the currently available blade sizes (9.4 mm, 13 mm) have been used. Although the procedure has been effective in most, some residual obstruction has been evident in some, particularly among those with left atrial outflow obstruction. Among the latter, the gradient was 3 mm Hg or less in two-thirds, and surgical septectomies were necessary in the others within days. Those with gradients of 3 mm Hg or less have shown no evidence of restenosis at echocardiographic examination during some months of follow-up.

Closure Techniques

Coil Embolization of Aortopulmonary Collaterals

Aortopulmonary collateral vessels are encountered frequently in patients with tetralogy of Fallot and rarely in patients with other forms of congenital heart disease. Their anatomy is highly variable; they may arise from head and neck vessels, the abdominal aorta, or coronary arteries, as well as from the descending thoracic aorta. Their courses within the thorax are unpredictable as well, and intraoperative recognition may be difficult. Vessels that arise from the descending aorta usually need to be approached from a posterior thoracotomy. As a result, most aortopulmonary collaterals are not closed at the time of reparative surgery; if they are, a second incision is needed.

In contrast, catheter techniques[36,86] can close most aortopulmonary collaterals at the time of diagnostic catheterization and eliminate the need for a second operation. Multiple angiograms can be used to identify anatomy quite precisely; success rates are high, morbidity low, and recanalization rare.

Technique. Precise angiographic definition is mandatory to identify the optimum coil size and location. Because the course of the vessel is often tortuous, multiple views and selective injections are needed. The authors have tried to avoid closing collaterals where no second source of blood to the affected lung is evident. However, even when a collateral is the only source, closure has been well tolerated. Coils are chosen to be 10–30% larger than the diameter of the vessel to be closed; smaller coils are nonocclusive and larger coils may extrude back into the aorta (Fig. 27). Frequently, multiple coils are needed to close high-flow lesions; larger coils are used as a framework and smaller coils, subsequently, to retard flow. The vessels are closed using a retrograde percutaneous technique with catheters that provide a straight course to the vessel and allow careful control of the tip during coil placement.

Results. Of 65 collaterals larger than 2 mm, closure was attempted in 58; among the other 7 vessels, 4 were too short and 3 could not be securely cannulated. Closure was complete or virtually complete in 50 of 58, partial in 7, and unsuccessful in 1. On late angiography, 1 of 18 previously closed vessels had recanalized, and 4 of 7 partially closed

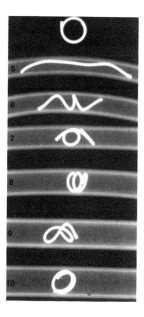

Figure 27. Coils placed in tubes of varying size. Oversized coils (**top**) will be nonocclusive; undersized coils (**bottom**) will encircle in mid-channel and allow flow on either side.

vessels had become completely closed. No patient had evidence of late coil migration.

Complications. There was no mortality associated with the procedure. Inadvertent coil embolization to the lung occurred in five cases; in two the coil was retrieved without difficulty, and in three the coils were left *in situ* in a distal lobular vessel. In each of these three cases, the incorrectly positioned coil caused neither vascular occlusion nor symptoms and has remained without causing clinical difficulties for as long as 4 years.

Less common cases of morbidity have included femoral pulse loss and extravascular injections of contrast material while trying to cannulate tortuous vessels (two patients).

Coil Embolization of Other Vessels

In addition to their use in aortopulmonary collaterals, coils have been useful for closing Blalock-Taussig shunts, systemic arteriovenous fistulas, pulmonary arteriovenous fistulas producing cyanosis, and venous malformations producing right-to-left shunts. Although each use, by itself, is not common, in aggregate they demonstrate the versatility of coils to achieve vessel closure.

Technique. The use of coils to close these various lesions is similar to that described for aortopulmonary collaterals. It should be noted that the coils need to be 10–30% larger than the stretched diameter of the vessel. The vessel will not stretch if it is a modified synthetic Blalock shunt; it may stretch by 50% or more if it is a systemic vein draining to the left atrium. The stretched diameter of the vessel always should be determined before dilatation by test occlusion with a balloon catheter.

Results. At The Boston Children's Hospital 7 of 10 Blalock-Taussig shunts (classic and modified) were closed successfully. These shunts are more difficult to close than most vessels because of their short length, proximity to cephalic vessels, and unobstructed course.

Feeding vessels to those arteriovenous malformations that cause heart failure in infancy can be closed relatively easily, even in neonates, using small-bore catheters and the newly developed Gianturco "mini-coils."[37] Because these malformations may develop collateral feeders after main feeding vessels are closed, successful technical embolization may not produce biologic success. For these reasons, transcatheter embolization of hepatic arteriovenous malformations is reserved for infants who have failed medical management.

Closure of venous channels which cause cyanosis has been quite successful, although most such channels are too large to close with coils, and require umbrella closure (see below).

Complications. No deaths occurred as a result of attempted embolization. However, in an attempt to partially occlude flow through a 4-mm shunt in an infant with single ventricle, severe ventricular dysfunction, and valve regurgitation, flow was reduced using a deliberately oversized coil. Although this succeeded, the patient developed a microangiopathic anemia several days after partial closure, which contributed, ultimately, to his death. Other complications included an asymptomatic pulmonary embolism and pulse loss.

Umbrella Closure of Patent Ductus Arteriosus

Although the transvascular plug method to close patent ductus arteriosus is more than two decades old,[87] its use was restricted by the need for a femoral arterial cutdown and, in younger children, by the size of the catheter. Rashkind's development of the double umbrella plug[90] allowed a much smaller delivery system (as small as 8F) and extended the transcatheter closure of patent ductus arteriosus to the young child and infant. Although initially a procedure with limited clinical success, because of modifications made by Mullins and others, closure is now achieved in more than 95% of cases.[92,114] Undoubtedly, further experience will improve results.

Although long-term experience with this technique is limited, late problems from device migration, embolic phenomena, or endocarditis have not been encountered. Significantly, the late follow-up of transarterial plug closure in several hundred cases[115] has been favorable also. If favorable late follow-up continues, it seems likely that transcatheter closure will become the therapy of choice for patent ductus arteriosus.

Technique.[114] A 7F femoral venous line is placed percutaneously, and a smaller (4–5F) arterial pigtail is inserted. After the briefest of hemodynamic studies, biplane aortography demonstrates the precise location, anatomy, and size of the patent ductus. For smaller defects, a 12-mm umbrella (requiring an 8F sheath) is used, whereas for defects more than 4 mm in diameter, a 17-mm umbrella (an 11F sheath) is required. Under general anesthesia, the patent ductus is crossed from the venous direction, the long sheath is advanced through the ductus over a guiding wire and the umbrella is delivered so that the distal arms open in the aorta and the proximal arms open in the pulmonary artery (Fig. 28). Angiography confirms correct placement and the device is released. To eliminate transductal flow, an inflated balloon is held against the thrombin-soaked and incompletely closed umbrella for a few minutes after release. The use of heparin is avoided in these procedures. Once closure appears optimal, the catheters are removed and the patient is observed for 4–6 hours before discharge, usually the same day.

Results. The results of patent ductus arteriosus closure in patients with restrictive and nonrestrictive patent ductus arteriosus have been analyzed separately. Attempts to close a restrictive patent ductus arteriosus (pulmonary artery pressure less than aortic pressure) were made in 48 infants, children, and adults (3/12 to 76 years, 4–55 kg). Among the first eight children, only three closures were complete; two closures were partial, and the umbrella embolized to the left pulmonary artery in the other three, necessitating operative removal. With technical modifications,[114] umbrellas have been implanted successfully in 39 of 40 patients; one had a tiny (less than 1 mm) patent ductus arteriosus that could not be crossed by any catheters larger than 4F. Each patent ductus arteriosus has been completely closed on clinical follow-up, although very small shunts have been seen on late color Doppler studies in some. Similar tiny jets occurring after surgical ligation of patent ductus arteriosus has led us to reconsider the importance of such a finding. Through 1989 more than 120 patients have undergone ductal closure using umbrella devices. On late follow-up, there have been no episodes of umbrella migration or erosion, endocarditis, or emboli.

The results in a much smaller series of nonrestrictive patent ductus arteriosus are much less satisfactory. Umbrella embolization occurred in two of five attempts and complete or subtotal closure was not achieved in any patient. Of four patients with residual shunts, two required subsequent surgical ligation. Thus, in our experience, a nonrestrictive patent ductus arteriosus is not likely to be completely closed with the transcatheter umbrella technique.

Complications. There have been no deaths and very few complications associated with this tech-

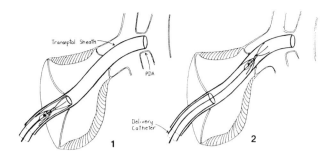

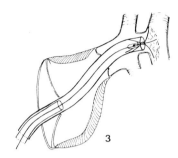

Figure 28. The sheath-extension technique developed by Dr. Charles Mullins for umbrella closure of a pulmonary ductus arteriosus.

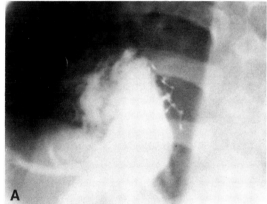

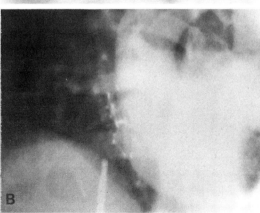

Figure 29. Umbrella closure of an atrial septal defect. **A,** Right atrial angiogram shows no right-to-left shunt. **B,** Levophase shows no left-to-right shunt.

nique. One patient had a transient pulse loss which resolved overnight after heparin therapy and one infant with a nonrestrictive patent ductus arteriosus needed to have her misplaced umbrella removed at cardiopulmonary bypass.

Transcatheter Closure of Atrial Septal Defects

Like patent ductus arteriosus, an atrial septal defect was first closed using ingenious transcatheter techniques more than 15 years ago by King and Mills.[51] Despite several initial successes, the catheter size was prohibitively large (23F) and the success rate was not high enough to permit widespread clinical use.

The more recent single umbrella device of Rashkind[90] could be advanced via a smaller sheath (15F), allowing its use in the pediatric age range. Small 2-mm hooks were used to attach the umbrella to the left atrial side of the septum. These hooks could attach incorrectly to the left atrial free wall and/or pulmonary veins; once attached, the hooks could not be repositioned, thus reducing the success rate of this procedure.

A clam-shell umbrella approach has been devised recently that allows further miniaturization (11–13F sheaths), eliminates the need for hooks, and allows the umbrella to be centered over the defect during placement (Fig. 29). This device has ben used successfully to close atrial defects in animals, and is now being used in children.

Technique. A most important step in transcatheter atrial septal defect closure is accurate assessment of the number, size, and location of the atrial septal defects. Defects larger than 25 mm, multiple defects including those outside the fossa ovalis, sinus venosus defects extending into the vena cavae, and defects with tissue rims less than 3–6 mm from

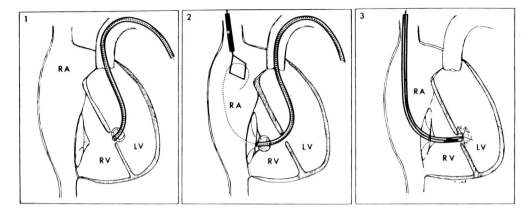

Figure 30. Original technique for transcatheter closure of ventricular septal defects. Recent experience suggests that this will become the treatment of choice for apical muscular ventricular septal defects.

the tricuspid valves or right pulmonary veins may be difficult to close without producing injury to adjacent structures. For patients with suitable defects, a balloon inflated in the defect confirms the location and stretched diameter. The umbrella should be 80% larger than the stretched diameter of the defect. The distal arms are opened in the left atrium and pulled slowly but firmly to bow the septum rightward. The right-sided arms are then opened, the umbrella readvanced to a neutral position, the proper location confirmed, and the umbrella released. Patients are monitored overnight, discharged the next day, and maintained on antibiotic prophylaxis for 6–9 months.

Results. Through 1987, the atrial septal defects closed in children and young adults[70] were patent foramina ovale associated with cyanosis or small atrial defects in postoperative patients (10 patients). Experimental studies on larger defects in animals, using the clam-shell septal occluder, resulted in six successful closures in eight attempts with good late results. Subsequently, through 1990, more than 70 patients have had atrial defects closed.

Complications. In this series there have been no deaths.

Transcatheter Closure of Ventricular Septal Defects

Most ventricular septal defects are near the aortic or tricuspid valves and require precise patch placement under direct operative vision. Some defects (i.e., in the muscular ventricular septum) may be difficult to close surgically and are remote from valvar structures. These congenital or postinfarction muscular defects have now been successfully closed in a small number of patients using transcatheter double-umbrella techniques.[63] Although preliminary, these results suggest that transcatheter closure of ventricular septal defects will prove useful in selected patients.

Technique. Ventricular septal defects are crossed in a retrograde fashion, from the left ventricle, using flow-directed balloon-tipped catheters. From the right ventricular side of the atrium the catheter or a 400-cm guide wire is snared from either the jugular or femoral vein, depending on the location of the ventricular septal defect (Fig. 30). With the long guide wire stabilized at both ends, a balloon is used to estimate the size of the ventricular septal defect. An 11F long Mullins sheath and dilator are advanced over the guide wire and into the left ventricle via a venous approach. The long sheath is used to direct the double-umbrella device to the ventricular defect.

Results. Attempts have been made in 10 patients to close ventricular septal defects with the transcatheter procedure. The ventricular septal defect was crossed in each patient; in two, the ventricular septal defect was too large for closure. In a third, the ventricular septal defect was too close to the aortic valve (following a Rastelli operation) to allow safe closure. In the other seven, the umbrella was properly placed across the ventricular septal defect. At the initial attempt to close a 13-mm defect (a postinfarction ventricular septal defect) with a 17-mm device; the device remained in position for a few seconds, but was swept into the pulmonary artery. The patient's extreme clinical condition prior to catheterization, precluded further therapy.

All other defects were substantially or completely closed by the umbrella. Clinical closure was less certain; several patients had more than one defect, resulting in incomplete clinical success. In patients with postinfarction ventricular septal defects, infarct extension in the first days after umbrella placement contributed to deteriorating clinical condition and ultimate patient demise. In patients with congenital, residual, or postoperative defects, transcatheter ventricular septal defect closure was clinically useful, and even lifesaving.

Complications. Other than the umbrella dislodgement noted above, there were no complications due to closure of the ventricular septal defect. The incidence of such potential complications as endocarditis, late migration of the device, or embolic phenomena must await longer term studies.

REFERENCES

1. Almen T: Development of nonionic contrast media. Invest Radiol 20(Suppl):2–9, 1985.
2. Al Zaibag M, Al Kasab S, Ribeiro PA, et al: Percutaneous double balloon valvotomy for rheumatic mitral-valve stenosis. Lancet 1:757–761, 1986.
3. Ansell G: Adverse reactions to contrast agents: scope of the problem. Invest Radiol 5:374–385, 1970.
4. Ansell G, Tweedie MRK, West CR, et al: The current status of reactions to intravenous contrast media. Invest Radiol 15:s32–s39, 1980.
5. Anthony CL, Tonkin ILD, Marin-Garcia J, et al: A double-blind randomized clinical study of the safety, tolerability and efficacy of Hexabrix in pediatric angiocardiography. Invest Radiol 19(Suppl):s335–s343, 1985.
6. Arnold LW, Keane JF, Kan JS, et al: Transient unilateral pulmonary edema after successful balloon dilation of peripheral pulmonary artery stenosis. Am J Cardiol 62:327–330, 1988.
7. Babic UU, Pejcic P, Djurisic Z, et al: Percutaneous transarterial balloon valvuloplasty for mitral valve stenosis. Am J Cardiol 57:1101–1104, 1986.
8. Balter S, Sones FM, Brancato R: Radiation exposure to the operator performing cardiac angiography with U-arm systems. Circulation 58:925–932, 1978.
9. Bargeron LM, Elliot LP, Soto B, et al: Axial cineangiography in congenital heart disease. I. Concept, technical and anatomic considerations. Circulation 56:1075–1083, 1977.
10. Beitzke A, Suppan C, Justich E: Complications in 1000 cardiac catheter examinations in childhood. Rontgenblatter 35:430–437, 1982.
11. Bettmann MA: Angiographic contrast agents: conventional and new media compared. AJR 139:787–794, 1982.
12. Bogren HG, Bursch JH: Digital angiography in the diagnosis of congenital heart disease. Cardiovasc Intervent Radiol 7:180–188, 1984.
13. Brannon ES, Weens HS, Warren JV: Atrial septal defect: study of hemodynamics by the technique of right heart catheterization. Am J Med Sci 210:480–491, 1946.
14. Buonocore E, Pavlicek W, Modic MT, et al: Anatomic and functional imaging of congenital heart disease with digital subtraction angiography. Radiology 147:647–654, 1983.
15. Cohn HE, Freed MD, Hellenbrand WF, et al: Complications and mortality associated with cardiac catheterization in infants under one year: a prospective study. Pediatr Cardiol 6:123–131, 1985.
16. Cournand AF, Ranges HS: Catheterization of the right auricle in man. Proc Soc Exp Biol Med 46:42, 1941.
17. Cribier A, Savin T, Berland J, et al: Percutaneous transluminal balloon valvuloplasty of adult aortic stenosis: report of 92 cases. J Am Coll Cardiol 9:381–386, 1987.
18. Cumberland DC: Hexabrix—a new contrast medium in angiocardiography. Br Heart J 45:698–702, 1981.
19. Cumberland DC: Metrizamide in pediatric angiography. Ann Radiol 24:99–104, 1981.
20. Curry TS, Dowdy JE, Murry RC: Christensen's Introduction to the Physics of Diagnostic Radiology, 3rd ed. Philadelphia, Lea & Febiger, 1984.
21. Dawson P: New contrast agents: chemistry and pharmacology. Invest Radiol 19(Suppl):293–300, 1985.
22. Dawson P: Chemotoxicity of contrast media and clinical adverse effects: a review. Invest Radiol 20(Suppl):84–91, 1985.
23. DeLezo JS, Pan M, Sancho M, et al: Percutaneous transluminal balloon dilation for discrete subaortic stenosis. Am J Cardiol 58:619–621, 1986.
24. Driscoll DJ, Hesslein PS, Mullins CE: Congenital stenosis of individual pulmonary veins: clinical spectrum and unsuccessful treatment by transvenous balloon dilation. Am J Cardiol 49:1767–1772, 1982.
25. Elliot LP, Bargeron LM, Bream PR, et al: Axial cineangiography in congenital heart disease. II. Specific lesions. Circulation 56:1084–1093, 1977.
26. Engles PHC, Ludwig JW, Verhoeven LAJ: Left ventricle evaluation by digital video subtraction angiocardiography. Radiology 144:471–474, 1982.
27. Fellows KE, Keane JF, Freed MD: Angled views in cineangiography of congenital heart disease. Circulation 56:484–490, 1977.
28. Fischer HW: Hemodynamic reactions to angiographic media: a survey and commentary. Radiology 91:66–73, 1968.
29. Forssmann W: Die Sondierung des rechten Herzens. Klin Wschr 8:2085, 1929.
30. Freed MD, Keane JF, Rosenthal A: The effect of heparinization to prevent arterial thrombosis after percutaneous cardiac catheterization in children. Circulation 50:565–569, 1974.
31. Freed MD, Nadas AS, Norwood WI, et al: Is routine preoperative cardiac catheterization necessary before repair of secundum and sinus venosus atrial septal defects? J Am Coll Cardiol 4:333–336, 1984.
32. Freed MD, Miettinen OS, Nadas AS: Oxymetric detection of intracardiac left-to-right shunts. Br Heart J 42:690–694, 1979.
33. Freeman LM, Blaufox MD (eds): Physician's Desk Reference for Radiology and Nuclear Medicine 1979/1980. Oradell, NJ, Medical Economics Co., 1979.
34. Friesinger G, Adams DF, Bourassa MG, et al: Report of the Inter-society Commission for Heart Disease Resources. Optimal resources for examination of the heart and lungs: cardiac catheterization and radiographic facilities. Circulation 68:893a–930a, 1983.
35. Friesinger G, Schaffer J, Cooley, JM, et al: Hemodynamic consequences of the injection of radiopaque material. Circulation 31:730–738, 1965.
36. Fuhrman BP, Bass JL, Castaneda-Zuniga W, et al: Coil embolization of congenital thoracic vascular anomalies in infants and children. Circulation 70:285–289, 1984.
37. Gianturco C, Anderson JH, Wallace S: Mechanical devices for arterial occlusion. AJR 124:428–435, 1975.
38. Gorlin R, Gorlin SG: Hydraulic formula for calculation of area of stenotic mitral valves, other cardiac valves and central circulatory shunts. Am Heart J 41:1–29, 1951.
39. Hales S: Statical Essays Containing Haemastaticks. West end of St. Paul's, London, W. Innys and R. Manby, 1733.
40. Hall EJ: Radiation and Life, 2nd ed. New York, Pergamon Press, 1987.
41. Hayward R, Dawson P: Contrast agents in angiocardiography. Br Heart J 52:361–368, 1984.
42. Helgason H, Keane JF, Fellows KE, et al: Balloon dilation of the aortic valve: studies in normal lambs and in children with aortic stenosis. J Am Coll Cardiol 9:816–822, 1987.

43. Higgins CB, Norris BL, Gerber KH: Quantitation of left ventricular dimensions and function by digital video subtraction angiography. Radiology 144:461–469, 1982.
44. Inoue K, Owaki T, Nakamura T, et al: Clinical application of transvenous mitral commissurotomy by a new balloon catheter. J Thorac Cardiovasc Surg 87:394–402, 1984.
45. Iseri L, Kaplan A, Evans MJ, et al: Effect of concentrated contrast media during angiography on plasma volume and plasma osmolality. Am Heart J 69:154–158, 1965.
46. Kan JS, White RI, Mitchell SE, et al: Percutaneous balloon valvuloplasty: a new method for treating congenital pulmonary valve stenosis. N Engl J Med 307:540–542, 1982.
47. Keane JF, Fellows KE, Lang P, et al: Pediatric arterial catheterization using a 3.2 French catheter. Cathet Cardiovasc Diagn 8:201–208, 1982.
48. Keane JF, Freed MD, Fellows KE, et al: Pediatric cardiac angiography using a 4 French catheter. Cathet Cardiovasc Diagn 3:313, 1979.
49. Keane JF, Fyler DC, Nadas AS: Hazards of cardiac catheterization in children with primary pulmonary vascular obstruction. Am Heart J 96:556–558, 1978.
50. Keane JF, Lang P, Newburger J, et al: Iliac vein inferior caval thrombosis after cardiac catheterization in infancy. Pediatr Cardiol 1:257–261, 1980.
51. King TD, Mills NL: Secundum atrial septal defect: nonoperative closure during cardiac catheterization. JAMA 235:2506–2509, 1976.
52. Kveselis DA, Rocchini AP, Beekman R, et al: Balloon angioplasty for congenital mitral stenosis. J Am Coll Cardiol 57:348–350, 1986.
53. Lababidi ZA, Daskalopoilos DA, Stoeckle H: Transluminal balloon coarctation angioplasty: experience with 27 patients. Am J Cardiol 5:1288–1291, 1986.
54. Lababidi Z, Wu JR: Percutaneous pulmonary valvuloplasty. Am J Cardiol 52:560–562, 1983.
55. Lababidi Z, Wu J, Walls JT: Percutaneous balloon aortic valvuloplasty: results in 23 patients. Am J Cardiol 53:194–197, 1984.
56. Lasser EC: A coherent biochemical basis for increased reactivity to contrast material in allergic patients: a novel concept. AJR 149:1281–1285, 1987.
57. Leibovic SJ, Fellows KE: Patient radiation exposure during pediatric cardiac catheterization. Cardiovasc Intervent Radiol 6:150–153, 1983.
58. Levin D, Dunham L: Angiography: principles underlying proper utilization of radiologic and cineangiographic equipment. In Grossman W (ed): Cardiac Catheterization and Angiography, 2nd ed. Philadelphia, Lea & Febiger, 1980.
59. Levin DC, Schapiro RM, Boxt LM, et al: Digital subtraction angiography: principles and pitfalls of image improvement techniques. AJR 143:447–454, 1984.
60. Lloyd TR, Marvin WJ Jr, Mahoney LT, et al: Balloon dilation valvuloplasty of bioprosthetic valves in extracardiac conduits. Am Heart J 114:268–274, 1987.
61. Lock JE, Bass JL, Amplatz K, et al: Balloon dilation angioplasty of coarctations in infants and children. Circulation 68:109–116, 1983.
62. Lock JE, Bass JL, Castaneda-Zuniga W, et al: Dilation angioplasty of congenital or operative narrowings of venous channels. Circulation 70:457–464, 1984.
63. Lock JE, Block PC, McKay RG, et al: Transcatheter closure of ventricular septal defects. Circulation 78:361–368, 1988.
64. Lock JE, Castaneda-Zuniga WR, Fuhrman BP, et al:

65. Lock JE, Cockerham JT, Keane JF, et al: Transcatheter umbrella closure of congenital cardiac defects. Circulation 75:593–599, 1987.
66. Lock JE, Keane JF, Fellows KE: Diagnostic and Interventional Catheterization in Congenital Heart Disease. Boston, Martinus Nijhoff, 1987.
67. Lock JE, Khalilullah M, Shrivastava S, et al: Percutaneous catheter commissurotomy in rheumatic mitral stenosis. N Engl J Med 313:1515–1519, 1985.
68. Lock JE, Niemi T, Burke BA, et al: Transcutaneous angioplasty of experimental aortic coarctation. Circulation 66:1280–1286, 1982.
69. Lock JE, Niemi T, Einzig S, et al: Transvenous angioplasty of experimental branch pulmonary artery stenosis in newborn lambs. Circulation 64:886–893, 1981.
70. Lock JE, Rome JJ, Davis R, et al: Transcatheter closure of atrial septal defects: experimental studies. Circulation 79:1091–1099, 1989.
71. Lurie PR, Fujita M, Neustein HB: Transvascular endomyocardial biopsy in infants and children: description of a new technique. Am J Cardiol 42:453–457, 1978.
72. Mandell VS, Lock JE, Mayer JE, et al: The "laid-back" aortogram: an improved angiographic view for demonstration of coronary arteries in transposition of the great arteries. Am J Cardiol 65:1379–1383, 1990.
73. Marvin WJ, Mahoney LT, Rose EF: Pathologic sequelae of balloon dilatation angioplasty for unoperated coarctation of the aorta in children (abstract). J Am Coll Cardiol 7:117A, 1986.
74. Matthews RA, Park SC, Neches WH, et al: Iliac venous thrombosis in infants and children after cardiac catheterization. Cathet Cardiovasc Diagn 5:67–74, 1979.
75. McClennan BL: Low osmolality contrast media: premises and promises. Radiology 162:1–8, 1987.
76. McKay RG, Safian RD, Lock JE, et al: Balloon dilation of calcific aortic stenosis in elderly patients: postmortem, intraoperative, and percutaneous valvuloplasty studies. Circulation 74:119–125, 1986.
77. McKay RG, Safian RD, Lock JE, et al: Assessment of left ventricular function following balloon aortic valvuloplasty. Circulation 75:192–203, 1987.
78. McKay RG, Lock JE, Safian RD, et al: Balloon dilation of mitral stenosis in adult patients: postmortem and percutaneous mitral valvuloplasty studies. J Am Coll Cardiol 9:723–731, 1987.
79. Miller SW, Castronove FP: Radiation exposure and protection in cardiac catheterization laboratories. Am J Cardiol 55:177–182, 1985.
80. Moore RE: The Physics of Cardiac Angiography. Riverside, CA, Myrle Co. Enterprises, Inc., 1985.
81. Morrow WR, Vick GW III, Nihill MR, et al: Balloon dilation of unoperated coarctation of the aorta: short- and intermediate-term results. J Am Coll Cardiol 11:133–138, 1988.
82. Park SC, Neches WH, Zuberbuhler JR, et al: Clinical use of blade atrial septostomy. Circulation 58:600–606, 1978.
83. Park SC, Neches WH, Mullins CE, et al: Blade atrial septostomy: collaborative study. Circulation 66:258–266, 1982.
84. Perry SB, Keane JF, Lock JE: Interventional catheterization in pediatric congenital and acquired heart disease. Am J Cardiol 61:109G–117G, 1988.
85. Perry SB, Lang P, Keane JF, et al: Creation and maintenance of an adequate interatrial communication in patients with left atrioventricular valve atresia or stenosis. Am J Cardiol 58:622–626, 1986.

86. Perry SB, Radtke W, Fellows KE, et al: Coil embolization to occlude aortopulmonary collaterals and shunts in patients with congenital heart disease. J Am Coll Cardiol 13:100–108, 1989.

87. Porstmann W, Wierny L, Warnke H, et al: Catheter closure of patent ductus arteriosus: 62 cases treated without thoracotomy. Radiol Clin North Am 9:203–218, 1971.

88. Przybojewski JF: Endomyocardial biopsy: a review of the literature. Cathet and Cardiovasc Diagn 11:287–330, 1985.

89. Radtke W, Keane JF, Fellows KE, et al: Percutaneous balloon valvotomy of congenital pulmonary stenosis using oversized balloons. J Am Coll Cardiol 8:909–915, 1986.

90. Rashkind WJ: Transcatheter treatment of congenital heart disease. Circulation 67:711–716, 1983.

91. Rashkind WJ, Miller WW: Creation of an atrial septal defect without thoractomy: a palliative approach to complete transposition of the great arteries. JAMA 196:991–992, 1966.

92. Rashkind WJ, Mullins CE, Hellenbrand WE, et al: Nonsurgical closure of patent ductus arteriosus: clinical application of the Rashkind PDA occluder system. Circulation 75:583, 1987.

93. Reagan K, Bettman MA, Finkelstein J, et al: Double-blind study of a new nonionic contrast agent for cardiac angiography. Radiology 167:409–413, 1988.

94. Reuter FG: Physician and patient exposure during cardiac catheterization. Circulation 58:134–135, 1978.

95. Richman AH, Chen B, Katz M: Effectiveness of lead lenses in reducing radiation exposure. Radiology 121:357–359, 1976.

96. Ring JC, Bass JL, Marvin W, et al: Management of congenital branch pulmonary artery stenosis with balloon dilation angioplasty: report of 52 procedures. J Thorac Cardiovasc Surg 90:35–45, 1985.

97. Ring JC, Kulik TJ, Burke BA, et al: Morphologic changes induced by dilation of the pulmonary valve annulus with overlarge balloons in normal newborn lambs. Am J Cardiol 55:210–214, 1985.

98. Rios B, Nihill MR, Mullins CE: Left ventricular endomyocardial biopsy in children with the transseptal long sheath technique. Cathet Cardiovasc Diagn 10:417–423, 1984.

99. Rubio-Alvarez V, Limon RL: Comisurotomia tricuspidea por medio de un cateter modificado. Arch Inst Cardiol Mexico 25:57–69, 1955.

100. Rubio-Alvarez V, Limon RL, Soni J: Valvulotomias intracardias por medico de un cateter. Arch Inst Cardiol Mexico 23:183–192, 1953.

101. Rudolph AM: Congenital Diseases of the Heart. Chicago, Year Book Medical Publishers, 1974, pp. 49–167.

102. Rupprath G, Neuhaus KL: Percutaneous balloon aortic valvuloplasty in infancy and childhood. Am J Cardiol 55:1855–1856, 1985.

103. Sagy M, Aladjem M, Shem-Tov A, et al: The renal effect of radiocontrast administration during cardioangiography in two different groups with congenital heart disease. Eur J Pediatr 141:2336–2339, 1984.

104. Saul JP, Keane JF, Fellows KE, et al: Balloon dilation angioplasty of postoperative aortic obstructions. Am J Cardiol 59:943–948, 1987.

105. Shapiro J: Radiation Protection: A Guide for Scientists and Physicians. Cambridge, Harvard University Press, 1972.

106. Shehadi WH: Adverse reactions to intravascularly administered contrast media: a comprehensive study based on a prospective survey. AJR 124:145–152, 1975.

107. Shehadi WH: Contrast media adverse reactions. Occurrence, recurrence and distribution patterns. Radiology 43:11–17, 1982.

108. Sholler GF, Keane JF, Perry SB, et al: Balloon dilation of congenital aortic stenosis: results and influence of technical and morphologic features on outcome. Circulation, 78:351–360, 1988.

109. Soto B, Coghlan CH, Bargeron LM: Present status of axially angled angiocardiography. Cardiovasc Intervent Radiol 7:156–165, 1984.

110. Stoermer J, Hentrich F, Galal D, et al: Risks der Herzkatheterisierung und angiokardiographic in sauglings und kindersalter. Klin Padiatr 196:191–194, 1984.

111. Swanson DP, Thrall JH, Shetty PC: Evaluation of intravascular low-osmolality contrast agents. Clin Pharm 5:877–891, 1986.

112. Waller BF, Girod DA, Dillon JC: Transverse aortic wall tears in infants after balloon angioplasty for aortic valve stenosis. J Am Coll Cardiol 4:1235–1241, 1984.

113. Wessel DL, Keane JF, Fellows KE, et al: Fibrinolytic therapy for femoral arterial thrombosis following cardiac catheterization in infants and children. Am J Cardiol 58:347–351, 1986.

114. Wessel DL, Keane JF, Parness I, et al: Outpatient closure of the patent ductus arteriosus. Circulation 77:1068–1071, 1988.

115. Wierny L, Plass R, Porstmann W: Transluminal closure of patent ductus arteriosus: long-term results of 208 cases treated without thoractomy. Cardiovasc Intervent Radiol 9:279–285, 1986.

116. Wolf GL, Draft L, Kilzer K: Contrast agents lower ventricular fibrillation threshold. Radiology 129:215–217, 1978.

117. Wren C, Sullivan I, Bull C, et al: Percutaneous balloon dilatation of aortic valve stenosis in neonates and infants. Br Heart J 58:608–612, 1987.

118. Yeager SB: Balloon selection for double balloon valvotomy. J Am Coll Cardiol 9:467–468, 1987.

119. Zeevi B, Keane JF, Fellows KE, et al: Balloon dilation of critical pulmonary stenosis in the first week of life. J Am Coll Cardiol 11:821–824, 1988.

Chapter 15

ASSESSMENT OF VENTRICULAR AND MYOCARDIAL PERFORMANCE

Steven D. Colan, M.D.

The evaluation of myocardial performance in children with congenital and acquired heart disease has assumed increasing importance because of the ever-improving medical and surgical therapeutic options now available. For most forms of structural heart disease, excellent surgical options exist, making such issues as the optimal type and timing of surgical intervention of critical importance. Because of the potential for myocardial injury as a result of the hemodynamic abnormalities associated with most forms of congenital heart disease, accurate assessment of the state of health of the myocardium is an important part of this process. Similarly, the expanding number of potent pharmacologic agents that are used in the therapy of cardiovascular disease necessitates the ability to evaluate both peripheral and myocardial effects to optimize therapy. The importance of this aspect of cardiovascular care is attested to by the large number of diagnostic modalities that have been applied to the measurement of ventricular function. Congenital heart disease remains one of the most challenging areas for the evaluation of ventricular performance because of complicating factors such as: (1) age- and size-related changes in myocardial and vascular performance, (2) the nearly universal presence of abnormal volume and/or pressure loads in structural heart disease, and (3) technical issues related to the increased risk and difficulty in obtaining invasive data from these patients, the need for sedation in small children, and the limited ability of infants and children to cooperate. The intent of this discussion is to review the general issues related to the assessment of myocardial contractility and loading conditions and to focus attention on those aspects of particular importance to the field of congenital heart disease. The technical aspects of data acquisition and methods of measurement for the various techniques are well covered elsewhere and will not be presented in detail here. Rather, the physiologic basis for the analysis and interpretation of the data will be emphasized, independent of the particular method by which flow, volume, pressure, or velocity data are acquired.

MYOCARDIAL VERSUS VENTRICULAR FUNCTION

The heart may be viewed as a pump designed to move blood from a low pressure venous reservoir to the high pressure arterial tree.[136,103] From this perspective, the critical aspects of cardiac performance relate to the maintenance of adequate flow rates at acceptable venous and arterial pressures. This can be likened to a "black box" approach, wherein the external aspects of the cardiac unit are examined with no attention to the internal workings of the machine. To a certain degree (that is, ignoring hormonal and autonomic control systems), this is the approach taken by the dependent organ systems. This attitude is reflected by the somewhat tongue-in-cheek attitude of the nephrologist who describes the organism as composed of kidneys and the renal-support system. To a large degree, the kidneys are unaware of the state of health of the heart, as long as an adequate renal arteriovenous pressure gradient is maintained while the kidneys allow passage of whatever nutrient flow they require. The success of this approach to cardiac performance is attested to by the common practice of monitoring arterial and venous pressures with cardiac output in the postoperative intensive care unit. Unfortunately, this view of the heart (as a pump) provides no direct information about the status of the myocardium (the heart viewed as a muscle). In fact, it is commonly observed that relatively severe myocardial dysfunction may coexist with normal arterial and venous pressures and normal cardiac output. From the point of view of the heart as a muscle, the function of the myocardium is to variably lengthen and shorten against a load. This can be effectively divided into diastole, during which the muscle must attain a certain length by

225

the application of a physiologically tolerable force, and systole, during which an adequate magnitude of shortening and force generation is required. The assessment of these two phases of the cardiac cycle will be considered individually, although the intimate relationship between systolic and diastolic performance makes their separate consideration somewhat artificial.

ASSESSMENT OF SYSTOLIC PERFORMANCE

In spite of recent advances in the understanding of myocardial mechanics, the percent of systolic fiber shortening (the absolute amount of systolic fiber shortening normalized for the end-diastolic fiber length) assessed clinically as percent of volume change (ejection fraction) or percent of change in dimensions (fractional shortening), remains the most common means for clinical evaluation of ventricular performance. Percent of shortening is a global descriptor of pump performance which incorporates arterioventricular and venoventricular interactions as well as the inotropic state, and, as such, has become firmly entrenched as a clinically useful tool. Although it is widely understood that the magnitude of shortening is the final product of a complex interplay of factors, which include vascular and hormonal influences, cardiac hypertrophy and geometry, and myocardial function,[13,35,102,138] nevertheless it is common clinical practice to equate the percent of shortening with myocardial contractility. Among the various factors that may account for this simplification is the observation that depressed contractility is the most common clinical cause of reduced percent of fiber shortening. Although a reduced percent of fiber shortening severe enough to cause congestive heart failure may be noted in the normal contractile state[27] and, conversely, a normal percent of shortening may be present in spite of abnormal contractility, these situations are less common. Hence,

for the majority of patients, use of more complex methods of evaluating ventricular performance may appear to be unnecessary. Nevertheless, it is clear that assessment of shortening alone fails to accurately reflect the contractile state of the myocardium in all subjects because of the additional effects of preload and afterload on the process of fiber shortening.[13]

Factors Influencing Fiber Shortening

Frequently, the terms "afterload," "preload," and "contractility" are used with only vague reference to their original meaning. Understanding how these terms are used in studies of isolated cardiac muscle is useful in conceptualizing their meaning when applied to the physiology of the intact heart. Much of our understanding of cardiac muscle physiology derives from studies performed using isolated strips of cardiac muscle. In experiments designed to assess the properties of isolated cardiac muscle, a strip of muscle is attached at one end to a movable lever to monitor muscle length and is fixed at the other end to a force transducer that records the strength and speed of contraction.[116] The lever system transmits an adjustable load to the muscle, which consists of two components. Weight is added to the trough to stretch the muscle to the desired length prior to the onset of contraction, and is therefore labelled the "preload." The amount of stretch induced by any preload depends on the distensibility or stiffness of the muscle. After the desired precontraction length is attained, a mechanical stop is attached to prevent further stretch. Any weight that is added thereafter will be encountered by the muscle only after the onset of shortening and, thus, represents the external force which resists shortening, or "afterload." It should be noted that in this experimental setup, there is a direct 1:1 relationship between the weight and the load. That is, the muscle shortens linearly and the weight is moved linearly

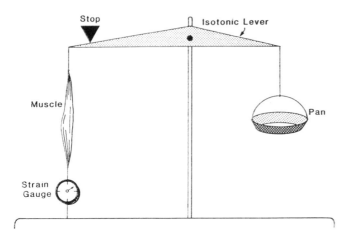

Figure 1. Setup for study of length-tension relationships in isolated cardiac muscle strips. The muscle is attached at one end to a movable lever to monitor muscle length and is fixed at the other end to a force transducer that records the strength and speed of contraction. Weight added to the pan exerts stretch on the muscle until the stop is attained. Further weight represents the afterload inasmuch as it does not affect the muscle until after the onset of contraction.

against gravity to an equal degree. Therefore, calculations of force, distance, work, etc. are direct and simple and necessitate no geometric assumptions. As will be discussed later, this simplicity is lost when the muscle fiber is assessed within the wall of the ventricle.

The isolated muscle preparation has generated a wealth of information. Reproducible relationships between the speed, strength, and degree of shortening and the loading conditions (afterload and preload) can be obtained using this system. The response to changes in afterload and/or preload are considered to represent external factors, whereas effects not ascribable to altered load are assumed to reflect intrinsic properties of the muscle which are incorporated in the somewhat intuitive notion of "contractility." This very useful working definition must be modified to accommodate experimental observations which indicate that loading status and contractility are not entirely independent factors, as will be discussed later. Nevertheless, for conceptual clarity it is useful to proceed initially from these straightforward distinctions.

Preload

In the isolated muscle, preload refers to the force needed to attain the desired precontraction length. Increasing this length while other conditions (afterload and contractility) are held constant results in increased total shortening, increased peak generated force, and higher peak velocity of shortening.[116] At the ultrastructural level, the explanation for the preload effect which has been commonly accepted is based on the sliding-filament model of contraction, in which the preload effect is believed to be due to length-dependent variation in the number of interacting cross bridges between contractile proteins.[91,1] Accordingly, an increase in end-diastolic fiber length alters the degree of myofilament overlap and increases the extent of shortening proportionally, much as the extent of recoil for a spring depends on the degree of stretch prior to release. However, experiments in isolated hearts have shown that changes in sarcomere length cannot fully account for the relation between length and force.[52,62,71,122] If the preload effect were entirely related to the mechanical effect of an increase in fiber length, the change in shortening should be precisely proportional to the increase in end-diastolic fiber length. In fact, the increase in shortening is in excess of what is anticipated, so that, for example, a 10% increase in end-diastolic fiber length results in more than a 10% increase in shortening. This phenomenon ("length-dependent activation") appears to be secondary to enhanced excitation-contraction coupling at longer muscle lengths,[62] implying that preload modulates the contractile state.

Regardless of the molecular mechanisms involved, at the fiber level preload is best repre-
sented by the end-diastolic fiber length. Extrapolation of this representation to the intact ventricle entails certain problems. Although preload in the intact ventricle is often estimated by parameters such as end-diastolic pressure, volume, or wall stress, each of these fails as a true representation of fiber length under certain conditions. Under normal circumstances, a rise in end-diastolic pressure results in greater end-diastolic fiber length. If there are external constraints (e.g., pericardial effusion or constriction or restrictive cardiomyopathy), this pressure-length relationship will be disturbed. Perhaps more problematic is the variability of pressure-volume relationships (that is, chamber compliance), making pressure an unreliable parameter for comparing preload among patients. Although atrial filling pressures are usually monitored in the postoperative period, in part as a measure of preload status, it is particularly under these circumstances that pressure may not reflect end-diastolic fiber length because of (1) altered myocardial compliance after cardiopulmonary bypass, (2) abnormal external constraint (mechanical ventillation, mediastinal edema, pericardial effusion), or (3) increased ventricular interaction due to elevation in right ventricular pressure (reactive pulmonary hypertension).

End-diastolic volume more directly reflects end-diastolic fiber length over the short term, but the ability of the ventricle to remodel and add fibers in series prevents this from being a useful index for comparing patients or assessing the same patient over long periods. End-diastolic stress provides a measure of the force distending the ventricle, providing true transmural pressure is measured. Because this is rarely possible in the clinical setting, the presence of significant external constraints invalidates the use of this index of preload. Perhaps more importantly, the primary assumption that underlies the estimation of end-diastolic fiber length from end-diastolic stress is that of a normal myocardial compliance (stress-strain relationship). Numerous conditions are known to invalidate this assumption (ischemia, fibrosis, drug therapy, effects of cardiopulmonary bypass). Thus, except under very well-controlled circumstances, each of these indices fails as an adequate measure of preload. Because end-diastolic fiber length cannot be directly measured *in vivo*, some alternative approach must be taken. An approach that will be presented in more detail subsequently relies on measuring the functional consequences of the existing preload conditions. In brief, because the magnitude of shortening depends on afterload, preload, and contractility, if afterload, contractility, and shortening can be directly measured, then preload can be calculated. Stated more intuitively, if the degree of shortening can be adjusted for the other factors that influence the contraction process, then the adjusted shortening will directly represent the end-diastolic fiber length, or preload.

Afterload

In the isolated muscle preparation, afterload refers to the weight or load that is faced by the contracting muscle, that is, the force resisting shortening. Although this force can be readily and directly measured in this experimental situation, when residing in the ventricle the force exerted by the muscle fibers is not directly measurable.[50] Frequently, the arterial pressure, resistance, or impedance is used as a measure of afterload.[16] However, these parameters fail to account for the geometric relationship between sarcomere shortening and force generation. It is possible to estimate this force based on the Laplace relationship between wall tension (T), pressure (P), and the radius of curvature (R) for thin-walled circular chambers where $T = P \times R$ (Fig. 2). Because there are multiple fibers across the ventricular wall and we are interested in obtaining the force on each fiber, the force must be adjusted for wall thickness (h) by calculating wall stress (force per unit area) as stress $= T/h = (P \times R)/h$. This, of course, is a mathematical simplification, because the radius of curvature of the inner wall in a thick-walled vessel is different from that of the outer wall. Therefore, it is customary to use mid-wall radius and to calculate the stress as a mean transmural value.

The heart is also nonspherical, so the radius of curvature is not uniform and, in fact, is different in the short-axis (circumferential) and long-axis (meridional) directions (Fig. 3). Certain geometric assumptions are necessary before a representative value for meridional and circumferential stress can be estimated, and several formulas have been proposed.[50,80,81,85,141] Although quantitatively dissimilar, yielding different absolute values for wall stress, the relative values obtained with these methods are comparable, undergoing parallel

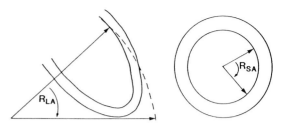

Figure 3. Although the short-axis radius of curvature (right figure) is uniform around the circumference of the ventricle, the long-axis radius of curvature varies continuously over the length of the ventricle.

changes with alterations in ventricular size and configuration.[51] Thus, it appears to be of greater importance to consider the assumptions made in the derivation rather than the exact formula that is employed. In each instance, the primary data from which these calculations are performed are the transmural pressure, the radius of curvature of the wall, and wall thickness. The radius and thickness data can be obtained from any of several modalities, including cineangiographic or radionuclide ventriculograms, echocardiograms, or magnetic resonance imaging. Similarly, pressure data can be obtained from either invasive or noninvasive means. Noninvasive aortic pressure can be obtained by recording indirect carotid (or axillary in young children) pulse waveforms calibrated with peripheral blood pressure.[20,21,23] The calibration is performed by assignment of systolic pressure to the peak of the tracing and diastolic pressure to the nadir, with simple linear interpolation to the intervening points (Fig. 4). If arterial pressure is not representative of left ventricular pressure because of aortic stenosis, end-systolic pressure in the aorta and left ventricle are still equal and, therefore, end-systolic stress can still be calculated.[11] In addition, Doppler measurement

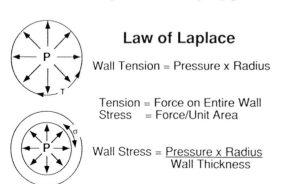

Law of Laplace

Wall Tension = Pressure x Radius

Tension = Force on Entire Wall
Stress   = Force/Unit Area

Wall Stress = $\dfrac{\text{Pressure x Radius}}{\text{Wall Thickness}}$

Figure 2. The Laplace relationship describes the relationship between the radius of curvature, transmural pressure, and wall tension. Division of tension by wall thickness provides a measure of the force per unit of cross sectional area.

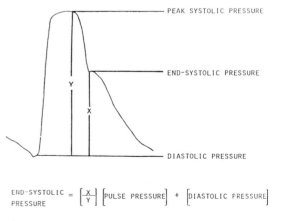

$$\begin{array}{l}\text{END-SYSTOLIC} \\ \text{PRESSURE}\end{array} = \left[\frac{X}{Y}\right]\left[\text{PULSE PRESSURE}\right] + \left[\text{DIASTOLIC PRESSURE}\right]$$

Figure 4. Estimation of end-systolic pressure from the carotid pulse tracing is performed by assignment of systolic pressure to the peak of the tracing and diastolic pressure to the nadir, with linear interpolation to the intervening points.

in the ascending aorta can be used to calculate the instantaneous transvalvar pressure gradient which, when added to aortic pressure, equals left ventricular pressure.[112] Thus, even in the presence of aortic stenosis it is possible to calculate wall stress throughout systole.

Of course, there are alternative approaches to assessing afterload. In particular, if one is interested in characterizing the pump performance of the heart, the arterial impedance (that is, the force resisting ejection) would provide more meaningful information.[69] However, recognizing that it may seem rather counterintuitive to characterize afterload in terms of measurements performed on the ventricle itself, it is worthwhile emphasizing that the intent is to quantify the factors that control myocardial performance, and hence we are interested in determining the afterload faced by the myofibrils rather than the ventricle as a whole. For the myocardium, it is the force opposing shortening within the wall which is the most direct measure of afterload. It is true that factors external to the heart (vascular resistance, capacitance, compliance, etc.) affect ventricular performance secondarily, but the means by which they affect myocardial performance is through their influence on wall stress.[64]

The transition from afterload as a constant weight in the isolated muscle preparation to afterload as wall stress in the intact ventricle introduces another level of complicity to the analysis, because wall stress is not constant during the course of the cardiac cycle. As shown in Figure 5, with the rise and fall of ventricular pressure, the decrease in ventricular dimension, and the increase in wall thickness during the contraction phase, wall stress rises rapidly to a peak value in early ejection, falls in a near-linear fashion to the end of ejection, and then drops more rapidly to diastolic levels. Therefore, the instantaneous afterload is a dynamic variable, leading naturally to the question as to which

phase of the process of stress development and decay is most physiologically relevant. Various investigators have used peak, mean, total systolic (stress-time integral) and end-systolic stress as indices of afterload. Each of these components has a different physiologic significance, and the appropriate index of afterload depends on the question that is to be addressed. That is, because myocardial oxygen consumption correlates more closely with total stress (stress-time integral) than with other stress indices,[68,121,126,135] this is the appropriate index when using wall stress to predict myocardial substrate utilization. Similarly, peak wall stress correlates most closely with the magnitude of hypertrophy[11,26,33,40,44,45] and, thus, is the appropriate stress index when assessing a stimulus to hypertrophy or the adequacy of hypertrophy. However, the measure of afterload which relates most closely to systolic performance is the stress at the end of systole. That is, end-systolic stress is the force that determines the extent of systolic shortening and is the index of afterload that is most relevant to the assessment of ventricular function. Because this is by no means intuitively obvious and because alternative measures of afterload are frequently used in assessing ventricular performance, it is worthwhile reviewing the evidence that this is in fact the case. A series of observations in isolated muscle preparations and whole ventricles have revealed several fundamental properties of cardiac muscle which are relevant to this discussion.

End-systolic stress determines end-systolic length at a constant contractile state. Isometric contractions in isolated muscle preparations at a constant inotropic state demonstrate a linear relation between length and peak force generation such that increasing the length of the muscle leads to a proportional increase in force generation (Fig. 6).[53,116,117] Because muscle length is constant, it cannot be determined whether this is an effect of end-

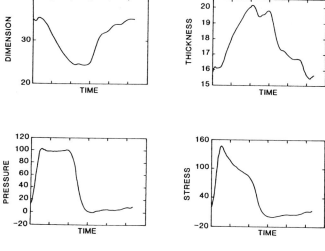

Figure 5. With the rise and fall of ventricular pressure, the fall in ventricular dimension, and the rise in wall thickness during the contraction phase, wall stress rises rapidly to a peak value in early ejection, falls in a near-linear fashion to end-ejection, and then drops more rapidly to diastolic levels.

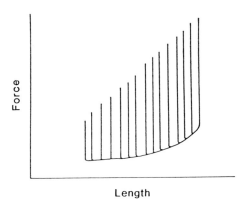

Figure 6. Isometric contractions in isolated muscle preparations at a constant inotropic state demonstrate a linear relation between length and peak force generation such that increasing the length of the muscle leads to a proportional augmentation of force generation.

diastolic length (preload) or end-systolic length. When the muscle is allowed to shorten isotonically (Fig. 7) or shortens against a variable load from a fixed end-diastolic length (Fig. 8), the determinant of this relation is the end-systolic length, because a linear end-systolic force-length relation is maintained independent of the end-diastolic length. Equivalent relationships are present in the intact ventricle, where a linear end-systolic stress-volume or pressure-volume relation is found in both isovolumic and ejecting ventricles.[123,128,131,137] Conceptually, the myocardium continues to contract until the critical force-length relation is encountered, at which time relaxation ensues. The force-length relation is relatively independent of the events earlier in the cardiac cycle (the ejection force-length trajectory), or, in other words, it is relatively history-independent.[128] The limitations on this history-independence will be discussed later, but within the confines of these limits, end-

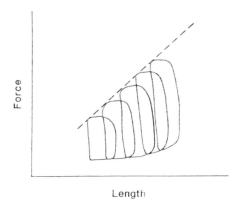

Figure 7. When the muscle is allowed to shorten isotonically, the determinant of the rise in force is seen to be the end-systolic length, because a linear end-systolic force-length relation is maintained independent of the end-diastolic length.

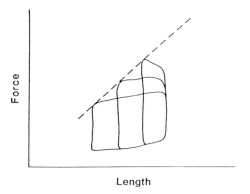

Figure 8. When the muscle shortens against a variable load from a fixed end-diastolic length, the same linear end-systolic-force-length relation is maintained.

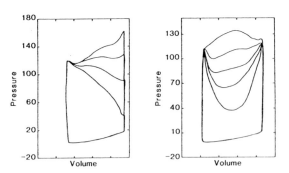

Figure 9. When isolated heart preparations are held at a fixed end-systolic and end-diastolic volume (and therefore by necessity end-systolic and end-diastolic wall thicknesses are also invariant), the ejection conditions can be varied widely and the same end-systolic pressure is attained. Thus, wall stress varies substantially at all points in the cardiac cycle without affecting end-systolic volume and ejected volume, providing end-systolic pressure is constant. (Modified from Suga H, et al.,[128] with permission.)

systolic force is the determinant of end-systolic length for any constant contractile state.

Wall stress at all phases of systole except end-systole can be altered without associated change in myocardial shortening. When isolated heart preparations are held at a fixed end-systolic and end-diastolic volume (therefore, by necessity, end-systolic and end-diastolic wall thicknesses are constant also), the ejection conditions can be varied widely and the same end-systolic pressure will be attained (Fig. 9).[128] Thus, end-systolic wall stress is constant as long as shortening is constant, even though peak and mean ejection pressure and peak, mean, and total wall stress are variable, indicating that shortening is independent of peak, mean, and total wall stress. Stated from the opposite perspective, a variable ejection resistance does not alter total shortening as long as end-systolic pressure is constant. Again, this means that peak, mean, and total wall stress can vary without affecting shortening.

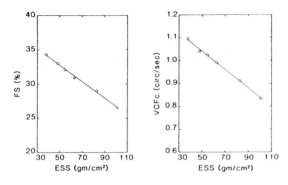

Figure 10. Data obtained in a single individual during infusion of the alpha-adrenergic agent, methoxamine. End-systolic stress and ventricular performance, assessed by either fractional shortening or the velocity of shortening, are closely related in an inversely linear fashion.

End-systolic stress and ventricular performance are closely related in an inversely linear fashion, whereas performance does not correlate with peak, mean, or total wall stress. In any individual, elevation of afterload by the infusion of the pure alpha-adrenergic agonist methoxamine results in a linear relationship between end-systolic stress and both the velocity and magnitude of shortening (Fig. 10).[10,22]

A similar relationship is noted when the results from a large number of individuals are combined (Fig. 11) with slope values for individuals which parallel the population slope (Fig. 12). The correlation between either index of function and peak, mean, and total wall stress is poor and relates only to the normal close association (colinearity) between end-systolic stress and stress at other points in the cardiac cycle.[11] This relationship has been confirmed also in patients with cardiac and noncardiac disease.[11,26,27,29,36,41,42,63,65,66,101] Thus, the force resisting shortening at the completion of contraction determines when shortening ceases. End-systolic wall stress is the quantitative measure of the force that is faced by the muscle at this point in the cardiac cycle, and is therefore the measure

of afterload, which is most relevant to ventricular function.

As would be expected, there are limits to the degree to which end-systolic force determines end-systolic fiber length. In particular, if the isometric end-systolic length-tension relationship is compared with the end-systolic length-tension relationship found when shortening is permitted, the end-systolic length is longer in the latter situation.[78,113,124,128,129] In essence, the length attained when the muscle shortens is less than would be predicted based on the isometric relation. This phenomenon has been labeled "shortening deactivation" and represents an actual loss of the maximum force-generating capacity (contractility) of the muscle caused by the process of shortening.[62] Because this fall in contractility is proportional to the overall magnitude of shortening, and because shortening is dependent on end-systolic stress, this represents at least a potential means by which changes in afterload may alter contractility. Of course, this disturbs the conceptual framework of afterload, preload, and contractility as independent determinants of ventricular function. Similarly, the preload-related phenomenon of "length-dependent activation" is representative of a process by which loading conditions may modulate contractile state. Although the magnitude of these effects is not clear, in the intact heart length-dependent activation and shortening deactivation appear to counterbalance each other to a large extent.[5,52,56,132]

Contractility

As previously defined, contractility refers to the intrinsic properties of cardiac muscle, that is, those contractile characteristics that are not secondary to afterload or preload. Although this distinction is somewhat artificial inasmuch as preload and afterload may, in fact, influence contractility under certain circumstances, the concept is very useful in the understanding of cardiovascular physiology, providing the limits are understood. The search for a precise, load-independent measure of contractility has been likened to the quest for the holy

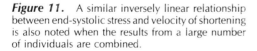

Figure 11. A similar inversely linear relationship between end-systolic stress and velocity of shortening is also noted when the results from a large number of individuals are combined.

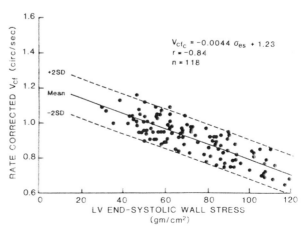

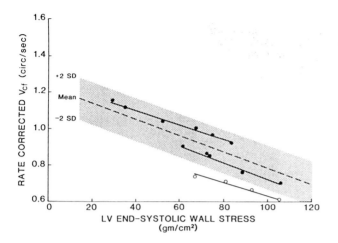

Figure 12. The slope of the stress-velocity relationship in any individual (solid lines) runs parallel to the slope of other individuals and to the slope of the population regression.

grail, and great skepticism exists as to the existence of such an index. In fact, the understanding of myocardial physiology has been enormously expanded by these efforts, as the usefulness and limits of each of these various indices of cardiac performance have been explored. The chronology of these efforts has been recounted in a number of excellent reviews[14,57,103] and will not be repeated here. Rather, an attempt will be made to present the approach that we have found to be the most clinically informative and useful, as well as a brief discussion of the strengths and weaknesses of several indices in common clinical use.

Ventricular Pressure-Volume Relationships. Much of our current understanding of the physiology of myocardial contractility is based on examination of myocardial force-length relationships and their equivalent in the intact heart and in the ventricular pressure-volume and stress-volume curves. As detailed in the discussion of afterload, for any given contractile state, there is a unique end-systolic force-length (or pressure-volume) relationship that is linear, at least within the physiologic range of ventricular volumes. When the contractile state is augmented (for example, during catecholamine infusion), the degree of shortening is increased for any end-systolic pressure, and the attained end-systolic pressure is higher for any end-systolic volume.[131] In effect, the end-systolic pressure-volume relation (ESPVR) is shifted to the left (Fig. 13). In addition, the slope of the ESPVR is more steep. The opposite effect is seen with a fall in contractility, which results in a rightward shift and a shallower slope to the ESPVR. Because the ESPVR is independent of the preload (within limits to be discussed subsequently) and because afterload is directly incorporated, the ESPVR provides a relatively load-independent measure of the contractile state.[107,130]

Calculation of the ESPVR involves the collection of pressure-volume or pressure-dimension data over a range of end-systolic pressures at a constant

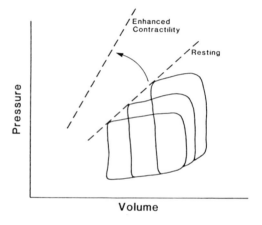

Figure 13. When the contractile state is augmented (for example, during catecholamine infusion), the end-systolic pressure-volume relation (ESPVR) is shifted to the left with a higher slope.

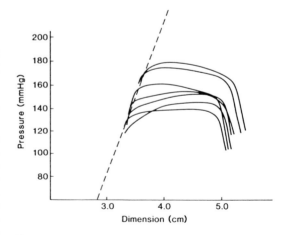

Figure 14. The end-systolic pressure-volume relation can be obtained clinically, either invasively or noninvasively, by collecting pressure-volume or pressure-dimension data over a range of end-systolic pressures at a constant contractile state.[27]

contractile state (Fig. 14). Alteration of end-systolic pressure can be performed by several methods, including transient occlusion of the inferior vena cava, pharmacologic manipulation of load with vasoconstrictors or vasodilators, or partial aortic occlusion. Although several invasive and noninvasive methods for clinical assessment of the ESPVR have been reported, several problems with this analysis have not been fully overcome. The ESPVR, although linear and load-independent in the isolated dog heart model,[123,131,133] has been shown to be nonlinear under other conditions, both from a theoretical approach[84] and from experimental observations,[17,56,75,122] and it is not entirely load-independent.[5,31,38,78,118] Because the degree of nonlinearity is variable, data must be gathered over a wide range of pressure values for any meaningful curve-fitting calculations. Although the position and steepness of the relation can be used to detect changes in contractile state in the same subject,[27] the slope of the ESPVR is dependent on absolute ventricular size,[8,127] making comparison of subjects with differences in ventricular size uncertain. Because data must be obtained over a range of end-systolic pressures, there is considerable opportunity for reflex alteration in autonomic tone in response to the elevation or reduction of blood pressure, thereby potentially altering the inotropic state during data collection, which would invalidate the data analysis. The need for pressure manipulation prevents frequent repetition of the test, precludes reassessment over short intervals, and renders the test, at best, cumbersome and, at worst, unusable for routine clinical use. Finally, assessment of contractility by this technique does not yield a direct measurement of loading status.

Several indices, theoretically based on the endsystolic pressure-volume relationship but obtainable without the need for afterload manipulation, have been reported. If the assumption is made that the line of the end-systolic pressure-volume relationship passes through the origin (Fig. 15), then any single end-systolic pressure-volume ratio can be used as an index of contractility. Although this type of single-point analysis has been used by many investigators, the limitations should be recognized. Essentially, this type of comparison forces the endsystolic pressure-volume relation through zero. The error incurred is the greatest in large ventricles, where a steep ESPVR with a large volume intercept will be misrepresented as a shallow ESPVR (Fig. 15), leading to the misdiagnosis of reduced contractility.

Stress-shortening and Stress-Velocity Analysis. As an alternative to methods for assessing contractility which rely on load manipulation, the possibility of fully accounting for the influence of loading conditions on ejection performance has been explored. Both percent of fractional shortening (FS) and the mean velocity of shortening (VCF) are in-

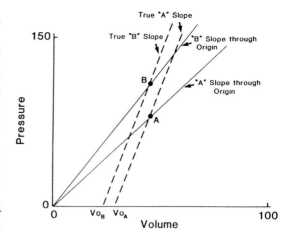

Figure 15. Potential error is incurred by the use of the end-systolic pressure-volume ratio as an index of contractility. Use of this index assumes that the end-systolic pressure-volume relationship passes through the origin. When the single end-systolic pressure-volume value is used to estimate Emax, the conclusion is reached that the contractile state for point B is better than for point A, because the slope through the origin is steeper (solid lines). However, the possibility also exists that these represent ventricles with different zero-pressure volumes, but equal contractility because the true Emax values (dotted lines) are equal.

dices of contractility known to be dependent on loading status. When end-systolic stress is used to assess afterload, FS and VCF are found to fall in an inversely linear fashion during afterload augmentation.[22] Of particular interest, the slopes of the stress-velocity and stress-shortening relations are the same in different individuals, and the slope in any individual parallels the mean population regression. The stress-shortening and stress-velocity relationships are sensitive to contractility (Fig. 16) and, thus, represent indices of contractility which incorporate afterload. Numerous examples of the clinical application of these indices have been reported.[11,26,27,29,36,41,42,48,63,65,66]

Although either of these indices permits assessment of contractility independent of afterload effects, it is through the combination of the two that a complete description of the factors influencing cardiac performance can be obtained because of the differential effects of preload on VCF and FS. Increased preload is known to augment fiber shortening and therefore FS. The effect of changes in preload on the stress-shortening relation is predictable (Fig. 17) and mimics the effect of changes in contractility. Thus, the stress-shortening relation fails to distinguish the effects of altered preload from altered contractility. In contrast, VCF is not dependent on preload.[22,76,90,99,100] Although there are almost certainly limits to the extent of this preload-independence, variations in preload within the physiologic range do not significantly alter VCF. The lack of effect of end-diastolic fiber length

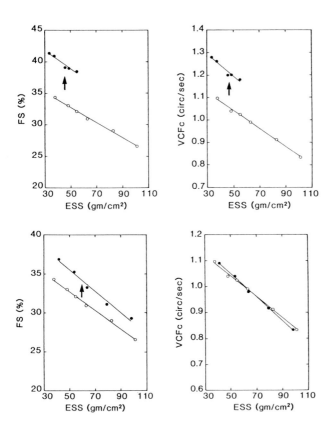

Figure 16. Infusion of dobutamine results in an upward shift of the stress-shortening and stress-velocity relationships. Thus, for any level of afterload, enhanced contractility results in higher magnitude and velocity of shortening.

Figure 17. The effect of preload augmentation on the stress-shortening and stress-velocity relationships in one subject is shown. The effect of changes in preload on the stress-shortening relation is predictable and mimics the effect of changes in contractility. The lack of effect of end-diastolic fiber length on both end-systolic stress and VCF accounts for the preload independence of the stress-velocity relation.

on both end-systolic stress and VCF accounts for the preload-independence of the stress-velocity relation (Fig. 17).[22] Thus, the stress-velocity relation represents a preload-independent index of contractility which incorporates afterload. When stress-velocity analysis is combined with stress-shortening analysis, abnormalities in fiber shortening not related to afterload or contractility (as assessed by the stress-velocity relation) can be recognized as being secondary to preload effects.

It is also possible to address these calculations in a more analytic fashion. Because percent of fiber shortening depends on the end-diastolic fiber length (preload), the force resisting shortening (afterload), the frequency of contraction (heart rate), and contractility, it should be possible to express quantitatively the percent of fiber shortening (Δl) as a function (f) of preload (λ), afterload (σ), heart rate (v), and contractility (c) as follows:

$$(1) \qquad \Delta l = f(\lambda, \sigma, v, c)$$

The effect of the frequency of contraction on shortening appears to be mediated primarily through effects on contractility, whereby it is possible to express observed contractility (c') as a function (f') of heart rate and the rate-independent contractile state (c):

$$(2) \qquad c' = f'(v, c)$$

and formula (1) can be rewritten as:

$$(3) \qquad \Delta l = f(\lambda, \sigma, c')$$

Because VCF is a function (f'') of afterload (σ) and contractility (c):

$$(4) \qquad VCF = f''(\sigma, c)$$

Afterload can be calculated as end-systolic stress and VCF can be measured directly; this equation can be solved for c and this value for contractility can be substituted in formula (3):

$$(5) \qquad \Delta l = f(\lambda, \sigma, c)$$

Because σ (afterload) is obtained as end-systolic stress and Δl is a measured value, this yields λ (preload) directly.

The stress-shortening relation has been used as an index of contractility by a number of authors[19,46,108] without adjustment for preload effects. This simplification can be justified when preload effects are unlikely to be significant. Under normal circumstances, the left ventricle operates near the peak of the Frank-Starling mechanism, particularly when measurements are performed with the patient in the supine position.[95] This accounts for the absence of preload augmentation during supine exercise, in contrast to the utilization of preload reserve which accompanies upright exercise.[98] Thus, the assumption has been made that preload effects are negligible under usual physiologic circumstances in humans.[95,104] Certainly, there are circumstances under which this assumption is invalid. For example, during hemodialysis there is a striking reduction in preload manifested as a disproportionate fall in shortening compared with changes in the velocity of shortening (Fig. 18).[27] Similarly, long-distance runners manifest a reduction in the stress-adjusted shortening fraction secondary to reduced preload when assessed at rest.[26] This finding can be understood as a ventricle adapted to a large volume load which is assessed when the volume load is not present, that is, in the preload-reduced state. Postoperative patients whose fluids are restricted and who are treated with diuretics manifest a reduced preload.[29] Preload-related changes in myocardial shortening have been shown to have a significant impact on the assessment of ventricular performance in the presence of aortic or mitral regurgitation.[83] Although it may be possible to define those physiologic states

in which preload effects can safely be ignored, it is almost certainly preferable to measure them directly through the use of combined stress-shortening and stress-velocity analysis.

Noninvasive Stress-Velocity and Stress-shortening Methods. Although the data necessary to calculate stress-shortening and stress-velocity indices can be obtained from invasive as well as noninvasive studies, it is the ease with which noninvasive assessment can be performed which allows wide applicability. Noninvasive estimation of end-systolic pressure from the carotid or axillary pulse tracing has been verified against invasive measurements.[20,21,23] It can be argued that in some subjects there will be a difference between the carotid and aortic root pressure contours due to peripheral wave reflections and differences in transmission rate of pressure harmonics.[79] At The Boston Children's Hospital, we have not found these effects to introduce more than a 3–7% error in the pressure measurement or stress calculation,[21,23] although we have not investigated subjects with peripheral vascular disease. In some subjects definition of the dicrotic notch may be difficult. We have encountered this difficulty in subjects with severe aortic regurgitation in whom the descent of the aortic pulse contour is virtually undisturbed by aortic valve closure. There are also subjects in whom multiple notches are found on the pulse descent because of reflected waves superimposed on the primary pulse contour. In these instances the ejection time can be obtained from the aortic valve M-mode or Doppler examination of the aorta and then used to obtain the exact time of end-systole on the pulse contour. Although several investigators have used peak pressure to estimate end-systolic stress, this is clearly not justifiable when the normal ratio of peak to end-systolic pressure fails to hold. It is not possible to recognize with certainty the situations in which peak and end-systolic pressure diverge without measuring end-systolic pressure (in which case the approximation is no longer needed!). Even the assumption that the approximation is valid for repeated measurements in the same individual is not valid if hemodynamic conditions are not constant.[27,79]

The calculations for both wall stress and the indices of ventricular function (FS and VCF) assume a symmetric ventricular configuration and pattern of contraction. In the normally shaped ventricle, the radius of curvature of the posterior wall along both the major and minor axes can be measured directly from long- and short-axis imaging data. If there are regional abnormalities in shape or if the ventricle is distorted because of septal displacement (right ventricular pressure or volume overload) the major and minor axes will not accurately reflect the radius of curvature of the posterior wall and the standard formulas for calculation of wall stress cannot be used. In any case, under these

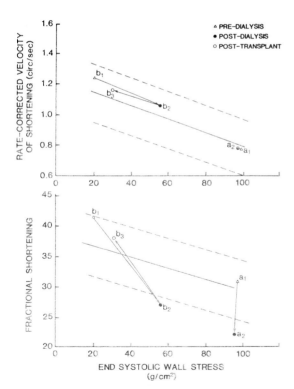

Figure 18. Two subjects evaluated before and after dialysis and/or transplantation. Subject 'a' experienced a marked reduction in fractional shortening in spite of little change in afterload (end-systolic stress is unchanged) and no change in contractility (the stress-velocity relation is unchanged). These findings are consistent with preload effects alone. Subject 'b' experienced a rise in afterload (higher end-systolic stress) after dialysis with secondary and proportional reduction in the velocity of shortening, indicating no change in contractility. The disproportionate fall in fractional shortening is indicative of reduced preload.

circumstances the marked variance in fiber load and shortening will invalidate global shortening characteristics as an adequate index of ventricular performance.

The assumptions concerning ventricular geometry which underlie the stress calculations are equally applicable to the indices of ventricular performance. The calculation of either percent or mean velocity of shortening as a global parameter relies on a symmetric pattern of contraction and a circular cross-sectional configuration. That is, because these calculations use changes in dimension to estimate alteration in fiber length, there must be a constant and known geometric relation between circumference and dimension. Although these indices have been calculated in subjects in whom the left ventricular configuration and change in systolic shape during contraction are clearly abnormal,[77] there is no reliable relation to myofiber shortening or contractility in this situation.

In addition to the fact that tests provide accurate data of value to patient care, the feasibility of performing and repeating a test is a major consideration for its clinical utility. From a practical point of view, there are few patients in whom these data cannot be obtained. There is no risk to the patient and there are no concerns about distortion of the hemodynamic state by the test itself. At The Boston Children's Hospital, we have found that sedation of infants is often necessary, but this is a part of our laboratory routine and does not add an additional burden. The ability to perform the test without disturbing the baseline hemodynamics also enables critically ill patients to be evaluated in the intensive care unit. The frequent repeatability of the test provides a particularly valuable contribution in this setting. Also, data have been collected from hundreds of normal subjects, including more than a hundred less than 4 years of age. This is a nearly impossible task when interventions must be performed, invasive data are needed, or radiographic procedures are included.

Application of Stress-Velocity and Stress-shortening Analysis. One of the primary reasons for considering the clinical use of more complex indices of myocardial performance is the assumption that the data that are obtained provide more useful information than the data obtained from the percent of fiber shortening alone. Stress-velocity and stress-shortening analyses have been used to address a number of clinically important issues that could not be adequately addressed using shortening data alone. For example, like many other investigators, we at The Children's Hospital in Boston have found that reversible abnormalities in shortening fraction are commonly seen in subjects with chronic renal failure. However, we found that even severely depressed FS and VCF in these subjects were entirely due to altered load rather than to abnormal contractility (Fig. 18).[27] Similarly, we

found that the reduced systolic function found in some endurance athletes and the enhanced function noted in others could be fully accounted for by altered load,[26] without the need to hypothesize either reduced or enhanced contractility as has been suggested by other investigators. The enhanced function characteristic of congenital aortic stenosis was found to be related to reduced afterload, whereas the reduced function commonly noted in hypertension secondary to coarctation of the aorta derives from the combination of excess afterload and reduced contractility.[11] Using these methods, the enhanced systolic ventricular performance typical of subjects with hyperthyroidism was shown to represent a true increase in contractility rather than the secondary effects of altered rate or load.[36] Both the acute fall in preload with diuretic therapy and the rise in contractility after administration of digitalis could be recognized in early postoperative patients in spite of the nearly balancing effects of these changes on the percent of fiber shortening.[29] In each of these situations, combined stress-shortening and stress-velocity analysis provided insight into the cardiovascular status which either was not detectable or was misrepresented by analysis of the percent of fiber shortening alone.

Recently, at The Children's Hospital in Boston, we have had the opportunity to examine a number of adolescents with Duchenne's muscular dystrophy who were scheduled to undergo spinal fusion for severe scoliosis. We found, as have others in the past, that the percent of fiber shortening was reduced in the majority (66%) of these patients. However, as shown in Figure 19, the reduction in systolic performance was predominantly due to excess afterload without significant reduction in con-

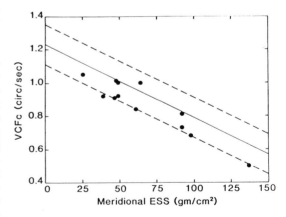

Figure 19. Stress-velocity relationships in a group of adolescents with Duchenne's muscular dystrophy who were scheduled to undergo spinal fusion for severe scoliosis. Reduced systolic performance was common and was secondary to excess afterload (elevated end-systolic stress) without significant reduction in contractility (the stress-velocity relation is normal).

tractility. The increase in afterload was due to reduced ventricular mass without chamber enlargement or systemic hypertension. Pathologically, this disease is characterized by myofibril dropout and fatty or fibrous replacement. The stress-velocity analysis is consistent with the pathologic findings of reduced working muscle, but implies near-normal performance of the residual myocardium. Studies based on shortening fraction alone, without assessment of loading status, have concluded that impaired contractility is typical of this disease when, in fact, this does not appear to be the case.

As a final example of the utility of this method, infants and young children commonly are observed to have increased systolic performance, but the cause (increased contractility or altered load) is not known. The changes in FS and VCF with age are presented in Figure 20. Without adjustment for load, there appears to be a dramatic age-related

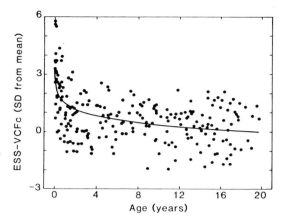

Figure 22.   The stress-shortening relation falls with age, with the most prominent effect in the first two years of life. This is consistent with age-modulation of contractility.

decline in contractility. However, in actuality, there is a substantial rise in afterload with growth (Fig. 21) which accounts for much of the observed change in ventricular performance. Nevertheless, even when load is considered, there is still a measurable fall in contractility with age, with the most prominent effect in the first 2 years of life (Fig. 22).[28]

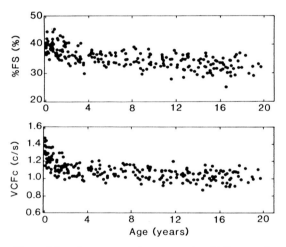

Figure 20.   There is a significant age-related fall in systolic performance, measured as fractional shortening or the velocity of shortening in normal children.

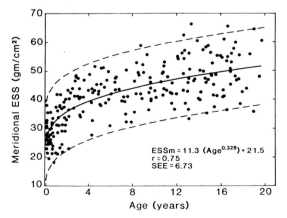

$$ESSm = 11.3 \ (Age^{0.328}) + 21.5$$
$$r = 0.75$$
$$SEE = 6.73$$

Figure 21.   There is a significant age-related rise in afterload in normal subjects.

ASSESSMENT OF DIASTOLIC PERFORMANCE

Abnormalities of ventricular filling, although less commonly recognized than systolic dysfunction, constitute an active area of basic and clinical investigation. It has become apparent in recent years that the failure to recognize diastolic dysfunction is more frequently due to inadequate means of detection and quantification than to the rarity of the disorder. Although the available methods for assessing diastolic function are expanding, clinical assessment of diastole still has not attained the level of ease, accuracy, and routine associated with evaluation of systolic function. This situation is likely to change as the level of understanding and the available methods improve. In fact, because of the intimate relationship between systolic and diastolic function, an adequate understanding of systolic abnormalities necessitates an improved approach to diastole.

Typically, diastole is taken to encompass that period from cessation of ejection (just prior to aortic valve closure) to the onset of the rapid rise in pressure during contraction. Hemodynamically, this period encompasses protodiastole, isovolumic relaxation, rapid filling, diastasis, and atrial contraction. From the aspect of myocardial mechanics, the primary event is muscle lengthening in response to a combination of effects which either inhibit or promote lengthening. It is customary to divide discussions about diastole into an early, active phase of relaxation, when changes in force and length are primarily the result of changes within the myocardium, and a later, passive phase, during which changes in force and length are primarily the result of external forces. Therefore, abnormalities of diastolic performance are generally related to the corresponding processes of active relaxation and passive myocardial compliance.[74] These represent distinct properties of the myocardium which may vary independently from each other.[47] However, because the process of relaxation is not completed until after the onset of filling, these events overlap in time to a variable degree. Although it is instructive to discuss relaxation and compliance as separate phenomena, it must be recognized also that this period of overlap is of considerable importance when clinical indices of diastolic performance are considered.

Ventricular Relaxation

Abnormal relaxation has been identified in association with a number of cardiac disorders. In particular, ischemia has been noted to result in profound alteration in the rate at which pressure falls during isovolumic relaxation.[43,87,105] In the presence of ischemia, abnormalities of relaxation are detectable prior to any changes in systolic performance, a finding that is not unexpected when the energetics of contraction and relaxation are considered.[58] The mechanisms involved in relaxation of cardiac muscle are believed to relate to both activation-controlled and load-controlled decay mechanisms. The activation-controlled loss of force within the ventricular wall which occurs early in diastole is an active, energy-consuming process, accounting for as much as 15% of the total energy utilized by the beating heart.[67,88] Although the precise relationship between Ca^{++} uptake and the changes in muscle length and tension which occur during diastole are not completely understood, it is generally agreed that the initiating event in relaxation is a reduction of cytosolic Ca^{++} by the calcium pump of the sarcoplasmic reticulum. It appears that adenosine triphosphate-dependent calcium sequestration by the sarcoplasmic reticulum results in actin-myosin dissociation caused by reduction of the Ca^{++} concentration in the region of the myofilament below the level needed for myofibrillar adenosine triphosphatase activation. In isolated muscle preparations, there are also substantial effects of load on the process of relaxation.[15,16] In contrast to the inactivation-controlled relaxation process, which relates to sequestration of Ca^{++} by the sarcoplasmic reticulum, the effect of load on relaxation is believed to be related to load-induced forcible detachment of the cross bridges which occurs when the stretching forces exceed the force level that the sum of the cross bridges are capable of sustaining.[15]

Indices of Relaxation

Generally, the measurement of relaxation in the intact ventricle is based on indices calculated from ventricular pressure-time relations during isovolumic relaxation. During this period of the cardiac cycle, ventricular volume is constant, and therefore, it may be assumed that dimension and wall thickness are also constant. If these assumptions are valid, decreases in wall tension, wall stress, and pressure are parallel processes and changes in pressure accurately reflect changes in force. In fact, because of alteration of ventricular conformation during isovolumic relaxation, changes in pressure and stress are not strictly equivalent. That is, as discussed earlier, wall stress relates to the local radius of curvature. During systole, the ventricle shortens proportionally more in the short than in the long axis, assuming a more elliptical shape. Diastolic lengthening is temporally and spatially nonuniform,[72,109] resulting in some change in shape even during isovolumic diastole. However, because the change in shape is small compared with the change in pressure, it is generally neglected. The pressure-based indices that have been employed are based on the observation that during isovolumic relaxation pressure falls in an exponential fashion. Because the peak rate of pressure decrease $[(dP/dt)_{min}]$ nearly always occurs after completion of ejection, the pressure trace from $(dP/dt)_{min}$ to the time of mitral valve opening (pressure crossover point for left atrial and left ventricular pressure) can be fit to a curve of the form:

$$P_t = P_o e^{-t/\tau} + P_b$$

where P_t = pressure as a function of time, P_o = pressure at the time of $(dP/dt)_{min}$, t = time, τ = time constant of relaxation, and P_b = asymptotic pressure. Thus, the time constant τ represents the time required for pressure at $(dP/dt)_{min}$ to be reduced by $1/e$.

Figure 23 represents the differences between several of the methods that have been suggested to calculate τ. Nonlinear, iterative, curve-fitting methods yield an excellent fit, but the solution obtained is not unique because it depends on estimates of the initial parameter and on convergence criteria. By assuming a zero asymptote (P_b), the resulting simplification can be fit to a curve of the form $ln\ P = ln\ P_o - \tau/t$ by standard linear methods. This assumption is not always correct and will incorrectly predict a change in relaxation in the presence of a baseline shift.[114] Alternatively, the first derivative of pressure with respect to time (dP/dt) can be fit to an equation of the form:

$$dP/dt = -(1/\tau)(P_t - P_b)$$

This method accounts for changes in the asymptotic pressure, but the time constant is not equiv-

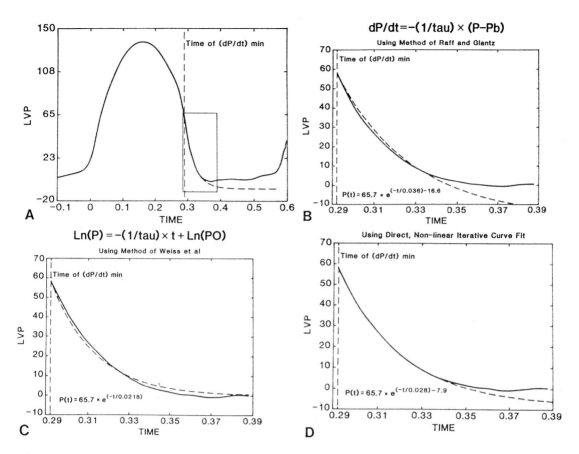

Figure 23. Differences obtained with the various methods of calculating the time constant of relaxation. **A,** Left ventricular pressure for a single cardiac cycle. The isovolumic relaxation period and the early portion of cardiac filling are the time periods of interest, as indicated by the boxed region. **B, C,** and **D,** The goodness of fit for the derived equation using several of the published methods. In each case, the original pressure tracing (solid line) is shown with the predicted pressure tracing (interrupted line) calculated using the Tau value obtained by the indicated method. The method of Weiss et al. assumes a zero asymptote, distorting the early portion of the curve fit as shown in panel C. The incorporation of a non-zero asymptote in the method of Raff and Glanz (**B**) improves the fit, but the residual variance is still high, as indicated by the visible difference between predicted and measured pressure. In contrast, a direct nonlinear iterative solution provides an excellent modeling of the isovolumic relaxation period, as shown in **D,** where deviation of the predicted from the measured value occurs only after onset of filling.

alent to the original definition. In addition, the use of time derivatives calculated from analog or digital signals introduces considerable and unpredictable noise amplification. In view of these issues, at The Boston Children's Hospital, we have elected to use iterative, nonlinear, curve-fitting techniques. Although the solution obtained by these methods depends on estimates of the initial parameter and on the iterative termination criterion, if the initial parameter estimates are based on a method with a single solution (such as a linear fit) and the convergence criterion is held constant, the solution will be unique.

Factors Affecting Relaxation

Differentiation of intrinsic myocardial relaxation abnormalities from those secondary to external influences requires a consideration of the factors that are known to influence this process. Most promi-

nent among these are load-dependent mechanisms of relaxation which have been extensively described in isolated muscle preparations. Although the presence of load-controlled decay mechanisms in cardiac muscle has been widely documented, the physiologic importance of these mechanisms for the intact ventricle remains controversial. In principle, the effects of load-dependent control of relaxation could be mediated by hemodynamic loading during late ejection, during isovolumic relaxation, and during the period of rapid filling. There has been substantial disagreement concerning the effect of altered load on ventricular relaxation in animal studies,[119] with relatively few studies available in humans. However, in a study by Starling and associates,[119] moderate alterations in load were not found to affect the process of isovolumic relaxation in humans. Similarly, because ventricular relaxation indices rely on the global parameter of chamber pressure rather than on events at the sarcomere level, nonuniform contraction and relaxation causes prolongation of τ and altered early filling patterns in animals[73] and humans.[9,61]

Usually, changes in contractility and systolic shortening are associated with significant changes in relaxation and appear to act through a similar mechanism. Because the inactivation mechanism is distinct from the activation mechanism involved in contraction, changes in relaxation may not always parallel changes in contractility. Thus, isoproterenol increases both contractility and the rate of relaxation, but an increase in calcium concentration impairs relaxation while augmenting contractility. The number of cross bridges and the duration of their cycle can be altered by various mechanisms which, in turn, play a major role in determining the decline in force during relaxation. These mechanisms act either by "sensitizing the contractile protein," resulting in a slower and later decline in force, or by "desensitization of the contractile protein," resulting in an earlier and faster decline in force.[139] In addition to pharmacologic agents, some mechanical control mechanisms, such as the magnitude of shortening, may also act in this fashion. In isolated muscle preparations, the affinity of troponin-C for calcium appears to relate inversely to the magnitude of shortening.[6,49,94] The reduction in bound calcium which results from the process of shortening enhances the rate of relaxation and the load-induced rapid lengthening. Thus, the rate of relaxation is dependent on the total magnitude of shortening, whether altered by preload, afterload, or contractility. The physiologic significance of shortening enhancement of relaxation, independent of changes in contractility, is uncertain. Changes in contractility have a measurable effect on the time constant of relaxation, whereas load-induced changes in systolic performance at a constant contractile state do not alter relaxation rate reliably.

An additional factor that plays an important role early in diastole is elastic recoil. The ventricle is capable of generating negative pressures early in diastole, thereby facilitating filling through a process of diastolic suction.[18,48,89,125,140] The degree of negativity attained is inversely proportional to the end-systolic volume.[48] In this regard, the phenomenon appears to be secondary to elastic forces stored during systole which are manifest as restoring forces early in diastole.[140] The importance of restoring forces varies with respect to the hemodynamic and the myocardial status.[48,130] Under normal conditions, elastic recoil appears to be a major determinant of the peak rate of fiber relengthening.[18] In the presence of myocardial dysfunction with an elevated end-systolic volume, the stored forces are relatively less and recoil plays a reduced role in ventricular filling. Elastic recoil is one of the forces which acts during the period of isovo-lumic relaxation. Therefore, the process of relaxation as quantitated by τ includes the effects of both inactivation and restoring forces.

Ventricular and Myocardial Compliance

In contrast to the active process of inactivation in the early part of diastole, the pressure-volume relation of the ventricle late in diastole is predominantly determined by the passive elastic properties of the myocardium. However, there are a number of nonmyocardial factors which contribute, and the distinction between chamber and myocardial properties is essential. Chamber stiffness (change in pressure/change in volume = dP/dV) or compliance (change in volume/change in pressure = dV/dP) refers to analysis of the pressure-volume relation of the ventricle and, as such, encompasses a variety of factors including myocardial properties, ventricular geometry, pericardial restraint, coronary filling, incomplete relaxation, and interventricular interaction.[39] The magnitude of the influence of each of these features under various hemodynamic circumstances has been the subject of considerable study.[39] Although chamber stiffness and compliance are measures of the ability of the ventricle to distend under pressure, myocardial stiffness refers to the ability of the muscle to stretch when exposed to a lengthening force. The force can be quantitated as wall stress (σ), as detailed earlier. Strain (ϵ) is defined as the change in length with respect to a reference length, ideally with the reference being the resting length, that is, length at a stress of zero. Thus, chamber properties are represented by the pressure-volume relation and myocardial properties are represented by the stress-strain relation, with myocardial stiffness = $d\sigma/d\epsilon$ and myocardial compliance = $d\epsilon/d\sigma$. If the myocardium were a purely elastic material, the change in length would depend only on the elongating force. However, the force required to induce rapid changes in length exceeds that required for more gradual stretching. Thus, myocardial stress is a function of both strain and strain rate (rate of change in length) and the myocardium is, therefore, a viscoelastic material. The viscous properties are most evident during periods of rapid lengthening, such as the rapid filling phase and atrial systole. Although the magnitude of the viscous effects is controversial, most investigators have either incorporated viscous effects in their mathematical models or have limited the analysis to periods in diastole when viscous effects are expected to be minimal (at the middle and end of diastole).

Myocardial Compliance Indices

A number of approaches to quantitative analysis of myocardial compliance have been described. In general, a mathematical model developed from predicted material properties and geometric considerations is used to calculate the best-fit equation for the pressure-volume or stress-strain data in mid and late diastole. For example, if an exponential stress-strain relationship is assumed, the equation for a purely elastic material is:

$$\sigma = \alpha(e^{\beta\epsilon} - 1)$$

If a viscoelastic model is used, it becomes necessary to incorporate strain rate $(d\epsilon/dt)$ into the equation, such as:

$$\sigma = \alpha(e^{\beta\epsilon} - 1) + \eta(d\epsilon/dt)$$

In this analysis, α and β are constants that describe the myocardial exponential stress-strain property and η accounts for the magnitude of the viscous properties. Although this approach has been used by a number of authors,[86] there is substantial controversy as to the correct method for the calculation of stress and the stress-strain analysis.[82] These controversies relate to the correct equation used to describe the material properties of the myocardium and the correct method for normalizing forces and dimensions to account for differences in geometry. Regardless of which equations are employed, several methodologic problems are common to the stress-strain calculations:

1. The reference length for strain calculations is best taken at zero stress, that is at a transmural pressure of zero. Because this is difficult to obtain as a static measurement (to eliminate viscous effects) in clinical situations, it is generally estimated by extrapolation of the observed stress-strain relationship or else another reference point is selected.

2. Adjustment for the non-zero external constraining forces from the pericardium and thorax is necessary to obtain myocardial compliance, necessitating either direct or indirect measurement of transmural pressure. Both in animals[115] and humans[134] right atrial pressure has been found to provide a good estimate of pericardial pressure. Studies of this sort have not been performed in patients with congenital heart disease, in whom the right ventricular transmural filling pressure would be expected to be non-zero because of the frequent finding of right ventricular hypertrophy in these patients.

3. The available methods for determining ventricular volume yield relatively few data points per beat, with sampling every 25–35 msec. The number of data points available for the curve fit is small, particularly at high heart rates. Few data points result in large variance and broad confidence intervals for the derived indices, particularly when nonlinear curve fits are used. In infants and young children, diastolic periods of 60–80 msec may be encountered (Fig. 24), precluding any meaningful mathematical analysis of pressure-volume data.

4. One must either include viscous effects in the model or exclude periods of rapid filling from the analysis. The latter approach further limits the number of data points per beat available for the curve fit, augmenting the problem referred to in paragraph 3.

5. The full range of physiologic stress-strain relations should be included for the most meaningful analysis, because extrapolation beyond the observed data range introduces large errors. To obtain the full physiologic range for end-diastolic pressure, interventions that raise and lower left ventricular filling pressure must be performed.

Overlap of Active and Passive Periods of Diastole

The amount of fiber lengthening that occurs during isovolumic relaxation is minimal, allowing the passive myocardial properties to be neglected during this portion of diastole. In mid to late diastole, relaxation should be complete and only passive myocardial properties are influential. Although normally complete shortly after mitral valve opening, in some pathologic conditions relaxation may not be completed until much later. Even in the normal heart, pressure continues to decline during early rapid filling in spite of increasing dimension, indicating that both active and passive processes are influential during this time. Pasipoularides and coworkers[96] postulated that measured left ventricular pressure represents the summation of components due to relaxation and passive filling. Potentially, an analytic approach of this sort could account for the observed pressure-volume or stress-strain relation throughout diastole. A meaningful model for the period of diastole during which active and passive myocardial properties interact is clearly desirable because it coincides with rapid filling, during which most of the filling occurs. In addition to potential confounding effects from viscous properties of the myocardium, there may be some influence of lengthening on relaxation. In isolated muscle, a load applied after relaxation ensues results in augmentation of relaxation.[16] In contrast, a provocative study in canine ventricles found that relaxation was slower during filling compared with nonfilling beats.[89] Thus, there appear to be many significant issues to be addressed concerning potential interaction, as well as overlap of active and passive diastolic properties, if a model is to be developed that can account for the observed pressure-volume relationship throughout diastole.

Diastolic Filling

The major physiologic consequences of abnormal relaxation and/or compliance are mediated through altered or impaired filling. At the whole organ level, filling is the primary event during diastole, and diastolic dysfunction is primarily of importance

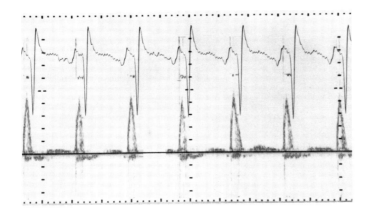

Figure 24. Mitral valve Doppler tracing in an infant with critical aortic stenosis, illustrating the very short diastolic filling periods (50–60 msec) that may be encountered in this age group.

when disordered filling is the result. Most of the available methods for noninvasive assessment of diastolic function are based on assessment of the pattern of diastolic filling. Although normal or abnormal patterns of filling are relatively easy to document using these methods, it must be understood that because of the interaction of relaxation and compliance and the influence of external factors, abnormal filling may occur in spite of normal relaxation and compliance, and normal filling may occur in spite of abnormal myocardial function. This section will focus on diastolic filling dynamics and their relation to myocardial properties and external factors.

Diastolic Mitral Inflow

The timing of diastolic filling events has been studied by a number of authors.[30,92,120] The onset of filling begins with unloading of the mitral valve during isovolumic relaxation. At moderate heart rates, this process is readily visible on 2-D echocardiography, where the frame preceding mitral valve opening shows some apical movement of the anterior mitral leaflet without separation of the valve leaflets. When ventricular pressure falls below left atrial pressure (first atrioventricular pressure crossover), rapid filling ensues. Ventricular pressure continues to decline during early rapid filling as the relaxation rate continues to exceed the filling force. After minimum pressure is attained, the effect of filling exceeds that of relaxation and ventricular pressure begins to rise. At or near the time of the peak rate of mitral inflow, ventricular pressure exceeds atrial pressure (second atrioventricular pressure crossover), and deceleration of the early filling wave begins. At lower heart rates, atrial filling from venous flow leads to a rise in atrial pressure until mid-diastolic atrial and ventricular pressure are essentially equal, and transmitral flow nearly ceases (diastasis). The late filling wave is due to atrial systole, which at higher heart rates merges with the early filling wave. Finally, the onset of ventricular contraction leads to

ventricular pressure in excess of atrial pressure, subsequent valve closure, and cessation of flow.

The pattern of diastolic filling can be quantitatively assessed by several invasive and noninvasive means, including angiography,[110] computed tomography,[106] radionuclide scintigraphy,[4,55] 2-D[143] and M-mode echocardiography,[24,29] and Doppler ultrasonography.[92] With the exception of Doppler, each of these methods provides a measure of the relation of left ventricular volume or dimension to time, from which the rate of change of volume or dimension can be obtained as a measure of flow rate. These volumetric methods all rely on some means of identification of ventricular borders in a user-interactive fashion. Because the time-volume curve is the measured data and the first derivative is a calculated result, there is substantial and unpredictable amplification of any error in measurement. In general, the measurement error is assumed to be random and its impact on the derived variables is reduced by filtering techniques such as fitting the data to a polynomial curve, from which the first and second derivatives are obtained analytically. Therefore, the accuracy of the calculation of the first derivative is dependent on the number of data samples which are obtained during the period of interest. Unfortunately, with the exception of M-mode echocardiography, the sampling rate for the other methods is 30–40 frames per second, with a sampling interval of 25–35 msec. This sampling rate is often marginal at slow heart rates, but at the higher heart rates which are common in infants and young children diastolic filling may persist for only 50–60 msec (Fig. 24), making these methods inadequate for an accurate curve fit. This is not a limitation for M-mode echocardiography, for which the time resolution is superb (1000 samples/sec).

More recently, Doppler ultrasonography has been used to measure left ventricular filling velocity directly. The sampling interval for pulsed and continuous-wave Doppler is 5 msec or less, providing at least 200 samples/sec. In addition, the rate of filling is obtained directly, so the problems involved in the calculation of the time derivative to obtain flow are eliminated. The velocity data can be converted to volume flow by multiplication by the orifice area. The time-velocity curve provides an accurate representation of the flow pattern, provided the area of the mitral orifice is relatively constant at the level of velocity measurement. Because the area of the orifice at the level of the mitral leaflets changes dynamically throughout diastole, the velocity just above the mitral annulus must be used.

The peak rate of flow, the time to peak flow, and some ratio of early and late filling are indices derived from all of these techniques. In addition, a number of variables derived from the Doppler time-velocity curve have been examined, including the ratio of the peak early vs the peak late velocity, the ratio of early vs late flow, the rate at which peak early flow is attained (acceleration time) and the rate of deceleration. It should be noted that although indices based on the ratio of early diastolic-to-late diastolic events have received a great deal of attention, at the higher heart rates that are normal in infants and children these events may merge (Fig. 24), precluding these calculations. Because the volume of flow varies, depending on absolute ventricular volume,[24,25] some means of normalization must be employed if subjects are to be compared with each other. Often, end-diastolic volume is used for the volumetric methods, although this remains controversial.[24,25,37] Similarly, the Doppler peak filling rate can be normalized to total transmitral flow.[12] Although the Doppler and volumetric methods provide comparable information concerning ventricular inflow and filling patterns, the Doppler technique has the advantage of providing a direct measure of flow, with excellent temporal resolution. In addition to the technical issues concerning the accuracy of data acquisition, if filling patterns are to be used to recognize abnormalities of diastolic relaxation and/or compliance, there must be a direct relationship between the observed filling patterns and these mechanical factors. As will be discussed subsequently, this does not appear to be the case. Thus, although these indices provide a clinically useful means by which abnormal patterns of filling can be detected, they do not provide a reliable measure of abnormal diastolic properties of the myocardium.

Relation Between Diastolic Filling and Myocardial Properties

Rather than devoting an extensive discussion to each of the many indices of diastolic function that have been derived from observation of filling patterns, a more general physiologic understanding can be reached by dividing these indices into two primary categories. Abnormalities of early rapid filling can be quantitatively assessed by any of a number of measures based on the early filling period (such as peak early velocity or flow, rate of acceleration or deceleration of flow) and rate indices based on determining time intervals (such as isovolumic relaxation, early filling time, time to a fixed percent of filling, etc.). The other major approach that has been taken is to examine an index based on the ratio of early vs late filling and/or velocities. Using these methods, abnormal diastolic filling patterns have been recognized to be a common finding in many forms of heart disease. Unfortunately, the clinical significance of these abnormalities is less well understood. At least three potential implications have been proposed:

1. Because filling abnormalities precede changes in systolic function in some disease categories, they may provide a tool for early diagnosis of cardiac involvement.

2. The observed abnormalities in diastolic filling may have physiologically important consequences related to elevation of pulmonary venous pressure which are due to elevated diastolic pressure and/or a reduction in systolic performance due to reduced preload.

3. Filling patterns may provide a means by which abnormal myocardial diastolic properties (impaired relaxation and/or compliance) can be detected.

It appears that early diagnosis is the least controversial of these potential applications. Although the net clinical utility of early recognition must be established on a disease-specific basis, there are a number of disorders for which abnormal filling appears to be a useful marker of myocardial involvement, which may well influence management.[2,7,32,34,60,142] Using the analysis of filling patterns for recognition of other diastolic disorders, such as constrictive pericardial disease, has also been documented.[2,4,60] Going beyond the issue of diagnosis, the physiologic consequences of an altered filling pattern depend on the magnitude of involvement. Severely abnormal relaxation can produce congestive heart failure, but the mild abnormalities that are commonly found are not known to be associated with increased morbidity or mortality. Nevertheless, it is likely that even mild abnormalities may be physiologically important during exercise or at rapid heart rates.[111] It is the potential for these methods reliably to detect the presence or absence of abnormal myocardial diastolic properties which has attracted the most interest, because the relevance to diagnosis and management would then be maximized. However, it is in this category that the most caution must be exercised because of the complex relationship between ventricular filling characteristics and mechanical properties of the myocardium.

Using the simplest model of ventricular diastolic mechanics, early diastolic ventricular pressure is largely determined by the rate of ventricular relaxation, whereas late diastolic ventricular pressure primarily manifests passive myocardial properties. Thus, abnormal early filling has been interpreted as an indication of impaired relaxation, and abnormal late filling (as recognized by abnormalities in the early vs late filling ratio) has been taken as an indication of abnormal compliance. Because of the shift of flow from one portion of diastole to another, filling during the less affected portion of diastole should be augmented and the early-to-late filling ratio should be even more abnormal. In fact, increasing chamber stiffness has been associated with decreased late filling and a proportional increase in the early filling phase.[3,120] Conversely, delayed relaxation is associated with diminished early diastolic filling and an increased contribution of the atrial phase filling.[3,54,120] The shift in relative filling is lost when both relaxation and compliance are impaired, as indicated by a lack of relationship between chamber stiffness and filling rate with impaired relaxation,[120] and normalization of early diastolic filling rates in spite of abnormal relaxation when filling rates are elevated.[3,93,110]

This model obviously represents a vast oversimplification of the relationship between the diastolic mechanical properties of the left ventricle and ventricular filling patterns. The transmitral pressure gradient, in addition to responding to the independent chamber determinants of the atrial and ventricular pressure-volume relationships, is also influenced by the acceleration and deceleration of inflow which result from the dynamic fluid behavior (inertial and viscous properties) of the blood and mitral valve. During early filling, the left atrial pressure reflects the passive compliance of the atrial chamber and the rate of atrial emptying. In contrast, the ventricular pressure is determined by dissipation of force within the ventricular wall and the passive diastolic properties of the ventricle. Each of these is responsive to changes in the ventricle's operating environment. Contraction of the ventricle to a volume less than equilibrium results in storage of elastic energy. Under these circumstances, release of the stored elastic energy increases the rate of decrease in ventricular pressure and speeds early diastolic filling. The other major determinant of the loss of active force within the wall is the rate of relaxation. Chamber compliance is determined by passive myocardial properties, but it also reflects the interaction of the left ventricle with the other cardiac chambers, the pericardium, and the lungs. Similarly, the characteristics of late diastolic filling are determined by the interaction of the independent properties of the atrial and ventricular chambers and the dynamic behavior of the fluid.

The numerous determinants of ventricular filling which interact with the diastolic mechanical properties of the myocardium prevent an accurate recognition of abnormal relaxation and/or compliance, using indices based solely on analysis of the filling pattern. In addition to the fact that the filling pattern tends to be normalized by combined abnormalities of compliance and relaxation, any of the nonmyocardial factors that affect chamber compliance or left atrial pressure result in altered filling characteristics. For example, altered preload can mimic abnormal compliance.[54,92] During therapeutic interventions, a shift of the relative early-to-late filling ratio toward a more normal ratio may be due to improved relaxation, but may also represent reduced pericardial constraint.[59,70,97] Thus, at present, it appears unlikely that analysis of filling alone will provide an accurate means by which to assess diastolic myocardial constituent properties.

REFERENCES

1. Abe H, Holt W, Watters TA, et al: Mechanics and energetics of overstretch: The relationship of altered left ventricular volume to the Frank-Starling mechanism and phosphorylation potential. Am Heart J 116:447–454, 1988.
2. Appleton CP, Hatle LK, Popp RL: Demonstration of restrictive ventricular physiology by Doppler echocardiography. J Am Coll Cardiol 11:757–768, 1988.
3. Appleton CP, Hatle LK, Popp RL: Relation of transmitral flow velocity patterns to left ventricular diastolic function: New insights from a combined hemodynamic and Doppler echocardiographic study. J Am Coll Cardiol 12:426–440, 1988.
4. Aroney CN, Ruddy TD, Dighero H, et al: Differentiation of restrictive cardiomyopathy from pericardial constriction: assessment of diastolic function by radionuclide angiography. J Am Coll Cardiol 13:1007–1014, 1989.
5. Baan J, Van der Velde ET: Sensitivity of left ventricular end-systolic pressure-volume relation to type of loading intervention in dogs. Circ Res 62:1247–1258, 1988.
6. Babu A, Sonnenblick E, Gulati J: Molecular basis for the influence of muscle length on myocardial performance. Science 240:74–76, 1988.
7. Balfour IC, Covitz W, Arensman FW, et al: Left ventricular filling in sickle cell anemia. Am J Cardiol 61:395–399, 1988.
8. Belcher P, Boerboom LE, Olinger GN: Standardization of end-systolic pressure-volume relation in the dog. Am J Physiol 249:H547–H553, 1985.
9. Bonow RO, Vitale DF, Bacharach SL, et al: Effects of aging on asynchronous left ventricular regional function and global ventricular filling in normal human subjects. J Am Coll Cardiol 11:50–58, 1988.
10. Borow KM, Green LH, Grossman W, et al: Left ventricular end-systolic stress-shortening and stress-length relations in human. Normal values and sensitivity to inotropic state. Am J Cardiol 50:1301–1308, 1982.
11. Borow KM, Colan SD, Neumann A: Altered left ventricular mechanics in patients with valvular aortic stenosis and coarctation of the aorta: effects on systolic performance and late outcome. Circulation 72:515–522, 1985.
12. Bowman LK, Lee FA, Jaffe CC, et al: Peak filling rate normalized to mitral stroke volume: a new Doppler echocardiographic filling index validated by radionuclide angiographic techniques. J Am Coll Cardiol 12:937–943, 1988.

13. Braunwald E, Ross, J: Control of cardiac performance. In Berne RM, Sperclakis N, Geiger SR (eds): Handbook of Physiology, Section 2: The Cardiovascular System, Vol. 1. Baltimore, Williams & Wilkins Co., 1979.

14. Brutsaert DL: Cardiac contractility: physiologic basis in isolated cardiac muscle, limitations in intact heart. Adv Cardiovasc Phys 5:1–13, 1983.

15. Brutsaert DL, Housmans PR, Goethals MA: Dual control of relaxation. Its role in the ventricular function in the mammalian heart. Circ Res 47:637–652, 1980.

16. Brutsaert DL, Rademakers FE, Sys SU: Triple control of relaxation: implications in cardiac disease. Circulation 69:190–196, 1984.

17. Burkhoff D, Sugiura S, Yue DT, et al: Contractility-dependent curvilinearity of end-systolic pressure-volume relations. Am J Physiol 252:H1218–H1227, 1987.

18. Caillet D, Crozatier B: Role of myocardial restoring forces in the determination of early diastolic peak velocity of fibre lengthening in the conscious dog. Cardiovasc Res 16:107–112, 1982.

19. Carabello BA, Green LH, Grossman W, et al: Hemodynamic determinants of prognosis of aortic valve replacement in critical aortic stenosis and advanced congestive heart failure. Circulation 62:42–48, 1980.

20. Colan SD, Fujii A, Borow KM, et al: Noninvasive determination of systolic, diastolic and end-systolic blood pressure in neonates, infants and young children: comparison with central aortic pressure measurements. Am J Cardiol 52:867–870, 1983.

21. Colan SD, Borow KM, MacPherson D, et al: Use of the indirect axillary pulse tracing for noninvasive determination of ejection time, upstroke time, and left ventricular wall stress throughout ejection in infants and young children. Am J Cardiol 53:1154–1158, 1984.

22. Colan SD, Borow KM, Neumann A: Left ventricular end-systolic wall stress-velocity of fiber shortening relation: a load-independent index of myocardial contractility. J Am Coll Cardiol 4:715–724, 1984.

23. Colan SD, Borow KM, Neumann A: Use of the calibrated carotid pulse tracing for calculation of left ventricular pressure and wall stress throughout ejection. Am Heart J 109:1306–1310, 1985.

24. Colan SD, Borow KM, Neumann A: Effects of loading conditions and contractile state (methoxamine and dobutamine) on left ventricular early diastolic function in normal subjects. Am J Cardiol 55:790–796, 1985.

25. Colan SD, Sanders SP, MacPherson D, et al: Left ventricular diastolic function in elite athletes with physiologic cardiac hypertrophy. J Am Coll Cardiol 6:545–549, 1985.

26. Colan SD, Sanders SP, Borow KM: Physiologic hypertrophy: effects on left ventricular systolic mechanics in athletes. J Am Coll Cardiol 9:776–783, 1987.

27. Colan SD, Sanders SP, Ingelfinger JR, et al: Left ventricular mechanics and contractile state in children and young adults with end-stage renal disease: effect of dialysis and renal transplantation. J Am Coll Cardiol 10:1085–1094, 1987.

28. Colan SD, Sanders SP, Parness IA, et al: Evidence of enhanced contractility in normal infants compared to older children and adults (abstract). J Am Coll Cardiol 13:135A–135A, 1989.

29. Colan SD, Trowitzsch E, Wernovsky G, et al: Myocardial performance after arterial switch operation for transposition of the great arteries with intact ventricular septum. Circulation 78:132–141, 1988.

30. Courtois M, Kovacs SJ, Ludbrook PA: Transmitral pressure-flow velocity relation: importance of regional pressure gradients in the left ventricle during diastole. Circulation 78:661–671, 1988.

31. Crottogini AJ, Willshaw P, Barra JG, et al: Inconsistency of the slope and the volume intercept of the end-systolic pressure-volume relationship as individual indexes of inotropic state in conscious dogs: presentation of an index combining both variables. Circulation 76:1115–1126, 1987.

32. De Bruyne B, Lerch R, Meier B, et al: Doppler assessment of left ventricular diastolic filling during brief coronary occlusion. Am Heart J 117:629–635, 1989.

33. Dodge HT, Stewart DK, Frimer M: Implications of shape, stress, and wall dynamics in clinical heart disease. In Fishman AP (ed): Heart Failure. Washington, DC, Hemisphere Publishing, 1978, pp. 43–54.

34. Douglas PS, Berko B, Lesh M, et al: Alterations in diastolic function in response to progressive left ventricular hypertrophy. J Am Coll Cardiol 13:461–467, 1989.

35. Elzinga G, and Westerhof N: How to quantify pump function of the heart. The value of variables derived from measurements on isolated muscle. Circ Res 44:303–308, 1979.

36. Feldman T, Borow KM, Sarne DH, et al: Myocardial mechanics in hyperthyroidism: importance of left ventricular loading conditions, heart rate and contractile state. J Am Coll Cardiol 7:967–974, 1986.

37. Fifer MA, Borow KM, Colan SD, et al: Early diastolic left ventricular function in children and adults with aortic stenosis. J Am Coll Cardiol 5:1147–1154, 1985.

38. Freeman GL, Little WC, O'Rourke RA: The effect of vasoactive agents on the left ventricular end-systolic pressure-volume relation in closed-chest dogs. Circulation 74:1107–1113, 1986.

39. Gilbert JC, Glantz SA: Determinants of left ventricular filling and of the diastolic pressure-volume relation. Circ Res 64:827–852, 1989.

40. Gould KL, Lipscomb K, Hamilton GW, et al: Relation of left ventricular shape, function, and wall stress in man. Am J Cardiol 34:627–634, 1974.

41. Graham TP, Franklin RCG, Wyse RKH, et al: Left ventricular wall stress and contractile function in childhood: normal values and comparison of Fontan repair versus palliation only in patients with tricuspid atresia. Circulation 74:I-61–I-69, 1986.

42. Graham TP, Franklin RC, Wyse RK, et al: Left ventricular wall stress and contractile function in transposition of the great arteries after the Rastelli operation. J Thorac Cardiovasc Surg 93:775–784, 1987.

43. Greenberg MA, Menegus MA: Ischemia-induced diastolic dysfunction: new observations, new questions. J Am Coll Cardiol 13:1071–1072, 1989.

44. Grossman W, Carabello BA, Gunther S, et al: Ventricular wall stress and the development of cardiac hypertrophy and failure. In Albert NR (ed): Perspectives in Cardiovascular Research: Myocardial Hypertrophy and Failure. New York, Raven Press, 1983, pp. 1–18.

45. Grossman W, Jones D, McLaurin LP: Wall stress and patterns of hypertrophy in the human left ventricle. J Clin Invest 56:56–64, 1975.

46. Gunther S, Grossman W: Determinants of ventricular function in pressure-overload hypertrophy in man. Circulation 59:679–688, 1979.

47. Hoit BD, Lew WYW, LeWinter M: Regional variation in pericardial contact pressure in the canine ventricle. Am J Physiol 255:H1370–H1377, 1988.

48. Hori M, Yellin EL, Sonnenblick EH: Left ventricular diastolic suction as a mechanism of ventricular filling. Jpn Circ J 46:124–129, 1982.

49. Housemans PR, Lee NKM, Blinks JR: Active shortening retards the decline of the intracellular calcium

transient in mammalian heart muscle. Science 221:159–161, 1983.

50. Huisman RM, Elzinga G, Westerhof N, et al: Measurement of left ventricular wall stress. Cardiovasc Res 14:142–153, 1980.

51. Huisman RM, Sipkema P, Westerhof N, et al: Comparison of models used to calculate left ventricular wall force. Med Biol Eng Comput 18:133–144, 1980.

52. Hunter WC: End-systolic pressure as a balance between opposing effects of ejection. Circ Res 64:265–275, 1989.

53. Huntsman LL, Rondinone JF, Martyn DA: Force-length relations in cardiac muscle segments. Am J Physiol 244:H701–H707, 1983.

54. Ishida Y, Meisner JS, Tsujioka K, et al: Left ventricular filling dynamics: influence of left ventricular relaxation and left atrial pressure. Circulation 74:187–196, 1986.

55. Iskandrian AS, Heo J, Segal BL, et al: Left ventricular diastolic function—evaluation by radionuclide angiography. Am Heart J 115:924–929, 1988.

56. Kass DA, Beyar R, Lankford E, et al: Influence of contractile state on curvilinearity of in situ end-systolic pressure-volume relations. Circulation 79:167–178, 1989.

57. Katz AM: Regulation of myocardial contractility 1958–1983: an odyssey. J Am Coll Cardiol 1:42–51, 1983.

58. Katz AM: Sarcoplasmic reticular control of cardiac contraction and relaxation. In Grossman W, Lorell BH (eds): Diastolic Relaxation of the Heart. Boston, Martinus Nijhoff, 1988, pp. 11–16.

59. Kingma I, Smiseth OA, Belenkie I, et al: A mechanism for the nitroglycerin-induced downward shift of the left ventricular diastolic pressure-diameter relation. Am J Cardiol 57:673–677, 1986.

60. Klein AL, Hatle LK, Burstow DJ, et al: Doppler characterization of left ventricular diastolic function in cardiac amyloidosis. J Am Coll Cardiol 13:1017–1026, 1989.

61. Kumada T, Katayama K, Matsuzaki M, et al: Usefulness of negative dP/dt upstroke pattern for assessment of left ventricular relaxation in coronary artery disease. Am J Cardiol 63:60E–64E, 1989.

62. Lakatta EG: Starling law of the heart is explained by an intimate interaction of muscle length and myofilament calcium activation. J Am Coll Cardiol 10:1157–1164, 1987.

63. Lang RM, Borow KM, Neumann A, et al: Adverse cardiac effects of acute alcohol ingestion in young adults. Ann Intern Med 102:742–747, 1985.

64. Lang RM, Borow KM, Neumann A, et al: Systemic vascular resistance: an unreliable index of left ventricular afterload. Circulation 74:1114–1123, 1986.

65. Lang RM, Borow KM, Neumann A, et al: Role of the beta$_2$ adrenoceptor in mediating positive inotropic activity in the failing heart and its relation to the hemodynamic actions of dopexamine hydrochloride. Am J Cardiol 62 (Suppl 5):46C–52C, 1988.

66. Lang RM, Fellner SK, Neumann A, et al: Left ventricular contractility varies directly with the blood ionized calcium. Ann Intern Med 108:524–529, 1988.

67. Langer GA: Ion fluxes in cardiac excitation and contraction and their relation to myocardial contractility. Physiol Rev 48:708–757, 1968.

68. Laskey WK, Reichek N, St John Sutton M, et al: Matching of myocardial oxygen consumption to mechanical load in human left ventricular hypertrophy and dysfunction. J Am Coll Cardiol 3:291–300, 1984.

69. Latham RD, Rubal BJ, Sipkema P, et al: Ventricular/vascular coupling and regional arterial dynamics in the chronically hypertensive baboon: correlation with cardiovascular structural adaptation. Circ Res 63:798–811, 1988.

70. Lavine SJ, Campbell CA, Held AC, et al: Effect of nitroglycerin-induced reduction of left ventricular filling pressure on diastolic filling in acute dilated heart failure. J Am Coll Cardiol 14:233–241, 1989.

71. Lew WYW: Time-dependent increase in left ventricular contractility following acute volume loading in the dog. Circ Res 63:635–647, 1988.

72. Lew WYW, LeWinter MM: Regional circumferential lengthening patterns in canine left ventricle. Am J Physiol 245:H741–H748, 1983.

73. Lew WYW, Rasmussen CM: Influence of nonuniformity on rate of left ventricular pressure fall in the dog. Am J Physiol 256:H222–H232, 1989.

74. Link KM, Weesner KM, Formanek AG: MR imaging of the criss-cross heart. Am J Roentgenol Radium Ther Nuc Med 152:809–812, 1989.

75. Little WC, Cheng C-P, Peterson T, et al: Response of the left ventricular end-systolic pressure-volume relation in conscious dogs to a wide range of contractile states. Circulation 78:736–745, 1988.

76. Mahler F, Ross J, O'Rourke RA, et al: Effects of changes in preload, afterload, and inotropic state on ejection and isovolumic phase measures of contractility in the conscious dog. Am J Cardiol 35:626–634, 1975.

77. Maroto E, Fouron JC, Douste-Blazy MY, et al: Influence of age on wall thickness, cavity dimensions and myocardial contractility of the left ventricle in simple transposition of the great arteries. Circulation 67:1311–1317, 1983.

78. Maughan WL, Sunagawa K, Burkhoff D, et al: Effect of arterial impedance changes on the end-systolic pressure-volume relation. Circ Res 54:595–602, 1984.

79. McDonald DA: Blood Flow in Arteries, 2nd ed. London, Edward Arnold Ltd., 1974, p. 309.

80. Mirsky I: Left ventricular stress in the intact human heart. Biophys J 9:189–199, 1969.

81. Mirsky, I: Review of various theories for evaluation of left ventricular wall stresses. In Mirsky I, Chiston DN, and Sander J (eds): Cardiac Mechanics: Physiological, Chemical and Mathematical Considerations. New York, John Wiley & Sons, 1974, pp. 381–409.

82. Mirsky I: Assessment of diastolic function: suggested methods and future considerations. Circulation 69:836–841, 1984.

83. Mirsky I, Corin WJ, Murakami T, et al: Correction for preload in assessment of myocardial contractility in aortic and mitral valve disease: application of the concept of systolic myocardial stiffness. Circulation 78:68–80, 1988.

84. Mirsky I, Tajimi T, Peterson KL: The development of the entire end-systolic pressure-volume and ejection fraction-afterload relations: a new concept of systolic myocardial stiffness. Circulation 76:343–356, 1987.

85. Moriarity TF: The law of Laplace: its limitations as a relation for diastolic pressure, volume, or wall stress of the left ventricle. Circ Res 46:321–331, 1980.

86. Nakamura T, Abe H, Arai S, et al: The stress-strain relationship of the diastolic cardiac muscle and left ventricular compliance in the pressure-overload canine heart. Jpn Circ J 46:76–83, 1982.

87. Nakamura Y, Sasayama S, Nonogi H, et al: Alterations in left ventricular relaxation, early diastolic filling and passive viscoelastic properties during postpacing ischemia. Am J Cardiol 63:72E–77E, 1989.

88. Nayler WG, Williams AJ: Relaxation in the mammalian heart muscle: some ultrastructural and biochemical considerations. Fourth Workshop on Contractile Be-

havior of the Heart, Utrecht, The Netherlands. Eur J Cardiol 7(Suppl):35, 1978.

89. Nikolic S, Yellin EL, Tamura K, et al: Passive properties of canine left ventricle: diastolic stiffness and restoring forces. Circ Res 62:1210–1222, 1988.

90. Nixon JV, Murray RG, Leonard PD, et al: Effect of large variations in preload on left ventricular performance characteristics in normal subjects. Circulation 65:698–703, 1982.

91. Noble MIM, Pollack GH: Molecular mechanisms of contraction. Circ Res 40:333–342, 1977.

92. Norman A, Thomas N, Coakley J, et al: Distinction of Becker from limb-girdle muscular dystrophy by means of dystrophin cDNA probes. Lancet 1:466–468, 1989.

93. Otto CM, Pearlman AS, Amsler LC: Doppler echocardiographic evaluation of left ventricular diastolic filling in isolated valvular aortic stenosis. Am J Cardiol 63:313–316, 1989.

94. Pan BS, Howe ER, Solaro J: Calcium binding to troponin-C in loaded and unloaded myofilaments of chemically skinned heart muscle preparations. Fed Proc 42:574, 1983.

95. Parker JO, Case RB: Normal left ventricular function. Circulation 60:4–12, 1979.

96. Pasipoularides A, Mirsky I, Hess OM, et al: Myocardial relaxation and passive diastolic properties in man. Circulation 74:991–1001, 1986.

97. Plotnick GD, Kahn B, Rogers WJ, et al: Effect of postural changes, nitroglycerin and verapamil on diastolic ventricular function as determined by radionuclide angiography in normal subjects. J Am Coll Cardiol 12:121–129, 1988.

98. Poliner LR, Dehmer GJ, Lewis SE, et al: Left ventricular performance in normal subjects: a comparison of the responses to exercise in the upright and supine positions. Circulation 62:528–534, 1980.

99. Quinones MA, Gaasch WH, Alexander JK: Influence of acute changes in preload, afterload, contractile state and heart rate on ejection and isovolumic indices of myocardial contractility in man. Circulation 53:293–302, 1976.

100. Quinones MA, Gaasch WH, Cole JS, et al: Echocardiographic determination of left ventricular stress-velocity relations in man. With reference to the effects of loading and contractility. Circulation 51:689–700, 1975.

101. Rajfer SI, Borow KM, Lang RM, et al: Effects of dopamine on left ventricular afterload and contractile state in heart failure: Relation to the activation of beta$_1$-adrenoceptors and dopamine receptors. J Am Coll Cardiol 12:498–506, 1988.

102. Ross J: Afterload mismatch and preload reserve: A conceptual framework for the analysis of ventricular function. Prog Cardiovasc Dis 18:255–264, 1976.

103. Ross J: Cardiac function and myocardial contractility: a perspective. J Am Coll Cardiol 1:52–62, 1983.

104. Ross J: Mechanism of cardiac contraction. What roles for preload, afterload, and inotropic state in heart failure. Eur Heart J 4(Suppl A): 19–28, 1983.

105. Ross J: Is there a true increase in myocardial stiffness with acute ischemia. Am J Cardiol 63:87E–91E, 1989.

106. Rumberger JA, Weiss RM, Feiring AJ, et al: Patterns of regional diastolic function in the normal human left ventricle: an ultrafast computed tomographic study. J Am Coll Cardiol 14:119–126, 1989.

107. Sagawa K, Suga H, Shoukas AA, et al: End-systolic pressure/volume ratio: a new index of ventricular contractility. Am J Cardiol 40:748–753, 1977.

108. Schulman DS, Remetz MS, Elefteriades J, et al: Mild mitral insufficiency is a marker of impaired left ven-

tricular performance in aortic stenosis. J Am Coll Cardiol 13:796–801, 1989.

109. Shapiro B, Marier DL, St. John Sutton MG, et al: Regional non-uniformity of wall dynamics in normal left ventricle. Br Heart J 45:264–270, 1981.

110. Sheikh KH, Bashore TM, Kitzman DW, et al: Doppler left ventricular diastolic filling abnormalities in aortic stenosis and their relation to hemodynamic parameters. Am J Cardiol 63:1360–1368, 1989.

111. Sholler GF, Colan SD, Sanders SP: Effect of isolated right ventricular outflow obstruction on left ventricular function in infants. Am J Cardiol 62:778–784, 1988.

112. Sholler GF, Colan SD, Sanders SP, et al: Noninvasive estimation of the left ventricular pressure waveform throughout ejection in young children with aortic stenosis. J Am Coll Cardiol 12:492–497, 1988.

113. Shroff SG, Janicki JS, Weber KT: Evidence and quantitation of left ventricular systolic resistance. Am J Physiol 249:H358–H370, 1985.

114. Slinker BK, Ditchey RV, Bell SP, et al: Right heart pressure does not equal pericardial pressure in the potassium chloride-arrested canine heart in situ. Circulation 76:357–362, 1987.

115. Smiseth OA, Frais MA, Kingma I, et al: Assessment of pericardial constraint: the relation between right ventricular filling pressure and pericardial pressure measured after pericardiocentesis. J Am Coll Cardiol 7:307–314, 1986.

116. Sonnenblick EH: Implications of muscle mechanics in the heart. Fed Proc 21:975–990, 1962.

117. Sonnenblick EH: Instantaneous force-velocity-length determinant in contraction of heart muscle. Circ Res 16:441–451, 1965.

118. Spratt JA, Tyson GS, Glower DD, et al: The end-systolic pressure-volume relationship in conscious dogs. Circulation 75:1295–1309, 1987.

119. Starling MR, Montgomery DG, Mancini J, et al: Load independence of the rate of isovolumic relaxation in man. Circulation 76:1274–1281, 1987.

120. Stoddard MF, Pearson AC, Kern MJ, et al: Left ventricular diastolic function: comparison of pulsed Doppler echocardiographic and hemodynamic indexes in subjects with and without coronary artery disease. J Am Coll Cardiol 13:327–336, 1989.

121. Strauer BE: Myocardial oxygen consumption in chronic heart disease: role of wall stress, hypertrophy, and coronary reserve. Am J Cardiol 44:730–740, 1979.

122. Su JB, Crozatier B: Preload-induced curvilinearity of left ventricular end-systolic pressure-volume relationships: effects on derived indexes in closed-chest dogs. Circulation 79:431–440, 1989.

123. Suga H, Sagawa K: Instantaneous pressure-volume relationships and their ratio in the excised, supported canine left ventricle. Circ Res 35:117–126, 1974.

124. Suga H, Yamakoshi K: Effects of stroke volume and velocity of ejection on end-systolic pressure of canine left ventricle. End-systolic volume clamping. Circ Res 40:445–450, 1977.

125. Suga H, Goto Y, Igarashi Y, et al: Ventricular suction under zero source pressure for filling. Am J Physiol 251:H47–H55, 1986.

126. Suga H, Goto Y, Nozawa T, et al: Force-time integral decreases with ejection despite constant oxygen consumption and pressure-volume area in dog left ventricle. Circ Res 60:797–803, 1987.

127. Suga H, Hisano R, Goto Y, et al: Normalization of end-systolic pressure-volume relation and Emax of different sized hearts. Jpn Circ J 48:136–143, 1984.

128. Suga H, Kitabatake A, Sagawa K: End-systolic pressure determines stroke volume from fixed end-diastolic vol-

ume in the isolated canine left ventricle under a constant contractile state. Circ Res 44:238–249, 1979.

129. Suga H, Sagawa K, Demer L: Determinants of instantaneous pressure in canine left ventricle: time and volume specification. Circ Res 46:256–263, 1980.

130. Suga H, Sagawa K, Kostiuk DP: Controls of ventricular contractility assessed by pressure-volume ratio, Emax. Cardiolvasc Res 10:582–592, 1976.

131. Suga H, Sagawa K, Shoukas AA: Load independence of the instantaneous pressure-volume ratio of the canine left ventricle and effects of epinephrine and heart rate on the ratio. Circ Res 32:314–324, 1973.

132. Sugiura S, Hunter WC, Sagawa K: Long-term versus intrabeat history of ejection as determinants of canine ventricular end-systolic pressure. Circ Res 64:255–264, 1989.

133. Taylor RR, Covell JW, Ross J: Volume-tension diagrams of ejecting and isovolumic contractions in left ventricle. Am J Physiol 216:1097–1102, 1969.

134. Tyberg JV, Taichman GC, Smith ER, et al: The relationship between pericardial pressure and right atrial pressure: an intraoperative study. Circulation 73:428–432, 1986.

135. Weber KT, Janicki JS: Myocardial oxygen consumption—the role of wall force and shortening. Am J Physiol 233:H421–H477, 1977.

136. Weber KT, Janicki JS: The heart as a muscle-pump system and the concept of heart failure. Am Heart J 98:371–384, 1979.

137. Weber KT, Janicki JS, Hefner LL: Left ventricular force-length relations of isovolumic and ejecting contractions. Am J Physiol 231:337–343, 1976.

138. Weber KT, Janicki JS, Hunter WC, et al: The contractile behavior of the heart and its functional coupling to the circulation. Prog Cardiovasc Dis 24:375–400, 1982.

139. Winegrad S: Regulation of cardiac contractile proteins: correlation between physiology and biochemistry. Circ Res 55:565–574, 1984.

140. Yellin EL, Hori M, Yoran C, et al: Left ventricular relaxation in the filling and nonfilling intact canine heart. Am J Physiol 250:H620–H629, 1986.

141. Yin FCP: Ventricular wall stress. Circ Res 49:830–842, 1981.

142. Zarich SW, Arbuckle BE, Cohen LR, et al: Diastolic abnormalities in young asymptomatic diabetic patients assessed by pulsed Doppler echocardiography. J Am Coll Cardiol 12:114–120, 1988.

143. Zoghbi WA, Rokey R, Limacher MC, et al: Assessment of left ventricular diastolic filling by two-dimensional echocardiography. Am Heart J 113:1108–1113, 1987.

Chapter 16

EXERCISE TESTING

Steven D. Colan, M.D.

Clinical and laboratory cardiovascular assessment is performed initially with the patient recumbent and motionless. Although ideal for anatomic description, the physiologic information gathered under these conditions does not accurately predict the response to usual or stressful activity. Complex multisystem changes are engendered by the transition from rest to exercise. Intracardiac shunts that are predominantly left-to-right at rest may reverse and become predominantly right-to-left. Pulmonary artery pressures and transvalvar gradients that are only mildly abnormal at rest may become critical at high flow rates. Mild to moderate myocardial dysfunction may cause no abnormalities with resting pressure or flow but may severely limit exercise tolerance. Although the obvious solution is to measure the response to exercise directly, interpretation of findings during exercise testing is frequently more complex than interpretation of measurements performed at rest. Thus, an abnormal increase in oxygen consumption may be due to a number of factors, including an inadequate test, abnormal cardiac response, abnormal vascular response, respiratory disease, abnormalities of the autonomic nervous system, or poor cardiovascular conditioning. To decipher exercise test results, the measured parameters must be appropriate to the clinical situation and to the particular question being addressed. In addition, the implication of any observed abnormality indicating the presence or absence of disease must take into account the frequency of that particular disease process in the population under consideration. Because all clinically useful tests have a certain false-positive and false-negative rate, the likelihood that a particular test result will correctly identify disease status depends on how often the disease is present in the relevant population. This important, and not entirely intuitive, observation precludes the wholesale application of standards developed in older adult populations to children and young adults. Because age- and disease-appropriate frequency data often are not available, it simply is not possible

to interpret accurately certain findings on exercise tests performed in children in spite of the fact that these same test results might be considered unequivocally abnormal in adults.

PHYSIOLOGY OF EXERCISE

Change in Cardiac Output with Dynamic Exercise

Heart rate increases early in exercise and continues to rise linearly with respect to oxygen consumption until exhaustion.[47,82] Initially, the predominant mechanism of cardio-acceleration is vagal withdrawal, with sympathetic activity dominating during more intense exercise.[103]

During upright exercise there is a 20–30% increase in **stroke volume** due to an increase in end-diastolic volume and a decrease in end-systolic volume.[79,96,115] With supine exercise the change in end-diastolic volume is attenuated or absent, resulting in little or no change in stroke volume. Thus, preload augmentation (Frank-Starling mechanism) plays a role in upright but not in supine exercise. The change in end-systolic volume reflects an increase in contractility due to augmented sympathetic nerve activity and circulating catecholamines.[48,96,115]

The net change in cardiac output is determined by the changes in heart rate and stroke volume; there may be as much as a four- to fivefold increase in trained individuals during exercise (from 5–25 liters per minute). Because the ability of the stroke volume to respond to increasing demand is so limited, rate increase is the principal mechanism of increasing systemic flow, accounting for 75–80% of the increase in cardiac output during upright exercise and 95–100% of the change during supine exercise. The dependence of exercise capacity on the ability to increase heart rate is well illustrated by the age-associated decrease in the maximal attainable heart rate, which fully accounts for the age-related decrease in maximal cardiac output and maximal oxygen consumption.[61,105]

Peripheral Factors

Simultaneously with muscle contraction, local metabolites induce dilatation of the small (resistance) blood vessels. The increase in flow is proportional to the strength of the muscle contraction and is predominantly under local control, because it is not altered by sympathectomy. In spite of vascular dilatation, flow is phasic because of the mechanical impedance imposed by muscular contraction, and the amplitude of the flow oscillations is proportional to the strength of the muscular contraction.[6] Overall there is a net decrease in systemic vascular resistance, but the increase in flow is out of proportion to the decrease in resistance, causing blood pressure to rise. Typically, there is a 50% rise in systolic pressure with only a small or no rise in diastolic pressure.[47] Functionally, this rise in pressure is necessary to provide an adequate driving force during the flow intervals and, therefore, is correspondingly greater when the flow interval is reduced at peak dynamic exercise and during sustained contractions (as with isometric exercise).

Neurohumoral Changes

The autonomic nervous system acts to coordinate the systemic resistance and capacitance of vessels with cardiac output. Failure of this system results in severe limitation of exercise due to an inadequate rise in blood pressure, as is seen in patients with idiopathic orthostatic hypotension.[80] Central neural mechanisms, along with reflex mechanisms involving skeletal muscle mechanicoreceptors, are responsible for initiating the cardiovascular response to exercise. During exercise, vasodilatation in some regional beds due to local mechanisms must be balanced by centrally mediated vasoconstriction of other vascular beds to maintain adequate perfusion pressure. As exercise progresses, the need for dissipation of heat increases, eliciting cutaneous vasodilatation, which is similarly balanced by centrally mediated regional vasoconstriction. Also, there is a powerful system neurohumoral response with tenfold increases in norepinephrine and epinephrine in plasma as well as smaller increases in renin activity and arginine vasopressin levels.[32,48,67,74] It is believed that these neurohumoral factors contribute to the enhancement of myocardial contractility and improved delivery of blood to working muscle and heart, although this has not been proved. The net beneficial[67] or detrimental[111] impact of the neurohumoral response is an issue of some importance, because many of the agents used in the therapy of congestive heart failure (beta-adrenergic blockers, angiotensin-converting enzyme inhibitors, direct vasodilators) impede these control mechanisms.

Myocardial Oxygen Consumption

Cardiac response to exercise involves changes in **preload** (that is, an increase in end-diastolic volume, as is seen with upright exercise), **afterload** (the force resisting muscle shortening which increases because of the rise in blood pressure), **contractility** (in response to the increase in catecholamines) and **heart rate.** With increased heart rate and contractility, the velocity of contraction is more rapid and systolic ejection time is shortened. The decrease in systolic time is proportional to the square root of the R-R interval and, therefore, there is a proportionately greater decrease in diastolic time, resulting in a decrease in diastolic coronary perfusion time. The compensating mechanisms that serve to maintain myocardial perfusion include coronary vasodilatation ("coronary reserve") and the increase in driving pressure. The demand side of this supply-demand equation is represented by the myocardial oxygen consumption, which depends on heart rate, the force of contraction (total systolic wall stress), and myocardial contractility.[123] Wall stress, in turn, is dependent on intracavitary dimensions, wall thickness, and pressure (see ch. 15).[28] Because of the increases in diastolic volume and arterial blood pressure during exercise, wall stress increases dramatically. Thus, all the determinants of myocardial oxygen consumption (wall stress, heart rate, and contractility) are greatly increased during exercise.

Although wall stress and contractility cannot be directly measured noninvasively during exercise, two of the contributing factors (pressure and heart rate) are measured routinely and their product (pressure × heart rate) provides a good estimate of the change in myocardial oxygen consumption during exercise.[55] When the arterial oxygen content is normal, coronary blood flow must increase from about 60 ml/100 gm at rest to about 240 ml/100 gm at peak exercise.[24] These flow rates can be attained in the normal individual during progressive exercise, but there is some evidence that normal individuals involved in sudden, high-intensity exercise may, indeed, develop myocardial ischemia.[16,45,46] This suggests that the healthy myocardial vasculature is capable of adapting to the high levels of coronary flow during vigorous exercise, but this adaptation may not occur rapidly enough to prevent ischemia during bursts of intense exercise.

Exercise Response of the Pulmonary Circulation

Table 1 lists certain cardiovascular parameters obtained in a group of normal volunteers during exercise. In both the systemic and pulmonary circulations there is an increase in pressure with a decrease in resistance. Although the absolute increase in pulmonary pressure is small, the proportional increase is twice that of the systemic cir-

Table 1. Systemic and Pulmonary Hemodynamic Changes in Response to Exercise in 12 Normal Men

	HR	CI	MAP	SVR	LVSWI	MPP	PVR	RVSWI
Rest	85	4.0	86	1640	59	15	260	9
Exercise	150	8.0	105	970	74	30	215	22
% change	76%	100%	41%	−40%	25%	100%	−17%	144%

HR = heart rate, CI = cardiac index, MAP = mean arterial pressure, SVR = systemic vascular resistance, LVSWI = left ventricular stroke work index, MPP = mean pulmonary pressure, PVR = pulmonary vascular resistance, RVSWI = right ventricular stroke work index.

culation (100% vs 40%). Because ventricular work is determined by the pressure-flow product, there is an overall 144% increase in right ventricular work compared with a 25% increase in left ventricular work during cardiovascular adaptation to this level of exercise. This excess demand on the right ventricle is demonstrated in chronically exercised animals in whom right ventricular hypertrophy exceeds that of the left ventricle.[7] Thus, one would anticipate that the status of the right ventricle might be of particular importance with respect to exercise capacity. Indeed, right ventricular, but not left ventricular, function correlates with exercise capacity.[12] This difference between the two circulations is of particular importance in subjects with congenital heart disease, in whom right ventricular abnormalities are common. In subjects who have undergone a right ventricular bypass procedure (Fontan operation), it is unlikely that a doubling of pulmonary pressures could be attained during exercise, thereby inherently limiting the increase in cardiac output. Further complicating this issue for subjects with congenital heart disease is the observation that in the presence of pulmonary hypertension without a ventricular communication, the increase in pulmonary pressure during exercise is excessive, further augmenting the exercise burden on the pulmonary ventricle.[43,75]

Indices for Measuring Cardiovascular Fitness

To compare test results among individuals requires an objective measure of cardiovascular capacity that is reproducible, sensitive, and readily obtainable. There are four indices of exercise fitness in common use:

1. Heart Rate Response. The response of the heart rate to any given exercise load may be the simplest and most commonly used measure, and is predicated on the linear relationship between heart rate and oxygen consumption.[23] Unfortunately, in patients with heart disease this relationship either fails to hold or is not comparable to that of normal individuals.[22]

2. Total Exercise Capacity. Total exercise capacity is determined routinely in most exercise laboratories, where performance on a standard exercise protocol is compared with age-matched healthy persons. The major limitation to this index

is a strong dependence on motivation and compliance, reducing the objectivity and reproducibility of the index. In addition, comparison can be made only between tests performed using the same test protocol and the same mode of exercise.[63,65,102,118,127]

3. Maximum Oxygen Consumption. Maximum oxygen consumption ($\dot{V}O_2max$) may be defined as the plateau in oxygen consumption that occurs during incremental exercise despite an increasing workload. Under ideal conditions, $\dot{V}O_2max$ is a highly reproducible measure of cardiovascular fitness that shows little day-to-day variability.[59,81,124] Although the $\dot{V}O_2max$ may not be obtainable in all cases because the subject must exercise to exhaustion, the failure to attain true $\dot{V}O_2max$ can be readily recognized.

4. Anaerobic Threshold. The anaerobic threshold has been gaining in popularity as an index of cardiovascular fitness. Conceptually, there exists a level of oxygen consumption at which the oxygen requirement of exercising muscle exceeds oxygen supply, resulting in an increased reliance on anaerobic glycolysis for the generation of energy. Thus, the anaerobic threshold is viewed as a critical measurement during exercise because it provides an index of the point at which oxygen delivery fails to keep up with metabolic demand.[122] This index appears to be very reproducible both in normal persons and patients with congestive heart failure.[9] Methods for determining anaerobic threshold have been adequately verified and its clinical usefulness is currently being explored.[97,100,122] However, there remains some controversy concerning the accuracy with which this index can be measured.

The index that is selected depends on the clinical situation. If a test is performed to detect exercise-induced arrhythmia, heart rate response is probably more critical than a precise measure of cardiovascular fitness. Although the total exercise capacity is a useful measurement in routine clinical assessment, in patients who are capable of cooperating with the more demanding process of exhaled gas analysis, measurement of $\dot{V}O_2max$ and anaerobic threshold provides desirable additional data. In particular, if the efficacy of a therapeutic intervention, such as surgery, balloon valvoplasty, or afterload reduction therapy, is to be assessed, an increase in $\dot{V}O_2max$ is the best indicator of a favorable response. Because the data that are requisite to anaerobic threshold determination are obtained simultaneously, it can be calculated as well, although this method is considered to be investigational because of the methodologic controversies surrounding its measurement.

Cardiovascular Adaptation to Chronic Exercise

Cardiovascular adaptation to regular exercise has been studied by many investigators. Frequent participation in aerobic exercise (isotonic) results in higher $\dot{V}O_2$max, a higher anaerobic threshold, reduced heart rate, and a reduced blood pressure response to any given level of exercise, thereby reducing myocardial oxygen consumption for an equivalent work load. Alterations in cardiac structures have long been noted to accompany the trained state, with left ventricular dilatation and a proportional increase in wall thickness observed most commonly. Various normal or diminished ejection parameters have been reported.

Anaerobic vs. Aerobic Exercise. Subjects who engage in predominantly anaerobic (isometric) exercise, such as weight lifting, do not experience the general training effects noted above. In these subjects the left ventricle does not dilate, but moderate to severe increase in wall thickness is noted, with normal to supranormal shortening characteristics. These changes can be understood best in terms of the physiologic alterations associated with each type of exercise.[29] Weight lifters are known to experience a large pressure load during exercise (intra-arterial pressures as high as 480 mm Hg have been measured!)[77] with a relatively small increase in cardiac output. The ventricular hypertrophy necessary to accommodate this pressure load results in excess hypertrophy and, therefore, high shortening characteristics are observed when these subjects are assessed in the resting state. In contrast, aerobically trained individuals experience a large increase in cardiac output during exercise with relatively minor pressure loads, resulting in ventricular dilatation without disproportionate hypertrophy. When examined in the resting state with the volume load removed, the ventricle appears preload-reduced, with low shortening characteristics. As a further consequence of this, aerobically trained individuals also demonstrate a dramatic increase in preload reserve, that is, they demonstrate an augmented increase in end-diastolic dimension during exercise.[33]

Exercise Programs for Cardiac Patients. These recognized benefits of aerobic exercise (improved peripheral response, improved cardiac preload, and afterload reserve) have prompted the widespread recommendations concerning exercise rehabilitation programs for patients recovering from myocardial infarction, and it is clear that even patients with chronic congestive heart failure are able to benefit from a controlled exercise pro-

gram.[42,112,117,119] Compared with the experience reported for adults with heart disease, there is relatively little information available concerning congenital heart disease.[107] It is interesting that most recommendations concerning exercise participation by patients with congenital heart disease emphasize what these patients should *not* do[50,57,116] rather than offer advice or encouragement as to what they should do! Generally, the purpose of these recommendations is to prevent adverse consequences from intense, competitive exercise.

Actually, the results of rehabilitation programs indicate that in the absence of ongoing, acute ischemia or inflammation (as would be anticipated in acute myocardial infarction, unstable angina, endocarditis, or acute pericarditis or myocarditis), the measurable benefits of exercise participation outweigh any theoretical adverse effects, even in subjects with severe ventricular dysfunction.[30,117] Thus, although complete exercise avoidance has been recommended in the presence of congestive heart failure because of the increased risk of sudden death,[37] recent studies would indicate that a controlled exercise program is, in fact, cardioprotective, even in these subjects. Generally, subjects with recognized abnormalities (such as severe aortic stenosis or anomalous origin of the coronary artery) who await a surgical intervention have not been evaluated and are not considered to be candidates for exercise programs.

Sudden Death during Exercise. Excluding the few, well-defined patient categories in whom exercise may cause direct myocardial injury, the recommendation of exercise avoidance generally is based on clinical associations rather than proven benefits. For example, the observation that one of the principal associations with sudden death during intense exercise in adolescents and young adults is hypertrophic cardiomyopathy[87] has resulted in the frequent recommendation that these patients avoid all but the mildest forms of exercise. The implicit assumption is that activity avoidance will prevent or reduce the occurrence of sudden death in these patients. Although, at first, this may seem a reasonable assumption, it is worth noting that there is *no* evidence that this intervention is effective in reducing the incidence of sudden death. In fact, there are reasons to believe that avoiding regular exercise may *increase* the risk of sudden death and there are certainly other adverse effects of exercise proscription.

The presumed mechanism of sudden death during exercise is arrhythmia related to the exercise-associated increases in catecholamine levels, myocardial oxygen consumption, and heart rate. Because the trained individual manifests lower levels of exercise-related catecholamine release, myocardial oxygen demand, and tachycardia, training in fact appears to reduce the risk of exercise-related arrhythmias[121] and sudden death.[113] Lack of routine exercise results in a lowering of the individual's threshold so that everyday activities, such as stair-climbing, become his or her maximal activity, an activity for which he or she is ill prepared.

Although specific evaluation of the risks and benefits of exercise in the less common disease categories has not been reported, available evidence suggests that a carefully planned program of aerobic exercise at an intensity level appropriate to the level of cardiovascular compromise can be beneficial to nearly all patients. The practice of recommending exercise limitation has adverse effects on the level of family anxiety, negative self-image, social isolation, and other problems that are more manifest in childhood. In the author's opinion, although providing firm direction toward more desirable forms of exercise is clearly warranted, the clinician is rarely justified in excluding exercise absolutely.

TYPES OF EXERCISE TESTING

Cardiac Catheterization

Exercise testing in the catheterization laboratory permits direct measurement of intra-arterial and intraventricular pressure and flow, data that are applicable to assessing the severity of valvar lesions, the degree of left ventricular dysfunction, alterations in shunts and pressure, coronary blood flow, and myocardial metabolism, among other things. The price of these additional data is the risk involved in exercising the subject in a supine position with relative immobilization and additional dangers involving potential catheter dislodgement, bleeding, and contamination. Even with unconstrained maximal supine exercise, the attained $\dot{V}O_2$, heart rate and blood pressure are lower than with upright exercise.[118] Under the conditions usually found in the catheterization laboratory, it is common to attain, at most, a doubling of cardiac output. This response may be adequate for hemodynamic assessment of valvar disease but does not permit characterization of cardiovascular fitness and may not adequately stress left ventricular reserve.

Type of Exercise

Although hand-grip exercise is used occasionally in situations in which the cardiovascular response to a pressure load is desired (hypertensive subjects, coronary artery disease, aortic insufficiency), generally, cardiovascular testing is performed with dynamic exercise on a treadmill, bicycle, or arm ergometer. The cardiovascular response to exercise is proportional to the amount of working muscle until at least 50% of the total muscle mass is involved, beyond which there is little change in cardiovascular stress with the addition of more muscle

mass.[76] Generally, the decision concerning the mode of exercise relates to the ease of data collection and test administration, considering the patient population, age, and the type of data to be collected.

Treadmill. The treadmill has become the standard instrument in most laboratories, providing a familiar form of exercise which elicits the highest attainable oxygen consumption rate because of involvement of arm, leg, and torso musculature. The work rate is directly controllable and is proportional to body size and the treadmill settings, thus demanding a minimum degree of attention by the exercising subject. The principal disadvantages to treadmill exercise relate to the amount of movement involved. Blood pressure measurement is more difficult and the electrocardiographic tracing contains more artifact than is present with bicycle ergometer recordings. Measurement of exhaled gases is cumbersome because of the amount of head movement that must be allowed to attain maximal exertion. Finally, studies that involve intravascular catheters, scintillation cameras, or echocardiographic imaging cannot be done.

Bicycle. Ease of data collection is the major advantage associated with bicycle ergometry. The electrocardiographic tracings are clean, blood pressure can be measured easily, catheters and the expired gas mouthpiece can be held in place, and echocardiographic or radionuclide data can be collected. Although the maximum oxygen consumption attained is less than for treadmill exercise, adequate cardiovascular stress usually can be achieved. Unfortunately, some subjects find this form of exercise less comfortable and performance is more variable. The mechanical bicycles rely on the patient to adjust to the desired workload, thereby demanding complete subject cooperation to maintain a constant work rate. This is a particular problem when working with children. The constant-workload electronic ergometer overcomes this problem by incorporating a variable resistance element to force a constant total workload regardless of pedaling speed. Unfortunately, as the subject tires this increase in resistance leads to fatigue and confusion and some subjects may stop prematurely.

Arm Ergometer. Certain patients who are incapable of bicycle or treadmill testing (amputees, paraplegics, certain patients with muscular dystrophy) must be stressed with arm ergometry. At any submaximal workload, arm exercise produces a higher heart rate and arterial pressure than leg exercise does, whereas maximum heart rate and oxygen uptake are lower.[108] These differences have been shown to be related to the smaller muscle mass involved in arm exercise. Because chronotropic and pressure stresses are similar to those for leg exercise, this is an effective exercise method to document myocardial ischemia. However, peak workloads attained during arm and leg exercise are not correlated, making it impractical to use maximum arm work as an index of cardiovascular fitness. Cardiac output is closely related to oxygen uptake without significant differences between modes of exercise, implying that measurements of $\dot{V}O_2$ and anaerobic threshold do provide valid comparative data among patients.

Exercise Protocol

Generally, the goal of the exercise test is to determine cardiovascular response to near-maximal levels of exertion. Because the level that is appropriate to each individual is not known prior to the examination, most procedures involve a progressive change from minimal exertion to levels sufficient to challenge even the most trained individuals. Because there is a time lag between the onset of a new level of work and the steady-state physiologic response, there must be sufficient time devoted to each level of exercise to attain this plateau if data of this type are being measured.[97] Thus, at any given workload the steady-state $\dot{V}O_2$ response is reached after 3–6 minutes. However, if maximal exertion is to be attained, the individual levels must be sufficiently brief that fatigue does not occur prematurely. The most common compromise is to use 3-minute stages, such as the **Bruce treadmill protocol.**[21] Employing standard protocols has the additional benefit of measuring an exercise tolerance that can be compared with published results. By permitting a rest period between work levels, it is possible to determine the cardiovascular response to each workload without the confounding factor of cumulative fatigue from prior levels. Although this provides the most accurate information, the time needed to perform these tests makes them impractical for routine clinical use.

Alternatively, the response to a rapidly escalating workload with minimal time periods provides a near-continuous progression that completely ignores the issues concerning steady-state measurements. It has been suggested that if the variable of interest has a reasonably invariant time-lag or is normalized to another variable with a similar time lag (for example, expressing the anaerobic threshold relative to the $\dot{V}O_2$), this type of study will indeed provide data that can be compared between patients.[97,122] This approach may have particular applicability in children in whom the tolerance to fatigue is often the limiting factor in obtaining maximal exertion. Finally, a flexible plan can be devised by which the workload on subsequent stages is based on the performance to that point.[109] In this case, the performance must be assessed by using a measure such as $\dot{V}O_2$max, because direct comparison of exercise duration is not possible.

In studies for which exhaled gas analysis is not desired or possible, the standard Bruce protocol is used in our laboratory.[21] This permits comparison of results with a vast body of previously published, age-adjusted standards for exercise capacity, and can be performed even in very young patients. For more sensitive assessment of cardiovascular fitness, a rapidly escalating (1 minute at each level) bicycle protocol designed to parallel the change in workload involved in the stages of the Bruce protocol is coupled with analysis of exhaled gases for $\dot{V}O_2$max and the anaerobic threshold. This makes it possible to attain $\dot{V}O_2$max in most subjects prior to the onset of extreme muscle fatigue. Finally, for patients for whom limitation of exercise capacity, based on clinical status or prior exercise testing, is expected, the protocol is revised to a slower rate of increase to permit a graded testing prior to cardiovascular exhaustion.

ABNORMALITIES OF MEASURED PARAMETERS (Exhibit 1)

Heart Rate

The change in heart rate with exercise is the principal determinant of the ability to augment cardiac output, because changes in stroke volume are relatively small. Therefore, primary abnormalities of rate response (sick sinus syndrome, congenital heart block) usually are accompanied by a reduced $\dot{V}O_2$max. In patients with structural defects, although the change in stroke volume with exercise may be abnormal,[35,83] limited exercise capacity is more commonly due to a reduced maximum heart rate.[4,14,15,60,101] Measurement of alternative indices of aerobic capacity, such as the anaerobic threshold, is necessary to distinguish between limited cardiovascular and/or chronotropic reserve.[101]

Blood Pressure

Although a subnormal increase in blood pressure with exercise is associated with many congenital cardiac defects,[2,4,17,56,62] a fall in blood pressure during exercise to levels below resting value is distinctly uncommon, occurring in <1% of normal

Exhibit 1

Boston Children's Hospital Experience **Treadmill Tests for the Year 1989 (N = 263)***	
Reason for Testing	% Tests
Exercise tolerance	43
Chest pain	24
Arrhythmias	47
ST and T wave changes	26
Blood pressure response	12
Other	24
*Over the preceding five years, an average of 314 treadmill stress tests were performed each year.	

adults[58,84] and even more rarely in children. Exertional hypotension is found most commonly in adult patients with severe coronary artery disease and generally is associated with evidence of regional and global ventricular dysfunction.[54,58,84] Although occasionally encountered in children with congenital heart disease,[2,17] its exact significance is less clear. In 1022 consecutive treadmill studies at The Boston Children's Hospital, exertional hypotension has been noted on only 12 occasions. In nine of these, the fall in blood pressure coincided with the onset of a significant sustained ventricular or atrial arrhythmia. The other three patients had severe cardiomyopathy with chronic congestive heart failure.

An excess rise in blood pressure during exercise occurs commonly after repair of coarctation of the aorta,[51] and may be a useful predictor of the adequacy of the repair. Although higher than normal values are associated also with certain other forms of heart disease, such as aortic regurgitation,[56] it is in the assessment and prediction of systemic hypertension that exertional hypertension has received the most attention. In addition to the exaggerated rise in blood pressure during exercise in subjects with hypertension,[71,110] several long-term studies have demonstrated a higher incidence of late development of hypertension in healthy volunteers who exhibited an exaggerated blood pressure response to exercise.[34,40]

Unfortunately, the usefulness of blood pressure measurements during exercise is limited by the accuracy with which they can be obtained. It is difficult to perform auscultatory measurements after the first three or four stages of the Bruce treadmill protocol because of patient movement. It is possible to limit motion during bicycle ergometry, and, generally, pressures are more accurately obtained. Often, the first postexercise pressure is taken as the peak value. Although several automated devices are currently available, attempts to document their accuracy generally have relied on comparison with mercury manometer methods.[3,53,64] Until comparison with intra-arterial recordings are available, their accuracy must remain somewhat suspect.

Changes in the Electrocardiographic S-T Segment

Often, exercise-induced changes in the electrocardiogram are used to diagnose myocardial ischemia and, by inference, a reduced coronary reserve. Typically, elevation of the S-T segment is taken to represent a transmural process, whereas depression of the S-T segment represents subendocardial ischemia or infarction.

The S-T segment is that portion of the electrocardiogram extending from the termination of the QRS complex (the J point) to the onset of the T wave. At this point in the cardiac cycle all myocardial cells are depolarized, there is no transmembrane current, and, therefore, the S-T segment is isoelectric. The position of the S-T segment is usually compared with that of the segment between the termination of the T wave and the beginning of the P wave (T-P segment) and that of the P-R segment, and is described as elevated or depressed relative to these other portions of the cardiac cycle that are normally isoelectric (Fig. 1). Subendocardial ischemia is associated with a loss of intracellular potassium (K^+), resulting in a diastolic current of injury. The repolarized myocardium ceases to be isoelectric, resulting in an elevation of the T-P and P-R segments relative to the baseline. Depolarization results in obliteration of the current of injury, and the S-T segment, although isoelectric, is depressed relative to the elevated diastolic baseline.[18] Thus, depression of the S-T segment is probably more correctly described as T-Q elevation.

The range of normal for the position of the S-T

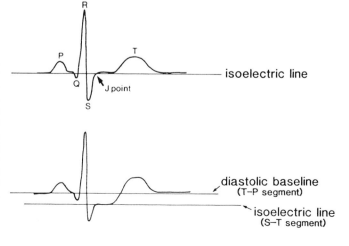

Figure 1. Illustration of electrocardiographic timing intervals and the nature of S-T segment depression. Under usual circumstances (panel A), the heart is isoelectric between beats (T-P interval), after atrial depolarization (P-Q interval) and after ventricular depolarization (S-T interval). With ischemia, (panel B) a diastolic "current of injury" that is absent after ventricular depolarization results in elevation of the T-P and P-Q segments relative to the S-T segment, a phenomenon that is generally described as S-T depression.

segment is from −0.5 to 2.0 mm relative to the T-Q segment. During exercise, the P-R interval shortens and the P wave amplitude and atrial repolarization wave increase with secondary downward displacement of the P-Q junction. The atrial repolarization may extend through the QRS complex and into the S-T segment, resulting in J point depression. Therefore, this J point depression, with a rapidly upsloping S-T segment that returns to baseline within 40–60 msec after the J point, is considered a normal finding (Fig. 2). The recommended location for measuring significant S-T depression is between 60 and 80 msec after the J point. Because the population variability of the shape and position of the S-T segment represents a continuum rather than a discontinuous function, it is necessary to define criteria for changes in the S-T segment, whereby the detection of an abnormal response is maximized and the false-positive rate is minimized. Several significant problems are encountered in this process.

Obtaining Accurate Electrocardiograms. The first problem encountered is that of obtaining accurate electrocardiograms. During exercise, there is considerably more noise in the electrocardiogram due to motion artifact, increased respiratory motion, and skeletal muscle contractions. The electrocardiogram becomes much more difficult to decipher, and establishing a stable baseline from which to measure elevation or depression of the S-T segment for individual beats is often not possible. Fortunately, most of the unwanted signal is either random noise or is periodic signal out of phase with the cardiac fundamental. Therefore, beat averaging provides effective filtering capability. Most electrocardiographic equipment used for exercise provides the ability to obtain averaged beats over a specified time period, yielding a clean image with improved diagnostic capacity. Determination of the diastolic baseline, J point position, and S-T segment slope can also be automated by most of these instruments (Fig. 3). The device must be capable of rejecting abnormal beats (premature or aberrantly conducted) from the averaging algorithm, but the averaged beats must still be viewed with caution in the presence of marked arrhythmias when "normal" beats constitute less than 50% of the total.

Criteria for Abnormal Responses. Changes in the S-T segment associated with ischemia are closely mimicked by other causes, including abnormal activation (pre-excitation syndromes, bundle branch block), drug therapy (digitalis), and electrolyte disturbances. Perhaps more importantly, S-T segment depression of 1.5 mm at 80 msec after the J point is seen in 6–30% of normal adults and children.[11,120,125] More stringent criteria for defining an abnormal response results in fewer false negatives but also leads to a decreased detection rate. In studies performed in adults with suspected coronary artery disease, the best trade-off between sensitivity and specificity occurs using the criteria of an S-T segment depression >1.5 mm at 80 msec after the J point. Efforts to improve on the discriminatory capability of the test by alternative analysis of changes in the S-T segment, such as correction of the S-T segment slope for heart rate, R-wave amplitude, exercise time, and integration of the area of the S-T segment depression, appear to yield somewhat higher diagnostic accuracy[26,38,44,73,88,120] at the expense of considerable additional computational complexity. Finally, rather than using depression of the S-T segment as a simple normal-abnormal dichotomy, reporting the S-T segment as a continuous variable, with more severe depression imparting a greater likelihood and greater severity of disease, adds significantly to the accuracy of the test.[39] In fact, this is general practice in any case, because most cardiologists would react more strongly to a 5-mm drop in the S-T segment than to a 1 or 1.5 mm change.

Application of Criteria to Congenital Heart Disease. There are at least two major problems in the direct application of these criteria to the young patient with congenital heart disease suspected of ischemia during exercise.

First, the end point in the validation studies has not been direct evidence of ischemia, but rather the finding of angiographically significant coronary artery disease. That is, the sensitivity and specificity of the test for diagnosing anatomically significant coronary artery disease have been examined, but more specific testing to determine if, in fact, there is biochemical evidence of ischemia which relates to these changes in the S-T segment

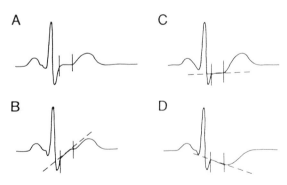

Figure 2. Patterns of changes in the J point and S-T segment with exercise. For each of the four beats, the J point and the end of the 60 msec interval after the J point are indicated with vertical tics, and an interrupted line is drawn to indicate the direction of the slope of the S-T segment in this interval. The horizontal S-T segments at rest (**A**) may not change during exercise but often J point depression, with upsloping of the S-T segment (**B**), is seen in normal individuals. The pattern associated with a good predictive capacity for ischemic heart disease involves persistent depression of the S-T segment at least 60 msec after the J point (**C**) or actual downsloping of the S-T segment (**D**).

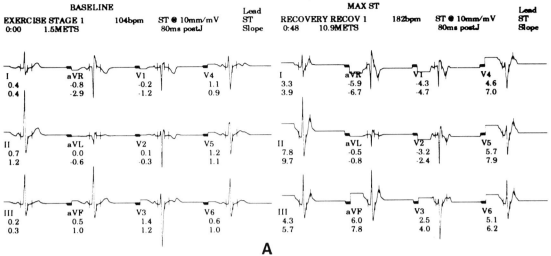

A

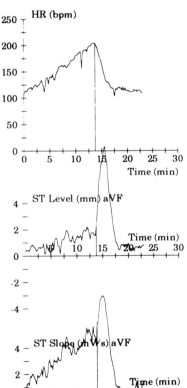

B

Figure 3. The effect of beat averaging on signal quality for the exercise electrocardiogram is shown. **A,** A 12-lead electrocardiogram at rest (BASELINE on the left) and at recovery following maximal exercise (RECOVERY on the right). The averaged waveforms are shown with the machine-derived timing for onset of the Q wave, the J point, and the end of the ST segment (vertical lines on each complex). The lead, the ST elevation, and the ST slope are indicated beneath each complex. **B,** This type of automated, graphic display is possible on most exercise electrocardiographic equipment. For example, the pattern of J point depression or elevation and the angle of the ST segment relative to the baseline can be rapidly visualized as a function of exercise level. HR (bpm), heart rate (beats per minute); ST level, ST elevation or depression relative to baseline; ST slope, slope from the J point to 80 msecs after J. Note the dramatic changes in ST level and ST slope which occur at the beginning of recovery in this patient.

has not been performed. Generally, for the young patient with congenital heart disease, one is interested in detecting ischemia, not atherosclerotic coronary artery disease. Even in studies comparing changes in the S-T segment with quantitative thallium imaging, the accuracy of both methods for predicting angiographic severity of coronary artery disease has been the end point of the study.[44]

Second, studies examining the predictive value of changes in the S-T segment during exercise have been performed in adult populations being evaluated for coronary artery disease, where the incidence of true positives is relatively high. The predictive value for any test (which equals true positive/[true positives + false positives]) depends on the sensitivity and specificity of the test but also on the prevalence of the disease in the population being studied (Table 2). Generally, in the case of adult patients with coronary artery disease, it is possible to estimate the age-adjusted incidence of the disease and, therefore, to calculate the probability of disease in any subject with a "positive" test. For the young patient suspected of experiencing ischemia, the incidence rate simply is not known, because there is no documentation that changes in the S-T segment are, in fact, related to ischemia in these patients. It is not correct to conclude that, simply because ischemia can cause changes in the S-T segment, all S-T segment changes are due to ischemia. For example, in patients with marked depression of the S-T segment during paroxysmal supraventricular tachycardia, no biochemical evidence of an inadequate myocardial oxygen supply was found.[86] Therefore, although so-called "ischemic" changes frequently are reported in patients with congenital heart disease,[27,126] such interpretation of the meaning of an "abnormal" exercise test is little better than a guess.

It is possible to define certain situations in which ischemia is likely to be a problem in the pediatric population. Obviously, coronary flow reserve may be inadequate in the presence of abnormalities of the coronary vasculature (coronary atherosclerosis, anomalous origin of a coronary artery, coronary artery stenoses or aneurysms), but even in the presence of normal coronary reserve, ischemia may result from excess demand. Thus, high intracavitary pressure, secondary to obstruction to ventricular outflow or vascular hypertension, is associated with an excess increase in wall stress and a resulting abnormal increase in myocardial oxygen consumption during exercise. A low arterial oxygen content due to cyanotic heart disease or pulmonary disease may reduce oxygen delivery and may worsen with exercise. Occasionally, reduced oxygen transport capacity due to anemia or hemoglobin defects may cause myocardial ischemia. The coronary perfusion pressure may be reduced because of either low arterial pressure or elevated ventricular diastolic pressure.

A remarkable number of congenital cardiac defects may be associated with one or more of these conditions. For example, in the presence of aortic stenosis, total myocardial oxygen consumption is elevated during exercise because of an excessive increase in total systolic wall stress, whereas coronary perfusion pressure is diminished because of a subnormal rise in arterial pressure with an abnormal rise in ventricular diastolic pressure.[66,114] The coronary microvasculature also appears to be abnormal in this disease, as reflected by abnormal coronary reserve even in the presence of angiographically normal coronary arteries.[93] A similar reduction in coronary reserve has been noted in response to pathologic ventricular hypertrophy, whether secondary to hypertension, hypertrophic cardiomyopathy, or aortic valve disease.[10,25,93,94] There are insufficient data to conclude whether hypertrophy occurring early in life in association with congenital heart disease has similar implications. Nevertheless, the potential for cardiac ischemia clearly exists in many subjects with various forms of congenital or acquired heart disease.

It is fair to say that the current methods for recognizing ischemia in patients with congenital heart

Table 2. Factors Used to Determine the Diagnostic Value of a Test

Sensitivity	$100 \times \dfrac{TP}{TP + FN}$	The percent of abnormal tests in subjects with disease
Specificity	$100 \times \dfrac{TN}{FP + TN}$	The percent of normal tests in subjects without disease
Predictive value	$100 \times \dfrac{TP}{TP + FP}$	The percent of subjects with an abnormal test who have disease
Relative risk	$\dfrac{\dfrac{TP}{TP + FP}}{\dfrac{FN}{TN + FN}}$	The relative rate of disease in those with an abnormal test compared with those with a normal test

TP = true positive, FP = false positive, TN = true negative, FN = false negative.

disease are inadequate, and their results must be treated with a great deal of skepticism. In the absence of better data, it appears prudent to interpret depression of the S-T segment in the vast majority of children and young adults with congenital heart disease as, at most, suggestive of ischemia. Nor should the absence of a positive test elicit much in the way of reassurance. The association of chest pain or more marked depression of the S-T segment probably justifies a higher level of suspicion. At The Boston Children's Hospital exercise thallium testing is advised in subjects in whom the probability of a true positive test is high, but clearly this test is most sensitive to regional perfusion abnormalities and may miss the presence of global ischemia.

Arrhythmias

This topic is covered in detail in chapter 27.

Ejection Fraction

Radionuclide angiography can be used to determine the ejection fraction at rest and during exercise. This method has been applied to a number of clinical situations[13,19,31,35,36,52,70,72,78,85,89,91,98,99] as an index of ventricular function and myocardial reserve. In general, application of this method to congenital heart disease has relied on the standards developed for adults suspected of having coronary artery disease and, therefore, the results must be examined again with these limitations in mind. During exercise, there are complex changes in afterload, preload, and contractility, the net result of which are quite difficult to predict in any individual. In general, any change in ejection fraction during exercise can be due to myocardial systolic or diastolic properties, but may also be related to vascular, autonomic, hormonal, positional, or pericardial factors. Therefore, it is not surprising that the normal ejection fraction response to exercise is highly variable.[20,68,69,90,98,99,106] Although there is difficulty in interpreting changes in ejection fraction during exercise among adults, studies performed in subjects with congenital heart disease introduce another level of uncertainty.[92,98,99] Therefore it appears that, although the change in ejection fraction during exercise provides some useful physiologic information and may be particularly valuable in population studies, the interpretation of individual test results is too problematic to permit it to be a useful clinical tool.

Other Parameters

Measurements of maximal tolerance, $\dot{V}O_2$, $\dot{V}O_2$max, anaerobic threshold, and cardiac output all provide useful information concerning the overall cardiovascular state of the individual. Serial assessment is particularly helpful for subjects at risk for cardiac injury (such as volume overload lesions of the left ventricle) and for critical evaluation of reported symptoms. Values before and after interventions, such as surgery, interventional catheterization, or drug therapy, enable therapeutic benefits to be monitored objectively in a global fashion. Interpretation of abnormal results for any of these indices of cardiovascular function must take into consideration that none of them is able to differentiate among the myriad of potential causes. Thus, for example, an abnormal anaerobic threshold may be related to ventricular dysfunction, but could also be due to anemia, poor conditioning, arterial desaturation, etc. Therapeutic decisions based on abnormalities or changes in any of these indices must be made with particular consideration to the numerous potentially related factors. Nevertheless, when the response to an acute intervention such as afterload reduction therapy is to be assessed, and other conditions are unlikely to have changed substantially, measurement of $\dot{V}O_2$max, and probably of the anaerobic threshold, may provide the best evidence of net physiologic benefit.

SAFETY OF EXERCISE TESTING

Although it is generally known that exercise testing can be performed safely in the vast majority of patients, it is more useful to consider those circumstances in which the risk may be higher and additional precautions may be warranted.[37] Stratification according to identifiable risk factors such as diagnosis or clinical condition can improve time and resource allocation in addition to providing optimal patient safety. As is often the case, the limited amount of data available from pediatric laboratories must be supplemented with data from studies in adults before any realistic conclusions can be reached. Decisions concerning safety must be made with well-defined end points. Thus, although ventricular tachycardia, chest pain, hypotension, and syncope have been reported as complications,[5] each of these events also qualifies as a diagnostically useful event, which warrants additional precautions but does not preclude testing. However, the possibility of death, myocardial infarction, or some other irreversible event must be considered as complications that would contraindicate testing if they constitute a reasonable expectation.

Suspected ischemic heart disease is the major referral diagnosis in most studies of the safety of exercise stress testing[41,104] and is the cause of most reported deaths during exercise testing.[8,104] Most centers involved in these studies have excluded patients with serious arrhythmias or recent myocardial infarction; therefore safety in these situations cannot be evaluated. No specific adverse predictors were identified in a large study of 170,000 tests with 16 deaths (about 1 per 10,000).[104]

Exercise testing is commonly performed for detection of arrhythmias and assessment of antiarrhythmic efficacy, and arrhythmias (ventricular fibrillation, ventricular tachycardia, or bradycardia) are reported to occur in 2.3% of the patients.[128] The major predictors were the presence of coronary artery disease and a history of exercise-associated arrhythmias. Of interest, ventricular dysfunction and the severity of arrhythmias on Holter monitoring were not predictive. No deaths or irreversible events were reported in 1377 tests. Thus, even though these subjects have a high incidence of induced arrhythmias warranting prompt intervention, they do not experience an unacceptable complication rate.[1,95]

Although congestive heart failure has been suggested as an absolute contraindication to exercise testing,[37] large studies have failed to support this contention, reporting no serious complications in as many as 2200 tests in subjects with congestive heart failure.[119] Arrhythmias are common, with 6% of subjects experiencing ventricular tachycardia, but even patients with leg edema and pulmonary edema were able to be tested safely.

Although few studies have reported complication rates subdivided in a manner that permits conclusions concerning other forms of heart disease, death has occurred during exercise testing in a subject with aortic stenosis.[8] Included among the reported 2% of complications in children were chest pain, syncope, hypotension, and potentially hazardous arrhythmias, none of which necessitated intervention, and there were no reported deaths.[5,49] Thus, safety issues should not preclude exercise testing in any child.

REFERENCES

1. Allen BJ, Casey TP, Brodsky MA, et al: Exercise testing in patients with life-threatening ventricular tachyarrhythmias: results and correlation with clinical and arrhythmia factors. Am Heart J 116:997–1002, 1988.
2. Alpert BS, Bloom KR, Newth CJ, et al: Hemodynamic responses to supine exercise in children with left-sided cardiac disease. Am J Cardiol 45:1025–1032, 1980.
3. Alpert BS, Flood NL, Balfour IC, et al: Automated blood pressure measurement during ergometer exercise in children. Cathet Cardiovasc Diagn 8:525–533, 1982.
4. Alpert BS, Moes DM, Durant RH, et al: Hemodynamic responses to ergometer exercise in children and young adults with left ventricular pressure or volume overload. Am J Cardiol 52:563–567, 1983.
5. Alpert BS, Verrill DE, Flood NL, et al: Complications of ergometer exercise in children. Pediatr Cardiol 4:91–96, 1983.
6. Andersen P, Saltin B: Maximal perfusion of skeletal muscles in man. J Physiol (Lond) 366:233–249, 1985.
7. Anversa P, Ricci R, Olivetti G: Effects of exercise on the capillary vasculature of the rat heart. Circulation 75:I-12–I-18, 1987.
8. Atterhog JH, Jonsson B, Samuelsson R: Exercise testing: A prospective study of complication rates. Am Heart J 98:572–579, 1979.
9. Aunola S, Rusko H: Reproducibility of aerobic and anaerobic thresholds in 20–50 year old men. Eur J Appl Physiol 53:260–266, 1984.
10. Bache RJ, Dai XZ, Alyono D, et al: Myocardial blood flow during exercise in dogs with left ventricular hypertrophy produced by aortic banding and perinephric hypertension. Circulation 76:835–842, 1987.
11. Bairey CN, Rozanski A, Levey M, et al: Differences in the frequency of ST segment depression during upright and supine exercise: assessment in normals and in patients with coronary artery disease. Am Heart J 114:1317–1323, 1987.
12. Baker BJ, Wilen MM, Boyd CM, et al: Relation of right ventricular ejection fraction to exercise capacity in chronic left ventricular failure. Am J Cardiol 54:596–599, 1984.
13. Baker EJ, Jones OD, Joseph MC, et al: Radionuclide measurement of left ventricular ejection fraction in tricuspid atresia. Br Heart J 52:572–574, 1984.
14. Barber G, Danielson GK, Heise CT, et al: Cardiorespiratory response to exercise in Ebstein's anomaly. Am J Cardiol 56:509–514, 1985.
15. Barber G, Danielson GK, Puga FJ, et al: Pulmonary atresia with ventricular septal defect: preoperative and postoperative responses to exercise. J Am Coll Cardiol 7:630–638, 1986.
16. Barnard RJ, MacAlpin JR, Kattus AA, et al: Ischemic response to sudden strenuous exercise in healthy men. Circulation 48:936–942, 1973.
17. Barton CW, Katz B, Schork MA, et al: Value of treadmill exercise test in pre- and postoperative children with valvular aortic stenosis. Clin Cardiol 6:473–477, 1983.
18. Becker RC, Alpert JS: Electrocardiographic S-T segment depression in coronary heart disease. Am Heart J 115:862–868, 1988.
19. Benson LN, Burns R, Schwaiger M, et al: Radionuclide angiographic evaluation of ventricular function in isolated congenitally corrected transposition of the great arteries. Am J Cardiol 58:319–324, 1986.
20. Bonow RO, Green MV, Bacharach SL: Radionuclide angiography during exercise in patients with coronary artery disease: diagnostic, prognostic and therapeutic implications. Int J Cardiol 5:229–233, 1984.
21. Bruce RA, Blackmon JR, Jones JW, et al: Exercise testing in adult normal subjects and cardiac patients. Pediatrics 32:742–756, 1963.
22. Bruce RA, Fisher LD, Cooper MN, et al: Separation of effects of cardiovascular disease and age on ventricular function with maximal exercise. Am J Cardiol 34:757–763, 1974.
23. Bruce RA, Kusumi F, Hosmer D: Maximal oxygen intake and normographic assessment of functional aerobic impairment in cardiovascular disease. Am Heart J 85:546–562, 1973.
24. Cannon PJ, Weiss MB, Sciacca RR: Myocardial blood flow in coronary artery disease: Studies at rest and during stress with inert gas washout techniques. Prog Cardiovasc Dis 20:95–120, 1977.
25. Cannon RO, III, Rosing DR, Maron BJ, et al: Myocardial ischemia in patients with hypertrophic cardiomyopathy: contribution of inadequate vasodilator reserve and elevated left ventricular filling pressures. Circulation 71:234–243, 1985.
26. Chaitman BR: The changing role of the exercise electrocardiogram as a diagnostic and prognostic test for chronic ischemic heart disease. J Am Coll Cardiol 5:1195–1210, 1986.

27. Chandramouli B, Ehmke DA, Lauer RM: Exercise-induced electrocardiographic changes in children with congenital aortic stenosis. J Pediatr 87:725–730, 1975.

28. Colan SD, Borow KM, Neumann A: Left ventricular end-systolic wall stress-velocity of fiber shortening relation: a load-independent index of myocardial contractility. J Am Coll Cardiol 4:715–724, 1984.

29. Colan SD, Sanders SP, Borow KM: Physiologic hypertrophy: effects on left ventricular systolic mechanics in athletes. J Am Coll Cardiol 9:776–783, 1987.

30. Conn EH, Williams RS, Wallace AG: Exercise responses before and after physical conditioning in patients with severely depressed left ventricular function. Am J Cardiol 49:296–300, 1982.

31. Cornyn JW, Massie BM, Greenberg B, et al: Reproducibility of rest and exercise left ventricular ejection fraction and volumes in chronic aortic regurgitation. Am J Cardiol 59:1361–1365, 1987.

32. Covertino VA, Keil LC, Bernauer EM, et al: Plasma volume, osmolality, vasopressin, and renin activity during graded exercise in man. J Appl Physiol 50:123–128, 1981.

33. Crawford MH, Petru MA, Rabinowitz C: Effect of isotonic exercise training on left ventricular volume during exercise. Circulation 72:1237–1243, 1985.

34. Criqui MH, Haskell WL, Heiss G, et al: Predictors of systolic blood pressure response to treadmill exercise: the Lipid Research Clinics Program Prevalence Study. Circulation 68:225–233, 1983.

35. Del Torso S, Kelly MJ, Kalff V, et al: Radionuclide assessment of ventricular contraction at rest and during exercise following the Fontan procedure for either tricuspid atresia or single ventricle. Am J Cardiol 55:1127–1132, 1985.

36. DePace NL, Iskandrian AS, Hakki AH, et al: Value of left ventricular ejection fraction during exercise in predicting the extent of coronary artery disease. J Am Coll Cardiol 1:1002–1010, 1983.

37. Detrano R, Froelicher VF: Exercise testing: uses and limitations considering recent studies. Prog Cardiovasc Dis 31:173–204, 1988.

38. Detrano R, Salcedo E, Passalacqua M, et al: Exercise electrocardiographic variables: a critical appraisal. J Am Coll Cardiol 8:836–847, 1986.

39. Diamond GA, Hirsch M, Forester JS: Application of information theory to clinical diagnostic testing. Circulation 63:915–921, 1981.

40. Dlin RA, Hanne N, Silverberg DS, et al: Follow-up of normotensive men with exaggerated blood pressure response to exercise. Am Heart J 106:316–320, 1983.

41. Doyle JT, Kinch SH: The prognosis of an abnormal electrocardiographic stress test. Circulation 41:545–553, 1970.

42. Ehsani AA, Biello DR, Schultz J, et al: Improvement of left ventricular contractile function by exercise training in patients with coronary artery disease. Circulation 74:350–358, 1986.

43. Epstein SE, Beiser GD, Goldstein RE, et al: Hemodynamic abnormalities in response to mild and intense upright exercise following operative correction of an atrial septal defect or tetralogy of Fallot. Circulation 42:1065–1075, 1973.

44. Finkelhor RS, Newhouse KE, Vrobel TR, et al: The ST segment/heart rate slope as a predictor of coronary artery disease: comparison with quantitative thallium imaging and conventional ST segment criteria. Am Heart J 112:296–304, 1986.

45. Foster C, Anholm JD, Hellman CK, et al: Left ventricular function during sudden strenuous exercise. Circulation 63:592–596, 1981.

46. Foster C, Dymond DS, Carpenter J, et al: Effect of warm-up on left ventricular response to sudden strenuous exercise. J Appl Physiol 53:380–383, 1982.

47. Francis GS, Goldsmith SR, Ziesche S, et al: Relative attenuation of sympathetic drive during exercise in patients with congestive heart failure. J Am Coll Cardiol 5:832–839, 1982.

48. Francis GS, Goldsmith SR, Ziesche SM, et al: Response of plasma norepinephrine and epinephrine to dynamic exercise in patients with congestive heart failure. Am J Cardiol 49:1152–1156, 1982.

49. Freed MD: Exercise testing in children: a survey of techniques and safety (abstract). Circulation 64:IV278, 1981.

50. Freed MD: Recreational and sports recommendations for the child with heart disease. Pediatr Clin North Am 31:1307–1320, 1989.

51. Freed MD, Rocchini A, Rosenthal A, et al: Exercise-induced hypertension after surgical repair of coarctation of the aorta. Am J Cardiol 43:253–258, 1979.

52. Freeman AP, Giles RW, Berdoukas VA, et al: Early left ventricular dysfunction and chelation therapy in thalassemia major. Ann Intern Med 99:450–454, 1983.

53. Garcia-Gregory JA, Jackson AS, Studeville J, et al: Comparison of exercise blood pressure measured by technician and an automated system. Clin Cardiol 7:315–321, 1984.

54. Gibbons RJ, Hu DC, Clements IP, et al: Anatomic and functional significance of a hypotensive response during supine exercise radionuclide ventriculography. Am J Cardiol 60:1–4, 1987.

55. Globel FL, Nordstrom LA, Nelson RR, et al: The rate-pressure product as an index of myocardial oxygen consumption during exercise in patients with angina pectoris. Circulation 57:549–556, 1978.

56. Gumbiner CH, Gutgesell HP: Response to isometric exercise in children and young adults with aortic regurgitation. Am Heart J 106:540–547, 1983.

57. Gutgesell HP, Gessner IH, Vetter VL, et al: Recreational and occupational recommendations for young patients with heart disease. A statement for physicians by the Committee on Congenital Cardiac Defects of the Council on Cardiovascular Disease in the Young, American Heart Association. Circulation 74:1195A–1198A, 1986.

58. Hammermeister KE, DeRouen TA, Dodge HT, et al: Prognostic and predictive value of exertional hypotension in suspected coronary heart disease. Am J Cardiol 51:1261–1266, 1983.

59. Hansen JE, Sue DY, Oren A, et al: Relation of oxygen uptake to work rate in normal men and men with circulatory disorders. Am J Cardiol 59:669–674, 1987.

60. Hesslein PS, Gutgesell HP, Gillette PC, et al: Exercise assessment of sinoatrial node function following the Mustard operation. Am Heart J 103:351–357, 1982.

61. Higginbotham MB, Morris KG, Williams RS, et al: Physiologic basis for the age-related decline in aerobic work capacity. Am J Cardiol 57:1374–1379, 1986.

62. Hirschfeld S, Tuboku Metzger AJ, Borkat G, et al: Comparison of exercise and catheterization results following total surgical correction of tetralogy of Fallot. J Thorac Cardiovasc Surg 75:446–451, 1978.

63. Hossack KF, Bruce RA, Green B, et al: Maximal cardiac output during upright exercise: approximately normal standards and variations with coronary heart disease. Am J Cardiol 46:204–212, 1980.

64. Hossack KF, Gross BW, Ritterman JB, et al: Evaluation of automated blood pressure measurements during exercise testing. Am Heart J 104:1032–1038, 1982.

65. Hossack KF, Kusumi F, Bruce RA: Approximate normal standards of maximal cardiac output during upright exercise in women. Am J Cardiol 47:1080–1086, 1981.

66. Hossack KF, Neilson GH: Exercise testing in congenital aortic stenosis. Aust NZ J Med 9:169–173, 1979.

67. Huang AH, Feigl EO: Adrenergic coronary vasoconstriction helps maintain uniform transmural blood flow distribution during exercise. Circ Res 62:286–289, 1988.

68. Iskandrian AS, Hakki AH: Radionuclide evaluation of exercise left ventricular performance in patients with coronary artery disease. Am Heart J 110:851–856, 1985.

69. Iskandrian AS, Hakki AH, Kane-Marsch S: Left ventricular pressure/volume relationship in aortic regurgitation. Am Heart J 110:1026–1032, 1985.

70. Iskandrian AS, Heo J: Radionuclide angiographic evaluation of left ventricular performance at rest and during exercise in patients with aortic regurgitation. Am Heart J 111:1143–1149, 1986.

71. Iskandrian AS, Heo J: Exaggerated systolic blood pressure response to exercise: a normal variant or a hyperdynamic phase of essential hypertension. Int J Cardiol 18:207–217, 1988.

72. Kavey RE, Thomas FD, Byrum CJ, et al: Ventricular arrhythmias and biventricular dysfunction after repair of tetralogy of Fallot. J Am Coll Cardiol 4:126–131, 1984.

73. Kligfield P, Okin PM, Ameisen O, et al: Evaluation of coronary artery disease by an improved method of exercise electrocardiography: the ST segment/heart rate slope. Am Heart J 112:589–598, 1986.

74. Kotchen TA, Hartley LH, Rice TW, et al: Renin, norepinephrine, and epinephrine response to graded exercise. J Appl Physiol 31:178–184, 1971.

75. Kulik TJ, Bass JL, Fuhrman BP, et al: Exercise induced pulmonary vasoconstriction. Br Heart J 50:59–64, 1983.

76. Lewis SF, Taylor WF, Graham RM, et al: Cardiovascular responses to exercise as functions of absolute and relative work load. J Appl Physiol 54:1314–1323, 1983.

77. MacDougall JD, Tuxen D, Sale DG, et al: Arterial blood pressure response to heavy resistance exercise. J Appl Physiol 58:785–790, 1985.

78. Manno BV, Hakki AH, Eshaghpour E, et al: Left ventricular function at rest and during exercise in congenital complete heart block: a radionuclide angiographic evaluation. Am J Cardiol 52:92–94, 1983.

79. Manyari DE, Kostuk WV, Purves PP: Left and right ventricular function at rest and during bicycle exercise in the supine and sitting position in normal subjects and patients with coronary artery disease: assessment and radionuclide ventriculography. Am J Cardiol 51:36–42, 1983.

80. Marshall RJ, Schirger A, Shepherd JT: Blood pressure during supine exercise in idiopathic orthostatic hypotension. Circulation 24:76–81, 1961.

81. Marx GR, Hicks RW, Allen HD, et al: Noninvasive assessment of hemodynamic responses to exercise in pulmonary regurgitation after operations to correct pulmonary outflow obstruction. Am J Cardiol 61:595–601, 1988.

82. McElroy PA, Janicki JS, Weber KT: Physiologic correlates of the heart rate response to upright isotonic exercise—relevance to rate-responsive pacemakers. J Am Coll Cardiol 11:94–100, 1988.

83. Mocellin R, Bastanier C, Hofacker W, et al: Exercise performance in children and adolescents after surgical repair of tetralogy of Fallot. Eur J Cardiol 4:367–374, 1976.

84. Morris SN, Phillips JF, Jordan JW, et al: Incidence and significance of decrease in systolic blood pressure during graded treadmill exercise testing. Am J Cardiol 41:221–226, 1978.

85. Murphy JH, Barlai-Kovach MM, Mathews RA, et al: Rest and exercise right and left ventricular function late after the Mustard operation: assessment by radionuclide ventriculography. Am J Cardiol 51:1520–1526, 1983.

86. Nelson SD, Kou WH, Annesley T, et al: Significance of ST segment depression during paroxysmal supraventricular tachycardia. J Am Coll Cardiol 12:383–387, 1988.

87. Northcote RJ, Ballantyne D: Cardiovascular implications of strenuous exercise. Int J Cardiol 8:3–12, 1985.

88. Okin PM, Kligfield P, Ameisen O, et al: Identification of anatomically extensive coronary artery disease by the exercise ECG ST segment/heart rate slope. Am Heart J 115:1002–1013, 1988.

89. Palmeri ST, Bonow RO, Myers CE, et al: Prospective evaluation of doxorubicin cardiotoxicity by rest and exercise radionuclide angiography. Am J Cardiol 58:607–613, 1986.

90. Parrish MD, Boucek RJ Jr, Burger J, et al: Exercise radionuclide ventriculography in children: normal values for exercise variables and right and left ventricular function. Br Heart J 54:509–516, 1985.

91. Parrish MD, Graham TP Jr, Bender HW, et al: Radionuclide angiographic evaluation of right and left ventricular function during exercise after repair of transposition of the great arteries. Comparison with normal subjects and patients with congenitally corrected transposition. Circulation 67:178–183, 1983.

92. Peterson RJ, Franch RH, Fajman WA, et al: Noninvasive determination of exercise cardiac function following Fontan operation. J Thorac Cardiovasc Surg 88:263–272, 1984.

93. Pichard AD, Gorlin R, Smith H, et al: Coronary flow studies in patients with left ventricular hypertrophy of the hypertensive type. Am J Cardiol 47:547–554, 1981.

94. Pichard AD, Smith H, Holt J, et al: Coronary vascular reserve in left ventricular hypertrophy secondary to chronic aortic regurgitation. Am J Cardiol 51:315–320, 1983.

95. Podrid PJ, Venditti FJ, Levine PA, et al: The role of exercise testing in evaluation of arrhythmias. Am J Cardiol 62(Suppl 12):24H–33H, 1988.

96. Poliner LR, Dehmer GJ, Lewis SE, et al: Left ventricular performance in normal subjects: a comparison of the responses to exercise in the upright and supine positions. Circulation 62:528–534, 1980.

97. Rajfer SI, Nemanich JW, Shurman AJ, et al: Metabolic responses to exercise in patients with heart failure. Circulation 76:VI46–VI53, 1987.

98. Ramsay JM, Venables AW, Kelly MJ, et al: Right and left ventricular function at rest and with exercise after the Mustard operation for transposition of the great arteries. Br Heart J 51:364–370, 1984.

99. Reduto LA, Berger HJ, Johnstone DE, et al: Radionuclide assessment of right and left ventricular exercise reserve after total correction of tetralogy of Fallot. Am J Cardiol 45:1013–1018, 1980.

100. Reybrouck T, Dumoulin M, Van der Hauwaert LG: Cardiorespiratory exercise testing after venous switch operation in children with complete transposition of the great arteries. Am J Cardiol 61:861–865, 1988.

101. Reybrouck T, Weymans M, Stijns H, et al: Exercise testing after correction of tetralogy of Fallot: the fallacy of a reduced heart rate response. Am Heart J 112:998–1003, 1986.

102. Riopel DA, Taylor AB, Hohn AR: Blood pressure, heart rate, pressure-rate product and electrocardiographic changes in healthy children during treadmill exercise. Am J Cardiol 44:697–704, 1979.

103. Robinson BF, Epstein SE, Beiser GD, et al: Control of heart rate by the autonomic nervous system. Studies in man on the interrelation between baroreceptor mechanisms and exercise. Circ Res 19:400–411, 1966.

104. Rochmis P, Blackburn H: Exercise tests. A survey of procedures, safety, and litigation experience in approximately 170,000 tests. JAMA 217:1061–1066, 1971.

105. Rodeheffer RJ, Gerstenblith G, Becker LC, et al: Exercise cardiac output is maintained with advancing age in healthy human subjects: cardiac dilation and increased stroke volume compensate for a diminished heart rate. Circulation 69:203–213, 1984.

106. Rozanski A, Diamond GA, Jones R, et al: A format for integrating the interpretation of exercise ejection fraction and wall motion and its application in identifying equivocal responses. J Am Coll Cardiol 5:238–248, 1985.

107. Ruttenberg HD, Adams TD, Orsmond GS, et al: Effects of exercise training on aerobic fitness in children after open heart surgery. Pediatr Cardiol 4:19–24, 1983.

108. Sawka MN, Glasner RM, Wilde SW, et al: Metabolic and circulatory responses to wheelchair and arm crank exercise. J Appl Physiol 49:784–788, 1980.

109. Schauer JE, Hanson P: Usefulness of a branching treadmill protocol for evaluation of cardiac functional capacity. Am J Cardiol 60:1373–1377, 1987.

110. Schieken RM, Clarke WR, Lauer RM: The cardiovascular responses to exercise in children across the blood pressure distribution: The Muscatine study. Hypertension 5:71–78, 1983.

111. Seitelberger R, Guth BD, Heusch G, et al: Intracoronary alpha-adrenergic receptor blockade attenuates ischemia in conscious dogs during exercise. Circ Res 62:436–442, 1988.

112. Shabetai R: Beneficial effects of exercise training in compensated heart failure. Circulation 78:775–776, 1988.

113. Siscovick DS, Weiss NS, Fletcher RH, et al: The incidence of primary cardiac arrest during vigorous exercise. N Engl J Med 311:874–877, 1984.

114. Smucker ML, Tedesco CL, Manning SB, et al: Demonstration of an imbalance between coronary perfusion and excessive load as a mechanism of ischemia during stress in patients with aortic stenosis. Circulation 78:573–582, 1988.

115. Steingart RM, Wexler J, Slagle S, et al: Radionuclide ventriculographic responses to graded supine and upright exercise: critical role of the Frank-Starling mechanism at submaximal exercise. Am J Cardiol 53:1671–1677, 1984.

116. Strauzenberg SE: Recommendations for physical activity and sports in children with heart disease. A statement by the Scientific Commission of the International Federation of Sports Medicine (FIMS) approved by the Executive Committee of the FIMS. J Sports Med 22:401–406, 1982.

117. Sullivan MJ, Higginbotham MB, Cobb FR: Exercise training in patients with severe left ventricular dysfunction: hemodynamic and metabolic effects. Circulation 78:506–515, 1988.

118. Thadani U, Parker JO: Hemodynamics at rest and during supine and sitting bicycle exercise in normal subjects. Am J Cardiol 41:52–59, 1978.

119. Tristani FE, Hughes CV, Archibald DG, et al: Safety of graded symptom-limited exercise testing in patients with congestive heart failure. Circulation 76:VI54–VI58, 1987.

120. Vergari J, Hakki H, Heo J, et al: Merits and limitations of quantitative treadmill exercise score. Am Heart J 114:819–826, 1988.

121. Viitasalo MT, Kala R, Eisalo A: Ambulatory electrocardiographic recording in endurance athletes. Br Heart J 47:213–220, 1982.

122. Wasserman K: Determinants and detection of anaerobic threshold and consequences of exercise above it. Circulation 76:VI29–VI39, 1987.

123. Weber KT, Janicki JS: Myocardial oxygen consumption—the role of wall force and shortening. Am J Physiol 233:H421–H477, 1977.

124. Weber KT, Janicki JS, McElroy PA: Determination of aerobic capacity and the severity of chronic and circulatory failure. Circulation 76:VI40–VI45, 1987.

125. Wetherbee JN, Bamrah VS, Ptacin MJ, et al: Comparison of ST segment depression in upright treadmill and supine bicycle exercise testing. J Am Coll Cardiol 11:330–337, 1988.

126. Whitmer JT, James FW, Kaplan S, et al: Exercise testing in children before and after surgical treatment of aortic stenosis. Circulation 63:254–263, 1981.

127. Wolthus RA, Froelicher VF Jr, Fischer J, et al: The response of healthy men to treadmill exercise. Circulation 55:153–157, 1977.

128. Young DZ, Lampert S, Graboys TB, et al: Safety of maximal exercise testing in patients at high risk for ventricular arrhythmia. Circulation 70:184–191, 1984.

Chapter 17

COMPUTING

Donald C. Fyler, M.D.

The remarkable value of computers to society, science, medicine, and to cardiologists is readily documented.[3-5] Sophisticated software[1] is available for word processing, data collection, data analysis, data storage, statistics, graphics, scheduling, accounting, and almost any imaginable purpose in cardiology. From a purely scientific point of view, the value of computers is emphasized by the number of papers presented at the International Computers in Cardiology meetings[2] and the hundreds of papers on computing in cardiology that have been published in recent years.

Although the Cardiology Department of the Boston Children's Hospital uses about 50 computers (mostly personal computers) for a variety of purposes (mainly word processing), the department has had a major interest in systematic accumulation of readily retrievable medical data about our patients for scientific purposes. There are some scheduling functions, but the system is not designed for business or administrative purposes.

The Information Systems Department of The Children's Hospital handles the administrative work of the Cardiology Department; cardiologists' billings are handled by a local firm. Although there were many false starts and mistakes, a working system of data management for cardiology patients has evolved over the past 20 years.

PURPOSE

The purpose of this system is to store and retrieve patient information. While the old system of maintaining card indexes, lists, and punch cards worked, the difficulty of reviewing data on a selected topic was sufficient to discourage browsing through the information. An ideal data-handling system allows the physician to pose a question and get a likely answer without having to rely on his or someone else's memory. **Retrieval** of factual information is the desired result. This is not a trivial point. Most available computing systems will accept and store almost unlimited amounts of data,

but no computer software presently on the market provides completely satisfactory retrieval, because the physician must understand the structure of the file, know the definitions used, and participate in developing the algorithms needed for output.

DATA COLLECTION

All reports produced by the department are typed into computer terminals, printed, and sent to the hospital chart. The input is interactively controlled by software, which adds precision; the resulting data are magnetically stored and maintained as a source of copies of reports and a resource for study (Table 1).

On input, software extracts key information (demographic, procedural, and diagnostic data) to update a summary file for each patient. Some information concerning clinic visits and surgical operations is entered directly into the patient summary file, there being no computed report to the hospital record. In each division of the cardiology department that produces information for the summary file, the data are handled according to the responsible physicians' convenience. For the most part, data are available for review within hours or days of entry.

Patient Summary File

The patient summary file was established so that the usually required information about a patient could be readily retrieved from a file uncluttered with nonessential material. The file is organized much like a hospital chart, being composed of event information in chronologic order, and can be described as an extract of key cardiac information about each patient (Fig. 1).

Selection of Data for Summary File. It is obvious that the success of such a procedure depends on what data are considered essential for inclusion in the summary. Clearly, not all physicians would agree on the key facts to be stored. The tendency to store excessive information must be resisted.

Table 1. Data Available for Analysis

Reports Available for Detailed Analysis	Data in Patient Summary File	Beginning Date
Cardiac catheterization	Diagnoses	1950
	Procedures	1982
	Complications	1982
Echocardiography	Diagnoses	1984
Electrocardiography	Selected diagnoses	1980
Surgery	Procedures	1950
	Complications	1973
Death	Diagnoses	
	Autopsy	1950
	Death certification no autopsy	1973
Stress tests	Diagnoses	1986
Clinic visit	Diagnoses (usually as Dx unchanged)	1973
Demographic data	Name, sex, birth date	1950

Although the computer can store virtually unlimited data, it is apparent that physicians (perhaps I should say human beings) cannot intellectually process unlimited amounts of data. Physicians cannot, without considerable expense and help, maintain the integrity of a large amount of data. However, it is possible to maintain a reliable summary file.

Generally, when faced with a computerized morass of data, the first order of business is to narrow down the data to hard facts by winnowing out soft and meaningless information. Only then can useful analysis begin. The theory behind the patient summary file is that carefully selected information can be reliably collected prospectively and used for searches or as core data for a retrospective study later.

At the same time, the original data, e.g., catheterization reports, echocardiographic reports, etc., can be searched for specific factual information and reviewed at a terminal.

Coding. To have a useful retrieval file, the data should be as unambiguous as possible. Coding the data as numbers helps to ensure consistency. When there is a limited number of acceptable codes, the amount of vague, confusing, or nonstandard language that slips into the file is diminished.

Clinic visits rarely produce new facts. In practice, when something new and important is discovered during a clinic visit, it is documented by reports of the tests that are ordered. Hence, the most important information obtained from a usual clinic visit is that the patient was alive on that day, vital information in calculating actuarial tables. Even though it is possible to change a diagnostic impression based solely on a clinic visit, this is a rare occurrence, and even then it is likely to be viewed as unsubstantiated data without a confirming event of some other type.

Clinical observations, such as varying intensity of a murmur, the size of the liver, or the respiratory rate, are useful observations in follow-up and management of the patient but contribute little to the diagnosis that is not better documented by other techniques. Chest x-rays pose a similar difficulty. While a pulmonary artery sling malformation might be recognized on the chest x-ray and the patient even referred to surgery without further evaluation, the fact that an operation was done to correct the malformation identifies that patient without doubt. For this reason the results of chest x-rays are not extracted for the patient summary file. Similarly, only a few items of electrocardiographic data are worth noting. There is little concern about the P-R interval, but an episode of ventricular tachycardia is of great interest.

Negative Information. It is important to record negative information. For example, ventricular defects that have closed spontaneously or diagnoses proposed by one diagnostic modality but ruled out by another are important facts. Without being confidant that we have the best method, we use a change in a single digit of a 6-digit diagnostic code to express the idea that the diagnosis has been ruled out. Although this may seem to be a slick answer to the problem, it requires that every search for a given diagnosis must consider this fact. Otherwise a list including patients in whom the diagnosis was ruled out might be produced. Furthermore, the diagnosis may be correct at one point and ruled out later, e.g., spontaneous closure of a ventricular septal defect. The system must allow accurate discovery of the facts in sequence, but the difficulty of managing the concept of "ruled out" should not be underestimated.

Functional Status of Surgical Procedures. Surgical procedures that are no longer functional pose a similar problem. An inadequate shunting procedure is an important fact. In this case, a digit allowing gradation of function, e.g., of a shunt operation or an artificial valve, is used with problems similar to negative information.

```
        CARDIOLOGY PATIENT SUMMARY        RECORD NO.    00-00-00-00
                                          NAME:         Test Case
                                          SEX:          M
                                          BIRTH DATE:   08/05/81

    EVENT     DATE     AGE AT EVENT         DXCODE       DIAGNOSIS
                        yr/mo/day
    CATH    08/07/81    00/00/03            120080       COARC (RO)
                                            141100       AS-VAL
                                            145080       AR (RO)
                                            202000       PFO
                                            240000       PHT
                                            340200       CHF
                                            153000       MR
                                                                    (AC/TH)
    SURG    08/07/81    00/00/03            141003       AS, SEVERE
                                    PR      660210       *AO-VALVOT
                                                                    (ARC)
    CLNC    02/08/82    00/06/05            141003       AS, SEVERE
                                                                    (DCF)
    CATH    04/25/83    01/08/20            141141       AS-VAL, RESID, MILD
                                            145031       AR, IATRO, MILD
                                            153001       MR, MILD
                                                                    (FS/PL)
    CLNC    05/07/84    02/09/02            382100       DX-UNCHNGED
                                                                    (DCF)
    ECHO    08/26/87    06/00/21            140100       AO-VAL-BICSPD
                                            141102       AS-VAL, MODERATE
                                            142101       AS-SUBVAL-DISCRET, MILD
                                            145001       AR, MILD
                                            153300       MVP
                                            153001       MR, MILD
                                            181380       LV DYSFUNC GLOBAL (RO)
                                                                    (DCF)
    CLNC    09/18/90    09/01/14            382100       DX-UNCHNGED
                                                                    (JFK)
```

Figure 1.   Modified from an actual patient summary. Events that are not shown but might be recorded include diagnoses reported on a electrocardiogram, results of an exercise test, death, catheterization procedures, and complications of cardiac catheterization or surgery. Codes are listed for ease in future entries. Diagnoses are abbreviated using local conventions. PR or (*) indicates a procedure performed on that date; RO, diagnosis ruled out; letters in parentheses are physicians' initials.

Outside Hospital Observations. For the most part, the data of interest for this book are those from The Boston Children's Hospital. Critical information may have been revealed by an echocardiogram, a catheterization, or an operation done elsewhere. Two methods are used to handle such information. First, an event accomplished elsewhere may be entered and identified by location. Unfortunately, the details of such an entry are sometimes difficult to gather. Often the dates, and sometimes the precise data, are not known. In this case prior operative procedures are entered as diagnostic codes. Such an entry indicates a prior operation—equivalent to the common notation "s/p" or status post. Unfortunately, outside data arrive via several routes so that arranging for systematic entry of this type of data is difficult.

Catheterization Procedures. Catheterization procedures, such as balloon valvuloplasty, are listed under the same codes as surgical procedures with a one-digit difference. As with surgical procedures, catheterization procedures may be listed as a diagnosis indicating status post, or listed as an event performed elsewhere.

Fetal Echocardiography. Fetal echocardiograms are a problem. At first the information is entered under the mother's name, and only after the baby is born is the infant's record established. For obvious reasons this is less than satisfactory, but a satisfactory answer is yet to be devised.

Length of Record. There is no limit to the chronologic length of a patient's summary file, nor is there any limit to the amount of summary data that may be stored as a single event. This makes it useful for special studies. A new file of demographic and other items of interest can be easily produced, ready for the addition and analysis of new study data. The file of data can be exported to someone's favorite spread-sheet for analysis.

Present Size of the Patient Summary File. The file now contains more than 40,000 patient records concerning over 100,000 events. About 10,000 of these patients have no known cardiac disease and represent patients seen once for evaluation of possible heart disease. When these patients, as well as those with mitral valve prolapse, are ignored, there are in the order of 18,000 patients who have significant congenital heart disease (1973–1990).

Errors. Computing systems are crippled by ridiculously simple errors. Errors in equal exponential garbage out. Accurate identification of patients has been the largest problem.

Errors in Record Numbers. Patient record numbers must be unique and completely reliable. If not, computing can become a nightmare. As with all things about computing, absolute precision is required. Our answer to this problem is to use the record number assigned by the hospital, in part to crosscheck readily with another computer file and, in part, to provide future access to useful information that may be in the hospital system, i.e., recovery of data about admissions of cardiac patients to other services in the hospital. In the future it is expected that the cardiology patient computer will be connected to the hospital network.

A common error is to have two record numbers for the same patient because of one incorrect digit. (One in 20 six-digit record numbers are in error as the result of one incorrect key stroke per 120.) Therefore, storing two records for the same patient with one digit difference in the record number is a problem. Mixing entries between two cardiac patients is not a common problem, because any random number accidentally typed as part of a six-digit record number will be an acceptable hospital record number, but most likely will not be the number of another cardiac patient and, therefore, will not be in the file.

Coding Errors. Diagnostic and procedural coding errors occur. In general there are fewer errors if the responsible physician does the coding at the time the report is completed. Often these errors are discovered when a copy of the data is put in front of the physician at the next patient visit or when a study of patients with that problem is undertaken. Whenever a question arises, the original data can be reviewed at a computer terminal.

Incorrect Dates. Incorrect dates are not common, in part, because all information is dated and the computer will not accept a date that is out of order for that patient and, in part, because age (based on the birth date) and the date of the event are printed with all output, where they may attract attention of the users.

Detection of Errors. The methods used to detect and correct errors are:

1. Maximal day-to-day use of the computer files by physicians and other knowledgeable people who will recognize errors is emphasized. Liberal provision for monthly summaries, case summaries, and searches of the file helps to reveal discrepancies. The more the file is used, the more the errors are recognized; or, the more useful the file, the fewer errors creep in!

2. Regular comparison to the demographic files maintained by the hospital uncovers most errors in the record numbers and also updates demographics.

3. A program that regularly searches the entire file for patients with nearly identical names or birth dates and with one-digit variation in record number finds others.

4. Printouts of patients on an alphabetical list points out patients with the same name. When these observations are crosschecked against birth dates, diagnoses, and procedures, some errors are glaringly obvious.

Clearly, crosschecking of data is an ongoing process that must be pursued vigilantly. It is obvious that the file of a child with a large number of observations, each confirming the same diagnosis, provides the most reliable information. To put this another way, the longer the follow-up of the patient and the more varied the kinds of confirmatory data received, the more reliable the information becomes.

Revisions of the Coding System

The coding system has passed through several revisions. Given modern computing, the shift from one coding system to another has been a matter of appropriate algorithms to cover the translations needed.

The urge to have everyone use the same coding system as a way to provide better communication among physicians is understandable, but this form of restriction is scarcely necessary because it is possible for any coding system to be readily translated into any other whenever the need arises. It is the author's conviction that attempting to limit the coding system to somebody's favorite classification is counterproductive, because limitation of language leads to limitations of thought that are sometimes not readily apparent.

From a purely scientific point of view, it would be best if a coding system were sharply defined and used indefinitely. The futility of this idea becomes apparent after 5–10 years, when changing concepts and new information naturally force change. Although precision and consistency are desirable, it is also important not to stifle progress with outmoded concepts.

The requirement for precision in computing influences the coding system. Codes based on some profound, physiologic, or embryologic theory that requires judgmental decisions about coding negate the entire process unless all of the coding is done by the same individual. Because our system depends on many physicians from different disciplines entering data, it is necessary to make the principal codes as unequivocal—as nonjudgmental—as possible. Such descriptions as "virtually intact septum," "possible," "malalignment," "mild hypoplasia," "near pulmonary atresia," or "mild mitral prolapse," although understandable to the originator, serve only to clutter a computer file. Fuzzy thinking leads to fuzzy data. Fuzzy data, inherent in all systems, are unavoidable; the goal is to keep them at a minimum. The problem is largely controlled if the central features (main diagnoses, procedures, and demographics) have the greatest possible precision. Ill-defined subcategories of information can always be accommodated but must not be allowed to confuse the basic system. To state this another way, important data should be handled with precision, and unimportant items of fuzzy information can be managed by a computer but are useful primarily to the originator.

Although some years ago it was impossible to handle data in English words because of the difference in storage expense between numbers and letters, today, because enormous amounts of data can be stored at minimal cost, the possibility of simply using English diagnoses may seem attractive. After all, a computer can recognize "ventricular septal defect" as easily as a number. English is fine so long as one person describes the diagnosis or surgical procedure. Use by numerous persons soon leads to slight variations in the terms or the spelling, which can be crippling. For this reason both numeric codes and English words are recorded and can be included simultaneously in a search. Generally, the numeric code helps to find the case, whereas words may explain nuances.

SEARCHES

There has been confusion about the data available in the computer. Somehow it does not seem possible to some physicians, usually older ones, that the computer produces exactly the same data found in the hospital chart and the very same data found in Cardiology Department reports. That the computer largely functions as a fancy crossfiling system seems simplistic and the result almost magical. There is concern that somehow the computer might mix it all up. The incredible precision that is the very foundation of computing is frightening.

A review of cases, using a computer, is the equivalent of an old-fashioned chart review; indeed, probably it is more precise because judgmental decisions about individual case selection, an inherently human frailty, are less likely. An algorithm defined by the physician selects the patients uniformly, whereas an individual may variably select cases with built-in prejudices. The errors that are encountered are largely administrative and are fewer in number than the expected errors that are usually found in hospital records.

All Cardiology Department files may be searched using similar programs. Multivectorial searches are possible, e.g., looking for a patient with a particular diagnosis, seen during a selected time period, who had a cardiac surgical procedure, by a particular surgeon. The search may be conducted by codes or as searches for strings of characters such English words or abbreviations. Because of the size of the patient summary file (40,000 records), the usual practice is to make a list based on a single factor, e.g., the patients seen in a given time period or with a particular diagnosis or operation. Further analysis of the data is then based

on that list. Generalized formatting programs can be used to show the information extracted. A variety of programs have been developed that provide for specific types of output, but it should be emphasized that user friendliness has not been a major goal. Rather it has been our philosophy that true browsing through data requires the direct participation of a knowledgeable physician posing questions in response to the answers obtained from the prior question in a truly interactive fashion. This can be done through a programmer, but surely the future holds better than that. Nonetheless, user-friendly programs that will someday anticipate the physician's every need are an unrealistic dream.

DATA ANALYSIS FOR THIS BOOK

Case Selection

The patient must have been seen between January 1, 1973 and January 1, 1988. Patients seen during this period but who were known to this department before that time are included. A minimum possible follow-up of 1 year for all patients was selected, in part, to ensure the precision afforded by multiple observations and, in part, to provide the possibility of a 1 year minimum follow-up of survivors (Exhibit 1). As a consequence of this decision, the earliest date for beginning data analysis for this book was January 1, 1989. Occasionally information developed after January 1, 1988 is presented if it seems of special interest. The data generated from this file have not been published in this form before and, therefore, are new to authors and are sometimes surprising.

Diagnostic Categorization of Patients

Ignoring the administrative entries such as "diagnosis unchanged," the diagnoses listed for any event were generalized to a single diagnosis for that event, using a hierarchical system of assigning a label (Table 2). The hierarchical order of categorical diagnoses was designed, as much as possible, to mimic the general usage of these terms in the Cardiology and Cardiac Surgery Departments of the Children's Hospital in Boston. These

Exhibit 1

Boston Children's Hospital Experience	
Patients Seen Between 1/1/73 and 1/1/88 (N = 23,638)	
Heart disease 16,429	No heart disease (includes administration entries and diagnosis of no disease) 7,209
Patients with heart disease First seen before 1973 2,677	Patients with heart disease First seen after 1973 13,752

Table 2. Diagnostic Hierarchy

1. Malpositions	15. Aortic valve abnormalities
Dextrocardia with situs solitus	Aortic stenosis valvar
Visceral heterotaxy	Subaortic stenosis
Cantrell's syndrome	Supravalvar aortic stenosis
Polysplenia	Aortic regurgitation
Ectopic cordis	16. Pulmonary valve abnormalities
2. Mitral atresia or aortic atresia	Pulmonary stenosis
Hypoplastic left heart	Valvar stenosis
Left atrioventricular valve atresia	Subvalvar stenosis
3. Tricuspid atresia	Double-chamber right ventricle
Right atrioventricular valve atresia	Peripheral pulmonary stenosis
4. Single ventricle	17. Tricuspid valve abnormality
5. Truncus arteriosus	Tricuspid regurgitation
Truncus	Tricuspid stenosis
Hemitruncus	Ebstein's disease
Aortopulmonary window	18. Mitral valve abnormalities
6. Double-outlet right ventricle	Mitral stenosis
7. D-transposition of the great arteries	Mitral regurgitation
8. L-transposition of the great arteries	19. Myocardial disease
9. Total anomalous pulmonary venous return	Myocarditis
10. Pulmonary atresia with intact septum	Inborn errors
11. Tetralogy of Fallot	Idiopathic hypertrophic cardiomyopathy
Pulmonary atresia	Friedreich's cardiomyopathy
Tetralogy of Fallot with endocardial cushion defect	Duchenne's and Becker's cardiomyopathies
12. Endocardial cushion defects	20. Pericardial disease
Atrial defect primum	21. Atrial septal defect secundum
Atrioventricular canal	Partially anomalous pulmonary veins
Common atrium	22. Patent ductus arteriosus
13. Coarctation of aorta	23. Aneurysms
Coarctation with intact ventricular septum	24. Fistulas
Coarctation with ventricular septal defect	Systemic
Interrupted aortic arch	Pulmonary
14. Ventricular defect	25. Pulmonary hypertension
With pulmonary vascular disease	26. Systemic hypertension
With aortic regurgitation	27. Miscellaneous
With aortic stenosis	
With mitral valve abnormality	
With pulmonary stenosis	
With pulmonary regurgitation	

diagnoses were recorded for all events for each patient and were compared and used to assign an overall categorical diagnosis for that patient. Eighty-five percent of the patients had concordant generalized event diagnoses. If there was discordance among event diagnoses, the combination of data from cardiac catheterization, echocardiograms, surgery, or autopsy was used to provide the best possible diagnosis. If there was still discordance, the diagnosis based on the most recent information was used. Up to this point categorization of the case material was accomplished using computer programs based on algorithms describing the above process.

Finally, there were variably conflicting data for approximately 300 patients whose summary data were printed out and sight-reviewed. Decisions, sometimes arbitrary, were made to describe each on an individual basis. When these questionable cases were compared with better documented cases, using the other diagnostic features, the age distribution, and other measures of comparability,

there was no obvious difference within the selected category.

Unusual and unexpected output was further sight-checked through examination of the detailed reports available via the computer. Very rarely, hospital charts were used to confirm apparent results that might influence generalizations about a particular topic.

The entire file of selected patients was divided into groups based on the assigned categorical diagnoses. Subsequently, each diagnostic group was reviewed in detail as each chapter was written.

Patients were considered in terms of their categorical diagnosis or the diagnosis without respect to categories. Thus, there were patients whose primary diagnosis (categorical diagnosis) was coarctation of the aorta and at the same time there were many others with coarctation of the aorta associated with some other important diagnosis, e.g., transposition of the great arteries.

Some error is inescapable. Clearly, exceptions must be made to cover the unique or rare cases that are included in this filing system; often these are listed under miscellaneous codes or ambiguous English and require review on a case-by-case basis.

The degree of diagnostic confusion can be quantified by simply comparing the entries of various events. If multiple surgical, echocardiographic, or catheterization entries are in diagnostic conflict, the degree of conflict can be expressed as a percent of the ultimately assigned categorical diagnosis. There was notable conflict in the malposition category. Analysis of this category of cardiac disease is better handled with the time-honored chart-by-chart review, at least until we know a better way. For this reason, patients with this group of diagnoses have been separated from all others. Therefore, a child with dextrocardia and tetralogy of Fallot is considered different from others with tetralogy of Fallot simply because, on the average, the chance for confusion is greater than for tetralogy of Fallot without malposition. All other cases with conflicting data represent less than 5% of the total number of children in each diagnostic category.

Calculation of **actuarial curves** is based on the date when the patient was first seen or, in the case of surgery, when an operation of a given type is first performed. Patients first seen before 1973 were excluded from these calculations. Most actuarial curves are plotted for 18 months, because systematic follow-up for actuarial purposes has not been done. Except for topics of particular interest, long-range follow-up has been deemed to cost too much to be done routinely for all cases.

Hospital mortality following surgery is defined as death between the first day the chest was opened to perform a given operation and 30 days later, and it is labeled 30-day mortality.

The tables and curves produced in these studies are presented as **exhibits** in each chapter, as appropriate.

COST OF COMPUTING

At some point in the academic practice of cardiology, the cost of computing must be considered. The degree of accuracy of the data ultimately determines the cost. Once a computer is available and a management system has been adopted, data analysis is the least expensive item unless a programmer is required. (Not all physicians have the academic interest or desire to study clinical data using a computer; hence, the added expense and inconvenience of a programmer may be unavoidable.) The author finds data analysis relatively easy and is convinced that methods already available can be improved and made more user friendly. Data storage becomes increasingly inexpensive as the technology for storage improves with time. The major expenditure is for personnel costs related to data collection. Someone must be responsible for the entry and accuracy of each datum. The number of items is less important than the accuracy. Each small increment in accuracy is associated with an exponential increase in cost.

Based on this reasoning we have arranged to accept and store the entry of the usual hospital reports with virtually no added expense, because these reports would be generated anyway. The added expense of initial programming and development of programs is now largely behind us. With the initial purchase and development completed, the main operational expense is the cost of personnel to maintain a reliable patient summary file, which is useful as a resource for academic and management information. In our scheme this operational cost is sufficiently diffuse that we can only guess at the day-to-day expense. The author believes that it is in the order of 2% of the departmental operational budget.

REFERENCES

1. Cardiovascular Software Directory. American College of Cardiology, Bethesda, Maryland, 1988.
2. Computers in Cardiology. Abstracts, Thirteenth Annual Scientific Sessions, Boston, October 7, 1986.
3. Geiser EA, Skorton DJ (eds): Seminar on computer applications for the cardiologist—I. J Am Coll Cardiol 8:930–948, 1986.
4. Geiser EA, Skorton DJ (eds): Seminar on computer applications for the cardiologist—II. J Am Coll Cardiol 8:1211–1217, 1986.
5. Geiser EA, Skorton DJ (eds): Seminar on computer applications for the cardiologist—III. J Am Coll Cardiol 9:204–214, 1987.

Section VII
Prevalence

Chapter 18

TRENDS

Donald C. Fyler, M.D.

PREVALENCE OF PEDIATRIC HEART DISEASE

The prevalence of congenital heart disease has been remarkably constant throughout the world and over the years (Table 1).[2–7,9–11,13] There is no reason to suspect a change in recent times. Not only is the incidence of congenital heart disease relatively predictable, but the relative frequency of the various congenital cardiac defects varies little (Table 2). An exception is subpulmonary ventricular septal defect, a lesion that is more common in Asia;[1] other than this, there is little to suggest a different prevalence overall or among the many defects. What variation is encountered can usually be ascribed to the vagaries of classification or the inadequacies of enumeration.

Worldwide, heart disease in children continues to be a major public health problem. Largely this is because of rheumatic heart disease, although in China myocardial disease is reported to be an important problem in children.[12] The incidence of rheumatic disease seems to be directly related to social circumstances (see ch. 22), and where poverty exists it is common. In the United States congenital heart disease accounts for almost all heart disease in children.

Perhaps of more interest than the total number of children born with heart disease is the number of babies who will require special medical facilities because of heart disease. The New England Infant Cardiac Program[7] reported that, excluding premature infants with patent ductus arteriosus, 3 infants of every 1000 live births will need cardiac catheterization and/or surgery and/or will die with congenital heart disease in early infancy. Approximately 5/1000 live births will require specialized

facilities at some time during their lives. The trained personnel and special equipment needed to manage the diagnostic questions about heart disease, to document hemodynamically unimportant cardiac lesions, to follow repaired patients, and to manage such problems as Kawasaki's disease or the dyslipidemias will vary with local interest. All together, about 10/1000 live births, or about 1% of children born each year, make up the patient material of pediatric cardiology in the United States.

CARDIAC LESIONS

The rank order of cardiac defects seen at the Children's Hospital in Boston has varied somewhat over time, reflecting the changing interests of the department (Table 3). The recent increase in atrial septal defects is probably related to local interests in closing these defects with devices introduced during cardiac catheterization (Fig. 1). The increase in the number of patients with heterotaxy (see ch. 37) is caused not only by an absolute increase in numbers but also by the fact that these patients now survive and return. It is predictable that the number of encounters with patients with heterotaxy will increase. The explanation for the increasing number of new patients with heterotaxy is less obvious.

The increase in the number of patients with myocardial problems was not anticipated and deserves attention (Table 3). The classification of myocardial disease has varied so much over the years that concern about the reliability of the data is justified. The disappearance of the disease called subendocardial fibroelastosis emphasizes this point. Clearly, this disease did not disappear; it was just renamed. Our present nomenclature and the prev-

Table 1. Prevalence of Congenital Heart Disease*

Author	Ferencz[6]	Fyler[7]	Calgren[3]	Mitchell[13]
Years of study	1981–1982	1969–1977	1941–1950	1956–1965
Reference population	Resident births, Marland and Washington, DC metropolitan area	Resident births, 6 New England states	Resident births, Gothenburg, Sweden	Selected pregnancies, 12 clinical centers, USA
Birth cohort: length of follow-up	1 year	1 year	7–16 years	1 month–9 years
No. of congenital heart disease cases	664	2,251	369	420
No. of livebirths	179,697	1,528,686	58,105	54,765
Prevalence per 1,000 livebirths				
Conotruncal and major septation defects				
Transposition of great arteries	0.211 (0.211)	0.215	0.379	0.201
Tetralogy of Fallot	0.262 (0.190)	0.214	0.310	0.292
Double outlet right ventricle	0.056 (0.056)	0.033		0.073
Truncus arteriosus	0.056 (0.056)	0.034	0.069	0.128
Endocardial cushion defects	0.362 (0.251)	0.118	0.172	0.274
Total anomalous pulmonary venous return	0.083 (0.083)	0.058	0.052	
Atresias				
Tricuspid atresia	0.039 (0.034)	0.057	0.086	0.091
Pulmonary atresia	0.083 (0.077)	0.071	0.069	0.091
Hypoplastic left heart syndrome	0.267 (0.205)	0.164	0.103	0.237
Valve and vessel lesions				
Pulmonic stenosis	0.189 (0.080)	0.073	0.275	0.657
Aortic stenosis	0.111 (0.083)	0.041	0.344	0.292
Coarctation of aorta	0.239 (0.200)	0.185	0.620	0.511
Septal defects				
Ventricular septal defect	0.863 (0.345)	0.379	1.699	2.264
Atrial septal defect	0.317 (0.094)	0.073	0.241	0.566
Patent ductus arteriosus	0.089 (0.062)	0.138	0.602	0.639
Other	0.468 (0.349)	0.177	0.396	0.950
Unable to classify			0.964	0.402
Total	3.70 (2.38)	2.03	6.35	7.67
Clinical diagnosis only			37%	48%
Rate of confirmed congenital heart disease	3.70 (2.38)	2.03	4.00	3.99

*From Ferencz C, Rubin JD, McCarter RJ, et al: Congenital heart disease: prevalence at live birth; the Baltimore-Washington Infant Study. Am J Epidemiol 121:31–36, 1984, with permission.

Table 1. Prevalence of Congenital Heart Disease *(Continued)*

Hoffman[10]	Feldt[5]	Dickinson[4]	Bound[2]	Laursen[11]
1959–1966	1950–1969	1960–1969	1957–1971	1963–1973
Members of Kaiser Foundation Health Plan	Resident births, Olmstead County, MN	Resident births, Liverpool, England	Resident births, Blackpool, England	Livebirths, Denmark
5–13 years	1–10 years	3–12 years	School age	Birth–15 years
163	179	884	338	5,249
19,044	32,393	160,480	56,982	(Approximately 855,000)
0.315	0.432	0.27	0.333	0.29
0.315 0.053	0.278	0.32	0.509	0.36
0.210 0.315	0.247	0.06 0.13	0.070 0.439	0.09 0.15
0.053		0.07	0.123	
	0.185	0.09	0.088	0.05
0.053		0.04		0.04
0.053	0.247	0.16	0.193	0.18
1.155		0.42	0.158	0.36
0.315	0.340	0.28	0.246	0.29
0.473	0.309	0.35	0.333	0.43
2.678	1.914	1.80	1.667	1.48
0.525	0.401	0.32	0.491	0.58
0.473	0.587	0.65	0.386	0.77
1.575	0.587	0.35	0.895	0.49
		0.18		0.58
8.56	5.53	5.51	5.93	6.14
52%	32%	32%	31%	30%
4.11	3.76	3.75	4.09	4.30

Table 2. Listing of Diseases by Hierarchical Diagnosis*

Diagnosis (1973–1987)	No. of Patients
Ventricular septal defect	3322
Pulmonary valve abnormality	1500
Tetralogy of Fallot	1403
Aortic valve abnormality	1060
Secundum atrial septal defect	891
Patent ductus arteriosus	866
Coarctation of the aorta	826
D-loop transposition	755
Endocardial cushion defect	717
Ventricular dysfunction	369
Malposition (heterotaxy)	335
Mitral valve abnormality	296
Hypoplastic left ventricle	287
Double-outlet right ventricle	224
Single ventricle	192
Tricuspid atresia	154
Pulmonary hypertension	135
Total anomalous pulmonary venous return	118
Pericardial abnormality	111
Truncus arteriosus	107
Rheumatic fever or rheumatic heart disease	102
L-loop transposition	90
Pulmonary atresia and intact ventricular septum	83
Systemic hypertension	76
Tricuspid valve abnormality	76
Ebstein's disease	75
Systemic artery anomaly	70
Systemic arteriovenous fistula	34
Cardiac tumor	32
Anomalous coronary artery from pulmonary artery	29
Aorto-pulmonary window	19
Origin of right pulmonary artery from aorta	10
Aneurysm, artery	13
Primary arrhythmia	883
Bicuspid aortic valve	71
Mitral valve prolapse	367
Patent foramen ovale	65
Questionable heart disease	63
No significant heart disease	6743
Noncardiac anomaly	577
No data†	466
TOTAL	23612

*Each patient listed once.
†A file was begun but no data entered.

alence of various myocardial problems at the present time at the Children's Hospital in Boston are presented in Table 4.

Over the past 15 years there has been a steady increase in the number of patients with primary myocardial problems. At present, this diagnosis ranks as the fourth most common form of heart disease, in the same range as patent ductus arteriosus, D-transposition of the great arteries, tetralogy of Fallot, and aortic valve disease. Some of this increase is the result of the increasing use of echocardiography and, thereby, the recognition of my-

ocardial dysfunction, which might otherwise have been unsuspected. Increasing numbers of patients survive neoplastic disease because of treatment with doxorubicin and are now being followed because of myocardial damage (Table 4). The acquired immunodeficiency syndrome (AIDS) further contributes to the number of patients with myocardial problems, and the Kawasaki syndrome contributes some more. There is no way to determine whether this increase is a local phenomenon, although it seems unlikely.

The management of children with the Kawasaki syndrome now includes examination of the coronaries to discover and manage the coronary aneurysms and myocardial problems that are part of this disease.

In the past 4 years the number of children referred for lipid evaluation because of positive screening tests or because of a positive family history has reached 500 per year. The level at which this will stabilize is a matter of interest for planners.

AGE WHEN FIRST SEEN

For some years it has been a matter of conviction at The Children's Hospital in Boston that the earliest discovery, diagnosis, and surgical treatment produces the best long-term results for patients with congenital heart disease. As a result, over the years the average age at surgery has decreased until recently, when it has stabilized and even risen slightly.

A survey of hospitalized patients in the past 2–3 years shows a bimodal age distribution of patients admitted with congenital heart disease. Infants newly discovered to have a cardiac problem constitute one group, whereas older children and adolescents with rhythm problems contribute to the second peak.

EFFECTS OF CHANGING TECHNOLOGY ON THE PRACTICE OF CARDIOLOGY

An increasing number of patients is being seen each year at The Children's Hospital in Boston (Table 5). Although some of this increase can be accounted for by the recently increasing birth rate, much of it can be accounted for by referral of patients for specialized techniques not formerly available, such as electrophysiologic studies, fetal echocardiography, new surgical techniques, and interventional cardiac catheterizations.

Patients who ultimately are proved to have no significant cardiac problem may undergo echocardiography as part of their examination, but studies that establish the absence of heart disease make up less than 15% of the workload. In any case, these patients do not contribute greatly to the cost of care, because follow-up is rarely needed.

Table 3. Relative Incidence of the Most Common Cardiac Problems in Recent Years

Year First Seen					
1982–1984 (n = 3073)		1985–1987 (n = 3654)		1988–1990 (n = 5512)	
Dx	%	Dx	%	Dx	%
VSD	17.7	VSD	17.3	VSD	14.1
TF	6.5	TF	7.2	ASD2	8.8
PS	5.8	PS	6.7	PS	6.8
ASD2	5.5	DTGA	6.5	MYO	6.4
ECD	5.3	ASD2	6.5	PDA	6.3
AS	5.0	AS	6.5	TF	6.3
COARC	5.0	PDA	4.9	DTGA	6.0
PDA	4.6	ECD	4.8	AS	5.9
DTGA	4.4	COARC	4.7	ECD	4.4
MIT	4.4	MIT	4.7	MIT	4.0
HLV	3.3	MYO	3.3	COARC	3.8
MYO	2.9	HLV	3.1	HLV	3.3
MAL	2.2	MAL	2.0	MAL	3.3

Abbreviations: VSD, ventricular septal defect; TF, tetralogy of Fallot; PS, pulmonary stenosis; ASD2, secundum atrial septal defect; ECD, endocardial cushion defect; AS, aortic stenosis; COARC, coarctation of the aorta; PDA, patent ductus arteriosus; DTGA, D-transposition of the great arteries; MIT, mitral valve disease; HLV, hypoplastic left heart syndrome; MYO, primary myocardial disease; MAL, malposition.

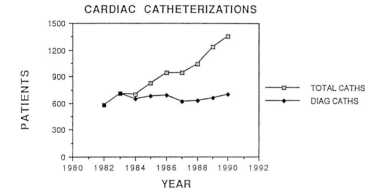

Figure 1. The increase in the total number of cardiac catheterizations is directly related to the increase in interventional procedures. (Courtesy Dr. M. Freed.)

Table 4. Primary Myocardial Disease in Infants and Toddlers Two Years Old or Less, 1982–1990

N = 346	
Category	Percent
Ventricular dysfunction due to ischemic damage	32
Idiopathic cardiomyopathy or myocarditis	31
Toxic cardiomyopathy (doxorubicin)	12
Kawasaki cardiomyopathy	9
Acquired Immunodeficiency Syndrome	7
Bacterial Sepsis	6
Glycogen and mucopolysaccharide storage cardiomyopathy	3

Courtesy Dr. A. Matitiau.

It was anticipated that the increasing number of echocardiograms (Table 5) would result in decreased numbers of diagnostic cardiac catheterizations. When considering only the patients who are ultimately proved to have heart disease, there is a trend compatible with this theory (Table 6). For the average patient the likelihood that cardiac catheterization will be needed has decreased somewhat, even though the absolute number of cardiac catheterizations is rising. Similarly, it was thought that the increasing number of interventional cardiac catheterizations would result in fewer cardiac operations. This also seems to be the case, because the proportion of patients undergoing cardiac surgery has decreased. Nonetheless, the absolute number of surgical procedures is increasing.

Despite these encouraging thoughts, the new procedures are technically more involved, require more physician time, and use more expensive equipment. The result is that the care of patients with congenital heart disease is becoming more expensive, even though the number of procedures per patient is not changing. The expected savings resulting from interventional catheterization procedures have yet to be realized, largely because the insurance bureaucracy is mired in its own paper.

It seems that many patients with congenital heart disease who survive will require medical supervision indefinitely; hence the average number of patients being followed will increase over the years (Table 7).

Who will take care of surviving patients is a matter of practical concern. Internists' lack of experi-

Table 5. Number of Procedures in Patients with Heart Disease by Year*

	1985	1986	1987	1988	1989	1990
Echocardiography						
Patients	1002	1610	1983	2073	2632	2993
Procedures	1834	2539	3254	3592	4297	4954
Catheterization						
Patients	716	770	734	839	912	1040
Procedures	838	949	954	1043	1181	1275
Surgery						
Patients	506	531	541	620	734	784
Procedures	724	734	748	819	912	963
Totals						
All patients	1422	1943	2173	2314	2817	3167
All procedures	3396	4222	4956	5454	6390	7192
Deaths	136	108	132	120	71	108
Percent Mortality	9.6	5.6	6.1	5.2	2.5	3.4

*Patients with no significant heart disease, mitral valve prolapse, and administrative problems excluded.

Table 6. Number of Procedures per Cardiac Patient*

Procedures	1985	1986	1987	1988	1989	1990
Echocardiograms	1.29	1.31	1.50	1.55	1.52	1.56
Catheterizations	0.58	0.48	0.42	0.44	0.41	0.40
Cardiac operations	0.51	0.38	0.35	0.36	0.33	0.30
Total procedures	2.38	2.17	2.27	2.35	2.26	2.26

*Considers patients established to have heart disease. Patients with no significant heart disease, mitral valve prolapse, or only bicuspid aortic valve were not included.

Table 7. Incremental Increase in Patients Undergoing Procedures Each Year

Patient Category	1985	1986	1987	1988	1989	1990
New patients	1109	1291	1265	1677	1897	1947
Patients carried over from previous years	313	652	908	637	920	1220
Total patients	1422	1943	2173	2314	2817	3167

ence with congenital heart disease is readily comprehended. One needs only to divide the number of probable survivors by the number of internists to recognize that each physician may have one surviving adult who could have had any of a variety of strange congenital cardiac lesions and/or major surgical procedures virtually unknown in adult practice. The average internist will find these patients interesting and often baffling. Some attention to this problem will be necessary.

Echocardiography

Because echocardiography can be performed with mobile equipment, without exposure to X-radiation, and can be repeated as often as needed, this diagnostic technique is being used increasingly. Fetal echocardiograms are performed at the request of ultrasonographers when there is concern about the anatomy of the fetal heart on routine obstetric screening; the number of such examinations has stabilized.

Intraoperative echocardiography, although somewhat cumbersome, is useful occasionally in specific situations. Perhaps more practical is the recent use of esophageal echocardiography in complex diseases to evaluate ongoing progress during cardiac surgery. Just how valuable this will be in the future remains to be determined.

The use of esophageal echocardiography to guide the placement of intracardiac devices during interventional cardiac catheterization is now an established procedure. The proximity of the echo transducer to the heart allows better definition of structures (particularly of the devices themselves) than does fluoroscopy. With better definition the likelihood of more precise placement is readily appreciated.

Cardiac Catheterization

The steady improvement in diagnosis by echocardiography results in fewer diagnostic cardiac catheterizations. Yet, because of interventional procedures, the number of cardiac catheterizations has reached an all-time high (Fig. 1). The numbers and types of interventional catheterization procedures continue to expand (see exhibit 2, ch. 14). Patent ductus arteriosus of suitable size and secundum atrial defects of suitable size and location

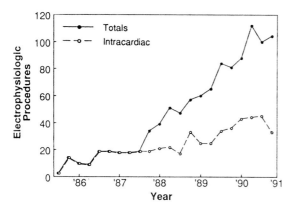

Figure 2. While the number of intracardiac electrophysiologic studies has increased gradually, the number of esophageal electrophysiologic studies has increased dramatically and accounts for most of the electrophysiologic studies at the present time. (Courtesy Dr. E. Walsh.)

are now (1991) closed routinely at cardiac catheterization. New interventions that are promising include the use of stents to reinforce the dilated vessels, particularly in patients with peripheral pulmonary stenosis. Equally interesting is the use of clamshell devices to close multiple ventricular septal defects. The possibility that these devices may not only replace a surgical procedure but actually be more satisfactory seems likely. One device may cover several adjacent holes, and the use of several devices to cover multiple holes in a patient with a ventricular defect of the Swiss cheese type has been accomplished.

Electrophysiologic Studies

It is becoming obvious that patients with congenital heart disease, with or without surgery, may develop important rhythm problems as they survive longer. The number of patients requiring evaluation, either by intracardiac or esophageal electrophysiologic study or by inpatient observation is increasing (Fig. 2). The more surgical success, the more patients survive, and the more often rhythm problems are encountered.

In the past few years a small number of patients have undergone surgical division of bypass tracts responsible for recurrent arrhythmias. More recently, catheter ablation techniques have been used successfully and give promise of replacing the surgical approach.[14]

Steady improvement in generators, lead wires, and batteries has resulted in less reservation about the use of pacemakers. More than 358 patients have had implantable pacemakers at The Children's Hospital in Boston, more than 50% of these in the past 10 years.[8]

Surgery

Even though many patients with conditions formerly corrected by surgical operations are now being treated with interventional catheter techniques, the number of surgical operations being performed at Children's Hospital is increasing (Table 5). Clearly, some of the least complicated cardiac defects are being managed by catheter techniques, with the result that the average cardiac surgical operation is becoming more difficult and dangerous.

Improved understanding of the hemodynamics involved in the Fontain principle has led to newer surgical methods that achieve better results. Artificial valves are avoided, right atrial-to-right ventricular connections, and right atrial-to-main pulmonary artery anastomoses have been largely

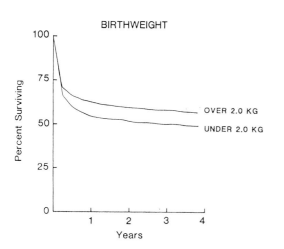

Figure 3. Effect of low birth weight on the survival of children with congenital heart disease. (Based on data from The New England Infant Cardiac Program.[7])

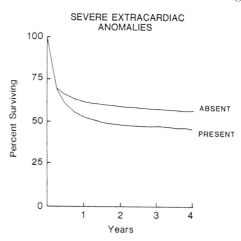

Figure 4. Effect of severe extracardiac anomalies on the survival of children with congenital heart disease. Severe extracardiac anomalies are defined as those which influence life and well-being and are not reparable. (Based on data from The New England Infant Cardiac Program.[7])

Table 8. Rank Order of Diagnoses Among Survivors with Congenital Heart Disease
by Age When Last Seen, 1973–1990

	1 Year (n = 4073)		1–9 Years (n = 8169)		10–19 Years (n = 5243)		More than 20 Years (n = 3015)	
Rank	Dx	%	Dx	%	Dx	%	Dx	%
1	VSD	27	VSD	21	VSD	14	VSD	16
2	PDA	11	PS	8	PS	11	TF	12
3	DTGA	8	ASD2	8	AS	11	AS	11
4	PS	7	TF	8	TF	6	PS	10
5	ASD2	6	AS	5	ASD2	5	ASD2	7
6	TF	6	DTGA	5	COARC	5	COARC	5
	Other	35	Other	45	Other	48	Other	39

Abbreviations: VSD, ventricular septal defect; PDA, patent ductus arteriosus; DTGA, D-transposition of the great arteries; PS, pulmonary stenosis; ASD2, secundum atrial septal defect; TF, tetralogy of Fallot.

abandoned. Rather, connections, single or multiple, between the superior vena cavae and the right and left pulmonary arteries are favored (see ch. 54, Fig. 5). Whatever means provides the greatest access of systemic venous blood to the pulmonary arteries is the goal. In some patients with borderline indications for a Fontan operation, an opening that allows some venous blood to enter the systemic circulation in support of the cardiac output is helpful (fenestrated Fontan) and, in others, a bidirectional Glenn operation may be preferable. Despite the attendant systemic arterial oxygen unsaturation, an upper limit to the right atrial pressure is thought to reduce the likelihood of postoperative pleural effusion. The resulting hemodynamics are better than might be expected. This improved understanding of the implications of the Fontan principle has led to a larger number of patients who are candidates for this kind of surgery and a much improved overall survival rate. The recent surgical mortality has been less than 4% whether a modified Fontan, a fenestrated Fontan, or a bidirectional Glenn operation is chosen.

SURVIVAL

Overall survival with congenital heart disease has improved in the past 20 years. Whereas mortality among infants with transposition of the great arteries was formerly nearly 100%, today it is minimal. Cardiac surgeons will have difficulty in maintaining low levels of mortality, because the least complicated surgical procedures, with the lowest mortalities, are now managed with interventional cardiac catheterization. On the average, increasingly difficult patients are being referred to the surgeons. A greater percentage of loss with surgery seems likely but is yet to be manifest.

Survival is dependent on the anatomic diagnosis and the possibility of successful correction. The improved survival with surgery for transposition of the great arteries has begun to show up in survival analyses, and survivors with tetralogy of Fallot are found with increasing frequency in older age groups (Table 8). Aortic stenosis is increasingly more prominent in the older age groups, and it is the most common congenital cardiac defect after the age of 30, at least in our group of survivors.

The negative influence of low birth weight and/or extracardiac anomalies on survival of patients with congenital heart disease is documented in Figures 3 and 4.

REFERENCES

1. Ando M, Takao A: Anatomic variabilities between races in some major cardiac anomalies (abstract). Teratology 12:194, 1975.
2. Bound JP, Logan WFWE: Incidence of congenital heart disease in Blackpool, 1957–1971. Br Heart J 39:445–450, 1977.
3. Carlgren LE: The incidence of congenital heart disease in Gothenburg. Proc Assoc Eur Paediatr Cardiol 5:2–8, 1969.
4. Dickinson DF, Arnold R, Wilkinson JL: Congenital heart disease among 160,480 liveborn children in Liverpool, 1960 to 1969. Br Heart J 46:55–62, 1981.
5. Feldt RH, Avasthey P, Yoshimasu F, et al: Incidence of congenital heart disease in children born to residents of Olmsted County, Minnesota, 1950–1969. Mayo Clin Proc 46:794–799, 1971.
6. Ferencz C, Rubin JD, McCarter RJ, et al: Congenital heart disease: prevalence at live birth; the Baltimore-Washington Infant Study. Am J Epidemiol 121:31–36, 1984.
7. Fyler DC, Buckley LP, Hellenbrand WE, et al: Report of the New England Regional Infant Cardiac Program. Pediatrics 65 (Suppl):376–460, 1980.
8. Gamble W: Personal communication.
9. Grabitz RG, Joffres MR, Collins-Nakai RL: Congenital heart disease: incidence in the first year of life. The Alberta Heritage Pediatric Cardiology Program. Am J Epidemiol 128:381–388, 1988.
10. Hoffman JIE, Christianson R: Congenital heart disease in a cohort of 19,502 births with long term follow-up. Am J Cardiol 42:641–647, 1978.
11. Laursen HB: Some epidemiologic aspects of congenital heart disease in Denmark. Acta Paediatr Scand 69:619–624, 1980.
12. Liu Ge Li, Yeh Min-Teh: Personal communication. (Tianjin Children's Hospital, Tianjin, China, 1990.)
13. Mitchell SC, Korones SB, Berendes HW: Congenital heart disease in 56,109 births. Circulation 43:323–332, 1971.

Section VIII
ACQUIRED HEART DISEASE

Chapter 19

INNOCENT MURMURS

Jane W. Newburger, M.D., M.P.H.

Innocent heart murmurs occur in approximately 50% of all children.[10,33] They occur in the absence of either anatomic or physiologic abnormalities of the heart and are not associated with subsequent cardiovascular disease.[3,4,29] The differentiation of innocent from organic murmurs for purposes of therapy, prognosis, and insurability is the leading cause for referral to a pediatric cardiologist (Exhibit 1). To distinguish innocent from organic murmurs requires knowledge of the auscultatory findings in the various structural cardiac abnormalities, as well as of the characteristic findings of innocent murmurs. Innocent murmurs can be recognized using skilled auscultation and bedside maneuvers, without the need for extensive diagnostic testing.[18,28]

PREVALENCE

The reported prevalence of murmurs in the neonatal period varies widely, from 1.7–77.4%, with varying estimates probably attributable to differences in the frequency and timing of examinations, examining conditions, auscultatory skill, and the threshold for the inclusion of very soft murmurs.[2,32] Overall, the majority of studies report a high incidence of murmurs in the first week of life. A heart murmur noted in the first 24 hours of life carries a 1:12 risk of congenital heart disease; one heard first at six months, a 1:7 risk; and one heard first at 12 months, only a 1:50 risk.[32] The only group with a predominance of organic murmurs (3:5) was that in which murmurs detected at birth persisted for 12 months.

After infancy, the reported prevalence of innocent heart murmurs ranges between 17 and 66%, with most authors reporting between 40 and 60%

(see ch. 18).[10,14,31,33,35,42] With exercise or with the use of phonocardiography, approximately 90% of children have murmurs.[19,25,35] Even in reviews from cardiology referral centers, the majority of children with newly referred murmurs have no significant heart disease.[11,12]

CLINICAL MANIFESTATIONS

General Characteristics

Innocent heart murmurs are always associated with normal heart sounds. The murmurs occur in systole, with the exception of the venous hum, which is continuous. Whereas organic murmurs may be of any length, innocent murmurs are usually very brief, peaking in the first half of systole. Organic murmurs often have widespread transmission, with a pattern determined by the lesion, whereas innocent murmurs are often well localized, usually along the left sternal border. It is unusual for the grade of an innocent murmur to be greater than 3 (on a scale of 1 to 6). The murmur's intensity often changes with position and, occasionally, from examination to examination. With the exception of venous hums, there are no innocent thrills. Of course, cyanosis should never accompany an innocent murmur. The quality of the innocent murmur is often vibratory and musical, or sometimes blowing, in contrast to the harsh quality of many organic murmurs. The most common innocent heart murmurs are described below.

Still's Murmur

Still's murmur[3,41] is most commonly heard in patients between the ages of 2 and 7 years. Char-

Exhibit 1

	Boston Children's Hospital Experience 1973–1987			
Age When Patients with a Murmur Were First Referred to a Cardiologist				
Age First Seen (years)	Congenital Heart Disease n = 14,012	No Significant Heart Disease n = 6,647	Mitral Valve Prolapse n = 366	Bicuspid Aortic Valve n = 71
0–1	44.9	16.0	3.3	8.6
1–5	21.8	27.3	8.5	18.6
5–10	14.9	24.5	16.4	38.6
10–15	9.9	19.3	38.0	18.6
15–20	5.1	10.7	28.7	11.4
20+	3.4	2.2	5.2	4.3
% Male	55.3	53.4	48.4	72.5
% Female	44.7	46.6	51.6	27.5

acteristically, it is a grade 1 to 3, vibratory, buzzing, or twanging systolic ejection murmur, the quality of which is similar to that of a tuning fork (Fig. 1). It is usually maximal in the third intercostal space, is much louder in the supine position than in the sitting position, and is characteristically louder with exercise, excitement, or fever. The intensity of ejection murmurs has been demonstrated by invasive phonocardiography to be greater above the aortic valve than above the pulmonary valve.[40] The association of Still's murmur with false chordae tendineae in the left ventricle is controversial, with some authors finding a strong relationship[30,44] and others finding a high prevalence of both Still's murmurs and false tendons in healthy hearts, but no association.[43] The cardiac index of children with Still's murmur is similar to

that of children without murmurs.[38] However, individuals with Still's murmur have been reported to have a significantly smaller mean ascending aortic diameter relative to body surface area, with higher average peak velocities in the ascending and descending aorta than are found in children and young adults without murmurs. These observations suggest that the origin of Still's murmur is related to a small ascending aortic diameter with concomitant high velocity of the aortic blood flow.[34]

The Innocent Pulmonic Systolic Murmur

The innocent pulmonic systolic murmur, also called the physiologic ejection murmur, is identical in quality to the murmur of an atrial septal defect, comprising a murmur caused by excess flow through the normal pulmonic valve but associated with a normal second sound. Using phonocardiography, this murmur may be detected in most normal subjects.[16] It is a grade 1 to 3, blowing, rather high-pitched, diamond-shaped murmur that always peaks in the first half of systole and is maximal in intensity in the second left intercostal space, without wide transmission. Like the Still's murmur, it is louder when the patient is in the supine position, and is accentuated by exercise, fever, or excitement. The innocent pulmonic systolic murmur may be heard in children of any age and frequently occurs in children with asthenic builds who have narrow anteroposterior diameters or who have pectus excavatum. Studies with intracardiac phonocatheters have demonstrated that the innocent pulmonic systolic murmur is located in the main pulmonary artery and is associated with the ejection of blood into the pulmonary artery.[6,37]

The Cervical Venous Hum

The cervical venous hum[4] is a continuous murmur with diastolic accentuation that may be elicited almost universally in normal children. It is located in the low anterior part of the neck, more often on the right than the left. This murmur is loudest with the patient in the sitting position and disappears or diminishes in the supine position.

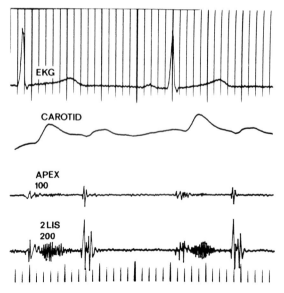

Figure 1. An innocent murmur at the second left interspace. Note the even, harmonic quality of a musical sound. (From Nadas AS, Fyler DC: Pediatric Cardiology, Philadelphia, W. B. Saunders Company, 1973, p. 101, with permission.)

Usually the venous hum is accentuated by turning the patient's head away from the side of the murmur and elevating the chin. The murmur may be obliterated by pressing lightly over the jugular vein with the stethoscope or a finger. The mechanism of the venous hum has not been definitively delineated, although it has been postulated to be secondary to turbulence of venous flow in the internal jugular veins and, occasionally, in the external jugular veins.[6,7,8,12,20,23,27,36]

The Supraclavicular Arterial Bruit

The supraclavicular arterial bruit is a crescendo-decrescendo systolic murmur heard best just above the clavicles, usually on the right side more than on the left. It radiates better to the neck than below the clavicles and, very occasionally, can generate a faint carotid thrill. The bruit may be accentuated by exercise, but is not affected by posture and respiration. It can be distinguished from the murmur of aortic stenosis by the disappearance of the supraclavicular murmur with the manuever of hyperextension of the shoulders[29] or compression of the subclavian artery against the first rib. Supraclavicular systolic murmurs have been postulated to arise from the major brachiocephalic arteries near their aortic origins.[5,6,13,17,49]

MINOR LABORATORY TESTS

In children newly referred for evaluation of a heart murmur, the results of diagnostic tests are not likely to change the clinical diagnosis of "no heart disease" when it has been made by a person trained in cardiac auscultation.[28] However, the qualifications of the examiner have been shown to have a major bearing on the power to distinguish innocent from organic murmurs in children.[26] Thus, these findings may not be generalizable to examinations performed by physicians less skilled in pediatric cardiology. Diagnoses made by less-experienced physicians may be influenced by test results. Insofar as such examiners equate "negative" test results with the absence of heart disease, a large proportion of cases of heart disease will be missed, because the false-negative rates for the tests are high.[26] If such examiners equate positive test results with the presence of heart disease, a high proportion of the positive diagnoses will be false because of the rarity of heart disease among the children tested. Thus, the use of laboratory tests cannot supplant a skilled auscultation in distinguishing between innocent and organic murmurs.

Many pediatric cardiologists obtain an electrocardiogram and chest x-ray or echocardiogram in children newly referred for murmur evaluation. Although such test results may have little influence on the immediate management of patients with innocent murmurs found by auscultation, they may have other uses, such as reassuring families and referring physicians or providing a baseline for comparison if the possibility of heart disease is raised again later. Diagnostic testing should be tailored to the clinical situation. However, the author believes that the majority of children older than 1 year of age can be evaluated with history, physical examination, and an electrocardiogram alone.

MANAGEMENT

For children less than 2 years old in whom the diagnosis of innocent murmur is first made, the author recommends reevaluation after 2 or 3 years if the murmur persists. Children more than 2 years old do not require reevaluation unless some uncertainty exists (for example, because of suboptimal patient cooperation or a possible abnormality on a diagnostic test).

It is of the utmost importance to reassure the family of a child with an innocent murmur. The label of heart disease may have profound adverse effects on the child and the family.[15,21] Even temporary mislabeling may increase the morbidity from cardiac nondisease.[1]

PROGNOSIS

Without cardiac catheterization or autopsy, the "innocence" of a heart murmur cannot be proved. However, the reliability of the impression on initial evaluation is supported by published follow-up and actuarial studies. Follow-up studies of series of patients diagnosed as having innocent murmurs have confirmed the original diagnosis in 97–100% of the patients.[22,24] Furthermore, actuarial data on people with systolic murmurs thought to be innocent show no deviation from the expected mortality—a discovery that led to a decision to remove restrictions on insurance and employment for those with innocent murmurs.[9]

REFERENCES

1. Bergman AB Stamm SJ: The morbidity of cardiac nondisease in schoolchildren. N Engl J Med 276:1008–1013, 1967.
2. Braudo M, Rowe RD: Auscultation of the heart—early neonatal period. Am J Dis Child 101:575–586, 1961.
3. Caceres CA, Perry LW: Still's murmur. In The Innocent Murmur: A Problem in Clinical Practice. Boston, Little, Brown & Co., 1967, pp. 115–160.
4. Caceres CA, Perry LW: The cervical venous hum. In The Innocent Murmur: A Problem in Clinical Practice. Boston, Little, Brown & Co., 1967, pp. 181–192.
5. Cassels DE: Cardiovascular murmurs in infants and children. Med Clin North Am 41:75–88, 1957.
6. Castle RF: Clinical recognition of innocent cardiac murmurs in infants and children. JAMA 177:1–5, 1961.

7. Cutforth R, Wiseman J, Sutherland RD: The genesis of the cervical venous hum. Am Heart J 80:488–492, 1970.

8. Edwards EA, Levine H: Peripheral vascular murmurs: mechanism of production and diagnostic significance. Arch Intern Med 90:284–300, 1952.

9. Engle MA: Insurability and employability: congenital heart disease and innocent murmurs. Circulation 56:143–145, 1977.

10. Epstein N: The heart in normal infants and children. J Pediatr 32:39–45, 1948.

11. Ferencz C, Craft J, Sultz H: Cardiac disease in children: an epidemiologic assessment of a specialty service as a basis for planning pediatrics. Pediatrics 52:395–401, 1973.

12. Fogel DH: The innocent systolic murmur in children: a clinical study of its incidence and characteristics. Am Heart J 59:844–855, 1960.

13. Fowler NO: The innocent murmur. In Physical Diagnosis of Heart Disease. New York, Macmillan, 1962, pp. 49–61.

14. Friedman S, Robie WA, Harris TN: Occurrence of innocent-adventitious cardiac sounds in childhood. Pediatrics 4:782–789, 1949.

15. Glaser HH, Harrison GS, Lynn DB: Emotional implications of congenital heart disease in children. Pediatrics 33:367–379, 1964.

16. Groom D and Sihvonen YT: A high sensitivity pickup for cardiovascular sounds. Am Heart J 54:592–601, 1957.

17. Kawabori I, Stevenson JG, Dooley TK, et al: The significance of carotid bruits in children: transmitted murmur of vascular origin, studied by pulsed Doppler ultrasound. Am Heart J 98:160–167, 1979.

18. Lembo NJ, Dell'Italia LJ, Crawford MH, et al: Bedside diagnosis of systolic murmurs. N Engl J Med 318:1572–1578, 1988.

19. Lessof M, Brigden W: Systolic murmurs in healthy children and in children with rheumatic fever. Lancet 2:673–674, 1957.

20. Levine SA, Harvey WP: Clinical Auscultation of the Heart. Philadelphia, W.B. Saunders, 1959.

21. Linde LM, Rasof B, Dunn OJ, et al: Attitudinal factors in congenital heart disease. Pediatrics 38:92–101, 1966.

22. Lynxwiler CP, Donahoe JL: Evaluation of innocent murmurs. South Med J 48:164–166, 1955.

23. Mannheimer E: Phonocardiography in children. Advances in Pediatrics. Chicago, Year Book Medical Publishers, 1955.

24. Marienfeld CJ, Telles N, Silvera J, et al: A 20-year follow-up study of "innocent" murmurs. Pediatrics 30:42–48, 1962.

25. McKee MH: Heart sounds in normal children. Am Heart J 16:79–87, 1938.

26. Miller RA, Stamler J, Smith JM: The detection of heart disease in children: results of mass field trials with use of tape recorded heart sounds. Circulation 32:956–965, 1965.

27. Moscovitz HL: The venous hum. Am Heart J 62:141–142, 1961.

28. Newburger JW, Rosenthal A, Williams RG, et al.: Non-invasive tests in the initial evaluation of heart murmurs in children. N Engl J Med 308:61–64, 1983.

29. Perloff JK: Normal or innocent murmurs. In The Clinical Recognition of Congenital Heart Disease, 3rd ed. Philadelphia, W.B. Saunders, 1987, pp. 8–18.

30. Perry LW, Ruckman RN, Shapiro SR, et al: Left ventricular false tendons in children. Am J Cardiol 52:1264–1266, 1983.

31. Rauh LW: Cardiac murmurs in children. Ohio State Med J 36:973–974, 1940.

32. Richards MR, Merritt KK, Samuels MH, et al: Frequency and significance of systolic cardiac murmurs in the first year of life. Pediatr 15:169–179, 1955.

33. Sampson JJ, Hahman PT, Halverson WL, et al: Incidence of heart disease and rheumatic fever in school children in their climatically different California communities. Am Heart J 29:178–204, 1945.

34. Schwartz ML, Goldberg SJ, Wilson N, et al: Relation of Still's murmur, small aortic diameter and high aortic velocity. Am J Cardiol 57:1344–1348, 1986.

35. Schwartzman J.: Cardiac status of adolescents. Arch Pediatr 58:443–452, 1941.

36. Segal BL: Innocent murmurs. In The Theory and Practice of Auscultation. Philadelphia, F.A. Davis, 1964, pp. 168–179.

37. Segal BL, Novack P, Kasparain H: Intracardiac phonocardiography. Am J Cardiol 13:188–197, 1964.

38. Sholler GF, Celermajer JM, Whight CM: Doppler echocardiographic assessment of cardiac output in normal children with and without innocent precordial murmurs. Am J Cardiol 59:487–488, 1987.

39. Stapleton JF, El-Hajj MM: Heart murmurs simulated by arterial bruits in the neck. Am Heart J 61:178–183, 1961.

40. Stein PD, Sabbah NH: Aortic origin of innocent murmurs. Am J Cardiol 39:655–671, 1977.

41. Still GF: Common Disorders and Diseases of Childhood. London, Frowde, Hodder & Stoughton, 1909, 731 pp.

42. Thayer WS: Reflections on the interpretation of systolic cardiac murmurs. Am J Med Sci 169:313–321, 1925.

43. Van Oort A, Van-Dam I, Heringa A, et al: The vibratory innocent heart murmur studied by echo-Doppler. Acta Paediatr Scand 329 suppl:103–107, 1986.

44. Wessel A, Beyer C, Pulss W, et al: False chordae tendineae in the left ventricle: echo and phonocardiographic findings. Z Kardiol 74:303–307, 1985.

Chapter 20

DYSLIPIDEMIA IN CHILDHOOD AND ADOLESCENCE

Jane W. Newburger, M.D., M.P.H.

Abnormalities in plasma lipoproteins are an important cause of premature coronary artery disease. The risk of this disease increases exponentially with plasma concentrations of total cholesterol; there is a substantial increase in risk with levels higher than 200 mg/dl. Furthermore, interventions that lower LDL or raise HDL-cholesterol levels lower the risk of coronary artery disease; a 1% reduction in the cholesterol level leads to a 2% reduction in coronary artery disease, whereas a 1% increase in HDL cholesterol leads to a 4% decrease in coronary artery disease.[14,21] As epidemiologic and pathologic investigations have introduced the concept of a presymptomatic phase of cardiovascular disease, efforts to prevent symptomatic disease have centered around the modification of plasma lipid concentrations in childhood and adolescence.

LIPID BIOCHEMISTRY

Lipids normally function as building blocks and fuels in the human body. Cholesterols are necessary components of cell membranes and associated structures like myelin and are needed as well for hormone synthesis. Triglycerides are a major source of energy. Lipoproteins are spherical particles with a surface composed of free cholesterol, phospholipids, and protein, and a core containing predominantly cholesterol esters and triglycerides. Lipoproteins are categorized by their relative density, composition, and electrophoretic mobility into four broad classes: chylomicrons, very low-density lipoproteins (VLDL), low-density lipoproteins (LDL), and high-density lipoproteins (HDL). The synthesis and catabolism of lipoproteins (Fig. 1) have been well described.[27]

Chylomicrons are large triglyceride-rich particles produced in the intestine in response to dietary fat and are carried by lymph from the gut through the thoracic duct to the venous system. They are the principal triglyceride-carrying lipoproteins in the nonfasting state. The primary apoproteins in chylomicrons are apoproteins B and C-II; the latter is responsible for triggering the action of lipoprotein lipase in the capillary endothelium of adipose tissue. The main function of chylomicrons is to deliver dietary triglycerides to adipose and other tissues.

VLDL transports triglycerides, which are endogenously synthesized, primarily in the liver and, to a lesser extent, in the intestine. VLDL contains apoproteins B100 and E. In the fasting state, most plasma triglycerides are carried by VLDL. Like chylomicrons, they deliver triglycerides to adipose and other tissues. In the process, VLDL is reduced first to intermediate-density particles and subsequently to low-density lipoproteins.

LDL is the major cholesterol-carrying lipoprotein in plasma. It delivers cholesterol to hepatocytes and peripheral cells for the synthesis of cell membranes and steroid hormones. Apoprotein B100, contained in LDL particles, is responsible for binding to the LDL receptor. The plasma level of LDL cholesterol is directly associated with the risk of coronary artery disease.

HDL serves as an acceptor of lipid, especially free cholesterol, from various tissues. It is produced directly by the liver and the intestine and is derived as well from chylomicron and VLDL catabolism. The major proteins of HDL are apoproteins A-I and A-II. HDL cholesterol acts as a mechanism for the removal of cholesterol from various tissues; its plasma level is inversely related to the risk of coronary artery disease.

Plasma levels of LDL and HDL cholesterol are not significantly different in the fasting and nonfasting states, but triglyceride levels can increase several fold after eating. After a fast of 12–14 hours, dietary triglycerides carried by chylomicrons are usually absent. In the fasting state, if plasma triglyceride is less than 500 mg/dl, the level of VLDL cholesterol is approximately equal to the triglyc-

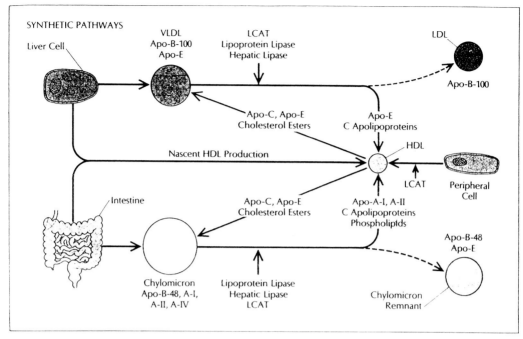

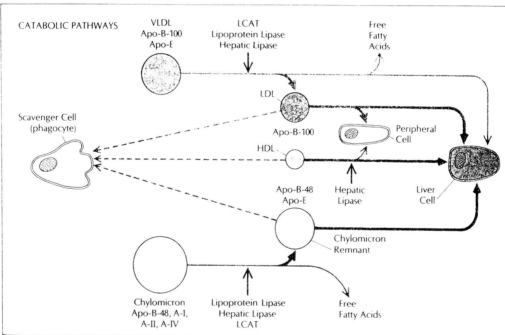

Figure 1. Schema of normal lipoprotein metabolism. Synthetic pathways originating in the liver and intestine are shown in the upper panel. Chylomicrons are produced in the intestine from dietary fat. VLDL synthesis occurs in the liver. Direct production of HDLS occurs in both liver and intestine. HDL constituents are also derived from chylomicrons and VLDL catabolism. As shown in the lower panel. LDLs can be catabolized in various cell types by both receptor-independent mechanisms. When plasma lipoproteins are elevated or abnormal in composition, they may be taken up by scavenger cells in tissues (with resultant xanthoma formation, lymphadenopathy, or hepatosplenomegaly). (From Schaefer EJ: When and how to treat the dyslipidemias. Hosp Pract 15:57–72, 1988, © Alan Iselin, with permission.)

eride level divided by five. Therefore, LDL cholesterol (LDL-C) can be estimated from total cholesterol (TC), HDL cholesterol (HDL-C), and triglycerides (TG), measured in the fasting state, by the following formula:

$$LDL\text{-}C = TC - HDL\text{-}C - TG/5$$

RATIONALE FOR LIPID MODIFICATION IN CHILDHOOD

The rationale for the modification of cholesterol in childhood is based on postmortem and epidemiologic data. Studies at autopsy suggest that, in some cases, the lesions of coronary artery disease begin to develop before adulthood. Fatty streaks in the aorta are found almost universally in children by the age of 3 years; the extent of such streaks has been reported to be highly correlated with levels of LDL cholesterol in the plasma.[24] However, fatty streaks in the aorta are poorly predictive of the prevalence of coronary artery disease. In contrast, fatty streaks in the coronary arteries may be detected in children as young as 10–14 years and are almost always seen in individuals over the age of 20 years.[29] Their frequency parallels that of atherosclerosis in different populations or cultures. Fibrous plaques in the coronary arteries rarely occur in the late teens, but increase rapidly over the next two decades in men. Corresponding changes occur approximately 20 years later in women. Autopsies of young men in the U.S. Armed Forces in the Vietnam and Korean wars demonstrated evidence of early atherosclerotic lesions by late adolescence and early adulthood.[12,23,31]

Further evidence of the importance of cholesterol in pediatrics comes from epidemiologic investigations in children across and within different populations. In cross-population studies, children from countries with a high incidence of coronary artery disease in adults have higher cholesterol levels than children from countries where adults have a low incidence of coronary artery disease.[18,37] Among children, the highest mean serum cholesterol has been found in Finland, with mean values in the United States and Western European countries following close behind. Within populations, elevated levels of total and LDL cholesterol in children have been strongly correlated with the occurrence of coronary artery disease in adult family members. In a study of the progeny of young victims of ischemic heart disease, 51% had abnormal levels of lipids or lipoproteins.[20]

The tracking of total cholesterol and LDL cholesterol support the importance of monitoring lipid levels in childhood.[7,13] In four cross-sectional school screens, the Muscatine Study[7] sampled school children repeatedly over a 6-year period. The 6-year correlation for cholesterol was 0.61 compared with 0.74 for height and weight and 0.30 for systolic blood pressure. A significant proportion of children with initially high cholesterol values demonstrated consistently high values throughout the study; of those children initially in the highest quintile, approximately half remained in the highest quintile after a 6-year interval. The Bogalusa Heart Study[13] evaluated the rankings of serum lipids and lipoproteins over an 8-year period, with race- and sex-specific correlations for LDL-cholesterol rank ranging from 0.55 to 0.71. The correlations for rankings of the levels of HDL cholesterol and VLDL cholesterol over the 8-year period were considerably lower, i.e., 0.25 to 0.43 and 0.31 to 0.48, respectively.

Recently, longitudinal observations were reported in a population whose cholesterol levels were first measured at ages 8–18 years and then reexamined more than a decade later (age range 20–31 years).[19] Correlations of childhood levels of total cholesterol with adult levels of total cholesterol, LDL cholesterol, and LDL/HDL cholesterol were all statistically significant ($p<0.05$). These data demonstrated the tracking of peer rank order of cholesterol from childhood to adult life, as well as that cholesterol measurements in childhood are predictors of future levels of LDL and LDL/HDL cholesterol. The probability of having a plasma cholesterol level in the upper decile of the adult distribution was negligible for those whose childhood levels were less than the 50th percentile. For those with childhood cholesterol levels above the 50th percentile, the risk of having a plasma cholesterol level in the upper decile as an adult increased exponentially with the childhood cholesterol level. Thus, cholesterol in childhood is a major predictor for cholesterol in the adult population.

Although these data demonstrate an association between childhood lipid values and later development of coronary artery disease, they do not prove that alteration of lipids in childhood through diet or pharmacologic management can influence the later development of coronary artery disease.

Current recommendations for the screening and treatment of dyslipidemias in childhood balance the potential adverse effects of lipid-lowering therapies (insignificant for temperate diet modification and exercise) with their presumed benefits based on histopathologic and epidemiologic data.

MEASUREMENT OF LIPIDS

The methods most commonly used for determination of serum cholesterol in clinical laboratories are enzymatic assays based on cholesterol esterase and oxidase.[2] Desk-top instruments that rely on capillary blood obtained by fingerstick have recently been marketed; generally, these also use an enzymatic method. A chemical colorimetric method was used in the large population studies on which guidelines for intervention are based. Serum cholesterol determinations in clinical laboratories may vary markedly, either higher or lower, from those obtained by reference laboratories on which normative data are based. Most experts believe that this variability is due mainly to the standards used for calibration of the instruments and the controls used to monitor the determinations, rather than to the instruments or the methods themselves.

Other sources of variability in lipid measurements include biologic variation, acute illness, ongoing weight loss, pregnancy, or use of certain medications. Furthermore, cholesterol concentrations may be affected by posture and by stasis: ideally, blood should be drawn from patients who have been sitting for at least 5 minutes, and the tourniquet should be applied just before blood is drawn.[26]

Cholesterol levels measured in serum are 3% higher than those measured in plasma. When cholesterol concentration is measured in serum, the blood should be allowed to clot at room temperature and the clot detached from the tube before centrifugation. When the measurement is made from plasma, the collection tube should be placed on ice and spun down in a refrigerated centrifuge.[26]

Screening for Dyslipidemia

There has been considerable debate about the virtues of selective screening of so-called high-risk children versus universal screening.

Selective Screening Strategy. The most recent guidelines from the American Heart Association recommend that, as a minimum, children should undergo measurement of total cholesterol, HDL cholesterol, and triglycerides after an overnight fast (usually 14 hours) if there is a positive family history (parents or grandparents) of premature cardiovascular disease (males under 50 years and females under 60 years), hyperlipidemia, sudden death, or xanthomas. In addition, children who, themselves, have risk factors (e.g., obesity, diabetes, or a history of Kawasaki disease) should undergo screening. Finally, in children with recurrent abdominal pain or postprandial irritability, chylomicrons and total triglycerides should be measured because of their association with pancreatitis. Screening is first performed at the age of 2 years.

Proponents of selective screening believe that universal screening (1) is too expensive, (2) will result in mislabeling of some children, and (3) will have limited value, in that the current recommendations for a prudent diet are being applied universally to all children.

Universal Screening Strategy. Recent reports have built a strong case for universal screening. Fewer than half of well-educated American adults currently know their serum cholesterol levels. Indeed, family histories are frequently incomplete. Approximately half of the children with elevated cholesterol levels would be missed if screening were performed only on those children with a positive family history.[10,15,16] Recently, investigators from the Bogalusa Heart Study examined the relation of parental history to children's lipid profiles.[10] White children with a parental history of heart attack or diabetes are significantly more likely to have elevated levels of total cholesterol and LDL cholesterol. In black children, however, parental history of cardiovascular disease has not been found to predict elevated levels of total or LDL cholesterol. Rather, older black children with a parental history of heart attack, hypertension, or diabetes have been reported to be approximately five times more likely than those without such a history (p<0.05) to have low levels of HDL cholesterol. Thus, increased familial risk appears to be associated with different risk factors in black persons versus white persons. Furthermore, although children with positive family histories were at increased risk for lipid and lipoprotein abnormalities, not all children with extreme levels were identified by family history. Indeed, only 40% of white children and 21% of black children with elevated levels of LDL cholesterol had a parent with a history of vascular disease.

Family history as a predictive screening for childhood hypercholesterolemia was also investigated using a population seen for routine care in eight office practices in the Chicago area.[16] The findings were similar to those obtained by the Bogalusa Group, with maternal and paternal histories of hypercholesterolemia being significantly associated with elevated LDL cholesterol, but having extremely low sensitivities. Family history factors most commonly recommended as criteria for cholesterol screening in children did not identify half of all children with LDL cholesterol and did not selectively identify the most severely affected children.

It is clear that the most effective strategy for detection of children with dyslipidemia would be through universal screening. Although the total cholesterol level can be measured easily and inexpensively, it has a low positive predictive value in detecting elevated LDL cholesterol or low HDL cholesterol in pediatric and adolescent patients.[11] The efficacy of screening procedures requires further evaluation before universal screening can be widely recommended.

NORMAL PLASMA LIPID AND LIPOPROTEIN LEVELS IN CHILDHOOD AND ADOLESCENCE

The distribution of plasma lipid and lipoprotein levels in children and adolescents, as determined in seven North American Lipid Research Clinics,[34] are displayed in Tables 1 and 2. Recent surveys[10,11,15,16] have suggested that total cholesterol levels may be higher than originally suggested at the Lipid Research Clinics, indicating the need for development of more flexible guidelines for determining risk status in children, including factors such as age, race, ethnicity, and sex.

SECONDARY CAUSES OF DYSLIPIDEMIA

Although dyslipidemia most commonly results from a combination of genetic and dietary factors, it may also be secondary to other systemic disorders. Indeed, the lipid profile may be affected by a wide variety of medications, endocrine and metabolic disorders (for example, diabetes mellitus, hypothyroidism), pregnancy, obstructive liver disease, and renal disease.[27] Furthermore, both viral and bacterial infections, so common in childhood, may have profound effects on the lipid profile in the month after the onset of infection.[25] In the first year of life, the most common causes of secondary hyperlipidemia are glycogen storage disease and congenital biliary atresia.[4] Endocrine disorders (such as hypothydroidism or diabetes mellitus) and renal disease are the most common secondary causes later in childhood. Exogenous causes, including medication and alcohol, are exceedingly common throughout childhood and adolescence.

In patients referred for evaluation of hyperlipidemia, secondary causes are often evident from a careful review of medical history and use of medications, together with a physical examination. When a secondary cause is not apparent, it may be appropriate to obtain a urinalysis and to measure blood levels of thyroid-stimulating hormone, alkaline phosphatase, serum glutamate pyruvate transaminase, albumin, and fasting glucose to rule out occult secondary causes.

FAMILIAL DYSLIPIDEMIAS

After secondary causes of dyslipidemia have been excluded, it is valuable to screen family members to determine whether the disorder is genetic (familial) or sporadic. Although delineation of the type of genetic disorder may not affect the treatment of an individual patient, such screening is especially important because other family members at high risk for premature coronary artery disease may be identified. Approximately half of individuals with premature atherosclerotic heart disease have underlying genetic disorders of lipid metabolism.[26] The major categories of familial dyslipidemia are briefly summarized below.[1,27]

Familial Hypercholesterolemia (FH). This autosomal codominant disorder is caused by an inherited defect in the gene encoding for the LDL receptor.[5] The heterozygous state (i.e., one defective gene) occurs in 1 of 500 people (0.2%) in the general population, but in 5% of survivors of myocardial infarction under the age of 60 years.[26] Total cholesterol levels usually exceed 300 mg/dl, and there is often a strong family history of hypercholesterolemia and premature coronary artery disease. In affected adults, tendinous xanthomas and corneal arcus are common, but children with heterozygous FH almost always have normal physical examinations. Patients with heterozygous FH rarely respond to dietary management alone; although they should adhere to a "Step 2" diet, it is not necessary to wait for 6 months before beginning pharmacologic therapy.

Homozygous FH is a rare disorder associated with total cholesterol levels greater than 600 mg/dl. Such patients may have tuberous as well as tendinous xanthomas; myocardial infarction may occur in childhood and adolescence. Pharmacologic therapy is not successful,[35] and treatment requires liver transplantation or continuous-flow plasmapheresis.[4]

Familial Combined Hyperlipidemia. This disorder occurs in approximately 1% of the population and in 15% of patients under the age of 60 who have survived myocardial infarction.[26] The underlying genetic defect is not known. The condition is characterized by multiple lipoprotein phenotypes within a single affected family, including increases in VLDL alone, increases in LDL alone, or elevations of VLDL and LDL. Overproduction of apolipoprotein B is a frequent finding, with or without an accompanying elevation in LDL cholesterol. When first-degree family members are not available for testing, combined hyperlipidemia can be diagnosed from measurements of elevated LDL cholesterol (greater than 160 mg/dl) together with a fasting triglyceride level exceeding 160 mg/dl. Regardless of phenotype, all patients with familial combined hyperlipidemia are at risk for premature coronary artery disease.

Polygenic (Severe Primary) Hypercholesterolemia. This is characterized by a severe, persistent elevation of LDL cholesterol in individuals without familial hypercholesterolemia or familial combined hyperlipidemia, and occurs in approximately 1% of the population. This disorder probably results from a variety of disturbances in LDL metabolism.

Familial Dysbetalipoproteinemia (Type 3 Hyperlipoproteinemia). This condition has an incidence of 1 in 5000 and is associated with defective catabolism of VLDL remnants and chylomicrons. It is secondary to an abnormality in the structure

Table 1. Normal Plasma Lipid Concentrations in the First Two Decades of Life (mg/L)

Age (yrs)	No.	Cholesterol			Triglycerides		
		Percentile			Percentile		
		5th	mean	95th	5th	mean	95th
0–4							
Males	238	114	155	203	29	56	99
Females	186	112	156	200	34	64	112
5–9							
Males	1253	121	160	203	30	56	101
Females	1118	126	164	205	32	60	105
10–14							
Males	2278	119	158	202	32	66	125
Females	2087	124	160	201	37	75	131
15–19							
Males	1980	113	150	197	37	78	148
Females	2079	120	158	203	39	75	132

Adapted from the Lipid Research Clinics Population Studies Data Book, I. The Prevalence Study, Lipid Metabolism Branch, Division of Heart and Vascular Diseases, National Heart Lung and Blood Institute, Public Health Service, National Institutes of Health, NIH publication No. 8–1527, Government Printing Office, 1980.

Table 2. Normal Plasma Lipoprotein Concentrations in the First Two Decades of Life (mg/L)

Age (yrs)	HDL Cholesterol				LDL Cholesterol				VLDL Cholesterol			
	No.	Percentile			No.	Percentile			No.	Percentile		
		5th	mean	95th		5th	mean	95th		5th	mean	95th
5–9												
Males	145	38	56	75	132	63	93	129	132	0	8	18
Females	127	36	53	73	114	68	100	140	113	1	10	24
10–14												
Males	298	37	55	74	288	64	97	133	288	1	10	22
Females	248	37	52	70	245	68	97	136	245	2	11	23
15–19												
Males	300	30	46	63	298	62	94	130	297	2	13	26
Females	297	35	52	74	295	59	96	137	295	2	12	24

Adapted from The Lipid Research Clinics Data Book (1980) (see Table 1).

of apolipoprotein E, which interferes with normal binding of remnant lipoproteins to liver cells and results in accumulation of modified VLDL remnants (beta-VLDL). The principal plasma lipid abnormalities include high serum triglyceride levels (greater than 400 mg/dl) together with cholesterol levels higher than 300 mg/dl. Patients with this disorder have an increased risk for premature coronary artery disease and peripheral vascular disease; as adults, they often have glucose intolerance, hyperuricemia, obesity, and tuberous and palmar xanthomas.

Familial Hypertriglyceridemia. This autosomal codominant disorder occurs in 1% of the general population and in 5% of victims of premature myocardial infarction.[26] The principal lipid abnormalities usually include a moderate elevation of triglycerides (less than 500 mg/dl) and VLDL cholesterol, with normal LDL-cholesterol and decreased HDL-cholesterol levels. When family screening cannot be performed, a patient is classified as having primary hypertriglyceridemia when the lipid profile shows an elevation of VLDL triglycerides without an accompanying elevation of LDL cholesterol.

Severe Hypertriglyceridemia. When this disorder occurs in children and adolescents it usually results from abnormal chylomicron metabolism secondary to deficiency in lipoprotein lipase or its activator protein (apo-CII). Serum triglyceride levels are usually greater than 1000 mg/dl and are secondary to accumulations of chylomicrons but not to VLDL. This condition is not associated with coronary artery disease, but may cause recurrent pancreatitis. Effective therapy requires severe reduction in the intake of dietary fat.

Familial Hypoalphalipoproteinemia (Reduced HDL Cholesterol). This autosomal dominant disorder is highly associated with increased risk for premature coronary artery disease. The genetic causes are still poorly understood. In some families, this condition may result from variations in the allele for Apo-A-I (the principal protein for HDL).

MANAGEMENT

The treatment of dyslipidemias may include diet modification, increased aerobic exercise, weight loss, and pharmacologic therapy. The cutoff values for LDL cholesterol at which policy-setting societies recommend beginning dietary and lifestyle interventions range from above the 75th percentile[8,9,32] to above the 95th percentile.[4] Varying normative data in different populations and regions further complicate the decision of which children to treat.

Diet. Patients with hyperlipidemia should first undergo dietary therapy, with the aim of reducing LDL-cholesterol levels while maintaining adequate nutrition for normal growth. Intakes of saturated fat and cholesterol are progressively reduced in two steps of therapy. In the first level of dietary modification recommended by the American Heart Association (the so-called Step 1 diet), fats provide 30% of the total calories, and the fat content is evenly divided among saturated, polyunsaturated, and monounsatuated fats. Dietary cholesterol is restricted to 100 mg/1000 calories, not to exceed 300 mg/day. Children who do not respond to this diet after a trial period (usually 3 months at The Children's Hospital in Boston) are advanced to a "Step 2" American Heart Association diet, in which saturated fatty acids should be reduced to less than 7% of the calories, with the remainder of total fat intake being supplied by polyunsaturated and monounsaturated fatty acids. Dietary cholesterol is reduced to less than 200 mg/day. A minimum of 6 months of intensive diet therapy is usual before initiating drug therapy.

In adults, dietary treatment of hypercholesterolemia may result in as much as a 15% lowering of total cholesterol levels.[21] Individual patients vary considerably in response to restriction of fat and cholesterol intake. Special caution must be used in families with low levels of HDL cholesterol, where rigorous restriction of dietary fat intake may further lower the serum HDL cholesterol and adversely effect the LDL/HDL ratio. Many families who are referred for lipid management have recently experienced death or myocardial infarction in a family member. Frequently, the stress within these families is considerable, and the diet of the children can easily become the focus of tension and conflict. Group sessions with hands-on experience can be especially helpful in diet counseling. In addition, success in teaching diet modification to children is dependent on tailoring programs to the child's age. Formal counseling with a nutritionist who has expertise both in dyslipidemia and in the requirements for growth in pediatric patients is recommended.

Lipid-lowering Drugs. When dietary measures fail to control high cholesterol concentrations, lipid-lowering drugs may be prescribed for selected patients. The development of criteria for pharmacologic treatment of childhood dyslipidemias has been hindered by the inability to measure treatment efficacy. Measurement of the early preclinical phase of coronary artery disease is not feasible with current technology. Furthermore, cardiovascular morbidity and mortality secondary to dyslipidemia are exceedingly rare in children and adolescents, and prospective clinical trials of pharmacologic interventions in childhood will require decades of observation. These handicaps, together with concern about known and unknown adverse effects of lipid-lowering agents in children, must be balanced by epidemiologic and postmortem studies indicating an association of childhood dyslipidemias with adult coronary artery disease. It is not surprising, therefore, that individual physicians vary considerably in their approach to pharmacologic therapy of childhood dyslipidemias. In general, pharmacologic therapy is not used in children with levels of LDL cholesterol less than 190 mg/dl unless the HDL cholesterol is exceedingly low or other significant risk factors are present.

Among the various lipid-lowering agents commonly prescribed for adults, those summarized below are most frequently used in children and adolescents.

Bile-acid Binding Resins. Cholestyramine and cholestipol reduce LDL-cholesterol levels by increasing receptor-mediated LDL catabolism.[28] These agents are not absorbed systemically and have the longest track record of safety for pediatric use. The average reduction in LDL cholesterol is dose-dependent; with an optimal dose regimen and exellent compliance, LDL cholesterol may be reduced by approximately 30%.[36] However, long-term compliance with the use of cholestyramine is low, with only 55% of patients complying after 6 years of treatment and 48% after 8 years. Better compliance is observed in children who begin therapy under the age of 10 years. The average dose of cholestyramine for a child is 4 gm t.i.d. (or 6 gm b.i.d.), and for an adult, 8 gm t.i.d. (or 12 gm b.i.d.) (the maximum recommended dose in an adult is 32 gm/day). Adverse effects include constipation and abdominal pain, often with flatulence, nausea, and vomiting. Such side effects may be less common in children. Laboratory data, including tests for liver function, hematocrit, chloride, and serum concentrations of vitamins A, D, and E, and folate, are evaluated annually. For children with familial hyperlipidemia, it is often necessary to use resin binders in combination with niacin.[17,22]

Niacin. Niacin decreases triglycerides, total cholesterol, and LDL cholesterol, and it increases HDL cholesterol by modifying the synthesis or secretion of VLDL and LDL.[3] At The Children's Hospital in Boston, niacin is used as the drug of choice in postpubertal patients with a lipid profile characterized by a high triglycerides and low HDL cholesterol. In addition, niacin is frequently used in combination with bile-acid sequestrants for children with heterozygous familial hypercholesterolemia. In men with previous myocardial infarction, niacin (3 gm/day) has been shown to reduce both further nonfatal myocardial infarctions[33] and mortality rate.[6] Niacin combined with cholestipol reduces the progression of old atheromata and the formation of new ones; it fosters regression of atherosclerosis in both native arteries and grafts (compared with placebos) in men with previous coronary artery bypass surgery.[5] Niacin is administered three times a day and increased gradually to a total daily dose of 25–50 mg/kg. In older children, therapy with a timed-release or long-acting preparation of niacin is usually begun at a dose of 125 mg or 250 mg b.i.d. and slowly increased to a total daily dose of 1500 mg. The average daily dose in an adult is 3 gm/day. Common adverse effects include flushing, pruritus, and gastrointestinal distress; these can be reduced by increasing the drug dose gradually, by giving the drug with meals, and by premedication with aspirin (300 mg) 30 minutes before each dose of niacin.[3] Other adverse effects include hepatotoxicity, glucose intolerance, hyperuricemia, dry eyes, and hyperpigmentation. Serum biochemistries, including tests for liver function, glucose, and uric acid, as well as a complete blood count, should be monitored once every 6 months in patients receiving niacin. Niacin is contraindicated in patients with liver disease or ulcers.

Lovastatin. Lovastatin is currently the most effective pharmacologic agent for reduction of LDL-cholesterol concentrations, achieving its effect through inhibition of HMG CoA reductase, the enzyme that catalyzes the rate-limiting step in cholesterol synthesis.[3] Use of lovastatin in a limited sample of adolescents with severe heterozygous familial hypercholesterolemia has been found to achieve substantially greater reductions in total cholesterol and LDL cholesterol than either resin binders or resin binders plus niacin.[30]

The usual dose of lovastatin in adults is 20 to 40 mg twice daily. As the long-term safety of lovastatin has not been demonstrated, its use at the present time should be restricted to postpubertal children with severe dyslipidemia who do not respond to other lipid-lowering agents.

REFERENCES

1. Hyperlipoproteinemia. Scientific American Medicine 9:1–10, 1986.
2. Serum cholesterol determinations. Med Lett Drugs Ther 29:41–42, 1987.
3. Choice of cholesterol-lowering drugs. Med Lett Drugs Ther 30:81–84, 1988.
4. A Joint Statement for Physicians by the Committee on Atherosclerosis and Hypertension in Childhood of the Council of Cardiovascular Disease in the Young and Nutrition Committee, American Heart Association. Diagnosis and treatment of primary hyperlipidemia in childhood. Circulation 74:1181A–1188A, 1986.
5. Brown MS, Goldstein JL: A receptor-mediated pathway for cholesterol homeostasis. Science 232:34–47, 1986.
6. Canner PL, Berge KG, Wenger NK, et al: Fifteen-year mortality in coronary drug project patients: long-term benefit with niacin. J Am Coll Cardiol 8:1245–1255, 1986.
7. Clarke WR, Schrott HG, Leaverton PE, et al: Tracking of blood lipids and blood pressures in school age children: The Muscatine Study. Circulation 58:626–634, 1978.
8. Committee on Nutrition: Indications for cholesterol testing in children. Pediatrics 83:141–142, 1989.

9. Consensus Development Conference: Lowering blood cholesterol to prevent heart disease. JAMA 253:2080–2086, 1985.
10. Dennison BA, Kikuchi DA, Srinivasan SR, et al: Parental history of cardiovascular disease as an indication for screening for lipoprotein abnormalities in children. J Pediatr 115:186–194, 1989.
11. Dennison BA, Kikuchi DA, Srinivasan SR, et al: Serum total cholesterol screening for the detection of elevated low-density lipoprotein in children and adolescents: The Bogalusa Heart Study. Pediatrics 85:472–479, 1990.
12. Enos WF, Beyer JC, Holmes A: Pathogenesis of coronary disease in American soldiers killed in Korea. JAMA 158:912–914, 1955.
13. Freedman DS, Shear CL, Srinivasan SR, at al: Tracking of serum lipids and lipoproteins in children over an 8-year period: The Bogalusa Heart Study. Prev Med 14:203–216, 1985.
14. Frick MH, Elo O, Haapa K, et al: Helsinki Heart Study: primary prevention trial with gemfibrozil in middle-aged men with dyslipidemia. N Engl J Med 317:1237–1245, 1987.
15. Garcia RE, Moodie DS: Routine cholesterol surveillance in childhood. Pediatrics 84:751–754, 1989.
16. Griffin TC, Christoffel KK, Binns HJ, et al: Pediatric Practice Research Group. Family history evaluation as a predictive screen for childhood hypercholesterolemia. Pediatrics 84:365–373, 1989.
17. Kane JP, Malloy MJ, Tun P, et al: Normalization of low-density-lipoprotein levels in heterozygous familial hypercholesterolemia with a combined drug regimen. N Engl J Med 304:251–258, 1981.
18. Knuiman JT, Hermus RJJ, Hautvast JG: Serum total and high-density lipoprotein cholesterol concentrations in rural and urban boys from 16 countries. Atherosclerosis 36:529–537, 1980.
19. Lauer RM, Lee J, Clarke WR, et al: Cholesterol screening in childhood. In Roche AF (ed): Prevention of Adult Atherosclerosis During Childhood. Columbus, OH, Ross Laboratories, pp. 97–102, 1988.
20. Lee J, Lauer RM, Clarke WR: Lipoproteins in the progeny of young men with coronary artery disease. Children with increased risk. Pediatrics 78:330–337, 1986.
21. Lipid Research Clinics Program: The Lipid Research Clinics Coronary Primary Prevention Trial results. II. The relationship of reduction in incidence of coronary heart disease to cholesterol lowering. JAMA 251:365–374, 1984.
22. Malloy MJ, Kane JP, Kunitake ST, et al: Complementarity of cholestipol, niacin, and lovastatin in treatment of severe familial hypercholesterolemia. Ann Intern Med 107:616–623, 1987.
23. McNamarra JJ, Molot MA, Stremple JF, et al: Coronary artery disease in combat casualties in Vietnam. JAMA 216:1185–1187, 1971.
24. Newman WP III, Freedman DS, Voors AW, et al: Relation of serum lipoprotein levels and systolic blood pressure to early atherosclerosis. N Engl J Med 314:138–144, 1986.
25. Sammalkorpi K, Valtonen V, Kerttula Y, et al: Changes in serum lipoprotein pattern induced by acute infections. Metabolism 37:859–865, 1988.
26. Schaefer EJ: When and how to treat the dyslipidemias. Hosp Pract 15:57–72, 1988.
27. Schaefer EJ, Levy RI: Pathogenesis and management of lipoprotein disorders. N Engl J Med 312:1300–1310, 1985.
28. Shepherd J, Packard CJ, Bicker S, et al: Cholestyramine promotes receptor-mediated low-density-lipoprotein catabolism. N Engl J Med 302:1219–1222, 1980.
29. Stary HC: Evolution and progression of atherosclerosis in the coronary arteries of children and adults. In Bates SR, Gangloff EC (eds): Atherogenesis and Aging. New York, Springer-Verlag, 1987, pp, 20–36.
30. Stein EA: Treatment of familial hypercholesterolemia with drugs in children. Arteriosclerosis Suppl I:I-145–I-151, 1989.
31. Strong JP: Coronary atherosclerosis in soldiers: a clue to the natural history of atherosclerosis in the young. JAMA 256:2863–2866, 1986.
32. Strong WB, Dennison BA: Pediatric preventive cardiology: atherosclerosis and coronary heart disease. Pediatr Rev 9:303–314, 1988.
33. The Coronary Drug Project Research Group: Clofibrate and niacin in coronary heart disease. JAMA 231:360–381, 1975.
34. U.S. Department of Health, Education and Welfare: Manual of Laboratory Operations. Lipid Research Clinics Program. Bethesda, MD, National Institutes of Health, 1974, pp. 75–628.
35. Uauy R, Vega GL, Grundy SM, et al: Lovastatin therapy in receptor-negative homozygous familial hypercholesterolemia: lack of effect on low-density lipoprotein concentrations or turnover. J Pediatr 113:387–392, 1988.
36. West RJ, Lloyd JK, Leonard JV: Long-term follow-up of children with familial hypercholesterolaemia treated with cholestyramine. Lancet 2:873–875, 1980.
37. Wynder EL, Williams CL, Laakso K, et al: Screening for risk factors for chronic disease in children from 15 countries. Prev Med 10:121–132, 1981.

Chapter 21

SYSTEMIC ARTERIAL HYPERTENSION

J.R. Ingelfinger, M.D.

That hypertension is a risk factor for cardiovascular disease, stroke and/or organ damage (e.g., renal disease) has been appreciated for some time.[18,46] Data on which this conclusion is based stem from many careful observations in predominantly male adults. Although severe pediatric hypertension may result in morbidity and mortality[28] if untreated, data linking childhood hypertension of mild or moderate degree to subsequent diseases are much less persuasive. Nevertheless, especially as "primary" systemic arterial hypertension often occurs in families, the prevailing opinion of most physicians evaluating and treating children is that hypertension in childhood, even if mild, bears watching and often warrants therapy. Although mild-to-moderate elevation of blood pressure in children most frequently results from early "primary" hypertension, a fair number of individuals with secondary causes for hypertension may be discovered through screening. Definitive therapy for such children, including careful pharmacologic management, results in less morbidity and mortality later. This chapter presents some of the features of normal and abnormal blood pressure in children and adolescents.

NORMAL VERSUS ABNORMAL BLOOD PRESSURE

Data on normal blood pressure have been widely available in the United States and other countries for the past 15 years. The present "normal blood pressure curves" from the Task Force on Blood Pressure Control in Children are culled from nine compatible studies on more than 72,000 children.[50] The norms for the 90th percentile are shown in Table 1 and should be used when examining children in an office setting. Graphic presentation of similar data showing all percentiles is provided in Figure 1. It is less clear that these norms, obtained in the seated position, are useful for random blood pressures determined under other circumstances. It is well known that blood pressure is a variable

measurement with a clear circadian rhythm and pattern. Blood pressure tends to be lowest in the morning and highest in the late afternoon and evening.[34] Blood pressure also changes with exercise, stress, and alterations in circulatory homeostasis (e.g., volume loading or hemorrhage).

A word about how to measure blood pressure seems in order.[50] Because normative data are derived from the seated position (or supine position in babies), the same techniques ought to be used during routine determination of blood pressure. The blood pressure cuff itself should easily encircle the arm, the inner bladder should go more than half way around the arm (optimally two-thirds to three-fourths of the way around), and the width should go from the antecubital fossa to two-thirds of the distance to the shoulder. Using too small a blood pressure cuff causes artifactual increases in blood pressure, but too large a cuff will not produce artifactually low pressures. If a stethoscope is used, firm but not heavy pressure should be placed on the antecubital fossa with the arm at the level of the heart. The cuff should be pumped up at least 30 mm above the expected pressure. Young children will become uncomfortable and uncooperative if the blood pressure cuff is inflated to 200 mm Hg. (If Korotkoff sounds are not heard, the blood pressure cuff should be inflated to a higher pressure so that one does not overlook a very high blood pressure reading.) Deflating the cuff at a rate of approximately 1–2 mm every second permits an accurate reading. It is important to be aware of factors that may adversely affect accurate measurement of blood pressure (Table 2). Appropriate cuff sizes must be used (Table 3). Automatic blood pressure devices such as the Dinamap, which is based on a plethysmographic technique, may be extremely helpful in providing multiple blood pressure measurements automatically. Although intra-arterial blood pressure measurements are certainly performed at cardiac catheterization or, in the very sick child, in an intensive care unit, the Dinamap is useful for most blood pressure monitoring pur-

Table 1. Age-specific Blood Pressure Measurements (90th Percentile)

	Age in Months												
	0	1	2	3	4	5	6	7	8	9	10	11	12
Boys													
Systolic blood pressure	87	101	106	106	106	105	105	105	105	105	105	105	105
Diastolic blood pressure	68	65	63	63	63	65	66	67	68	68	69	69	69
Height (cm)	51	59	63	66	68	70	72	73	74	76	77	78	80
Weight (kg)	4	4	5	5	6	7	8	9	9	10	10	11	11
Girls													
Systolic blood pressure	76	98	101	104	105	106	106	106	106	106	106	105	105
Diastolic blood pressure	68	65	64	64	65	65	66	66	66	67	67	67	67
Height (cm)	54	55	56	58	61	63	66	68	70	72	74	75	77
Weight (kg)	4	4	4	5	5	6	7	8	9	9	10	10	11

	Age in Years																	
	1	2	3	4	5	6	7	8	9	10	11	12	13	14	15	16	17	18
Boys																		
Systolic blood pressure	105	106	107	108	109	111	112	114	115	117	119	121	124	126	129	131	134	136
Diastolic blood pressure	69	68	68	69	69	70	71	73	74	75	76	77	77	78	79	81	83	84
Height (cm)	80	91	100	108	115	122	129	135	141	147	153	159	165	172	178	182	184	184
Weight (kg)	11	14	16	18	22	25	29	34	39	44	50	55	62	68	74	80	84	86
Girls																		
Systolic blood pressure	105	105	106	107	109	111	112	114	115	117	119	122	124	125	126	127	127	127
Diastolic blood pressure	67	69	69	69	69	70	71	72	74	75	77	78	78	81	82	81	80	80
Height (cm)	77	89	98	107	115	122	129	135	142	148	154	160	165	168	169	170	170	170
Weight (kg)	11	13	15	18	22	25	30	35	40	45	51	58	63	67	70	72	73	74

Modified from the Report of the Second Task Force on Blood Pressure Control in Children—1987. Pediatrics 79:1, 1987. Copyright 1987 by the American Academy Pediatrics.

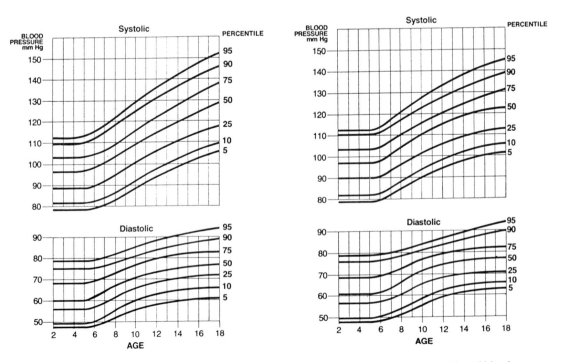

Figure 1. **A,** Percentiles of blood pressure measurement in boys (right arm, seated). **B,** Percentiles of blood pressure measurement in girls (right arm, seated). (From Blumenthal S, et al: Report of the task force on blood pressure control in children. Pediatrics 59[Suppl]:797, 1977. Copyright American Academy of Pediatrics 1977.)

Table 2. Sources for Error in Blood Pressure Measurement

Patient Problems
Patient not in basal state, e.g.,
  anxious
  clenched arms
  full bladder
  arm not at heart level

Observer Problems
Observer introduces bias, e.g.,
  rounds off numbers
  hears poorly
  doesn't read correctly, due to parallax

Technical Problems
Instrumentation problems, e.g.,
  calibration inaccurate
  cuff worn out
Measurement problems, e.g.,
  cuff size inappropriate
  cuff applied incorrectly
  arm not at heart level
  cuff inflated or deflated inaccurately
  stethoscope applied too firmly, bell not used
  Korotkoff sounds not recorded
  pressure not taken in arms and legs
  failure to note patient position
  too few measurements taken

Table 3. Cuff Sizes to Use for Blood Pressure Measurement*

Age Group	Bladder Width (cm)	Bladder Length (cm)
Neonate	2.5–4.0	5.0–9.0
Infant	4.0–6.0	11.5–18.0
Child	7.5–9.0	17.0–19.0
Adult	11.5–13.0	22.0–26.0
Large adult	14.0–15.0	30.5–33.0
Thigh	18.0–19.0	36.0–38.0

*A child of a certain age may not necessarily use the corresponding cuff size for that age group. Large adult thigh cuffs should be used for individuals with especially large arms.

Table 4. Normal Blood Pressure and Pulse Rate in Various Positions and with Various Activities

Activities	Blood Pressure	Pulse Rate
Systolic		
Seated cf.* supine	↑	—
Standing cf. supine	↑	—
Dynamic exercise cf. at rest	—	↑
Isometric exercise cf. at rest	—	↑
Diastolic		
Seated cf. supine	—	—
Standing cf. supine	—	—
Dynamic exercise cf. at rest	— or ↓	↑
Isometric exercise cf. at rest	↑	↑
Mean Arterial Pressure		
Seated cf. supine	↑	—
Standing cf. supine	↑	—
Dynamic exercise cf. at rest	↑	↑
Isometric exercise cf. at rest	↑	↑
At Rest Trained vs. Untrained		
Dynamic exercise	↓	↓
Isometric exercise	↓	↓

*cf. = compared to.

poses. The correlation between the Dinamap machine and intra-arterial pressure seems good.[8]

Ambulatory blood pressure monitoring is feasible in a cooperative child of school age or older.[15] Using this technique, in which blood pressures are recorded on an ambulatory device and downloaded into a computer, may be helpful in determining the percentage of blood pressure readings that are elevated in a child thought to have hypertension or to determine whether a child has true hypertension at all.

Blood pressure varies with posture.[32] Table 4 shows the usual pattern of blood pressure and pulse with posture. Certain patients with "primary" hypertension appear to have a fall in mean arterial pressure on assuming the erect from the supine posture. Even though this fall in mean arterial pressure is not a sensitive or specific finding, it may be sufficiently prevalent to suggest subsequent evaluation of any elevation in a child's blood

pressure. Blood pressure levels also change with exercise.[22,37] During dynamic exercise systolic pressure normally rises to levels that, at rest, would be thought to be hypertensive. For example, exercise to exhaustion on a stationary bicycle produces systolic blood pressure levels as high as 200 or 210 mm Hg in normal subjects. A hypertensive child doing dynamic exercise has a similar response pattern. Generally, during dynamic exercise the diastolic pressure stays the same or even decreases. In contrast, both systolic and diastolic blood pressures generally rise during isometric exercise. For this reason, isometric exercise usually is not recommended for the hypertensive youngster. However, available information suggests that resting blood pressure is decreased in the trained youngster who does either dynamic or isometric exercise. More studies are needed to determine the appropriate recommendation for the child with hypertension who is committed to doing isometric exercise (see p. 252).

The question of what constitutes a normotensive or a hypertensive child is often difficult to answer. Generally, severe elevation of blood pressure is simple to diagnose, and a ready explanation is usually found. However, in a youngster with mildly elevated blood pressure, diagnosis and management may be more difficult. The present Task Force norms (Table 1) list the 90th percentile for height and weight as well as for blood pressure. It is recommended that if a youngster has a blood pressure level between the 90th and 95th percentiles for age, the blood pressure should be taken again on three different occasions. If the child is overweight, the apparent elevation in blood pressure may be due to body size. Although loss of weight may be helpful in lowering blood pressure, an overweight child with a markedly elevated blood pressure should be evaluated further even prior to weight loss.

REGULATION OF BLOOD PRESSURE

Blood pressure levels at any given moment are regulated by a complex combination of hormonal and physical factors.[21] If blood pressure is thought of as the product of cardiac output and peripheral resistance, a variety of physical factors that may affect systemic arterial blood pressure should be considered, including heart rate and stroke volume, as well as blood flow factors. Resistance is affected not only by physical factors but, within given vascular beds, by a variety of hormones.

One of the most cogent and clear schemes for conceptualizing control of blood pressure was put forward some years ago by Guyton and colleagues.[20,21] Figure 2 shows a summary of this work, in which some factors controlling blood pressure act rapidly, whereas others act in a more sustained fashion to respond to changes in physical and biochemical factors that occur when an organism has to respond to changes in physiology.[20,21] For example, changes in blood volume or changes in catecholamine secretion due to stress all result in a complex pattern of responses which alters blood pressure (Fig. 2).

A variety of hormones and vasoactive factors affect blood pressure levels, the most influential of these being the renin-angiotensin system.[14] The major end-product of the renin-angiotensin system is the peptide "angiotensin II," a potent vasoconstrictor in a variety of vascular beds, the peripheral

vasculature and the kidney, where it affects renal plasma flow. With situations such as severe salt restriction or volume depletion the kidney releases renin, which acts on angiotensinogen (renin substrate) to produce angiotensin I, which in turn is converted by angiotensin-converting enzyme to angiotensin II. Although this circulating system is controlled primarily by renin from the kidney, renin substrate (angiotensinogen) produced in the liver, and converting enzyme produced in the lung, it is increasingly evident that multiple renin-angiotensin systems also exist in local tissue and that these are of key importance in the regulation of blood pressure in individual organ systems. A variety of stimuli increase or decrease renin levels and the activity of this system (Table 5).

Other hormonal systems are also important in blood pressure regulation (Table 6).[24] In the short term, catecholamine secretion normally contributes to blood pressure control; in pathologic hypercatecholamine states (such as pheochromocytoma or neuroblastoma) it may cause severe hypertension. Both mineralocorticoids and glucocorticoids are involved in maintenance of blood pressure. In cases of adrenal hypertrophy, or tumor, these hormones may reach very high levels, resulting in severe secondary hypertension. Less well-known hormonal systems also may play a role, still to be defined, in blood pressure regulation (e.g., atrial peptin,[4] ouabain-like hormones, or a vasoconstrictor peptide called endothelin[26]). Still other hormones such as prolactin, thyroid hormone, vasoactive intestinal peptide, and antidiuretic hormone, may play a role. Table 5 lists a number of these hormones and their effects.

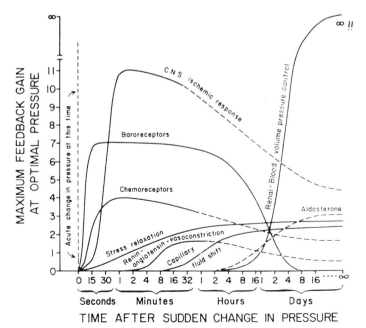

Figure 2. Potency of various arterial pressure control mechanisms at different time intervals after the onset of a disturbance to the arterial pressure. Note especially the infinite gain of the renal–body fluid pressure control mechanism that occurs after a few days' time. (From Guyton AC: Textbook of Medical Physiology, 6th ed. Philadelphia, W.B. Saunders, 1961, p. 248, with permission.)

Table 5. Factors that Stimulate or
Inhibit Release of Renin

Stimulating Factors	Inhibiting Factors
Circulatory	**Circulatory/Ionic**
Hemorrhage	Volume loading
Volume depletion	Salt loading
(actual or effective)	↑ K^+
Hypotension	↑ Ca^{2+}
Salt depletion	↑ Cl^-
Hormonal	**Hormonal**
Glucagon	Mineralocorticoids
Parathyroid hormone	Angiotensin II
Adrenocorticotropic	Antidiuretic hormone
hormone	
Norepinephrine and other	
catecholamines	
Drugs	**Drugs**
Vasodilators	Mineralocorticoids
Diuretics	Beta blockers
Alpha stimulators	Alpha stimulators

Table 6. Hormonal Systems Affecting
Blood Pressure

Hormonal System	Blood Pressure Effect
Major Effectors	
Renin-angiotensin system	↑
Catecholamines	↑
Glucocorticoids	↑
Mineralocorticoids	↑
Prostaglandins	
Vasodilatory	↓
Vasoconstrictor	↑
Kinins	↑ or ↓
Renomedullary relaxing substance	↓
Atrial peptin (atrial natriuretic factor)	↓ ?
Endothelin	↑ ?
Other Effectors	
Thyroid hormone	SBP* ↑
Parathyroid hormone	↑
Serotonin	↓ or ↑
Vasoactive intestinal peptide	↓ or ↑
Prolactin	↓ ?
Antidiuretic hormone	↓ ?

*SBP = systolic blood pressure.

CAUSES OF HYPERTENSION

Primary Hypertension

Primary hypertension is still a diagnosis of exclusion.[19,50] In addition, it is increasingly obvious that primary hypertension is a syndrome, multiple forms of which remain to be defined. Among individuals with primary hypertension a number of features commonly include family pattern, sensitivity to high-salt intake (in about half), and failure to modulate renal blood flow and adrenal sensitivity to angiotensin II in response to a high- or low-salt diet.[30,56] Much has been written about the epidemiology and course of primary hypertension, and the reader is referred to several general reviews.[5,30,43,56]

Secondary Hypertension

In unselected populations a random child with an elevated blood pressure is far more likely to have primary hypertension, whereas in referral centers, where children with more elevated blood pressures are likely to be seen, secondary hypertension is much more common. The proportion of diagnoses of secondary hypertension in given categories is fairly uniform: about 8 of 10 children with secondary hypertension have renal parenchymal disease, and 1 of 10 has renovascular disease.[29] Roughly 2% of children with secondary hypertension have coarctation of the aorta; about 0.5% have pheochromocytoma or neural crest tumors. Other forms of secondary hypertension, although important to identify, are less common. Table 7 lists the major forms of secondary hypertension. This is not meant to be an exhaustive list, as additional entities are always being uncovered. Some of the major categories of secondary hypertension will be discussed briefly.

Renal Parenchymal Disease with Hypertension. Many types of renal parenchymal disease are associated with elevated blood pressure. Among these, chronic pyelonephritis or reflux nephropathy with pyelonephritic scars, glomerulonephritis of various sorts, renal obstructive disease, and polycystic kidney disease are among the most common.[29,45] The reasons for blood pressure elevation in these entities is complicated, although activation of the renal renin-angiotensin system often is involved. In the case of glomerulonephritis, decreased renal function and renal perfusion lead to increased secretion of renin from the juxtaglomerular apparatus, which initiates a cascade of events when there is angiotensin II-mediated hypertension. In addition, when the glomerular filtration rate is decreased, volume loading results in a failure to excrete the increased plasma water, which may result in increased plasma volume and hypertension on that basis as well. In pyelonephritis, interstitial scarring may lead to changes in intrarenal plasma flow, which also may activate the renin-angiotensin system. During episodes of severe acute pyelonephritis there may be sufficient interstitial swelling to add to activation of this system.

Most individuals with obstructive uropathy do not have hypertension. Generally, hypertension occurs with fairly acute worsening of renal function. The hypertension in obstructive uropathy may be transient, and the diagnosis of obstruction may be made because of the acute hypertension. Treating the obstruction often greatly improves or cures the hypertension. (This does not occur invariably, as scarring may make it difficult to have normal renal plasma flow.)

The mechanism of hypertension in polycystic kidney disease is not well established, although

Table 7. Forms of Secondary Hypertension

Renal
- Acute glomerulonephritis
- Hemolytic uremic syndrome
- Bilateral obstructive uropathy
- Congenital defects: polycystic kidneys, Ask-Upmark kidney, hypoplastic disorders
- Unilateral renal disorders
  - Renal artery abnormalities, stenosis, neurofibromatosis, thrombosis, trauma, fistula, fibromuscular dysplasia, external compression
  - Unilateral parenchymal disease, pyelonephritis, congenital defects, obstructive uropathy, radiation nephritis, infarction
  - Perirenal masses
- Anaphylactoid purpura (Henoch-Schönlein) nephritis
- After renal transplantation (rejection, steroid-related)
- Acute renal failure
- Following blood transfusions or volume expansion in patients with renal disease
- After genitourinary surgery
- After renal biopsy
- Tumors of the kidney (Wilms' tumor, juxtaglomerular cell tumors, tuberous sclerosis)
- Collagen disease (periarteritis, lupus erythematosus, dermatomyositis)
- Chronic glomerulonephritis and chronic pyelonephritis
- Heavy metal poisoning
- Amyloidosis (familial form)
- Fabry's disease (angiokeratoma corporis diffusum)
- Familial nephritis (Alport's syndrome, medullary cystic disease)
- Renal tubular acidosis with nephrocalcinosis

Vascular
- Coarctation of the aorta
- Polycythemia
- Anemia (systolic only)
- Pseudoxanthoma elasticum
- Takayasu's arteritis
- Radiation aortitis
- Patent ductus arteriosus (systolic only)
- Arteriovenous fistula (systolic)
- Leukemia
- Subacute bacterial endocarditis
- Cardiac problems (heart block, aortic insufficiency)

Endocrine
- Pheochromocytoma
- Congenital adrenal hyperplasia
- Hyperthyroidism (systolic only)
- 17-Hydroxylase deficiency
- Aldosteronism (primary)
- Neuroblastoma
- Cushing's disease
- Liddle's syndrome
- Hyperparathyroidism
- Ovarian tumors

Metabolic
- Diabetes mellitus (renal involvement)
- Gouty nephropathy
- Acute intermittent porphyria
- Hypercalcemia
- Hypernatremia

Neurologic
- Dysautonomia (Riley-Day syndrome)
- Neurofibromatosis
- Increased intracranial pressure (of any cause, especially tumors, infection, trauma)
- Guillain-Barré syndrome
- Poliomyelitis

Drug-related
- Steroid administration (corticosteroids and desoxycorticosterone acetate)
- Heavy metals (mercury and lead)
- Reserpine overdose
- Amphetamine overdose
- Following intravenous alpha-methyldopa
- Following sympathomimetic drugs (nose drops, cough medicine, cold preparations)
- Excessive ingestion of licorice
- Use of birth control pills

Miscellaneous
- Burns
- Stevens-Johnson syndrome
- Cyclic vomiting with dehydration
- Hypertension related to stretching of the femoral nerve (leg traction)
- Renoprival hypertension

activation of the renin-angiotensin system has been invoked. Yet, other factors such as renomedullary-relaxing substance, vasodilatory prostaglandins, and other hormones may be involved in the pathogenesis.

Control of renal parenchymal hypertension is important for the preservation of renal function. It is important to use hypotensive agents that achieve this with minimal side effects (converting enzyme inhibitors or beta blockers are advocated).

Renovascular Disease. Renovascular disease may occur at several times during childhood.[11,48] In infancy, usually in the sick newborn,[1] one of the most common types of hypertension is caused by renovascular accidents such as thrombosis or thromboembolism related to umbilical artery catheters or by spontaneous thrombotic episodes. Medical management with hypotensive agents is

the treatment of choice in these infants. Often, after a stormy initial period it is possible to discontinue hypotensive medication, because the hypoperfused renal tissue may infarct, and the remaining tissue may be either improved in function or be completely recovered.

In older children stenosis of the renal arteries (either isolated or involving multiple renal vessels) may occur because of a variety of causes. A large proportion of youngsters afflicted with this stenosis have other systemic diseases, such as tuberous sclerosis or neurofibromatosis.[11,45,51] In such instances the arterial abnormalities may progress so that, ultimately, multiple vessels may be involved even though only one or two were involved initially. Other apparent causes of renovascular disease and stenosis of the renal arteries may be related to poorly understood syndromes, such as

Williams syndrome, or to the sequelae of viral diseases such as congenital rubella. In addition, hypertension due to renal artery stenosis may be caused by compression of renal vessels by fibrous bands (as in neurofibromatosis), enlarged lymph nodes (as with tumors), or by scar tissue following surgical or other trauma. Finally, stenosis of the renal arteries may occur in a child with renal transplantation.

It is well to remember that abnormalities of the renal arteries may occur in concert with other vascular abnormalities.[11,45] In the child with neurofibromatosis it is not uncommon to find that multiple peripheral vessels are involved—an example is stenosis of the superior mesenteric artery or a hypoplastic aorta. General aortitis may involve the aorta and renal vessels at the same time.[10,54] There are also poorly understood syndromes in which there may be maldevelopment of the abdominal aorta along with stenosis of the renal arteries.

The therapy of renal artery disease is interventional.[52] Transluminal angioplasty is increasingly available for children and is the preferred mode when possible.[7] Secondary therapies include reconstruction of renal vessels and, sometimes, autotransplantation of the affected kidney.[23] Long-term follow-up of any of these modalities often is satisfactory. However, because arterial disease is so frequently progressive, the ultimate prognosis is guarded. In view of this last fact, preservation of renal parenchyma is of prime importance.

Coarctation of the Aorta. Coarctation of the aorta is an important cause of secondary hypertension in childhood (see ch. 34). In most centers, aortic coarctation is discovered early and treated surgically sooner than was the case in previous eras. The pathogenesis of hypertension in coarctation of the aorta is complicated. The mechanical obstruction results in some of the hypertension; in addition, multiple hormonal systems, including the renal-angiotensin system, are activated because of the change in the pattern of blood flow in the major conducting artery of the body (see ch. 34).[2]

Endocrine Hypertension. Endocrine hypertension may be due to exogenous causes, such as administration of glucocorticoid,[53] or to anabolic steroid (usually self-administered).[33] Endocrine-related hypertension also may occur spontaneously.[6,25] Hypertension related to the pituitary gland may occur with primary Cushing's syndrome owing to chromophobe adenoma. In the latter instance, increased ACTH stimulates the adrenal gland to produce steroids, ultimately resulting in hypertension. Thyroid-related hypertension, usually systolic, may occur with hyperthyroidism. Whenever there is isolated systolic hypertension, hyperthyroidism should be considered.

Adrenal hypertension may occur because of adrenal medullary hyperactivity, as in pheochromocytoma, where increased catecholamines are secreted.[27,49] Chromaffin tissue elsewhere in the body also may become adenomatous and result in a pheochromocytoma. Adrenal cortical hyperplasia, adenoma, or adenocarcinoma may result in primary hypercorticism and Cushing's syndrome. In these instances treating the tumors or the hyperplasia with suppressive therapy is indicated.

Hypertension also may occur because of hypercalcemia related to parathyroid adenomas, but is extremely rare in children and adolescents. Occasionally, abnormalities in the synthesis of steroid hormones caused by inborn errors of metabolism may result in definable hypertension.[36] An example is the 11-beta hydroxylase-deficiency form of congenital adrenal hyperplasia.

Central Nervous System–mediated Hypertension. Hypertension of the central nervous system is not well understood. Increases in intracranial pressure from almost any cause are associated with hypertension, usually acute.[3,40] However, problems that may cause changes in the vasomotor centers of the brain or in the functioning of various neural interconnections between basal ganglia have also been associated with hypertension. On occasion, the syndrome of absent corpus callosum is associated not only with electrolyte abnormalities, but with hypertension as well. It is known that in addition to the production of an ouabain-like substance (in the central nervous system), there is a complete renin-angiotensin system. Other vasoactive hormones may be involved also. There is some evidence that some forms of primary hypertension are associated with abnormalities of the central nervous system; these have yet to be fully defined in humans.

Iatrogenic and Other Forms of Hypertension. A host of pharmacologically active agents may be involved in acute or sustained hypertension.[33] Some of these are listed in Table 7, and should always be considered when hypertension is discovered. Because patients and their families may be unwilling or unable to pinpoint some of the substances that would cause acute or sustained hypertension, a puzzling case of hypertension, especially acute, necessitates obtaining a toxic screen.

Acute Hypertension, Accelerated Hypertension, and Hypertensive Crisis. The causes of sudden or acute hypertension are listed in Table 8. Acute hypertensive episodes may occur in the course of evaluation and management of sustained hypertension and may be sudden and transient.[16] Mechanisms are variable, ranging from neurally-mediated hypertension to renin-mediated hypertension.

A variety of agents are available for the treatment of hypertensive crisis (see Appendix). The advantages and disadvantages of these various therapeutic drugs are also noted in the Appendix.

Table 8.   Causes of Acute (Often Transient) Hypertension

Volume expansion	Sodium-containing agents, steroids, non-steroids, oral contraception
Autonomic effects	Antihypertensive drug-drug interaction, amphetamines, phencyclidine Monoaminooxidase inhibitors plus dietary or drug indiscretion, anti- depressants, sympathomimetics, ergot alkaloids
Rebound hypertension	Drug-drug interaction (clonidine, methyldopa, beta blockers)
Accidents and surgery	Burns, orthopedic accidents, orthopedic surgery, urologic surgery, trauma
Nephropathies	Hemolytic uremic syndrome Acute postinfectious nephritis Acute nephritis (non-postinfectious): anaphylactoid purpura, systemic lupus, membranoproliferative glomerulonephritis Pyelonephritis
Renovascular disease	Renal artery stenosis, segmental renal artery stenosis, post-transplanta- tion hypertension
Tumors	Pheochromocytoma, neuroblastoma (renin-secreting)
Central nervous system	Increased intracranial pressure—any cause

DIAGNOSTIC STUDIES IN THE HYPERTENSIVE CHILD[12,13,50]

It goes without saying that a careful history, including recent events and family history, is essential in the evaluation of a child or adolescent with elevated blood pressure. A careful history may alert the clinician to the appropriate direction for hypertensive evaluation. For instance, a history of antecedent sore throat and rather darkish urine over several preceding days would certainly point in the direction of acute nephritis; an astute history of a youngster's activity might lead to the discovery of self-medication. A positive family history of primary hypertension, endocrinopathy, or systemic disease such as Von Recklinghausen's syndrome may be very valuable in the evaluation of the child with hypertension.

Physical examination as a diagnostic test is at least equally important. Blood pressure readings in four extremities are necessary to rule out coarctation, as is examination for radial-femoral delay and strength of the pulse. Examination of each organ system may give a hint as to the etiology of the hypertension and as to end-organ damage.

Once physical examination is completed, the evaluation of the hypertensive child involves, first, a set of screening examinations followed by various phases of increasingly invasive studies. Every patient should have a urinalysis and culture, and tests for blood urea nitrogen and creatinine, as well as total CO_2 and electrolytes. If primary hypertension is suspected on the basis of a relatively moderate increase in blood pressure and positive family history, the Task Force for Blood Pressure Control in Children recommends obtaining a cholesterol level, or possibly a lipoprotein electrophoresis, to rule out other risk factors. If all of these studies are negative and the blood pressure elevation is mild or moderate, nonpharmacologic therapy should be considered, except in the very young child.

If blood pressure still does not come under control, a second set of evaluations should be performed. Ninety percent of secondary hypertension is renal or renovascular in origin; this necessitates imaging of the genitourinary system.[47] Most sources agree that the combination of radionuclide renal scintiscanning, with or without ultrasound, is superior to the intravenous urogram for identifying renal and renovascular hypertension. However, the Task Force for Blood Pressure Control in Children recommends using the imaging study with which a given center has the most experience.[50] Recently, radionuclide renal scanning after converting-enzyme inhibition has been found superior to scanning alone because the converting-enzyme inhibitor accentuates differences in blood flows.[31,55] If there is a high index of suspicion for renovascular disease, angiography should be considered next. A venous injection with digital-subtraction angiography gives reasonable imaging of the main renal vessels. However, definitive transluminal angioplasty cannot be done through this route, and small children or any individual with a substantial abnormality of the small branches of the renal arteries will require an arterial injection. Formal arteriography is best reserved for the patient for whom there is a very high index of suspicion of renovascular disease and for whom interventional radiology will be used.

Cardiac evaluation is important in the assessment of a hypertensive child. In addition to a careful physical examination, echocardiography[9] (see ch. 13) provides an excellent indicator of left ventricular wall thickness and function. In addition, formal exercise testing may be helpful in determining whether a hypertensive youngster should have pharmacologic therapy prior to participation in sports.[38]

Part of the evaluation of hypertension should be the identification of individuals with labile hypertension, individuals who are salt sensitive, and those who are stress reactors. A variety of studies are helpful in this area. In the office, stress tests are simple to perform and require no special equipment. Three easy-to-perform stresses include serial subtraction from 100, ice water immersion of an extremity, and isometric hand-grip exercise. Blood pressure is monitored while any of these stresses is performed. An increase in blood pressure of more than 20 mm diastolic and 30 systolic indicates a stress reactor. The lability of blood pressure and also the percentage of blood pressure readings above the norm for age may be determined by 24-hour ambulatory blood pressure monitoring. The information learned from such an evaluation may be helpful in determining whether there is truly hypertension, whether pharmacologic therapy would be efficacious, and whether there is a change in the normal circadian rhythm of the blood pressure level. Salt sensitivity[30,56] may be assessed by putting the patient on a no-added salt diet (first choice), by increasing salt in the diet (which may make a patient more hypertensive), or by administering diuretics for a therapeutic trial. Salt sensitivity generally suggests primary hypertension unless there are obvious renal abnormalities.

THERAPY FOR SUSTAINED HYPERTENSION

Nonpharmacologic therapy is recommended for mild hypertension as a first approach.[50] Even moderate hypertension in an older child or adolescent may respond to diet, exercise, or stress reduction techniques. Of the various dietary therapies for hypertension, only two have enough data backing them to warrant recommendation for children with hypertension. Because many individuals are sensitive to salt, a no-added salt diet seems sensible and will not be harmful in most patients.[35,39] (Notable exceptions: a child with salt-losing nephropathy or a child with congenital adrenal hyperplasia. Generally, these conditions are easy to diagnosis in advance.) An additional dietary manipulation is a calorie-restricted diet for the overweight child.[41,42] Exercise as an adjunct for blood pressure control is worthwhile, although exercise testing should be done in the severely hypertensive child prior to the initiation of an exercise program. Dynamic rather than static exercise should be recommended. For the motivated child, stress reduction techniques, such as a non-cult relaxation technique, may be helpful. In our experience the patient must want to comply with these therapies or they are totally ineffectual.

Pharmacotherapy in hypertension should be used only in the youngster with moderate-to-marked elevation of blood pressure.[44,50] A large variety of agents are now available, although many are not formally approved for use in children. The classes of pharmacologic agents are listed in the Appendix. A pragmatic approach to the selection of pharmacologic therapy ought to be employed. It makes sense to use the agents with which one is most familiar because there are large numbers of agents available in several classes (for example, numerous beta blockers). Rather than step-care therapy, popularized in the 1970s, monotherapy should be used as long as it is practical. The majority of youngsters with hypertension are adolescents, and compliance is a major difficulty. For this reason a polypharmaceutical approach is practically doomed to failure. Once blood pressure has been well controlled for a period of 3–6 months, it makes sense to try to decrease medication or even discontinue it. This concept, popularized as step-down therapy[17] makes eminent good sense in the child with hypertension.

REFERENCES

1. Adelman RD: The hypertensive neonate. Clin Perinatol 15:567–585, 1988.
2. Alpert RS, Bain HH, Balfe JW, et al: Role of the renin-angiotensin-aldosterone system in hypertensive children with coarctation of the aorta. Am J Cardiol 43:828–834, 1979.
3. Amery A, VanAken H (eds): A symposium: acute blood pressure and the brain. Am J Cardiol 63:1C–50C, 1989.
4. Atlas SA: Atrial natriuretic peptide: a new factor in hormonal control of blood pressure and electrolyte homeostasis. Annu Rev Med 37:397–414, 1986.
5. Berenson GS, Cresanta JL, Webber LS: High blood pressure in the young. Annu Rev Med 35:535–560, 1984.
6. Bryan TB, Brouhard BH: Hypertension in children: endocrine aspects. Nephron 23:106–111, 1979.
7. Chevalier RL, Tegtmeyer CJ, Gomez RA: Percutaneous transluminal angioplasty for renovascular hypertension in children. Pediatr Nephrol 1:89–98, 1987.
8. Colan S, Fujii A, Borow K, et al: Noninvasive determination of systolic, diastolic and end-systolic blood pressure in neonates, infants and young children. Comparison with central aortic pressure measurements. Am J Cardiol 52:867–875, 1983.
9. Culpepper WS: Cardiac anatomy and function in juvenile hypertension: current understanding and further concerns. Am J Med 75:57–61, 1983
10. Danaraj TJ, Wang HO, Thomas MA: Primary arteritis of the aorta causing renal artery stenosis and hypertension. Br Heart J 25:153–165, 1963.
11. Daniels SR, Loggie JMH, McEnery PT: Clinical spectrum of intrinsic renovascular hypertension in children. Pediatrics 80:698–704, 1987.
12. DeSanto NG, Trevisan M, Capasso G, et al: Blood pressure and hypertension in childhood: epidemiology, diagnosis, and treatment. Kidney Int 25:S115–118, 1988.
13. Dillon MJ: Blood pressure. Arch Dis Child 63:347–349, 1988.
14. Dzau VJ, Pratt RE: Renin-angiotensin system: biology, physiology and pharmacology. In Haber E, Morgan H, Katz A, et al (eds): Handbook of Experimental Cardiology. New York, Raven Press, 1986, pp. 1631–1661.
15. Egger M, Bianchetti MG, Gnadinger M, et al: Twenty-four hour intermittent, ambulatory blood pressure monitoring. Arch Dis Child 62:1130–1135, 1987.

16. Farine M, Arbus GS: Management of hypertensive emergencies in children. Pediatr Emerg Care 5:51–55, 1989.

17. Finnerty FA Jr: Step-down therapy in hypertension: its importance in long-term management. JAMA 246:2593–2596, 1981.

18. Gordon T, Kannel WB (eds): An epidemiological investigation of cardiovascular disease: The Framingham Study. U.S. DHEW, Sec. 1–27, 1968–1971.

19. Gruskin AB et al: Primary hypertension in the adolescent: facts and unresolved issues. In Loggie JMH et al (eds): NHLBI Workshop on Juvenile Hypertension. New York, B.M.I., 1984, pp. 305–333.

20. Guyton AC: Short-term regulation of mean arterial pressure: nervous reflex and hormonal mechanisms for rapid pressure control and long term regulation of mean arterial pressure. In Guyton AC: Textbook of Medical Physiology, 6th ed. Philadelphia, W.B. Saunders, 1981, pp. 246–273.

21. Guyton AC, Coleman TG, Crowley AW, et al: Arterial pressure regulation overriding dominance of the kidneys in long-term regulation and in blood pressure. Am J Med 52:584–594, 1972.

22. Hagberg JM, Ehsani AA, Goldring D, et al: Effect of weight training on blood pressure and hemodynamics in hypertensive adolescents. J Pediatr 104:147–151, 1984.

23. Hendren WH, Kim SH, Herrin JR, et al: Surgically correctable hypertension of renal origin in childhood. Am J Surg 143:432–442, 1982.

24. Ingelfinger JR: The renin-angiotensin system and other hormonal systems in the control of blood pressure. In Ingelfinger JR: Pediatric Hypertension. Philadelphia, W.B. Saunders Co., 1982, pp. 45–63.

25. Ingelfinger JR: Endocrine causes of hypertension. In Ingelfinger JR: Pediatric Hypertension. Philadelphia, W.B. Saunders Co., 1982, pp. 185–203.

26. Inoue A, Yanagisawa M, Kimura S, et al: The human endothelin family: Three structurally and pharmacologically distinct isopeptides predicted by three separate genes. Proc Natl Acad Sci 86:2863–2867, 1989.

27. Lewis D, Dalton N, Ridger S: Phaeochromocytoma: report of three cases. Pediatr Nephrol 1:46–49, 1987.

28. Lloyd-Still J, Cottom DG: Severe hypertension in childhood. Arch Dis Child 42:34–39, 1967.

29. Londe S: Causes of hypertension in the young. Pediatr Clin North Am 25:55–65, 1978.

30. Luft FC, Miller JZ, Cohen SJ, et al: Heritable aspects of salt sensitivity. Am J Cardiol 61:1H–6H, 1988.

31. Majid M, Potter BM, Guyetta PC, et al: Captopril enhanced renal scintigraphy for detection of renal artery stenosis—an update (abstract). J Nucl Med 27:962(A), 1986.

32. McGrory WW, Klein AA, Rosenthal RA: Blood pressure, heart rate and plasma catecholamines in normal and hypertensive children and their siblings at rest and after standing. Hypertension 4:507–513, 1982.

33. Messerli FH, Frohlich ED: High blood pressure: a side effect of drugs, poisons and food. Arch Intern Med 139:682–687, 1979.

34. Millar-Craig MW, Bishop CN, Raftery EB: Circadian variation of blood pressure. Lancet 1:795–797, 1978.

35. Morgan T, Gillies A, Morgan G, et al: Hypertension treated by salt restriction. Lancet 1:227–230, 1978.

36. New MI, Levine LS: Adrenocortical hypertension. Pediatr Clin North Am 25:67–81, 1978.

37. Nudel DB, Gootman N, Brunson SC, et al: Exercise performance of hypertensive adolescents. Pediatrics 65:1073–1078, 1980.

38. Olin R: Blood pressure response to dynamic exercise in healthy and hypertensive youths. Pediatrician 13:34–43, 1986.

39. Parijs J, Joosins J, Van der Linden L, et al: Moderate sodium restriction and diuretics in the treatment of hypertension. Am Heart J 85:22–34, 1973.

40. Reis DJ: The brain and hypertension: reflections on 35 years of inquiry into the neurobiology of the circulation. Circulation 70:III31–45, 1984.

41. Reisin E, Abel R, Modon M, et al: Effect of weight loss without salt restriction on the reduction of blood pressure in overweight hypertensive patients. N Engl J Med 298:1–6, 1978.

42. Rocchini AP, Katchy V, Anderson J, et al: Blood pressure in obese adolescents: effect of weight loss. Pediatrics 82:16–23, 1988.

43. Rosenbaum PA, Elston RC, Srinivasan SR, et al: Cardiovascular risk factors from birth to 7 years of age: The Bogalusa Heart Study. Predictive value of parental measures in determining cardiovascular risk factor variables in early life. Pediatrics 80:807–816, 1987.

44. Roy LP: Drug therapy in childhood hypertension. Indian J Pediatr 55:359–371, 1988.

45. Scharer K: Renal hypertension in childhood. Annales Nestle 42:1–18, 1984.

46. Shurtleff D: Some characteristics related to the incidence of cardiovascular disease and death: The Framingham Study, 18 year follow-up. U.S. DHEW, Pub. No (NIH) 74-599, Sec. 30, 1974.

47. Siegel MJ, St. Armour TE, Siegel BA: Imaging techniques in the evaluation of pediatric hypertension. Pediatr Nephrol 1:76–88, 1987.

48. Stanley JC: Renal vascular disease and renovascular hypertension in children. Urol Clin North Am 11:451–463, 1984.

49. Stackpole RH, Melicow MM, Uson AC: Pheochromocytoma in children: report of 9 cases and review of the first 100 published cases with follow-up studies. J Pediatr 63:315–330, 1963.

50. Task Force on Blood Pressure Control in Children—National Heart, Lung and Blood Institute: Report of the second task force on blood pressure control in children—1987. Pediatrics 79:1–25, 1987.

51. Tilford DL, Kelsch RC: Renal artery stenosis in childhood neurofibromatosis. Am J Dis Child 126:665–668, 1973.

52. Watson AR, Balfe JW, Hardy BE: Renovascular hypertension in childhood: a changing perspective in management. J Pediatr 106:366–372, 1985.

53. Whitworth JA: Mechanisms of glucocorticoid-induced hypertension. Kidney Int 31:1213–1224, 1987.

54. Wiggelinkhuizen J, Cremin BJ: Takayasu arteritis and renovascular hypertension of childhood. Pediatrics 62:209–217, 1978.

55. Willems CD, Shah V, Uchiyama M, et al: Captopril as an aid to diagnosis in childhood hypertension. Clin Exp Hypertens [A]8:747–749, 1986.

56. Williams GH, Hollenber NK: "Sodium-sensitive" essential hypertension: emerging insights into pathogenesis and therapeutic implications. Contemp Nephrol 3:303–331, 1985.

Chapter 22

RHEUMATIC FEVER

Donald C. Fyler, M.D.

DEFINITION

Rheumatic fever is a poorly understood "auto-immune" reaction to group A, beta-hemolytic, streptococcal pharyngitis. It is a self-limited disease that involves the joints, skin, brain, serous surfaces, and the heart. Were it not for cardiac valve damage, the disease would be of little practical consequence.

PREVALENCE

"In the 1920's rheumatic fever was the leading cause of death in individuals between 5 and 20 years of age . . . In 1938 there were more than a thousand deaths in New York City alone . . . In New England, childhood rheumatism accounted for nearly half of adult heart disease and in Boston's crowded North End hardly a family was spared"[3] (Fig. 1).

Now, in developed countries, rheumatic fever and rheumatic heart disease have become uncommon (Exhibit 1).[13] Whether measured as attacks or deaths from acute rheumatic fever, or numbers of patients with rheumatic heart disease, the problem is vanishing in the United States.[2,14,30,33] In stark contrast, it remains a devastating problem in developing countries. It is estimated that there are 15 to 20 million new cases of rheumatic fever in the world each year, and this could be an underestimate.[55]

Several terms, e.g., "developing," "third world," "disadvantaged," "semi-tropical," or "tropical" are accurate generalized descriptions of the countries in which rheumatic fever is common. It is a disease of the socially disadvantaged; it is associated with poverty. Still, it must be remembered that these are only generalizations. Pockets of rheumatic fever are reported in developed, first world, advantaged, countries with cool climates (e.g., the Navajos in the United States[9] and the Maoris in New Zealand[43]), as well as in Polynesia[35] and Hawaii.[7] To those familiar with the era when patients

were sent to warm climates ("safely free of rheumatic fever") to recover,[19] the irony of the situation is sobering. It is now apparent that the prevalence data from that period were seriously flawed and, one suspects, that even today they still are. Estimates of the prevalence of rheumatic fever in the U.S. in the recent past vary by 100-fold,[20] even in this well-to-do country where devotion to numbers and computers is a way of life.

Why are the figures for the precise prevalence of rheumatic fever and rheumatic heart disease so elusive? In part, it is because there is no specific test for rheumatic fever, and in part, because an attack of rheumatic fever may cause so few symptoms that an episode of active disease may be overlooked. There was so much confusion about the diagnosis of rheumatic fever among military personnel during World War II that criteria were invented to provide a rational basis for management of patients.[18,44] Those labeled as having had rheumatic fever who did not meet Jones criteria often exceeded those who did. In the past, before modern knowledge of mitral valve prolapse as a cause of mitral regurgitation or bicuspid aortic valves as a cause of aortic regurgitation, surveys counted many of these patients as having rheumatic heart disease. Still, admitting the obvious confusion, if the main features of rheumatic disease are consid-

---

Exhibit 1

Boston Children's Hospital Experience
1973–1987

Rheumatic Fever or Rheumatic Heart Disease

In the years 1973–1987, 102 patients with a diagnosis of rheumatic fever or rheumatic heart disease were referred to the cardiology department of the Children's Hospital. This does not represent the entire experience of this hospital during this period. Rather, it includes those patients who needed cardiac evaluation, or cardiac surgery, or were somehow matters of interest to the cardiology department. It is our impression that a significant number were recent immigrants and not natives of New England.

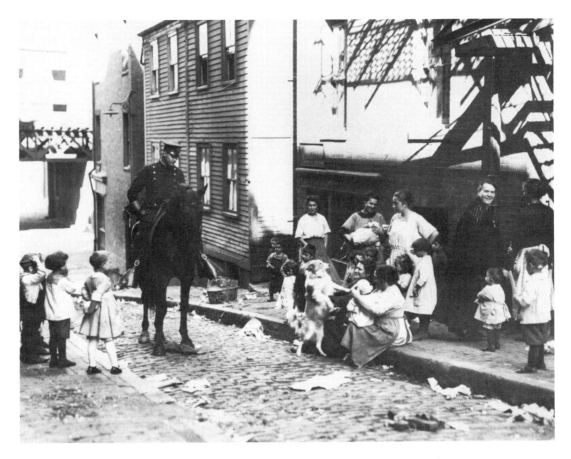

Figure 1.   Foster Street, North End, Boston, 1905. (Courtesy of Gates and Tripp.)

ered, rheumatic fever has nearly disappeared from our country in our lifetime. To emphasize this situation, one needs only to go to a disadvantaged country in which rheumatic fever and rheumatic heart disease are common to get a sensation of déjà vu.

However, just when we are beginning to feel comfortable about the disease, it is reappearing in parts of the United States in sufficient numbers to warrant concern.[21] There are mounting numbers of reports from all parts of the United States: Ohio,[16,8] the Rocky Mountain states,[51] Pennsylvania,[52] Hawaii,[7] and Florida.[46]

PATHOGENESIS

A "Social Disease"

Rheumatic fever is found mainly in poverty-stricken populations. In the past, in the United States, it seemed to be predominantly a disease of the Caucasian ghettos (Fig. 1); now it is a disease of blacks.[14] Whether this is because of poor nutrition, crowding, or unavailability of medical services is not known. There is good reason to believe that prevalence may simply depend on the availability of penicillin.[33]

Group A Streptococcal Pharyngitis

Since Cheadle's[6] Harveian lectures 100 years ago, physicians have noted that pharyngitis often occurs a week or so before the onset of rheumatic fever, and that, at least in temperate climates, there is a seasonal incidence of rheumatic fever. Throat cultures often grew beta-hemolytic streptococci. Still, it was not generally accepted until 35 years ago that group A, beta-hemolytic, streptococcal infection invariably preceded an attack of acute rheumatic fever.[44] The convincing evidence was the high and rising levels of streptococcal antibodies (antistreptolysin O) in the sera of children with active rheumatic fever. With the acceptance of group A, beta-hemolytic, streptococcal pharyngitis as being inextricably involved in the pathogenesis of rheumatic fever, research focused sharply on the streptococcus as a causative agent.

The following observations must be reconciled in any theory of the causation of rheumatic fever:

1. From the clinical point of view it is established that infants with beta-hemolytic, streptococcal infections do not get rheumatic fever. The youngest age at which rheumatic fever occurs is approximately 2 years, with the disease being rare in the third year. The average age at which a child has a first attack of acute rheumatic fever is 8 years.

2. There is a latent period from the onset of streptococcal pharyngitis to the onset of rheumatic fever (average, 18 days).[39]

3. At most, during an epidemic of beta-hemolytic, streptococcal pharyngitis, rheumatic fever occurs in 3% of untreated patients.[40]

4. Chorea may be manifest without evidence of preceding streptococcal infection; yet it may be followed some years later by mitral stenosis.

5. The dramatic response to ACTH or cortisone (the clinical course is reversed in days) suggests that an immunologic mechanism is involved in the pathogenesis.[48–50]

6. Rheumatic fever damages primarily the mitral valve, to a lesser extent the aortic valve, rarely the tricuspid valve, and extremely rarely the pulmonary valve. Why one valve is more prone to rheumatic damage than another is unknown. At the worst, 50–60% of patients with acute rheumatic fever develop damaged valves. The relation between mitral valve prolapse and rheumatic fever requires further study.[28]

7. Group A, beta-hemolytic, streptococcal pharyngitis in a child who has recovered from rheumatic fever is likely to reactivate the disease; indeed, the second attack is likely to mimic the first in its manifestations.[12,41] Whether recurrent streptococcal infection with the original M type will produce a second attack is unknown.

8. Group A, beta-hemolytic, streptococcal impetigo is *not* followed by rheumatic fever.[53] Why the patient must have pharyngitis to stimulate rheumatic fever is unknown. Perhaps the weak antibody response to streptococcal skin infection compared with pharyngeal infection is a clue to understanding this difference.[22] The difference in recognizable "rheumatic antigens" on blood cells versus cells from the tonsils of patients with rheumatic heart disease compared with controls may provide further understanding.[15] Equally mysterious is that impetigo may trigger glomerulonephritis but not rheumatic fever. A limited number of specific group A streptococcal M types cause glomerulonephritis; only rarely do both acute rheumatic fever and acute glomerulonephritis occur together. In contrast, no M-type specificity for rheumatic fever has been found.[54] There are about 80 M types of group A, beta-hemolytic streptococci, many of which have been associated with epidemics of rheumatic fever.

That particularly virulent (mucoid) strains of streptococci may be required to cause rheumatic fever is an attractive hypothesis that is difficult to prove.

Extensive studies of group A, beta-hemolytic streptococcus have focused largely on the layer of the capsule (Fig. 2) that contains the M proteins, used to identify streptococcal types, and to a lesser extent on the carbohydrate layer, used to group the streptococci. The M protein is structurally similar to the heart muscle protein, tropomyosin.[34] There is cross-reactivity of heart muscle antigens derived from the myocardial sarcolemma with streptococcal antigens.[23–26] Streptococcal antibodies can be identified in the caudate nucleus of patients who have had chorea[17] and the sera of patients with rheumatic fever react with heart tissues, but not when the antibodies have been absorbed by streptococcal antigens.[55]

Genetic Factors

The familial incidence of rheumatic fever has been mentioned in the literature for nearly 100 years. Numerous studies of siblings and relatives have been carried out, largely confirming the impression that a familial factor plays a role.[29] An alloantigen has been demonstrated on B-cells in 75% of patients with rheumatic fever, whereas it is noted in only about 16% of nonrheumatic patients.[36] Others have suggested that the HLA-DR antigen is a marker for patients known to have rheumatic heart disease.[38] These observations tend to confirm the idea that there is a genetic background for rheumatic fever, but laboratory demonstration of a host factor in rheumatic fever is still less than completely convincing.

Pathogenetic Hypothesis

The current hypothesis, which reconciles the disparate group of observations, may be stated as follows: In a genetically susceptible individual, repeated, untreated, streptococcal infections in early life sensitize the child to the possibility of rheumatic fever. Sometime after the age of 2, a beta-hemolytic, group A, streptococcal pharyngitis sets off an unusually high antibody response. After recovery from the pharyngitis there is a 10-day latent period of relative well-being, following which an autoimmune response involving the excess streptococcal antibodies begins, lasts many weeks, and gradually damages the left heart valves. Later, a recurrent streptococcal infection may reactivate the disease. There is continuing valve damage after clinical evidence of rheumatic activity has subsided. How much of this is caused by recurrent rheumatic fever, by smoldering activity, or by hemodynamic factors causing scarring is unknown. It is known that Aschoff nodules (accepted by most as a sign of rheumatic activity) are found in the biopsied heart structures at cardiac surgery years after the known attack.[45]

PATHOLOGY

There are inflammatory lesions in the heart, blood vessels, brain, and serous surfaces of the joints and pleura. The pathologic picture is characterized by a distinctive and pathognomonic granuloma, consisting of perivascular infiltration of cells

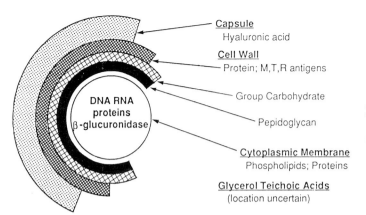

Figure 2. Group A Streptococcus cell wall. (From Markowitz M, Gordis L: Rheumatic Fever, 2nd ed. Philadelphia, W.B. Saunders, 1972, with permission.)

and fibrinoid protoplasm (Aschoff body) (Fig. 3). Aschoff bodies are found in all patients with clinical rheumatic activity, in those who have died of fulminant rheumatic fever, and in many with chronic rheumatic valvar abnormalities as well,[45] suggesting that many patients with this disease have subclinical, active, rheumatic fever smoldering for years. To account for the observed association of rheumatic mitral disease and mitral valve prolapse, it has been suggested that mitral valve prolapse develops because of smoldering rheumatic fever.[28,47]

As many as 50% of patients with a first attack of rheumatic fever have valve involvement. The mitral valve is most commonly involved, being at first incompetent and, later, in some patients, becoming stenotic. When first involved the aortic valve becomes incompetent, but unlike the mitral valve, almost never becomes stenotic. Aortic regurgitation does occur as a solitary lesion (5% of patients), but is more often seen in combination with mitral

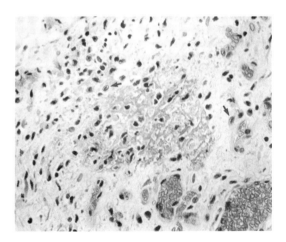

Figure 3. Pericardial Aschoff nodule. There is a discrete area of fibrinoid degeneration with inflammatory, poorly formed, granulomatous reaction. "Anitschkow's" cells are present at the periphery of the nodule (arrow). Hematoxylin and eosin. (Courtesy of Antonio Perez, M.D., Children's Hospital, Boston, MA.)

regurgitation. Mitral regurgitation alone or associated with aortic regurgitation is by far the most common lesion, so much so that the diagnosis of rheumatic heart disease without mitral disease is suspect. Incompetent and even stenotic tricuspid valves are seen (Fig. 4) and rarely an incompetent pulmonary valve is reported.

CLINICAL MANIFESTATIONS

A history of pharyngitis is reported by about half of the patients with acute rheumatic fever. Pharyngitis ranges from typical symptoms of streptococcal, pharyngeal infection to vague symptoms of an upper respiratory illness. With spontaneous subsidence of the sore throat there is a latent period when the child is afebrile and seems well. About 10 days later the child becomes ill again. At this point elevation of the antistreptolysin-O titer is demonstrable and throat culture may produce beta-hemolytic streptococci, which prove to be group A.

The fever associated with acute rheumatic fever is not high, rarely over 103°F. It may be so low as to be recognized only with systematic recording on a temperature chart. Much has been made of tachycardia being out of proportion to fever as a sign of rheumatic fever. In our experience this has not been a prominent feature in the usual case of active disease except when there is congestive heart failure, a more than adequate explanation for tachycardia. A child with active rheumatic fever who is febrile is rarely flushed—more often pale.

Polyarthritis

The majority of patients have some joint symptoms (Table 1).[27,32] Several joints may be intermittently involved (polyarthritis), ranging from vague arthralgia to florid swelling, heat, redness, and demonstrable joint fluid. Occasionally, it is difficult to elicit objective evidence of arthritis; intermittent limping and other limitations of function to guard painful joints may be the only historical data. When

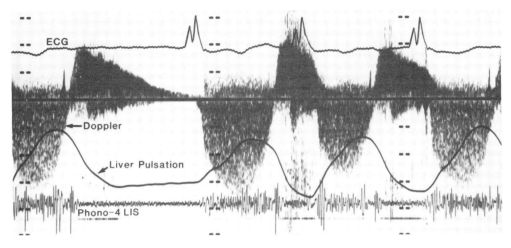

Figure 4. These tracings were obtained from a 16-year-old Grenadan girl who had severe rheumatic mitral and tricuspid disease. Tricuspid regurgitation is demonstrated by the Doppler tracing and coincident pulsation of a grossly enlarged liver.

there is active involvement (swollen, red, or tender joints), there is fever. The joints most involved are the knees, hips, ankles, elbows, wrists, and shoulders; characteristically the joint symptoms are migratory, rarely involving a single joint for more than 2 days. Unlike joint involvement in rheumatoid arthritis, the small joints of the hands and feet, the temporomandibular joints, and sternoclavicular joints are not commonly involved in polyarthritis. The pain can be exquisite, the child reacting to any contact with the inflamed joint, including the weight of bed sheets. A swollen joint that is not tender results from some disease other than rheumatic fever. The stage of acute arthritis associated

with obvious fever is self-limited, commonly subsiding within a few days and rarely lasting longer than a month.

It is a striking clinical observation that chorea and acute polyarthritis never occur together. This is readily believable because the combination of these two problems would produce memorable difficulties.

Carditis

Although roughly half of patients with acute rheumatic fever have evidence of carditis on first examination, symptoms of congestive heart failure are relatively uncommon. When there is congestive failure the patients are sometimes very ill with dyspnea, hepatomegaly, vomiting, tachycardia, and fever, as well as florid joint involvement.

When there is pericardial effusion, there may be a cough and often precordial or left shoulder pain that varies with position.

Carditis is mainly manifested by the appearance of murmurs. By far the most common cardiac observation is the presence of an apical systolic murmur. The murmur of mitral regurgitation is characteristically blowing, of high frequency, and transmits to the axilla. It extends through most of systole, beginning with the first sound. Often there is a short, apical, mid-diastolic rumble (Carey-Coombs murmur) that does not signify mitral stenosis. The presystolic crescendo of mitral stenosis is not encountered in a first attack of acute rheumatic fever. A repeated, careful search for an early diastolic blowing murmur is required, because there may be aortic insufficiency. Occasional irregularity can be documented with a variable 2:1 block. A friction rub indicates pericarditis. With pancarditis there may be gross congestive heart

Table 1. Principal Manifestations of Rheumatic Fever in 457 Initial Attacks, Exclusive of Cases of Pure Chorea

Manifestations	Cases	%
Significant murmurs	240	53
Pericarditis	29	6
Congestive heart failure	36	8
Prolonged P-R interval	115	25
Subcutaneous nodules	54	12
Erythema marginatum	48	11
Chorea (exclusive of pure chorea)	61	13
Fever	405	89
Elevated sedimentation rate	421	92
Fever and/or elevated sedimentation rate	442	97
Antistreptolysin-O titer of 400 units or more	376	82
Joint pain	412	90
Syndrome of joint pain, fever and/or elevated sedimentation rate, and elevated antistreptolysin-O titer	338	74
Total cases	457	

From Massell BF, Fyler DC, Roy SB: Am J Cardiol 1:436–449, 1958,[32] with permission.

failure, a tender, enlarged liver, visible pulsating neck veins when the patient is in the sitting position, shortness of breath, and pulmonary rales.

Erythema Marginatum

In a small percentage of patients with active rheumatic fever, a distinctive rash, erythema marginatum, may be observed. When present it is virtually a certain sign of active rheumatic fever (Fig. 5). It is an irregular, geometric, circinate, marginate, red rash over the torso that is evanescent. This rash may be brought out by hot baths and does not itch.

Subcutaneous Nodules

Firm nodules over hard bony surfaces such as the elbows, wrists, shins, knees, ankles, vertebral column, and occiput are seen occasionally in patients with active rheumatic fever (Fig. 6). On microscopy these structures resemble Aschoff nodules and almost invariably signify rheumatic activity. This phenomenon is uncommon in first attacks, generally being seen in patients who already have well-established heart disease. Nodules are best detected under side-lighting when the skin is slowly moved over the bony surfaces such as the elbows or knees. Nodules are more often seen than palpated, and are small, nontender, lumps attached to the underlying bone. It is interesting that injections of small amounts of the patient's own blood into these bony surfaces will often produce nodules similar in appearance and on histologic examination. Production of nodules by Massell's method has been used as a test of rheumatic activity.[1] These observations support the suggestion that nodules are the result of trauma to the hard bony areas in patients who have active disease.

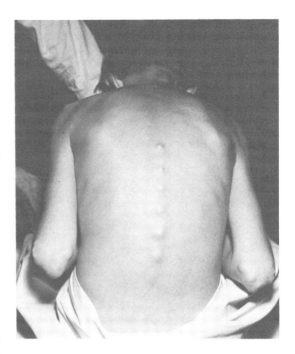

Figure 6. This is an extreme example of nodules selected because the nodules are readily seen. (Courtesy of Benedict F. Massell, M.D.)

Chorea

Sydenham's chorea (St. Vitus' dance) is a distinctive clinical entity with virtually no differential diagnosis. There are purposeless, choreiform movements, aggravated by stress, in an emotionally labile child or young adolescent (usually female). Chorea is less common in older adolescents and is not seen in adults. There may be slurred speech, grotesque facial grimacing, or illegible penmanship. The outstretched hands assume a characteristic "spooning" position; asked to show the tongue, it flicks out and in like a snake's tongue; a fine tremor is palpable in the outstretched hands. In a severe attack the child may be unable to feed herself, and the thrashing movements of the extremities may result in bruises. The more the parents chastise the child about spilling food, nervousness, and dropping things, the more the child's equanimity and coordination disintegrate. Often the onset of chorea is reported to have followed some major psychological trauma such as a bad automobile accident.

Chorea may exist in two circumstances. It simply may be part of an otherwise active rheumatic process (almost never with simultaneous arthritis), in which case there is an elevated sedimentation rate, fever, and evidence of a preceding streptococcal infection; or it may be an isolated phenomenon, pure chorea, without other evidence of rheumatic activity.

Pure Chorea. The number of patients with pure

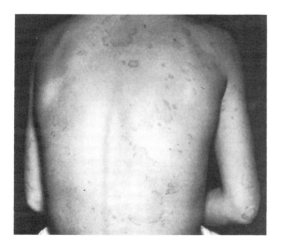

Figure 5. Erythema marginatum. (Courtesy of Benedict F. Massell, M.D.)

chorea is variable. As many as 10% of rheumatic patients may have pure chorea. The choreiform movements, labile mood, and coordination problems are indistinguishable from those in patients who have chorea associated with active rheumatic fever. However, with pure chorea all other manifestations of rheumatic fever are absent. There is no fever and there may be no evidence of a preceding streptococcal infection by history, throat culture, or antistreptolysin titer. There is no evidence of cardiac involvement and no elevation of the sedimentation rate.

Occasionally a patient will have unilateral chorea (hemichorea), all features being characteristic except that abnormal movements are confined to one side. It is probably pure chance that the author's experience with hemichorea has been of the pure form, without other evidence of rheumatic activity. With observation hemichorea often extends to involve the other side; indeed, with careful observation many patients with bilateral chorea have more pronounced signs on one side.

Whether a child has chorea or not can usually be determined in the first minutes of the physical examination, because the disease is readily recognized if it has ever been seen before. If a question remains, the performance of the child should be observed under varying circumstances. The outstretched hands, the movements of the tongue, the ability to pronounce Methodist-Episcopal or some other equally difficult phrase, the response to irritation (usually the examination alone is irritating enough), and the inability to write may resolve the question.

Abdominal Pain

At intervals, in the past, children were hospitalized for abdominal pain with fever and ended up with abdominal exploration for appendicitis, after which it was discovered that the child had acute rheumatic fever. Whether this abdominal pain is a consequence of pericardial effusion or inflammation of abdominal serous surfaces is not clear. However, it has occurred often enough to be reasonably well documented in the author's experience. Nevertheless, if the patient fulfills the criteria for abdominal exploration, it is safer to go ahead with surgery than to assume that the pain results from rheumatic fever.

ANCILLARY STUDIES

Minor Laboratory Tests

A throat culture from an untreated patient often grows hemolytic streptococci. The antistreptolysin-O titer is elevated and may continue to rise, sometimes to remarkably high levels, as the period of observation continues. Other streptococcal antibodies may be elevated.

The sedimentation rate is almost invariably elevated, as is the C-reactive protein. The possibility of finding a normal sedimentation rate in a child with a severely congested liver should be kept in mind, but is rarely seen in practice. The sedimentation rate must be corrected for anemia, because anemia is common in these patients. There is a plethora of modern-day nuclear scans and enzyme determinations that might be of value in a patient with acute rheumatic fever, but for obvious reasons there has not yet been sufficient experience with these.

Electrocardiogram

The electrocardiogram is not particularly useful in the diagnosis of acute rheumatic fever. Roughly 20% of patients have a prolonged PR interval, particularly if repeated electrocardiograms are taken. Atropine shortens the prolonged PR interval to normal. Occasionally patients have intermittent 2:1 block, and rarely complete heart block has been reported. Nonspecific changes in the T wave and ST segment are seen but are neither common nor specific to this diagnosis.

Chest X-ray

The heart size may be variably enlarged if there is carditis (Fig. 7).

Echocardiogram

Where rheumatic fever is common, echocardiographers report that many patients with acute rheumatic fever, including some patients with pure chorea, have evidence of mitral regurgitation, even in the absence of a mitral regurgitant murmur.[51] The high incidence of mitral valve prolapse in patients with rheumatic heart disease has piqued the interest of echocardiographers.[28] In the acute attack there may be evidence of myocardial depression with reduced shortening fraction and dilation of the left ventricle. Chronic valvar incompetence can be readily evaluated using two-dimensional echocardiography and Doppler techniques, the evaluation of valvar incompetence proceeding as for valvar incompetence of any cause.

Echocardiograms are the method of choice in evaluating the presence and amount of pericardial fluid. It may be that this tool will become particularly useful in the diagnosis and treatment of rheumatic heart disease. At the present time, in Boston, we have had too little experience to comment further.

Cardiac Catheterization

There is no need for cardiac catheterization in patients with acute rheumatic fever.

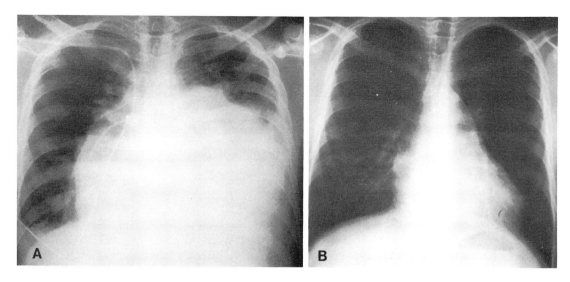

Figure 7. These chest x-rays are from a native American boy who lived his entire life in Massachusetts. He developed active rheumatic fever that remained active for 8 months despite steroid and salicylate therapy. (There was insignificant pericardial fluid.) Because of gross congestive heart failure (**A**), the mitral and aortic valves were replaced. There was dramatic improvement (**B**). (Courtesy of Williams & Wilkins.)

DIAGNOSIS

There being no specific tests for rheumatic fever, T. Duckett Jones, in 1944,[18] published clinical criteria for the diagnosis of rheumatic fever that have come into widespread use in a slightly modified

Table 2. Jones Criteria (Revised) for Guidance in the Diagnosis of Rheumatic Fever*

Major Manifestations	Minor Manifestations
Carditis	**Clinical**
Polyarthritis	Previous rheumatic fever or
Chorea	rheumatic heart disease
Erythema marginatum	Arthralgia
Subcutaneous nodules	Fever
	Laboratory
	Acute phase reactions
	Erythrocyte sedimentation
	rate, C-reactive protein,
	leukocytosis
	Prolonged P-R interval

Plus
Supporting evidence of preceding streptococcal infections (increased ASO or other streptococcal antibodies; positive throat culture for group A streptococcus; recent scarlet fever)

From Stollerman GH, Markowitz M, Taranta A, et al: Jones criteria (revised) for guidance in diagnosis of rheumatic fever. Circulation 32:664–668, 1965, by permission of the American Heart Association, Inc.

*The presence of two major criteria, or of one major and two minor criteria, indicates a high probability of the presence of rheumatic fever if supported by evidence of a preceding streptococcal infection. The absence of the latter should make the diagnosis doubtful, except in situations in which rheumatic fever is first discovered after a long latent period from the antecedent infection (e.g., Sydenham's chorea or low-grade carditis).

form (Table 2).[44] Further modification may be desirable.[11] In Jones' scheme, two major or one major and two minor criteria are required to make the diagnosis of rheumatic fever. The use of his criteria in the diagnosis of acute rheumatic fever is straightforward for the majority of patients. There are, however, two groups of patients who cause some confusion.

1. Chorea. For practical purposes the presence of chorea alone proves the diagnosis of acute rheumatic fever. Confusion often arises when there is hemichorea or when the physician has not seen this disease. Usually the diagnosis is self-evident.

2. Probable Rheumatic Fever. There is a sizable group of patients who have arthritis, fever, and evidence of a preceding streptococcal infection who are labeled as having probable rheumatic fever. For some of these patients the diagnosis is ultimately shown to be erroneous, but the group as a whole tends to develop valvar damage in significant numbers over the years.

Arthralgia alone is not sufficient to suggest the diagnosis of acute rheumatic fever, regardless of positive ancillary laboratory results. Obviously, such patients are encountered. However, if all such patients were labeled as being prone to rheumatic fever (and all that designation implies), the large number of mistaken diagnoses could scarcely be justified.

Similarly, while in theory a patient with acute rheumatic fever might have monoarticular arthritis, this entity is sufficiently rare, and other forms of monoarticular arthritis are sufficiently common that a diagnosis of acute rheumatic fever based on involvement of one joint is most often an error. The authors believe that the minimal joint involvement needed to label a patient as a "rheumatic," with its life-long implications, is a single "objective" joint and at least one other joint with arthralgia. Anything observed by someone other than the patient is taken as an objective sign, i.e., limping, swelling, redness, or inability to use an arm to lift objects. Arthritis without tenderness is not acceptable. Using this as the minimal acceptable evidence of joint involvement, there are a number of patients with joint involvement, evidence of recent streptococcal infection, and an elevated sedimentation rate. We believe these children should be considered to have rheumatic fever and observed for the late development of valvar disease. With follow-up, only a small percentage have turned out to have other diseases, most commonly, rheumatoid arthritis or lupus erythematosus.

Differential Diagnosis

Myocardial Disease. The differential diagnosis between rheumatic fever and acute myocardial disease is a common clinical problem. Often there is good evidence for a myocardial or pericardial disorder but no evidence of valvar disease. It is an important principle that **there is no rheumatic heart disease without valvar involvement. There must be a murmur to diagnose rheumatic heart disease.** An obvious difficulty arises in the patient with no murmur and echocardiographic evidence of mitral regurgitation. Over the years it has become accepted that a murmur is required to diagnose rheumatic carditis. Echo-Doppler demonstration of mitral regurgitation in the absence of a murmur does not change this dictum. On the other hand, inability to demonstrate mitral regurgitation by echo-Doppler, in the presence of a murmur, is taken as virtual proof of the absence of mitral regurgitation, and some other explanation of the murmur should be sought. It is evident that some years of observation will be required to learn the full value of echocardiography in the diagnosis and management of rheumatic fever.

Rheumatoid Arthritis. Rheumatoid arthritis can be confused with acute rheumatic fever in two ways. With continued follow-up, the syndrome of arthritis, elevated antistreptolysin titer, and elevated sedimentation rate may turn out to be rheumatoid arthritis. One should be wary of this possibility, particularly if the joints involved are the small joints of the hands and feet. In any case follow-up usually solves this problem.

A more pressing differential difficulty occurs when the patient has pericardial effusion, fever, evidence of a prior streptococcal infection, and an elevated sedimentation rate. Without murmurs typical of rheumatic heart disease these patients have most often turned out to have rheumatoid arthritis or, rarely, lupus erythematosus.

Other Joint Diseases. Rarely there may be more than one joint involved with septic arthritis. This differential resolves itself in days with observation. Trauma and aseptic forms of arthritis are almost invariably monoarticular and are usually readily recognized. For practical purposes, monoarticular arthritis is not rheumatic fever.

Sickle Cell Disease. Sickle cell disease may mimic acute rheumatic fever in many respects, including cardiomegaly, systolic and diastolic murmurs, and joint pain. A family history may provide a clue, and a sickle cell preparation and electropheresis of the hemoglobin will confirm the diagnosis. All black patients in whom the diagnosis of acute rheumatic fever or rheumatic heart disease is under consideration, should be studied for sickle cell anemia before treatment for rheumatic fever is begun.

Infective Endocarditis. Infective endocarditis may be the cause of fever in a child who has murmurs compatible with rheumatic heart disease. Differentiation between infective endocarditis and active rheumatic fever may be difficult because both diseases cause murmurs and may be associated with elevated sedimentation rates and arthritis or arthralgia. Observation over a few days generally makes it possible to distinguish between the two possibilities. Any question of infective endocarditis is a mandatory indication for multiple blood cultures. It is said that active rheumatic fever and bacterial endocarditis do not occur together; the authors cannot deny this from their own experience.

MANAGEMENT

Acute Attack

After throat cultures have been obtained, **penicillin therapy is begun.** The doses used are therapeutic (600,000–900,000 U of benzathine penicillin intramuscularly for children, and 1,200,000 U for adolescents [or penicillin, 200,000 U orally; four times daily and continued until the patient has been treated 10 days[29]]). At that time a preventive maintenance dose of penicillin is begun (200,000 U orally, twice daily, every day). Management of a patient with clearly active rheumatic fever or suspected rheumatic fever without the use of antibiotics is an unconscionable error, because continued streptococcal infection can be expected to aggravate the disease. Despite the absence of demonstrable streptococci or an elevated antistreptolysin titer, patients with chorea are given penicillin as all others with acute rheumatic fever.

The hoary recommendation that all physical activity for patients with active rheumatic fever should be rigidly limited has dwindled into obscurity. No longer do we limit activity as a means to prevent further heart damage. The idea that rheumatic cardiac involvement is different from other types of myocardial disease, or that exercise is more likely to cause scarring simply has no basis in fact. Limitation of activity is managed as it is in everyone else with a febrile illness or congestive heart failure or both. Avoidance of vigorous activity is ordinarily left to the patient who, when sick, scarcely feels like moving around anyway. Rigorous attention to eradication and prevention of streptococcal infection is a much more rewarding enterprise.

Salicylates are used for control of pain and suppression of rheumatic activity in patients who do not have carditis or have only questionable evidence of cardiac involvement (Table 3). On the other end of the spectrum, it is mandatory that the child with pancarditis and congestive heart failure receive prednisone as a life-saving measure. There is room for debate about the use of prednisone for the child with valvulitis that is not life-threatening, because unassailable evidence that further valve damage can be prevented is lacking. One can find data to support whatever course of treatment is proposed.[48–50] In our view, the risks of prednisone therapy are outweighed, even in this intermediate group, by the possibility that valve damage may be reduced. Consequently, for all children with acute active disease and unequivocal valve involvement, we use steroid therapy initially and later switch to salicylates (Table 3). As mentioned, the discovery of mitral regurgitation by echocardiography, without a murmur, is considered equivocal evidence, at least until more data become available.

How long treatment should be continued is perhaps even more controversial. There is an initial response of joint symptoms, fever, and sedimentation rate to treatment with prednisone or salicylates. Demonstrable response, often dramatic, occurs in 48–72 hours and complete suppression in 7–10 days. The sedimentation rate returns to normal sooner when prednisone is used. After 2–3 weeks without clinical or laboratory evidence of activity, the dose of prednisone can be tapered and aspirin added while observing the response. Sometimes there is a reappearance of symptoms or laboratory findings (rebound phenomenon) despite this weaning process. The dose then should be increased until suppression is again attained. In any case, treatment is rarely needed beyond 12–16 weeks.

Management of congestive heart failure is usually best accomplished with diuretics. Digoxin is also used but requires caution because digoxin in the presence of an inflamed myocardium is known to precipitate dangerous rhythm problems, fortunately rarely.

Rheumatic pericardial effusion tends to accumulate slowly and rarely causes tamponade even with a large accumulation.

Although chorea is a self-limited disease, the emotional distress can be alleviated with phenobarbital or valium. With an improved mood, the choreiform movements are less marked. If chorea is associated with other manifestations of rheumatic activity, particularly if there is valvar involvement, corticosteroids may provide measurable improvement, although we do not use prednisone for pure chorea. In severe cases, hospitalization may be needed, if for no other reason than to assist the child in eating and to prevent injury from flailing movements.

Table 3.   Treatment of Acute Rheumatic Fever

Treatment and prophylaxis of group A, hemolytic, streptococcal infection:

Benzathine penicillin, 1.2 million units intramuscularly every month

Suppressive therapy

With no heart involvement:

Aspirin 100 mg/kg/day in four divided doses.

Reduce dose if salicylate level exceeds 25 mg/100 ml
Reduce dose if symptoms of salicylism (tinnitus)
Reduce dose by 25% after 1 week if good clinical response and continue for 6–8 weeks, tapering the dose in the last 2 weeks.

With valvar involvement:

Prednisone, 2.0 mg/kg/day for 2 weeks, then taper for 2 weeks.

With good response begin aspirin 75 mg/kg/day in the 3rd week and continue until the 8th week, tapering in the final 2 weeks.

Increase suppressive dose if symptoms return or sedimentation rate rises.

From Markowitz M, Gordis L: Rheumatic Fever, 2nd ed. Philadelphia, W.B. Saunders, 1972, with permission.

Course

Untreated active rheumatic fever lasts from a few weeks to several months, averaging between 8 and 16 weeks for rheumatic activity as measured by the presence of an elevated sedimentation rate, congestive failure, nodules, erythema marginatum, or continued chorea. Rheumatic activity persists longer in patients who have carditis.

At the time of initial presentation, as many as 50% of children with rheumatic fever already have a significant murmur. As the days and weeks go by, under appropriate therapy, some children lose the murmur, whereas others develop murmurs for the first time (Table 4). These changes are less frequent the longer the disease lasts, but the cardiac status never completely stabilizes; some individuals first develop new cardiac murmurs 20 years later (Table 5).[4] Young women who had pure chorea as children tend to develop pure mitral stenosis; there is only a presystolic crescendic murmur and no murmur of mitral regurgitation.

Individuals with mitral or aortic regurgitation,

Table 4. Incidence of Development of Significant Murmurs at Various Intervals after the Onset of 206 Initial Attacks of Rheumatic Fever

Duration of illness (days)	Patients developing murmurs during interval		
	Number	Percent of patients with carditis	Percent of total patients
1–7	78	76	38
8–14	7	6.8	3.4
15–28	4	3.9	1.9
29–42	3	2.9	1.4
43–91	4	3.9	1.9
More than 91	7	6.8	3.4
Total	103	100	50

From Massell BF, Fyler DC, Roy SB,[32] with permission
*Data for patients observed between 1941 and 1951.

Table 5. Prognosis of Rheumatic Fever in 1000 Patients

Initial examination	347 with no heart disease	653 with heart disease
20-year follow-up	4/7 without heart disease	1/6 without heart disease
	3/7 with heart disease	2/6 with heart disease
	10 died	3/6 died

or both may experience worsening of the existing valvar damage as the years go by. Although this may be the result of recurrent rheumatic fever, it also may simply be a result of the hemodynamics (**mitral regurgitation begets mitral regurgitation**). Mitral stenosis (Fig. 8) usually requires years to develop, sometimes as many as 20 years, although it has occurred as early as 2–3 years after the ap-

parent onset of rheumatic fever. In countries in which rheumatic fever is common, mitral stenosis develops more rapidly, being seen in small children. Biopsies of the atrial appendages in patients undergoing mitral valve surgery show Aschoff nodules in high frequency the nearer the surgery is to the attack of active rheumatic fever, but they are still present in some patients many years later. The presence of Aschoff nodules is taken as evidence of smoldering, low-grade, rheumatic activity.

When chorea is associated with other signs of activity, the incidence of ultimate valve damage is comparable to that caused by active rheumatic fever without chorea. When there is chorea with no other signs of rheumatic activity (pure chorea), ultimate heart damage is less frequent, appears late, and is most often pure mitral stenosis without preceding mitral regurgitation (Table 5).

Recurrent Rheumatic Fever

A second attack of rheumatic fever represents a failure of secondary prevention. Most often there has been a lapse of penicillin prophylaxis; less often, oral penicillin has been ineffective. It is usually possible to document the intervening streptococcal infection by throat culture and by a rise in antibodies. The first order of business is to eliminate oral streptococci and re-establish adequate prevention. If the recurrence appeared while the patient was receiving oral penicillin, a switch to monthly injections is required. In all other respects the treatment of a recurrent attack of acute rheumatic fever is the same as for a first attack. The question of adequate prophylaxis must be examined. Perhaps a switch to intramuscular benzathine penicillin is needed. Perhaps the interval between

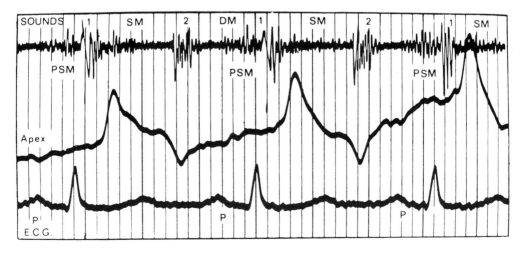

Figure 8. Typical presystolic crescendic murmur in a patient with rheumatic heart disease and mitral valve involvement. Tracing recorded at cardiac apex. Prominent first heart sound, 1; moderately split second heart sound, 2; decrescendic medium-frequency moderate-intensity systolic murmur, SM; mid-diastolic murmur, DM; presystolic crescendic murmur, PSM. (From Nadas AS, Fyler DC: Pediatric Cardiology. Philadelphia, W.B. Saunders, 1973, with permission.)

doses of intramuscular penicillin should be shortened to 3 weeks instead of 4.

A recurrent attack usually resembles the earlier attack, although valvar involvement may be extended. The appearance of congestive heart failure in a rheumatic child is always interpreted as evidence of active disease and, by implication, involvement of the myocardium as well as the valves. Although this is a useful working hypothesis, some patients develop sufficient valvar deformity within months of the apparent first onset of the disease to be the main cause of congestive heart failure (Fig. 7).[41] The problem may necessitate a decision between treating active myocardial involvement or advanced valvar disease as the cause of the congestive heart failure. Echocardiography usually solves this question, but cardiac catheterization may be needed for a confident decision about surgery. When there is valvar deformity sufficient to cause congestive heart failure, surgery may be needed and may be lifesaving, despite associated myocardial damage. When in doubt, surgery is probably the best choice, because any myocardial problem is only aggravated by the valvar abnormality. The idea that cardiac surgery is specifically prohibited in the face of active rheumatic disease is no longer tenable.

Primary Prevention

The idea that rheumatic fever could be prevented through control of streptococcal infection was proposed as early as 1937,[31] but sulfanilamide was ineffective. During World War II it was possible to document the spread of streptococcal infection through military camps and to establish that adequate and timely treatment of streptococcal pharyngitis prevents rheumatic fever.[5] Based on these studies, it was determined that treatment of streptococcal pharyngitis begun as late as 9 days after onset will prevent rheumatic fever. It was recommended that group A streptococcal infection be treated for a full 10 days (Table 6).

The practical question is the management of pharyngitis in modern-day pediatric practice. Surely, children with febrile sore throats should have throat cultures, and if these are positive for hemolytic streptococci, antibiotic therapy should be continued for 10 days, even in this era of declining rheumatic fever in the U.S.[10,42]

Where there is organized throat culturing and central reporting of beta-hemolytic streptococcal recovery, community physicians respond to this information, resulting in a reduction in the spread of streptococcal infection and elimination of rheumatic fever.[37] Even more rapid methods of streptococcal identification based on examination of throat swabs may prove superior.

The possibility that a streptococcal vaccine might prevent rheumatic fever is a natural thought, but there is concern that such a vaccine based on streptococcal products might, in susceptible individuals, actually aggravate rather than prevent rheumatic fever. For this reason research in this area is expected to proceed with caution.

Secondary Prevention

A patient who has had acute rheumatic fever is susceptible to recurrent rheumatic fever for the rest of his life. **Once a rheumatic, always a rheumatic.** The likelihood of recurrence is greater the shorter the time interval since rheumatic activity, and when there has been valve damage. Recurrences are more common among children than adults, especially when there has already been a preceding recurrence.[30]

Table 6. Primary Prevention of Rheumatic Fever (Treatment of Streptococcal Tonsillopharyngitis)

Agent	Dose	Mode	Duration
Benzathine penicillin G	600,000 units for patients 60 lb 1,200,000 units for patients >60 lb	Intramuscular	Once
Penicillin V (phenoxymethylpenicillin)	250 mg 3 times daily	Oral	10 days
For individuals allergic to penicillin:			
Erythromycin estolate	20–40 mg/kg/day 2–4 times daily (maximum 1 g/day)	Oral	10 days
	or		
Ethylsuccinate	40 mg/kg/day 2–4 times daily (maximum 1 g/day)	Oral	10 days

The following agents are acceptable but usually not recommended: amoxicillin, dicloxacillin, oral cephalosporins, and clindamycin.

The following are not acceptable: sulfonamides, trimethoprim, tetracyclines, and chloramphenicol.

From Dajani AS, Bisno AL, Chung KJ, et al: Prevention of rheumatic fever. Circulation 78:1082–1086, 1988, by permission of the American Heart Association, Inc.

Table 7. Secondary Prevention of Rheumatic Fever (Prevention of Recurrent Attacks)

Agent	Dose	Mode
Benzathine penicillin G	1,200,000 units	Intramuscularly every 4 weeks*
	or	
Penicillin V	250 mg twice daily	Oral
	or	
Sulfadiazine	0.5 g once daily for patients 60 lb 1.0 g once daily for patients >60 lb	Oral

For individuals allergic to penicillin and sulfadiazine:

Erythromycin	250 mg twice daily	Oral

From Dajani AS, Bisno AL, Chung KJ et al: Prevention of rheumatic fever. Circulation 78:1082–1086, 1988, by permission of the American Heart Association, Inc.

*In high-risk situations, administration every 3 weeks is advised.

Although oral penicillin V (250 mg) administered twice each day will prevent secondary attacks of rheumatic fever, compliance with this routine is often less than optimum. For more reliable coverage the use of benzathine penicillin G (1,200,000 units intramuscularly every 4 weeks) is more dependable, although more painful (Table 7). Some problems with oral penicillin have been traced to mouth organisms that produce penicillinase, but most are a result of forgetfulness or active rebellion.

Any patient who has had a known attack of rheumatic fever should be followed for at least 5 years (the time of greatest recurrence), and those with valvar damage should be followed indefinitely. When following these patients, it is useful to record the antistreptolysin-O titer, as well as the sedimentation rate, to serve as a baseline if subsequent concern about rheumatic activity arises.

REFERENCES

1. Bhattacharya S, Reddy KS, Sundaram KR, et al: Differentiation of patients with rheumatic fever from those with inactive rheumatic heart disease using the artificial subcutaneous nodule test, myocardial reactive antibodies, serum immunoglobulin and serum complement levels. Int J Cardiol 14:71–78, 1987.
2. Bisno AL, Shulman ST, and Dajani AS: The rise and fall (and rise?) of rheumatic fever. JAMA 259:728–729, 1988.
3. Bland EF: The way it was. Circulation 76:1190–1195, 1987.
4. Bland EF and Jones TD: Rheumatic fever and rheumatic heart disease. A twenty-year report on 1000 patients followed since childhood. Circulation 4:836–843, 1951.
5. Catanzaro FJ, Stetson CA, Morris AJ, et al.: The role of the streptococcus in the pathogenesis of rheumatic fever. Am J Med 17:749–756, 1954.
6. Cheadle WB: Harveian Lectures on the various manifestations of the rheumatic state as exemplified in childhood and early life. Lancet 1:821–827, 871–877, 921–927, 1889.
7. Chun LT, Reddy V, and Yamamoto LG: Rheumatic fever in children and adolescents in Hawaii. Pediatrics 79:549–552, 1987.
8. Congeni B, Rizzo C, Congeni J, et al: Outbreak of acute rheumatic fever in northeast Ohio. J Pediatr 111:176–179, 1987.
9. Coulehan J, Grant S, Reisinger K, et al: Acute rheumatic fever and rheumatic heart disease on the Navajo reservation, 1962–1977. Pub Health Rep 95:62–68, 1980.
10. Dajani AS, Bisno AL, Chung KJ, et al: Prevention of rheumatic fever. A statement for health professionals by the committee on rheumatic fever, endocarditis, and Kawasaki disease of The Council on Cardiovascular Disease in the Young, the American Heart Association. Circulation 78:1082–1086, 1988.
11. Denny FW: T Duckett Jones and rheumatic fever in 1986. T Duckett Jones memorial lecture. Circulation 76:963–970, 1987.
12. DiSciascio G, and Taranta A: Rheumatic fever in children. Am Heart J 99:635–655, 1980.
13. Editorial: Decline in rheumatic fever. Lancet 2:647–648, 1985.
14. Gordis L: The virtual disappearance of rheumatic fever in the United States: lessons in the rise and fall of disease. Circulation 72:1155–1162, 1985.
15. Gray ED, Regelmann WE, Abdin Z, et al: Compartmentalization of cells bearing "rheumatic" cell surface antigens in peripheral blood and tonsils in rheumatic heart disease. J Infect Dis 155:247–252, 1987.
16. Hosier DM, Craenen JM, Teske DW, et al: Resurgence of acute rheumatic fever. Am J Dis Child 141:730–733, 1987.
17. Husby G, van de Rijn I, Zabriskie JB, et al: Antibodies reacting with cytoplasm of subthalamic and caudate nuclei neurons in chorea and acute rheumatic fever. J Exp Med 144:1094–1110, 1976.
18. Jones TD: The diagnosis of rheumatic fever. JAMA 126:481–484, 1944.
19. Jones TD, White PD, Roche CF, et al: The transportation of rheumatic fever patients to a subtropical climate. JAMA 109:1308–1310, 1937.
20. Kaplan EL: Acute rheumatic fever. Symposium on Pediatric Cardiology. Pediatr Clin North Am 25.4:817–829, 1978.
21. Kaplan EL, Hill HR: Return of rheumatic fever: consequences, implications, and needs. J Pediatr 111:244–246, 1987.
22. Kaplan EL, Anthony BF, Chapman SS, et al: The influence of the site of infection on the immune response to group A streptococci. J Clin Invest 49:1405–1414, 1970.
23. Kaplan MH, Craig JM: Immnologic studies of heart tissue: VI. Cardiac lesions in rabbits associated with autoantibodies to heart induced by immunization with heterologous heart. J Immunol 90:725–733, 1963.
24. Kaplan MH, Suchy ML: Immunologic relation of streptococcal and tissue antigens. II. Cross-reaction of antisera to mammalian heart tissue with a cell wall constitutent of certain strains of group A streptococci. J Exp Med 119:643–650, 1964.
25. Kaplan MH, and Svec KH: Immunologic relation of streptococcal and tissue antigens. III. Presence in human sera of streptococcal antibody cross-reactive with heart tissue. Association with streptococcal infection,

rheumatic fever, and glomerulonephritis. J Exp Med 119:651–666, 1964.

26. Kaplan MH, Meyeserian M, Kushner I: Immunologic studies of heart tissue. IV. Serologic reactions with human heart tissue as revealed by immunofluorescent methods: isoimmune, Wassermann and autoimmune reactions. J Exp Med 113:17–36, 1961.

27. Lahiri K, Rane HS, Desai AG: Clinical profile of rheumatic fever: A study of 168 cases. J Trop Pediatr 31:273–275, 1985.

28. Lembo NJ, Dellitalia LJ, Crawford MH, et al: Mitral valve prolapse in patients with prior rheumatic fever. Circulation 77:830–836, 1988.

29. Markowitz M, Gordis L: Rheumatic Fever, 2nd ed. Philadelphia, W.B. Saunders, 1972.

30. Markowitz M: The decline of rheumatic fever: role of medical intervention. J Pediatr 106:545–550, 1985.

31. Massell BF: Studies on the use of prontylin in rheumatic fever. N Engl J Med 216:487, 1937.

32. Massell BF, Fyler DC, Roy SB: The clinical picture of rheumatic fever: diagnosis, immediate prognosis, course and therapeutic implications. Am J Cardiol 1:436–449, 1958.

33. Massell BF, Chute CG, Walker AM, et al: Penicillin and the marked decrease in morbidity and mortality from rheumatic fever in the United States. N Engl J Med 318:280–286, 1988.

34. Mische SM, Manjula BN, Fischetti VA: Relation of streptococcal M protein with human and rabbit tropomyosin the complete amino acid sequence of human cardiac alpha tropomyosin, a highly conserved contractile protein. Biochem Biophys Res Commun 142:813–818, 1987.

35. Neutze JM: The third international conference on rheumatic fever and rheumatic heart disease: Rheumatic fever and rheumatic heart disease in the western Pacific region. N Z Med J 101:404–406, 1988.

36. Patarroyo ME, Winchester RJ, Vejerano A, et al: Association of B-cell alloantigen with susceptibility to rheumatic fever. Nature 278:173–174, 1979.

37. Phibbs B, Taylor J, and Zimmerman RA: A community-wide streptococcal control project. The Natrona County Primary Prevention Program, Casper, Wyoming. JAMA 214:2018–2024, 1970.

38. Rajapakse CNA, Halim K, Al-Orainey I, et al: A genetic marker for rheumatic heart disease. Br Heart J 58:659–662, 1987.

39. Rammelkamp CH Jr, Stolzer BL: The latent period before the onset of acute rheumatic fever. Yale J Biol Med 34:386–398, 1961.

40. Rammelkamp CH, Wannamaker LW, Denny FW: The epidemiology and prevention of rheumatic fever. Bull NY Acad Med 28:321–334, 1952.

41. Sanyal SK, Berry AM, Duggal S, et al: Sequelae of the initial attack of acute rheumatic fever in children from North India: a prospective 5-year follow-up study. Circulation 65:375–379, 1982.

42. Shulman ST (ed): Pharyngitis: Management in an Era of Declining Rheumatic Fever. New York, Praeger, 1984.

43. Stanhope JM: New Zealand trends in rheumatic fever, 1885–1971. N Z Med J 82:297–299, 1975.

44. Stollerman GH, Markowitz M, Taranta A, et al: Jones criteria (revised) for guidance in diagnosis of rheumatic fever. Circulation 32:664–668, 1965.

45. Thomas WA, Averill JH, Castleman B, et al: The significance of Aschoff bodies in the left atrial appendage: a comparison of 40 biopsies removed during mitral commissurotomy with autopsy material from 40 patients dying from rheumatic fever. N Engl J Med 249:761–765, 1983.

46. Tolaymat A, Goudarzi T, Soler GP, et al: Acute rheumatic fever in north Florida. South Med J 77:819–823, 1984.

47. Tomaru T, Uchida Y, Mohri N, et al: Post inflammatory mitral and aortic valve prolapse: a clinical and pathological study. Circulation 76:68–76, 1987.

48. United Kingdom and U.S. Joint Report on Rheumatic Fever: The treatment of acute rheumatic fever in children: a cooperative clinical trial of ACTH, cortisone and aspirin. Circulation 11:343–377, 1955.

49. United Kingdom and U.S. Joint Report on Rheumatic Fever: The evolution of rheumatic heart disease in children: five-year report of a cooperative clinical trial of ACTH, cortisone and aspirin. Circulation 22:503–515, 1960.

50. United Kingdom and U.S. Joint Report on Rheumatic Heart Disease: The natural history of rheumatic fever and rheumatic heart disease: ten-year report of a cooperative clinical trial of ACTH, cortisone and aspirin. Circulation 32:457–476, 1965.

51. Veasy LG, Wiedmeier SE, Orsmond GS, et al: Resurgence of acute rheumatic fever in the intermountain area of the United States. N Engl J Med 316:421–427, 1987.

52. Wald ER, Dashefsky B, Feidt C, et al.: Acute rheumatic fever in western Pennsylvania and the tristate area. Pediatrics 80:371–374, 1987.

53. Wannamaker LW: The chain that links the heart to the throat. Circulation 48:9–18, 1973.

54. Zabriskie JB: Rheumatic fever: a streptococcal-induced autoimmune disease? Pediatr Annu 11:383–396, 1982.

55. Zabriskie JB: Rheumatic fever: the interplay between host, genetics, and microbe. Circulation 71:1077–1086, 1985.

Chapter 23

KAWASAKI SYNDROME

Jane W. Newburger, M.D., M.P.H.

DEFINITION

Kawasaki syndrome is a disease of unknown etiology marked by acute vasculitis that occurs predominantly in infancy and early childhood. It is characterized by fever, bilateral nonexudative conjunctivitis, erythema of the lips and oral mucosa, changes in the extremities, rash, and cervical lymphadenopathy. Coronary artery aneurysms or ectasia develop in approximately 15–25% of children with the disease and may lead to myocardial infarction, sudden death, or chronic coronary artery insufficiency.[28,29,69] In the United States, Kawasaki syndrome is a leading cause of acquired heart disease in children.

PREVALENCE

First described in Japan in 1967, Kawasaki syndrome is now known to occur in both endemic and community-wide epidemic forms in North America, Europe, and Asia, in children of all races,[30,47] but is markedly more prevalent in Japan and in children of Japanese ancestry.[49] The cumulative number of documented cases of Kawasaki syndrome reported in Japan by the end of 1984 was greater than 60,000.[77] In the United States, an increase in the number of new cases reported to the Centers for Disease Control between 1981 and 1985 suggested a rising incidence rate.[58] In the United States prevalence is highest among Orientals, is intermediate in Blacks, and is lowest in Caucasians.[58] Sporadic cases and community-wide epidemics have been reported in widely distant parts of the United States, with outbreaks most common in the late winter and spring. In recent outbreaks in Boston and in Rochester, New York, the incidence of Kawasaki syndrome in children under the age of 5 years rose from 1.6 and 5.6 per 100,000 per year, respectively, to 66 and 179 per 100,000 per year in the three- to four-month epidemic periods.[3] The minimum annual incidence in Asian-American children less than 5 years old has

been estimated as 24.4/100,000, a significantly greater rate than for other racial groups.[65] Kawasaki syndrome occurs overwhelmingly in young children, with its peak incidence occurring in infants 1 to 2 years of age and with 85% of the cases occurring in children less than 5 years old. The male-to-female ratio of cases is approximately 1.5:1. Children with this syndrome belong to families of higher socioeconomic status than would be expected, based on community census data. In Japan, its recurrence rate has been reported to be 3.9% and the proportion of sibling cases, 1.4%.[77]

ETIOLOGY AND PATHOGENESIS

The cause of Kawasaki syndrome is unknown. Antecedent viral infections of the upper respiratory tract and exposure to freshly cleaned carpets have been associated with the disease.[58,59] Immunoregulatory abnormalities may contribute to its pathogenesis. During the acute phase, there is a marked deficiency of suppressor T-cells, helper T-cells become activated, and there are increased numbers of B-cells spontaneously secreting IgG and IgM antibodies.[39] Recent investigations have explored the possibility that this high level of immune activation could be associated with endothelial damage. Recently, it was demonstrated that IgM antibodies in the sera of children with acute Kawasaki syndrome cause complement-mediated killing of gamma interferon–treated, cultured, human vascular endothelial cells.[41] In addition, IgG and IgM antibodies in sera from patients with acute disease have been reported to cause lysis of cultured human vascular endothelial cells stimulated with interleukin-1 or tumor necrosis factor.[42] These observations suggest that mediator secretion by activated T-cells and macrophages could promote vascular injury in Kawasaki syndrome.

PATHOLOGY

The mortality in cases of Kawasaki syndrome is approximately 0.3%, with virtually all deaths occurring secondary to the cardiac sequelae of this disease.[18] The first week of the illness is characterized by acute perivasculitis and vasculitis of the microvessels and small arteries and by acute perivasculitis and endarteritis of the three major coronary arteries. Pericarditis, myocarditis, inflammation of the atrioventricular conduction system, and endocarditis with valvulitis may be present. During this early period, death may be caused by arrhythmia or myocarditis. Not until the second or third week is panvasculitis of the coronary arteries and aneurysm formation with thrombosis found. In cases seen at autopsy approximately 1 month after onset of the illness, granulation of the coronary arteries and disappearance of inflammation in the microvessels are seen. Severe stenosis of the major coronary arteries often is evident in late death. The causes of sudden death are myocarditis and arrhythmia in stage I; ischemic heart disease, rupture of aneurysms and myocarditis, including lesions of the conduction system, in stage II; and ischemic heart disease in stages III and IV. The peak mortality occurs 15–45 days after the onset of fever, during which time well-established coronary vasculitis occurs concomitantly with marked elevation of the platelet count and a hypercoagulable state. However, sudden death from myocardial infarction may occur many years later in children with aneurysms and stenoses of the coronary artery. Deaths occurring later than 1 month after onset of the illness are almost always secondary to coronary artery aneurysms or stenosis and consequent ischemic heart disease. Although at autopsy the coronary arteries are virtually always involved, Kawasaki syndrome consists of a generalized systemic vasculitis involving all small and medium-sized blood vessels. Aneurysms are reported in the femoral, iliac, renal, axillary, and brachial arteries.

CLINICAL MANIFESTATIONS

By definition of the Centers for Disease Control,[47] the child with Kawasaki syndrome must have fever lasting 5 or more days without other reasonable explanation and satisfy at least four of the following five criteria: (1) bilateral conjunctival injection; (2) at least one of the following mucous membrane changes: injected or fissured lips, injected pharynx, or "strawberry tongue"; (3) at least one of the following extremity changes: erythema of the palms or soles, edema of the hands or feet, or periungual desquamation; (4) polymorphous exanthem that is rarely vesicular or bullous and is often accentuated in the perineum, where it may be associated with local desquamation; and (5) acute nonsuppurative cervical lymphadenopathy (at least one node 1.5 cm or larger in diameter). Conjunctival hyperemia associated with anterior uveitis can be identified by slit-lamp examination

in approximately 83% of patients examined within the first week of illness.[5] The slit-lamp examination may be extremely useful in differentiating Kawasaki syndrome from other pediatric illnesses characterized by fever, rash and conjunctivitis.

In addition to these principal symptoms, many other significant symptoms and signs frequently are present in children with Kawasaki syndrome. Arthralgia and arthritis occur in approximately one-third of patients.[46,58] Arthritis of the small joints usually occurs early in the acute phase, and involvement of large weight-bearing joints becomes manifest in the second and third week of the illness. Urethritis associated with sterile pyuria is recognized by the presence of white cells on microscopic urinalysis. Because the white cells are mononuclear rather than polymorphonuclear, the dipstick test for myeloperoxidase activity (i.e., white blood cell enzyme) will be negative. Aseptic meningitis usually is associated with a mild mononuclear pleocytosis in the cerebrospinal fluid and with normal glucose and protein. Hydrops of the gallbladder may be present, with or without obstructive jaundice.[67,68] Diarrhea, vomiting, and abdominal pain may also be presenting symptoms.

The conventional diagnostic criteria should be viewed as guidelines that are particularly useful in preventing overdiagnosis but they may result in failure to recognize incomplete forms of the illness. Signs and symptoms of Kawasaki syndrome may be particularly subtle or absent in infants less than 6 months of age,[6] the subgroup at highest risk for coronary lesions. The reported occurrence of coronary artery involvement among children with incomplete criteria[11,62,64] suggests that echocardiography should be performed in all children with prolonged unexplained fever and some signs of Kawasaki syndrome, especially if associated with subsequent peripheral desquamation or if the child is younger than 6 months.

Tachycardia and gallop rhythm are more prominent than would be expected from the degree of fever and anemia. These findings are thought to be secondary to myocarditis, a universal feature of early Kawasaki syndrome.[18,79] The severity of myocarditis does not appear to be associated with the risk of coronary artery aneurysm.[1,23]

Pericardial effusion may develop toward the latter part of the acute phase and is secondary to myopericarditis; it only rarely progresses to tamponade, and resolves spontaneously in most instances.

Minimal aortic regurgitation and mitral regurgitation can be documented in a small number of patients. Usually these are transient findings in the acute stage, though late onset has been reported.[21,22,52]

Congestive heart failure may occur secondary to myocarditis in the acute phase. During the subacute stage, congestive heart failure usually is caused by myocardial dysfunction secondary to ischemia or infarction, with or without valvar regurgitation.

Coronary artery ectasia or aneurysms occur in 15–25% of children with Kawasaki syndrome.[28,29,69] Echocardiography may reveal dilatation of the coronary arteries, beginning 7 days after the first appearance of fever, usually peaking 3 or 4 weeks after onset of the illness. Several scoring systems have been developed to identify children at highest risk for formation of coronary artery abnormalities.[9,50] Other reported risk factors include male gender, age under 1 year, hemoglobin less than 10 gm/dl, a white cell count greater than 30,000/mm³, an erythrocyte sedimentation rate greater than 101 mm/hr (Westergren), elevated C-reactive protein, and persistence of elevation of C-reactive protein or sedimentation abnormality for more than 30 days. The duration of fever, presumably reflecting the severity of ongoing vasculitis, has been confirmed as a powerful predictor of coronary artery aneurysms in other studies.[13,25,34] During the first week of the illness children who will develop aneurysms cannot be clearly distinguished from those who will remain unaffected.

Laboratory Data

Laboratory findings in the acute stage of Kawasaki syndrome include a high leukocyte count with a left shift. A normocytic, normochromic anemia is present early and persists until the inflammatory process begins to subside.[46] Increased platelet turnover occurs, together with marked hypercoagulability in the acute phase.[4] Thrombocytosis peaks typically in the third or fourth week after onset of the fever. Elevation of liver transaminases, usually two- to threefold, is common in the acute phase, usually with a cholestatic profile of elevated bilirubin and alkaline phosphatase. Early in the disease, increases in acute phase reactants and erythrocyte sedimentation rate are characteristic. Indeed, elevation of the latter typically persists after resolution of the fever, a feature that may help to distinguish Kawasaki syndrome from common viral illnesses.

Electrocardiography

The electrocardiogram in acute Kawasaki syndrome may show mild abnormalities consistent with myocarditis, most commonly a prolonged P-R interval and nonspecific changes in the S-T segment and T waves.

Chest X-ray

The x-ray findings are nonspecific.

Echocardiography

Echocardiographic examination should be performed in the first, second, and third to fourth weeks of the disease. Additional examinations may be necessary in some patients who have persistent fever or abnormalities on earlier examination. Uncooperative young patients should be sedated to obtain optimal visualization of the coronary arteries. Views of the right, the left main, the left anterior descending, and circumflex coronary arteries should be obtained, together with Doppler interrogation of the mitral and aortic valve and quantitative assessment of left ventricular function.

The caliber of the coronary artery in normal children varies.[2] However, the following simple working definition, proposed by the Japanese Ministry of Health,[31] should correctly categorize most vessels. A coronary artery with a lumen at least 3 mm in diameter (measured inside to inside) in a child less than 5 years of age, or 4 mm in a child at least 5 years old, is considered abnormal. Additionally, if the internal diameter of a segment measures at least 1.5 times that of an adjacent segment, that segment is considered abnormal. Also, a coronary artery whose lumen is clearly irregular is classified as abnormal even if its greatest internal diameter is less than 3 mm.

Cardiac Catheterization

Selective coronary arteriography provides definitive delineation of coronary artery anatomy (Fig. 1). Because of the potential morbidity and mortality associated with angiography, it is performed only in patients with persistent echocardiographic evidence of aneurysms. Using a percutaneous femoral approach, right and left heart studies are performed. Then selective coronary angiograms (using specially formed 4.5-French pediatric coronary artery catheters) are obtained in at least two projections for each coronary artery. Large volume injections of nonionic contrast (up to 0.5 cc/kg) may be necessary to obtain the best images.

Coronary artery aneurysms imaged at angiography are classified as either localized or extensive.[31,71] Localized aneurysms, confined to one arterial segment, are further classified as either fusiform (spindle-shaped) or saccular (showing abrupt transition from the normal to the dilated state, e.g., spherical, dumbbell-shaped, triangular, or sack-like). Extensive aneurysms involve more than one segment and may be either ectatic (uniformly dilated) or segmented (having multiple dilated segments joined by normal or stenotic segments). Coronary aneurysms that appear early in Kawasaki syndrome usually occur in the proximal segments of the major coronary vessels;[29] aneurysms that occur distally are almost always associated with proximal coronary abnormalities. Aneurysms may occur also in arteries outside the coronary system, most commonly the subclavian, brachial, axillary, iliac, or femoral vessels, and oc-

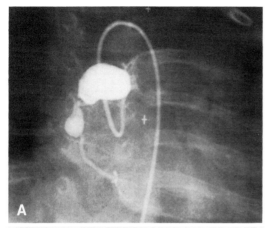

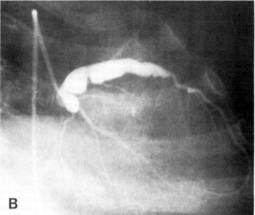

Figure 1. **A,** Selective right coronary arteriogram in the right anterior oblique projection demonstrating a segmented giant aneurysm of the right coronary artery. **B,** Selective left coronary arteriogram in the right anterior oblique projection demonstrating a fusiform aneurysm of the left anterior descending coronary, with the irregular inferior border of the most distal segment resulting from thrombus formation. There is also a saccular aneurysm of the proximal circumflex artery.

casionally in the abdominal aorta and renal arteries.[69] For this reason, abdominal aortography and subclavian arteriography often are performed in patients undergoing coronary arteriography for Kawasaki syndrome.

MANAGEMENT

Salicylates

Conventional therapy for Kawasaki syndrome includes aspirin as an anti-inflammatory and antithrombotic agent. The ideal regimen of aspirin is controversial and inadequately studied.[13,25,35,36,38,78] At Children's Hospital in Boston, children in the acute phase of Kawasaki syndrome are usually treated with 80–100 mg of aspirin per kilogram per day, divided into four doses, for its antipyretic and

anti-inflammatory effects, monitoring the serum aspirin level only to exclude toxicity. As soon as possible after defervescence, the aspirin dose is lowered to 3–5 mg/kg/day as a single dose to optimize its antiplatelet effect. If painful arthritis develops, aspirin may be maintained at the anti-inflammatory dosage. Salicylate therapy has never been proved in a prospective therapeutic trial to reduce the prevalence of aneurysms.

Intravenous Gamma Globulin

High doses of gamma globulin administered intravenously have been demonstrated to be safe and effective in reducing the incidence of coronary artery abnormalities when given early in the course of Kawasaki syndrome.[19,20,48,56] The prevalence of coronary artery abnormalities among children treated with high doses of intravenous gamma globulin and aspirin compared with that in children treated with aspirin alone is reduced by approximately threefold at 2 weeks and by fivefold at 7 weeks after diagnosis and initiation of therapy. Furthermore, intravenous gamma globulin reduces the incidence of giant aneurysms, the most serious form of coronary abnormality caused by the disease.[61]

Abnormalities of left ventricular systolic function and contractility improve more rapidly in children treated in the acute phase with high doses of intravenous gamma globulin, together with aspirin, than in those treated with aspirin alone.[55] The effect of gamma globulin on myocardial mechanics is especially interesting because few therapeutic agents have been shown to reverse rapidly the ventricular dysfunction associated with myocarditis due to other causes.

Finally, high doses of intravenous gamma globulin reduce fever and laboratory indicators of the acute-phase response.[56] The mechanism by which gamma globulin ameliorates the vasculitis of Kawasaki syndrome is unknown. Children treated with gamma globulin had a significant reduction in circulating activated T-cells and in the number of antibody-producing B-cells compared with children treated with aspirin alone.[40] These data suggest that gamma globulin works, in part, by blocking immune activation.

Antithrombotic Therapy

Paradoxically, the risk of coronary artery thrombosis is greatest after the acute phase subsides, when well-established coronary vasculitis occurs concomitantly with marked elevation of the platelet count and a hypercoagulable state. Low doses of aspirin (3–5 mg/kg/day, given as a single dose) are the mainstay of antithrombotic therapy in Kawasaki disease. Dipyridamole (3–6 mg/kg/day, in three divided doses) may be substituted for aspirin when salicylates are contraindicated (e.g., in the event of chickenpox or influenza). For children without evidence of coronary artery ectasia or aneurysms, antiplatelet therapy is usually discontinued approximately 2 months after onset of the illness.

Children with coronary artery abnormalities require long-term antithrombotic therapy, usually with low doses of aspirin. Sometimes dipyridamole is added to aspirin therapy, although its value when added to aspirin is controversial.[14] The risk of coronary thrombosis and myocardial infarction is especially great in children who show a rapid increase in coronary size or who have giant aneurysms during the subacute phase.[15,51,75] During this period some investigators advocate treatment with heparin, together with an antiplatelet agent.[51] For chronic antithrombotic therapy, options include antiplatelet therapy with aspirin (with or without dipyridamole), anticoagulant therapy with warfarin, or a combination of anticoagulant and antiplatelet therapy (usually warfarin with dipyridamole or sulfinpyrazone). No prospective data exist to guide the clinician in choosing an optimal regimen; the regimen that is currently most popular is that of aspirin with dipyridamole because of its safety and ease of administration.

Thrombolytic Therapy

Despite the use of antithrombotic agents, myocardial infarction, secondary to thrombotic occlusion of coronary aneurysms, may develop in some children, especially those with giant aneurysms. In others, the presence of a coronary artery thrombus may be detected on serial 2-D echocardiography (Fig. 2). Treatment with thrombolytic agents, mainly urokinase and streptokinase, either intravenous or intracoronary, has been used with variable success.[7,27,76] Thrombolytic therapy for coronary artery thrombosis is most effective if begun within 3–4 hours of the onset of symptoms.[43] Following clot lysis, heparin, together with aspirin, followed by a long-term oral antithrombotic regimen (e.g., aspirin and dipyridamole or warfarin and dipyridamole), is recommended after successful reperfusion of coronary occlusion, but the ideal long-term antithrombotic regimen has not been established.[27,44]

Surgical Management

Surgical management of the Kawasaki syndrome consists primarily of bypass grafts for obstructive lesions of the coronary artery,[24,26,32,33,57,70,72] although mitral valvuloplasty or mitral valve replacement is necessary occasionally in children with papillary muscle dysfunction or valvulitis. A coronary bypass graft should be considered when stenosis has been demonstrated to be progressive, when the myocardium to be perfused through the graft is still viable, and when no appreciable lesions

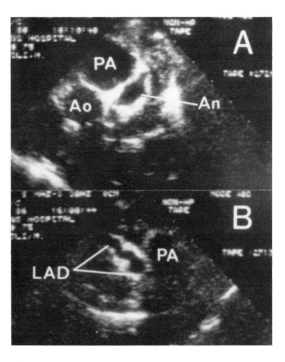

Figure 2. **A**, Echocardiogram in a short-axis parasternal view showing a fusiform aneurysm (An) of the proximal left anterior descending coronary artery. **B**, Parasternal long-axis view, angled to the left, showing a dilated and tortuous left anterior descending coronary artery (LAD). Pa, pulmonary artery; Ao, aorta. (From Newburger JW, Takahashi M, Burns JC, et al: The treatment of Kawasaki syndrome with intravenous gamma globulin. N Engl J Med 315:341–347, 1986, with permission.)

are present in the artery peripheral to the planned graft site. When these conditions are satisfied, Suzuki and associates[70] propose that coronary bypass grafts be considered for patients in whom more than one of the following four arteriographic findings are observed:

1. Stenosis of the left main coronary artery has progressed to critical severity.

2. Occlusions are present in two or more vessels.

3. Collateral vessels of an occluded coronary artery arise from the peripheral portion with progressive localized stenosis.

4. Segmental stenosis or critical localized stenosis in the right coronary artery occurs together with progressive localized stenosis in the left anterior descending coronary artery.

Isolated stenotic lesions in the proximal left anterior descending artery or in the right coronary artery are not considered to be an indication for bypass grafting.

Recently Kitamura and colleagues[33] reported improved results with the use of internal mammary artery grafts in pediatric patients. In a series of 9 patients, the internal mammary artery was used for 12 coronary arteries (most frequently for the left anterior descending coronary) with bilateral internal mammary grafts placed in 3 patients. In comparison, 10 autologous saphenous vein grafts were used for 10 coronary arteries. The early (within 1 month) and later patency rates for the saphenous vein grafts were 84% and 68% respectively, compared with early and late patency rates for the internal mammary artery grafts of 100% each. Furthermore, the diameter and length of the internal mammary grafts increased with the general somatic growth of the children, whereas the saphenous vein grafts tended to shorten somewhat over time. After surgery, on exercise, patients showed improvement in the electrocardiogram, in thallium-20 myocardial scans, and in the response of stroke volume to the increase in end-diastolic pressure. Greater patient accrual and further follow-up are necessary to assess the long-term results of coronary bypass surgery for obstructive lesions associated with Kawasaki syndrome.

Other Considerations

Children who have had Kawasaki syndrome, especially those with active or regressed coronary lesions, should be monitored and treated aggressively for other risk factors pertaining to adult atherosclerotic vascular disease (e.g., hyperlipidemia or hypertension).

COURSE

Regression and Evolution of Coronary Artery Lesions

The arterial lesions of Kawasaki syndrome gradually transform with the passage of time, sometimes with apparent partial or total regression of aneurysms and sometimes with the development of stenosis or occlusions.[8] Therefore, coronary angiography should be repeated at intervals of 1–5 years in some patients with multiple severe coronary lesions, especially in those for whom future surgical management is contemplated. Angiograms have shown resolution of aneurysms 1–2 years after onset of the disease in approximately one-half to two-thirds of coronary arteries.[29,71] The likelihood of resolution of the aneurysm appears to be determined in large measure by its initial size, with smaller aneurysms having a greater likelihood of regression.[15,53] Other factors positively associated with regression of aneurysms include age less than 1 year, saccular (rather than fusiform) aneurysm morphology, and location of the aneurysm in a distal coronary segment.[71] Vessels that do not undergo resolution of abnormalities may show persistence of aneurysmal morphology, development of stenosis or occlusion, or abnormal tortuosity. Although the size of the aneurysm tends to diminish over time, stenotic lesions secondary to marked myointimal proliferation frequently are progressive.[69]

Children with so-called giant aneurysms (i.e., those with a maximum diameter greater than 8 mm) have the worst prognosis. Few of these aneurysms regress and most progress to stenosis or obstruction, usually within 1–3 years.[53,74,75] Patients with giant aneurysms are at highest risk for myocardial infarction, and nearly all late deaths from Kawasaki syndrome occur in this subgroup.[16,51]

Myocardial Infarction

Myocardial infarction caused by thrombotic occlusion in an aneurysmal and/or stenotic coronary artery is the principal cause of death in Kawasaki syndrome. Among 195 patients with myocardial infarction 142 (72.8%) suffered infarction in the first year after onset of the disease; 77 of these had a myocardial infarction within 3 months of onset.[28]

Mortality from the first myocardial infarction was 22%. Most fatal attacks were associated with obstruction either in the left main coronary artery or in both the right main and left anterior descending coronary arteries. In survivors, obstruction frequently was present in a single vessel, most commonly in the right coronary artery.

The clinical course after myocardial infarction is variable, and these children may have a greater capacity for recovery of myocardial function than adults, a phenomenon noted in children with myocardial infarction secondary to anomalous origin of the left coronary artery from the pulmonary trunk[60] and to surgical complications of the arterial switch procedure in transposition of the great arteries.[12] Of 152 survivors of a first myocardial infarction, 16% had a second myocardial infarction, with a mortality of 62.5%. A third attack occurred in 6 of the 9 survivors, with only 1 patient surviving.[28]

Patients with Spontaneous Regression of Aneurysm

Angiography indicates that resolution of aneurysms may occur by marked myointimal proliferation or by organization of thrombus.[17,18,63,73] Healed axillary aneurysms have been reported to exhibit histologic characteristics similar to those seen in early atherosclerosis.[63] Pathologic examination of coronary artery aneurysms that have regressed reveal fibrous intimal thickening despite normal artery diameter. The histologic abnormalities in arteries with aneurysm regression have raised concerns that such segments may be predisposed to accelerated atherosclerosis.[63,71,73] Furthermore, coronary artery segments in which aneurysms have regressed also show abnormalities in vascular reactivity.[37,45,66]

Course after Kawasaki Syndrome without Detectable Coronary Lesions

Myocardial Function. The universal presence of myocarditis and the frequent documentation of diminished left ventricular function and contractility during the acute phase of Kawasaki syndrome form the basis for concern about long-term effects on myocardial function. Biopsies of the right ventricular myocardium have shown histologic abnormalities, including fibrosis and disarrangement, abnormal branching, and hypertrophy of myocytes, which can be detected from 2 months to 11 years after onset of the disease; their severity was unrelated to the presence of coronary artery abnormalities.[73] Thus, the histologic sequelae of myocarditis appear to persist.

The occurrence of late abnormalities of left ventricular function among children without coronary artery lesions has been controversial. In several studies[10,23] resolution of left ventricular dysfunction was noted within 2 months of onset of the disease, whereas long-term abnormalities of both left ventricular size and of systolic and early diastolic function have been described by others. In the author's experience, early abnormalities of left ventricular contractility and myocardial function generally resolve within 1–3 years.[55] Assessment of the full impact of the Kawasaki syndrome on heart function must await the follow-up of these children into adulthood.

Valvar Regurgitation. Delayed dysfunction of the mitral and aortic valves, unrelated to myocardial ischemia, has been reported as a rare complication of Kawasaki syndrome.[21,22] At Children's Hospital in Boston, 2 children (among 178 patients with Kawasaki syndrome who are actively followed) have had delayed aortic valve regurgitation, neither having evidence of congenital malformation or of other causes for the regurgitation.

Coronary Artery Status. Data concerning the long-term status of the coronary arteries in children who never had demonstrable abnormalities are meager and inconclusive.[17,37,73] Generalized endothelial cell dysfunction has been suggested by late metabolic abnormalities, including altered lipid profiles,[54] which persist beyond clinical resolution of the disease. From the purely clinical perspective, children without known cardiac sequelae during the first month of Kawasaki syndrome appear to return to their previous, usually excellent, state of health, without signs or symptoms of cardiac impairment. At Children's Hospital in Boston such children are evaluated every 3–5 years after recovery from the acute illness. Meaningful knowledge about long-term coronary artery status in this population must await their careful surveillance over the coming decades.

REFERENCES

1. Anderson TM, Meyer RA, Kaplan S: Long-term echocardiographic evaluation of cardiac size and function in patients with Kawasaki disease. Am Heart J 110:107–115, 1985.
2. Arjunan K, Daniels SR, Meyer RA, et al: Coronary artery caliber in normal children and patients with Kawasaki disease but without aneurysms: an echocardiographic and angiographic study. J Coll Cardiol 8:1119–1124, 1986.
3. Bell DM, Brink EW, Nitzkin JL, et al: Kawasaki syndrome: description of two outbreaks in the United States. N Engl J Med 304:1568–1575, 1981.
4. Burns JC, Glode MP, Clarke SH, et al: Coagulopathy and platelet activation in Kawasaki syndrome: identification of patients at high risk for development of artery aneurysms. J Pediatr 105:206–211, 1984.
5. Burns JC, Joffe L, Sargent RA, et al: Anterior uveitis associated with Kawasaki syndrome. Pediatr Infect Dis J 4:258–261, 1985.
6. Burns JC, Wiggins JW Jr, Toews WH, et al: Clinical spectrum of Kawasaki disease in infants younger than 6 months of age. J Pediatr 109:381–384, 1986.
7. Burtt DM, Pollack P, Bianco JA: Intravenous streptokinase in an infant with Kawasaki's disease complicated by acute myocardial infarction. Pediatr Cardiol 6:307–311, 1986.
8. Butler DF, Hough DR, Friedman SJ, et al: Adult Kawasaki syndrome. Arch Dermatol 123:1356–1361, 1987.
9. Capannari TE, Daniels SR, Meyer RA, et al: Sensitivity, specificity and predictive value of two-dimensional echocardiography in detecting coronary artery aneurysm in patients with Kawasaki disease. J Am Coll Cardiol 7:355–360, 1986.
10. Chung KJ, Brandt L, Fulton DR, et al: Cardiac and coronary arterial involvement in infants and children from New England with mucocutaneous lymph node syndrome (Kawasaki disease). Angiocardiographic-echocardiographic correlations. Am J Cardiol 50:136–142, 1982.
11. Cloney DL, Teja K, Lohr JA: Fatal case of atypical Kawasaki syndrome. Pediatr Infect Dis J 6:297–299, 1987.
12. Colan SD: Personal communication.
13. Daniels SR, Specker B, Capannari TE, et al: Correlates of coronary artery aneurysm formation in patients with Kawasaki disease. Am J Dis Child 141:205–207, 1987.
14. Fitzgerald GA: Dipyridamole. N Engl J Med 316:1247–1257, 1987.
15. Fujiwara T, Fujiwara H, Hamashima Y: Size of coronary aneurysm as a determinant factor of the prognosis in Kawasaki disease: clinicopathologic study of coronary aneurysms. Prog Clin Biol Res 250:519–520, 1987.
16. Fujiwara T, Fujiwara H, Hamashima Y: Frequency and size of coronary arterial aneurysm at necropsy in Kawasaki disease. Am J Cardiol 59:808–811, 1987.
17. Fujiwara T, Fujiwara H, Nakano H: Pathological features of coronary arteries in children with Kawasaki disease in which coronary arterial aneurysm was absent at autopsy. Circulation 78:345–350, 1988.
18. Fujiwara H, Hamashima Y: Pathology of the heart in Kawasaki disease. Pediatrics 61:100–107, 1978.
19. Furusho K, Kamiya T, Nakano H, et al: High–dose intravenous gammaglobulin for Kawasaki disease. Lancet 2:1055–1058, 1984.
20. Furusho K, Kamiya T, Nakano H, et al: Japanese gammaglobulin trials for Kawasaki disease. Prog Clin Biol Res 250:425–432, 1987.

21. Gidding SS: Late onset valvular dysfunction in Kawasaki disease. Prog Clin Biol Res 250:305–309, 1987.

22. Gidding SS, Shulman ST, Ilbawi M, et al: Mucocutaneous lymph node syndrome (Kawasaki disease): delayed aortic and mitral insufficiency secondary to active valvulitis. J Am Coll Cardiol 7:894–897, 1986.

23. Hiraishi S, Yashiro K, Oguchi K, et al: Clinical course of cardiovascular involvement in the mucocutaneous lymph node syndrome: Relation between clincal signs of carditis and development of coronary arterial aneurysm. Am J Cardiol 47:323–330, 1981.

24. Hirose H, Kawashima Y, Nakano S, et al: Long-term results in surgical treatment of children 4 years old or younger with coronary involvement due to Kawasaki disease. Circulation 74:177–181, 1986.

25. Ichida F, Fatica NS, Engle MA, et al: Coronary artery involvement in Kawasaki syndrome in Manhattan, New York: risk factors and role of aspirin. Pediatrics 80:828–835, 1987.

26. Ino T, Iwahara M, Boku H, et al: Aortocoronary bypass surgery for Kawasaki disease. Pediatr Cardiol 8:195–197, 1987.

27. Kato H, Ichinose E, Inoue O, et al: Intracoronary thrombolytic therapy in Kawasaki disease: treatment and prevention of acute myocardial infarction. Prog Clin Biol Res 250:445–454, 1987.

28. Kato H, Ichinose E, Kawasaki T: Myocardial infarction in Kawasaki disease: clinical analyses in 195 cases. J Pediatr 108:923–927, 1986.

29. Kato H, Ichinose E, Yoshioka F, et al: Fate of coronary aneurysm in Kawasaki disease: serial coronary angiography and long-term follow-up study. Am J Cardiol 49:1758–1766, 1982.

30. Kawasaki T: Acute febrile mucocutaneous lymph node syndrome: clinical observations of 50 cases. Jpn Allergol 16:178, 1967.

31. Killip T, Fisher LD, Moch MB, (eds): National Heart, Lung and Blood Institute Coronary Artery Surgery Study (CASS). Circulation 63:I-1–I-81, 1981.

32. Kitamura S: Surgical treatment for coronary arterial lesions in Kawasaki disease. Prog Clin Biol Res 250:455–458, 1987.

33. Kitamura S, Kawachi K, Oyama C, et al: Kawasaki heart disease treated with an internal mammary artery graft in pediatric patients: a first successful report. J Thorac Cardiovasc Surg 89:860–866, 1985.

34. Koren G, MacLeod SM: Difficulty in achieving therapeutic serum concentrations of salicylate in Kawasaki disease. J Pediatr 105:991–995, 1984.

35. Koren G, Lavi S, Rose V, et al: Kawasaki disease: review of risk factors for coronary aneurysms. J Pediatr 108:388–392, 1986.

36. Koren G, Schaffer F, Silverman E, et al: Determinants of low serum concentration of salicylates in patients with Kawasaki disease. J Pediatr 112:663–667, 1988.

37. Kurisu Y, Azumi T, Sugahara T, et al: Variation in coronary arterial dimension (distensible abnormality) after disappearing aneurysm in Kawasaki disease. Am Heart J 114:532–538, 1987.

38. Kusakawa S, Tatara K: Efficacies and risks of aspirin in the treatment of Kawasaki disease. Prog Clin Biol Res 250:401–413, 1987.

39. Leung DY: Immunologic abnormalities in Kawasaki syndrome. Prog Clin Biol Res 250:159–165, 1987.

40. Leung DY, Burns JC, Newburger JW: Reversal of lymphocyte activation in vivo in the Kawasaki syndrome by intravenous gammaglobulin. J Clin Invest 79:468–472, 1987.

41. Leung DY, Collins T, Lapierre LA: Immunoglobulin M antibodies present in the acute phase of Kawasaki syndrome lyse cultured vascular endothelial cells stimulated by gamma interferon. J Clin Invest 77:1428–1435, 1986.

42. Leung DY, Geha RS, Newburger JW, et al: Two monokines, interleukin 1 and tumor necrosis factor, render cultured vascular endothelial cells susceptible to lysis by antibodies circulating during Kawasaki syndrome. J Exp Med 164:1958–1972, 1986.

43. Marder VJ, Sherry S: Thrombolytic therapy: current status (first of two parts). N Engl J Med 318:1512–1520, 1988.

44. Marder VJ, Sherry S: Thrombolytic therapy: current status (second of two parts). N Engl J Med 318:1585–1595, 1988.

45. Matsumara K, Okuda Y, Ito T, et al: Coronary angiography of Kawasaki disease with the coronary vasodilator dipyridamole: assessment of distensibility of affected coronary arterial wall. Angiology 39:141–147, 1988.

46. Melish ME: Kawasaki syndrome: a 1986 perspective. Rheum Dis Clin North Am 13:7–17, 1987.

47. Morens DM, Anderson LJ, Hurwitz ES: National surveillance of Kawasaki disease. Pediatrics 65:21–25, 1980.

48. Nagashima M, Matsushima M, Matsuoka H, et al: High-dose gammaglobulin therapy for Kawasaki disease. J Pediatr 110:710–712, 1987.

49. Nakamura Y, Yanagawa I, Kawasaki T: Temporal and geographical clustering of Kawasaki disease in Japan. Prog Clin Biol Res 250:19–32, 1987.

50. Nakano H: Predictive factors of coronary aneurysm in Kawasaki disease—correlation between coronary arterial lesions and serum albumin, cholinesterase activity, prealbumin, retinol-binding protein and immature neutrophils. Prog Clin Biol Res 250:535–537, 1987.

51. Nakano H, Nojima K, Saito A, et al: High incidence of aortic regurgitation following Kawasaki disease. J Pediatr 107:59–63, 1985.

52. Nakano H, Saito A, Ueda K, et al: Clinical characteristics of myocardial infarction following Kawasaki disease: report of 11 cases. J Pediatr 108:198–203, 1986.

53. Nakano H, Ueda K, Saito A, et al: Repeated quantitative angiograms in coronary arterial aneurysm in Kawasaki disease. Am J Cardiol 56:846–851, 1985.

54. Newburger JW, Burns JC, Shen G, et al: Altered lipid metabolism following Kawasaki syndrome (abstract). Circulation 76:515, 1987.

55. Newburger JW, Sanders SP, Burns JC, et al: Left ventricular contractility and function in Kawasaki syndrome: effect of intravenous gamma globulin. Circulation 79:1237–1246, 1989.

56. Newburger JW, Takahashi M, Burns JC, et al: The treatment of Kawasaki syndrome with intravenous gamma globulin. N Engl J Med 315:341–347, 1986.

57. Nishida H, Endo M, Hayashi H, et al: Early occlusion of saphenous vein grafts due to marked intimal proliferation in Kawasaki disease. Prog Clin Biol Res 250:527–528, 1987.

58. Rauch AM: Kawasaki syndrome: Critical review of U.S. epidemiology. Prog Clin Biol Res 250:33–44, 1987.

59. Rauch AM: Kawasaki syndrome: Review of new epidemiologic and laboratory developments. Pediatr Infect Dis J 6:1016–1021, 1987.

60. Rein AJJT, Colan SD, Parness IA, et al: Regional and global left ventricular function in infants with anomalous origin of the left coronary artery from the pulmonary trunk: preoperative and postoperative assessment. Circulation 75:115–123, 1987.

61. Rowley AH, Duffy CE, Shulman ST: Prevention of giant coronary aneurysms in Kawasaki disease by intravenous gamma globulin therapy. J Pediatr 113:290–294, 1988.

62. Rowley AH, Gonzalez-Crussi F, Gidding SS, et al: Incomplete Kawasaki disease with coronary artery involvement. J Pediatr 110:409–413, 1987.

63. Sasaguri Y, Kato H: Regression of aneurysms in Kawasaki disease: a pathological study. J Pediatr 100:225–231, 1982.

64. Schuh S, Laxer RM, Smallhorn JF, et al: Kawasaki disease with atypical presentation. Pediatr Infect Dis J 7:201–203, 1988.

65. Shulman ST, McAuley JB, Pachman LM, et al: Risk of coronary abnormalities due to Kawasaki disease in urban area with small Asian population. Am J Dis Child 141:420–425, 1987.

66. Spevak PJ, Newburger JW, Keane J, et al: Reactivity of coronary arteries in Kawasaki syndrome: an analysis of function. (abstract) Am J Cardiol 60:640, 1987.

67. Sty JR, Starshak RJ, Gorenstein L: Gallbladder perforation in a case of Kawasaki disease: image correlation. JCU 11:381–384, 1983.

68. Suddleson EA, Reid B, Woolley MM, et al: Hydrops of the gallbladder associated with Kawasaki syndrome. J Pediatr Surg 22:956–959, 1987.

69. Suzuki A, Kamiya T, Kuwahara N, et al: Coronary arterial lesion of Kawasaki disease: cardiac catheterization findings of 1100 cases. Pediatr Cardiol 7:3–9, 1986.

70. Suzuki A, Kamiya T, Ono Y, et al: Indication of aortocoronary bypass for coronary arterial obstruction due to Kawasaki disease. Heart Vessels 1:94–100, 1985.

71. Takahashi M, Mason W, Lewis AB: Regression of coronary aneurysms in patients with Kawasaki syndrome. Circulation 75:387–394, 1987.

72. Takeuchi Y, Suma K, Shiroma K, et al: Surgical experience with coronary arterial sequelae of Kawasaki disease in children. J Cardiovasc Surg 22:231–238, 1981.

73. Tanaka N, Naoe A, Masuda H, et al: Pathological study of sequelae of Kawasaki disease (MCLS): with special reference to the heart and coronary arterial lesions. Acta Pathol Jpn 36:1513–1527, 1986.

74. Tatara K, Kusakawa S: Long-term prognosis of giant coronary aneurysms in Kawasaki disease. Prog Clin Biol Res 250:579, 1987.

75. Tatara K, Kusakawa S: Long-term prognosis of giant aneurysm in Kawasaki disease: an angiographic study. J Pediatr 111:705–710, 1987.

76. Terai M, Ogata M, Sugimoto K, et al: Coronary arterial thrombi in Kawasaki disease. J Pediatr 106:76–78, 1985.

77. Yangawa H, Kawasaki T, Shigematsu I: Nationwide survey on Kawasaki disease in Japan. Pediatr 80:58–62, 1989.

78. Yokoyama T, Kato H, Ichinose E: Aspirin treatment and platelet function in Kawasaki disease. Kurume Med J 27:57–61, 1980.

79. Yutani C, Okano K, Kamiya T, et al: Histopathological study on right endomyocardial biopsy of Kawasaki disease. Br Heart J 43:589–592, 1980.

Chapter 24

CARDIOMYOPATHIES

Steven D. Colan, M.D., Philip J. Spevak, M.D.,
Ira A. Parness, M.D., and Alexander S. Nadas, M.D.

DEFINITION

Arbitrarily, the term cardiomyopathy includes all entities in which myocardial pathology is the dominant feature and there is no gross structural basis for cardiac disability.

CLASSIFICATION

Most authorities discussing cardiomyopathies accept the revised World Health Organization physiologic classification[406] of: (1) dilated, (2) hypertrophic, and (3) restrictive myopathies. The etiology may be known or unknown, and any one patient, in time, may show characteristics of more than one category.

1. Dilated cardiomyopathies are characterized by congestive heart failure caused by impaired biventricular systolic function (left ventricular hypokinesis usually dominating). In rare instances, arrhythmias or conduction disturbances may be the presenting signs.

2. Hypertrophic cardiomyopathy, in contrast to the dilated type, almost never produces congestive heart failure as a first symptom, although rarely this may occur much further along in the disease. Initial symptoms may include dyspnea, angina, palpitations, syncope, and even unexpected death. Physiologically, systolic function is not impaired, even hyperkinetic, whereas diastolic dysfunction is progressive. The left ventricle is stiff, and an outflow gradient may be present at rest or on effort. Often there is mitral incompetence. The anatomic basis of these abnormalities is ventricular hypertrophy.

3. Restrictive cardiomyopathies are characterized by impaired diastolic function (poor compliance) similar to that seen in constrictive pericarditis but usually limited to the left ventricle. The cavity of the left ventricle is small; systolic function is preserved. Clinically, there is dyspnea and right-sided heart failure.[43] Pediatric patients rarely show evidence of restrictive cardiomyopathy; consequently, this problem will not be discussed further.

PREVALENCE

At the present time there are no reliable data on the prevalence of cardiomyopathies in children. A review of experience with primary myocardial disease (dilated cardiomyopathy, including myocarditis, and autopsy-proven endocardial fibroelastosis) at The Children's Hospital of Boston in a 30-year period (1945–74)[139] found 161 patients who met clinical criteria (cardiomegaly, no murmur, echocardiographic changes, and no coarctation of the aorta), representing less than 1% of the total cardiac admissions. In the more recent 15–year period (1973–87), 367 patients (2.5%) were categorized as having primary myocardial disease. A report from the Mayo Clinic,[366] in 1985 listed 24 children who were seen over a 10-year period.

The National Center for Health Statistics reported 10,345 deaths from cardiomyopathy in 1982,[124] with the majority caused by dilated cardiomyopathy (87%). Hypertrophic cardiomyopathy was present in only 2% of males and 6% of females. Death rates were lowest in childhood (1–14 years) but relatively higher in infants (less than 1 year). In the Regional Infant Cardiac Program the highest incidence of cardiomyopathies was in the first week of life.[114] Data from the National Center for Health Statistics showed a significant increase (two- or threefold) in reported deaths attributed to cardiomyopathy between 1970 and 1982. There has been no explanation of this increase. Others have estimated that 0.7% of all cardiac deaths (mostly adults) could be attributed to cardiomyopathy; more than 90% of these could be categorized as dilated.[1]

ETIOLOGY

As of 1990 the etiology of cardiomyopathy in most patients cannot be determined, even though the reported causes are numerous and diverse (Tables 1 and 2).

Table 1. Classification of
Primary Cardiomyopathies

Diseases Related to Energy Creation or Utilization
Fatty Acid Transport
  Primary carnitine deficiency (DH)[40,154,180,238,301,363,378,386,393]
    Biosynthetic defect[298]
    Absorption defect[393]
    Transport defect[299,300]
    Excessive urinary loss[61,65,393]
  Secondary carnitine deficiency (DHI)
    Dietary deficiency
    Excessive urinary losses
    Liver disease
    Dehydrogenase enzyme deficiencies
    Organic acidurias
      Blutaric aciduria type II
      Isovaleric aciduria
      Methylmalonic aciduria
      Propionic aciduria
      Homocystinuria
    Other metabolic disorders
      Cytochrome disorders (HI)
      Kearns-Sayre (H−)[55]
      X-linked mitochondrial disease (D)[23]
  Transferase enzyme disorders (D)[125]

Glucose Utilization
  Glycolysis (N)
  Glycogenolysis
    Glycogen storage disease type 2
      (Pompe's) (H)[25,37,51,54,94,123,146,216,287,340]
      Normal acid maltase, "type 2-like disease"[19]
      Cardiac phosphorylase kinase deficiency (H)[96,335]
      Glycogen storage disease, type 3 (Cori) (H)[96,251,278,309]
  Glycogen synthesis
    Glycogen storage disease, type 4 (Anderson's) (D)[336,353]

Protein Metabolism
  Amino acid degradation
    β-ketothiolase deficiency (D−)[161]

Disorders of Mitochondrial Function
  Fatty acid oxidation
    Short chain acyl CoA dehydrogenase deficiency (N)
    Medium chain acyl CoA dehydrogenase deficiency (N)
    Long chain acyl CoA dehydrogenase deficiency (H)[147,267]
    Multiple chain acyl CoA deydrogenase deficiency
      Glutaric aciduria type II (I)[272]
  Pyruvate metabolism[30]
    Pyruvate dehydrogenase complex disorder (H−)
    Pyruvate carboxylase deficiency (H−)
    Leigh's Disease (H−)[199,313,332]
  Citric acid cycle (N)
  Oxidative phosphorylation
    Complex 1 deficiency (I−)[259]
    Complex 2 deficiency (N)
    Complex 3 (Cytochrome C reductase) deficiency
      (I)[195,281]
      Histiocytoid cardiomyopathy-(I)[41,49,103,244,297,314,404]
    Complex 4 (Cytochrome C oxidase) deficiency-
      (I)[195,281,303,334,394]
  Idiopathic (suspected mitochondrial) "Cardiomyopathy
    plus syndromes"
    X-linked inheritance (D)[23,270]
    Congenital cataract (H)[75,333]
    Ophthalmoplegia (A−)[55]
    Brain infarcts (AI−)[35]
    Vermal atrophy/lactic acidosis (I−)[63]
    Skeletal muscle weakness (HI−)[110,175]
    Oncocytic (AI)[345]

Table 1. Classification of
Primary Cardiomyopathies *(Continued)*

Disorders of Lysosomal Enzymes
Mucopolysaccharidoses[250]
  Type 1H Hurler (CV; usually −)
  Type 1S Scheie (CV−)
  Type 1S/H Hurler-Scheie (I−)
  Type 2 Hunter (CV; usually −)
  Type 4 Morquio (V−)
  Type 6 Maroteaux-Lamy (CIV)[252]
  Type 7 Sly (CIV)[268]
Mycolipidoses
  Type 2 I-cell disease (I)[351]
  Type 3 Pseudo-Hurler polydystrophy (V−)
Glycoproteinoses
  Fucosidosis (I)[92]
  Aspartylglycosaminuria (VI−)
  Sialidosis (VI−)[306]
  Mannosidosis (IA−)
Ceramidase deficiency
  Farber's lipogranulomatosis (VA)[260]
Sphingomyelin lipidoses
  Niemann-Pick disease (VIM)[398]
Glucosylceramide lipodoses
  Gaucher's disease (HRI−)[292]
Gangliosidoses
  G$_{M1}$ gangliosidoses (D)[66,200,306]
  G$_{M2}$ gangliosidoses
    Tay-Sachs (E)
    Sandhoff's (VDI)[31]

Other Metabolic Disorders
Ethanolaminosis (I)[387]
Phytanic acid storage disease (Refsum's) (ED−)[302]

A = Arrhythmia without cardiomyopathy
C = Coronary artery disease
D = Dilated cardiomyopathy
E = Electrocardiographic manifestations alone reported
H = Hypertrophic cardiomyopathy
I = Cardiac disease reported but inadequately characterized
M = Microscopic findings reported, not necessarily with
      clinical manifestations
N = No cardiac disease reported
      Report of cardiac involvement not described in in-
      fancy
R = Restrictive cardiomyopathy
V = Valvar disease

From Moller JH, Neal WA: Fetal, Neonatal, and Infant
Cardiac Disease. East Norwalk, CT, Appleton-Lange, 1990,
with permission.

PATHOLOGY

Except for hypertrophic forms of cardiomyopathy, the pathology of myocardial disease may be
described (with few exceptions) as follows: Gross
examination typically reveals considerable ventricular enlargement of one or both ventricles.[102] The
left ventricular mass is often increased but not disproportionately, as in hypertrophic myopathy, and
not sufficiently to return the mass/volume ratio to
normal. Frequently the thickness of the ventricular
wall is increased, but it may be normal or even
decreased. There may be areas of softening. The
greater the dilatation of the ventricle, the less likely
are the walls to be thickened.[81] Sometimes, in in-

Table 2. Classification of Secondary Myocardial Disease

Infectious
Viral (see p. 335)
Septicemia (D)
Postmyocarditis (D)
Acquired immune deficiency syndrome[191]

Nutritional
Thiamine deficiency (D)
Kwashiorkor
Pellagra
Selenium deficiency (D)

Endocrine
Hypo- and hyperthyroidism (DH)
Hypoparathyroidism (D)
Pheochromocytoma (D −)[178]
Infant of a diabetic mother (H)
Hypoglycemia (D)
Tyrosinemia (H)[93]

Neuromuscular
Friedreich's ataxia (H −)[343] (see p. 348)
Duchenne's dystrophy (see p. 349)

Collagen
Lupus erythematosus

Drugs/Toxins
Anthracyclines (D)
Steroids/ACTH (H)[11,362]
Catecholamines (D)
Iron overload

Other
Beckwith-Wiedemann syndrome (M)[193]
Noonan syndrome (H)[7]
Multiple lentigines (H)[7]
Epidermolysis bullosa (D −)[48]
Turner syndrome (D −)[58]
Kawasaki (see ch. 23)
Rheumatic fever (see ch. 22)

Note: key is the same as in Table 1.
From Moller JH, Neal WA: Fetal, Neonatal, and Infant Cardiac Disease. East Norwalk, CT, Appleton-Lange, 1990, with permission.

fants with cardiomyopathy, there may be endocardial thickening (i.e., endocardial fibroelastosis).[104] Mural thrombi are found at postmortem examination in at least a third of patients.[18,304] Clots are most often found in the apex of the left ventricle and in the left atrial appendage. Often there is dilatation of the atrioventricular valve rings,[81,304] and jet lesions are noted in the atria from atrioventricular valve regurgitation.

Microscopically, there is considerable variation among specific disease processes. Often there is degeneration of the sarcolemma or myocytolysis.[136,304] Some consider evidence of myocytolysis a constant feature.[81] The remaining cells may have more variability in size than normal, and often the muscles fibers are longer than normal. Usually the mean muscle fiber diameter is reduced.[81] Intracellular organelles are often abnormal; the nuclei may be hyperchromatic.[81] There is often an increase in interstitial connective tissue unrelated to preexisting necrosis.[101] Fibrosis is more typically

seen in the subendocardium and papillary muscles.[229]

CLINICAL MANIFESTATIONS

The initial symptoms of dilated cardiomyopathy are generally those of respiratory distress secondary to congestive heart failure.[139,140,326,366] Parents of infants and small children note pallor, irritability, tachypnea, sweating, and easy fatigability, particularly during feeding.[109] The rate of growth may fall off. Less often (10–20% of children), the initial symptoms include: arrhythmia (usually ventricular ectopic activity);[91] syncope; cardiomegaly noted incidentally on the chest x-ray; neurologic problems, such as seizure or delayed development; gastrointestinal complaints, such as vomiting or abdominal pain; or fever. In some series, a nonspecific acute febrile illness has occurred in as many as 50% of children with cardiomyopathy within 3 months of the onset of symptoms of heart failure, but cardiac biopsy has not demonstrated evidence of myocarditis.[366] Occasionally acute myocardial disease is associated with viral encephalitic symptoms and sometimes with hepatitis.

In the largest reported series of infants and children with cardiomyopathy, approximately half of the patients were first seen in infancy;[139,140,366] roughly 25% had been symptomatic for 24 hours or less. Often, a superimposed respiratory illness precipitates hospital admission. The clinical presentation of hypertrophic cardiomyopathy is much more likely to be prompted by the detection of a heart murmur than by the manifestations of congestive failure.[232,325]

Because the manifestations of myocarditis may be nonspecific, a high index of suspicion for this disease must be applied to the evaluation of unexplained tachypnea and tachycardia and to a new onset of sustained arrhythmia. Fever is not a universal finding but often accompanies classic myocarditis. A history of upper respiratory symptoms is so nonspecific that, despite often being present, it does not help establish a diagnosis. Chest pain is a clue to the involvement of the pericardium.

Family history is positive in as many as 25% of children more than 2 years of age.[14,21,129,139,140,194,258, 275,307,308,328,366,383] Among 184 children and adults undergoing heart transplantation for end-stage dilated cardiomyopathy, 9% had a familial etiology, and there were 5 sibling pairs.[384]

Physical Examination

Signs of congestive heart failure are common and include tachypnea, tachycardia, sweating, hepatomegaly, pallor, and, in some advanced cases, hypotension and shock. If the child has been in congestive failure for some time, there may be failure to thrive. Generally the patient is not cyanotic, although the oxygen saturation may be reduced if there is pulmonary edema. Wheezes may be heard in the lung fields; however, rales are rare in infants.

On cardiac examination, the heart sounds may be muffled and an S_3 or (much more commonly) an S_4 gallop is present. An apical murmur of mitral regurgitation is unusual. In some lysosomal storage diseases, aortic regurgitation may be heard.

Because myocardial disease is seen within the framework of syndromes, it is important to look for characteristic features (for example, hypothyroidism, hyperthyroidism, muscular dystrophy, nutritional deficiency, drug or toxin exposure, and maternal diabetes). There may be clues to their presence on physical examination.

Several of the mitochondrial myopathies and lysosomal storage diseases are associated with prominent neurologic features, including hypotonia, seizures, and developmental delay. Mitochondrial myopathies often are associated with ophthalmologic lesions, including cataracts and retinal abnormalities. Patients with lysosomal storage diseases have particularly striking, coarse facial features (Hurler's syndrome).

Various tachyarrhythmias or conduction defects may be associated with congestive failure or may even dominate the clinical presentation. Pediatric patients, from infancy throughout adolescence, may be seen because of refractory ventricular tachycardia or atrial flutter;[264,388] myocarditis should always be suspected in this setting. Complete heart block is another presenting arrhythmia.[213] Bundle branch[354] or fascicular blocks occur as well.

Electrocardiography

Changes in the S-T segments and T waves are present in the majority of children, particularly in the lateral and left precordial leads. These abnormalities typically include flattening or inversion of T waves with depressed S-T segments.[368] Generalized low voltage is sometimes seen.[109] More than 50% of infants with dilated cardiomyopathy may have left ventricular hypertrophy and 85% have an inferior QRS axis.[139,140] Occasionally, focal myocarditis may mimic infarction, with localized Q-wave abnormalities and elevation of the S-T segment.[72,135,315]

At the outset, arrhythmias, such as atrioventricular (AV) block, bundle branch or fascicular block, or consecutive atrial or ventricular ectopy, may be manifest; these have been noted in approximately 15% of infants with cardiomyopathy. Greenwood found that 42% had ventricular ectopy (from single ventricular premature beats to ventricular tachycardia), 31% had supraventricular tachycardia, and 12% had either second-degree AV block or AV dissociation.[139]

Certain diseases have almost specific electrocardiographic abnormalities. In carnitine deficiency, huge T waves (as large as 60–80 mm)[378,393] or elevated S-T segments are present.[238] In Pompe's disease, the features are a short P-R interval, very large left precordial voltages, and sometimes findings consistent with the Wolff-Parkinson-White syndrome.[25,51,94,123]

Chest X-ray

The heart is usually enlarged and there may be signs of pulmonary venous congestion, although this may be deceptive, especially in fulminant myocarditis when the ventricle has not had time to dilate. Such patients will have bilateral infiltrates of pulmonary edema (sometimes mistaken for pneumonia) with only borderline heart enlargement. More typically, however, the cardiac silhouette is clearly enlarged, occasionally massively so, with a "water-bottle" configuration of pericardial effusion.

In many of the lysosomal storage diseases there are skeletal abnormalities known as dysostosis multiplex: widening of the medial end of the clavicle; premature closure of the sutures, sometimes resulting in scaphocephaly; shallow orbits; and rounded and relatively immature vertebral bodies.[250]

Echocardiography

The two-dimensional echocardiogram usually demonstrates a dilated, thin-walled, and globally hypokinetic left ventricle.[290] M-mode analysis with quantification of wall stress allows load-independent assessment of contractility and is useful in serial follow-up, especially after introduction of afterload reduction therapy. Often, the right ventricle is not obviously dilated or dysfunctional, although rarely, right ventricular dysfunction is the dominant abnormality.[240] In some cases of acute myocarditis, the left ventricle is severely hypokinetic despite the absence of dilatation. No echocardiographic features differentiate myocarditis from other dilated cardiomyopathies. An "overshoot" phase of ventricular hypertrophy has been noted during recovery from myocarditis. Thrombi may be present in the left side of the heart and should be carefully sought.

Color flow mapping has become indispensable for excluding other causes of global left ventricular dysfunction, such as anomalous origin of the left coronary artery.[317] The Doppler examination commonly discloses associated mitral and/or tricuspid regurgitation. Continuous-wave Doppler interrogation of the tricuspid regurgitant jet allows diagnosis of associated pulmonary hypertension.

An echocardiographic study of 37 children with dilated cardiomyopathy found ventricular dimensions increased by approximately 50% above the mean predicted.[120] Ejection parameters were decreased to 25–50% in the same patients. In another study of children with clinically suspected, postmyocarditis cardiomyopathy, ejection parameters were decreased by a similar amount.[128] Other investigators have reported comparable abnormalities in ventricular dimensions and systolic function.[140,366] Decreased segmental wall motion has been reported in 64% of adults with dilated cardiomyopathy; these patients carry a better prognosis than those with diffuse wall-motion abnormalities.[395]

Doppler interrogation has been used to examine left ventricular ejection dynamics.[204] Typically, in dilated cardiomyopathy, peak velocity and peak acceleration are decreased, both at rest and with peak exercise. In addition, the preejection period is prolonged, whereas ejection time is decreased. Like other ejection parameters, these flow measurements are dependent on loading conditions.

Echocardiographic follow-up of children with dilated cardiomyopathy is limited. Of infants who are first seen with severe congestive failure, approximately 70% survive 1 year.[140,366] Of the survivors, approximately half will show little improvement (in terms of normalization of ventricular dimensions and ejection parameters), 25% will improve but remain abnormal, and 25% will normalize.[120,385] Recent data suggest a somewhat better outcome.[237]

Loading conditions may be markedly abnormal in dilated cardiomyopathy. In adults with cardiomyopathy, elevations in both peak and end-systolic wall stress are typical.[115,145,167,256] Because measures of function, such as shortening fraction, are afterload dependent, the functional abnormalities reported are due in part to the afterload mismatch. Furthermore, there may be large fluctuations in preload. In adults with dilated cardiomyopathy, end-diastolic wall stress is typically increased, which (if myocardial and chamber stiffness are normal) reflects increased preload.[115,145,166,167,256] In this regard, infants seem to be different.[237]

The left ventricular shape and the distribution of wall stress may help to predict survival. In infants and adults with dilated cardiomyopathy, poor prognostic factors included a more spherical configuration of the left ventricle and a more even distribution of wall stress in meridional and circumferential planes.[88,237]

Besides its usefulness in evaluating ventricular function, echocardiography can be helpful in ruling out obstructive structural lesions, such as aortic valve disease or coarctation, that cause decreased left ventricular function.

An important anomaly which may be recognized by echocardiography is anomalous origin of the left coronary artery arising from the pulmonary artery; adequate images can be obtained in most infants to show the normal origin of the coronary arteries (see ch. 51). Sometimes the presence of normal antegrade flow can be seen with color Doppler. Also, the absence of retrograde flow into the pulmonary artery is evidence against an anomalous coronary origin. When there is an anomalous left coronary artery, the diameter of the right coronary artery is increased.[201]

Cardiac Catheterization

In patients with myocardial disease, cardiac catheterization may be needed for hemodynamic assessment, angiography (primarily to help rule out a structural defect), or myocardial biopsy.

Hemodynamics. The left- and, often, right-sided filling pressures are frequently increased, although at rest, if the child is sedated, or if the patient has been aggressively treated with diuretics, the filling pressure may be relatively normal. As the cardiomyopathy becomes more severe, cardiac output declines. Eventually, mixed venous oxygen saturation will decrease, reflecting low cardiac output. The arterial oxygen saturation is normal unless there is pulmonary edema. There is often an increase in both systemic and pulmonary resistance, the latter resulting in increased pulmonary artery pressure. As the systolic dysfunction becomes more severe, the left ventricular pressure tracing has a less rapid upstroke and downstroke.[144] In addition, with end-stage disease, the peak left ventricular and aortic pressures decline.

Angiography. It is crucial to exclude the presence of an anomalous origin of the coronary artery in an infant with dilated cardiomyopathy. An aortogram may be necessary if the coronary artery anatomy cannot be determined by ultrasound. However, if meticulously sought, especially with Doppler color flow mapping, anomalies of the coronary may be excluded without angiography.

In some cases angiography may be necessary to exclude structural heart disease. Ventriculograms are sometimes useful as part of a functional assessment, so that ventricular volumes and ejection fractions can be determined. The degree of valvular regurgitation can also be assessed.

Myocardial Biopsy. While endomyocardial biopsy can be performed relatively safely, even in hemodynamically compromised infants (see ch. 14), the role and value of the information obtained are not clear.[106,111,211,271,327] When biopsies are obtained, examination by both light and electron microscopy is mandatory. In addition, specimens should be frozen in case metabolic studies are later necessary. In general, it is desirable to perform the procedure early in the course of the disease to maximize the possibility of identifying an etiologic agent.

Endomyocardial biopsy may be of value in some metabolic diseases. Hart reported a case of dilated cardiomyopathy associated with carnitine deficiency in which serum carnitine levels were normal, yet skeletal and cardiac tissue levels were decreased.[154] Also, in one form of glycogen storage disease (a deficiency of cardiac phosphorylase kinase), glycogen deposition is confined to the heart, as is the kinase abnormality. Consequently, cardiac tissue is necessary to make the diagnosis. Matitiau found the results of biopsy to be predictive of the outcome in infants with congestive cardiomyopathy.[237]

Laboratory Tests

Arterial blood gases often reveal respiratory alkalosis and mild hypoxemia resulting from pulmonary edema. Mixed acid-base disturbances with metabolic acidosis signal low cardiac output and are an indication for intensive inotropic or mechanical cardiopulmonary support.

Nuclear Scans

Gallium scanning in adult patients[184,241,276] has been reported to be helpful in the diagnosis of myocarditis, but its utility is controversial. More recently, radiolabeled, monoclonal, antimyosin antibody scans[85,186] have been applied in centers reporting on adults, with promising results. It has been suggested that these nuclear scans might be more sensitive than endomyocardial biopsy, which suffers from sampling error. In support of this, these centers report a higher response to immunosuppressive therapy in patients with positive scans. The authors have no experience with these techniques in pediatric patients and there are no pediatric data in the literature. More experience will be required to assess the usefulness of nuclear scanning in myocarditis and other cardiomyopathies.

MANAGEMENT

Treatment of dilated cardiomyopathy associated with congestive heart failure includes vigorous use of all available means for support of the myocardium and circulation. The possibilities for recovery from congestive heart failure caused by myocardial disease contrast sharply with those from congestive heart failure resulting from structural damage, where ultimate success depends on surgical repair.

The usual anticongestive medications are employed. Digitalis derivatives are used with some caution, because digitalis may produce an arrhythmia in an inflamed myocardium. Diuretics, oxygen, electrolyte manipulation, afterload reduction, artificial ventilation, and sedation can all be used effectively. Antiarrhythmic drugs are used as needed, keeping in mind dangerous cross-drug effects (see ch. 27).

Cardiac transplantation is considered when all else fails.

It is important to emphasize that the hypertrophic cardiomyopathies must not be managed in the same way as the dilated forms (see p. 342). There are important risks in using positive inotropic agents and in manipulation of blood volume in these patients.

COURSE

There are relatively few reports of the natural history of cardiomyopathy in infants and children. In a retrospective review of "primary myocardial disease,"[139] poor prognostic factors included pulmonary vascular congestion on the x-ray, a cardiac index of less than 3 L/min/m², and a superior and rightward QRS axis on the electrocardiogram. Factors that did not predict a poor outcome included presentation as a neonate and the presence of heart failure, arrhythmia, or left ventricular hypertrophy. This study confirmed the longstanding clinical impression that one-third die, one-third survive with permanent damage, and one-third recover to be virtually normal.

In a recent review of 24 patients less than 18 years old,[366] the survival rates were 63% at 1 year, 50% at 2 years, and 34% at 5 years. Overall, 63% of the patients died during a mean follow-up period of 33 months. The mortality rate among the 10 infants was 30%. Severe mitral regurgitation was a bad prognostic sign, whereas viral symptoms within 3 months of presentation were associated with a better survival. Factors that were not of prognostic significance included the cardiothoracic ratio; electrocardiographic evidence of left ventricular hypertrophy, ventricular arrhythmias, and abnormalities of the S-T segment and T wave; decreased function shown on the echocardiogram; and diminished cardiac index or elevated left ventricular end-diastolic pressure at catheterization. Intracardiac thrombosis was noted in 23% of the patients and systemic arterial embolism occurred in 8%.

In a recent review of 24 infants less than 2 years old who had congestive cardiomyopathy that was not related to toxic drugs or storage diseases, 70% survived (60% recovered completely). Death was predicted by the severity of left ventricular dysfunction, globular shape of the left ventricle, and endocardial fibroelastosis. Myocardial biopsy was useful in the prognosis as well as the diagnosis.[237] In another study of 12 surviving children less than 2 years old at the onset of dilated cardiomyopathy,[140] 25% died during a mean follow-up period of 3.9 years. Three patients died suddenly and two patients died of intractable congestive failure. All 20 who were more than 2 years old at onset died; the mean time period between onset of symptoms and death was 2 years. Besides age, predictors of a poor outcome were persistent cardiomegaly and the development of atrial fibrillation or ventricular arrhythmias. Thromboembolic events occurred in 9% of the patients, none of whom was anticoagulated at the time.

In an autopsy series of 9 infants with cardio-myopathy,[87] the duration of symptoms was 2 months or less in all patients. In a series of 22 children with congestive cardiomyopathy who were first seen in infancy and who survived more than 2 years, 15 continued to have increased left ventricular dimensions, and 7 had diminished function as indicated by a shortening fraction measured at echocardiography.[385]

SPECIFIC PROBLEMS

Myocarditis

Definition. Myocarditis (like other dilated car-diomyopathies) is an incompletely understood and ill-defined group of related diseases. In 1899, Fiedler[189,190] described the pathologic and clinical findings of isolated interstitial cardiac inflamma-tion, usually with a fulminant course, which was not associated with the then known causes of my-ocardial inflammation. The histologic findings of profuse, interstitial round-cell infiltration and my-ocyte degeneration he described remain the most universally accepted criteria for the diagnosis of myocarditis. Literally, myocarditis means inflam-mation of myocardium, but most clinicians assume that infection,[187] even if it cannot be documented, is the cause of the inflammation. Although often true, the situation is really much more complicated because myocarditis may have noninfectious causes, such as collagen vascular diseases. Con-versely, certain infectious cardiomyopathies (such as diphtheritic) do not satisfy the literal definition of myocarditis insofar as the primary mechanism of injury involves circulating toxin rather than my-ocardial inflammation. However, for the purposes of this discussion, myocarditis is considered to in-clude only histologically confirmed inflammatory disease, irrespective of etiology. This does not belie the difficulty in obtaining premortem histologic confirmation, especially late in the course of the disease.[196] The common association of pericarditis has led some authors to use the term "myoperi-carditis" for this disease. Pancarditis seen with rheumatic fever includes myocarditis but, follow-ing convention, rheumatic fever is treated as a sep-arate entity and is discussed elsewhere (see ch. 22).

Myocarditis has been classified[16,242] based on the particular histologic picture; the type of interstitial infiltrate may occasionally help the clinician to for-mulate a differential diagnosis (Table 3). A partic-ular histologic appearance may have prognostic im-plications; for example, idiopathic "giant cell"[80,82,403] myocarditis characterizes a syndrome of fulminant and frequently fatal myocarditis that commonly af-flicts adolescents and young adults.

From a clinical standpoint, myocarditis may be broadly divided into infectious or noninfectious categories. Nearly every known infectious agent, including viruses, protozoa, fungi, rickettsiae, and bacteria, has been implicated (with variably con-vincing evidence) as a cause. The most common agents[405] identified in human disease are entero-viruses,[257] particularly Coxsackie viruses.[141,168,310] Coxsackie virus is also the most intensively studied pathogen in animal models. More recently, atten-tion has been focused on myocarditis caused by the human immunodeficiency virus.[142,215]

Noninfectious myocarditis is diagnosed when myocardial inflammation is observed in the ab-sence of evidence of recent infection. Usually it is associated with autoimmune diseases (e.g., Tak-ayasu's arteritis,[367] Kawasaki disease)[112,411] or an al-lergic (usually, drug associated) reaction with eo-sinophilic infiltrate.[365]

Viral Myocarditis. There are two major levels of uncertainty in the diagnosis of "viral" myocar-ditis. First, the firm diagnosis of this condition is difficult—clinical diagnosis may often be at odds with the currently accepted, albeit somewhat ques-tionable,[69,214,339] standard of histologic diagnosis, usually obtained by transcatheter endomyocardial biopsy.[28,60,64,91,111,207,211,217,326,409] Second, even when the diagnosis of myocarditis is unequivocally estab-lished by histologic criteria, the etiology frequently remains obscure or is supported only by circum-stantial evidence of recent viral infection, such as paired serum viral titers. With currently available clinical tools, the etiology of even thoroughly in-vestigated myocarditis is most likely to be "idio-pathic."

Still, a great deal is known about Coxsackie virus myocarditis in animal models; histologically proved human myocarditis is seen in the setting of well-documented Coxsackie virus infection, and it is presumed to be the etiology, even though the virus cannot be recovered from the myocardium. How-ever, recent advances in molecular biology[42,95,377] may allow the identification of viral genomes in biopsy material, facilitating the etiologic diagnosis.

Pathology. Myocardial histology is variable, de-pending on the state of illness and the age of the patient.[405] In the first 5 days of illness in neonates, polymorphonuclear cells predominate, whereas in adolescents and adults, at all stages of illness poly-morphonuclear cells are rare. By day 5, mono-morphonuclear cells predominate, consisting of eosinophils and macrophages, but mostly lympho-cytes. The mononuclear cellular collections may be focal or diffuse, perivascular or interstitial, and as-sociated with varying degrees of edema and my-ocyte necrosis.

Because of interobserver variability and contro-versies surrounding the histologic definition of my-ocarditis, a group of pathologists met to formulate histologic criteria that could be applied to a multi-center study of the disease. The resultant "Dallas criteria"[16,17,84] have gained widespread acceptance. Briefly, these criteria require the presence of in-

Table 3.   Differential Diagnosis of Myocardial Infiltrates*

Causes of Lymphocytic Infiltrate	Causes of Eosinophilic Infiltrate
Idiopathic	(Drug) Hypersensitivity
Infection (most commonly viral; also, fungal, protozoal, rickettsial, chlamydial, mycoplasmal)	Hypereosinophilic syndrome (e.g., Loeffler's endomyocardial disease)
Aberrant immune response (post-infectious, Kawasaki disease, other collagen vascular diseases)	Parasitic infestation
	Wegener's granulomatosis
Lymphoma	Severe cardiac allograft rejection
(Associated with granulomatous infiltrate, see below)	Idiopathic
(Associated with eosinophilic infiltrate, see below)	
Granulomatous ("Giant Cell") Infiltrate	**Neutrophilic Infiltrate**
Idiopathic	Viral infection (early phase)
Collagen vascular diseases (rheumatic fever, idiopathic early-phase rheumatoid arthritis, Wegener's granulomatosis)	Bacterial infection
	Toxic (diphtheria)
Proliferative disorders of the phagocyte system (juvenile xantho-granuloma, malignant histiocytosis)	Infarction
	Pressor effect
Metabolic disorders (granulomatous disease of childhood, gout oxalosis)	
Sarcoidosis	
Infection (bacterial, mycobacterial, fungal, parasitic, rickettsial)	
Hypersensitivity reactions	
Foreign body reactions	

*From Aretz HT, Billingham ME, Edwards WD, et al: Myocarditis: a histolopathologic definition and classification. Am J Cardiovasc Pathol 1:3–14, 1986, with permission.

terstitial inflammation surrounding necrotic myocytes for the definite histologic diagnosis of myocarditis.

Clinical Manifestations. The clinical manifestations of myocarditis are similar to those of most other dilated myocardiopathies.

Laboratory Tests. Some laboratory tests are useful in understanding myocarditis. For example, the MB fraction of the muscle enzyme "creatine phosphokinase (CPK)" may be elevated if there is significant myocyte necrosis, just as it is in the setting of infarction.[157] Other muscle or liver enzymes, such as glutamic oxaloacetic transferase and lactic dehydrogenase, may be elevated because of associated hepatitis or injury resulting from congestive heart failure. The erythrocyte sedimentation rate and other acute phase reactants are elevated in some patients. The spinal fluid analysis may reveal evidence of associated meningitis or encephalitis.

Paired sera for acute and convalescent viral titers are often performed to screen for recent viral infection. There are many problems with this approach, not the least of which is that infections with Coxsackie and other viruses are common in childhood, whereas the prevalence of myocarditis is very low. Thus, a fourfold rise in viral titers does not prove causation. In general, viral cultures of myocardial tissue have not been successful. Newer molecular biology technologies are likely to soon be transferred from the research laboratory into the clinical arena.

Management. Supportive therapy for acute severe myocarditis includes bed rest, sedation, cardiovascular support with intravenous inotropes, vasodilators, and diuretics, and antiarrhythmic therapy as necessary. Overwhelming cardiovascular collapse can be treated with intraaortic balloon counterpulsation and even extracorporeal membrane oxygenator support or other cardiac assist devices. Because even the most critically ill can recover, every possible means of support should be brought to bear.

It has been shown in murine models that exercise after infection with Coxsackie virus causes a higher mortality,[119] prompting recommendations for bed rest after recovery from this disease for an arbitrary period of weeks or months.

Specific antiviral therapy for the Coxsackie virus is not available. Presumably, most clinical disease is seen after the viral replication phase, and thus antiviral therapy may be of little value. Ribavirin and interferon therapies have been investigated in murine myocarditis models. The transfer of passive immunity with gamma globulin therapy has not been investigated in Coxsackie viral myocarditis. High doses of gamma globulin improve myocardial dysfunction in acute Kawasaki disease, but it has not been shown histologically that this is due to resolution of the myocarditis.

Articles about immunosuppressive therapy for myocarditis appeared as early as 1953, although the initial report of ACTH therapy was in an unproved case.[4,118,389] The first use of immunosuppressive therapy for myocarditis, which was guided by histology, was reported in 1980.[235] The approach was adapted from the Stanford protocols for treatment of cardiac allograft rejection, to which the histologic picture of myocarditis bears a striking resemblance. Subsequently, numerous reports of immunosuppressive therapy for myocarditis have been published, either as anecdotal case reports or in nonrandomized studies; some have suggested that immunosuppressive therapy works in a subgroup of patients;[4] others have found no benefit. The potential detrimental effects of immunosuppression were suggested experimentally by murine models of myocarditis that showed a worsened outcome if infection was preceded by steroid treatment of the animals. More recently, similar adverse effects have been reported for nonsteroidal anti-inflammatory drugs as well.

Anecdotally, newer immunosuppressive therapies have been tried for myocarditis, including cyclosporine and monoclonal anti-OKT3 antibody. Overall, convincing evidence of the efficacy of immunosuppressive therapy is lacking. A multicenter randomized trial of immunosuppression sponsored by the National Institutes of Health is under way, but the trial does not include pediatric patients. A similar study in pediatric patients would be required to settle the controversy. Based on studies of murine models, immunosuppression in the early febrile stage of the disease is likely to be dangerous and should not be undertaken. Immunosuppressive therapy for patients with biopsy-proven myocarditis may be tried cautiously in the setting of persistent left ventricular dysfunction, as long as the physician and patient understand the risks and benefits of the approach. The authors have used a regimen of cyclosporine and low-dose prednisone for 6 months following a 2-week period during which a high dose of prednisone is gradually reduced; this is similar to the regimen used to treat cardiac allograft rejection.

Cardiac transplantation may be undertaken in desperately acutely ill individuals, but it should be understood that even the most critically ill can recover from this illness. Deciding when to proceed with transplantation is a difficult decision. There is also a report suggesting that, in adults, active myocarditis at the time of transplantation may be a risk factor for poor outcome, mostly because of an increased incidence of rejection. There should be no evidence of ongoing viral sepsis at the time of transplantation.

Outcome. The outcome for pediatric patients with myocarditis in the modern era is unknown. In children less than 2 years old, 6 of 8 with biopsy-confirmed disease survived, most with full recovery of ventricular function.[237] Even those with life-threatening arrhythmias and/or severe congestive heart failure requiring intravenous inotropic support recovered fully. Whether this experience can be repeated remains to be seen.

Defects of Myocardial Energy Metabolism

In the fetus approximately 60% of the myocardial energy requirements are met by lactate extraction while the remaining energy needs are satisfied by glucose metabolism via the citric acid cycle (glycolysis).[105] After birth, free fatty acids become the predominant energy source, accounting for nearly 70% of basal myocardial energy requirements. Glucose is the next most important substrate for the heart, with lactate, pyruvate, and ketone bodies serving as backup substrates.

Fatty Acid Metabolism. Fat obtained from the diet or manufactured by the body is stored in adipose cells as triglycerides. Utilization requires lipases, which hydrolyze the triglycerides to free fatty acids. Oxidation of free fatty acids occurs within the mitochondrial matrix. Transport across the mitochondrial membranes must be preceded by conversion to fatty acyl CoA compounds on the outer surface of the mitochondrial membrane.

Depending on the length of the carbon chain, fatty acids are termed short (shorter than C_8), medium (C_8 or C_{10}), or long-chain (longer than C_{10}). Activated short- and medium-chain fatty acids can cross the inner mitochondrial membrane freely; however, long-chain fatty acids require a special transport system that is located on the inner membrane. Carnitine is an important cofactor involved in transport, during which the acyl group of free fatty acyl CoA is transferred to carnitine. The reaction is catalyzed by fatty acyl CoA/carnitine fatty acid transferase, which is specific for the length of the carbon chain of the free fatty acid. Once inside the inner mitochondrial matrix, the fatty acids can be oxidized.

Primary Carnitine Deficiency. Defects in transport related to a deficiency of the transferase enzyme cofactor, carnitine, have been associated with infantile cardiomyopathy. Two clinical forms of carnitine deficiency have been described.[289] A myopathic pattern is characterized by normal levels of carnitine in serum and cardiac muscle but low levels in skeletal muscle. Weakness of skeletal muscle is typical, and primary cardiac disease is not usually present. The myopathic form typically affects older children and young adults.

Systemic carnitine deficiency sometimes,[40,61,65,154,180,238,363,378,386,393] but not always,[99] is associated with myocardial disease.[243] This form is termed systemic because usually the levels of carnitine in the plasma as well as those in the tissues are depressed. In its most severe form there is cardiomyopathy, weakness of skeletal muscle, episodes of nonketotic hypoglycemia sometimes associated with seizures, and encephalopathy. Typically, patients are seen within the first few years of life, although systemic disease has developed later, during early childhood.[40]

There are few morphologic descriptions of the cardiac disease in systemic carnitine deficiency, with case reports of both dilated and hypertrophic cardiomyopathy.[154,180] Besides cardiomyopathy, cardiac involvement has also included the development of mitral insufficiency, sinus arrest, and nodal escape rhythms.[378]

There may be several mechanisms for depressed carnitine levels in primary carnitine deficiency. Some cases have been attributed to excessive renal losses of carnitine[61,393] and others to a defect in gastrointestinal absorption of carnitine.[393] However, not all patients with systemic carnitine deficiency display these abnormalities.[100] No reports of primary systemic disease have been related to abnormal carnitine biosynthesis.[298]

Some cases of carnitine deficiency have seemed to improve coincident with the administration of carnitine supplementation.[61,378] Improvement in systolic ventricular function and exercise capacity have been reported.[378] L-carnitine has usually been administered at a dose of 75–175 mg/kg/day. Some patients have been treated with DL-carnitine at doses of 2–3 gm/day,[154,238] but not all responded to treatment.[154]

Secondary Carnitine Deficiency and Carnitine Transferase Enzyme Disorders. Carnitine levels may be depressed secondary to other primary metabolic errors, because carnitine acts as a buffer for other acyl groups besides fatty acyl CoA. In addition, important transferase enzymes are required to transport long-chain fatty acids into the mitochondria for beta oxidation.[125,329]

Glycogen Storage Disease Type 2. There are three clinical forms of type 2 glycogen storage disease: infantile (type 2A or Pompe's disease), infantile/juvenile (type 2B), and adult (type 2C). Pompe's disease is seen in the first 6 months of life, with profound hypotonia, congestive heart failure, and muscle weakness.[37,51,94,287] Death usually occurs by 1 year of age from cardiorespiratory failure, pneumonia, or aspiration.[174] Cardiomegaly is striking. Often, hepatomegaly is not present until congestive failure occurs. In some children, but not all, the tongue is enlarged.

Echocardiographically, there is marked concentric hypertrophy with preservation of systolic function.[146,340] Papillary muscles may also be hypertrophied. The left ventricular cavity may be nearly obliterated, and outflow tract obstruction occurs in approximately 20%.[287]

Electrophysiologic studies have been performed on 3 patients with Pompe's disease.[25,123] The short P-R interval on the electrocardiogram is probably due to a short A-H interval. In addition, the P-A interval is at the lower limits of normal and the H-V interval is slightly lengthened. Why the conduction properties are abnormal is unknown. The changes may be related to alteration of conduction by glycogen or alteration of the anatomic relationships secondary to the hypertrophy.

The diagnosis of Pompe's disease is established by finding increased intracellular glycogen and an acid maltase (alpha-1-4-glucosidase) deficiency. Leukocyte acid maltase can be measured; however, there can be interference by a renal isoenzyme present in leukocytes. The interfering activity can be removed during the assay or, more definitively, acid maltase activity can be assessed in fibroblasts.[174] There are reports of infants with clinical features typical of Pompe's disease who have normal acid maltase activity.[19] The defect in such patients has not been identified, although patients are typically male, suggesting an X-linked pattern of inheritance.[155]

Family studies of Pompe's disease are consistent with an autosomal recessive pattern of inheritance, and the structural gene for alpha-glucosidase has been located on chromosome 17.[216] Fibroblasts cultured from amniocentesis can be used for prenatal diagnosis.

There is no specific treatment for Pompe's disease.

Hypertrophic Cardiomyopathy

This disorder was first described by Teare in 1958,[370] and clinical interest in it has grown at a remarkable rate. In addition to the fascinating pathologic and physiologic findings in hypertrophic cardiomyopathy (HCM), the study of this disorder has implications for the control and consequences of secondary hypertrophy. Unfortunately, progress in improving the long-term outlook for this often fatal disorder has been more elusive.

Definition. Few aspects of this disease are free from controversy, and the definition itself is no exception. A major obstacle to understanding HCM is the lack of agreement as to what it is. Many names have been applied ("asymmetrical hypertrophy of the heart," "functional subaortic stenosis," "idiopathic hypertrophic subaortic stenosis," "asymmetrical septal hypertrophy," etc.),[221] each of which has generally reflected a particular clinical or pathologic aspect of the disease. However, with broader recognition of the disorder, and particularly since echocardiography has allowed recognition of abnormal cardiac hypertrophy in otherwise healthy individuals, it has become apparent that a rather broad spectrum of diseases may be encountered, and definitions based on regional differences in wall thickness or the presence of dynamic left ventricular outflow obstruction are inadequate. In the absence of a definitive marker, the working definition of hypertrophic cardiomyopathy is purely descriptive and is generally taken to consist of "abnormal ventricular hypertrophy without an identifiable primary cause." The hypertrophy may be localized or global, systolic function and cardiac output are normal, and potential causes of a hyperdynamic circulatory state (catecholamine-secreting tumors, hyperthyroidism) are absent.

Because it has been impossible to define limits, HCM has become synonymous with any form of idiopathic left ventricular hypertrophy. As a result, the clinical spectrum has become more and more diverse, and it is no longer possible to identify clinical characteristics which define the disorder. It appears that HCM represents a heterogeneous group of disorders that have in common the presence of unexplained hypertrophy. There is, however, a subset of patients who share a common constellation of findings and represent "typical" HCM. The pathology, physiology, and prognosis for these patients are well defined. The difficulty lies in knowing whether a particular patient belongs to this group and therefore carries the same guarded prognosis.

The inadequacy of this definition is particularly apparent when a mild-to-moderate stimulus for hypertrophy is known to be present, thereby excluding the diagnosis of HCM, but the magnitude and pattern of hypertrophy are typical for HCM. In some cases the chance coexistence of two diseases can be invoked. For example, in a child with a small ventricular septal defect, normal right ventricular pressure, and marked asymmetric septal hypertrophy typical for HCM, it is difficult to avoid the diagnosis. However, if a patient with moderate aortic stenosis is found to have severe ventricular hypertrophy far beyond what is usually seen in this situation, at what point should the additional diagnosis of HCM be considered? There is a subgroup of elderly patients with hypertension who manifest clinical and pathologic findings similar to those of HCM.[223,376] By the strict definition of the disease, these subjects are not considered to have HCM. Clinically, the definition of the disease is often extended to include subjects who manifest hypertrophy that is well out of proportion to the severity of the hemodynamic lesions, although extreme caution is warranted in this situation. This dilemma is by no means restricted to pathologic hypertrophy, as athletes with hypertrophy that is more marked than the usual physiologic response are often encountered. This group is additionally problematic, because many subjects with HCM are athletes and are first diagnosed after sudden death.

Prevalence. As would be anticipated from the foregoing discussion of the controversy concerning the definition of the disease, the reported prevalence depends on the definition and method of investigation. Studies that include asymptomatic individuals recognized only by echocardiographic screening or on autopsy report higher numbers than do studies restricted to clinically apparent disease. Because of this, the reported prevalence varies from 3.2 to 33 per 100,000.[29]

Genetics. The genetic transmission of HCM is generally felt to be autosomal dominant, with about 50% of cases representing new mutations. Reports of substantially less than the expected 50% incidence in offspring can probably be explained by failure to recognize asymptomatic cases[97] and by variation in the age at screening.[225] Because the disease may not be manifest during childhood, studies conducted in adults tend to find an incidence closer to the theoretical value of 50%

transmission[137,156] than do those that include children.

Association of HCM with numerous clinical disorders has been described. Although many of these are isolated case reports and, therefore, may well represent chance association, in at least three disorders HCM is seen with enough frequency to indicate that the two are related. Patients with Friedreich's ataxia have a 25–50% incidence of HCM (see p. 348); a syndrome with lentiginosis associated with HCM (and the interesting acronym of LEOPARD syndrome: **L**, lentigines; **E**, ECG abnormalities, primarily conduction defects; **O**, ocular hypertelorism; **P**, pulmonary stenosis and subaortic valvular stenosis; **A**, abnormal genitalia; **R**, retardation of growth; and **D**, deafness) has been described;[172,352] and Noonan's syndrome is often associated with HCM.[90] Finally, many genetic disorders are often accompanied by cardiac hypertrophy[53] but clearly represent disease outside the usual meaning of "typical" HCM.

Pathology. Gross pathology characteristically demonstrates increased heart weight, a nondilated left ventricle with maximal thickness of the septum greater than that of the free wall, a thickened mitral valve with mural endocardial plaque in the outflow portion of the septum in apposition to the anterior leaflet of the mitral valve, dilated atria, and, in some cases, grossly visible areas of scarring without significant narrowing of the epicardial coronary arteries. Although asymmetric hypertrophy is typical, equal but increased thickness of both the septum and free wall is not uncommon. Age-related differences include absence of septal endocardial plaque or myocardial scarring in subjects less than 10 years of age. Although it is not possible to determine on postmortem examination whether outflow obstruction was present, mural plaques are more common, and both free-wall and septal hypertrophy tend to be more marked in these cases.

Focal myocardial fiber disarray or disorganization within the ventricular septum is a feature of this disease that is observed in most cases. Although this is not unique to HCM, normal hearts or heart conditions other than HCM rarely show myocardial fiber disarray that involves more than 5% of the septum, whereas 90% of hearts with HCM have this finding in >5% of the septum.[220,227,228] Although similar focal disorganization may be observed in the free wall of the right and left ventricles, this is much less common.

Abnormal intramural coronary arteries are also reported in a high percentage of subjects with HCM. The abnormalities consist of an increase in the number and size of arteries with thickened walls and narrowed lumens. These abnormal vessels are most common in the ventricular septum but are also present in the left ventricular free wall.[233,369] The significance of these abnormal vessels is undetermined, although they may play a role in the reduced coronary reserve of HCM[362] and/or the occurrence of transmural infarction.[113] Similar abnormal coronary vessels have been observed in normal fetuses, in tunnel subaortic stenosis,[226] and in aortic atresia.[305] Thus, like asymmetric hypertrophy and focal myocardial disarray, the presence of abnormal intramural coronary arteries is not specific for HCM, but it is more marked and more common than in other diseases.

Physiology. *Left Ventricular Outflow Gradient.* It has been customary to classify HCM as obstructive or nonobstructive, depending on the presence of a pressure gradient between the left ventricle and aorta. The gradient can be present at rest or latent (provokable) and may demonstrate marked spontaneous lability. In nonobstructive HCM the gradient is absent, both at rest and with provocation. Although the pressure gradient is the criterion used in the classification with respect to obstruction, it is clear that some subjects have pressure gradients without obstruction. The pathophysiology of the pressure gradients between the left ventricle and ascending aorta which are commonly observed in this disease has been the subject of extensive investigation and numerous contentious and vociferous debates. From all of this has emerged a growing understanding of a complex situation. It is now clear that pressure difference between the left ventricle and the aorta is due to at least four different mechanisms in various patients with HCM.

The first mechanism represents an augmentation of the normal ejection process. At the onset of contraction, the ventricular wall imparts an impulse to the column of blood within the ventricular chamber, resulting in flow acceleration across the outflow tract. In the normal state, the intraventricular pressure gradient related to this phenomenon may be as high as 5–10 mm Hg, and in hypercontractile states even higher gradients are observed. In subjects with increased ventricular mass, such as HCM, the impulse is augmented and flow acceleration is higher than usual, resulting in an abnormally high gradient.[261] Two characteristics of this pressure gradient distinguish it from the other mechanisms. First, no anatomic obstruction is present. Second, because the pressure difference is present only during the flow acceleration phase, this is an early systolic phenomenon, resolving by midsystole as flow acceleration ceases. In contrast, each of the other mechanisms manifests a peak pressure difference late in systole.

The second mechanism whereby a pressure gradient is generated is the most commonly observed and relates to septal-mitral contact during ejection. With the onset of the more forceful than usual contraction and rapid flow acceleration through an outflow tract narrowed by septal hypertrophy, Venturi forces are produced that draw the anterior and/or posterior leaflet of the mitral valve toward the septum.[223,224] Septal-mitral apposition occurs, obstructing the outflow tract and often causing mitral regurgitation. This is the mechanism responsible for the widely recognized echocardiographic finding of systolic anterior motion (SAM) of the mitral valve. In this situation, true obstruction to flow is present and the stenosis is subvalvar, with high pressure in the inflow and apical areas and normal pressure in the outflow region. Flow continues, albeit after a slowing of the flow rate, resulting in the "spike-and-dome" configuration of the aortic pressure tracing, with 40–70% of ejection occurring after the onset of obstruction.[401] As is typical of obstruction to outflow, ejection time is prolonged. This form of obstruction tends to be dynamic, increasing with augmentation of the contractile force or reduction in chamber size. Many physiologic maneuvers have been described that cause the murmur and pressure gradient in the obstructive form of HCM to change. These changes are affected by changes in peripheral resistance, cardiac output, filling volume, contractility, or a combination of these, with secondary alterations in arterial pressure and the magnitude of left ventricular outflow obstruction. For example, angiotensin infusion leads to higher ventricular pressure without altered contractility. The induced rise in systolic volume decreases septal-mitral apposition, reducing or even abolishing the outflow gradient.[399]

The third mechanism that may cause a pressure difference in HCM is cavity obliteration with secondary catheter entrapment. In these subjects, the apical cavity obliterates early in systole.[143] If the pressure catheter is located in the apex, high pressure is recorded as the myocardial force is exerted directly on the catheter,[74] whereas normal pressure is found in the inflow and outflow portions of the left ventricle. Septal-mitral apposition is absent and flow from the high-pressure to the low-pressure area ceases, indicating that this does not represent true obstruction to flow.

Finally, occasionally, obstruction to outflow may occur at a position apical to the mitral valve leaflets, at the mid-ventricular level. In this situation the obstruction is at the level of the enlarged papillary muscle, with elevated apical pressure but normal pressure in the inflow and outflow portion of the ventricle. There is a distinguishable apical chamber that generally does not empty substantially once obstruction ensues in midsystole.[401,402]

Conflicting data exist concerning the influence of the presence of obstruction to left ventricular outflow on the course of the disease, with some authors noting no relation to symptoms or sudden death but others finding a direct relation between the gradient and the symptomatic status.[400] Surgical or pharmacologic reduction in the outflow gradient is usually associated with a reduction in symptoms, although apparently the incidence of sudden death is not improved.

Diastolic Dysfunction. By definition, systolic dysfunction is not a primary feature of HCM, although occasional progression to a dilated, congestive cardiomyopathy has been described. However, a large body of evidence has now accumulated, indicating that diastolic dysfunction is a prominent feature of HCM and often plays a substantial role in its physiologic consequences.[24,38,50,163,285,318,319,338,402] As discussed in chapter 15, diastole consists of two phases, relaxation and passive filling, both of which are disturbed in HCM. Several mechanisms probably contribute to the abnormalities in relaxation: (1) asynchronous activation and inactivation, (2) ischemia, and (3) a possible primary defect in cellular calcium handling. Similarly, abnormal passive properties are also multifactorial: (1) increased wall thickness alone decreases chamber compliance, regardless of whether myocardial compliance is impaired, and (2) myocardial fibrosis may also influence chamber stiffness through increased intrinsic myocardial stiffness. In addition to the congestive symptoms that result from the elevation in diastolic pressure, diastolic dysfunction also impairs myocardial blood flow, further predisposing the hypertrophied ventricle to ischemia.

Chest Pain. This is one of the most common complaints in HCM. The chest pain may have characteristics of angina but often is atypical, occurring at rest, having a variable threshold of onset, and perhaps being prolonged in duration. Although the similarity of the chest pain in some subjects with HCM to that in coronary artery disease suggests that ischemia may be responsible, most subjects with HCM are free of epicardial coronary artery disease. Thus, if the pain is ischemic, the mechanism is different from that in patients with coronary artery disease. In fact, multiple studies of symptomatic patients with HCM, with or without obstruction, have shown metabolic evidence of myocardial ischemia (decreased myocardial lactate uptake or net lactate production) during pacing or catecholamine infusion.[57,76,277,284,372] Patients without a history of chest pain do not manifest the same ischemic response to these stresses. Chest pain is common in children and teenagers with HCM; however, similar studies have not been performed in this group.

Several features of this disease could predispose to ischemia. As noted previously, abnormal intramural coronary arteries are often present. The absolute increase in mass requires higher net coronary flow. In many hypertrophic processes neovascularization fails to keep pace with growth of new myofibrils, resulting in increased diffusion distance. Whether abnormal neovascularization is present in HCM is not known, although reduced coronary reserve has been found, the magnitude of which correlated with left ventricular mass.[344] Elevated diastolic pressure and impaired relaxation interfere with diastolic coronary perfusion, and systolic compression of epicardial and septal perforator vessels interferes with systolic coronary flow.[288] The importance of these various mechanisms in any given patient is unknown.

Clinical Manifestations. *History.* In about half of these patients it is possible to elicit a history of another family member with HCM or a family history of sudden death at a young age. Although many young patients are asymptomatic, the full spectrum of symptoms associated with this disease may be present from early childhood. The chest pain is often not typical of angina, occurring at rest, lasting for several hours without enzymatic evidence of myocardial necrosis, and being unpredictable in onset. Subjects may have no pain on maximal exercise testing on one occasion and then experience severe pain early in exercise on another. Needless to say, this makes assessment of therapy difficult. Reduced exercise tolerance due to dyspnea is common, although congestive symptoms are not, at least beyond the age of 1 year. In contrast, infants with HCM often are brought to the clinic with symptoms more typical of congestive heart failure, with tachypnea, distended abdomen, and poor feeding and growth. Palpitations are common in adults but rarely noted by children. More frequently, episodes of paroxysmal tachycardia are reported, often with symptoms suggestive of hypotension. Syncope occurs in 15–25% of adult subjects but is less common in childhood. Generally, it is not related to documented arrhythmias but is strongly associated with the risk of sudden death, especially in the young.

Physical Examination. Most children and young adults appear remarkably healthy, and many patients are athletes. Although many physical findings have been described for this disease, most relate to dynamic ventricular outflow obstruction and are absent in subjects without obstruction. Therefore, a completely normal physical examination in a healthy patient, who may be athletic, does not exclude the presence of this potentially fatal disorder. This observation has led some observers to suggest echocardiographic screening as part of an evaluation prior to sports participation. The apical and parasternal cardiac impulses are often augmented but rarely displaced. Hepatomegaly is common in infants but rarely encountered beyond this age. In the presence of outflow obstruction, a bisferiens carotid pulse may be encountered, corresponding to the "spike-and-dome" aortic pulse contour. Parasternal and carotid systolic thrills are frequent in patients with left or right ventricular outflow obstruction. The murmur of dynamic left ventricular outflow obstruction may be noted, with a typical pattern of changes in response to maneuvers and extrasystoles.[203] Very loud systolic murmurs are usually found in subjects with subpulmonary stenosis, which is more common in infants and children with the disease than in adults. The murmur of mitral regurgitation is frequent, though difficult to separate from the loud outflow murmur. Aortic regurgitation may be heard but is less commonly encountered than in discrete subaortic stenosis.

Electrocardiography. Although very few patients with HCM and obstruction to left ventricular outflow have a normal electrocardiogram, about 25% of patients without obstruction have normal tracings. The most common abnormalities are left ventricular hypertrophy, changes in the S-T segment and T wave, and abnormal Q waves. These electrocardiograms can certainly be dramatic, although rarely diagnostic.

Chest X-ray. Usually, the chest x-ray is not helpful, demonstrating a normal cardiac silhouette and normal pulmonary vasculature. If cardiac enlargement is present it generally reflects the atrial enlargement that is usually seen in this disease.

Echocardiography. The echocardiogram has become the diagnostic standard in HCM because it allows one to visualize directly the ventricular size, thickness, and systolic function. Although numerous M-mode findings have been reported, the two-dimensional echocardiogram provides a full picture of the anatomic abnormalities and, when it is combined with Doppler interrogation, the physiology can generally be understood as well. Although certain patients cannot be adequately imaged by transthoracic echocardiography, with the advent of transesophageal techniques even this obstacle can be overcome. The entire heart can be visualized in multiple tomographic planes, allowing complete definition of regional hypertrophy. Several studies have documented the incidence of involvement of the various anatomic regions.[222,234,342,402] Localized hypertrophy of the anterior septum is seen in 10–15% of patients, and 20–35% of patients have involvement of both anterior and posterior portions of the septum. At least 50% of patients have involvement of the anterolateral free wall in addition to the septum. The incidence of isolated involvement of the posterior and apical portions of the septum or anterolateral free wall without hypertrophy of the anterior septum is as much as 20%. The reported incidence of concentric hypertrophy is variable but may be as much as 20%.

In addition to defining the location and extent of hypertrophy, echocardiography can also reveal other important features of the disease. The presence of anterior motion of the mitral apparatus can be seen, as well as the presence and extent of septal-mitral apposition.[224,255,402] Systolic fluttering and early closure of the aortic valve may be seen in patients with outflow obstruction.[202] Doppler echocardiography is useful in defining the site and extent of left and/or right ventricular outflow obstruc-tion,[70,274,324,357,371,408] as well as mitral and/or aortic regurgitation.

Both M-mode[150,319] and Doppler[68,121,183,198,230,364] echocardiographic techniques reveal abnormal filling characteristics in most patients. The peak rates of wall thinning and chamber expansion are often subnormal on digitized M-mode echocardiograms. Although early reports indicated that the mitral inflow Doppler patterns in this disease were most consistent with abnormal relaxation,[121,183,198] later reports have demonstrated that nearly any pattern, including normal flow contours, may be seen,[68,230,364] regardless of myocardial and chamber properties. It is now clear that when there are abnormalities of both relaxation and passive chamber properties, mitral inflow patterns tend to normalize, rendering this an unreliable technique for excluding diastolic dysfunction.

Cardiac Catheterization. The hemodynamic findings in this disorder depend on the presence or absence of obstruction. The pressure gradient may be absent, labile (varying between 0 and 200 mm Hg), or constant. The arterial pulse tracing may have a "spike-and-dome" configuration, reflecting midsystolic obstruction to flow. In the obstructive form of the disease, post-extrasystolic beats show a fall in arterial pressure in spite of a marked increase in ventricular pressure, reflecting the rise in contractility and secondary increase in dynamic obstruction. Mean atrial and atrial "a" wave pressures are elevated, as is the ventricular diastolic pressure. Because cavity size is normal or small, the ventricular diastolic pressure:volume relationship is abnormal, indicating reduced chamber compliance. The right ventricle may be involved, particularly in infants and children, with outflow gradients and elevated diastolic pressure. Left ventriculography shows a hypertrophied ventricle with obliteration of the cavity in systole. The enlarged papillary muscles may fill the cavity during systole, and anterior motion of the mitral leaflets into the outflow tract may be evident. Simultaneous right and left ventricular angiography in a cranially angulated, left anterior oblique projection is useful to display the size and configuration of the interventricular septum. In infants, the septum often impinges on the right ventricular outflow, and obliteration of the right ventricular cavity in systole may be noted.

Management. The goals of therapy in this disorder are to reduce symptoms and prolong survival. The symptoms of chest pain, dyspnea, and exercise intolerance can often be managed medically, although surgery has been successful in certain patient groups. The goal of medical management is to reduce ventricular filling pressure, either by improving diastolic function or by increasing chamber size secondary to a decrease in contractility. Digitalis is usually contraindicated unless atrial fibrillation occurs. Although dyspnea is a common symptom, diuretic therapy is usually not beneficial and may increase the outflow gradient because of a reduction in chamber volume. The beneficial effect of maintaining or expanding the circulating blood volume is illustrated by the response to pregnancy. Women with HCM tend to have substantial clinical improvement during the second and third trimesters, with reduction or abolition of outflow gradients related to the increase in blood volume during pregnancy.

The mainstay of therapy for many years was beta-adrenergic blockade. Chest pain and dyspnea are often relieved by propranolol, although increased exercise tolerance is seen less often. The response appears to be dose dependent and very high dosage levels have often been used. Unfortunately, side effects, such as fatigue and depression, are often encountered at these high dosage levels and may be intolerable. In spite of early improvement, symptoms often recur and may not respond to dose escalation. In spite of symptomatic improvement, many studies have failed to show a reduction in mortality in response to propranolol. It should be noted that these studies have invariably been uncontrolled, using historical controls for comparison. Nonetheless, it does not appear that the 3–5% annual mortality associated with this disease is substantially reduced by propranolol therapy.

More recently, calcium blockers in general, and verapamil in particular, have been used extensively in patients with HCM. Improved diastolic relaxation is generally noted in response to the administration of verapamil, with a secondary reduction in diastolic pressure and mean left atrial pressure. This is believed to be the mechanism for the reduction in dyspnea and increase in exercise capacity that occurs. Nearly all patients have substantial and sustained symptomatic improvement; this may be dramatic in some individuals. Some studies have documented a fall in the incidence of sudden death to 1–1.5% per year, but again, these are uncontrolled studies which rely on historical controls.

In patients with outflow obstruction, septal myotomy or myectomy can often relieve both the gradient and mitral regurgitation. Many patients experience striking relief of symptoms, in spite of the fact that symptoms are not generally correlated with the presence and degree of obstruction. However, the operation is associated with significant risk, with an operative mortality of 5–10% and frequent complications such as aortic regurgitation, iatrogenic ventricular septal defect, complete heart block, necessity for mitral valve replacement, and perioperative infarction. Postoperatively, the annual mortality appears to be unchanged. Consequently, surgery is generally reserved for patients with intractable and debilitating symptoms despite maximum medical therapy.

It is presumed that many or most of the instances of sudden death in HCM are arrhythmic events. Therefore, antiarrhythmic therapy appears to represent a rational alternative, but this has not proved highly effective. Although some patients have high-grade ventricular ectopy and are at increased risk of sudden death, this is the exception. In general Holter monitor recordings do not show ectopy in most pediatric patients. Amiodarone has been reported to reduce the incidence of sudden death in certain high-risk subgroups; pediatric experience is limited.

Avoidance of strenuous exercise is generally recommended for patients with HCM because sudden death often occurs during intense exercise. Unfortunately, it has not been shown that survival is improved for those who do not exercise, nor is it known what level of exercise represents a safe limit. The clinician is responsible for advising these patients and their parents as to the safe limits (short of permanent bed rest) for activity. Detraining and social stigmatization are particularly difficult problems for the adolescent who is excluded from the usual school activities and peer interactions. Competitive team sports elicit an emotional overlay that appears to increase the risk associated with the sport itself, in addition to demanding more intense exercise. Certain activities, such as weight lifting, are associated with high levels of circulating catecholamines that may predispose to arrhythmias and elicit a marked stimulus to eccentric cardiac hypertrophy. However, there is little evidence that low-level, aerobic exercise represents a significant risk to these patients, and it does provide measurable hemodynamic and psychological benefits.

Sudden Death. Numerous potential mechanisms exist for sudden death in HCM. Individual reports have described asystole, complete heart block, myocardial infarction, and supraventricular tachycardia with rapid ventricular response as antecedent events.[219,245,248] Hypotension with diminished coronary filling and secondary autonomic outflow would be expected to be particularly poorly tolerated in this disease and may represent a common initiating event. In adults, nonsustained ventricular tachycardia, on ambulatory monitoring, is a highly specific risk factor for sudden death. However, adolescent patients, who have the highest incidence of sudden death, are rarely found to have arrhythmias. The association of exercise with sudden death in patients with this disease may be related to abnormalities of autonomic control, which have been reported to cause exercise-induced hypotension in some subjects.

Course. The clinical course for HCM is highly age-dependent. Hypertrophic cardiomyopathy appears to carry a worse prognosis for infants than for older age groups; symptomatic infants generally manifest congestive heart failure and cyanosis and have a particularly poor outlook, with 9 of 11 in one series dying within the first 5 years.[232] Ventricular hypertrophy may develop during childhood or adolescence, but its appearance in a previously normal adult has not been described. The severity of hypertrophy may progress during periods of accelerated somatic growth in adolescents,[231] but progression does not appear to be a feature of the disease in adults.[246,350] It is not clear whether regression of the disease ever occurs, but if so it is rare. Systolic function does not generally change with time although the transition to a thin-walled congestive cardiomyopathy has been reported[245] in adult patients. In adults with obstruction, the pressure gradient is also generally stable, although progression does occur in children and adolescents. The natural history of diastolic function in HCM and its relation to the tendency toward progressive symptoms have not been adequately defined. Arrhythmias are not common in children; they increase in frequency with age. Although 50% of adult patients are symptomatic at the time of diagnosis, most cases of HCM in children and adolescents are discovered on the basis of screening examinations or abnormal physical findings. The usual course of the disease is slow progression of symptoms with a superimposed high incidence of sudden death. Sudden death results in an annual mortality of 3–5% in adults and 6–8% in children,[245,247,248] and reduction of sudden death is clearly the primary goal in this disease. Improved survival has been reported after surgery or treatment with verapamil and with some antiarrhythmics; however, negative results have also been reported for each of these therapeutic modalities. At this juncture, an effective therapeutic strategy, medical or surgical, which has more than salutary impact on the natural history of the disease, remains to be devised.

Doxorubicin Cardiomyopathy

The anthracycline antibiotics are valuable antitumor agents, and doxorubicin (Adriamycin), in particular, has the broadest spectrum of antitumor activity of available cancer chemotherapeutic agents. Thousands of children have received doxorubicin over the past 20 years, and the drug is used in the therapy of several of the most common pediatric oncologic disorders, including acute lymphocytic leukemia, non-Hodgkin's lymphoma, and osteogenic sarcoma. The usefulness of this agent is limited by a dose-related cardiomyopathy, with congestive heart failure developing in 2–20% of all patients treated with doxorubicin.[192] Because many recipients of doxorubicin are now long-term survivors, late residua from their therapy often represent their most important clinical problems. At Boston Children's Hospital, doxorubicin is the most common cause of chronic congestive cardiomyopathy in children.

Mechanism of Anthracycline-mediated Cardiac Injury. The pathogenesis of doxorubicin cardiotoxicity, although not completely understood, is thought to involve the generation of reactive oxygen species resulting from the reduction of doxorubicin to its semiquinone free-radical form.[3,266,373] Among the mechanisms that have been hypothesized to account for doxorubicin-induced cardiotoxicity, current evidence supports lipid peroxidation, oxidation of critical sulfhydryl groups, and/or release of calcium from sarcoplasmic reticulum.[2,197,279,294,346,347,414] These mechanisms need not be mutually exclusive. Thus, the long-term cumulative effect of doxorubicin may be related to free-radical induction, leading to the peroxidation of membrane phospholipids, thereby altering membrane permeability or calcium channel function.[71,153,171,375,390] Similarly, oxidation of critical thiol groups associated with the channel complex could alter channel function. The cardioselectivity of these actions may reflect an enhanced susceptibility of the heart to oxidant stress caused by low levels of superoxide dismutase, catalase, and glutathione peroxidase.[294] The clinical importance of these findings relates to the potential for reduced toxicity if the cardiac injury can be reduced without interference with antitumor activity. Although the mechanism of antitumor activity is also speculative, doxorubicin is known to bind to mammalian DNA and is believed to exert antitumor activity through DNA fragmentation and inhibition of DNA synthesis.[62] It appears that it may be possible in animal modes to reduce the severity of cardiac cell injury by mechanisms that reduce free-radical formation without altering the antitumor efficacy.[262] Although very promising, it has not yet been confirmed whether clinical cardiac toxicity in humans is amenable to such manipulation.

Histopathology of Anthracycline Cardiotoxicity. Numerous investigators have studied the histologic changes of doxorubicin cardiomyopathy in both animals and humans on postmortem tissues and endomyocardial biopsies.[45,46,182,192] The histologic abnormalities are not unique to doxorubicin cardiomyopathy but are distinguishable from the changes seen in response to radiation or ischemia. The lesions are typically disseminated yet focal, with normal tissue adjacent to damaged tissues. Microscopic examination of postmortem tissue reveals a rather distinctive appearance of vascular degeneration and interstitial edema without evidence of inflammatory changes. The intracellular vacuoles are due to distention and swelling of the sarcoplasmic reticulum, and the severity of the histologic injury increases as the total dose increases. Ultrastructurally, the damage to myocytes takes two forms: myofibrillar loss with intact mitochondria, and vacuolar degeneration, with the earliest manifestation being distention of the sarcoplasmic reticulum. Both lesions progress until myocyte death, at which point mitochondrial degeneration and cristolysis ensue. Many of the ultrastructural changes are nonspecific and occur in other forms of cardiomyopathy, including vacuolization and distention of the sarcoplasmic reticulum.

Clinical Manifestations. Clinically, the adverse effects of the anthracycline antibiotics can be divided into acute, subacute, and chronic toxicity.[13,47,122,192,212,410] Occasionally, supraventricular arrhythmias and ventricular premature beats are noted during, and shortly after, administration of doxorubicin, but these are rarely clinically important.[355] There are rare reports of a subacute syndrome of transient left ventricular dysfunction or a pericarditis/myocarditis syndrome.[47] However, it is the chronic effects of doxorubicin that represent the most significant clinical problem. Generally, the patient has a congestive cardiomyopathy with left ventricular dysfunction, elevated filling pressures, and reduced cardiac output, with onset 2–4 months after completion of therapy. The ventricular dysfunction is based on a cumulative myocardial insult and congestive failure is often delayed for a period of time after the last dose of the drug because of a time delay in the full cytotoxic effect of the drug.[185] The mean latency period has been reported to be 3–8 weeks,[26,253,254,295,391,392] with occasional reports of congestive heart failure appearing several years after the completion of therapy.[108,131,134] Although initial experience indicated that after the onset of symptoms doxorubicin-induced cardiomyopathy was rapidly progressive, irreversible, and always fatal, more recent reports describe survival for years after the onset of clinical cardiotoxicity, with occasional recovery of function.[210,316]

Most investigations have focused on the incidence of congestive heart failure in assessing late outcome after doxorubicin therapy. However, it has been well established that myocardial injury accompanies even relatively low cumulative doses, with histopathologic evidence of injury present after as little as 180 mg/m^2 of body surface area.[45] Although the morphologic damage is proportional to the total cumulative dose, there is considerable variability in the onset of histologic and functional changes. In fact, functional abnormalities correlate weakly with dose, and little or no clinical deterioration is noted until a certain patient-specific threshold dose is surpassed.[46] The incidence of clinical congestive heart failure is dose-related in a nonlinear fashion,[46] with 2–5% of patients experiencing symptomatic cardiotoxicity after cumulative doses of 400–500 mg/m^2. However, even with cumulative doses in excess of 1000 mg/m^2, no more than 50% of patients develop clinical congestive heart failure.[392] Thus, it is clear that symptomatic cardiac injury represents a poor measure of the true extent of doxorubicin cardiotoxicity.

Survivors of childhood cancer constitute a patient group of particular importance because of their long life expectancy and the superimposed influences of growth and development. At The Children's Hospital in Boston, the authors have evaluated a large, relatively homogeneous cohort of patients who were previously treated for acute lymphocytic leukemia. The children were evaluated 1–15 years (median = 6.4 years) after a total cumulative dose that varied from 45–550 mg/m^2 (median = 324 mg/m^2). Echocardiographic evidence of abnormal myocardial mechanics was found in 62% of the subjects, with 39% having elevated afterload, 7% having reduced contractility, and 16% having both excess afterload and reduced contractility. The 55% incidence of excess afterload was attributable mostly to abnormal ventricular wall thickness. Myocardial afterload (wall stress) is determined by ventricular dimension, wall thickness, and pressure. Pressure was not elevated in these patients and cavity dimension tended to be at most minimally increased. However, wall thickness was decreased, particularly when considered with reference to ventricular dimension. Thus, the left ventricular mass/volume ratio was abnormally low because of low mass. In patients in whom serial studies were available, 74% demonstrated a progressive rise in afterload over a mean period of 3.1 years. In these subjects, the increase in ventricular dimension was proportional to somatic growth, but wall thickness failed to increase proportionately. The clinical history was of limited use in evaluating these patients, because there was no relation between reported symptoms and any of the abnormalities on the echocardiogram or on exercise capacity during treadmill exercise testing.

Total cumulative dose, age at the time of doxorubicin therapy, and the length of time since completion of therapy were each related to the incidence of cardiac abnormalities. Excess afterload was most closely related to age at therapy and time since therapy, whereas abnormal contractility was determined predominantly by the total cumulative dose and was strongly related to depression of function early after completion of therapy. These differences, as well as the histologic findings, led to the conclusion that these abnormalities represent two different processes. Depressed contractility appears to represent the usual form of cardiotoxicity which has been commonly reported in pediatric and adult series of doxorubicin recipients. This injury appears to be relatively stable after completion of therapy. However, excess afterload is a particular risk for the patient less than 4 years old; it appears gradually over time and becomes manifest as inadequate myocardial growth compared with the rate of somatic growth. This form of doxorubicin-mediated cardiac injury appears to represent impaired growth capacity of the myocardium, a problem of particular importance to the small child.

Risk Factors for Doxorubicin Cardiotoxicity. Numerous clinical studies have identified certain factors that place patients at increased risk for the adverse cardiac effects of doxorubicin. Patients older than 70 years and younger than 4 years appear to be at increased risk.[296,392] Some investigators[45,46,295] (though not all)[392] have found prior or concurrent mediastinal irradiation to increase the risk. Coadministration of cyclophosphamide may be a risk factor,[379] but this was not confirmed in several large studies.[254,295,392] Although the use of several additional chemotherapeutic agents has been reported to increase the risk of doxorubicin cardiomyopathy, this risk has not been adequately confirmed for any except mitomycin. Preexisting hypertension or cardiac disease has been associated with increased risk.[46,295,392] However, the two factors that have been found to bear the strongest relationship to the incidence of cardiotoxicity are the total cumulative dose and the dosing regimen.

The relationship between the total cumulative dose of doxorubicin and symptomatic cardiotoxicity is nonlinear, with an inflection point somewhere between 400 and 600 mg/m^2. For example, in one study the incidence of doxorubicin cardiomyopathy was 7% in subjects who received less than 550 mg/m^2, increasing to 18% in the patients who received 750 mg/m^2.[392] Although there is some variation in the dose at which the incidence of congestive heart failure has been observed to rise, this general pattern has been observed in the numerous studies in which it has been examined.

A weekly dosing regimen is associated with less cardiotoxicity than the standard regimen of dosing every 3 weeks.[13,380] Smaller, more frequent dosing results in lower plasma concentrations. If free-radical formation is an important component in the mechanism of doxorubicin-induced cardiomyopathy, lower plasma levels would be less likely to exceed the tissue free-radical scavenger systems, resulting in less myofibrillar damage.[27] In support of this concept, a number of reports indicate that further reduction in toxicity can be achieved by continuous infusion therapy.[117,173,208,358] Furthermore, although studies to date indicate that there is a definite relationship between doxorubicin plasma levels and cardiotoxicity, no such relationship to therapeutic response has been shown.[77]

Prevention of Doxorubicin Cardiomyopathy. The approaches to toxicity reduction which have been used include altered dosing regimens with lower peak serum levels, coadministration of agents aimed at reducing oxygen radical injury, and dose reduction, either to a predetermined maximum or as dictated by one of several monitoring programs. As mentioned above, several studies indicate that continuous infusion therapy can successfully reduce cardiac injury. Several agents which might provide protection have been investigated, including vitamin E,[162,413] selenium (a cofactor for glutathione peroxidase),[86,179,265] N-acetylcysteine and cysteamine,[293] taurine,[148,149]

L-carnitine,[83] coenzyme Q10,[138,269] and ICRF 187.[8,33,158] Although many of these agents appear to reduce toxicity in animal models, with few exceptions[83,349] these results have not been duplicated in humans. Nevertheless, this preliminary work appears promising.

Programs based on dose restriction continue to be the most commonly employed means of attempting to prevent doxorubicin cardiomyopathy. In general, two approaches have been followed. Many centers have elected to limit the total cumulative dose to a level that results in an "acceptable" incidence of cardiomyopathy. For example, if a maximum cumulative dose of 400–500 mg/m^2 is chosen, congestive heart failure should occur in fewer than 5% of patients. However, the disadvantage to this approach is that regardless of the exact limit that is chosen, many patients could safely receive a higher dose of the drug because of marked differences in individual susceptibility to doxorubicin-induced cardiomyopathy. Consequently, monitoring programs have been widely employed that attempt to detect cardiotoxicity on an individual basis, thereby permitting individual dosing regimens, with dose reduction in patients with evidence of cardiac injury. It has been demonstrated that doxorubicin-induced myocardial injury can be detected by several different means, including endomyocardial biopsy,[45,46,182] cardiac catheterization,[45,46] echocardiography,[26,32,159,177] radionuclide angiography during rest and exercise,[6,9,67,209,249,280,291,330,356,359] and magnetic resonance relaxation properties.[374] In some cases, the accuracy of the test for prediction of congestive heart failure has been tested. Although various means have been employed to detect myocardial injury, in other regards the monitoring programs that have been recommended are quite similar. The basic approach is to evaluate patients periodically during doxorubicin therapy and to delay or discontinue the drug in patients who have abnormal test results.[9,26,32,45,67,209,249,291,330,356] Although conceptually simple, verification of the utility of this type of cardiac monitoring program introduces a number of complex issues that have not been fully addressed.

Treatment. 1. Treatment goals. It is often assumed that cardiotoxicity can be reduced without adversely affecting antitumor efficacy. Unless there is a direct correlation between myocardial damage and chemotherapeutic efficacy, or a higher than needed cumulative dose is planned, a program that, by design, reduces the total cumulative dose *must* decrease antitumor effect. Reduction in cardiotoxicity must be viewed as a tradeoff between cancer and cardiac disease. For example, if dose reduction in response to an abnormal cardiac test eliminates symptomatic heart disease but results in an increased relapse rate in children with leukemia, it is clear that a mild-to-moderate degree of cardiac compromise would represent a preferable alternative. Evaluation of the success of any cardiac monitoring program must include a decision as to how much cardiac injury is acceptable relative to the probable antitumor benefit from a given treatment regimen. At perhaps the most simplistic level, documentation of improved overall survival is needed. None of the monitoring programs published to date has documented improved survival, nor has the impact on antitumor effect been assessed.

2. Antitumor efficacy. Documentation of reduced chemotherapeutic efficacy is often hampered by methodologic limitations in assessment of antitumor activity. Thus, for palliative treatment of disseminated neoplasms there is often a limited ability to estimate the tumor burden, and curative treatment protocols may require years to evaluate changes in relapse rate. Most studies of the usefulness of cardiac monitoring programs have not used concurrent controls, relying on historical controls for cure rates. Rarely are the patient groups or treatment protocols similar enough in other respects to ensure that the monitoring program is solely responsible for observed differences.

3. Is monitoring superior to dose reduction? Because the cardiac monitoring lowers the total cumulative dose in a percent of patients, a reduced incidence of cardiomyopathy would be anticipated even if the dose reduction were randomly applied. Thus, the monitoring program may result in a sufficient number of patients having early drug discontinuation that the mean cumulative dose for a specific protocol is reduced from 550 to 450 mg/m^2. The monitoring program can be considered successful only if the result for both cardiotoxicity and antitumor efficacy are superior to nonselective dose reduction to a similar degree.

4. Effect of known risk factors. Several studies have shown that there are several identifiable risk factors for doxorubicin-associated cardiomyopathy. Nearly all children are free of the known risk factors, and the efficacy of the monitoring program appears to be substantially reduced in patients without known risk factors.

5. Specificity for congestive heart failure. Although many of these tests have proved sensitive for doxorubicin-induced cardiomyopathy, the false-positive rate is usually very high. The effect of this lack of specificity on the monitoring program is that 20–30% of patients who could, in fact, tolerate higher doses of the drug have inappropriate discontinuation of therapy because of the false-positive rate.[159,273] Although the overall incidence of congestive heart failure may be effectively diminished under these circumstances, the effect on antitumor treatment remains to be determined.

Nearly all these concerns could be addressed by comparison of late outcomes in a prospective, controlled study of cardiac monitoring. In one of the few efforts to employ a prospective, controlled study the reduction in incidence of congestive heart failure by a program of periodic endomyocardial biopsy and right heart catheterization was not significant, even in high-risk patients.[44] At present, the benefits of serial cardiac assessment for doxorubicin-induced cardiomyopathy as a means of dose adjustment in low-risk patients, such as children, remain enticing but unproven.

Prognosis. The long-term consequences of symptomatic and/or subclinical doxorubicin cardiomyopathy are poorly characterized. Although improvement in cardiac function has been reported after discontinuation of doxorubicin[210,316] abnormalities which are present several months after completion of therapy often do not improve, even if clinical status stabilizes.[130,133] Determining the outcome from doxorubicin-induced cardiomyopathy is complicated by the fact that many patients die from their underlying disease.[151] Symptomatic idiopathic cardiomyopathy is known to entail a high mortality. In one study, 63% of children survived for 1 year and 34% for 5 years.[366] In a more recent study in children more than 2 years of age with dilated cardiomyopathy, the 2-year survival rate was 20% and all 12 patients were dead by 9 years after onset of the illness, regardless of whether congestive heart failure was present at the time of diagnosis.[140] More data concerning the prognosis in congestive cardiomyopathy are available from studies in adults, where 15–60% annual mortality rates are reported and 60–75% are dead at 5 years after the onset.[236,381] The degree of ventricular dysfunction correlates closely in a hyperbolic fashion with survival, so that reduction of the ejection fraction from 60 down to 30% is associated with an increase in annual mortality of 10–20%.[282]

Elevated ventricular afterload is common in patients with ventricular dysfunction. At least 50% of recipients of doxorubicin have an abnormal elevation of afterload, with or without abnormal contractility, and the excess afterload appears to progress with time. Other investigators have also noted that the incidence of cardiac abnormalities in children previously treated with doxorubicin increases with time.[218] The secondary effects of increased left ventricular wall stress (afterload) include augmented normalized work load and increased myocardial oxygen consumption. The consequences of prolonged elevation of left ventricular wall stress are not clear, but there is some evidence that this is one factor contributing to the eventual myocardial deterioration associated with lesions causing left ventricular volume and pressure overload.[39] Years will be required to fully evaluate the long-term consequences of doxorubicin-induced abnormalities of myocardial mechanics in young survivors of childhood cancer.

Friedreich's Ataxia

Friedreich's ataxia is an autosomal recessive hereedofamilial disorder[12] characterized by progressive degeneration of the spinocerebellar tracts, including the dorsal columns, pyramidal tracts, and to some extent the cerebellum and medulla. In addition to the neurologic deficit, which is secondary to the dying-back neuropathy, there is muscular weakness in the majority of patients after the first few years, with initial involvement of the lower extremities and later development of weakness in the upper limbs. Diabetes and cardiomyopathy are present in most, if not all, patients with Friedreich's ataxia. The chief clinical expression is ataxia, which becomes manifest before adolescence, with incoordination of limb movements, nystagmus, dysarthria, absence of the deep tendon reflexes, impairment of sense of position, and progressive development of scoliosis, pes cavus, and hammer toe. Affected children frequently become wheelchair bound in the second or third decades of life, and scoliosis is found in nearly all.[10,78] Because of the association of pes cavus and awkward gait, the clinical findings are similar to those of peripheral neuropathies, particularly early in the disease. Cardiac abnormalities have been identified in nearly all subjects with Friedreich's ataxia.

Etiology. The etiology of Friedreich's ataxia is not known, nor has the genetic defect been identified. A deficiency of a mitochondrial malic enzyme has been found in Friedreich's ataxia.[360] Thus, the propensity toward neuropathy and cardiomyopathy could be attributed to the fact that activity of this enzyme is usually highest in these tissues, and this has been proposed as a unifying hypothesis in this disease.[22]

Cardiomyopathy. Abnormalities of the heart have been considered part of the disease since Friedreich's original description.[286]

Histopathology. Individual myocyte hypertrophy, widely scattered focal degeneration, and varying degree of interstitial fibrosis are the major features.[188,205,382] The marked disorganization of the hypertrophied muscle cells that is characteristic of hypertrophic cardiomyopathy is not a pathologic feature of the heart disease in Friedreich's ataxia.

Clinical Manifestations. The clinical manifestations of cardiac abnormalities in Friedreich's ataxia are usually noted during the late stages of the disease. The cardiac symptoms consist of exertional dyspnea, palpitations, chest pain, and pedal edema. Respiratory failure is the usual late outcome in Friedreich's ataxia, and it can be attributed to the combination of severe scoliosis and neuromuscular dysfunction.[52] In light of the skeletal deformity and neurologic disability, it is difficult to know when dyspnea is a manifestation of cardiac involvement in these patients.

Electrocardiography. Some abnormality of the electrocardiogram has been found in from 75–90% of patients.[5,59,132,286] Repolarization abnormalities, including diffuse T-wave inversion, are the most commonly reported findings, being seen in 40–90% of patients.[5,132,152,286] Interestingly, repolarization abnormalities are seen in some patients with echocardiographically normal hearts. Atrial tachycardia, particularly atrial flutter, or fibrillation, is the most common arrhythmia,[5,132,282,283,286] and is found in as many as 50% of patients before death.[164] Atrial dysrhythmias are generally a late manifestation and are usually associated with ventricular dysfunction and congestive heart failure.[5]

Echocardiography. Hypertrophy of varying degrees of severity and patterns of involvement has been observed in all studies. All patterns and gradation can be found, with concentric, asymmetric and no hypertrophy each seen in some percentage of patients.

Management. Supportive therapy is all that is available in 1991.

Course. The importance of the cardiac disease to the ultimate clinical course in Friedreich's ataxia is somewhat difficult to ascertain. There are no long-term prospective studies of the natural history of the disease. Although a number of more recent reports document cardiac dysfunction in occasional patients, establishing the overall clinical significance of the myocardial abnormalities associated with Friedreich's ataxia awaits studies that comprehensively examine the relationship of cardiac function to the commonly noted problem of dyspnea and/or respiratory insufficiency.

Similarities between the cardiac findings in Friedreich's ataxia and hypertrophic cardiomyopathy have led some investigators to suggest that hypertrophic cardiomyopathy is the characteristic cardiac manifestation of Friedreich's ataxia. This suggestion is based on observation of some patients with Friedreich's ataxia in whom there is a hypertrophied nondilated heart with asymmetric septal hypertrophy and dynamic left ventricular outflow tract obstruction.[34,73,116,312] Although there are certainly some cases with asymmetric septal hypertrophy, the predominant form of hypertrophy in Friedreich's ataxia appears to be concentric. This contrasts with hypertrophic cardiomyopathy, in which concentric hypertrophy is seen occasionally but asymmetric involvement is the norm. Myocardial disarray, the pathologic hallmark of hypertrophic cardiomyopathy, is absent in Friedreich's ataxia. Ventricular arrhythmias and sudden death, which are frequent in hypertrophic cardiomyopathy, are not commonly reported in Friedreich's ataxia. Thus, although the abnormal hypertrophy that is often seen in Friedreich's ataxia may represent a form of hypertrophic cardiomyopathy, the implications do not seem to be the same as those usually associated with this diagnosis.

Duchenne's and Becker's Muscular Dystrophies

With an incidence of about 1/30,000 live births,[98] the Duchenne form of muscular dystrophy is the most common and most severe type of childhood progressive muscular dystrophy. Transmission of the genetic defect is by an X-linked recessive gene, with approximately two-thirds of mothers of affected boys thought to be carriers. Although serum levels of creatinine kinase and other sarcoplasmic enzymes are elevated from birth, the first clinical manifestation is weakness, which becomes apparent when the child begins to walk, or between 2 and 6 years of age at the latest. Weakness progresses to an inability to walk by the end of the first decade, with the development of contractures, progressive deformity, and severe kyphoscoliosis in the later stages. Invariably there is an associated cardiomyopathy, although this is usually masked by the consequences of the skeletal myopathy. The average age at death is 18–19 years, with occasional survival to age 25 or 30.[263] Death is related to respiratory insufficiency in 90% of the cases. Although occasionally the cardiomyopathy is of clinical importance, the distinction between cardiac and pulmonary compromise has not been vigorously pursued because of the absence of available therapeutic options.

Molecular Basis. Substantial progress has been made in understanding the molecular basis for Duchenne's muscular dystrophy, with cloning of the affected gene and characterization of the missing protein product, dystrophin.[169,331] Dystrophin is predominantly localized in the plasma membrane of striated muscle cells and appears to be a component of the membrane cytoskeleton in myogenic cells.[397] The protein is normally present in the surface membrane of both skeletal and cardiac muscle, and it is absent in both locations in patients with Duchenne's muscular dystrophy.[15] The structure of dystrophin is similar to that of other cytoskeletal proteins and is thought to be important in maintaining the structural integrity of the plasma membrane. The proposed mechanisms whereby the absence of dystrophin leads to cell injury are either through increased susceptibility to mechanical injury to the sarcolemma during the application of the force of contraction or through excess cation permeability leading to excess Ca^{++} influx and secondary sarcolemma breakdown.[20,89,311]

Becker's dystrophy is a milder disease with similar clinical manifestations and slower progression. Because the genetic abnormalities that underlie these disorders have been defined, it has been possible to determine that these clinically distinct disorders actually represent variable abnormalities in the same gene. The unifying feature of these diseases is an abnormality of either the quantity or composition of dystrophin. Dystrophin is absent in nearly all patients with the Duchenne phenotype,[36] but in Becker's dystrophy there may be either reduced quantities of a normal protein or normal quantities of a structurally abnormal protein.[170] Cases with intermediate severity represent variable expression of these same gene defects. Dystrophin electrophoresis is diagnostically useful in this regard because it permits accurate distinction between cases with more serious and less serious prognoses.[170]

Histopathology. The absence of dystrophin in cardiac muscle results in a histologic pattern that is similar to that in skeletal muscle. Myocardial ultrastructural changes include loss of thick and thin myofilaments, ranging from having a motheaten appearance to total myofibrillar loss.[321] The heart shows multifocal degenerative changes of varying severity. Fibrosis is a prominent feature, with the epicardial regions showing more extensive changes.[107] The posterobasilar region of the left ventricle has been reported to be the most severely involved,[321] and the left ventricular free wall of the myocardium is generally described as showing diffuse but spotty involvement. The atria and right ventricle tend to be the least affected, with the interventricular septum somewhat more so. Involvement of the posterior papillary muscles probably accounts for the mitral valve prolapse that is often observed.[320]

Clinical Manifestations. *Electrocardiography.* The electrocardiogram in Duchenne's muscular dystrophy is characterized by tall, narrow R waves in the anterior precordial leads, and deep, narrow Q waves in the lateral leads. The Q waves are present from the earliest stages of the disease and do not progress over time. The same electrocardiographic pattern is noted in the asymptomatic female carriers of Duchenne's muscular dystrophy.

Persistent or labile sinus tachycardia is present from early in the disease. On 24-hour electrocardiographic recordings the rate may never fall below 100 beats per minute. In contrast to the normal age-related fall in heart rate, the tachycardia persists and may even progress with age.[323] The cause of the sinus tachycardia is unknown.

Echocardiography. Mitral valve prolapse has been reported in about 50% of subjects,[322,407] although these data were based on M-mode echocardiography studies for which the diagnostic criteria may be less reliable. At The Children's Hospital in Boston, echocardiographic studies, with an apical four-chamber, two-dimensional view, have shown prolapse of sufficient magnitude to result in displacement of mitral leaflets posterior to the mitral annulus in about 10% of patients. Factors that have been reported to be responsible for the increased incidence of mitral valve prolapse in Duchenne's muscular dystrophy include involvement of the subvalvar apparatus in the degenerative process, geometric changes due to reduction in atrial and ventricular dimensions, and distortion of left ventricular geometry related to the deformity of the thorax that is usually seen.[407]

Cardiac Catheterization. This is rarely indicated in these patients.

Myocardial Function. Most cardiac functional data are derived from echocardiographic and radionuclide studies. The thickness of the left ventricular posterior wall and the dimensions of the cavity are less than those of age-matched normal individuals.[126,127,239] The left ventricular free-wall thickness and short-axis dimension have been studied serially in patients with Duchenne's muscular dystrophy and were found to decrease inappropriately with age.[127,239] This pattern of "atrophic heart" was noted in those patients who were the most emaciated and showed the most motor impairment. However, even when compared with a group of wheelchair-bound controls the left ventricular measurements were reduced (Table 1).[127]

Likewise, most studies of ventricular function have noted abnormal systolic function with progressive abnormalities over time. Reduced shortening fraction[126,165,176,181] and velocity of shortening[165] have been found.

Because each of these ejection phase indices (systolic time intervals, ejection fraction, shortening fraction, mean velocity of shortening) is dependent on both contractility and load, it is not possible to determine what role is played by each of these factors. When the authors evaluated patients with Duchenne's muscular dystrophy who had a wide range of systolic performance, it was found that although contractility appeared lower than that in age-matched controls, the predominant factor that accounted for the fall in systolic function was excess afterload (Fig. 1). In these patients abnormal wall thickness was the single abnormal factor that accounted for the observed excess afterload.

Even in the presence of severe ventricular dysfunction, these patients do not manifest ventricular dilatation. This abnormal end-diastolic pressure/volume relation indicates reduced compliance, as would be seen in a restrictive myopathy. Additionally the marked fibrosis that is evident histologically would be expected to severely reduce myocardial and chamber compliance.

Management. Advances in the knowledge about the molecular basis for Duchenne's muscular dystrophy have not yet had an effect on the clinical management. Even recognition of cardiac involvement is not simple or routine. Clinical evaluation, electrocardiograms, isoenzyme determinations, and chest x-rays have not been helpful in assessing the degree of cardiac involvement.[79] The skeletal and cardiac involvement in Duchenne's muscular dystrophy may progress at different rates. Therefore, the extent of cardiac impairment cannot be deduced from assessment of skeletal muscle weak-

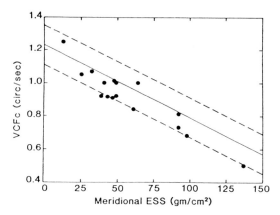

Figure 1. Relationship of rate-adjusted velocity of circumferential shortening (VCFc) to meridional end-systolic wall stress (ESS) in 16 teenage patients with Duchenne's muscular dystrophy evaluated prior to scoliosis surgery. The mean value for the normal population (solid line) and 95% confidence intervals (interrupted lines) for this relationship are shown. Although marked ventricular dysfunction was present in many, as indicated by the low VCFc values, this was mostly due to high afterload (ESS). After consideration of the effect of afterload, many subjects tended to be near the lower limits of normal (points near the lower confidence interval line); distinctly abnormal values (indicting abnormal contractility) were not found.

ness. The electrocardiographic abnormalities do not evolve with age, negating the potential usefulness of this tool. The heart does not dilate in spite of impaired function, limiting the utility of chest x-rays in detecting cardiac dysfunction. Thus, some means of specific assessment of cardiac performance must be used, such as echocardiography, or radionuclide ventriculography. At The Children's Hospital in Boston we have relied on echocardiographic assessment, although in our experience at least 25% of these subjects cannot be adequately evaluated by ultrasound once the nonambulatory phase of the disease is reached. We have had no personal experience with evaluation prior to initiation of assisted ventilation. However, many of these patients have major orthopedic surgical procedures performed in our institution and we have monitored our experience in these patients.

Surgery is known to be a somewhat dangerous prospect in patients with Duchenne's muscular dystrophy, leading some institutions to advise against it altogether. In the authors' opinion, if the risks are properly defined and appropriate precautions are taken, the truly high-risk patients can be excluded and surgery can be performed in the remainder with reasonable risk. Delivery of anesthesia is notoriously hazardous in these patients, with reports of hyperthermia, cardiac arrest, and acute rhabdomyolysis.[56,160,206,337,348,396] The heart in Duchenne's muscular dystrophy has been reported to be excessively sensitive to a number of non-anesthetic agents, including the calcium channel blocking agent, verapamil.[412] Thus, pharmacologic interventions must be carefully considered and creative therapy is to be avoided. In general, anesthetic regimens with the least cardiodepressent actions are used in these patients,[341] but in the presence of known cardiac dysfunction, additional intraoperative and postoperative monitoring is employed, with placement of systemic artery and pulmonary artery thermodilution catheters to continuously record cardiac output, pulmonary artery wedge pressure, and arterial pressure. Because such additional precautions are relatively easy to implement, this is generally a simple decision with little controversy.

The most difficult decision is faced when one attempts to define criteria by which patients should be excluded from surgery altogether. Certainly the nature of the contemplated procedure should influence this decision. Spinal fusion is one of the most common operations performed in the late stages of the disease. This operation causes the most extreme form of cardiovascular stress, with marked shifts in blood fluid, prolonged delivery of anesthesia, induced hypotension, and the use of multiple drugs. Although severe cardiomyopathy is believed to be a contraindication to spinal fusion in Duchenne's muscular dystrophy,[361] it is not known what level of the dysfunction represents an increased risk for this procedure. At Children's Hospital in Boston, after an unexpected intraoperative death that appeared to be related to cardiac failure in a patient not clinically recognized to have significant impairment, we have instituted a program of preoperative assessment that includes echocardiography and 24-hour ambulatory electrocardiographic monitoring. Based on the findings at the time of assessment, the procedure is judged to be of relatively low risk (normal echocardiogram), moderate risk (mild-to-moderate ventricular dysfunction), or high risk (severe ventricular dysfunction). In general, only emergency procedures are undertaken in the high-risk patient. In patients with a moderate risk, elective procedures, such as spinal fusion, are still pursued, but additional precautions are taken regarding anesthesia. Using these methods, spinal fusion has been successfully performed even in the presence of fairly marked ventricular dysfunction (shortening fraction < 20%) without incident. One patient with a fractional shortening < 5% was excluded from surgery because in our judgment this represented too extreme a risk. It should be noted that although we have the experience to suggest that nearly all of these patients can safely undergo procedures such as spinal fusion, we do not have data to define the level of ventricular function below which surgery should not be performed. For the present, this remains a decision based on clinical experience with other disorders.

REFERENCES

1. Abelmann WH, Lorell BH: The challenge of cardiomyopathy. J Am Coll Cardiol 13:1219–1239, 1989.
2. Abramson JJ, Buck E, Salama G, et al: Mechanism of anthraquinone-induced calcium release from skeletal muscle sarcoplasmic reticulum. J Biol Chem 263:18750–18758, 1988.
3. Afanasev IB, Korkina LG, Suslova TB, et al: Are quinones producers or scavengers of superoxide ion in cells. Arch Biochem Biophys 281:245–250, 1990.
4. Ainger LE: Acute aseptic myocarditis: corticosteroid therapy. J Pediatr 64:716–723, 1964.
5. Alboliras ET, Shub C, Gomez MR, et al: Spectrum of cardiac involvement in Friedreich's ataxia: clinical, electrocardiographic and echocardiographic observations. Am J Cardiol 58:518–524, 1986.
6. Alcan KE, Robeson W, Graham M, et al: Early detection of anthracycline-induced cardiotoxicity by stress radionuclide cineangiography in conjunction with Fourier amplitude and phase analysis. Clin Nucl Med 10:160–166, 1985.
7. Alday LE, Moreyra E: Secondary hypertrophic cardiomyopathy in infancy and childhood. Am Heart J 108:996–1000, 1984.
8. Alderton P, Gross J, Green MD: Role of (+ −)-1,2-bis (3,5-dioxyopiperazinyl-1-yl) propane (ICRF-187) in modulating free radical scavenging enzymes in doxorubicin-induced cardiomyopathy. Cancer Res 50:5136–5142, 1990.
9. Alexander J, Dainiak N, Berger HJ, et al: Serial assessment of doxorubicin cardiotoxicity with quantitative radionuclide angiocardiography. N Engl J Med 300:278–283, 1979.
10. Allard P, Dujaime M, Raso JV, et al: Pathomechanics and management of scoliosis in Friedreich's ataxia patients: preliminary report. Can J Neurol Sci 7:383–388, 1980.
11. Alpert BS: Steroid-induced hypertrophic cardiomyopathy in an infant. Pediatr Cardiol 5:117–118, 1984.
12. Andermann E, Remillard GM, Goyer C, et al: Genetic and family studies in Friedreich's ataxia. Can J Neurol Sci 3:287–301, 1976.
13. Anders RJ, Shane JG, Zeller FP: Lower incidence of doxorubicin-induced cardiomyopathy by once a week low dose administration. Am Heart J 111:755–759, 1986.
14. Anselmi A, Suarez JA, Anselmi G, et al: V. Primary cardiomyopathy in identical twins. Am J Cardiol 35:97–102, 1975.
15. Arahata K, Ishiura S, Ishiguro T, et al: Immunostaining of skeletal and cardiac muscle surface membrane with antibody against Duchenne muscular dystrophy peptide. Nature 333:861–863, 1988.
16. Aretz HT: Myocarditis: The Dallas Criteria. Hum Pathol 18:619–624, 1987.
17. Aretz HT, Billingham ME, Edwards WD, et al: Myocarditis: a histolopathologic definition and classification. Am J Cardiovasc Pathol 1:3–14, 1986.
18. Ashkenazi A, Frydman M, Weitz R, et al: Myocarditis and acute infantile hemiparesis. Helv Paediatr Acta 39:491–495, 1984.
19. Atkin J, Snow JW, Zellweger H, et al: Fatal infantile cardiac glycogenosis without acid matase deficiency presenting as congenital hydrops. Eur J Pediatr 142:150, 1984.
20. Baker MS, Austin L: The pathological damage in Duchenne muscular dystrophy may be due to increased intracellular oxy-radical generation caused by the ab-

sence of dystrophin and subsequent alterations in Ca²⁺ metabolism. Med Hypotheses 29:187–193, 1989.

21. Bansal RK, Bhardwaj RP, Thaper RK, et al: Familial dilated cardiomyopathy—study in two families. Indian Heart J 40:99–102, 1988.

22. Barbeau A: Friedreich's ataxia 1980: an overview of the physiopathology. Can J Neurol Sci 7:455–468, 1980.

23. Barth PG, Scholte HR, Berden JA, et al: An X-linked mitochondrial disease affecting cardiac muscle, skeletal muscle and neutrophil leucocytes. J Neurol Sci 62:327–355, 1983.

24. Betocchi S, Bonow RO, Bacharach SL, et al: Isovolumetric relaxation period in hypertrophic cardiomyopathy: assessment by radionuclide angiography. J Am Coll Cardiol 7:74–81, 1986.

25. Bharati S, Serratto M, DuBrow I, et al: The conduction system in Pompe's disease. Pediatr Cardiol 2:25–32, 1982.

26. Biancaniello T, Meyer RA, Wong KY, et al: Doxorubicin cardiotoxicity in children. J Pediatr 97:45–50, 1980.

27. Bielack SS, Erttmann R, Winkler K, et al: Doxorubicin: effect of different schedules on toxicity and antitumor efficacy. Eur J Cancer Clin Oncol 25:873–882, 1989.

28. Billingham ME: The safety and utility of endomyocardial biopsy in infants, children and adolescents (editorial comment). J Am Coll Cardiol 15:443–445, 1990.

29. Bjarnason I, Jonsson S, Hardarson T: Mode of inheritance of hypertrophic cardiomyopathy in Iceland echocardiographic study. Br Heart J 47:122–129, 1982.

30. Blass JP: Inborn errors of pyruvate metabolism. In Stanbury JB, Wyngaarden JB, Fredrickson DS, et al (eds): The Metabolic Basis of Inherited Disease, 5th ed. New York, McGraw-Hill, 1983, pp. 193–203.

31. Blieden LC, Desnick RJ, Carter JB, et al: Cardiac involvement in Sandhoff's disease. Am J Cardiol 34:83–88, 1974.

32. Bloom KR, Bini RM, Williwma CM, et al: Echocardiography in adriamycin cardiotoxicity. Cancer 41:1265–1269, 1978.

33. Blum RH, Walsh C, Green MD, et al: Modulation of the effect of anthracycline efficacy and toxicity by ICRF-187. Cancer Invest 8:267–268, 1990.

34. Boehm TM, Dickerson RB, Glasser SP: Hypertrophic subaortic stenosis in a patient with Friedreich's ataxia. Am J Med Sci 260:279–284, 1970.

35. Bogousslavsky J, Perentes E, Deruaz JP, et al: Mitochondrial myopathy and cardiomyopathy with neurodegenerative features and multiple brain infarcts. J Neurol Sci 55:351–357, 1982.

36. Bonilla E, Samitt CE, Miranda AF, et al: Duchenne muscular dystrophy: deficiency at the muscle cell surface. Cell 54:447–452, 1988.

37. Bonnici F, Shapiro R, Joffe HS, et al: Angiocardiographic and enzyme studies in a patient with type II glycogenosis (Pompe's disease). S Afr Med J 58:860–862, 1980.

38. Bonow RO, Vitale DF, Maron BJ, et al: Regional left ventricular asynchrony and impaired global left ventricular filling in hypertrophic cardiomyopathy: effect of verapamil. J Am Coll Cardiol 9:1108–1116, 1987.

39. Borow KM, Colan SD, Neumann A: Altered left ventricular mechanics in patients with valvular aortic stenosis and coarctation of the aorta: effects on systolic performance and late outcome. Circulation 72:515–522, 1985.

40. Boudin G, Mikol J, Guillard A, et al: Fatal systemic carnitine deficiency with lipid storage in skeletal muscle, heart, liver and kidney. J Neurol Sci 30:313–325, 1976.

41. Bove KE, Schwartz, DC: Focal lipid cardiomyopathy in an infant with paroxysmal atrial tachycardia. Arch Pathol 95:26–36, 1973.

42. Bowles NE, Richardson PJ, Olsen EGJ, et al: Detection of Coxsackie-B-virus-specific RNA sequences in myocardial biopsy samples from patients with myocarditis and dilated cardiomyopathy. Lancet 1:1120–1122, 1986.

43. Braunwald E: Heart Disease: A Textbook of Cardiovascular Medicine. Philadelphia, W. B. Saunders, 1980, pp. 1460–1472.

44. Bristow MR, Lopez MB, Mason JW, et al: Efficacy and cost of cardiac monitoring in patients receiving doxorubicin. Cancer 50:32–41, 1982.

45. Bristow MR, Mason JW, Billingham ME, et al: Doxorubicin cardiomyopathy: evaluation by phonocardiography, endomyocardial biopsy, and cardiac catheterization. Ann Intern Med 88:168–175, 1978.

46. Bristow MR, Mason JW, Billingham ME, et al: Dose effect and structure function relationships in doxorubicin cardiomyopathy. Am Heart J 102:709–718, 1981.

47. Bristow MR, Thompson PD, Martin RP, et al: Early anthracycline cardiotoxicity. Am J Med 65:823–832, 1978.

48. Brook MM, Weinhouse E, Jarenwattananon M, et al: Dilated cardimyopathy complicating a case of epidermolysis bullosa dystrophica. Pediatr Dermatol 6:21–23, 1989.

49. Bruton D, Herdson PB, Becroft DM: Histiocytoid cardiomyopathy of infancy: an unexplained myofibre degeneration. Pathology 9:115–122, 1977.

50. Brutsaert DL: Nonuniformity: a physiologic modulator of contraction and relaxation of the normal heart. J Am Coll Cardiol 9:341–348, 1987.

51. Bulkley BH, Hutchins GM: Pompe's disease presenting as hypertrophic myocardiopathy with Wolff-Parkinson-White syndrome. Am Heart J 96:246–252, 1978.

52. Bureau MA, Ngassam P, Lemieux B, et al: Pulmonary function studies in Friedreich's ataxia. Can J Neurol Sci 3:343–347, 1976.

53. Burn J, Bennett CP: Genetics of cardiomyopathy and disease of the myocardium. In Julian DG (ed): Disease of the Heart. London, Balliere-Tindall, 1989.

54. Busch HFM, Koster JF, van Weerden TW: Infantile and adult-onset acid maltase deficiency occurring in the same family. Neurology 29:415–416, 1979.

55. Butler IJ, Gadoth N: Kearns-Sayre syndrome: a review of a multisystem disorder of children and young adults. Arch Intern Med 136:1290–1293, 1976.

56. Buzello W, Huttarsch H: Muscle relaxation in patients with Duchenne's muscular dystrophy: use of vecuronium in two patients. Br J Anaesth 60:228–231, 1988.

57. Cannon RO, Schenke WH, Maron BJ, et al: Differences in coronary flow and myocardial metabolism at rest and during pacing between patients with obstructive and patients with nonobstructive hypertrophic cardiomyopathy. J Am Coll Cardiol 10:53–62, 1987.

58. Carmo I, Brites A, das Neves BS, et al: A case of Turner syndrome with dilated cardiomyopathy. Acta Med Port 1:223–226, 1988.

59. Casazza F, Ferrari F, Finocchiaro G, et al: Echocardiographic evaluation of verapamil in Friedreich's ataxia. Br Heart J 55:400–404, 1986.

60. Cassling RS, Linder J, Sears TD, et al: Quantitative evaluation of inflammation in biopsy specimens from idiopathically failing or irritable hearts: experience in

80 pediatric and adult patients. Am Heart J 110:713–720, 1985.

61. Cederbaum SD, Auestad N, Bernar J: Four-year treatment of systemic carnitine deficiency. N Engl J Med 310:1295–1396, 1984.

62. Cera C, Palumbo M: Anticancer activity of anthracycline antibiotics and DNA condensation. Anticancer Drug Res 5:265–271, 1990.

63. Challa VR, Markesbery WR, Baumann RJ, et al: Lactic acidosis associated with cerebellar vermal atrophy and cardiomyopathy. Neuropadiatrie 9:277–284, 1978.

64. Chandra RS: The role of endomyocardial biopsy in the diagnosis of cardiac disorders in infants and children. Am J Cardiovasc Pathol 1:157–172, 1987.

65. Chapoy PR, Angelnii C, Brown WJ, et al: Systemic carnitine deficiency—a treatable inherited lipid-storage disease presenting as Reye's syndrome. N Engl J Med 303:1389–1394, 1980.

66. Charrow J, Hvizd MG: Cardiomyopathy and skeletal myopathy in an unusual variant of GM1 gangliosidosis. J Pediatr 108:729–732, 1986.

67. Choi BE, Berger HJ, Scwartz PE, et al: Serial radionuclide assessment of doxorubicin cardiotoxicity in cancer patients with abnormal baseline resting left ventricular performance. Am Heart J 106:638–643, 1983.

68. Choong CY, Herrmann HC, Weyman AE, et al: Preload dependence of Doppler-derived indexes of left ventricular diastolic function in humans. J Am Coll Cardiol 10:800–808, 1987.

69. Chow LH, Radio SJ, Sears TD, et al: Insensitivity of right ventricular endomyocardial biopsy in the diagnosis of myocarditis. J Am Coll Cardiol 14:915–920, 1989.

70. Cooper M, Shaddy R, Silverman N, et al: Usefulness of Doppler echocardiography for determining hyperdynamic improvement with intravenous verapamil in hypertrophic cardiomyopathy. Am J Cardiol 56:201–202, 1985.

71. Cortes EP, Gupta M, Chou C, et al: Adriamycin cardiotoxicity: early detection by systolic time interval and possible prevention by coenzyme Q10. Cancer Treat Rep 62:887–891, 1978.

72. Costanzo-Nordin MR, O'Connell JB, Subramanian R, et al: Myocarditis confirmed by biopsy presenting as acute myocardial infarction. Br Heart J 53:25–29, 1985.

73. Cote M, Davignon A, Elias G, et al. Hemodynamic findings in Friedreich's ataxia. Can J Neurol 3:333–336, 1976.

74. Criley JM, Siegel RJ: Has "obstruction" hindered our understanding of hypertrophic cardiomyopathy? Circulation 72:1148–1154, 1985.

75. Cruysberg JR, Sengers RC, Pinckers A, et al: Features of a syndrome with congenital cataract and hypertrophic cardiomyopathy. Am J Ophthalmol 102:740–749, 1986.

76. Cuccurullo F, Mezzetti A, Lapenna D, et al: Mechanism of isoproterenol-induced angina pectoris in patients with obstructive hypertrophic cardiomyopathy and normal coronary arteries. Am J Cardiol 60:667–673, 1987.

77. Cummings J, Smyth JF: Pharmacology of adriamycin: the message to the clinician. Eur J Cancer Clin 24:579–582, 1988.

78. Daher YH, Lonstein JE, Winter RB, et al: Spinal deformities in patients with Friedreich's ataxia: a review of 19 patients. J Pediatr Orthop 5:553–557, 1985.

79. Danilowicz D, Rutkowski M, Myung D, et al: Echocardiography in Duchenne muscular dystrophy. Muscle Nerve 3:298–303, 1980.

80. Davidoff R, Palacios I, Southern J, et al: Giant cell versus lymphocytic myocarditis: a comparison of their clinical features and long-term outcome. In press.

81. Davies MJ: The cardiomyopathies: a review of terminology, pathology and pathogenesis. Histopathology 8:363–393, 1984.

82. Davies MJ, Pomerance A, Teare RD: Idiopathic giant cell myocarditis—a distinctive clinico-pathological entity. Br Heart J 37:192–195, 1975.

83. De Leonardis V, De Scalzi M, Neri B, et al: Echocardiographic assessment of anthracycline cardiotoxicity during different therapeutic regimens. J Clin Pharmacol Res 7:307–311, 1987.

84. Dec GW, Fallon JT, Southern JF, et al: "Borderline" myocarditis: an indication for repeat endomyocardial biopsy. J Am Coll Cardiol 15:283–289, 1990.

85. Dec GW, Palacios I, Yasuda T, et al: Antimyosin antibody cardiac imaging: its role in the diagnosis of myocarditis. J Am Coll Cardiol 16:97–104, 1990.

86. Dimitrov NV, Hay MB, Siew S, et al: Abrogation of adriamycin-induced cardiotoxicity by selenium in rabbits. Am J Pathol 126:376–383, 1987.

87. Doshi R, Lodge KV: Idiopathic cardiomyopathy in infants. Arch Dis Child 48:431–435, 1973.

88. Douglas PS, Morrow R, Ioli A, et al: Left ventricular shape, afterload and survival in idiopathic dilated cardiomyopathy. J Am Coll Cardiol 13:311–315, 1989.

89. Duncan CJ: Dystrophin and the integrity of the sarcolemma in Duchenne muscular dystrophy. Experiencia 45:175–177, 1989.

90. Duncan WJ, Fowler RS, Farkas LG, et al: A comprehensive scoring system for evaluating Noonan syndrome. Am J Med Genet 10:37–50, 1981.

91. Dunnigan A, Staley NA, Smith SA, et al: Cardiac and skeletal muscle abnormalities in cardiomyopathy: comparison of patients with ventricular tachycardia or congestive heart failure. J Am Coll Cardiol 10:608–618, 1987.

92. Durand P, Borrone C, Della Cella G: Fucosidosis. J Pediatr 75:665–674, 1969.

93. Edwards MA, Green A, Colli A, et al: Tyrosinaemia type I and hypertrophic obstructive cardiomyopathy (letter). Lancet 1:1437–1438, 1987.

94. Ehlers HK, Hagstrom JWC, Lukas DS, et al: Glycogen-storage disease of the myocardium with obstruction to left ventricular outflow. Circulation 25:96–109, 1962.

95. Eisenstein BI: The polymerase chain reaction: a new method of using molecular genetics for medical diagnosis. N Engl J Med 322:178–183, 1990.

96. Eishi Y, Takemura T, Sone R, et al: Glycogen storage disease confined to the heart with deficient activity of cardiac phosphorylase kinase: a new type of glycogen storage disease. Hum Pathol 16:193–197, 1985.

97. Emanuel R, Withers R, O'Brien K: Dominant and recessive modes of inheritance in idiopathic cardiomyopathy. Lancet 2:1065–1067, 1971.

98. Engel AG: Duchenne dystrophy. In Engel AG, Banker BQ (eds): Myology: Basic and Clinical. New York, McGraw Hill, 1986, pp. 1185–1240.

99. Engel AG, Banker BQ, Eiben RM: Carnitine deficiency: clinical, morphological, and biochemical observations in a fatal case. J Neurol Neurosurg Psychiatry 40:313–322, 1977.

100. Engel AG, Rebouche CJ, Wilson DM, et al: Primary systemic carnitine deficiency. II. Renal handling of carnitine. Neurology 31:819–825, 1981.

101. Factor SM, Sonnenlick EH: The pathogenesis of clinical and experimental congestive cardiomyopathies: recent concepts. Prog Cardiovasc Dis 27:395–420, 1985.

102. Ferrans VJ: Pathologic anatomy of the dilated cardio-myopathies. Am J Cardiol 64:9C–11C, 1989.
103. Ferrans VJ, McAllister HA, Haese WH: Infantile car-diomyopathy with histiocytoid change in cardiac mus-cle cells. Circulation 53:708–719, 1976.
104. Fishbein MC, Ferrans VJ, Roberts WC: Histologic and ultrastructural features of primary and secondary en-docardial fibroelastosis. Arch Pathol Lab Med 101:49–54, 1977.
105. Fisher DJ, Heymann MA, Rudolph AM: Myocardial oxygen and carbohydrate consumption in fetal lambs in utero and adult sheep. Am J Physiol 238:H399–H405, 1980.
106. Fowles RE, Mason JW: Role of cardiac biopsy in the diagnosis and management of cardiac disease. Prog Cardiovasc Dis 27:153–172, 1984.
107. Frankel KA, Rosser RJ: The pathology of the heart in progressive muscular dystrophy: epimyocardial fibro-sis. Hum Pathol 7:375–386, 1976.
108. Freter CE, Lee TC, Billingham ME, et al: Doxoru-bicin cardiac toxicity manifesting seven years after treatment. Am J Med 80:483–485, 1986.
109. Freundlick E, Munk J, Griffel B, et al: Primary my-ocardial disease in infancy. Am J Cardiol 13:721–733, 1964.
110. Fried K, Beer S, Vure E, et al: Autosomal recessive sudden unexpected death in children probably caused by a cardiomyopathy associated with myopathy. J Med Genet 16:341–346, 1979.
111. Fujita M, Neustein HB, Lurie PR: Transvascular en-domyocardial biopsy in infants and small children: my-ocardial findings in 10 cases of cardiomyopathy. Hum Pathol 10:15–30, 1979.
112. Fujiwara H, Hamashima Y: Pathology of the heart in Kawasaki disease. Pediatrics 61:100–107, 1978.
113. Fujiwara H, Onodera T, Tanaka M, et al: Progression from hypertrophic obstructive cardiomyopathy to typ-ical dilated cardiomyopathy-like features in the end stage. Jpn Circ J 48:1210–1214, 1984.
114. Fyler DC, Buckley LP, Hellenbrand WE, et al: Report of the New England Regional Infant Cardiac Program. Pediatrics 65:375–461, 1980.
115. Gaasch WH, Battle WE, Oboler AA: Left ventricular stress and compliance in man: with special reference to normalized ventricular function curves. Circulation 45:746–762, 1972.
116. Gach JV, Andriange M, Franck G: Hypertrophic ob-structive cardiomyopathy and Friedreich's ataxia: re-port of a case and review of literature. Am J Cardiol 27:436–441, 1971.
117. Garnick MB, Weiss GR, Steele GD Jr, et al: Clinical evaluation of long term continuous-infusion doxoru-bicin. Cancer Treat Rep 67:133–142, 1983.
118. Garrison RF, Swisher RC: Myocarditis of unknown etiology (Fiedler's?) treated with ACTH. J Pediatr 42:591–599, 1953.
119. Gatmaitan BG, Chason JL, Lerner AM: Augmentation of the virulence of murine Coxsackie virus B-3 my-ocardiopathy by exercise. J Exp Med 131:1121–1136, 1970.
120. Ghafour AS, Gutgesell HP: Echocardiographic eval-uation of left ventricular function in children with con-gestive cardiomyopathy. Am J Cardiol 44:1332–1338, 1979.
121. Gidding SS, Snider AR, Rocchini AP, et al: Left ven-tricular diastolic filling in children with hypertrophic cardiomyopathy: assessment with pulsed Dopper echo-cardiography. J Am Coll Cardiol 8:310–316, 1986.
122. Gilladoga AC, Manuel C, TAn CTC, et al: The car-diotoxicity of adriamycin and daunomycin in children. Cancer 37:1070–1078, 1976.
123. Gillette, PC, Nihill MR, Singer BD: Electrophysio-logical mechanism of the short PR interval in Pompe disease. Am J Dis Child 128:622–626, 1974.
124. Gillium RF: Idiopathic cardiomyopathy in the United States, 1970–1982. Am Heart J 111:752–755, 1986.
125. Glasgow AM, Engel AG, Bier DM, et al: Hypogly-cemia, hepatic dysfunction, muscle weakness, car-diomyopathy, free carnitine deficiency and long-chain acylcarnitine excess responsive to medium chain tri-glyceride diet. Pediatr Res 17:319, 326, 1983.
126. Goldberg SJ, Feldman L, Reinecke C, et al: Echocar-diographic determination of contraction and relaxation measurements of the left ventricular wall in normal subjects and patients with muscular dystrophy. Cir-culation 62:1061–1069, 1980.
127. Goldberg SJ, Stern LZ, Feldman L, et al: Serial left ventricular wall measurements in Duchenne's mus-cular dystrophy. J Am Coll Cardiol 21:136–142, 1983.
128. Goldberg SJ, Valdes, Cruz LM, et al: Two-dimensional echocardiographic evaluation of dilated cardio-myopathy in children. Am J Cardiol 52:1244–1248, 1983.
129. Goldblatt J, Melmed J, Rose AG: Autosomal recessive inheritance of idiopathic dilated cardiomyopathy in a Madeira Portuguese kindred. Clin Genet 31:249–254, 1987.
130. Goorin AM, Borow KM, Goldman A, et al: Congestive heart failure due to adriamycin cardiotoxicity. Cancer 47:2810–2816, 1981.
131. Goorin AM, Chauvenet AR, Perez-Atayde AR, et al: Initial congestive heart failure, six to ten years after doxorubicin chemotherapy for childhood cancer. J Pe-diatr 116:144–147, 1990.
132. Gottdiener JS, Hawley RJ, Maron BJ, et al: Charac-teristics of the cardiac hypertrophy in Friedreich's ataxia. Am Heart J 103:525–531, 1982.
133. Gottdiener JS, Mathisen DJ, Borer JS, et al: Doxo-rubicin cardiotoxicity: assessment of late ventricular dysfunction by radionuclide cineangiography. Ann In-tern Med 94:430–435, 1981.
134. Gottlieb SL, Edmiston A, Haywood LJ: Late doxo-rubicin cardiotoxicity. Chest 78:880–882, 1980.
135. Goudevenos J, Parry G, Gold RB: Coxsackie B4 viral myocarditis causing ventricular aneurysm. Int J Car-diol 27:122–124, 1990.
136. Gravanis MB, Ansari AA: Idiopathic cardiomyopathies: a review of pathologic studies and mechanisms of path-ogenesis. Arch Pathol Lab Med 111:915–929, 1987.
137. Greaves SC, Roche AH, Neutze JM, et al: Inheritance of hypertrophic cardiomyopathy: a cross-sectional and M mode echocardiographic study of 50 families. Br Heart J 58:259–266, 1987.
138. Greenberg S, Frishman WH: Co-enzyme Q10: a new drug for cardiovascular disease. J Clin Pharmacol 30:596–608, 1990.
139. Greenwood RD, Nadas AS, Fyler DC: The clinical course of primary myocardial disease in infants and children. Am Heart J 92:549–560, 1976.
140. Griffin ML, Hernandez A, Martin TC, et al: Dilated cardiomyopathy in infants and children. J Am Coll Car-diol 11:139–144, 1988.
141. Grist NR, Bell EJ: Coxsackie viruses and the heart. Am Heart J 77:295–300, 1969.
142. Grody WW, Cheng L, Lewis W: Infection of the heart by the human immunodeficiency virus. Am J Cardiol 66:203–206, 1990.
143. Grose R, Strain J, Spindola Franco H: Angiographic and hemodynamic correlations in hypertrophic car-

diomyopathy with intracavitary systolic pressure gradients. Am J Cardiol 58:1085–1092, 1986.

144. Grossman W: Cardiac Catheterization and Angiography, 3rd ed. Philadelphia, Lea & Febiger, 1986.

145. Grossman W, Jones D, McLaurin LP: Wall stress and patterns of hypertrophy in the human left ventricle. J Clin Invest 56:56–61, 1975.

146. Gussenhoven WJ, Busch HFM, Kleijier WJ, et al: Echocardiographic features in the cardiac type of glycogen storage disease. II. Eur Heart J 4:41–43, 1983.

147. Hale DE, Batshaw ML, Coates PM, et al: Long-chain acyl coenzyme a dehydrogenase deficiency: an inherited cause of nonketotic hypoglycemia. Pediatr Res 19:666–671, 1985.

148. Hamaguchi T, Azuma J, Awata N, et al: Reduction of doxorubicin-induced cardiotoxicity in mice by taurine. Res Commun Chem Pathol Pharmacol 59:21–30, 1988.

149. Hamaguchi T, Azuma J, Harada H, et al: Protective effect of taurine against doxorubicin-induced cardiotoxicity in perfused chick hearts. Pharmacol Res 21:729–734, 1989.

150. Hanrath P, Mathey DG, Siegert R, et al: Left ventricular relaxation and filling pattern in different forms of left ventricular hypertrophy: an echocardiographic study. Am J Cardiol 45:15–23, 1980.

151. Haq MM, Legha SS, Choksi J, et al: Doxorubicin induced congestive heart failure in adults. Cancer 56:1361–1365, 1985.

152. Harding AE, Hewer RL: The heart disease of Friedreich's ataxia: a clinical and electrocardiographic study of 115 patients, with an analysis of serial electrocardiographic changes in 30 cases. Q J Med 208:489–502, 1983.

153. Harris RN, Doroshow JH: Effect of doxorubicin enhanced hydrogen peroxide and hydroxyl radical formation on calcium sequestration by cardiac sarcoplasmic reticulum. Biochem Biophys Res Commun 130:739–745, 1985.

154. Hart ZH, Chang CH, DiMauro S, et al: Muscle carnitine deficiency and fatal cardiomyopathy. Neurology 28:147–151, 1978.

155. Hart ZH, Servidei S, Peterson PL, et al: Cardiomyopathy, mental retardation, and autophagic vacuolar myopathy. Neurology 37:1065–1068, 1987.

156. Haugland H, Ohm OJ, Boman H, et al: Hypertrophic cardiomyopathy in three generations of a large Norwegian family: a clinical, echocardiographic and genetic study. Br Heart J 55:168–175, 1986.

157. Heikkila J, Karjalainen J: Evaluation of mild acute infectious myocarditis. Br Heart J 47:381–391, 1982.

158. Hellmann K: ICRF 187. J Chemother 1:355–358, 1989.

159. Henderson IC, Sloss LJ, Jaffe N, et al: Serial studies of cardiac function in patients receiving adriamycin. Cancer Treat Rep 62:923–929, 1978.

160. Henderson WA: Succinylcholine-induced cardiac arrest in unsuspected Duchenne muscular dystrophy. Can Anaesth Soc J 31:444–446, 1984.

161. Henry CG, Strauss AW, Keating JP, et al: Congestive cardiomyopathy associated with β-ketothiolase deficiency. J Pediatr 99:754–757, 1981.

162. Hermansen K, Wassermann K: The effect of vitamin E and selenium on doxorubicin (adriamycin) induced delayed toxicity in mice. Acta Pharmacol Toxicol (Copenh) 58:31–37, 1986.

163. Hess OM, Grimm J, Krayenbuehl HP: Diastolic function in hypertrophic cardiomyopathy: effects of propranolol and verapamil on diastolic stiffness. Eur Heart J 4:47–56, 1983.

164. Hewer RL: The heart in Friedreich's ataxia. Br Heart J 31:5–14, 1969.

165. Heymsfield SB, Mcnish T, Perkins JV, et al: Sequence of cardiac changes in Duchenne muscular dystrophy. Am Heart J 95:283–294, 1978.

166. Hirota Y: A clinical study of left ventricular diastolic properties. Jpn Circ J 46:49–57, 1982.

167. Hirota Y, Furubayasi K, Kaku K, et al: Hypertrophic nonobstructive cardiomyopathy: a precise assesment of hemodynamic characteristics and clinical implications. Am J Cardiol 50:990–997, 1982.

168. Hirschman SZ, Hammer GS: Coxsackie virus myopericarditis. Am J Cardiol 34:224–231, 1974.

169. Hoffman EP, Brown RH Jr, Kunkel LM: Dystrophin: the protein product of the Duchenne muscular dystrophy locus. Cell 51:919–928, 1987.

170. Hoffman EP, Fishbeck KH, Brown RH, et al: Characterization of dystrophin in muscle-biopsy specimens from patients with Duchenne's or Becker's muscular dystrophy. N Engl J Med 318:1363–1368, 1988.

171. Holmberg SR, Williams AJ: Patterns of interaction between anthraquinone drugs and the calcium-release channel from cardiac sarcoplasmic reticulum. Circ Res 67:272–283, 1990.

172. Hopkins BE, Taylor RR, Robinson JS: Familial hypertrophic cardiomyopathy and lentiginosis. Aust NZ J Med 5:359–364, 1975.

173. Hortobagyi GN, Frye D, Buzdar AU, et al: Decreased cardiac toxicity of doxorubicin administered by continuous intravenous infusion in combination chemotherapy for metastatic breast carcinoma. Cancer 63:37–45, 1989.

174. Howell RR, Williams JC: The glycogen storage diseases. In Stanbury JB, Wyngaarden JB, Fredrickson DS, et al (eds): The Metabolic Basis of Inherited Disease, 5th ed. New York, McGraw-Hill, 1983, pp. 141–166.

175. Hubner G, Grantzow R: Mitochondrial cardiomyopathy with involvement of skeletal muscles. Virchows Arch [Pathol Anat] 399:115–125, 1983.

176. Hunsaker RH, Fulkerson PK, Barry FJ, et al: Cardiac function in Duchenne's muscular dystrophy: results of 10 year follow up study and noninvasive tests. Am J Med 73:235–238, 1982.

177. Hutter JJ, Sahn DJ, Woolfenden JM: Evaluation of the cardiac effects of doxorubicin by serial echocardiography. Am J Dis Child 135:653–658, 1981.

178. Imperato-McGinley J, Gautier T, Ehlers K, et al: Reversibility of catecholamine-induced dilated cardiomyopathy in a child with a pheochromocytoma. N Engl J Med 316:793–797, 1987.

179. Imura N, Naganuma A, Satoh M, et al: Depression of toxic effects of anticancer agents by selenium or pretreatment with metallothionine inducers. Sangyo Ika Daigaku Zasshi 9:223–229, 1987.

180. Ino T, Sherwood G, Benson LN et al: Cardiac manifestations in disorders of fat and carnitine metabolism in infancy. J Am Coll Cardiol 11:1301–1308, 1988.

181. Ishikawa K, Kanemitsu H, Ishihara T, et al: Echocardiographic study of the Duchenne type of progressive muscular dystrophy. Jpn Circ J 45:295–301, 1981.

182. Isner JM, Ferrans VJ, Cohen SR, et al: Clinical and morphological cardiac findings after anthracycline chemotherapy. Am J Cardiol 51:1167–1174, 1983.

183. Iwase M, Sotobata I, Takagi S, et al: Effects of diltiazem on left ventricular diastolic behavior in patients with hypertrophic cardiomyopathy: evaluation with exercise pulsed Doppler echocardiography. J Am Coll Cardiol 9:1099–1105, 1987.

184. Jacobs JC, Rosen JM, Szer IS: Lyme myocarditis diagnosed by gallium scan. J Pediatr 105:950–952, 1984.

185. Jaenke RS: Delayed and progressive myocardial lesions

after adriamycin administration in the rabbit. Cancer Res 36:2958–2966, 1976.

186. Jain D, Zaret BL: Antimyosin cardiac imaging in acute myocarditis (editorial comment). J Am Coll Cardiol 16:105–107, 1990.

187. James TN: Myocarditis and cardiomyopathy (editorial). N Engl J Med 308:39–41, 1983.

188. James TN, Cobbs BW, Coghlan HC, et al: Coronary disease, cardioneuropathy, and conduction system abnormalities in the cardiomyopathy of Friedreich's ataxia. Br Heart J 57:446–457, 1987.

189. Jarcho S: Fiedler on acute interstitial myocarditis (1989). Am J Cardiol 32:221–223, 1973.

190. Jarcho S: Fiedler on acute interstitial myocarditis (1989). Am J Cardiol 32:716–718, 1973.

191. Joshi VV, Gadol C, Connor E, et al: Dilated cardiomyopathy in children with acquired immunodeficiency syndrome: a pathologic study of five cases. Hum Pathol 19:66–73, 1988.

192. Kantrowitz NE, Bristow MR: Cardiotoxicity of antitumor agents. Prog Cardiovasc Dis 27:195–199, 1984.

193. Kapur S, Kuehl KS, Midgely FM, et al: Focal giant cell cardiomyopathy with Beckwith-Wiedemann syndrome. Pediatr Pathol 3:261–269, 1985.

194. Kariv I, Kreisler B, Sherf L, et al: Familial cardiomyopathy. Am J Cardiol 28:693–706, 1971.

195. Kennaway NG, Buist NR, Darley Usmar VM, et al: Lactic acidosis and mitochondrial myopathy associated with deficiency of several components of complex III of the respiratory chain. Pediatr Res 18:991–999, 1984.

196. Kereiakes DJ, Parmley WW: Myocarditis and cardiomyopathy. Am Heart J 108:1318–1326, 1984.

197. Kim DH, Landry AB III, Lee YS, et al: Doxorubicin induced calcium release from cardiac sarcoplasmic reticulum vesicles. J Mol Cell Cardiol 21:433–436, 1989.

198. Kitabatake, Inoue M, Asao M, et al: Transmitral blood flow reflecting diastolic behavior of the left ventricle in health and disease: a study by pulsed Doppler technique. Jpn Circ J 46:92–102, 1982.

199. Kluitmann G, Braumann HG, Kratz HW, et al: Acute course of Leigh syndrome with hypertrophic cardiomyopathy in a female infant. Monatsschr Kinderheilkd 133:688–693, 1985.

200. Kohlschutter A, Sieg K, Sieg K, et al: Infantile cardiomyopathy and neuromyopathy with β-galactosidase deficiency. Eur J Pediatr 139:75–81, 1982.

201. Koike K, Musewe NN, Smallhorn JF, et al: Distinguishing between anomalous origin of the left coronary artery from the pulmonary trunk and dilated cardiomyopathy: role of echocardiographic measurement of the right coronary artery diameter. Br Heart J 61:192–197, 1989.

202. Krajcer Z, Orzan F, Pechacek LW, et al: Early systolic closure of the aortic valve in patients with hypertrophic subaortic stenosis and discrete stenosis: correlation with preoperative and postoperative hemodynamics. Am J Cardiol 41:823–829, 1978.

203. Kramer DS, French WJ, Criley JM: The postextrasystolic murmur response to gradient in hypertrophic cardiomyopathy. Ann Intern Med 104:772–776, 1986.

204. Kussmaul WG, Kleaveland JP, Martin JL, et al: Effects of exercise and nitroprusside on left ventricular ejection dynamics in idiopathic dilated cardiomyopathy. Am J Cardiol 59:647–655, 1987.

205. LaMarche JB, Cote M, Lemieux B: The cardiomyopathy of Friedreich's ataxia: morphological observations in 3 cases. Can J Neurol Sci 7:389–396, 1980.

206. Lang SA, Duncan PG, Dupuis PR: Fatal air embolism in an adolescent with Duchenne muscular dystrophy during Harrington instrumentation. Anaesth Analg 69:132–134, 1989.

207. Leatherbury L, Chandra RS, Shapiro SR, et al: Values of endomyocardial biopsy in infants, children and adolescents with dilated or hypertrophic cardiomyopathy and myocarditis. J Am Coll Cardiol 12:1547–1554, 1988.

208. Legha SS, Benjamin RS, Mackay B, et al: Reduction of doxorubicin cardiotoxicity by prolonged continuous intravenous infusion. Ann Intern Med 96:133–139, 1982.

209. Lenzhofer R, Dudczak R, Gumhold G, et al: Noninvasive methods of the early detection of doxorubicin induced cardiomyopathy. J Cancer Res Clin Oncol 106:136–142, 1983.

210. Lewis AB, Crouse VL, Evans W, et al: Recovery of left ventricular function following discontinuation of anthracycline chemotherapy in children. Pediatr 68:67–72, 1981.

211. Lewis AB, Neustein HB, Takahashi M, et al: Findings on endomyocardial biopsy in infants and children with dilated cardiomyopathy. Am J Cardiol 55:143–145, 1985.

212. Lewis AB, Pilkington R, Takahashi M, et al: Echocardiographic assessment of anthracycline cardiotoxicity in children. Med Pedtr Oncol 5:167–175, 1978.

213. Liao PK, Seward JB, Hagler DJ, et al: Acute myocarditis associated with transient marked myocardial thickening and complete atrioventricular block. Clin Cardiol 7:356–362, 1984.

214. Lie JT: Myocarditis and endomyocardial biopsy in unexplained heart failure: a diagnosis in search of a disease (editorial). 109:525–528, 1988.

215. Lipshultz SE, Chanoock S, Sanders SP, et al: Cardiovascular manifestations of human immunodeficiency virus infection in infants and children. Am J Cardiol 63:1489–1497, 1989.

216. Loonen MCB, Busch HFM, Koster JF, et al: A family with different clinical forms of acid maltase deficiency (glycogenosis type II): biochemical and genetic studies. Neurology 31:1209–1216, 1981.

217. Lurie PR, Fujita M, Neustein HB: Transvascular endomyocardial biopsy in infants and small children: description of a new technique. Am J Cardiol 42:453–457, 1978.

218. Makinen L, Makipernaa A, Routonen J, et al: Long term cardiac sequelae after treatment of malignant tumors with radiotherapy or cytostatics in childhood. Cancer 65:1913–1917, 1990.

219. Maron BJ, Bonow RO, Cannon RO III, et al: Hypertrophic cardiomyopathy: interrelations of clinical manifestations, pathophysiology and therapy. II. N Engl J Med 316:844–852, 1987.

220. Maron BJ, Edwards JE, Moller JH, et al: Prevalence and characteristics of disproportionate ventricular septal thickening in infants with congenital heart disease. Circulation 59:126–133, 1979.

221. Maron BJ, Epstein SE: Hypertrophic cardiomyopathy: a discussion of nomenclature (editorial). Am J Cardiol 43:1242–1244, 1979.

222. Maron BJ, Gottdiener JS, Epstein SE: Pattern and significance of distribution of left ventricular hypertrophy in hypertrophic cardiomyopathy: a wide angle, two-dimensional echocardiographic study of 125 patients. Am J Cardiol 48:418–428, 1981.

223. Maron BJ, Gottdiener JS, Roberts WC, et al: Left ventricular outflow tract obstruction due to systolic anterior motion of the anterior mitral leaflet in patients with concentric left ventricular hypertrophy. Circulation 57:527–533, 1978.

224. Maron BJ, Harding AM, Spirito P, et al: Systolic anterior motion of the posterior mitral leaflet: a previously unrecognized cause of dynamic subaortic obstruction in patients with hypertrophic cardiomyopathy. Circulation 68:282–293, 1983.

225. Maron BJ, Nichols PF III, Pickle LW, et al: Patterns of inheritance in hypertrophic cardiomyopathy: assessment by M-mode and two dimensional echocardiography. Am J Cardiol 53:1087–1094, 1984.

226. Maron BJ, Redwood DR, Roberts WC, et al: Tunnel subaortic stenosis: left ventricular outflow tract obstruction produced by fibromuscular tubular narrowing. Circulation 54:404–416, 1976.

227. Maron BJ, Roberts WC: Quantitative analysis of cardiac muscle cell disorganization in the ventricular septum of patients with hypertrophic cardiomyopathy. Circulation 59:689–706, 1979.

228. Maron BJ, Roberts WC: Hypertrophic cardiomyopathy and cardiac muscle cell disorganization revisited: relation between the two and significance. Am Heart J 102:95–110, 1981.

229. Maron BJ, Roberts WC: Cardiomyopathies in the first two decades of life. Cardiovasc Clin 11:35–78, 1981.

230. Maron BJ, Spirito P, Green KJ, et al: Noninvasive assessment of left ventricular diastolic function by pulsed Doppler echocardiography in patients with hypertrophic cardiomyopathy. J Am Coll Cardiol 10:733–742, 1987.

231. Maron BJ, Spirito P, Wesley Y, et al: Development and progression of left ventricular hypertrophy in children with hypertrophic cardiomyopathy. N Engl J Med 315:610–614, 1986.

232. Maron BJ, Tajik AJ, Ruttenberg HD, et al: Hypertrophic cardiomyopathy in infants: clinical features and natural history. Circulation 65:7–17, 1982.

233. Maron BJ, Wolfson JK, Epstein SE, et al: Intramural ("small vessel") coronary artery disease in hypertrophic cardiomyopathy. J Am Coll Cardiol 8:545–557, 1986.

234. Martin RP, Rakowski H, French J, et al: Idiopathic hypertrophic subaortic stenosis viewed by wide angle, phased array echocardiography. Circulation 59:1206–1217, 1979.

235. Mason JW, Billingham ME, Ricci DR: Treatment of acute inflammatory myocarditis assisted by endomyocardial biopsy. Am J Cardiol 45:1037–1044, 1980.

236. Massie BM, Conway M: Survival of patients with congestive heart failure: past, present and future prospects. Circulation 75:IV–11–19, 1987.

237. Matitiau A, Colan SD, Perez A, et al: Infantile congestive cardiomyopathy: relation of outcome to LV function, hemodynamics and histology (abstract). Circulation, 1990.

238. Matsuishi T, Hirata K, Terasawa K, et al: Successful carnitine treatment in two siblings having lipid storage myopathy with hypertrophic cardiomyopathy. Neuropadiatrie 16:6–12, 1985.

239. Matsuoka S, Ii K, Akita H, et al: Clinical features and cardiopulmonary function of patients with atrophic heart in Duchenne muscular dystrophy. Jpn Heart J 28:687–694, 1987.

240. Matsuoka Y, Sennari E, Hayakawa K: Idiopathic myocarditis characterized by marked right ventricular dilation: report of two autopsy cases. Jpn Circ J 51:51–58, 1990.

241. Matsuura H, Ishikita T, Yamamoto S, et al: Gallium-67 myocardial imaging for the detection of myocarditis in the acute phase of Kawasaki disease (mucocutaneous lymph node syndrome): the usefulness of single photon emission computed tomography. Br Heart J 58:385–392, 1987.

242. McAllister HA: Myocarditis: some current perspectives and future directions (editorial). Tex Heart Inst J 14:331–334, 1987.

243. McGarry JD, Foster DW: Systemic carnitine deficiency. N Engl J Med 303:1413–1416, 1980.

244. McGregor CGA, Gibson A, Caves P: Infantile cardiomyopathy with histiocytoid change in cardiac muscle cells: successful surgical intervention and prolonged survival. Am J Cardiol 53:982–983, 1984.

245. McKenna WJ: The natural history of hypertrophic cardiomyopathy. Cardiovasc Clin 19:135–148, 1988.

246. McKenna WJ, Borggrefe M, England D, et al: The natural history of left ventricular hypertrophy in hypertrophic cardiomyopathy: an electrocardiographic study. Circulation 66:1233–1240, 1982.

247. McKenna WJ, Deanfield JE: Hypertrophic cardiomyopathy: an important cause of sudden death. Arch Dis Child 59:971–975, 1984.

248. McKenna WJ, Goodwin JF: The natural history of hypertrophic cardiomyopathy. Curr Prob Cardiol 6:1–26, 1981.

249. McKillop JH, Bristow MR, Goris ML, et al: Sensitivity and specificity of radionuclide ejection fraction in doxorubicin cardiotoxicity. Am Heart J 106:1048–1056, 1983.

250. McKusick V, Neufeld EF: The mucopolysaccharide storage diseases. In Stanbury JB, Wyngaarden JB, Fredrickson DS, et al (eds): The Metabolic Basis of Inherited Disease, 5th ed. New York, McGraw-Hill, 1983, pp. 751–777.

251. Miller CG, Alleyne GA, Brooks SE: Gross cardiac involvement in glycogen storage disease type 3. Br Heart J 34:862–864, 1972.

252. Miller G, Partridge A: Mucopolysaccharidosis type VI presenting in infancy with endocardial fibroelastosis and heart failure. Pediatr Cardiol 4:61–62, 1983.

253. Minow RA, Benjamin RS, Gottlieb JA: Adriamycin (NSC-123127) cardiomyopathy—an overview with determination of risk factors. Cancer Chemother Rep 6:195–201, 1975.

254. Minow RA, Benjamin RS, Lee ET, et al: Adriamycin cardiomyopathy—risk factors. Cancer 39:1397–1402, 1977.

255. Mintz GS, Kotler MN, Segal BL, et al: Systolic anterior motion of the mitral valve in the absence of asymmetric septal hypertrophy. Circulation 57:256–263, 1978.

256. Mirsky I, Cohn PF, Levine JA: Assessment of left ventricular stiffness in primary myocardial disease and coronary artery disease. Circulation 50:128–136, 1974.

257. Modlin JF: Perinatal echovirus and group B Coxsackievirus infections. Clin Perinatol 15:233–246, 1988.

258. Moller P, Lunde P, Hovig T, et al: Familial cardiomyopathy. Clin Genet 16:233–243, 1979.

259. Morgan Hughes JA, Hayes DJ, Cooper M, et al: Mitochondrial myopathies: deficiencies localized to complex I and complex III of the mitochondrial respiratory chain. Biochem Soc Trans 13:648–650, 1985.

260. Moser HW, Chen WW: Ceramidase deficiency: Farber's lipogranulomatosis. In Stanbury JB, Wyngaarden JB, Fredrickson DS, et al (eds): The Metabolic Basis of Inherited Disease, 5th ed. New York, McGraw-Hill, 1983, pp. 820–830.

261. Murgo JP, Alter BR, Dorethy JF, et al: Dynamics of left ventricular ejection in obstructive and nonobstructive hypertrophic cardiomyopathy. J Clin Invest 66:1369–1382, 1980.

262. Myers CE, McGuire WP, Liss RH, et al: Adriamycin: the role of lipid peroxidation in cardiac toxicity and tumor responses. Science 197:165–167, 1977.

263. Myokoyama M, Kondo K, Hizawa K, et al: Life spans

of Duchenne muscular dystrophy patients in the hospital care program in Japan. J Neurol Sci 81:155–158, 1987.

264. Nakagwa M, Hamaoka K, Okano S, et al: Multiform accelerated idioventricular rhythm (AIVR) in a child with acute myocarditis. Clin Cardiol 11:853–855, 1988.

265. Nakano E, Takeshige K, Toshima Y, et al: Oxidative damage in selenium deficient hearts on perfusion with adriamycin: protective role of glutathione peroxidase system. Cardiovasc Res 23:498–504, 1989.

266. Nakazawa H, Andrews PA, Callery PS, et al: Superoxide radical reactions with anthracycline antibiotics. Biochem Pharmacol 34:481–490, 1985.

267. Naylor EW, Mosovich LL, Guthrie R, et al: Intermittent non-ketotic dicarboxylic aciduria in two siblings with hypoglycaemia: an apparent defect in beta-oxidation of fatty acids. J Inherited Metab Dis 3:19–24, 1980.

268. Nelson A, Peterson L, Frampton B, et al: Mucopolysaccharidosis VII (β-glucuronidase deficiency) presenting as nonimmune hydrops fetalis. J Pediatr 101:574–576, 1982.

269. Neri B, Neri GC, Bandinelli M: Differences between carnitine derivatives and coenzyme Q10 in preventing in vitro doxorubicin related cardiac damage. Oncology 45:242–246, 1988.

270. Neustein HB, Lurie PR, Dahms B, et al: An X-linked recessive cardiomyopathy with abnormal mitochondria. Pediatrics 64:24–29, 1979.

271. Neustein HB, Lurie PR, Fugita M: Endocardial fibroelastosis found on transvascular endomyocardial biopsy in children. Arch Pathol Lab Med 103:214–219, 1979.

272. Niederewieser A, Steinmann B, Exner U, et al: Multiple acyl-Co A dehydrogenation deficiency (MADD) in a boy with nonketotic hypoglycemia, hepatomegaly, muscle hypotonia, and cardiomyopathy. Helv Paediatr Acta 38:9–26, 1983.

273. Nielsen D, Jensen JB, Dombernowsky P, et al: Epirubicin cardiotoxicity: a study of 135 patients with advanced breast cancer. J Clin Oncol 8:1806–1810, 1990.

274. Nishimura RA, Tajik AJ, Reeder GS, et al: Evaluation of hypertrophic cardiomyopathy by Doppler color flow imaging: initial observations. Mayo Clin Proc 61:631–639, 1986.

275. O'Connell JB, Fowles RE, Robinson JA, et al: Clinical and pathological findings of myocarditis in two families with dilated cardiomyopathy. Am Heart J 107:127–135, 1984.

276. O'Connell JB, Robinson JA, Henkin RE, et al: Immunosuppressive therapy in patients with congestive cardiomyopathy and myocardial uptake of gallium-67. Circulation 64:780–786, 1981.

277. Ogata Y, Hiyamuta K, Terasawa M, et al: Relationship of exercise or pacing induced ST segment depression and myocardial lactate metabolism in patients with hypertrophic cardiomyopathy. Jpn Heart J 27:145–158, 1986.

278. Olson LJ, Reeder GS, Noller KL, et al: Cardiac involvement in glycogen storage disease 3: morphologic and biochemical characterization with endomyocardial biopsy. Am J Cardiol 53:980–981, 1984.

279. Ondrias K, Borgotta L, Kim DH, et al: Biphasic effects of doxorubicin on the calcium release channel from sarcoplasmic reticulum of cardiac muscle. Circ Res 67:1167–1174, 1990.

280. Palmeri ST, Bonow RO, Myers CE, et al: Prospective evaluation of doxorubicin cardiotoxicity by rest and exercise radionuclide angiography. Am J Cardiol 58:607–613, 1986.

281. Papadimitriou A, Neustein HB, DiMauro S: Histiocytoid cardiomyopathy of infancy: deficiency of reducible cytochrome b in heart mitochondria. Pediatr Res 18:1023–1028, 1984.

282. Parmley WW: Factors causing arrhythmias in chronic congestive heart failure. Am Heart J 114:1267–1272, 1987.

283. Pasternac A, Krol R, Petitclerc R, et al: Hypertrophic cardiomyopathy in Friedreich's ataxia: symmetric or asymmetric? Can J Neurol Sci 7:379–382, 1980.

284. Pasternac A, Noble J, Streulens Y, et al: Pathophysiology of chest pain in patients with cardiomyopathies and normal coronary arteries. Circulation 65:778–789, 1982.

285. Paulus WJ, Lorell BH, Craig WE, et al: Comparison of the effects of nitroprusside and nifedipine on diastolic properties in patients with hypertrophic cardiomyopathy: altered left ventricular loading or improved muscle inactivation. J Am Coll Cardiol 2:879–886, 1983.

286. Pentland B, Fox KA: The heart in Friedreich's ataxia. J Neurol Neurosurg Psychiatry 46:1138–1142, 1983.

287. Pernot C, Loth P, Gautier M: The myocardiopathies of glycogenosis. Arch Mal Coeur 71:428–436, 1978.

288. Pichard AD, Meller J, Teichholz LE, et al: Septal perforator compression (narrowing) in idiopathic hypertrophic subaortic stenosis. Am J Cardiol 40:310–314, 1977.

289. Pierpoint ME, Tripp ME: Abnormalities of intermediary metabolism. In Pierpont ME, Moller JH (eds): Genetics of Cardiovascular Disease. Boston, Martinus Nijhoff, 1986, pp. 193–214.

290. Pinamonti B, Alberti E, Cigalotto A, et al: Echocardiographic findings in myocarditis. Am J Cardiol 62:285–291, 1988.

291. Piver MS, Marchetti DL, Parthasarathy KL, et al: Doxorubicin hydrochloride (adriamycin) cardiotoxicity evaluated by sequential radionuclide angiocardiography. Cancer 56:76–80, 1985.

292. Platzker Y, Fisman E, Pines A, et al: Unusual echocardiographic pattern in Gaucher's disease. Cardiology 72:144–146, 1985.

293. Powell SR, McCay PB: Inhibition of doxorubicin initiated membrane damage by N-acetylcysteine: possible mediation by a thioldependent, cytosolic inhibitor of lipid peroxidation. Toxicol Appl Pharmacol 96:175–184, 1988.

294. Powis G: Free radical formation by antitumor quinones. Free Radic Biol Med 6:63–101, 1989.

295. Praga C, Beretta G, Vigo PL: Adriamycin cardiotoxicity: a survey of 1,273 patients. Cancer Treat Rep 63:827–834, 1979.

296. Pratt CB, Ransom JL, Evans WE: Age related adriamycin cardiotoxicity in children. Cancer Treat Rep 62:1381–1385, 1978.

297. Radford DJ, Chalk SM: Infantile xanthomatous cardiomyopathy. Aust Paediatr J 16:123–125, 1980.

298. Rebouche CJ, Engel AG: Primary systemic carnitine deficiency. I. Carnitine biosynthesis. Neurology 31:813–818, 1981.

299. Rebouche CJ, Engel AG: Carnitine transport in cultured muscle cells and skin fibroblasts from patients with primary systemic carnitine deficiency. In Vitro 18:495–500, 1982.

300. Rebouche CJ, Engel AG: Kinetic compartmental analysis of carnitine metabolism in the human carnitine deficiency syndromes: evidence for alterations in tissue carnitine transport. J Clin Invest 73:857–867, 1984.

301. Regitz V, Hodach RJ, Shug AL: Carnitine deficiency:

a treatable cause of cardiomyopathy in children. Klin Wochenschr 60:393–400, 1988.

302. Richterich R, van Mechelen P, Rossi E: Refsum's disease (heredopathia atactica polyneuritiformis): an inborn tetramethyl hexadecanoic acid. Am J Med 39:230–236, 1965.

303. Rimoldi M, Bottacchi E, Rossi L, et al: Cytochrome-C-oxidase deficiency in muscles of a floppy infant without mitochondrial myopathy. J Neurol 227:201–207, 1982.

304. Roberts WC, Ferrans VJ: Pathologic anatomy of the cardiomyopathies. Hum Pathol 6:287–342, 1975.

305. Roberts WC, Perry LW, Chandra RS, et al: Aortic valve atresia: a new classification based on necropsy study of 73 cases. Am J Cardiol 37:753–756, 1976.

306. Rosenburg H, Frewen TC, Li MD, et al: Cardiac involvement in diseases characterized by β-galactosidase deficiency. J Pediatr 106:78–80, 1985.

307. Rosenquist M, Biorck G, de Faire U, et al: Familial cardiomyopathy—a 15-year follow-up. Eur J Cardiol 12:107–120, 1980.

308. Ross RS, Bulkley BH, Hutchins GM, et al: Idiopathic familial myocardiopathy in three generations: a clinical and pathologic study. Am Heart J 96:170–179, 1978.

309. Rossignol AM, Meyer M, Rossignol B, et al: Glycogenosis type III myocardiopathy. Arch Fr Pediatr 36:303–309, 1979.

310. Rozkovec A, Cambridge G, King M et al: Natural history of left ventricular function in natal Coxsackie myocarditis. Pediatr Cardiol 6:151–156, 1985.

311. Rudge MF, Duncan CJ: Ultrastructural changes in the cardiomyopathy of dystrophic hamsters and mice. Tissue Cell 20:249–253, 1988.

312. Ruschaupt DG, Thilenius OG, Cassels DE: Friedreich's ataxia associated with idiopathic hypertrophic subaortic stenosis. Am Heart J 84:95–102, 1972.

313. Rutledge JC, Haas JE, Monnat R, et al: Hypertrophic cardiomyopathy is a component of subacute necrotizing encephalomyelopathy. J Pediatr 101:706–710, 1982.

314. Saffitz JE, Ferrans VJ, Rodriguez VJ, et al: Histiocytoid cardiomyopathy: a cause of sudden death in apparently healthy infants. Am J Cardiol 52:215–217, 1983.

315. Saffitz JE, Schwartz DJ, Southworth W, et al: Coxsackie viral myocarditis causing transmural right and left ventricular infarction without coronary narrowing. Am J Cardiol 52:644–647, 1983.

316. Saini J, Rich MW, Lyss AP: Reversibility of severe left ventricular dysfunction due to doxorubicin cardiotoxicity. Ann Intern Med 106:814–816, 1987.

317. Sanders SP, Parness IA, Colan SD: Recognition of abnormal connections of coronary arteries using Doppler color flow mapping. J Am Coll Cardiol 13:922–926, 1989.

318. Sanderson JE, Gibson DG, Brown DJ, et al: Left ventricular filling in hypertrophic cardiomyopathy: an angiographic study. Br Heart J 39:661–670, 1977.

319. Sanderson JE, Traill TA, Sutton MG, et al: Left ventricular relaxation and filling in hypertrophic cardiomyopathy: an echocardiographic study. Br Heart J 40:595–601, 1978.

320. Sanyal SK, Johnson WW, Dische MR, et al: Dystrophic degeneration of papillary muscle and ventricular myocardium: a basis for mitral valve prolapse in Duchenne's muscular dystrophy. Circulation 62:430–438, 1980.

321. Sanyal SK, Johnson WW, Thapar MK, et al: An ultrastructural basis for electrocardiographic alterations associated with Duchenne's progressive muscular dystrophy. Circulation 57:1122–1129, 1978.

322. Sanyal SK, Leung RK, Tierney RC, et al: Mitral valve prolapse syndrome in children with Duchenne's progressive muscular dystrophy. Pediatrics 63:116–123, 1979.

323. Sanyal SK, Tierney RC, Rao PS, et al: Systolic time interval characteristics in children with Duchenne's progressive muscular dystrophy. Pediatrics 70:958–964, 1982.

324. Sasson Z, Yock PG, Hatle LK, et al: Doppler echocardiographic determination of the pressure gradient in hypertrophic cardiomyopathy. J Am Coll Cardiol 11:752–756, 1988.

325. Schaffer MS, Freedom RM, Rowe RD: Hypertrophic cardiomyopathy presenting before 2 years of age in 13 patients. Pediatr Cardiol 4:113–119, 1983.

326. Schmaltz AA, Apitz J, Hort W: Endomyocardial biopsy in infants and children: technique, indications and results. Eur J Pediatr 138:211–215, 1982.

327. Schmaltz AA, Apitz J, Hort W: Dilated cardiomyopathy in childhood: problems of diagnosis and long term follow-up. Eur Heart J 8:100–105, 1987.

328. Schmidt MA, Michels VV, Edwards WD, et al: Familial dilated cardiomyopathy. Am J Med Genet 31:135–143, 1988.

329. Scholte HR, Hulsmann WC, Luyt Houwen IE, et al: Carnitine palmityltransferase deficiencies. Biochem Soc Trans 13:643–645, 1985.

330. Schwartz RG, McKenzie WB, Alexander J, et al: Congestive heart failure and left ventricular dysfunction complicating doxorubicin therapy: seven year experience using serial radionuclide angiocardiography. Am J Med 82:1109–1118, 1987.

331. Scott MO, Sylvester JE, Heiman Patterson T, et al: Duchenne muscular dystrophy gene expression in normal and diseased human muscle. Science 239:1418–1420, 1988.

332. Seitz RJ, Langes K, Frenzel H, et al: Congenital Leigh's disease: panencephalomyelopathy and peripheral neuropathy. Acta Neuropathol (Berl) 64:167–171, 1984.

333. Sengers RCA, ter Haar BGA, Trijbels JMF, et al: Congenital cataract and mitochondrial myopathy of skeletal and heart muscle associated with lactic acidosis after exercise. J Pediatr 86:873–880, 1975.

334. Sengers RCA, Trijbels JMF, Bakkeren JAJM, et al: Deficiency of cytochromes b and aa3 in muscle from a floppy infant with cytochrome oxidase deficiency. Eur J Pediatr 141:178–180, 1984.

335. Servidei S, Metlay LA, Chodosh J, et al: Fatal infantile cardiopathy caused by phosphorylase b kinase deficiency. J Pediatr 113:82–85, 1988.

336. Servidei S, Riepe RE, Langston C, et al: Severe cardiopathy in branching enzyme deficiency. J Pediatr 111:51–56, 1987.

337. Sethna NF, Rockoff MA: Cardiac arrest following inhalation induction of anaesthesia in a child with Duchenne's muscular dystrophy. Can Anaesth Soc J 33:799–802, 1986.

338. Shaffer EM, Rocchini AP, Spicer RL, et al: Effects of verapamil on left ventricular diastolic filling in children with hypertrophic cardiomyopathy. Am J Cardiol 61:413–417, 1988.

339. Shanes JG, Ghali J, Billingham ME, et al: Interobserver variability in the pathologic interpretation of endomyocardial biopsy results. Circulation 75:401–405, 1987.

340. Shapir Y, Roguin N: Echocardiographic findings in Pompe's disease with left ventricular obstruction. Clin Cardiol 8:181–185, 1985.

341. Shapiro F, Sethna N, Colan S, et al: Spinal fusion in Duchenne muscular dystrophy: a multidisciplinary approach. Circulation (in press).

342. Shapiro LM, McKenna WJ: Distribution of left ventricular hypertrophy in hypertrophic cardiomyopathy: a two-dimensional echocardiographic study. J Am Coll Cardiol 2:437–444, 1983.

343. Sharratt GP, Jacob JC, Hobeika C: Friedreich's ataxia presenting as cardiac disease. Pediatr Cardiol 6:41–42, 1985.

344. Shimamatsu M, Toshima H: Impaired coronary vasodilatory capacity after dipyridamole administration in hypertrophic cardiomyopathy. Jpn Heart J 28:387–401, 1987.

345. Silver MM, Burns JE, Sethi RJ, et al: Oncocytic cardiomyopathy in an infant with oncocytosis in exocrine and endocrine glands. Hum Pathol 11:598–605, 1980.

346. Singal PK, Deally CM, Weinberg LE: Subcellular effects of adriamycin in the heart: a concise review. J Mol Cell Cardiol 19:817–828, 1987.

347. Singal PK, Tong JG: Vitamin E deficiency accentuates adriamycin-induced cardiomyopathy and cell surface changes. Mol Cell Biochem 84:163–171, 1988.

348. Smith CL, Bush GH: Anaesthesia and progressive muscular dystrophy. Br J Anaesth 57:1113–1118, 1985.

349. Speyer JL, Green MD, Kramer E, et al: Protective effect of the bispiperazinedione ICRF-187 against doxorubicin-induced cardiac toxicity in women with advanced breast cancer. N Engl J Med 319:745–752, 1988.

350. Spirito P, Maron BJ: Absence of progression of left ventricular hypertrophy in adult patients with hypertrophic cardiomyopathy. J Am Coll Cardiol 9:1013–1017, 1987.

351. Sprigz RA, Doughty RA, Spackman TJ, et al: Neonatal presentation of I-cell disease. J Pediatr 93:954–958, 1982.

352. St. John Sutton MG, Tajik AJ, Giuliani ER, et al: Hypertrophic obstructive cardiomyopathy and lentiginosis: a little known neural ectodermal syndrome. Am J Cardiol 47:214–217, 1981.

353. Stanbury JB, Wyngaarden JB, Fredrickson DS, et al: The Metabolic Basis of Inherited Disease, 5th ed. New York, McGraw-Hill, 1983.

354. Stapleton JF, Segal JP, Harvey WP: The electrocardiogram of myocardiopathy. Prog Cardiovasc Dis 13:217–239, 1970.

355. Steinberg JS, Cohen AJ, Wasserman AG, et al: Acute arrhythmogenicity of doxorubicin administration. Cancer 60:1213–1218, 1987.

356. Steinberg JSD, Wasserman AG: Radionuclide ventriculography for evaluation and prevention of doxorubicin cardiotoxicity. Clin Ther 7:660–667, 1985.

357. Stewart WJ, Schiavone WA, Salcedo EE, et al: Intraoperative Doppler echocardiography in hypertrophic cardiomyopathy: correlations with the obstructive gradient. J Am Coll Cardiol 10:327–335, 1987.

358. Storm G, Van Hoesel QG, Gittenberger-de Groot A, et al: A comparative study on the antitumor effect, cardiotoxicity and nephrotoxicity of doxorubicin given as a bolus, continuous infusion or entrapped in liposomes in the Lou/M Wsl rat. Cancer Chemother Pharmacol 24:341–348, 1989.

359. Strashun AM, Goldsmith SJ, Horowitz SF: Gated blood pool scintigraphic monitoring of doxorubicin cardiomyopathy: comparison of camera and computerized probe results in 101 patients. J Am Coll Cardiol 8:1082–1087, 1986.

360. Stumpf DA. Friedreich's disease: a metabolic cardiomyopathy. Am Heart J 104:887–888, 1982.

361. Swank SM, Brown JC, Perry RE: Spinal fusion in Duchenne's muscular dystrophy. Spine 7:484–491, 1982.

362. Tacke E, Kupferschmid C, Lang D: Hypertrophic cardiomyopathy during ACTH treatment. Klin Padiatr 195:124–128, 1983.

363. Taillard F, Mundler O, Tillous Borde, et al: Value of radionuclide assessment with thallium 201 scintigraphy in carnitine deficiency cardiomyopathy. Eur Heart J 9:811–818, 1988.

364. Takenaka K, Dabestani A, Gardin JM, et al: Left ventricular filling in hypertrophic cardiomyopathy: a pulsed Doppler echocardiographic study. J Am Coll Cardiol 7:1263–1271, 1986.

365. Talierco CP, Olney BA, Lie JT: Myocarditis related to drug hypersensitivity. Mayo Clin Proc 60:463–468, 1985.

366. Taliercio CP, Seward JB, Driscoll DJ, et al: Idiopathic dilated cardiomyopathy in the young: clinical profile and natural history. J Am Coll Cardiol 6:1126–1131, 1985.

367. Talwar KK, Chopra P, Narula J: Myocardial involvement and its response to immunosuppressive therapy in nonspecific aortoarteritis (Takayasu's disease)—a study by endomyocardial biopsy. Int J Cardiol 23:323–334, 1988.

368. Talwar KK, Radhakrishnan S, Chopra P: Myocarditis manifesting as persistent atrial standstill. Int J Cardiol 20:283–286, 1988.

369. Tanaka M, Fujiwara H, Onodera T, et al: Quantitative analysis of narrowing of intramyocardial small arteries in normal hearts, hypertensive hearts, and hearts with hypertrophic cardiomyopathy. Circulation 75:1130–1139, 1987.

370. Teare D: Asymmetrical hypertrophy of the heart in young adults. Br Heart J 20:1, 1958.

371. Teirstein PS, Yock PG, Popp RL: The accuracy of Doppler ultrasound measurement of pressure gradients across irregular, dual, and tunnel-like obstructions to blood flow. Circulation 72:577–584, 1985.

372. Thompson DS, Naqvi N, Juul SM, et al: Effects of propranolol on myocardial oxygen consumption, substrate extraction, and hemodynamics in hypertrophic obstructive cardiomyopathy. Br Heart J 44:488–498, 1980.

373. Thompson JA, Hess ML: The oxygen free radical system: a fundamental mechanism in the production of myocardial necrosis. Prog Cardiovasc Dis 28:449–462, 1986.

374. Thompson RC, Canby RC, Lojeski EW, et al: Adriamycin cardiotoxicity and proton nuclear magnetic resonance relaxation properties. Am Heart J 113:1444–1449, 1987.

375. Tiede R, Sareen S, Singal PK: Transferrin delays oxygen radical induced cardiac-contractile failure. Can J Physiol Pharmacol 68:480–485, 1990.

376. Topol EJ, Traill TA, Fortuin NJ: Hypertensive hypertrophic cardiomyopathy of the elderly. N Engl J Med 312:277–283, 1985.

377. Tracy S, Wiegand V, McManus B, et al: Molecular approaches to enteroviral diagnosis in idiopathic cardiomyopathy and myocarditis. J Am Coll Cardiol 15:1688–1694, 1990.

378. Tripp ME, Katcher ML, Peters HA, et al: Systemic carnitine deficiency presenting as familial endocardial fibroelastosis: a treatable cardiomyopathy. N Engl J Med. 305:385–390, 1981.

379. Ulmer HE, Ludwig R, Geiger H: Assessment of adriamycin cardiotoxicity in children by systolic time intervals. Eur J Pediatr 131:21–31, 1979.

380. Umsawasadi T, Valdivieso M, Booser DJ, et al: Weekly doxorubicin versus doxorubicin every 3 weeks in cyclophosphamide, doxorubicin, and cisplantic chemo-

therapy for non small cell lung cancer. Cancer 64:1995–2000, 1989.

381. Unverferth DV, Magorien RD, Moeschberger ML, et al: Factors influencing the one year mortality of dilated cardiomyopathy. Am J Cardiol 54:147–152, 1984.

382. Unverferth DV, Schmidt WR 2nd, Baker PB, et al: Morphologic and functional characteristics of the heart in Friedreich's ataxia. Am J Med 82:5–10, 1987.

383. Urie PM, Billingham ME: Ultrastructural features of familial cardiomyopathy. Am J Cardiol 62:325–327, 1988.

384. Valantine HA, Hunt SA, Fowler MB, et al: Frequency of familial nature of dilated cardiomyopathy and usefulness of cardiac transplantation in this subset. Am J Cardiol 63:959–963, 1989.

385. Van der Hauwaert LG, Denef B, Dumoulin M: Long-term echocardiographic assessment of dilated cardiomyopathy in children. Am J Cardiol 52:1066–1071, 1983.

386. Van Dyke DH, Griggs RC, Markesbery E, et al: Hereditary carnitine deficiency of muscle. Neurology 25:154–159, 1975.

387. Vietor KW, Havsteen B, Harms D, et al: Ethanolaminosis: a new recognized, generalized storage disease with cardiomegaly, cerebral dysfunction and early death. Eur J Pediatr 126:61–75, 1977.

388. Vignola PA, Aonuma K, Swaye PS, et al: Lymphocytic myocarditis presenting as unexplained ventricular arrhythmias: diagnosis with endomyocardial biopsy and response to immunosuppression. J Am Coll Cardiol 4:812–819, 1984.

389. Voigt GC: Steroid therapy in viral myocarditis. Am Heart J 75:575–576, 1968.

390. Von Herbay A, Dorken B, Mall G, et al: Cardiac damage in autologous bone marrow transplant patients: an autopsy study. Cardiotoxic pretreatment as a major risk factor. Klin Wochenschr 66:1175–1181, 1988.

391. Von Hoff DD, Layard M: Risk factors for the development of doxorubicin cardiotoxicity. Cancer Treat Rep 65(Suppl 4):19–24, 1982.

392. Von Hoff DD, Layard MW, Basa P, et al: Risk factors for doxorubicin-induced congestive heart failure. Ann Intern Med 91:710–717, 1979.

393. Waber LJ, Valle D, Neill C, et al: Carnitine deficiency presenting as familial cardiomyopathy: a treatable defect in carnitine transport. J Pediatr 101:700–705, 1982.

394. Wallace DC: Mitochondrial genes and disease. Hosp Pract [Off] 21:77–92, 1986.

395. Wallis DE, O'Connell JB, Henkin RE, et al: Segmental wall motion abnormalities in dilated cardiomyopathy: a common finding and good prognostic sign. J Am Coll Cardiol 4:674–679, 1984.

396. Wang JM, Stanley TH: Duchenne muscular dystrophy and malignant hyperthermia—two case reports. Can Anaesth Soc J 33:492–497, 1986.

397. Watkins SC, Hoffman EP, Slayter HS, et al: Immu-

noelectron microscopic localization of dystrophin in myofibers. Nature 333:863–866, 1988.

398. Westwood M: Endocardial fibroelastosis and Niemann-Pick disease. Br Heart J 39:1394–1396, 1977.

399. Wigle ED, Adelman AG, Auger P, et al: Mitral regurgitation in muscular subaortic stenosis. Am J Cardiol 24:698–706, 1969.

400. Wigle ED, Henderson M, Rakowski H, et al: Muscular (hypertrophic) subaortic stenosis (hypertrophic obstructive cardiomyopathy): the evidence for true obstruction to left ventricular outflow. Postgrad Med J 62:531–536, 1986.

401. Wigle ED, Rakowski H: Evidence for true obstruction to left ventricular outflow in obstructive hypertrophic cardiomyopathy (muscular or hypertrophic subaortic stenosis). Z Kardiol 76:61–68, 1987.

402. Wigle ED, Sasson Z, Henderson MA, et al: Hypertrophic cardiomyopathy: the importance of the site and the extent of hypertrophy. A review. Prog Cardiovasc Dis 28:1–83, 1985.

403. Wilson MS, Barth RF, Baker PB et al: Giant cell myocarditis. Am J Med 79:647–652, 1985.

404. Witzleben CL, Pinto M: Foamy myocardial transformation of infancy: "lipid" or "histiocytoid" myocardiopathy. Arch Pathol Lab Med 102:306–311, 1978.

405. Woodruff JF: Viral myocarditis. Am J Pathol 101:426–479, 1980.

406. World Health Organization: Report of the WHO/IFSC task force on the definition and classification of cardiac myopathies. Br Heart J 44:672–673, 1980.

407. Yazawa Y: Mitral valve prolapse related to geometrical changes of the heart in cases of progressive muscular dystrophy. Clin Cardiol 7:198–204, 1984.

408. Yock PG, Hatle L, Popp RL: Patterns and timing of Doppler detected intracavitary and aortic flow in hypertrophic cardiomyopathy. J Am Coll Cardiol 8:1047–1058, 1986.

409. Yoshizato T, Edwards WD, Alboliras ET, et al: Safety and utility of endomyocardial biopsy in infants, children and adolescents: a review of 66 procedures in 53 patients. J Am Coll Cardiol 15:436–442, 1990.

410. Young RC, Ozolos RF, Meyers CE: The anthracycline antineoplasmic drugs. N Engl J Med 305:139–153, 1981.

411. Yutani C, Go S, Kamiya T, et al: Cardiac biopsy of Kawasaki disease. Arch Pathol Lab Med 105:470–473, 1981.

412. Zalman F, Perloff JK, Durant NN, et al: Acute respiratory failure following intravenous verapamil in Duchenne's muscular dystrophy. Am Heart J 105:510–511, 1983.

413. Zidenberg-Cherr S, Keen CL: Influence of dietary manganese and vitamin E on adriamycin toxicity in mice. Toxicol Lett 30:79–87, 1986.

414. Zorzato F, Salviati G, Facchinetti T, et al: Doxorubicin induces calcium release from terminal cisternae of skeletal muscle. J Biol Chem 260:7349–7355, 1985.

Chapter 25

PERICARDIAL DISEASE

Donald C. Fyler, M.D.

DEFINITION

Virtually any pathologic process, ranging from viral or bacterial infections to tumors and collagen diseases, can involve the pericardium.

PREVALENCE

Primary pericardial disease is a rare problem in pediatrics. There were 95 individuals with a primary pericardial disease and 468 with secondary pericardial problems, usually following surgery, in Boston Children's Hospital experience between 1973 and 1987 (Exhibit 1).

PHYSIOLOGY

Normally, the pericardium places no significant limit on the amount of venous return that can be accommodated within the heart at rest and exercise. When there is pericardial effusion, the available space to handle venous return is reduced and if there is excessive pericardial fluid, there may be severe limitation of venous return and, therefore, of cardiac output.

The capacity of the pericardium is influenced by its natural stiffness. Rapid accumulation of fluid is tolerated less well than slow accumulation, which may allow large amounts of pericardial fluid to collect without producing symptoms. The stiffness of the pericardium is influenced by the disease process, and if there is thickening, as in bacterial infection, the ability of the pericardium to dilate may be less than normal. Finally, if the pericardium is thickened, scarred, and even calcified, it may become a rigid structure with an unyielding limit on the amount of venous return that can be accommodated.[6,7]

With increased pressure within the pericardial sac, the pressures in all chambers of the heart are elevated. In advanced stages, right and left atrial mean pressures and right and left ventricular end-

Exhibit 1

Boston Children's Hospital Experience 1973–1987		
Primary Diagnosis Pericardial Disease		
	1973–77	*1978–82*	*1983–87*
Number of Patients	22	18	67*

*44 of these patients were diagnosed by echocardiography only.

Types of Pericardial Problems

Problem	Primary Pericardial Disease n = 95	Secondary Pericardial Disease n = 468
Absent pericardium	5	7
Constrictive pericarditis	4	1
"Pericarditis"	35	48
Cardiac surgery	—	377
Postpericardiotomy syndrome	—	35
Pericardial effusion only discovered at echocardiography	44	—
Other	7	—

There were 95 children seen with primary pericarditis in the 15-year period between 1973 and 1987. Pericardial disease was encountered in 468 children with other cardiac problems, most of these (377) associated with surgery. There were 77 patients who had pericardial effusion associated with Fontan's operation. There was an increase in diagnosis of pericardial effusion with the advent of echocardiography

diastolic pressures are virtually identical with the intrapericardial pressure (Fig. 1).

The clinical features of pericardial disease are dependent, primarily, on the limitation of venous return and, secondarily, on limitation of cardiac output. Initially, there is restriction of increased cardiac output with exercise; later, symptoms of limited output may be observed at rest. When the

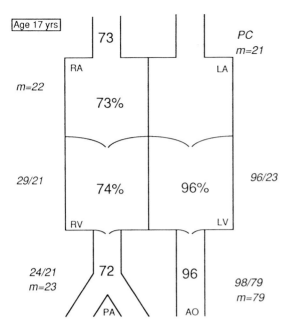

Figure 1. Physiologic diagram of a patient with constrictive pericarditis. Note the similarity of atrial, ventricular end-diastolic, and pulmonary diastolic pressures. This 17-year-old boy worked until a few days before admission, when his doctor insisted on hospitalization because of ascites which had developed over months. RA = right atrium, LA = left atrium, RV = right ventricle, LV = left ventricle, AO = aorta, PA = pulmonary artery, large bold numbers = oxygen percent saturation, italics = pressure.

pericardial fluid is under increased pressure, the cardiac output is depressed, the peripheral pulses and the pulse pressure are small, and the systolic blood pressure is low. Normal respiratory variation of blood pressure is increased when there is pericardial effusion. This is "pulsus paradoxus" which, in fact, is not paradoxical at all. Pulsus paradoxus is best documented by observing the variation in the blood pressure, and it is said to be present when there is variation in excess of 10 mm Hg in systole or diastole (see Fig. 2, ch. 11). The venous pressure is elevated, there is neck vein distention and liver enlargement, and, in advanced cases, there may be ascites and peripheral edema. Tamponade refers to the sudden accumulation of pericardial fluid, such as blood, sufficient to inhibit cardiac output. With rapidly accumulating pericardial effusion there may be cardiovascular collapse and death.

CLINICAL MANIFESTATIONS

Inflammation of the pericardium may cause precordial or left shoulder pain, often aggravated or relieved by changes in physical position. Sometimes, it is associated with a hacking cough that also varies with position; the patient commonly notes that sitting up and leaning forward improves the cough. Pericardial pain is related to *acute* pericardial distention; patients with a *chronic* large effusion often have no pain at all.

Signs of right-sided heart failure support the diagnosis of pericardial disease. The liver may be enlarged, and there may be peripheral edema and ascites. The neck veins are distended and estimates of venous pressure are in excess of normal.

Because pericardial effusion limits the amount of blood that can enter the heart, it is unusual to encounter evidences of pulmonary edema. Although the left atrial pressure is elevated, it equals and does not exceed the right atrial pressure and, therefore, pulmonary edema is unlikely. There are no rales; there is no dyspnea or tachypnea.

On auscultation, a friction rub may be audible. A friction rub is diagnostic of pericardial disease and, when discovered, makes the diagnosis. The "rub" sounds are best heard with the stethoscopic diaphragm and may be heard in systole and diastole. The sound may seem quite close to the ear and is sometimes misinterpreted as movement of the stethoscope on the chest surface. It may sound like two leather surfaces being rubbed together or like the sounds produced when hair is rubbed between the fingers. Whenever there is a large collection of pericardial fluid, the pericardial surfaces are not in direct contact and a friction rub is not likely. Generally speaking, pericardial friction rubs are a feature of pericarditis when there is neither excess fluid collection nor signs of tamponade.

When there is a large amount of pericardial fluid the heart sounds may be distant because the fluid collection attentuates the transmission of sound.

Electrocardiography

The electrocardiogram is not especially helpful in the diagnosis of pericardial disease. It may show generalized elevation of the S-T segment "pericardial pattern" but this is rarely clear cut (Fig. 2).

Chest X-Ray

Depending on the amount of pericardial fluid, there is generalized enlargement of the heart shadow. Evidences of individual chamber enlargement are not seen; rarely, calcification of the pericardium is visible.

Echocardiography

Pericardial thickening or pericardial fluid is readily identified by echocardiography. Viewed in multiple projections the thickness of the pericardium and the amount of fluid can be quantified accurately. Since echocardiograms became available, the recognition of pericardial fluid has increased. Fully two-thirds of all patients found to have pericardial fluid in the past 15 years at Chil-

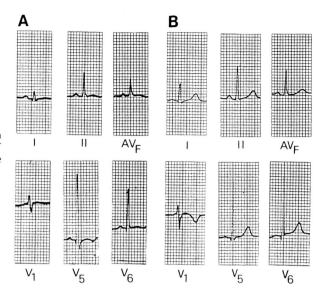

Figure 2. Electrocardiogram from a patient with pericarditis. **A,** Note the flattened and inverted T waves. **B,** The same patient 2 years later. Note the improvement in the T waves.

dren's Hospital in Boston were discovered with echocardiographic techniques, many postoperatively (see Fig. 28, p. 181).

Cardiac Catheterization

Cardiac catheterization is not required for the diagnosis of a pericardial disease. Occasionally, a patient with an unexplained cardiac problem comes to cardiac catheterization and is discovered to have generalized equilibration of diastolic pressures and atrial pressures (Fig. 1). When this occurs, the possibilities of constrictive pericarditis or restrictive myocarditis must be considered.

Pericardial tapping is usually accomplished in the catheterization laboratory because of the available equipment, particularly fluoroscopy.

Pericardiocentesis

A pericardial tap has about the same risk as a pleural tap and should be carried out as a diagnostic test in all patients with a pericardial effusion of unknown cause. This is especially important if there is any possibility that the underlying cause is bacterial infection, because drainage may be life-saving. There should be enough fluid to reasonably expect to remove some for diagnostic purposes. The child is placed in a semi-sitting position, roughly 45 degrees, and sedated or anesthetized as needed. Fluoroscopy or echocardiography should be available for deciding where to place the needle and for determining whether it is located where it ought to be.

A short, beveled, but sharp, needle is inserted beneath the xiphoid and angled upward and leftward toward the left shoulder. Sometimes, a pop is felt as the needle is passed into the pericardium. Attempts to withdraw fluid are made with each advance of the needle. If fluid is obtained, enough is removed to alleviate tamponade; a small amount

will provide significant benefit (20 ml is usually enough to produce improvement in an adult). If the fluid is grossly bloody, the possibility that the needle is in a cardiac chamber must be considered. A few drops on a towel are sometimes immediately convincing that the problem is blood-stained fluid and not pure blood. On other occasions, when there is debate, centrifugation of the fluid may show a hematocrit much lower than that of the blood.

Once it is established that the fluid obtained is being removed from the pericardium, all fluid that can be easily removed is taken out. Older patients undergoing tapping under sedation may report relief from symptoms at this point.

Whether or not to leave a drain in the pericardium depends on the probable diagnosis. When there is evidence of infection, a guide wire is passed into the pericardium; its position is confirmed by fluoroscopy or echocardiography, and then a catheter is passed over the wire into the pericardium as a drain. If there is dense fibrinoid material a large catheter may be needed. The drain should remain in place until there is no further drainage.

Once the diagnosis is established, often only after detailed examination of the fluid, definitive therapy can be undertaken.

SPECIFIC PROBLEMS

Bacterial Pericarditis

Children with bacterial pericarditis are acutely, often desperately, ill. They may have symptoms and signs of tamponade as well as evidences of overwhelming sepsis.[2] As soon as the diagnosis is suspected, relief of tamponade is undertaken. Removal of minimal amounts of fluid will relieve the danger, at least temporarily, and fluid for diagnosis and cultures will be available. A drain is left in the pericardium and appropriate heavy antibiotic therapy is begun.

Some bacterial infections may lead to constrictive pericarditis in a short time. With pericarditis caused by *Hemophilus influenzae*, this has occurred as early as a few weeks after onset. Serial echocardiograms are undertaken to evaluate this possibility. Sometimes as early as 1 month following onset, pericardiectomy has been necessary to relieve constriction. In general, however, bacterial pericarditis does not lead to constrictive pericarditis, and once therapy is undertaken, a permanent cure is anticipated.

Viral Pericarditis

Children with this disease have symptoms of a viral illness, including fever; usually the white count and differential blood count are normal, but because of pain in the chest or shoulder, or the presence of a friction rub, they are examined by echocardiography. When pericardial fluid has been demonstrated, the diagnosis is established. Management is expectant. Only rarely is pericardial drainage required. Most often patients with this type of pericarditis are discharged with a regimen of anti-inflammatory therapy such as aspirin or indomethacin; they should be followed for at least several months to monitor their progress.

Postpericardiotomy Effusions

Most patients have bloody pericardial fluid following cardiac surgery.[8] This is usually more a matter of interest than a problem requiring treatment, but in some patients, particularly following a Fontan operation, excess pericardial fluid may require attention as early as 7 days after operation, and sometimes it may persist for months.

Postpericardiotomy syndrome describes a pericardial effusion that appears following recovery from uncomplicated cardiac surgery.[1] Generally, it appears between 7 days to 2 months after the operation, and for this reason all patients who undergo cardiac surgery should have a chest x-ray 2 weeks after discharge to exclude this possibility. The child may have been progressing well in the postoperative period only to regress, lose appetite, seem sick, and complain of discomfort. An echocardiogram confirms the diagnosis. Occasionally, such a child will develop tamponade and require pericardial drainage of bloody serous fluid, but most are managed with anti-inflammatory agents such as aspirin, indomethacin and, rarely, prednisone for weeks to months following discovery of the problem.

Constrictive Pericarditis

Usually, the cause of constrictive pericarditis is not evident. Generally, there is an insidious onset of right-sided heart failure. Peripheral edema, ascites, hepatomegaly, and distention of the neck veins, with associated symptoms of fatigue and lassitude, are the classical symptoms but they appear gradually over a time. On chest x-ray, the heart is usually not large and may be normal in size (Fig. 3). Sometimes, but not necessarily, there may be visible calcification of the pericardium. On echocardiography there is thickening of the pericardium and limitation of cardiac motion. Cardiac catheterization is usually undertaken, in part to assess the contribution of myocardial dysfunction and, in part, simply to document the situation against future care.

Once a diagnosis is made, the surgeons are asked to remove as much of the thickened, stiff, sometimes adherent, pericardium as is possible.[3] Often, patients are not obviously improved in the immediate postoperative period. Residual evidence of congestive heart failure is common and improvement is slow. The theory that cardiac contraction has been compromised for a long period and, there-

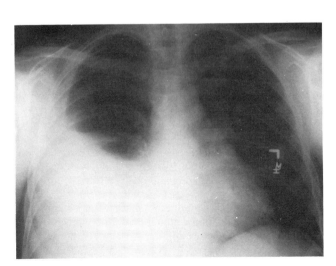

Figure 3. Chest x-ray of a 17-year-old boy with chronic constrictive pericarditis and ascites. Note the small size of the heart and the pleural effusion.

fore, the amount of cardiac muscle available for contraction is limited is not particularly convincing. It seems, rather, that there is associated myocardial damage as well as pericardial disease in these patients. In any case, careful follow-up of progress is needed and, with time, recovery often seems complete.

Rheumatic Fever

Acute rheumatic fever and rheumatic heart disease may be associated with accumulation of serous pericardial fluid. It is rare that tamponade develops, and it is unheard of to have rheumatic pericarditis without associated rheumatic murmurs (a useful and distinguishing diagnostic feature). Rarely, pericardial tapping is required.

Collagen Disease

Patients with lupus erythematosus, rheumatoid arthritis, scleroderma, or dermatomyositis may develop intrapericardial effusion. Only rarely is this massive, and very rarely is there tamponade. Usually the underlying disease is apparent, although occasionally, particularly in patients with lupus erythematosus or with rheumatoid arthritis, pericardial effusion may be the first problem presented. Unfortunately, if a diagnostic pericardial tap is done, the fluid is not characteristic. Generally, the disease declares itself with continued observation.

Idiopathic Pericarditis

Occasionally, one sees a patient in whom no cause for pericarditis is found. Sometimes such a patient will have recurrent pericardial effusion over months or years. Anti-inflammatory agents such as aspirin or indomethacin have been helpful in managing some of these patients.

Tuberculous Pericarditis

At Children's Hospital in Boston, the last patient with tuberculous pericarditis was seen more than 30 years ago. The combination of pericarditis and a positive history of tuberculosis, or a positive tuberculin test, should suggest this possibility. Modern antituberculous therapy should play a major role in managing this problem.

Tumor

Intrapericardial teratoma is a disease of newborn and small infants characterized by the recurrent accumulation of serous pericardial fluid (see p. 729).

Other Causes of Pericardial Effusion

Pericardial inflammation or pericardial effusion is described with hypothyroidism, nephrosis, uremia, Cooley's anemia, diseases associated with lymphedema, radiation damage, invasive tumors, and renal dialysis.

Absence of the Pericardium

Rarely, absence of a portion of the pericardium is recognized on a chest x-ray taken for some other

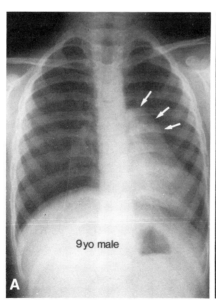
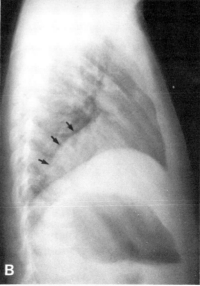

Figure 4. **A,** Anteroposterior chest x-ray of a patient showing the typical x-ray appearance of partial absence of the left pericardium. Note the unusual bump on the left heart border (arrows) which results from herniation of the left atrial appendage. **B,** Lateral view of the same patient showing an unusually large defect that causes herniation of the left ventricle as well (arrows).

reason (Fig. 4). The defect produces an atypical contour because of protusion of part of the heart into the defect. Syncope and sudden death have been described, presumably because of torsion of the cardiac structure, which is herniated through the defect.[5] Occasionally, it has been described as a familial anomaly. It has not been our practice to recommend surgery routinely to eliminate the possibility of herniation, but because of this concern, particularly when the disease is familial, surgery is sometimes inescapable.

REFERENCES

1. Engle MA, Zabriskie JB, Senterfit LB, et al: Viral illness and the postpericardiotomy syndrome: a prospective study in children. Circulation 62:1151–1158, 1980.
2. Feldman WE: Bacterial etiology and mortality of pu-rulent pericarditis in pediatric patients: review of 162 cases. Am J Dis Child 133:641–644, 1979.
3. McCaughan BC, Schaff HV, Piehler JM, et al: Early and late results of pericardiectomy for constrictive pericarditis. J Thorac Cardiovasc Surg 89:340–350, 1985.
4. Morgan RJ, Stephenson LW, Woolf PK, et al: Surgical treatment of purulent pericarditis in children. J Thorac Cardiovasc Surg 85:527–531, 1983.
5. Rowland TW, Twible EA, Norwood WI, et al: Partial absence of the left pericardium. Am J Dis Child 136:628–630, 1982.
6. Shabetai R, Fowler NO, Guntheroth WG: The hemodynamics of cardiac tamponade and constrictive pericarditis. Am J Cardiol 26:480–489, 1970.
7. Spodick DH: The normal and diseased pericardium: current concepts of pericardial physiology, diagnosis, and treatment. J Am Coll Cardiol 1:240–251, 1983.
8. Weitzman LB, Tinker WP, Kronzon I, et al: The incidence and natural history of pericardial effusion after cardiac surgery: an echocardiographic study. Circulation 69:506–511, 1984.

Chapter 26

INFECTIVE ENDOCARDITIS

Jane W. Newburger, M.D., M.P.H.

Recent advances in the diagnosis and therapy of infectious endocarditis have improved the mortality of this dreaded illness from nearly 100% in the preantibiotic era to approximately 10% in recent years.[36] Infectious endocarditis occurs almost exclusively in individuals with preexisting anatomic abnormalities of the cardiovascular system, with an incidence that varies with the specific lesion. In the pathogenesis of infectious endocarditis,[28] local turbulence is believed to promote a sterile network of fibrin and platelets on the endocardial surface, which is colonized later by microorganisms entering the bloodstream from a distant site. The infecting microorganisms are protected by the microthrombus from normal host defense mechanisms and from antibiotic penetration, necessitating the use of high-dose parenteral antimicrobial agents over a long period. The considerable morbidity and mortality of infectious endocarditis make its prompt diagnosis, management, and prevention a matter of great importance.

PREDISPOSING FACTORS

Structural Heart Disease

Cardiac malformation is the major factor predisposing to infective endocarditis. Although rheumatic heart disease has gradually declined as a substrate for endocarditis, the increased survival of children with congenital heart disease in the past two decades has increased the number and mean age of children susceptible to infective endocarditis. In general, lesions leading to a high velocity of blood flow through a heart valve, septal defect, or blood vessel are associated with increased susceptibility to endocarditis (Table 1).[8,11,13,16,17,25,30,34,37,39] The children at highest risk are those with cyanotic heart disease (e.g., tetralogy of Fallot) or ventricular septal defect with aortic regurgitation or obstruction, as well as those with prosthetic valves, and those who have had recent cardiac surgery. Endocarditis is exceedingly uncommon in individuals with isolated atrial septal defect secun-

Table 1. Incidence of Infective Endocarditis in Children with Specific Lesions

Cardiac Abnormality	Incidence*
Ventricular septal defect	1–1.8
Ventricular septal defect with aortic regurgitation	23
Patent ductus arteriosus	3.3
Valvar pulmonic stenosis	0.2
Coarctation of aorta	1.8–2.0
Tetralogy of Fallot	18

*Number per 1,000 patient-years.
From Johnson DH, Rosenthal A, Nadas AS: A forty-year review of bacterial endocarditis in infancy and childhood. Circulation 51:581–588, 1975, by permission of the American Heart Association, Inc.

dum and with mild pulmonic valve stenosis. Infective endocarditis occurs relatively infrequently in children without known preexisting heart disease (6% of the cases at The Children's Hospital, Boston, from 1963 to 1972);[20] approximately one-third of adults with infective endocarditis appear to have had normal hearts before the onset of illness.[3,4,28,32]

Dental Procedures and Dental Diseases

Dental procedures constitute the most frequent antecedent event prior to infective endocarditis. In retrospective reviews, the median frequency of history of recent dental procedure in patients with infective endocarditis is 16%. Among 141 patients with infective endocarditis at our institution, symptoms developed in eight (5.6%) within 7 days after dental procedures.[20] Such statistics are difficult to interpret, however, as no study has examined the frequency of dental visits during a comparable period in subjects without infective endocarditis. Indeed, the condition necessitating the dental procedure may, in itself, give rise to bacteremia or may increase the risk of bacteremia with the procedure. The oral hygiene of children with heart disease is usually poorer than that of normal children; this is particularly true for children with cyanotic congenital heart disease, who have a higher incidence of periodontal disease.[18,22]

Most cases of infective endocarditis due to

mouth organisms result from bacteremia not associated with dental procedures. Indeed, normal daily activities such as brushing teeth, use of dental floss and especially water irrigation devices, and even mastication are frequently followed by transient bacteremia (most commonly *Streptococcus viridans*).[3,14] The effect of these activities on the risk of developing infective endocarditis has never been studied, but it seems reasonable to assume that they play an important role.

Other Procedures

In addition to cardiac surgery and dental procedures, other surgical procedures followed by bacteremia have been associated with infective endocarditis. Such procedures include tonsillectomy, bronchoscopy, ventriculoatrial shunts for treatment of hydrocephalus, urologic surgery, and procedures such as placement of urinary catheters.[9] Cardiac catheterization precedes endocarditis in 2% of the cases (3 of 149 episodes of endocarditis) in our institution.[20] However, the risk of endocarditis following catheterization is small, especially if catheterization is performed using the percutaneous technique. Endocarditis may be a subtle complication of hemodialysis, with bacteremia resulting from infection of access sites.[26]

Extracardiac Infections

Infectious foci outside the heart may be the origin of bacteremia leading to infective endocarditis.[14] Among such lesions are infections of the skin (e.g., "boils"), pneumonia, acute pyelonephritis, sinusitis, osteomyelitis, and, of course, sepsis. Approximately half of the cases of endocarditis in infants occur secondary to sepsis in the absence of preexisting structural cardiac abnormalities.[21,42] Patients suffering from burns have increased susceptibility to endocarditis, often caused by *Staphylococcus aureus*.

Drug Addiction

Intravenous injection of drugs in addicts is associated with endocarditis. In such individuals, the most common causative organism is *Staphylococcus aureus*, and the right side of the heart is involved more often than the left.[9,27] In a number of cases, simultaneous involvement of several valves has been reported.

MICROBIOLOGY

Streptococcus viridans is the most common causative organism of infective endocarditis in children and adults.[4,9,20] Endocarditis caused by *Staphylococcal species* has become increasingly common, now accounting for approximately one-fifth of the cases.[4,9] Among patients without preexisting heart disease, *Staphylococcus aureus* is the most common causative organism.[9] A variety of other organisms may also be found. Gram-negative and fungal endocarditis occur most often following cardiac surgery or in debilitated patients. In approximately 10–15% of cases of infective endocarditis, blood cultures are negative.[9,20]

DIAGNOSIS

The diagnosis of infective endocarditis requires first that the clinician have a high index of suspicion. Infective endocarditis should be suspected in any child with structural heart disease who is seen with fever of unknown origin or other manifestations of infection. Diagnosis of infective endocarditis should meet one of the following three criteria: (1) pathologic evidence of endocarditis (e.g., at cardiac surgery, embolectomy), (2) at least two sets of blood cultures obtained by separate venipunctures positive for the same organism with no source of bacteremia other than the heart, or (3) a clinical course compatible with infective endocarditis. The child with fever and a new or changing murmur should be considered to have endocarditis unless proved otherwise.

The clinical course of infective endocarditis is determined by the virulence of the infecting organism and the resistance of the host. With organisms of low virulence, such as *Streptococcus viridans*, the onset of the disease may be insidious and the course, indolent (endocarditis lenta). Often, symptoms and signs of endocarditis are nonspecific; they include fever, anorexia, weight loss, pallor, night sweats, malaise, and myalgias. Signs attributable to embolic or immunologic phenomena include splinter hemorrhages, retinal hemorrhages, Janeway lesions, Osler nodes, splenomegaly, clubbing, arthralgias, arthritis, glomerulonephritis, and aseptic meningitis. Changing murmurs and development of congestive heart failure result from infection and consequent destruction of intracardiac structures. Neurologic symptoms are found in 20% of children with infective endocarditis[20] and include central nervous system emboli (7–12%),[5,20] hemorrhage, meningitis, toxic encephalopathy, and headache. Arterial embolization usually occurs late in the untreated course of the disease and may affect the lungs, kidneys, spleen, brain, or large vessels.[20,23]

Blood cultures are positive in approximately 85–90% of reported cases.[4,20,23] There are no differences between cultures obtained from peripheral arteries or veins. If the etiologic agent is to be isolated at all, it will be cultured in the first culture 77–86% of the time. After six cultures have been obtained, all patients who will be culture-positive will be detected. At Boston Children's Hospital three to six sets of blood cultures are obtained; usually multiple blood cultures are positive. The importance of separate venipuncture sites for each set of cultures and the need for strict sterile technique must be stressed. Each blood sample should be cultured in both aerobic and anaerobic media. If the patient has received an antibiotic in the preceding 48 hours, the culture bottles should contain resin, for antibiotic absorption, or enzyme, for antibiotic degradation. Blood cultures should be held for 3 weeks to permit the growth of fastidious organisms.

In addition to positive blood cultures, laboratory data in infective endocarditis often include anemia, leukocytosis, elevated sedimentation rate, hematuria, diminished complement component 3, and mildly elevated bilirubin. Formation of vegetations and myocardial abscess may be visualized sometimes by echocardiography.[40]

COMPLICATIONS

Most children with infective endocarditis have defervescence within 1 week after initiation of antibiotic therapy. Persistent or recurrent fever beyond this time requires investigation of a variety of potential causes including uncontrolled cardiac infection or metastatic suppuration, drug sensitivity, intercurrent infection, inflamed injection sites, thrombophlebitis (especially in adults), and arterial embolization.[12] The most common cause of fever is extensive infection of the valve ring and adjacent structures. Persistence of low-grade fever without positive blood cultures, or any other signs of activity, presents one of the most difficult problems in management of endocarditis, usually leaving the clinician to decide between the diagnoses of recurrent infection and drug sensitivity. Occasionally, discontinuation of antibiotic therapy may be necessary; this is a matter of clinical judgment.

Large arterial emboli arising from vegetations may be either suppurative or sterile; emboli do not necessarily indicate persistent infection. Symptoms and prognosis of embolization are related to the extent of infarction, the organ that is affected, and whether or not the embolus is suppurative.

Focal embolic and diffuse glomerulonephritis are the most frequent renal lesions associated with bacterial endocarditis.[41] Diffuse glomerulonephritis is thought to originate from deposition of immune complexes and complement in a "lumpy-bumpy" manner throughout the glomerulus. The immune-complex glomerulonephritis usually improves as infection is controlled. When renal function is decreased, nephrotoxic antibiotics, such as the aminoglycosides, should be used cautiously, with monitoring of serum levels.

Congestive heart failure is the leading cause of death during endocarditis and usually is associated with the development of hemodynamically significant valvar regurgitation, most often aortic.[38] Other less common causes include rupture of the sinus of Valsalva into the cardiac chambers, perforation of the ventricular or atrial septum, formation of an aortopulmonary window, or the development of myocarditis or myocardial abscesses. Frequently, development of congestive heart failure during endocarditis calls for prompt surgical intervention.

PREVENTION

Inasmuch as infective endocarditis cannot occur without preceding bacteremia, attempts at prevention have focused on the use of antibiotic prophylaxis for those procedures or conditions associated with a high frequency of bacteremia. The efficacy of the currently recommended antibiotic prophylaxis regimens has never been studied in man. Animal studies using indwelling cardiac catheters and intravenous injections of bacteria have provided a method for ranking the efficacy of antibiotic prophylaxis regimens *in vivo*. However, the presence of a foreign body and the use of a high inoculum of organisms limit the usefulness of this system as a model for infective endocarditis in man. The rare occurrence of infective endocarditis makes study of the efficacy of antibiotic prophylaxis through a prospective double-blind trial impractical because of the enormous number of patients required.

Nevertheless, we prescribe antimicrobial prophylaxis for all children with structural heart disease (with the exceptions of uncomplicated secundum atrial septal defect and ligated and divided patent ductus arteriosus) who are subjected to dental procedures or manipulations of the respiratory, gastrointestinal, urinary, or genital tracts. Antibiotic prophylaxis also should be given to patients who have had a previous episode of infective endocarditis, even in the absence of clinically detectable heart disease. Some experienced physicians do not use prophylaxis in patients with pure pulmonic stenosis. Although the risk of endocarditis is low, physicians may choose to use antibiotics in patients with ventriculoatrial shunts placed to relieve hydrocephalus.

Antibiotic Prophylaxis

The most recent American Heart Association recommendations for antibiotic prophylaxis are summarized below.[9]

Dental Procedures and Surgery of the Upper Respiratory Tract (e.g., Tonsillectomy, Bronchoscopy)

Antibiotic prophylaxis is recommended for all dental procedures that may cause gingival bleeding, including professional cleaning, and is directed against alpha hemolytic (viridans) strepto-cocci. In addition to antibiotic prophylaxis, children with structural heart disease should be strongly encouraged to maintain excellent oral hygiene practices and to keep routine dental appointments every 6 months to 1 year. Antibiotic prophylaxis is not necessary for shedding of deciduous teeth or for endotracheal intubation. Oral regimens are more convenient and safer. Parenteral regimens are more likely to be effective; they are recommended especially for patients with prosthetic heart valves, those who have had endocarditis previously, or others at high risk. In patients taking oral penicillin continuously for rheumatic fever prophylaxis or for other purposes, viridans streptococci relatively resistant to penicillin may be present in the oral cavity. Such patients should receive a parenteral regimen or erythromycin.

Dosage for Most Structural Heart Disease (Excluding Prosthetic Valves or Other High-Risk Lesions)

Penicillin Regimens. Oral. For patients weighing more than 60 pounds, use amoxicillin, 3 gm orally 1 hour before the procedure, then 1.5 gm 6 hours later. For children weighing less than 60 pounds, give 50 mg/kg orally 1 hour before, then 25 mg/kg 6 hours later.

Parenteral. For patients unable to take oral medications, use ampillicin, 2 gm intravenously or intramuscularly 30–60 minutes before a procedure, and 1 gm 6 hours later. For children under 60 pounds, use ampicillin, 50 mg/kg of body weight 30–60 minutes before the procedure, then 25 mg/kg 6 hours later.

Patients Allergic to Penicillin. Give erythromycin ethylsuccinate 800 mg, or erythromycin stearate 1 gm, orally 2 hours before, then half the dose 6 hours later. Alternatively, use clindamycin, 300 mg orally 1 hour before and half dose 6 hours later. For children, give erythromycin 20 mg/kg of body weight (maximum 1 gm) 2 hours before a procedure and 10 mg/kg (maximum 500 mg) 6 hours later, or clindamycin 10 mg/kg 1 hour before and half dose 6 hours later.

Dosage for Patients with Prosthetic Valves or at Very High Risk

Parenteral Ampicillin and Gentamicin. For adults, administer ampicillin, 2 gm intramuscularly or intravenously, plus gentamicin, 1.5 mg/kg of body weight intramuscularly or intravenously, 30 minutes before the procedure, followed by 1.5 gm of amoxicillin orally 6 hours later (as an alternative to the oral dose, the parenteral regimen may be repeated once 8 hours later). Pediatric doses are ampicillin, 50 mg/kg intramuscularly or intravenously, and gentamicin, 2.0 mg/kg intramuscularly or intravenously, both given 30 minutes before the procedure, followed by amoxicillin, 25 mg/kg,

given orally 6 hours later (the parenteral regimen may be repeated once 8 hours later instead of the oral dose).

Patients Allergic to Penicillin. Give vancomycin, 1 gm, intravenously slowly over 1 hour, beginning 1 hour before the procedure. The pediatric dose is 20 mg/kg of body weight intravenously (maximum 1 gm), infused slowly over 1 hour, beginning 1 hour before the procedure. No repeat dose is necessary.

Genitourinary and Gastrointestinal Tract Surgery or Instrumentation

The most common agent responsible for endocarditis following genitourinary and gastrointestinal tract surgery or instrumentation is enterococcus. Thus, antibiotic prophylaxis for these procedures is directed primarily against enterococci. Prophylaxis is recommended for cystoscopy, prostatic surgery, urethral catheterization (especially in the presence of infection), urinary tract surgery, vaginal hysterectomy, gallbladder surgery, esophageal dilation, sclerotherapy of esophageal varices, colonoscopy, upper gastrointestinal endoscopy with biopsy, or proctosigmoidoscopic biopsy. Other procedures more rarely followed by bacteremia or endocarditis include percutaneous liver biopsy, upper gastrointestinal endoscopy or proctosigmoidoscopy without biopsy, barium enema, uncomplicated vaginal delivery, and brief bladder catheterization with sterile urine. In the absence of infection, prophylaxis is not routinely required in the following gynecologic procedures: uterine dilatation and curettage, cesarean section, therapeutic abortion, sterilization procedures, or intrauterine device insertion or removal. However, it may be prudent to administer prophylactic antibiotics even for low-risk procedures to patients at high risk for endocarditis.

Standard Regimen. Parenteral Ampicillin and Gentamicin. For adults, give ampicillin, 2 gm intramuscularly or intravenously 30 minutes before the procedure, plus gentamicin, 1.5 mg/kg of body weight (not to exceed 80 mg) intravenously or intramuscularly 30 minutes before the procedure. For children, give ampicillin, 50 mg/kg intramuscularly or intravenously (maximum 2.0 gm) and gentamicin, 2.0 mg/kg intramuscularly or intravenously 30 minutes before the procedure. Amoxicillin, 25 mg/kg orally 6 hours later, or the parenteral dose may be repeated 8 hours later.

Patients Allergic to Penicillin. Vancomycin, 1 gm for adults (20 mg/kg of body weight to a maximum of 1 gm for children), given intravenously, slowly over 1 hour, *plus* gentamicin, 1.5 mg/kg intramuscularly or intravenously (2 mg/kg for children) given 1 hour before the procedure. These doses may be repeated once 8–12 hours later.

Oral Regimen for Minor or Repetitive Procedures in Low-risk Patients. Amoxicillin, 3 gm (50 mg/kg of body weight to a maximum of 3 gm for children) orally 1 hour before the procedure, and 1.5 gm (25 mg/kg to a maximum of 1.5 gm for children) 6 hours later.

Cardiac Surgery. At the time of cardiac surgery, prophylaxis should be directed primarily against staphylococci and should be of short duration. Most commonly, penicillinase-resistant penicillins or first-generation cephalosporins are selected. An antibiotic regimen should be chosen based on each hospital's antibiotic susceptibility data. Routinely, prophylaxis is started immediately before the operative procedure and continued for no more than 2 days postoperatively to minimize emergence of resistant organisms. Careful dental evaluation should be performed several weeks prior to elective cardiac surgery.

Other Considerations. Antibiotic prophylaxis should be prescribed for surgical procedures on any infected or contaminated tissues (e.g., incision and drainage of abscesses). The antibiotic regimen should be individualized but in most instances should include appropriate coverage for *Staphylococcus aureus*. Prophylactic antibiotics are not required for diagnostic cardiac catheterization and angiography, following which infective endocarditis is extremely uncommon.

The clinician should use his or her own judgment in determining the duration and choice of antibiotics under special circumstances, as it is impossible to make recommendations for all possible situations.

THERAPY

General Principles

Spontaneous cure of infective endocarditis rarely, if ever, occurs; rather, cure requires prompt diagnosis and institution of antibiotic therapy. All patients with endocarditis should be followed closely by a cardiologist and an infectious diseases specialist. To select the appropriate antibiotic, the causative organism must be isolated and its sensitivity to antimicrobial agents determined. In general, bactericidal drugs are more effective than bacteriostatic ones in eradicating infection. The effectiveness of antimicrobial therapy should be assessed by measuring the antibacterial activity of the patient's serum, at various intervals after antibiotic administration, against the infecting organisms, sometimes together with antimicrobial blood levels. Bactericidal effects should be seen at dilutions of 1–8 or greater for antibiotic therapy to be effective.[7]

Blood cultures should be obtained during the earliest days of therapy to ensure eradication of bacteremia. The duration of therapy necessary to effect cure is controversial. Generally, at Children's Hospital in Boston, we treat infective en-

docarditis caused by sensitive organisms such as *Streptococcus viridans* for a minimum of 4 weeks, but extend the treatment course to 6 weeks or more when infection is caused by *Staphylococcus aureus*, gram-negative organisms, or organisms that are less sensitive to antimicrobial therapy. Although a treatment course of 2 weeks has been reported to cure *Streptococcus viridans*, more data are needed before we would recommend this approach. In selected cases, patients with endocarditis may be treated with intravenous therapy at home after they are clinically stable and antibiotic therapy has been optimized.

Empirical Therapy

Delay in institution of therapy may be costly in patients with acute endocarditis; antibiotics should be given immediately after three to five cultures have been obtained in any child at risk for endocarditis who appears acutely ill and who has a compatible clinical picture. Examination of a buffy-coat smear may reveal the etiologic organism before blood culture results are available. As *Staphylococcus aureus* is frequently the etiologic agent in acute endocarditis and in endocarditis occurring early after cardiac surgery, initial therapy should include a penicillinase-resistant penicillin (e.g., oxacillin, methicillin), together with gentamicin and, occasionally, with ampicillin as well. If methicillin-resistant *Staphylococcus aureus* is a frequent hospital isolate, then vancomycin should be used. After identification of the causative organism, therapy should be changed according to the sensitivities of the causative organism. In children presenting with a subacute or chronic illness compatible with infective endocarditis, one may legitimately delay the start of therapy for 2 or 3 days while awaiting the results of blood cultures as, with few exceptions, initiation of antibiotic therapy commits the patient to a full course of treatment.

In approximately 10–15% of cases of infective endocarditis, blood cultures never yield growth, and the diagnosis must rest on a highly suggestive clinical picture. The factors that predispose to the culture-negative state are obscure in the majority of patients, although previous antibiotic use, technical variables in laboratory methods, and differences in criteria for diagnosis may play a role. In the examination of valvular tissue from patients with culture-negative endocarditis, the majority of patients have been found to have infection with common organisms or to have no organisms apparent within the vegetations, although unusual organisms have been noted occasionally.[33] Initial therapy for subacute infective endocarditis with negative blood cultures should include penicillin or ampicillin and an aminoglycoside to provide effective coverage against enterococcal species.

When *Staphylococcus aureus* seems likely (e.g., after cardiac surgery), a penicillinase-resistant penicillin or cephalosporin should be added to this regimen. In patients who respond rapidly with defervescence and an improved state of well-being, administration of antibiotics should be continued for a minimum of 4 weeks. If all studies continue to be negative and there has been no clinical improvement at the end of 1 week, serologic studies (e.g., Histoplasma and Aspergillus immunodiffusion, *Coxiella burnetti* and Chlamydia complement fixation, Brucella agglutinins, Candida antigens), and arterial blood cultures for fungi should be carried out. When these studies are negative, we continue an antibiotic regimen of penicillin, gentamicin, and oxacillin or nafcillin for a total course of 6 weeks. In selected patients, surgical intervention should be considered.[33]

Surgical Therapy

Although the majority of cases of infective endocarditis can be treated successfully with antimicrobial agents alone, certain patients continue to have high mortality. This is largely determined by the virulence of the etiologic organism, the site of intracardiac infection (e.g., prosthetic valve), and the degree of valve destruction. The most frequent indications for surgery in the treatment of infective endocarditis include (1) at least moderately severe or worsening congestive heart failure, (2) infection uncontrolled by antibiotics, (3) more than one serious systemic embolus, (4) local suppurative complications, including perivalvular and myocardial abscess with conduction system abnormalities, and (5) resection of a mycotic aneurysm. Prompt surgical intervention is mandatory in critically ill patients, even when antibiotic therapy has been minimal. Acute aortic regurgitation complicated by congestive heart failure has an especially high mortality with medical management alone. Virtually all patients with prosthetic valve endocarditis (except when late-onset endocarditis is caused by penicillin-sensitive *Streptococcus viridans*) will require valve replacement.

Prosthetic Valve Endocarditis

Infective endocarditis involving prosthetic materials (e.g., valves, conduits, patches) presents particularly difficult issues in management. Patients with early infection of prosthetic valves (i.e., less than 2 months following cardiac surgery) have an exceedingly high mortality, ranging from 68–88% in a series of adult patients. Causative organisms are often *Staphylococcus epidermidis*, *Staphylococcus aureus*, streptococci, gram-negative bacilli, diphtheroids, Candida species, and other opportunistic organisms.[1,2,10,19,24,29,31,35] Mortality in late prosthetic valve endocarditis is somewhat lower (36–53%) and the bacteriologic spectrum more closely resembles that occurring on native valves, with streptococci being the most commonly isolated species. Several investigators recommend combined early surgical and antimicrobial therapy for prosthetic valve endocarditis, although prompt and vigorous antibiotic treatment alone may be effective occasionally for late infections with *Streptococcus viridans*. Infection on mechanical valves is most often localized to the sewing ring, whereas endocarditis of porcine heterografts is localized more commonly on the cusps, causing leaflet destruction.[6,15]

Other Aspects of Management

All patients with infective endocarditis should have frequent physical examinations and continuity of care by at least one physician. Measures to relieve stress on the cardiovascular system include bed rest, control of fever, transfusion for severe anemia, and maintenance of fluid and electrolyte balance. A complete dental examination and any necessary dental procedures should be performed as soon as the patient's condition permits and satisfactory antibiotic serum bactericidal levels have been achieved. Implications of the illness and prolonged hospitalization should be discussed with the child and parents at the time of admission; psychological support is helpful during the lengthy hospitalization.

Discharge and Follow-up

Blood cultures should be obtained on several occasions during the 2 months after discontinuation of therapy. If the patient feels well and cultures are negative, all normal activities may be resumed. Elective surgery and catheterization should probably be deferred for 6 months following endocarditis.

REFERENCES

1. Aintablian A, Hilsenrath J, Hamby RJ, et al: Endocarditis in prosthetic valves. N Y State J Med 76:673–677, 1976.
2. Auger P, Marquis G, Dyra I, et al: Infective endocarditis update: experience from a heart hospital. Acta Cardiol 36:105–123, 1981.
3. Bayliss R, Clark C, Oakley CM, et al: The teeth and infective endocarditis. Br Heart J 50:506–512, 1983.
4. Bayliss R, Clarke C, Oakley CM, et al: The microbiology and pathogenesis of infective endocarditis. Br Heart J 50:513–519, 1983.
5. Blumenthal S, Griffiths SP, Morgan BC: Bacterial endocarditis in children with heart disease: a review based on the literature and experience with 58 cases. Pediatrics 26:993–1017, 1960.
6. Bortolotti U, Thiene G, Milano A, et al: Pathological study of infective endocarditis on Hancock porcine bioprostheses. J Thorac Cardiovasc Surg 81:934–942, 1981.
7. Carrizosa J, Kaye D: Antibiotic concentrations in serum, serum bactericidal activity, and results of therapy of streptococcal endocarditis in rabbits. Antimicrob Agents Chemother 12:479–483, 1977.
8. Cardelia JU, Befeler B, Hildner FJ, et al: Hypertrophic subaortic stenosis complicated by aortic insufficiency and subacute bacterial endocarditis. Am Heart J 81:543–547, 1971.

9. Committee on Rheumatic Fever and Infective Endcarditis: Prevention of bacterial endocarditis. JAMA 264:2919–2922, 1990.

10. Delgado DG, Cobbs CG: Infections of prosthetic valves and intravascular devices. In Mandell GL, Douglas RG Jr (eds): Principles and Practice of Infectious Diseases. New York, John Wiley and Sons, 1979, p 690.

11. Deucher D, Bescos LL, Chakorn S: Fallot's tetralogy: a 20-year surgical follow-up. Br Heart J 34:12–22, 1972.

12. Douglas A, Moore-Gillon J, Eykyn S: Fever during treatment of infective endocarditis. Lancet 1:1341–1343, 1986.

13. Epstein EJ, Coulshed N: Bacterial endocarditis in idiopathic hypertropic subaortic stenosis. Cardiologia 54:30–36, 1969.

14. Everett ED, Hirshmann JV: Transient bacteremia and endocarditis prophylaxis: a review. Medicine 56:51, 1977.

15. Ferrans VJ, Boyce SW, Billingham ME, et al: Infection of glutaraldehyde-preserved porcine valve heterografts. Am J Cardiol 43:1123–1136, 1979.

16. Frank S, Braunwald E: Idiopathic hypertropic subaortic stenosis. Clinical analysis of 126 patients with emphasis on the natural history. Circulation 37:759–788, 1968.

17. Gersony WM, Hayes CJ: Bacterial endocarditis in pulmonary stenosis, aortic stenosis and ventricular septal defect. Circulation 56(Suppl I):84–87, 1977.

18. Gould MSE, Picton DCA: The gingival condition of congenitally cyanotic individuals. Br Dent J 109:96, 1969.

19. Grignon A, Spencer H, Robson HG, et al: Prosthetic valve infections. Can J Surg 24:615–618, 1981.

20. Johnson DH, Rosenthal A, Nadas AS: A forty-year review of bacterial endocarditis in infancy and childhood. Circulation 51:581–588, 1975.

21. Johnson DH, Rosenthal A, Nadas AS: Bacterial endocarditis under two years of age. Am J Dis Child 129:183–186, 1975.

22. Kaner A, Losch PK, Green H: Oral manifestations of congenital heart disease. J Pediatr 29:269, 1946.

23. Kaplan EL, Rich H, Gersony W, et al: A collaborative study of infective endocarditis in the 1970's: emphasis on infections in patients who have undergone cardiovascular surgery. Circulation 59:327–335, 1979.

24. Karchmer AW, Dismukes WE, Buckley MJ: Late prosthetic valve endocarditis: clinical features influencing therapy. Am J Med 64:199–206, 1978.

25. Kato H, Hirose M, Fukuda H, et al: Natural history of ventricular septal defect. Jpn Circ J 36:814–818, 1972.

26. King LH Jr, Bradley KP, Shires DL Jr, et al: Bacterial endocarditis in chronic hemodialysis patients: a complication more common than previously suspected. Surgery 69:554–556, 1971.

27. Korzeniowski OM, Sande MA: The National Collaborative Endocarditis Study Group: Combination antimicrobial therapy for Staphylococcus aureus endocarditis in patients addicted to parenteral drugs and in nonaddicts: a prospective study. Ann Intern Med 97:496–503, 1982.

28. LevisonME: Pathogenesis of infective endocarditis. In Kaye D (ed): Infective Endocarditis. Baltimore, University Park Press, 1976, p. 29.

29. Magilligan DJ Jr, Quinn EL, Davila JC: Bacteremia endocarditis and the Hancock valve. Ann Thorac Surg 24:508–518, 1977.

30. Manning JA: Endocarditis prophylaxis in the child with congenital heart disease after surgery. 1975 (unpublished).

31. Masur H, Johnson WD Jr: Prosthetic valve endocarditis. J Thorac Cardiovasc Surg 80:31–37, 1980.

32. McKinney DS, Rafts TE, Bisno AL: Underlying cardiac lesions in adults with infective endocarditis: the changing spectrum. Am J Med 82:681–687, 1989.

33. Pesanti EI, Smith IM: Infective endocarditis with negative blood cultures. An analysis of 52 cases. Am J Med 66:43–50, 1989.

34. Rosenthal A: When to operate on congenital heart disease. In Chung EK (ed): Controversy in Cardiology. New York, Springer, 1976.

35. Rossiter SJ, Stinson EB, Oyer PE, et al: Prosthetic valve endocarditis: comparison of heterograft tissue valves and mechanical valves. J Thorac Cardiovasc Surg 76:795–803, 1978.

36. Sande MA, Kaye D, Root RK: Endocarditis. Contemporary Issues in Infectious Diseases, Vol. 2. New York, Churchill Livingstone, 1984.

37. Shah P, Sineh WSA, Rose V, et al: Incidence of bacterial endocarditis in ventricular septal defects. Circulation 32:127, 1966.

38. Stinson E: Surgical treatment of infective endocarditis. Prog Cardiovasc Dis 22:145–168, 1979.

39. Ukuda Y, Tsuneda T, Morishima A, et al: Right coronary artery to left ventricle fistula: the sixth case in the literature and discussion. Jpn Heart J 14:184–191, 1973.

40. Wann LS, Dillon JC, Weyman AE, et al: Echocardiography in bacterial endocarditis. N Engl J Med 295:135–139, 1976.

41. Wilson JW, Houghton DC, Bennett WM, et al: The kidney and infective endocarditis. In Rahimtoola SH (ed). Infective Endocarditis. Orlando, FL, Grune & Stratton, Inc., 1977.

42. Zakrewski T, Keith JD: Bacterial endocarditis in infants and children. J Pediatr 67:1179–1193, 1965.

Chapter 27

CARDIAC ARRHYTHMIAS

Edward P. Walsh, M.D., and J. Philip Saul, M.D.

The basic principles of cellular electrophysiology and recording theory are presented in chapter 12. This chapter is intended as a practical review of the diagnosis and treatment of cardiac arrhythmias in the pediatric age group. Whenever possible, topics have been arranged by clinical presentation, with primary emphasis on the surface electrocardiogram as the diagnostic tool most familiar to all practitioners.

PATHOPHYSIOLOGIC BASIS OF CARDIAC ARRHYTHMIAS

Arrhythmias may result from disorders of impulse generation (too fast or too slow), disorders of impulse conduction (block or reentry), or any combination thereof. These abnormalities are best understood by first examining their cellular genesis. Admittedly, some of the cellular models for cardiac arrhythmias discussed in this section have been derived from experimental preparations of isolated heart tissue and cannot always be verified as the exact cause of a clinical rhythm disorder in the intact human heart. Nevertheless, close correlation between these in vitro models, and the often stereotypic pattern of rhythm disorders in vivo, permits some intelligent speculation regarding the basic mechanism of an arrhythmia at the bedside.

Premature Beats and Tachycardias

Normally, by virtue of its rapid spontaneous depolarization, the sinus node can claim priority as the pacemaker of the heart. Premature beats and tachyarrhythmias may preempt sinoatrial activity secondary to disorders of either automaticity or reentry.

Abnormal Automaticity. Enhanced automaticity of a focus outside the sinoatrial node may result from any change in membrane condition that promotes early achievement of threshold potential (Fig. 1). A single abnormal discharge can generate an isolated ectopic beat, while, hypothetically, repetitive discharge from a focus can create a sus-

tained automatic tachycardia.[1] Abnormal automaticity of this type has been implicated as the possible mechanism for some unusual clinical arrhythmias in children, such as ectopic atrial tachycardia, junctional ectopic tachycardia, and some atypical ventricular arrhythmias. The clinical characteristics that suggest such a mechanism include: (1) inability to terminate the arrhythmia with cardioversion or pacing maneuvers, (2) wide variation in tachycardia rate (largely dependent on the autonomic state), (3) specific pharmacologic response, and (4) transient overdrive suppression following prolonged rapid pacing (similar to the recovery behavior of the sinoatrial node). Unfortunately, these clinical features are not in themselves absolute verification of an abnormal automatic focus; there is some overlap with other arrhythmia models, particularly "triggered" automaticity, as discussed below. In practice, one must be content with a diagnosis of "probable" abnormal automaticity, although the behavior of such arrhythmias is usually so consistent that the speculation about cellular mechanism may well be accurate, and at the very least it helps direct one toward a specific treatment plan.

Triggered Automaticity. A second form of automatic cellular depolarization is the phenomenon of triggered automaticity. The electrical triggers in this case are small oscillations that may occur during phase 3 ("early" afterdepolarizations) or phase 4 ("late" afterdepolarizations) of a cellular action potential (Fig. 2). If the oscillations are sufficiently high in amplitude, the threshold potential is exceeded and the cell may be triggered to undergo one or more rhythmic depolarizations. In experimental preparations, early afterdepolarizations[19] may be produced by hypokalemia, high levels of catecholamines, certain antiarrhythmic drugs, and hypoxic injury. The delayed type[85] has been produced by toxic levels of cardiac glycosides, acute hyponatremia, and exposure to norepinephrine.

Efforts to define clinical features that identify triggered automatic tachycardias in the intact heart

377

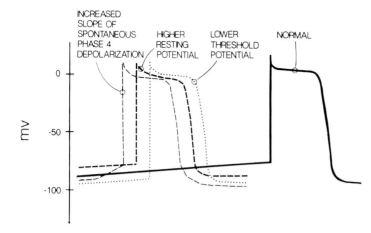

Figure 1. Theoretical changes in cellular conditions which can promote abnormal automaticity. The "normal" action potential in this example is a hypothetical Purkinje cell with gradual phase 4 depolarization that will eventually reach threshold potential and generator action potentials at slow rates. Changes in resting potential, threshold potential, or the slope of phase 4 can cause premature depolarization.

have been frustrating,[62] because there is wide overlap with characteristics of both abnormal automatic foci and reentry circuits. Features in common with abnormal automaticity include wide variation in rate (with "warm-up" at initiation and "cool down" at termination), as well as sensitivity to catecholamines. Features in common with reentry include ability to initiate and terminate tachycardia with pacing maneuvers and termination with DC shock. One of the few unique characteristics appears to be that the rate of discharge in triggered automaticity is quite dependent on the preceding rhythm and varies directly with the rate of the pacing drive train that initiates the arrhythmia. In classic reentry the rate of tachycardia is not influenced by antecedent rhythm and is determined solely by the conduction properties of the tissues constituting the reentry loop.

While it is tempting to assign the label of triggered automaticity to some typical clinical arrhythmias (such as premature beats occurring with digoxin toxicity, or some tachycardias due to catecholamine sensitivity), irrefutable in vivo evidence is still lacking. However, microelectrode studies of human atrial and ventricular tissue have, indeed, shown early and late afterdepolarizations in vitro.[58] Triggered activity is probably operative in some clinical rhythm disorders, but presently the technology for positive identification in the intact heart is lacking. This likely will change as recording techniques and our understanding of triggered activity improve.

Reentry. By far the most common mechanism for sustained tachyarrhythmias is the phenomenon of reentry (alternately referred to as "circus movement" or "reciprocation"). It is the one model for clinical tachyarrhythmias with unequivocal in vivo verification. Reentry implies that a single stimulus or excitation wave front can return and reactivate the same tissue from whence it came (Fig. 3). Because cardiac cells require a refractory period after initial depolarization, the return stimulus cannot simply walk backwards in its old footprints; there must be a second pathway in the circuit (limb B in Fig. 3), and the excitation must be sufficiently delayed at some point in the circuit to allow recovery of the original tissue (limb A in Fig. 3). An additional requirement is that the return limb

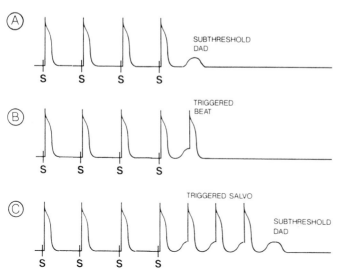

Figure 2. Diagrammatic demonstration of delayed afterdepolarization (DAD) and triggered activity. A cell is paced (s) to generate action potentials. At termination of the pacing drive train, there is a delayed oscillation of the cellular potential. If the oscillation is of low amplitude, triggering does not occur (**A**). If the oscillation exceeds threshold potential, it may trigger single beats (**B**) or a series of beats (**C**).

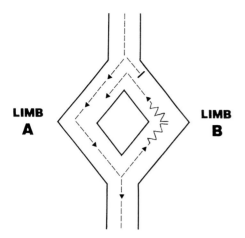

Figure 3. Diagram showing the three classic requirements for reentry: (1) dual pathways, (2) unidirectional, anterograde block in limb B, and (3) an area of slow conduction (wavy line in limb B) that allows time for limb A to recover from initial depolarization. The zone of slow conduction can be located anywhere along the circuit.

somehow be protected against the initial depolarization; i.e., there must be unidirectional anterograde block of the original stimulus in limb B so that it will not be refractory to retrograde conduction. When all three requisites (dual pathways, conduction delay, and unidirectional block) are met, single "echo" beats or a sustained reentrant arrhythmia can follow. Reentry is prevented if conduction in one limb can be sufficiently modified or interrupted.

The classic example of reentry occurs in the Wolff-Parkinson-White syndrome (WPW), utilizing the AV node and the accessory connection between the atrium and the ventricle (the so-called Kent bundle) as the two limbs of the circuit. This syndrome offered the first real proof that reentry was an operative mechanism in the intact heart, and it represents a natural laboratory for the study of the reentry phenomenon to the point of being called the "Rosetta Stone" of electrophysiology.[122] Apart from WPW syndrome, reentry also appears responsible for atrial flutter (reentry in atrial muscle), atrial fibrillation (possibly multiple atrial reentry circuits), SA-node and AV-node reentry, and probably most forms of ventricular tachycardia. The detailed physiology of these individual disorders is presented later in this chapter.

The general clinical features of reentry rhythms, in contradistinction to abnormal automatic foci, include: (1) ability to initiate and terminate tachycardia with appropriately timed premature beats, (2) a narrow range in the tachycardia rate with minimal beat-to-beat variation, (3) abrupt paroxysmal onset and termination, (4) specific pharmacologic response, (5) successful termination with DC shock, and (6) findings at electrophysiologic study that satisfy the strict definitions of "entrainment" (Fig. 4). Such characteristics can be used to assign the label of reentry to a clinical arrhythmia with reasonable certainty, but note once again that some overlap exists with features of triggered automaticity (Table 1). At present, the demonstration of entrainment appears to be the most exacting criterion for a reentry circuit.[71]

Bradycardia and Block

Abnormally slow heart rates result from depression of depolarization in pacemaker cells and/or block of electrical activation. When SA node automaticity is impaired, one of several latent pacemaker sites in the atrium or AV conducting tissue normally assumes responsibility for generating cardiac rhythm. The escape rate depends on the level of the new pacemaker; foci located in more distal portions of the conducting system have slower phase 4 depolarization and, thus, produce lower rates. Latent pacemakers (particularly those below the AV node) also lack the rich autonomic influence found at the SA node and may exhibit a blunted chronotropic response to exertion and stress.

Block may occur at any stage of the cardiac excitation process. This includes **exit block** (Fig. 5) and **entrance block** at a pacemaker focus, or **conduction block** of an established depolarization wave front at various levels of the heart. Block is a physiologic event if an initiating impulse is premature and arrives at a cardiac site during normal refractoriness, whereas pathologic block occurs in the setting of abnormally long refractory periods, abnormally slow conduction velocity, or complete electrical discontinuity.

There is some merit to a scheme that correlates patterns of block on the surface electrocardiogram with the specific type of cardiac cells involved in the event. Generally, slow-response cells of the SA node and AV node (mostly dependent on calcium channel activity) demonstrate a characteristic sequence of gradual and progressive conduction delay in response to an increasingly premature stimulus, culminating in eventual block of an impulse. This pattern is often described as "decremental conduction" or "Wenckebach periodicity" and is a hallmark of conduction delay in these tissues.[104] It is rather unusual to observe this same phenomenon in fast-response cells of either the His-Purkinje system, accessory pathways, or working muscle. With few exceptions,[29] because conduction through these areas tends to be "all or none," episodic block is an unheralded event. A familiar clinical example involves the distinction between atrioventricular conduction disturbances due to disease involving the AV node (Mobitz I block) vs. disease of the bundle of His (Mobitz II block). The former shows gradual lengthening of the P-R interval before a blocked P wave, whereas the latter usually shows an abrupt nonconducted beat (Fig. 6).

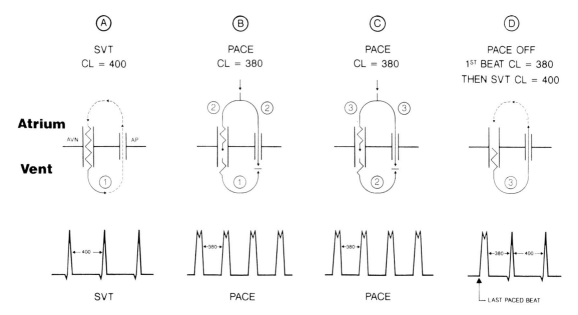

Figure 4. The concept of entrainment, demonstrated in a hypothetical reentry tachycardia involving the AV node (AVN) and an accessory pathway (AP) in the WPW syndrome. The tachycardia has a cycle length of 400 msec and is (initially) shown at a point in time (**A**) when beat #1 is traveling through the AV node. The atrium is then paced at a cycle length slightly shorter than tachycardia. Paced beat #2 depolarizes the atrium, the accessory pathway, and part of the ventricle and enters the zone of slow conduction in the AV node (**B**). This maneuver has interrupted the reentry circuit, but has not extinguished it completely because beat #1 is still "alive" in the lower regions of the circuit. As pacing is continued (**C**), the reentry circuit is fully entrained. When pacing is terminated (**D**), the first return beat (beat #3) is in fact generated by prior pacing and emerges at the faster paced cycle length. Tachycardia then resumes at its old rate. The observation of an early return beat is but one of several "rules of entrainment."

EVALUATION AND MANAGEMENT OF PREMATURE BEATS

Premature beats are common in the pediatric age group, with atrial ectopy predominating in infants or young children and ventricular ectopy during adolescence.[24] Although isolated premature beats are usually benign, they may serve as markers of more serious underlying pathology or as the initiating impulses for reentry tachycardias in susceptible individuals.

Atrial Premature Beats (APBs)

Atrial ectopy appears on the electrocardiogram as an early P wave with an axis and morphology differing from those of the normal sinus P wave. Atrial premature beats are usually followed by a

Table 1. Distinguishing Features of Cellular Tachycardia Mechanisms*

	Abnormal Automaticity	Triggered Activity	Reentry
Mode of initiation	Spontaneous	Spontaneous pacing and/or premature beats	Critically timed premature beats
Response to DC cardioversion	None	Usually terminates	Terminates
Response to overdrive pacing	Brief suppression but quickly resumes	Usually terminates	Terminates
"Entrainment" possible	No	No	Yes
Rate "warm-up" and "cool-down"	Yes	Yes	No
Rate varies directly with preceding rhythm	No	Yes	No
Response to catecholamines	Increase rate	Increase rate	None or slight increased rate
Response to drugs that prolong refractoriness	Variable	Variable	Slow or stop tachycardia

*Features listed for automaticity and triggered activity are largely conjecture based on in-vitro cell behavior.

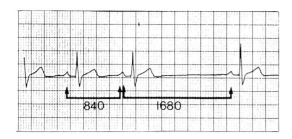

Figure 5. An example of probable exit block from the SA node. The resting cycle length for sinus node discharge is 840 msec. An abrupt pause in sinus rhythm is then observed, lasting exactly twice that interval. This presumably corresponds to block of conduction between the SA node discharge and atrial muscle.

Junctional Premature Beats (JPBs)

Ectopic beats arising from the AV node or proximal His-Purkinje system are rather rare. The ECG reveals an early normal QRS but no preceding P wave (Fig. 8). Prognostic and diagnostic considerations are generally similar to those for atrial premature beats. Occasionally, JPBs can affect atrioventricular conduction if their timing coincides with a normal atrial depolarization. Collision of the premature beat with a normal atrial impulse can mimic abrupt AV block by the mechanism of "concealed conduction" and, thus, JPBs may be considered in the differential diagnosis of some atypical AV conduction abnormalities.[115] In general, JPBs do not require treatment.

normal QRS (Fig. 7A), but when sufficiently early, they can conduct with QRS aberration (Fig. 7B) or become blocked at the AV node (Fig. 7C). If the patient is completely asymptomatic and the physical examination is otherwise normal, occasional atrial premature beats are most always benign and do not necessarily warrant further investigation. However, in a child with a past history of dizziness or sustained palpitations, atrial premature beats could be a manifestation of an underlying reentry circuit with the potential for supraventricular tachycardia. Therefore, testing with a Holter monitor or transesophageal electrophysiologic study is indicated for patients with atrial premature beats and any symptoms suggestive of supraventricular tachycardia.

In asymptomatic patients, the diagnostic evaluation is expanded if the beats are frequent and/or seem to arise from multiple foci (i.e., variable morphologies for the P wave on a rhythm strip). Hyperthyroidism, structural heart disease and cardiomyopathy need to be considered as possible causes. It is useful to include evaluation with thyroid function testing, a chest x-ray, and Holter monitoring for these patients.

Ventricular Premature Beats (VPBs)

Ventricular ectopy is characterized by an early beat with a wide and bizarre QRS complex, without a preceding P wave (Fig. 9). The T-wave axis is usually directed opposite to the QRS. Ventricular ectopy can usually be distinguished from atrial premature beats with aberrant conduction by the absence of a premature P wave and the presence of a fully "compensatory pause" (Fig. 10).

Ventricular premature beats are common. They are reported to occur in about 1–2% of all pediatric patients with ostensibly normal hearts, and clinical follow-up of such subjects has revealed a generally benign prognosis.[79] However, there does appear to be a definite age predilection for "benign" ventricular ectopy. From studies of Holter recordings, ventricular ectopy is clearly more common after puberty, occurring in only 1% of normal infants[134] and children[133] compared with 50–60% of healthy teenagers[144] and young adults.[9] The physiologic basis for this age distinction is not clear, but it does support the notion that VPBs may be of less concern during the adolescent years.

Unfortunately, ventricular ectopy on a routine

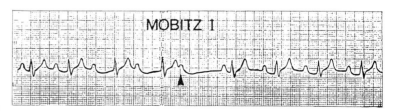

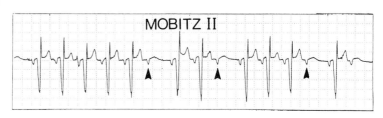

Figure 6. Comparison of conduction block in the slow response cells of the AV node (Mobitz I) and the fast response cells of the His Purkinje system (Mobitz II).

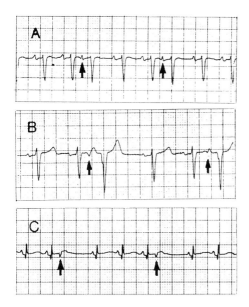

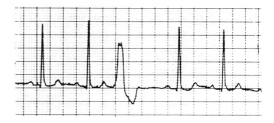

Figure 9. Ventricular premature beat showing distortion of the QRS and T wave.

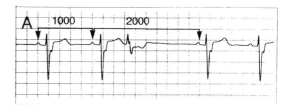

Figure 7. Atrial premature beats (marked by arrow) causing (**A**) normal QRS, (**B**) conduction with aberration, and (**C**) block.

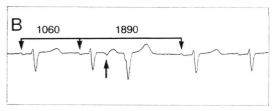

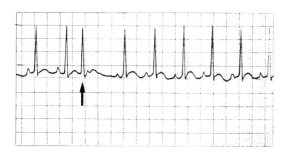

Figure 8. Junctional premature beat. Note that the early QRS is identical to a sinus beat, but is not preceded by a P wave.

Figure 10. Comparison of a ventricular premature beat (**A**) and an atrial premature beat with aberration (**B**). Note that the pause following ventricular ectopy is typically "compensatory" (i.e., the interval between P waves for the sinus beats flanking the ectopic beat is exactly twice that for sinus rhythm). The pause following atrial ectopy is "noncompensatory," and the premature P wave (arrow) can be seen.

ECG may be a manifestation of more serious underlying arrhythmias. For this reason, at Boston Children's Hospital, patients with VPBs usually undergo monitoring with 24-hour Holter recordings. The appearance of higher grade ectopic activity (Table 2) on long-term monitoring may indicate the need for an expanded diagnostic evaluation, including echocardiography and possible catheterization with electrophysiologic testing. Some reports suggest that suppression of ventricular premature beats with exercise testing indicates a benign condition,[79] although this is not universally true in the authors' experience.

Asymptomatic patients with isolated VPBs and normal hearts do not require treatment. The management of asymptomatic patients with high-grade ectopy will be discussed later in this chapter.

EVALUATION AND MANAGEMENT OF TACHYCARDIAS

The key to effective management of tachycardia is accurate identification of the underlying mechanism of the arrhythmia which must be understood in terms of both site of origin as well as electrophysiologic pathology (i.e., reentry vs. automaticity). First, it is helpful to review basic definitions and generate a useful classification scheme as an introduction to these diverse disorders.

Terminology and Classification

The terms **supraventricular tachycardia** (SVT) and **ventricular tachycardia** (VT) are practical starting points for describing a tachyarrhythmia, but they are sorely lacking in specificity. Supraventricular tachycardia is a broad category that includes any rapid rhythm arising from either the atrium, the atrioventricular junction, or an accessory pathway, whereas ventricular tachycardia refers to disorders that arise from cardiac site(s) below the bifurcation of the bundle of His. Because they

Table 2. Modified Lown Classification for Ventricular Ectopy and Common Synonyms Used for Description of Ventricular Arrhythmias on Long-term Monitoring

0	No ectopy		
1	Occasional VPBs (30/hour)	"Isolated"	Low grade
2	Frequent VPBs (>30/hour)		
3	Multiform VPBs		Moderate grade
4a	Couplets	"Repetitive"	
4b	VT or VF		High grade
5	Early VPB (R on T)		

VPB, ventricular premature beat; VT, ventricular tachycardia (≥3 consecutive beats); and VF, ventricular fibrillation.

convey little specific information regarding focus of origin or mechanism, these terms are often too imprecise for directing therapeutic decisions. Even less useful is the phrase **paroxysmal atrial tachycardia** (PAT), which is not only imprecise, but is often erroneously applied to tachycardias involving the AV node or accessory pathways.

By far the most meaningful nomenclature involves a classification that identifies tachycardias by specific mechanism and site of origin (Table 3). The list is long, but it underscores the diverse nature of clinical tachyarrhythmias, each of which requires a fairly unique approach to diagnosis and therapy.

Bedside Diagnosis of Tachycardia Mechanisms from the Surface Electrocardiogram

Although 18 tachycardia mechanisms are listed in Table 3, at the bedside it is necessary to narrow the differential to only one or two choices in order to plan therapy and organize further diagnostic testing. Often this can be accomplished with a careful review of the standard surface electrocardiogram.

The first step is to review a 12-lead tracing taken during tachycardia (a single-lead rhythm strip is

hopelessly inadequate) and to examine the duration and morphology of the QRS complex. When the QRS is narrow (i.e., identical to a conducted sinus beat in all 12 leads), it can be assumed that the ventricles are activated over the AV node and the His-Purkinje system, a finding that effectively eliminates ventricular tachycardia from the differential diagnosis. If a wide QRS is observed, ventricular tachycardia must be the primary consideration, but the differential also includes any SVT that is distorted by a disturbance of bundle branch conduction or involves anterograde conduction over a preexcitation pathway.

Differential Diagnosis of Narrow QRS Tachycardias. The possible mechanisms for narrow QRS tachycardias are shown in Figure 11. Each diagram is accompanied by a sample electrocardiogram (hypothetical lead II) that emphasizes the diagnostic clues to be found in the timing and axis of the P wave.

The first example is **sinus tachycardia,** which is the prototype "automatic" arrhythmia. Although not strictly pathologic, it is a good example of the behavior of an automatic focus, in that it accelerates and decelerates in a gradual manner ("warm-up" and "cool-down") and varies slightly in rate with respiration or changes in autonomic tone. Note in Figure 11 that P waves arising from the SA node

Table 3. Mechanisms for Tachycardia Listed by Site of Origin and Probable Cellular Pathophysiology

Site of Origin	Automaticity	Reentry
SA Node	Sinus tachycardia	SA node reentry
Atrial	Ectopic atrial tachy. Multifocal atrial tachy.	Atrial flutter Atrial fibrillation
A-V junction	Junctional ectopic tachy.	AV node reentry
WPW syndrome		Orthodromic reentry Antidromic reentry Preexcited A fib/A fl
"Concealed" accessory pathway		Orthodromic reentry Permanent junctional Reciprocating tachy.
Mahaim fiber		Antidromic reentry Preexcited A fib/A fl
Ventricle	Atypical VT	Ventricular tachycardia

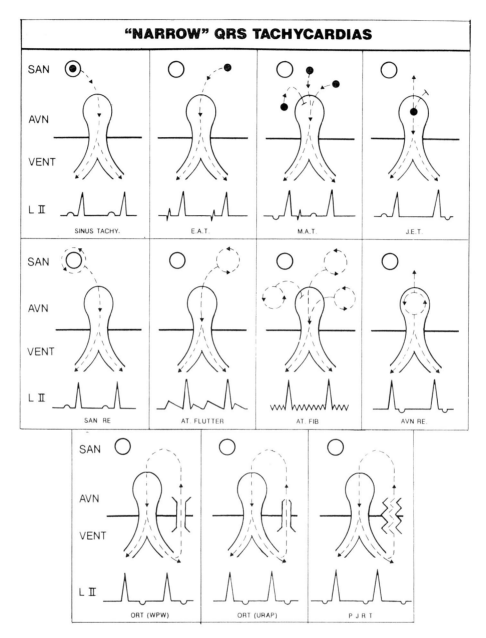

Figure 11. Mechanisms for "narrow" QRS tachycardia. Diagrams show the SA node (SAN) upper left, with the AV node (AVN) and bundle branches crossing to the ventricle (vent). Surface lead II emphasizes the P-wave timing and morphology.

register a normal axis of about +60° (i.e., upright in lead II). Because sinus tachycardia usually occurs under conditions of high circulating catecholamines, conduction at the AV node is generally robust, so the A:V ratio is 1:1 in most instances.

In **ectopic atrial tachycardia,** there is an abnormal atrial focus which generates rapid depolarization. Several features distinguish it from sinus tachycardia. First, the P-wave axis is abnormal because of eccentric atrial depolarization. Second, because catecholamine levels are not necessarily elevated and the mechanism does not directly in-

volve the AV node or ventricles, episodic block of AV-node conduction can often be observed without interruption of the arrhythmia, especially during vagal stimulation or sleep. **Multifocal atrial tachycardia** presents a similar picture, although in this instance multiple competing P-wave morphologies are observed.

Junctional ectopic tachycardia is a rare disorder that is seen almost exclusively in young children following congenital heart surgery, but occasionally may arise de novo. Note in Figure 11 that the focus of rapid discharge is centered in the AV node or the proximal bundle of His. As with other automatic tachycardias, the rate accelerates gradually and exhibits perceptible variation over time. However, the key feature here is possible dissociation of the P and QRS, a consequence of the fact that atrial tissue is not directly linked to the arrhythmia mechanism. In some patients there may be passive 1:1 retrograde atrial depolarization with a P axis of −120 degrees, whereas in others retrograde conduction may be intermittent or even absent altogether. Junctional ectopic tachycardia is the only narrow QRS tachyarrhythmia in which the ventricular rate can be faster than the atrial rate.

Automatic ectopic tachycardias are sometimes difficult to identify from a surface electrocardiogram alone, particularly when P-wave activity is not clearly seen. Perhaps their most notable characteristic is refractoriness to cardioversion, overdrive pacing, and conventional medications. Often, the diagnosis is made retrospectively after these remedies have been attempted unsuccessfully.

Reentry mechanisms are the most common cause of a narrow QRS tachycardia. Their most distinctive characteristics are abrupt paroxysmal onset and termination, as well as strictly regular rates.

Reentry in the vicinity of the SA node produces an electrocardiographic picture similar to that of sinus tachycardia (P-wave axis +60 degrees) except that it starts abruptly and demonstrates minimal variation in rate during maneuvers that augment or depress sympathetic tone. There may be variable atrioventricular block depending on the state of AV node conduction.

Reentry within atrial muscle produces two very familiar clinical arrhythmias: a single atrial reentry circuit referred to as **atrial flutter,** or multiple, small reentry circuits referred to as **atrial fibrillation.** Atrial fibrillation is readily recognized on the ECG, but atrial flutter is sometimes more difficult to identify. The rate in flutter (classically 300 beats per minute) may vary widely from patient to patient. Atrial rates as fast as 400/min may be seen in infants, and rates as slow as 140/min may occur in older patients with dilated hearts. The hallmark sawtooth pattern in leads II, III, and aV$_F$ may also be difficult to demonstrate at times, particularly during the 1:1 atrioventricular conduction of slower flutter rates or during 2:1 conduction when every other flutter wave is buried under a QRS. Careful electrocardiographic observation during vagal stimulation, which often modifies AV conduction, may uncover hidden flutter waves.

The final four circuits for narrow QRS tachycardia include reentry within the AV node and those tachycardias that reciprocate between the atrium and ventricle via an accessory pathway. In all four conditions, a strict 1:1 ratio must be maintained between the atrium and ventricle during SVT, and the atria are exclusively depolarized from below to produce a retrograde P-wave axis of approximately −120 degrees. These tachycardias start abruptly, operate at fixed and regular rates, and react to vagal stimulation with either minimal rate response, or abrupt termination. As shown in Figure 11, the timing of the retrograde P wave can be used as a fairly reliable marker to differentiate the disorders. In AV node reentry, the P wave is generated nearly simultaneously with the QRS—sometimes slightly before, sometimes superimposed, but most often immediately after (within 70 msec). In comparison, the reciprocating tachycardias that involve an accessory pathway must traverse a physically longer circuit, thus generating the P wave 70 msec or more after the QRS complex.

Further differentiation among these AV reciprocating circuits is possible by examining the electrocardiogram after tachycardia has been terminated. For AV node reentry, the electrocardiogram is usually normal between episodes. For a bidirectional accessory connection (i.e., WPW syndrome) the diagnosis is made by observing the delta wave and short P-R interval after sinus rhythm is restored. Concealed pathways, which function as unidirectional retrograde connections, may be harder to diagnose because the ECG in sinus rhythm is completely normal. Differentiation between AV-node and concealed-pathway reentry may require electrophysiologic study for final resolution. However, one variety of concealed pathway (the permanent form of junctional reciprocating tachycardia) can usually be diagnosed with certainty. As the name implies, this form of SVT is very difficult to terminate for more than a few beats and it exhibits a dramatically prolonged interval between the QRS and the P wave during the tachycardia, as shown in Figure 11.

A summary of the diagnostic clues for the differentiation of narrow QRS tachycardias is provided in Table 4.

Differential Diagnosis of Wide QRS Tachycardias. A wide QRS tachycardia **should always be managed as a VT until proven otherwise!** Often, the surface electrocardiogram offers no reliable features to eliminate VT from consideration and proof may come only from invasive electrophysiologic testing. Likewise, patient age and prior medical status should never persuade one to assume that a wide QRS rhythm is a relatively benign SVT. Although rare in the pediatric population, VT may occur at any age, even in previously healthy children.[4]

Figure 12 diagrams the possible mechanisms and ECG features of wide QRS tachycardias in pediatric patients. One of the most valuable diagnostic observations on an electrocardiogram is the presence of dissociation between the rapid QRS and a slower P wave. If the ventricles are seen to beat independently of the atrium, the differential di-

Table 4. Differential Diagnosis of Narrow QRS Tachycardia Mechanisms

	Sinus Tachy.	Ectopic Atrial Tachy.	Multifocal Atrial Tachy.	Junctional Ectopic Tachy.	SA Node Reentry	Atrial Flutter	Atrial Fib.	AV Node Reentry	Orthodromic Tachy. (WPW)	Orthodromic Tachy. ("concealed")	PJRT
Onset and termination	warm-up cool-down	warm-up cool-down	warm-up cool-down	warm-up cool-down	abrupt	abrupt	abrupt	abrupt	abrupt	abrupt	incessant
Atrial rate in SVT	variable	variable	variable	normal or variable	fixed	fixed		fixed	fixed	fixed	fixed
A:V ratio in SVT	1	≥1	≥1	<1	≥1	≥1	>1	1	1	1	1
P-wave axis	normal	"ectopic"	multiple	normal or retrograde variable	normal	"ectopic"	multiple	retrograde	retrograde	retrograde	retrograde
V-A time for retrograde P wave								<70 msec	>70 msec	>70 msec	>>>70 msec
Response to vagal stimulation	mild decr. rate	AV block	AV block	none	AV block	AV block	AV block	none or terminate	none or terminate	none or terminate	none or terminate
Response to DC cardioversion	none	none	none	none	terminate	terminate	terminate	terminate	terminate	terminate	transient terminate
ECG in sinus rhythm	normal	normal	normal	normal	normal	normal	normal	normal	WPW	normal	normal
Prevalence in infants		rare	rare	mostly postop.	rare	occasional	rare	rare	common	common	rare
Prevalence in older children		rare	rare	rare	rare	occasional	occasional	common	common	common	rare

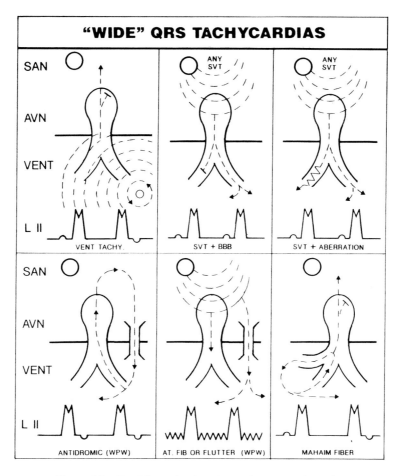

Figure 12. Possible mechanisms for "wide" QRS tachycardia.

agnosis is limited to either VT or Mahaim fiber reentry. Note, however, that **the absence of atrioventricular dissociation does not rule out these conditions;** there is frequently passive retrograde 1:1 atrial depolarization from VT or Mahaim reentry in a young patient. One of the potential consequences of AV dissociation is the finding of "fusion beats," caused by intermittent penetration of atrial impulses. Although fusion is fairly specific for a ventricular tachycardia, it may also occur during some arrhythmias in the WPW syndrome. After resumption of sinus rhythm the electrocardiogram provides additional diagnostic clues. If the patient is noted to have permanent bundle branch block at rest that is identical to the QRS in tachycardia, it is a fairly safe assumption that the primary arrhythmia was SVT. Similarly, if WPW syndrome (short P-R interval and delta wave) or Mahaim fiber activity (delta wave with normal P-R) is seen, these pathways are likely to have participated in the tachycardia. The most difficult differential diagnosis involves the choice between VT and SVT with rate-related QRS aberration. In children with SVT, aberration may involve either the right or left bundle

branch, often making the ECG indistinguishable from that of VT except by intracardiac electrophysiologic study.

The differential features of wide QRS tachycardia mechanisms are summarized in Table 5, but note that the degree of diagnostic resolution is much less exact than that possible for narrow QRS tachycardias on the basis of ECG findings alone.

Management of Specific Tachyarrhythmias

The preceding section was meant to serve as a rough road map for identification of a tachycardia mechanism at the bedside. Expanded discussion of the physiology and treatment of these individual disorders follows. The tachycardias have been divided into four major groups, including three varieties of supraventricular mechanisms ("automatic," and "reentry" with or without accessory pathways), and ventricular tachycardias.

Automatic Supraventricular Tachycardias

Ectopic Atrial Tachycardia (EAT). Ectopic atrial tachycardia is a primary atrial tachycardia which probably results from enhanced automaticity of a

Table 5. Differential Diagnosis of Wide QRS Tachycardia Mechanisms

	Ventricular Tachycardia	SVT with BBB	SVT with Aberration	Antidromic (WPW)	Preexcited A fib/A fl (WPW)	Antidromic Mahaim Reentry
Onset and termination	abrupt	abrupt	abrupt	abrupt	abrupt	abrupt
AV dissociation	sometimes	no	no	no	no	sometimes
BBB morphology in tachycardia	right/left may vary	right/left fixed	right/left may vary	right/left fixed	right/left usual vary	left BBB fixed
"Fusion" beats?	sometimes	no	QRS may narrow	no	yes	no
Response DC conversion	usually terminates	terminate	terminate	terminate	terminate	terminate
ECG in sinus rhythm	normal	BBB	normal	WPW	WPW	Mahaim
HBE in tachycardia	HV dissociation	normal HV	normal HV	negative HV	variable HV	negative HV
Prevalence in infants	occasional	mostly postop.	occasional	rare	rare	rare
Prevalence in older children	occasional	mostly postop.	occasional	occasional	occasional	rare

single non-sinus atrial focus (see Fig. 11). This arrhythmia accounts for only about 10% of cases of SVT,[52,80] but it is notoriously difficult to treat.

Clinical Manifestations and Electrophysiologic Features. Ectopic atrial tachycardia rarely causes acute symptoms. Its discovery is usually via routine physical examination or through detection of congestive heart failure secondary to longstanding arrhythmia. Indeed, it is not unusual for patients to present with dilated cardiomyopathy and what initially may be confused with sinus tachycardia. Ectopic atrial tachycardia may also be seen as a transient disorder following cardiac surgery.

The hallmark of the arrhythmia is an atrial rate that is inappropriately rapid for age and physiologic state, but varies on both a beat-to-beat and a long-term basis to a degree that excludes a reentrant mechanism. The P-wave morphology differs from sinus rhythm and depends on the site of the automatic focus, which may be anywhere in the right or left atrium. Because the arrhythmia mechanism is confined to atrial tissue, the ventricular response rate and the P-R interval are determined independently by the AV node. First- and second-degree AV block, as well as occasional bundle branch aberrancy, are common findings (Fig. 13).

The primary feature at electrophysiologic study is the fast atrial rate, with the earliest atrial activation arising from a point distant from the sinus node (Fig. 14). The tachycardia cannot be terminated with pacing or DC cardioversion; however, it usually exhibits at least brief overdrive suppression in response to rapid atrial pacing.

Management. Clinical symptoms may improve simply by lowering the ventricular rate, so that initial therapy can be directed at the AV node. Digoxin improves ventricular function, both

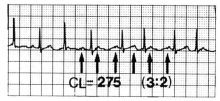

30 sec post exercise

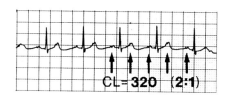

2 min post exercise

Figure 13. Lead II recording from a patient with ectopic atrial tachycardia. The upper strip was obtained after exercise and shows rapid atrial depolarization (arrows) at a cycle length of 275 msec, which conducts with 3:2 ratio. During rest (lower strip), both the atrial rate and A:V ratio are slower.

through its inotropic effect and through its vagally mediated enhancement of AV node block. In addition, digoxin may lower the atrial rate directly in rare cases. Although beta blockers must be used with care in patients with ventricular dysfunction secondary to EAT, they are often effective in slowing the atrial focus in this disorder and may even be the only necessary therapy for many patients. Verapamil, phenytoin, procainamide, flecainide, encainide, and amiodarone, as well as the investigational agents ethmozine[23] and sotalol,[118] may also be effective, but an empirical trial is necessary

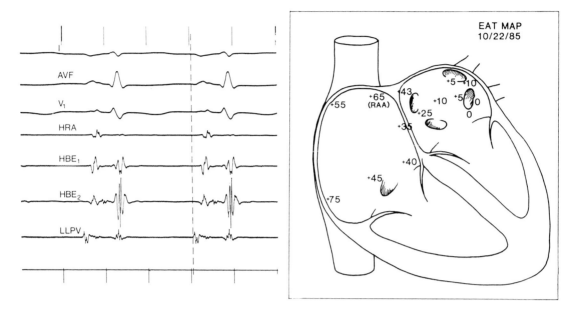

Figure 14. Intracardiac mapping of an ectopic atrial focus in the area of the left lower pulmonary vein (LLPV).

for each agent. In the authors' experience intravenous administration of phenytoin may be particularly effective for postoperative patients with transient ectopic atrial tachycardia.

Prevention. Ectopic atrial tachycardia in postoperative patients can usually be controlled medically and is usually transient. However, the chronic spontaneous variety may be refractory to all medical therapy except that directed at increasing the degree of AV block. In such cases, excision or cryoblation of the ectopic focus in the operating room may be attempted, although occasional failures have been reported due either to inability to localize the ectopic focus under anesthesia or to recurrence at a new focus postoperatively.[53] Transcatheter ablation has also been used successfully in some cases.[56]

Multifocal Atrial Tachycardia (MAT). Multifocal atrial tachycardia (also referred to as chaotic atrial rhythm) is a rare disorder in children which appears to be caused by multiple foci of enhanced atrial automaticity. The surface electrocardiogram demonstrates a variable P-wave morphology with highly variable P-P intervals that are short for the patient's age and physiologic state. The P-R intervals, R-R intervals and QRS morphology may also vary because of rate-related block in both the AV node and the His-Purkinje system (Fig. 15).

Although the exact cause is unknown, MAT has been associated with chronic lung disease in adults[120] and may be seen as a transient idiopathic disorder during infancy[94] or in the postoperative period after congenital heart surgery in children.

Treatment is difficult and usually involves medications which enhance AV block to decrease the maximum ventricular rate (digoxin, beta blockers,

or verapamil). Occasionally, verapamil may slow or eradicate this atrial tachycardia directly.[93] Instances of sudden death have been reported in some infants with poor rate control.[153]

Junctional Ectopic Tachycardia (JET). Junctional ectopic tachycardia likewise appears to be caused by enhanced automaticity, but in this case the focus is within the AV node or the bundle of His. It should not be equated with the normal junctional escape rhythm that may be seen in the setting of sinus node dysfunction or AV block (Fig. 16). At times, the rate of junctional ectopic discharge is only mildly to moderately accelerated and may be of little acute hemodynamic significance, but rapid rates (180–300/min) are poorly tolerated. Junctional ectopic tachycardia may occur as a congenital disorder with a definite familial tendency,[44] but more commonly it is seen as a transient arrhythmia (lasting 1–4 days) immediately following cardiac surgery.[64]

Clinical Manifestations and Electrophysiologic Features. Postoperatively, rapid JET can cause severe hemodynamic compromise. This situation may lead to an increase in the level of infused and endogenous beta-adrenergic agonists, which in turn further accelerates the tachycardia and may paradoxically exacerbate the patient's already poor condition. Prior to the recognition of effective therapies for rapid postoperative junctional ectopic tachycardia, the mortality rate was high. The congenital form of JET is rare, but it may likewise be associated with morbidity and mortality from either the hemodynamic stress of persistent tachycardias or episodic disturbances of AV conduction.[54]

The electrocardiographic pattern is distinctive. Junctional ectopic tachycardia is the only narrow

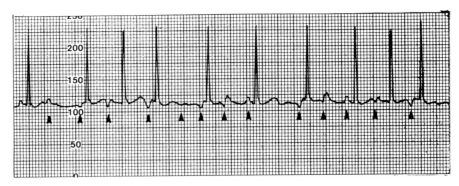

Figure 15. Multiple P-wave morphology (arrows) on surface ECG lead II from a teenager with multifocal atrial tachycardia.

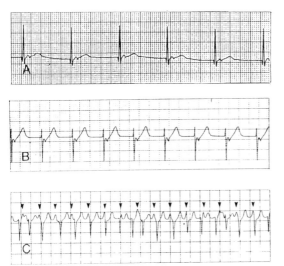

Figure 16. The spectrum of junctional rhythm. **A,** Slow junctional escape rhythm in a patient with sinus node dysfunction at 62 bpm. **B,** Mildly accelerated junctional rhythm in a stable postoperative patient at 100 bpm. **C,** Rapid junctional ectopic tachycardia at 200 bpm. Note slower P waves (arrows) and instances of "early" QRS due to occasional conduction of atrial depolarization.

complex SVT in which the rhythm is characterized by AV dissociation and a ventricular rate which is greater than the atrial rate. True AV block is not common in the postoperative form, as demonstrated by occasional atrial capture beats when sinus P waves are appropriately timed (Fig. 16C) and by the ability to establish AV synchrony by atrial pacing at a rate faster than the rate of the ectopic focus.

Management. For rapid postoperative JET, acute improvement in hemodynamics is best accomplished by both reestablishing AV synchrony and attempting to lower the junctional rate. AV synchrony alone (which can be provided by either fixed-rate atrial pacing at a rate higher than the tachycardia rate, or by atrial pacing triggered from the previous ventricular complex) may sometimes improve hemodynamics enough that the cycle of

adrenergic stimulation previously described gradually subsides.[138]

Therapy to directly slow the junctional rate is more difficult but is often necessary. Digoxin has been reported to be effective in some series, but in the authors' experience it rarely modifies JET and is limited by delayed onset of action. Equally poor results have been found with phenytoin, verapamil, propranolol, and procainamide. On the other hand, the use of induced hypothermia to 34° is remarkably effective,[2] and for refractory cases the addition of procainamide during hypothermia is usually successful in slowing JET to more physiologic ranges. Since 1986, using AV synchrony, followed by hypothermia to a minimum of 34°, with the addition of procainamide for refractory cases, all rapid junctional ectopic tachycardias in postoperative patients have been successfully controlled at our Center.[129]

"Reentrant" Supraventricular Tachycardias Not Involving Accessory Pathways

Sinus Node Reentry Tachycardia. *Clinical Manifestations and Electrophysiologic Features.* Sinus node reentry is rare. In most series, it accounts for between 5 and 10% of SVTs in children or adults. At The Children's Hospital in Boston it represented less than 1% of SVT seen over a 3-year period.

Reentry within the sinus node or perinodal tissue produces an abrupt onset of atrial tachycardia at a relatively fixed rate, with a surface P-wave morphology that is identical to that of sinus rhythm (Fig. 17). Variable first- and second-degree AV block can be seen.

At electrophysiologic study, the tachycardia can often be induced or terminated with atrial pacing, with neither critically dependent on AV conduction.[61] The P-R interval during tachycardia is relatively long and somewhat variable. Atrial mapping during tachycardia reveals the earliest activation to be near the junction of the superior vena cava and the right atrium.

Management. Vagal maneuvers or esophageal atrial pacing are often effective for acute conver-

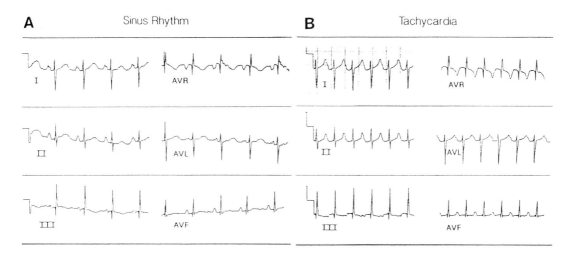

A   Sinus Rhythm   **B**   Tachycardia

Figure 17.   Sinus node reentry. P-wave morphology in all frontal leads is identical in sinus rhythm (**A**) and tachycardia (**B**). P waves are superimposed on the T wave during tachycardia. Unlike sinus tachycardia, this rhythm was strictly regular, could be easily and reproducibly initiated with atrial pacing, and eventually responded to therapy with digoxin.

sion. DC cardioversion is likewise successful, and pharmacologic conversions can sometimes be achieved with digoxin. Hypothetically, verapamil and beta blockers should be effective as well, but experience is limited.

Prevention. Chronic drug therapy begins with digoxin, both to increase AV block and to prevent recurrent reentry. Verapamil and beta blockers are probably reasonable alternatives to digoxin. SA-node reentry is rarely a chronic recurring disorder in children.

Atrial Flutter. Atrial flutter can be considered to involve a single reentry loop confined to atrial muscle. As with other primary atrial tachycardias, the ventricular rate is determined entirely by the response properties of the AV conducting system. The circuit may be small, on the order of a millimeter (micro-reentry), or large, on the order of centimeters (macro-reentry). Although abnormalities in the conduction and refractory periods of atrial tissue are often present, simple dispersion of the refractory periods of the atrial muscle is adequate to produce sustained reentry. The flutter rate is entirely dependent on the size of the reentry circuit and the average conduction velocity of the involved tissue. Thus, large reentry circuits that generally occur around anatomic obstacles, such as a surgical scar or abnormal atrial tissue, tend to have longer cycle lengths and slower rates (150 to 300 beats/min, often referred to as Type I flutter), whereas, smaller circuits in relatively normal atrial tissue, such as in newborn infants without structural heart disease, tend to have faster rates (300 to 500 beats/min, often called Type II flutter).

No distinction is made here between atrial muscle reentry and atrial flutter since the mechanisms are virtually identical. Atrial flutter is a diagnosis based on a characteristic appearance on the surface ECG in which the baseline looks like a sawtooth which is often most prominent in leads II, III, aV_F, and V_1 (Fig. 18). There is no obvious isoelectric segment in these leads, with the sawtooth pattern presumably corresponding to the electrophysiologic property of continuous activation of atrial tissue throughout the tachycardia cycle. Thus, the only difference between classic atrial flutter and other forms of reentry within atrial muscle is the electrocardiographic appearance. Otherwise, the clinical characteristics, ventricular response rate, and potential therapies are identical.

Clinical Manifestations and Electrophysiologic Features. The clinical presentation of atrial muscle reentry is largely dependent on the ventricular response rate, as determined by the conduction properties of the AV node. In the majority of cases the A:V ratio is >1, resulting in ventricular rates of 120–200/min. Thus, syncope due to 1:1 atrioventricular conduction is rare, whereas palpitations, decreased energy, weakness, and symptoms of mild congestive heart failure are common presenting symptoms.

Sometimes the tachycardia may be difficult to diagnose on the surface electrocardiogram during 2:1 block because of the superimposition of alternate flutter waves on the QRS-T complex (Fig. 19). In such cases, the clinical diagnosis usually can be made through either an increase or decrease in the degree of AV block induced by autonomic maneuvers.

Although the typical electrocardiographic appearance of atrial flutter, with a sawtooth baseline and inverted P waves in leads II, III, and aV_F, may be seen, many patients have more discrete P waves and a variety of P-wave axes. Obtaining an atrial electrogram via either an esophageal or intracar-

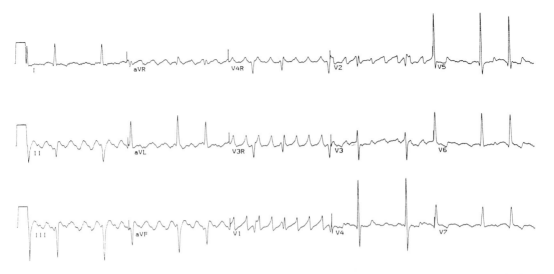

Figure 18. Surface ECG showing atrial flutter. Note sawtooth baseline in leads II, III, aV_F, and the right chest leads. The ventricular response rate varies from 2:1 to 4:1.

diac lead virtually always clarifies the diagnosis, revealing a strictly regular, rapid atrial rate.

Management. Although direct-current cardioversion with relatively low energy (¼ joule/kg) is almost always successful in terminating atrial reentry, at Boston Children's Hospital the treatment of choice has usually been atrial pacing via either an esophageal lead or endocardial/epicardial leads when available. This approach offers the advantage of providing immediate backup pacing if a long pause occurs at flutter termination, as is often seen in the setting of the sick sinus syndrome. Esoph-

ageal pacing can be successful in as many as 73% of cases (Fig. 20), while epicardial/endocardial pacing can be effective in 63%.[11] Transient atrial fibrillation, usually lasting a few seconds to minutes, often occurs prior to reversion to sinus rhythm with pacing techniques. In some cases fibrillation may persist, necessitating alternate therapy.

If DC shock or pacing cardioversion is not performed or not desirable, pharmacologic conversion may be attempted. Digoxin should be given initially to inhibit a rapid ventricular response, although digoxin alone will rarely convert atrial flut-

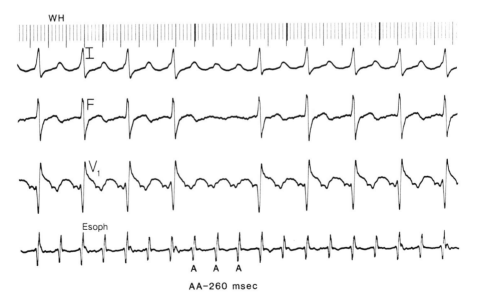

Figure 19. Esophageal recording of atrial flutter. Lead V_1 displays the typical sawtooth baseline but leads I and aV_F could easily be mistaken for sinus tachycardia when conduction is 2:1. Brief periods of higher grade A:V block, as in the middle of this trace, or an esophageal recording can confirm the diagnosis in difficult cases.

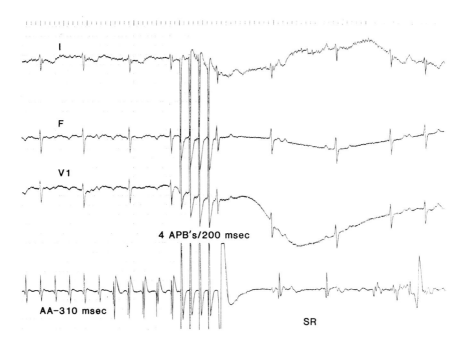

Figure 20. Conversion of atrial flutter with esophageal pacing. An atrial esophageal electrogram (bottom trace) confirmed the diagnosis of atrial flutter. A sensing artifact is present in atrial beats 8–12, then four pacing artifacts are present, followed by a 200-msec blanking period. After pacing, the first QRS is junctional and the second beat is sinus.

ter directly to sinus rhythm. More effective drugs for this purpose include procainamide, quinidine, flecainide, and amiodarone, all of which have the potential to terminate the arrhythmia by slowing atrial conduction velocity and lengthening the atrial refractory periods. Note, however, that paradoxical increases in ventricular response rate can occur with some of these second-line agents (particularly quinidine) because of slowing of the atrial rate as well as the vagolytic effects on the AV node.[108] They should not be commenced until digitalization is complete.

Prevention. Following a first episode of atrial flutter patients should be maintained on a drug such as digoxin, which will prevent a rapid ventricular response should the arrhythmia recur. For those with a documented recurrence, oral quinidine or procainamide in combination with digoxin is the next step. If, with adequate serum levels, these agents are unsuccessful, then flecainide, sotalol, or amiodarone may be tried. Alternatively an atrial antitachycardia pacing unit can be considered, particularly for patients with the sick sinus syndrome who require bradycardia pacing prior to institution of drug therapy, or for those whose tachycardia is unresponsive to drugs alone. Candidates for this device must demonstrate reproducible termination of their flutter with pacing maneuvers prior to a final decision regarding an implant.

Atrial Fibrillation. Atrial fibrillation is a primary atrial tachycardia, probably due to multiple small and constantly changing reentry circuits within one or both atria. Though common in adults, atrial fibrillation is rare in small children, possibly because of an atrial size that is inadequate to support multiple reentry circuits. The common clinical settings for atrial fibrillation in the pediatric age group include complex anatomic defects with advanced AV valve regurgitation, preexcitation syndromes (e.g., WPW), or the sick sinus syndrome. Atrial fibrillation may also be caused by hyperthyroidism, which should be investigated in new patients without obvious underlying heart disease.

Clinical Manifestations and Electrophysiologic Features. Patients with atrial fibrillation usually experience palpitations. Syncope due to a rapid ventricular response is rare in the absence of the WPW syndrome. Those with compromised ventricular function and particularly slow or fast ventricular response rates may experience weakness or congestive heart failure in addition to palpitations.

The electrocardiogram typically reveals a low-amplitude, irregular base-line alteration (Fig. 21) that at times may be difficult to differentiate from artifact or rapid atrial flutter. Ventricular response rates are generally between 80 and 150 beats/minute. An electrocardiographic hallmark is the nearly random variation in length of the R-R intervals (irregularly-irregular) due to chaotic atrial rates and variable AV-node conduction. Intermittent QRS aberration (Ashman's phenomenon) is also seen (Fig. 22).

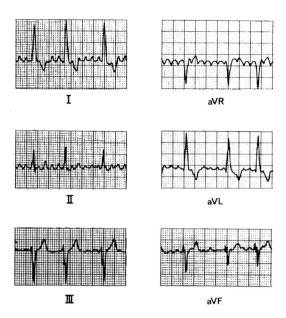

Figure 21. Atrial fibrillation that developed in a patient with tricuspid atresia. The ventricular response rate is about 90 bpm.

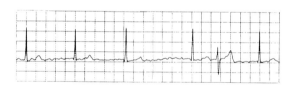

Figure 22. Ashman's phenomenon in a patient with atrial fibrillation. There is a relative pause between the 3rd and 4th QRS, followed by closer spacing between the 4th and 5th QRS (which is aberrant). Ashman's typically occurs after such "long-short" intervals.

Management. As for atrial flutter, initial therapy for atrial fibrillation should be directed at lowering the ventricular rate, usually with digoxin. Unlike atrial flutter, in atrial fibrillation atrial pacing is not useful in the conversion of atrial fibrillation to sinus rhythm. In adults, trials of pharmacologic conversion with agents such as quinidine and procainamide are successful in only 10 to 15% of patients.[156] Experience in children and adolescents has been similar. Thus, elective DC cardioversion is employed for most patients with sustained atrial fibrillation. Patients who have been in atrial fibrillation for more than a few days should be anticoagulated for at least 1 week prior to cardioversion in an attempt to minimize the chance of clot formation within poorly contracting atrial tissue.[99]

Prevention. Drug therapy for prevention of recurrent atrial fibrillation is similar to that for atrial flutter and may be difficult at times. Studies in adults reveal that, regardless of therapy, as few as 30–50% of patients will maintain sinus rhythm for 12 months after acute cardioversion.[156] Pediatric experience has been only slightly better.

AV-Nodal Reentrant Tachycardia (AVNRT). The presence of two discrete conduction pathways within the AV node probably underlies most forms of AV-nodal reentrant tachycardia. Typically, one of the pathways, known as the "slow" limb, exhibits slow conduction velocity but has a relatively short refractory period, whereas the "fast" pathway conducts much more rapidly but has a longer refractory time. Although there is no firm anatomic evidence to support this hypothesis, the functional evidence is convincing, including electrocardiographic recognition of spontaneous sudden changes in the P-R interval (Fig. 23) and the demonstration of a discontinuity in the AV-nodal conduction time (A-H interval) with atrial premature stimuli during electrophysiologic testing (Fig. 24).

Typically, during normal sinus rhythm both the slow and fast pathways conduct anterograde, but the wave front from the fast pathway is the first to reach the bundle of His and leads to a ventricular complex. The wave front in the slow pathway may be blocked by retrograde conduction from the ventricular end of the fast pathway, or it may simply find the distal AV node and His tissue refractory (Fig. 25A). When a premature atrial impulse occurs at an appropriate interval, conduction in the fast pathway is blocked because of its longer refractory period, allowing the impulse to return toward the atria, retrograde in the fast pathway, which is no longer refractory (Fig. 25B), thereby setting up "slow-fast" AV-node reentry. There is no *a priori* reason why the refractory characteristics of the two pathways might not be reversed, setting up a "fast-slow" form of tachycardia, but in practice, when tachycardia due to a concealed accessory pathway has been carefully ruled out, less than 10% of patients exhibit the fast-slow variety.

Clinical Manifestations and Electrophysiologic Features. AVNRT is rather unusual in young patients. It seems most likely to occur in children older than the age of 5 years. It is probable that the electrophysiologic substrate (i.e., dual AV–node paths) is present from birth, but is simply unmasked with age as both the autonomic influences and the refractory characteristics of the AV nodal tissue change with growth. By comparison AVNRT may be the most common mechanism for SVT in patients who are first seen in adulthood.[152]

The tachycardia rate in children with AVNRT is usually between 200 and 300/min, but may be as slow as 120/min. Severe hemodynamic compromise is rare with AVNRT, but feelings of anxiety, chest pain, and dizziness are frequent.

Dual AV nodal pathways can usually be demonstrated at electrophysiologic study by the presence of a discontinuous anterograde AV nodal conduction curve (defined as a more than 40 msec

Figure 23. Dual AV node pathways on the surface ECG. The P-R interval spontaneously changes from 320 msec to 180 msec when the heart rate slows, indicating a shift from the slow pathway with a shorter refractory period to the fast pathway with a longer refractory period.

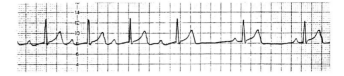

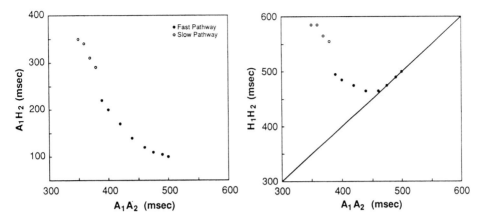

Figure 24. Electrophysiologic characteristics of dual AV-node pathways. As the A-A interval decreases during atrial extrastimulus testing, the A-H interval increases because of first-degree AV node block (**A**). The H-H interval decreases but the change is less than that for the A-A, yielding a slope of less than 1 in (**B**). At the effective refractory period of the fast pathway, a 75-msec jump occurs in both the A-H and H-H intervals with only a 10-msec decrease in A-A, meeting the functional criteria for dual AV node pathways.

increase in the A-H interval with a 10-msec decrease in the coupling interval of a premature atrial impulse [A_1–A_2]) caused by sudden block in the fast pathway. Similarly, a jump in the retrograde V-A time during premature ventricular stimulation can be used to demonstrate dual pathways. However, electrophysiologic criteria for dual AV nodal pathways may be found in as many as 35% of children who do not have spontaneous SVT.[14] Also, some patients with well-documented AVNRT do not meet the criteria for dual AV nodal pathways.

During the typical slow-fast AVNRT, the retrograde conduction time in the fast pathway (the H-A interval) is approximately equal to the H-V interval; thus, the ventricular and atrial depolarizations occur at approximately the same time. This finding corresponds to the P wave occurring nearly simultaneously with the QRS complex on the surface cardiogram (Fig. 26) and essentially rules out tachycardia involving an extranodal accessory pathway, which typically shows a delay of at least 70 msec between ventricular and atrial depolarization.

Management. In general, any maneuvers that enhance vagal activity (Fig. 27) and slow AV nodal conduction (such as the Valsalva maneuver, carotid sinus massage, excitation of the diving reflex, or elevation of arterial pressure produced by lying supine) may promote slowing and termination. If vagal maneuvers fail, pharmacologic therapy is usually successful in this disorder and should be directed at blocking AV nodal conduction with agents such as verapamil, esmolol, or adenosine.

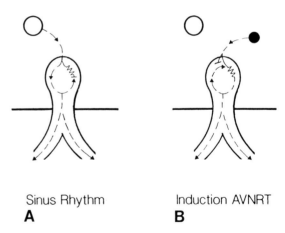

Sinus Rhythm

A

Induction AVNRT

B

Figure 25. Dual AV-node pathways. In sinus rhythm (**A**) antegrade conduction proceeds down both the slow and fast pathways simultaneously, but conduction in the fast pathway usually reaches the point where they merge again first. The fast pathway then excites the His-Purkinje system, and conduction may proceed retrograde up the slow pathway, blocking its antegrade conduction. Occasionally, slow pathway conduction is so slow that the distal AV node is no longer refractory when its wave front arrives, giving rise to two ventricular activations from a single atrial stimulus. Tachycardia may be induced (**B**) when conduction blocks first in the fast pathway because of its short refractory period, then proceeds down the slow pathway, and finally reenters retrograde in the fast pathway.

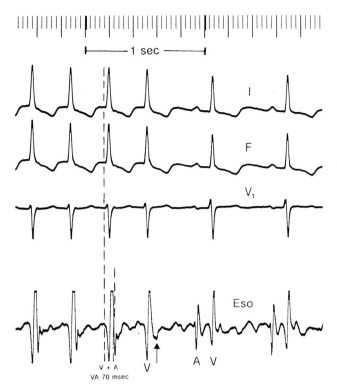

Figure 26. AV-node reentry tachycardia. Surface ECG leads I, aV_F, and V_1 demonstrate a regular, narrow complex tachycardia with an R-R interval of 320 msec, which spontaneously terminates. P waves are not clearly visible but there is the suggestion of a P wave at the end of the QRS leads I and aV_F. The esophageal recording (eso) during tachycardia shows a single complex that has an additional component when compared to the V complex in sinus rhythm, and to the final beat of tachycardia. This complex represents an early retrograde A, yielding a V-A interval of 70 msec.

If this is not effective, indirect enhancement of vagal tone with peripheral vasoconstrictors (such as phenylephrine or methoxamine) may be tried.

As an alternative technique, atrial pacing via an esophageal lead is virtually 100% effective in terminating AVNRT in patients of all ages, with no substantial risks. Similarly, DC cardioversion with ¼ to ½ joule/kg is also nearly uniformly effective, but presents the disadvantages of needing anesthesia and possibly repeated shocks if tachycardia recurs. Although digoxin has long been the cornerstone for both emergency and long-term treatment of SVT in infants and children, its delayed onset of action limits its use in acute management of AVNRT and most other forms of reentrant tachycardia.

Prevention. The goals of long-term treatment of AVNRT should be both to prevent the onset of tachycardia and minimize the duration of episodes once established. Patients who have infrequent episodes that terminate quickly are often best managed with the nonpharmacologic autonomic maneuvers described above, trading a few minutes of discomfort for the inconvenience and possible side effects of long-term drug treatment. Patients who suffer from prolonged, frequent bouts of tachycardia require chronic medical therapy. The most successful agents appear to be those that modify AV-node conduction characteristics and/or suppress ectopic beats that may serve as the initiating events for reentry (digoxin, beta blockers, or verapamil). When conventional therapy is unsuccessful,

class IA, IC, and III agents may sometimes be useful; however, at Boston Children's Hospital the potential side effects of these medications has led us to initiate therapy as an inpatient procedure and to document electrophysiologic efficacy, using programmed electrical stimulation, prior to discharge. Recently, both surgical[73] and catheter ablation techniques[63] for AV-node modification have been described; these may obviate the need for long-term medical therapy in selected patients.

Supraventricular Tachycardias Due to Accessory Pathways

In 1930, Wolff, Parkinson, and White described a syndrome that consisted of a short P-R interval, bundle branch block on the surface QRS complex, and paroxysmal tachycardia.[150] Although they were unaware of any electrophysiologic or anatomic correlates to this disorder, their report sparked further investigation that ultimately confirmed the notion that the WPW syndrome was caused by an extranodal AV connection, often referred to as a Kent bundle. It is now understood that these accessory connections may express themselves through a variety of electrocardiographic abnormalities and tachycardias, with the specific manifestations dependent on the refractory and conduction properties of the AV node and accessory connection.

Several varieties of accessory pathways or connections have now been identified, including: (1) the classic atrioventricular pathways of the WPW syndrome that are usually capable of both anter-

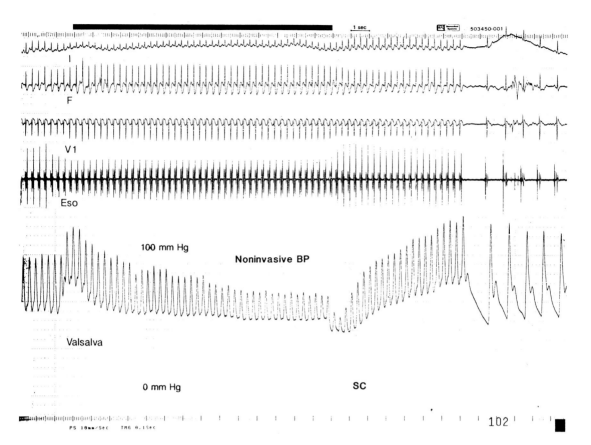

Figure 27. In some patients, as in this one with orthodromic reciprocating tachycardia, the Valsalva maneuver is reproducibly effective at terminating tachycardia. Here tachycardia terminates when the systolic blood pressure* reaches 130 mm Hg during phase IV of the Valsalva maneuver. Although difficult to see on this scale, the tachycardia terminates with an atrial deflection in the esophageal electrogram, suggesting block in the AV node. (*Finapress, Ohmeda Inc.)

ograde or retrograde conduction and may be located anywhere along the right or left atrioventricular groove, (2) concealed, accessory atrioventricular pathways that conduct only in the retrograde direction, again with varied location, and (3) Mahaim fibers that arise from the AV node or the bundle of His, and classically insert into the right ventricle. There is also variable evidence to support the existence of pathways running from the atrium to the bundle of His, so-called "James" fibers, which bypass the AV node and predispose to reentry tachyarrhythmias (the Lown-Ganong-Levine syndrome).

The characteristic appearance of the WPW syndrome on the surface ECG during sinus rhythm is that of a short P-R interval and a slurred initial QRS deflection, known as a **delta wave.** These findings reflect the fact that conduction from the atrium to the ventricle via the accessory connection is generally faster than conduction in the AV node. Thus, some segment of the ventricle is "**preexcited**" by the eccentric spread of activation from the accessory connection. The degree of preexcitation depends on the relative conduction velocities of the

AV node and the accessory connection (Fig. 28). Electrophysiologically, preexcitation is characterized by a short or negative H-V interval on a His bundle recording because ventricular activation occurs relatively early compared to the activation of the normal pathways (Fig. 29).

In agreement with the theoretical dipole model of surface electrocardiography in which the QRS complex is a projection of the heart vector on a particular lead orientation, the delta wave can be used to roughly identify the site of earliest ventricular activation and hence, the location of the accessory connection. Gallagher and coworkers[39] derived the algorithm for delta wave mapping shown in Figure 30, by comparing the polarity of the first 40 msec of the QRS in the 12 standard electrocardiogram leads to the location determined by epicardial activation mapping at surgery. This technique can be much more accurate than the simple Type A or B classification for WPW.

The most commonly observed tachyarrhythmias in the WPW syndrome are orthodromic reciprocating tachycardia (ORT), antidromic reciprocating tachycardia, and atrial fibrillation or flutter.

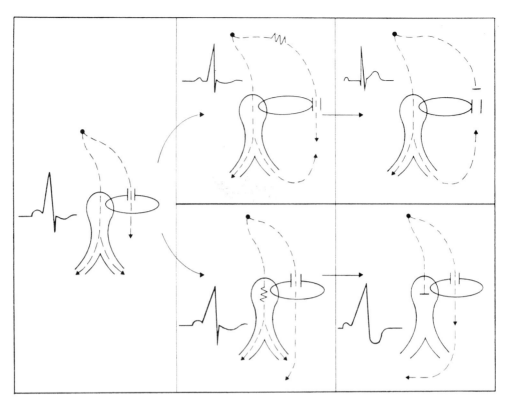

Figure 28. Origin of the delta wave in the WPW syndrome. During sinus rhythm the surface ECG appearance is influenced by the balance between ventricular depolarization through the AV node and the accessory pathway (AP), which depends on the relative conduction times from the atria to the ventricles through each pathway. Typically (far left panel), conduction reaches the ventricle first through the AP, yielding a short P-R interval, eccentric depolarization, and a delta wave, but conduction through the AV node also depolarizes a large amount of ventricle. The relative contribution of the accessory pathway may be small (upper panels), yielding relatively normal QRS and P-R intervals. By comparison, if conduction is delayed in the AV node (lower middle panel), more ventricular tissue is depolarized via the AP, yielding a shorter P-R and a more prominent delta wave. Rarely, the AV node may block while the AP remains excitable (lower right panel), yielding fully eccentric ventricular depolarization known as maximal preexcitation.

Clearly, this wide variety of arrhythmia mechanisms is a consequence of the capacity for either anterograde or retrograde conduction in the accessory pathway. By contrast, concealed pathways which conduct only in the retrograde direction from ventricle to atrium (i.e., no delta wave on the surface electrocardiogram) are incapable of supporting antidromic tachycardia or preexcited conduction of atrial fibrillation or flutter and participate only in ORT. In rare cases an accessory connection may conduct only anterograde so that ORT is not possible.

Orthodromic Reciprocating Tachycardia (ORT) due to the Wolff-Parkinson-White Syndrome. This tachycardia is by far the most common manifestation of WPW in the pediatric age group, accounting for 100% of the presenting symptoms in patients with WPW at The Children's Hospital in Boston who are less than 1 year of age and approximately 90% in those of all ages. The tachycardia circuit (see Fig. 11) includes anterograde conduction from the atrium to the ventricle through the AV node, yielding a normal, narrow QRS, and retrograde conduction from the ventricle to the atrium through an accessory connection, yielding a retrograde P-wave morphology (axis of −60 to −120°).

Clinical Manifestations and Electrocardiographic Features. As in AVNRT, severe acute hemodynamic compromise is rare in ORT, despite relatively high ventricular rates (200 to 320/min). The typical presentation is identical to that of AVNRT, with the exception that ORT occurs commonly in young infants and may go undetected for hours to days, sometimes resulting in congestive heart failure and even cardiovascular collapse.[51]

The surface electrocardiogram during ORT typically displays a narrow QRS morphology with a strictly regular rate; however, transient rate-related left or right bundle branch block may occur, particularly at the instant of tachycardia initiation. If the bundle branch block occurs ipsilateral to the side of the accessory connection, the tachycardia cycle length usually increases because of conduction delay in the ventricular muscle limb of the tachycardia circuit (Fig. 31). When this finding is

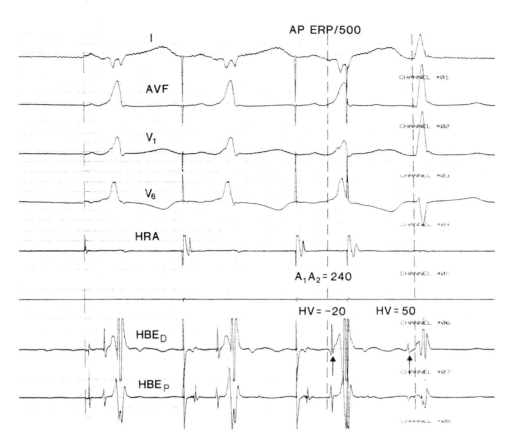

Figure 29. Electrophysiologic characteristics of the WPW syndrome. During sinus rhythm or atrial pacing, as shown here, ventricular activation occurs first through the accessory pathway (AP) so that the His activation (first arrow) occurs after the beginning of the surface QRS complex. A negative or short H-V interval during an atrial driven rhythm defines preexcitation. A premature atrial stimulus 240 msec after regular atrial pacing, with a 500 msec interval, causes block in the AP. The result is a long P-R interval, a normal QRS complex and a positive and normal H-V interval of 50 msec. Because the stimulus was the longest A-A interval that did not produce preexcitation, it is the AP effective refractory period (ERP), at a drive train of 500 msec.

observed, it helps to identify the location of the accessory pathway as either right- or left-sided.[84] Retrograde P waves typically occur during the T wave such that their visibility is variable between individuals. The initiating events for ORT can include sinus acceleration, atrial premature beats, junctional beats, or ventricular premature beats. The usual requirement for initiation is block of anterograde conduction in the accessory connection plus enough delay in AV nodal conduction to allow the accessory connection and atria to be excitable when the reentrant wave front reaches them.

Electrophysiologic Features. An atrial recording (either intracardiac or esophageal) during ORT demonstrates (1) an A:V ratio of unity, and (2) an interval from the earliest deflection of the QRS to the rapid deflection of the P wave (the V-A interval) greater than 70 msec. In addition, to prove that the tachycardia involves an extranodal accessory connection, other conditions must be met. Either the V-A interval in tachycardia must increase dur-

ing transient bundle branch aberration, or it must be possible to preexcite the atrium with a ventricular premature beat placed into tachycardia at a time when the bundle of His is refractory,[49] thus proving that the atrium was not activated via the AV node.

Initiation of tachycardia can usually be achieved with a critically timed atrial premature stimulus that blocks anterograde in the accessory connection and encounters an appropriate delay in the AV node. Thus, the atrial premature stimulus must occur at an interval shorter than the effective refractory period of an accessory connection. Termination of the tachycardia can be achieved almost uniformly with the placement of critically timed atrial premature stimuli. Once ORT is confirmed, the location of the accessory connection may be mapped by identifying the site of earliest retrograde atrial activation during ORT (Fig. 32). Left posterior and lateral pathways can be mapped accurately using a multielectrode catheter in the cor-

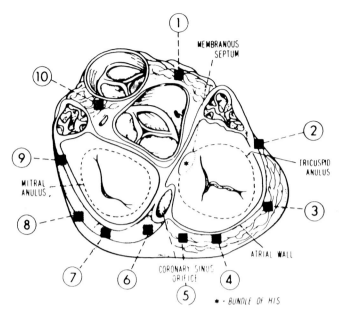

| | | I | II | III | AVR | AVL | AVF | V₁ | V₂ | V₃ | V₄ | V₅ | V₆ |

1. RIGHT ANTERIOR PARASEPTAL   6. LEFT POSTERIOR PARASEPTAL
2. RIGHT ANTERIOR   7. LEFT POSTERIOR
3. RIGHT LATERAL   8. LEFT LATERAL
4. RIGHT POSTERIOR   9. LEFT ANTERIOR
5. RIGHT PARASEPTAL   10. LEFT ANTERIOR PARASEPTAL

DELTA WAVE POLARITY

	I	II	III	AVR	AVL	AVF	V₁	V₂	V₃	V₄	V₅	V₆
①	+	+	+(±)	−	±(+)	+	±	±	+(±)	+	+	+
②	+	+	−(±)	−	+(±)	±(−)	±	+(±)	+(±)	+	+	+
③	+	±(−)	−	−	+	−(±)	±	±	±	+	+	+
④	+	−	−	−	+	−	±(+)	±	+	+	+	+
⑤	+	−	−	−(+)	+	−	±	+	+	+	+	+
⑥	+	−	−	−	+	−	+	+	+	+	+	+
⑦	+	−	−	±(+)	+	−	+	+	+	+	+	−(±)
⑧	−(±)	±	±	±(+)	−(±)	±	+	+	+	+	−(±)	−(±)
⑨	−(±)	+	+	−	−(±)	+	+	+	+	+	+	+
⑩	+	+	+(±)	−	±	+	±(+)	+	+	+	+	+

± = Initial 40 msec delta wave isoelectric
+ = Initial 40 msec delta wave positive
− = Initial 40 msec delta wave negative

Figure 30. Surface ECG delta wave in the WPW syndrome. The polarity of the delta wave, defined as the first 40 msec of the QRS, in each of the 12 standard ECG leads was compared with that of the accessory pathway (AP) location found by epicardial activation mapping at the time of surgical AP ablation. The results demonstrate typical delta wave polarity maps for 10 AP locations around the AV ring. (From Gallagher et al.,[39] with permission.)

onary sinus, while right-sided and septal pathways require more involved catheter manipulation for accurate localization.

Management. The anterograde limb of the tachycardia circuit in ORT, the AV node, is nearly identical to the anterograde limb of the tachycardia circuit in the slow-fast form of AVNRT. Consequently, with only a few exceptions, the therapeutic maneuvers for conversion of ORT to sinus rhythm are identical to those for AVNRT: (1) DC cardioversion if hemodynamically unstable; (2) supine position plus Valsalva maneuver for children, or ice bag for infants; (3) atrial pacing via the esophagus if available; (4) verapamil, esmolol, or adenosine, intravenously; (5) procainamide, intravenously; (6) digoxin (for stable infants); (7) elective DC cardioversion. Because verapamil and digoxin have the potential for accelerating the rate of atrial

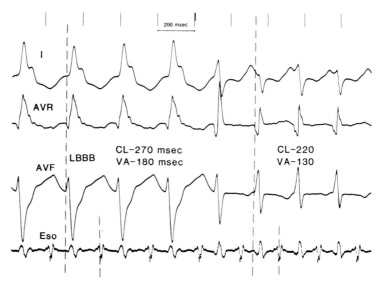

Figure 31. Orthodromic tachycardia. /Cycle length change with bundle branch block./ A change from transient left bundle branch block (LBBB) to a normal QRS complex during tachycardia led to a 50 msec decrease in the cycle length (CL), suggesting the diagnosis of orthodromic reciprocating tachycardia and the involvement of a left-sided accessory pathway.

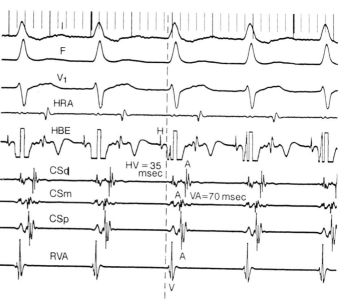

Figure 32. Electrophysiologic characteristics of orthodromic tachycardia. During orthodromic reciprocating tachycardia, the QRS complex is usually normal on the surface ECG, and the H-V interval is always normal or long (35 msec in the His bundle electrogram [HBE] here). The three coronary sinus electrograms (CS distal, CS mid, and CS proximal) contain the earliest atrial activations, preceding those in both the HBE lead and the high right atrial (HRA) lead. Atrial activation is earliest in the mid-CS lead, corresponding to a left posterior position in the coronary sinus (position 7 in Fig. 33), and agreeing with the delta wave polarity map in sinus rhythm. The shortest VA time was 70 msec.

impulse conduction in accessory connections, they are absolutely contraindicated as emergency therapy for patients with the WPW syndrome who are experiencing atrial fibrillation or flutter. However, both may be effective and safe for rapid termination of ORT, but extreme care should be taken to ensure that the diagnosis of a regular, **narrow** complex tachycardia is correct prior to their administration. The utility of digoxin is, once again, limited by delayed onset of action.

Prevention. The anterograde electrophysiologic properties of the accessory connection must be taken into account when preventive therapy is being considered for ORT in patients with WPW. Both digoxin[125] and verapamil[67] have the potential for enhancing anterograde conduction in the ac-

cessory connection. Consequently, both are contraindicated as long-term therapy for most patients with WPW. Although it is common practice to use digoxin in the treatment of infants with WPW because of their very low risk of atrial fibrillation, the theoretical risk of using digoxin in these infants (who typically have very rapid conducting accessory connections), combined with reports of infrequent sudden death in infants with WPW on digoxin,[20] has led the authors to recommend oral propranolol as an initial choice for all term infants requiring long-term therapy. Because of the possible role of propranolol in exacerbating hypoglycemia, apnea, and bradycardia, digoxin is still used for many premature infants. For older patients the following steps are recommended: (1) periodic vagal maneuvers; (2) a beta blocker to impair AV-node, and possibly accessory pathway conduction and to decrease premature beats that act as initiating events; (3) class IA, IC, or III agents with initiation of therapy while an inpatient, and electrophysiologic testing to assess arrhythmia inducibility; and (4) surgical or catheter ablation of the accessory connection.

When treatment with class I or III agents becomes necessary, follow-up electrophysiologic study should be used to assess the effect of each medication on the anterograde effective refractory period and on the minimum cycle length for 1:1 conduction of the accessory connection.

Antidromic Reciprocating Tachycardia in the Wolff-Parkinson-White Syndrome. This regular wide complex tachycardia in which the reentry circuit is exactly the opposite of that of ORT (see Fig. 12) is rather uncommon, accounting for less than 5% of the cases of pediatric SVT in the authors' experience.

Clinical Manifestations and Electrocardiographic Features. The tachycardia rate and, thus, the clinical presentation of antidromic reentry is usually similar to that of ORT. Because activation of the ventricle occurs entirely via the accessory pathway, the QRS complex is abnormal, demonstrating maximal preexcitation (Fig. 33). Retrograde conduction from the ventricles to the atria occurs through the AV node, yielding a retrograde P-wave axis of about −120°.

Electrophysiologic Features. Initiation of antidromic reentry requires that anterograde conduction is blocked in the AV node while it continues in the accessory pathway, i.e., the anterograde refractory period of the accessory pathway must be longer than that of the AV node. Maintenance of the tachycardia then requires that the retrograde refractory period of the AV node be less than the tachycardia cycle length. The relative infrequency of antidromic tachycardia seems to be due to difficulty in meeting both of these conditions. When antidromic tachycardia does occur, the H-V interval is markedly negative with the His bundle deflection occurring near the end of the QRS complex. Retrograde atrial activation, demonstrating a pattern of junctional origin, occurs after the His deflection and before ventricular activation.

Management. As with ORT, tachycardia maintenance is dependent on conduction in both the AV node and the accessory pathway. Consequently, if the diagnosis of antidromic tachycardia is firm, rapid conversion can be performed with an identical protocol to that described for ORT. If the episode is the first presentation of a regular wide complex tachycardia in a patient without a prior 12-lead electrocardiogram in sinus rhythm, the arrhythmia will need to be treated as described for ventricular tachycardia until proven otherwise. If any irregularity exists in the rate or QRS morphology, preexcited atrial fibrillation or flutter

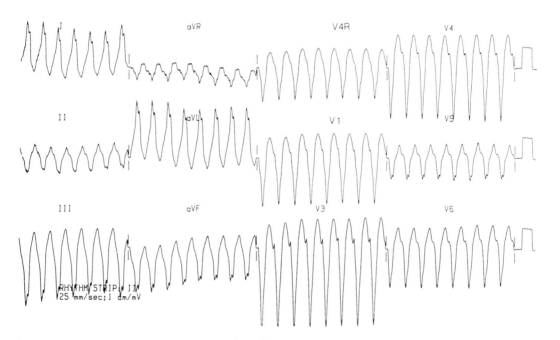

Figure 33. Surface ECG showing antidromic tachycardia. This regular, wide-complex tachycardia at a rate of 187 beats per minute was induced at electrophysiology study. P waves are not clearly visible. The initial QRS deflections were identical to those in sinus rhythm, strongly suggesting that these complexes represent maximal preexcitation. The electrophysiologic characteristics were those of antidromic reciprocating tachycardia involving a right, posterior accessory pathway.

must be considered and the patient treated accordingly.

Prevention. The long-term management of antidromic reentry is also similar to that for ORT in patients with the WPW syndrome. Once again digoxin and verapamil, both of which may enhance conduction in accessory pathways, should be avoided. Long-term beta blockers, as well as class IA, IC, and III drugs, are all acceptable for prevention. Because virtually all patients with antidromic tachycardia have a relatively rapidly conducting accessory pathway, follow-up electrophysiologic study is recommended to investigate the effects of the therapy on anterograde accessory pathway function in any patient who requires treatment with drugs other than beta blockers. More definitive ablation therapy should be considered if hemodynamic compromise is present or if repeated episodes of wide-complex tachycardia necessitating treatment in a facility unfamiliar with the patient may complicate medical care.

Preexcited Atrial Fibrillation or Flutter in the Wolff-Parkinson-White Syndrome. When an accessory AV connection with anterograde conduction is present, every beat of atrial origin may activate the ventricles through the AV node, the accessory pathway, both, or neither. Thus, during any rapid atrial tachycardia, the rate and pattern of ventricular activation depend on the conduction times and the refractory period of both the AV node and the accessory connection. In such a case, the normal protection of the ventricles from rapid conduction of atrial arrhythmias by the AV node is diminished by the presence of an accessory AV pathway. Thus, a rapid ventricular rate, and possibly ventricular fibrillation in response to atrial fibrillation or rapid flutter, is a potential cause of syncope and sudden death in patients with WPW.[86] Patients with the WPW syndrome are much more prone to episodic atrial fibrillation than is the general population. There is little doubt that the accessory pathway contributes directly to this tendency, because elimination of pathway conduction with medical or ablative therapy prevents such arrhythmias.[127]

A number of factors may be responsible for deterioration of the ventricular rhythm during atrial fibrillation: (1) the presence of multiple accessory pathways, (2) shortening of the accessory pathway refractory period in response to the sympathetic discharge induced by the initial tachycardia, (3) disorganized ventricular contraction and resultant hypotension due to the extreme irregularity of the rapid ventricular rhythm, and (4) activation of the ventricles via one AV pathway during the recovery period of activation from the other pathway (i.e., effective R-on-T). The presence of a rapid ventricular response to induced atrial fibrillation in the electrophysiology laboratory is somewhat predictive of those who will experience spontaneous syncope or sudden death; most patients who have had ventricular fibrillation have minimum ventricular cycle lengths during atrial fibrillation of about 200 msec or less.

Clinical Manifestations and Electrocardiographic Features. Because spontaneous atrial fibrillation is rare in children with WPW, and even more rare in infants, few pediatric patients come to the hospital with atrial fibrillation. However, the presence of extremely rapidly conducting accessory pathways in infants makes the potential for diaster high should atrial fibrillation occur. Most older patients with this particular arrhythmia come to the hospital with severe palpitations due to a rapid, irregular ventricular rate, or with hypotension and syncope.

With atrial fibrillation, the surface ECG always reveals an irregular rhythm with QRS complexes that typically vary in morphology because of variable fusion between AV-node and accessory-pathway conduction (Fig. 34). During atrial flutter the rhythm may be strictly regular (Fig. 35). The presence of two distinct aberrant QRS patterns suggests the possibility of multiple accessory pathways. Important prognostic features are the shortest R-R interval between any two preexcited beats and the average ventricular rate.[86]

Electrophysiologic Features. The typical findings during atrial fibrillation in WPW are a rapid irregular rate and variable preexcitation of conducted beats (Fig. 36). Unfortunately, the anterograde effective refractory period of the accessory pathway does not necessarily predict the ventricular response during atrial fibrillation. Thus, if atrial fibrillation does not occur spontaneously during an electrophysiologic study in a patient with WPW, attempts should be made to induce it to help evaluate the potential for rapid conduction.[145] In practice, atrial fibrillation may be difficult to induce in children, so the response of the accessory pathways to rapid atrial pacing may need to suffice.

Management. There are two goals in the initial treatment of atrial fibrillation in WPW: first, to reduce the ventricular response rate and, second, to terminate the atrial fibrillation. If severe hemodynamic compromise is present, synchronized DC cardioversion will accomplish both goals with the lowest risks and quickest results. If the patient is not severely compromised, medical therapy can be considered. Procainamide administered intravenously is probably the most effective drug, because it usually slows conduction over the accessory pathway and may also terminate atrial fibrillation directly. Although both digoxin and verapamil lower the rate of impulse conduction in the AV node, they may also enhance conduction in the accessory pathway, with the net result being an increase in the ventricular rate and potential degeneration of

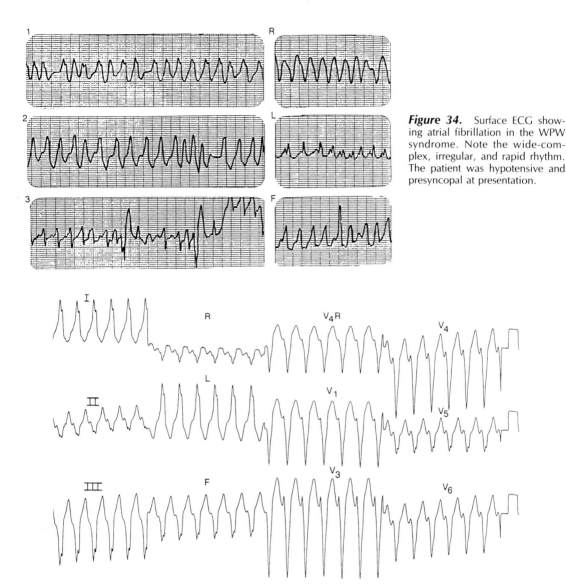

Figure 34. Surface ECG showing atrial fibrillation in the WPW syndrome. Note the wide-complex, irregular, and rapid rhythm. The patient was hypotensive and presyncopal at presentation.

Figure 35. Surface ECG showing atrial flutter in the WPW syndrome. The tachycardia was induced at electrophysiologic study in the same patient as in Figure 33. The QRS morphology is identical to that in Figure 33, but the rate is lower, 158 vs. 187 beats per minute. Intracardiac recordings demonstrated the diagnosis of atrial flutter with 2:1 AV conduction.

a stable ventricular rhythm to fibrillation. Consequently, both digoxin and verapamil are absolutely contraindicated in this setting.

Intravenous beta blockers are likely to reduce the ventricular rate by reducing conduction in both the AV node and the accessory pathway, but they should be used with caution in any patients with hemodynamic compromise. A short-acting beta blocker, such as esmolol, frequently lowers the ventricular rate through its effect on accessory pathway conduction. Thus, at the Boston Children's Hospital our treatment strategy involves: (1) DC cardioversion if the patient is hemodynamically unstable, (2) procainamide, intravenously, (3) a short-acting beta blocker, and (4) elective DC cardioversion.

Prevention. As with initial therapy, the goals of long-term treatment are twofold: to prevent recurrences of atrial fibrillation and to reduce the ventricular rate should atrial fibrillation recur. If the ventricular response to spontaneous atrial fibrillation is relatively slow, a trial of beta blockade may be considered. For patients in whom intravenous procainamide is helpful during the initial treatment, oral procainamide can be used. Other class IA and IC or III agents can also be considered, but proof of efficacy via electrophysiologic testing should be obtained. If either syncope or severe hemodynamic compromise occurred at presentation, medical therapy should be considered palliative, awaiting definitive surgical or catheter ablation of the accessory pathway.

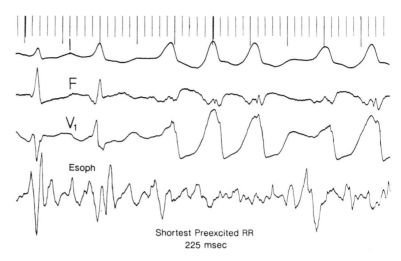

Figure 36. Atrial electrogram showing atrial fibrillation in the WPW syndrome. The esophageal recording demonstrates continuously irregular atrial activity, while surface recordings show an irregular rhythm with variable QRS morphology and a shortest preexcited R-R interval of 225 msec. The findings suggest the potential for spontaneous malignant arrhythmia in this 13-year-old with WPW and a history of syncope.

Shortest Preexcited RR
225 msec

Orthodromic Tachycardia Involving a Concealed Accessory AV Connection. Wolff, Parkinson, and White originally described a syndrome consisting of a delta wave in the QRS on a surface ECG during sinus rhythm (ventricular preexcitation) and paroxysmal tachycardia. Because the delta wave depends on the ability of the accessory connection to conduct anterograde, only patients with anterograde conduction in the accessory connection have true WPW syndrome. However, orthodromic tachycardia is not dependent on this anterograde conduction. Indeed, while more than 90% of infants with supraventricular tachycardia have arrhythmias consistent with ORT, only 35–40% of these have WPW.[25] When ORT occurs without evidence of ventricular preexcitation in sinus rhythm, the accessory AV connection is said to be a "concealed" or "unidirectional retrograde" accessory pathway. This fact bears only minimal significance for the presence and management of the ORT but importantly affects the risk of sudden death, because rapid anterograde conduction of atrial flutter/fibrillation is not possible.

ORT due to a concealed accessory pathway was the tachycardia mechanism in 62% of patients at Boston Children's Hospital who had regular narrow-complex tachycardia. Its clinical, electrocardiographic (Fig. 37), and electrophysiologic manifestations are identical to those of ORT in the presence of WPW, except that sinus rhythm, as seen on the ECG, and the anterograde response to atrial pacing are normal. Initial management of the arrhythmia is also identical to that of ORT with WPW. However, the fact that verapamil and digoxin are not contraindicated makes the recommendations for preventive care significantly different from those for patients with WPW. Consequently, for prevention, the following is recommended: (1) periodic vagal maneuvers; (2) digoxin, beta blocker, or verapamil to impair AV conduction; (3) class IA, IC, or III agent, with initiation

of therapy while an inpatient, and electrophysiologic testing to assess arrhythmia inducibility; (4) surgical or catheter ablation of the accessory connection.

Permanent Form of Junctional Reciprocating Tachycardia (PJRT). Once thought to represent the fast-slow form of AV-nodal reciprocating tachycardia, it is now clear[18] that most cases of this tachycardia are due to ORT involving a posterior-septal accessory connection with slow conduction properties similar to those of the AV node. This term is usually applied to incessant tachycardias that have a variable rate, a dramatically long R-P interval and a normal P-R interval, and that initiate and terminate on a single beat, suggesting a re-entrant mechanism. Although uncommon, accounting for only 1% of the cases of SVT seen at Boston Children's Hospital, the striking difficulty of controlling the arrhythmia makes it seem more prevalent.

Clinical Manifestations and Electrocardiographic Features. The relatively low rates of PJRT make palpitations unusual, with the presenting symptoms usually being congestive heart failure secondary to the incessant metabolic demand on the myocardium. Patients may first be seen as infants or children, but rarely past early adolescence. The unique electrophysiologic properties of the accessory pathway, which include AV node-like responses to autonomic stimuli, account for most of the electrocardiographic features. The fact that the accessory pathway is posterior-septal leads to atrial activation, which originates near the AV node, yielding a retrograde P wave with an axis of approximately −120°, whereas slow conduction in the accessory pathway leads to the long R-P interval (Fig. 38). The tachycardia may start and stop often, usually initiating with either sinus tachycardia or an atrial premature beat. Tachycardia cycle lengths are variable because conduction times in both the anterograde limb of the tachycardia circuit (the AV node) and the retrograde limb (the acces-

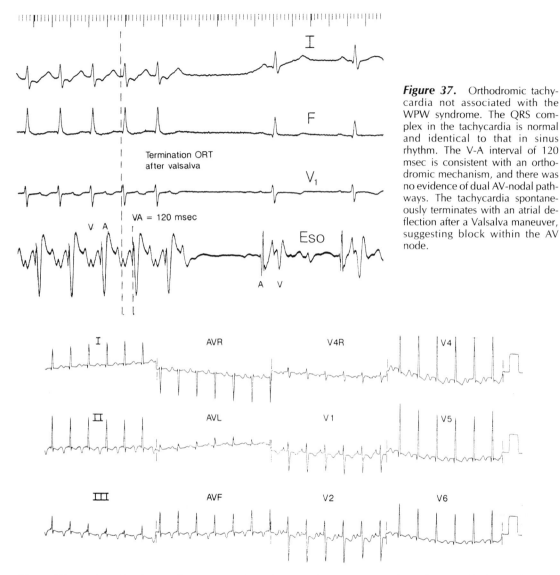

Figure 37. Orthodromic tachycardia not associated with the WPW syndrome. The QRS complex in the tachycardia is normal and identical to that in sinus rhythm. The V-A interval of 120 msec is consistent with an orthodromic mechanism, and there was no evidence of dual AV-nodal pathways. The tachycardia spontaneously terminates with an atrial deflection after a Valsalva maneuver, suggesting block within the AV node.

Figure 38. Surface ECG showing the permanent form of junctional reciprocating tachycardia. Note the slow tachycardia rate of 150 beats/minute, the retrograde P-wave axis of −100 degrees, the long R-P interval, and the normal P-R interval. The tachycardia was nearly incessant in this 10-year-old girl, and it had a highly variable rate.

sory pathway) are susceptible to autonomic state; thus, the tachycardia rate may vary as widely as 150–250/min in the same patient. Because anterograde conduction is always through the AV node during tachycardia, the QRS morphology is always that of sinus rhythm. Rate-related bundle branch block is unusual but sometimes seen. During sinus rhythm, the QRS complex is usually normal on the surface ECG, suggesting the absence of anterograde conduction in the accessory connections; however, QRS aberrancy consistent with anterograde conduction over a posterior-septal pathway has been noted after AV-node ablation in some patients with PJRT,[121] suggesting that the capacity for anterograde pathway conduction exists at least in some cases.

Electrophysiologic Features. Mapping of atrial excitation during tachycardia usually reveals a pattern that is indistinguishable from that of retrograde activation via the AV node (occurring earliest low in the right atrial side of the septum). In some cases, atrial activation at or near the mouth of the coronary sinus may precede that in the lower septum on the right atrial side. The V-A interval is generally long (>150 msec). The tachycardia is usually easy to initiate and terminate with placement of critically-timed atrial or ventricular premature beats.

Management. Although emergency therapy is rarely necessary because acute hemodynamic compromise is unusual, the protocol outlined for the more typical ORT is probably reasonable for PJRT.

The caveat to such a protocol is that the tachycardia is likely to recur as soon as the terminating stimulus is removed. Thus, maneuvers that enhance vagal activity, atrial pacing, and DC cardioversion may terminate the tachycardia for as little as one beat. Such a response is often more diagnostic than therapeutic. Thus, suppression of tachycardia with long-acting drugs is necessary for initial stabilization.

Prevention. Long-term therapy for PJRT may be both difficult and frustrating. Although one strives for complete suppression of tachycardia, with PJRT it may be necessary to settle for relative tachycardia control. Because both of the tachycardia limbs have properties similar to those of the AV node, long-term treatment begins with drugs which primarily affect AV conduction, e.g., digoxin, beta blockers, or verapamil. Various class IA and IC antiarrhythmic therapies have also been reported to be effective, with encainide being particularly effective at higher doses.[136] Because of the potential for proarrhythmicity with class I and III drugs, inpatient management is imperative when beginning or titrating therapy with these agents. Surgical division of the posterior accessory pathway may be effective but carries a small risk of AV block.[46] Catheter ablation techniques, using DC energy applied into the mouth of the coronary sinus as a marker of the posterior septum, have been effective in approximately 75% of cases.[109] More recently, radiofrequency energy has been used to ablate posterior-septal pathways, a technique that may be safer and very promising option. Our general scheme for progression of long-term therapy for PJRT is: (1) digoxin; (2) digoxin plus a beta blocker; (3) digoxin plus verapamil; (4) class IA or IC agent with inpatient assessment of tachycardia control and proarrhythmicity; (5) class III agent; and (6) surgical or catheter ablation of the accessory pathway.

The difficulty of controlling PJRT, combined with its effects on ventricular function, is leading to earlier surgical or catheter ablation for the prevention of this arrhythmia.

Mahaim Fibers. Mahaim fiber is the eponym given to accessory conduction pathways that arise from either the AV node (nodoventricular) or the His-Purkinje system (fasciculoventricular). The vast majority of such connections are directed to the right ventricle.

As in the Wolff-Parkinson-White syndrome, early ventricular activation results in the electrocardiographic appearance of a delta wave with a somewhat wide and distorted QRS. With Mahaim fibers, however, some portion of the AV node is interposed between the atrium and ventricle, such that nodal delay is preserved and the P-R interval appears normal (Fig. 39). Another feature in common with WPW is a dynamic balance between normal conduction over the His-Purkinje network and abnormal preexcitation over the Mahaim fiber, which varies according to the refractory characteristics and conduction velocity of the two limbs and is also modulated by the timing of the atrial depolarization. This results in a wide array of electrocardiographic appearances (Fig. 40) and ultimately can predispose to reentry arrhythmias.

Clinical Manifestations and Electrocardiographic Features. Functional Mahaim connections contributing to arrhythmias and electrocardiographic changes are rare in both the pediatric and adult populations. In the authors' limited experience with this disorder, the presenting complaint is usually nonsustained rapid palpitations in an otherwise healthy patient, but Mahaim fibers (like the WPW syndrome) have also been seen in some patients with Ebstein's anomaly.

The surface ECG in sinus rhythm is variable and at times quite normal. Indeed, the preexcitation pattern can wax and wane, depending on sinus rate or the presence of premature beats. Electrophysiologic study may be necessary to unmask Mahaim conduction in some patients. Because most Mahaim fibers insert distally into the right ventricle, the delta wave and ventricular activation are directed right to left, sometimes mimicking left bundle branch block or type B WPW.

The classic reentry tachycardia in this disorder is antidromic, with forward conduction over the Mahaim fiber and return over the normal His-Pur-

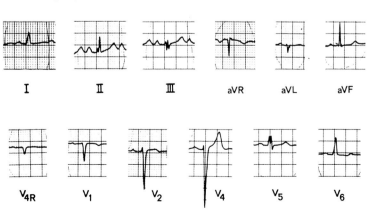

Figure 39. Surface ECG from a patient with a Mahaim fiber proven at intracardiac electrophysiologic study. Note the delta waves in many leads but a normal P-R interval.

I II III aVR aVL aVF

V_{4R} V_1 V_2 V_4 V_5 V_6

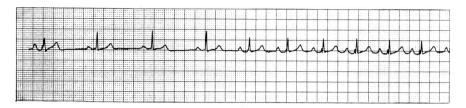

Figure 40. Lead II recording from same patient as in Figure 39, showing variability in the degree of preexcitation due to sinus arrhythmia and its effect on the relative contribution of conduction over the Mahaim-fiber and normal His-Purkinje pathways.

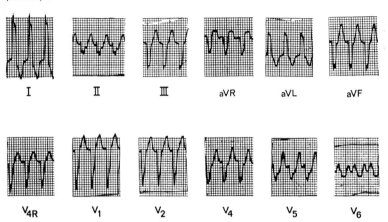

I   II   III   aVR   aVL   aVF

V4R   V1   V2   V4   V5   V6

Figure 41. Sustained wide QRS tachycardia in a patient with a Mahaim fiber proven at electrophysiologic testing. In an emergency setting, this tracing is indistinguishable from that of ventricular tachycardia or atypical WPW tachycardia.

kinje system (Fig. 41), resulting in a wide QRS tachyarrhythmia.[42] Because the atrium is not a necessary link in the circuit, AV dissociation may occasionally be observed. Less common arrhythmias include reentry within the AV node or within atrial muscle (flutter and fibrillation) where the Mahaim fiber provides bystander preexcitation of ventricular complexes.

Electrophysiologic Features. Positive identification of Mahaim conduction usually requires intracardiac electrophysiologic study. The diagnostic key is demonstration of a short or negative H-V interval for a preexcited beat (similar to that seen in WPW) but with gradual lengthening of the AV time (Fig. 42) in response to premature stimuli

(unlike WPW where the AV time remains fairly constant). During antidromic tachycardia, one may observe AV dissociation, or at least be able to demonstrate independence of atrial activation with premature ventricular and atrial stimuli during reentry. Some right anterior pathways in the WPW syndrome may be difficult to differentiate from Mahaim connections[87] unless AV dissociation is demonstrated.

Management. In an emergency setting, it should be remembered that Mahaim reentry simulates VT or antidromic tachycardia in the WPW syndrome on the surface ECG, and the diagnosis is usually entertained only after initial stabilization. Often, it is necessary to employ an emergency treatment

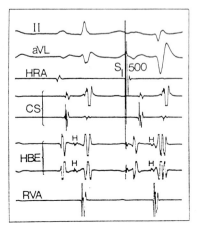

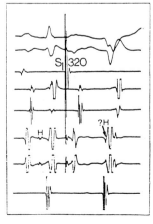

Figure 42. Intracardiac recordings during study of a patient with a Mahaim fiber. In the left panel a sinus beat displays a normal QRS, a normal P-R, and a normal HV. A premature atrial stimulus is then delivered at 500 msec and causes preexcitation with distortion of the QRS and shortening of the HV. In the right panel, an earlier stimulus at 320 msec increases the degree of preexcitation, with further widening of the QRS and a His spike that is now buried within the QRS. Note, however, that the stimulus-QRS time is increasing progressively, a finding that is not typically seen in the WPW syndrome, and that suggests the presence of Mahaim conduction.

strategy similar to that used for ventricular tachycardia. Specifically, reentry can be terminated with DC cardioversion and, often, with intravenous procainamide.

Prevention. Recurrent Mahaim fiber tachycardia can be treated with either pharmacologic trials or ablation techniques. The choice of drugs depends somewhat on the level of origin of the fibers. For nodoventricular connections, AV-node tissue participates in the reentry circuit, and initial therapy may involve agents that modify conduction at the nodal level (e.g., beta blocker, verapamil). Theoretically, a fasciculoventricular fiber is less likely to respond to these agents, and this may necessitate the use of class I or class III drugs. Because Mahaim tachycardias are rare, experience with pharmacologic response is somewhat limited, suggesting the need for serial electrophysiologic testing to confirm drug efficacy in every patient. For refractory cases, successful surgical[40] and transcatheter ablation[68] have been achieved.

Ventricular Tachycardia

Tachycardias that originate from myocytes or Purkinje cells below the bifurcation of the common bundle of His are grouped under the heading of VT. Although reentry mechanisms account for the majority of these disorders, automatic foci and triggered automaticity have been implicated as the cellular mechanism in select cases.[157]

In general, VT carries a more serious prognosis than SVT. This difference arises not only from the hemodynamic disadvantage of the fast ventricular rate but, more importantly, from the fact that VT typically occurs in abnormal myocardium with suboptimal function, which may also be vulnerable to degeneration into ventricular fibrillation.

Clinical Manifestations. The clinical presentation of VT is varied in the pediatric age group. For infants and young children, symptoms of congestive heart failure may be the first indication of a sustained arrhythmia. Indeed, younger patients seem able to tolerate incessant VT for long periods (several days on occasion); it may not degenerate to fibrillation unless low cardiac output leads to severe acidosis. In older children and teenagers, symptoms are more similar to those encountered in adults with ischemic heart disease. They include palpitations, dizziness, shortness of breath, a "full feeling" in the throat, syncope, and even cardiac arrest. Not all patients with ventricular arrhythmias are symptomatic. Occasionally a young patient may have high-grade ventricular ectopy first detected as an irregular pulse on a routine examination.

The causes of ventricular tachycardia in the young are diverse. The conditions most frequently associated with VT at Boston Children's Hospital are highlighted in Table 6.

Electrocardiographic Features. By convention,

Table 6. Conditions Associated with Ventricular Tachycardia in Young Patients

Congenital Myopathy
 Hypertrophic cardiomyopathy
 Carnitine deficiency
 Storage diseases
 Muscular dystrophy
 "Familial" myopathy

Acquired Myopathy
 Myocarditis (acute or remote)
 Adriamycin cardiotoxicity
 HIV infection
 Hemochromatosis
 Idiopathic dilated myopathy

Anatomic Cardiac Defects (before and/or after surgery)
 Tetralogy of Fallot
 Aortic stenosis
 Transposition (D and L forms)
 Ventricular septal defect
 Single ventricle
 Right ventricular dysplasia
 Mitral valve prolapse
 Cardiac tumors

Primary Electrical Disorders
 Prolonged Q-T (congenital and acquired)
 Diffuse conduction system disease
 Bradycardia conditioned (sick sinus and heart block)
 Idiopathic VT

Coronary Artery Disease
 Vasculitis
 Anomalous origin of left coronary from pulmonary artery
 Compression due to aberrant course of coronary off aorta
 Kawasaki's disease

Intoxications and Exposures
 Digoxin toxicity
 Antiarrhythmic drugs (class I and III)
 Tricyclic antidepressant overdose
 Organophosphate exposure
 Substance abuse

VT is defined as three or more consecutive ectopic beats of ventricular origin. The term "nonsustained" is applied to short sequences, whereas "sustained" VT usually implies an episode lasting longer than 30 seconds and/or causing hemodynamic instability.

The QRS complex during VT appears wide and bizarre with a P wave that is either dissociated or arises from passive retrograde conduction. There may be competition between the ventricular arrhythmia and episodic anterograde conduction over the AV node such that "fusion beats" may be noted (Figs. 43A and 43B).

Several varieties of VT may be distinguished by the appearance of the QRS complex during tachycardia. The term "monomorphic" is applied to a uniform QRS morphology; "bidirectional" denotes two alternating QRS types, "polymorphic" indicates a widely varying QRS (Fig. 43C), and "torsade de pointes" describes a specific pattern of positive and negative oscillation of the QRS direc-

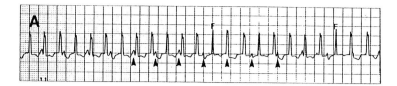

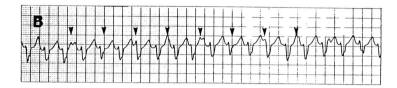

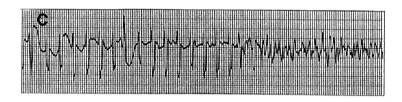

Figure 43. Example of ventricular tachycardia. **A,** Monomorphic VT from an infant with incessant tachycardia, showing dissociated P waves (arrows) and fusion beats (F). **B,** Monomorphic VT from a teenager with myocarditis, again showing A-V dissociation. **C,** Polymorphic VT from a postoperative patient, degenerating to ventricular fibrillation in the latter portion of the strip. **D,** Torsade de pointes from a patient being treated with quinidine.

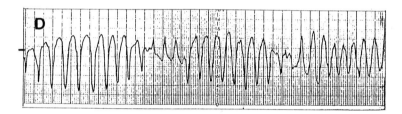

tion which seems to twist around the isoelectric line of the electrocardiogram (Fig. 43D).

Electrophysiologic Features. Intracardiac electrophysiologic study is commonly recommended for all patients with symptomatic or sustained VT. The goals of such testing are threefold: (1) to rule out atypical SVT as the true mechanism for the arrhythmia, (2) to attempt to recreate the arrhythmia to gain insight into its mechanism and focus of origin, and (3) to evaluate the response to antiarrhythmic drugs with intravenous testing and/or serial follow-up studies after the administration of oral agents.

Electrophysiologic evaluation begins with atrial stimulation, using the standard premature stimulus technique. Besides assessing general conduction parameters, atrial pacing may pinpoint an alternate explanation for the patient's tachycardia by unmasking preexcitation pathways or bundle branch aberration that may not always be apparent on a surface electrocardiogram during resting sinus rhythm. In rare instances, VT may be triggered with atrial stimulation alone.[50]

The crux of electrophysiologic testing for VT is programmed stimulation of the ventricle with an ordered sequence of premature beats in an attempt to recreate the patient's clinical arrhythmia. Stimulation protocols vary but usually involve a series of single, double, and triple stimuli, with and without a preceding eight-beat "drive train," delivered at increasingly premature intervals until the local ventricular tissue is refractory (see p. 157). Stimulation is usually performed at the right ventricular apex, but additional sites (e.g., right ventricular outflow and left ventricular apex) are sometimes employed. Repetition of the protocol during infusion of isoproterenol is needed occasionally to trigger a tachycardia.

The most useful response to ventricular stimulation is exact replication of the rate and QRS morphology of the patient's clinical arrhythmia. The data can then be used as an end-point against which follow-up stimulation can be compared while the patient is receiving antiarrhythmia therapy, both to verify drug efficacy and also to help rule out "proarrhythmic" effects (Fig. 44). Unfortunately, on occasion, nonspecific ventricular arrhythmias (including ventricular fibrillation) may be induced that bear no resemblance to the clinical arrhythmia, and the significance of such a response remains uncertain.

Emergency Management. Sustained ventricular

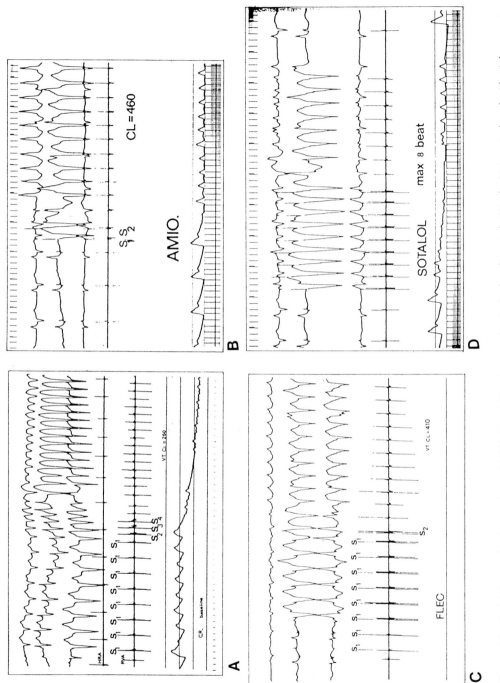

Figure 44. Serial drug testing in a patient with VT due to dilated myopathy. At the baseline study (**A**), the VT was induced with triple premature beats after an 8-beat drive train. After administration of flecainide (**B**) and amiodarone (**C**), sustained tachycardia was slower but easier to induce. After administration of sotalol (**D**), only slow nonsustained VT was induced.

tachycardia should be treated as an emergency. If the clinical situation permits, arterial blood pressure and perfusion should be assessed and a 12-lead electrocardiogram recorded. A brief history, with particular attention to medications and possible toxic exposures, should also be obtained.

Any patient who is unresponsive or significantly hypotensive should be treated with immediate DC shock of 1.0–2.0 joules/kg. The energy should be synchronized to the QRS if the VT is well organized and has sufficient amplitude, but an unsynchronized discharge is necessary for ventricular fibrillation or rapid polymorphic VT with low-voltage QRS complexes. If an initial shock is unsuccessful, the energy can be doubled and repeated for one or two additional trials.

If the patient is awake and stable, or if electrical conversion is unsuccessful, intravenous drug therapy should be initiated. Lidocaine, administered as a bolus and followed by a continuous infusion, is the safest first-line agent. Second-line choices depend somewhat on the electrocardiographic appearance and the cause of the VT. For most forms of VT procainamide is quite effective. If, however, the VT is of the torsade de pointes variety or occurs in the setting of digoxin toxicity, phenytoin may be a preferred second agent. A magnesium infusion is also remarkably effective in quieting some cases of torsade.[140] Additional intravenous drug trials with third-line agents, such as bretylium or esmolol, may be tried if necessary. As a general rule, there is no place for verapamil or digoxin in the emergency treatment of VT (or any tachycardia with a wide QRS for which the mechanism is uncertain).

Occasionally, a patient with sustained VT may be refractory to pharmacologic maneuvers, at which point a transvenous ventricular pacing wire may be inserted, which often allows repeated overdrive pacing to interrupt reentry arrhythmia. Ventricular pacing itself may also suppress recurrent torsade de pointes. Rare cases of incessant VT sometimes do not yield to this full treatment plan, at which point investigational drugs (e.g., intravenous amiodarone), surgical excision, or transcatheter electrical ablation may be attempted when all other measures have failed.[45]

Prevention. The most difficult aspect of long-term therapy for ventricular arrhythmias is deciding who to treat. On a case by case basis the following must be taken into account: (1) the patient's symptoms (or lack thereof), (2) the presence and degree of underlying cardiac pathology, (3) the rate, duration, and morphology of the VT, and (4) the known natural history of the specific disorder. The physician must constantly balance side effects of therapy (including negative inotropic properties and proarrhythmic potential of some drugs) against the ultimate risk of malignant arrhythmias.

As an aid in the decision making process, aggressive evaluation of cardiac structure and function is justified. Even when other clinical testing is normal, it is still recommended that patients with VT undergo cardiac catheterization for hemodynamics, angiography, and ventricular biopsy. Subtle pathologic processes such as right ventricular dysplasia,[116] coronary anomalies,[95] and myopathy,[26] may be uncovered only with these techniques. If cardiac structure and function are normal, selected patients with ventricular ectopy who are asymptomatic are often followed closely without therapy, whereas symptomatic patients (whether or not cardiac pathology is demonstrated) are usually treated. Unfortunately this leaves a large and complex "gray zone" of asymptomatic patients with varied degrees of cardiac pathology who may exhibit nonsustained, but high-grade ventricular ectopy. At Boston Children's Hospital, our institutional bias is not to begin prophylactic drug therapy in borderline cases if an aggressive ventricular stimulation protocol does not induce VT in the catheterization laboratory. Admittedly, we remain influenced by the findings on Holter monitoring and treadmill stress testing, and sometimes therapy is begun despite benign findings of programmed stimulation. Some forms of VT cannot be evaluated accurately with ventricular stimulation techniques.

Long-term therapy for ventricular arrhythmia is usually initiated in the hospital with continuous monitoring. The available drug options are varied (see pp. 419–424), each agent having its own less than perfect record for efficacy and safety. The success of such therapy can be gauged with serial electrophysiologic studies, Holter monitoring, and exercise testing. Ideally, an arrhythmia should be suppressed by all criteria. With electrophysiologic testing, success is defined as noninducibility with a full stimulation protocol in a patient who had reproducible initiation of VT prior to medications. Proarrhythmia may be suggested if the VT is induced with less aggressive stimulation and/or has become more malignant in terms of duration and rate compared to the control state. Using Holter monitoring and/or stress testing, effective therapy may be defined as elimination of all repetitive ectopy (couplets and VT), along with a reduction of isolated ventricular premature beats. Again, proarrhythmia is suggested if tachycardias are observed to be faster, more frequent, or of longer duration.

Drug therapy for VT is not always successful. Symptomatic patients at high risk may require surgical or catheter ablation if a discrete focus of origin can be localized. Automatic implantable cardiac defibrillators may have to be considered when conventional options have failed.

Ventricular Tachycardia in Childhood. *Incessant Ventricular Tachycardia with Congestive Failure.* This rare condition has been observed most frequently in infants.[45] The tachycardia is usually monomorphic and moderate in rate (Fig. 43A) but so protracted that ventricular function may ultimately become compromised. The cellular mechanism is poorly understood, but it exhibits many features typical for an automatic focus in that it often fails to respond to DC shock or interruption by overdrive pacing and may not be affected by conventional drugs. Some patients have required surgical excision of the VT focus, and the excised segment often shows pathologic features that suggest hamartomas of Purkinje cell origin.

In patients with advanced ventricular dysfunction, treatment is difficult. Intravenous procainamide is often successful in slowing the rate and, occasionally, may suppress it entirely. Other drugs may be tried on an empirical basis, but unfortunately, most antiarrhythmic medications have the potential to further depress function, so that arrhythmia mapping and surgery may need to be considered if the child cannot be stabilized quickly.

For incessant VT with preserved ventricular function, one has the luxury of multiple medication trials. In many such infants the VT is eventually controlled with drugs, with beta blockers being quite effective in the authors' experience.

Long Q-T Syndrome. A prolonged QTc interval on the electrocardiogram can be a marker for diffuse abnormalities of ventricular depolarization, which in turn may predispose to recurrent VT of the torsade de pointes variety.[123] A long Q-T may be seen as a congenital disorder, or it may be acquired from exposure to certain drugs, toxins, or electrolyte disturbances (Table 7).

The congenital forms deserve the most emphasis here. Although many cases are sporadic, a clear genetic pattern is evident in the Romano-Ward (autosomal dominant) and Jervell-Lange-Neilsen (autosomal recessive) syndromes. The dominant disorder has no clinical marker aside from the ar-

rhythmia, whereas the recessive syndrome carries hereditary nerve deafness as part of its presentation. Unfortunately, the Romano-Ward syndrome is often identified in a family only after a serious event has befallen one member.

The symptoms of long Q-T syndromes may surface at any age and usually involve episodic dizziness, palpitations, syncope, and even cardiac arrest. These symptoms have been well documented to correlate with episodes of torsade de pointes, and although the VT will often stop spontaneously, a prolonged episode can ultimately result in death. The condition may sometimes be confused with a neurologic disorder; for this reason **an electrocardiogram should be obtained as a routine part of the work-up for any patient with unexplained syncope or a first seizure.** The long Q-T syndrome may also be involved in some cases of sudden infant death.[141]

The diagnosis depends on demonstration of a Q-T interval that is prolonged beyond normal range when corrected for heart rate (Fig. 45). Ambulatory monitoring in classic cases reveals the emergence of ventricular premature beats and episodic torsade de pointes, usually occurring at times of stress and excitement. Programmed ventricular stimulation is generally not effective for triggering VT or predicting treatment response in the long Q-T syndrome,[77] and currently one must rely on patient symptoms and monitoring. Because of the strong hereditary tendency, all blood relatives should have screening electrocardiograms (regardless of symptom status) whenever an index case is identified.

The etiology of the congenital long Q-T syndrome is not well understood, but it relates at least in part to an abnormality of autonomic influence on ventricular repolarization, perhaps caused by an imbalance of control from the right vs. the left cervical sympathetic ganglia.[124] Most often, initial treatment involves beta blockade with high doses of propranolol. Second-line antiarrhythmic drugs are restricted to those that do not prolong the Q-T interval as part of their mechanism of action, effectively limiting the choices to lidocaine and phenytoin for intravenous use, or phenytoin, mexiletine, and tocainide for long-term oral administration. Sinus bradycardia and variable atrioventricular block may also be associated with this syndrome and may necessitate permanent pacemaker placement[27] both to relieve bradycardia and to reduce VT that may be conditioned by slow ventricular rates. Cases that remain refractory to these measures may be considered for cervical ganglion surgery[6] or an implanted defibrillator.

Ventricular Tachycardia and Congenital Heart Disease. Ventricular arrhythmias are often described as a complication of congenital anatomic defects both before and after surgical repair. Lesions most frequently associated with VT include

Table 7. Causes of Prolonged Q-T Interval

Congenital Long Q-T Syndromes
Romano-Ward
Jervell and Lange-Nielsen
Sporadic form
? Sudden infant death syndrome (SIDS)

Drugs and Toxins
Class I and III antiarrhythmic drugs
Phenothiazines
Tricyclic antidepressants
Organophosphate exposure
Pentamidine

Other Intrinsic Cardiac Disorders
Complete heart block
Dilated myopathy
Sick sinus syndrome

Miscellaneous
Hypocalcemia
Hypomagnesemia
Hypokalemia
? HIV infection
CNS injury

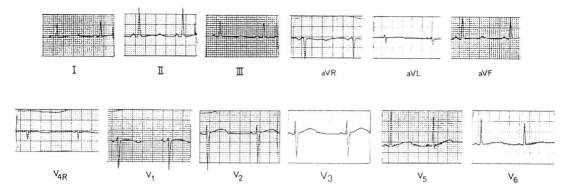

I   II   III   aVR   aVL   aVF

V$_{4R}$ V$_1$ V$_2$ V$_3$ V$_5$ V$_6$

Figure 45. Surface ECG from a patient with the long Q-T syndrome who experienced multiple episodes of torsade de pointes with syncope. The T wave has a terminal hump that may, in fact, be a prominent U wave. The calculation of the Q-T interval should include this terminal portion when it is this pronounced. The corrected Q-T-U interval at this heart rate was 0.56 msec.

tetralogy of Fallot and aortic stenosis; a lesser number of cases involve single ventricle, ventricular septal defect, and transposition of the great arteries (both D and L forms).

High-grade ventricular arrhythmias may appear even prior to intracardiac surgery in some patients,[22] lending support to the notion that surgical scarring is not always a direct causative factor. Additionally, there is growing evidence that patients undergoing complete repair of congenital defects early in life are less likely to develop ectopy at late follow-up.[147] Indeed, it may be that long-standing hemodynamic burdens from chronic cyanosis or ventricular pressure and volume loads are the primary etiology of these arrhythmias. Other factors correlated with ventricular ectopy and sudden death in the tetralogy population include older age at follow-up,[48] elevated systolic or end-diastolic right ventricular pressure,[48] and prior large palliative shunts (e.g., Potts).[81]

Both monomorphic and polymorphic VT can be observed in patients with congenital heart lesions. In most instances, patients who have experienced sustained VT will demonstrate reproducible initiation of their arrhythmia with programmed stimulation in the electrophysiology lab,[74] suggesting a cellular mechanism of either reentry or triggered automaticity. Mapping of the VT focus often reveals an origin near the areas of a surgical scar, but VT can also arise from areas that have not been directly traumatized.

Although it is universally agreed that patients with sustained VT and symptoms require therapy, decisions are more difficult in the absence of symptoms when lower grade ectopy is detected by routine surveillance monitoring. Currently, there is active debate regarding the justification for prophylactic therapy in the asymptomatic group. For example, it is argued that the presence of ventricular ectopy in tetralogy patients is an independent risk factor for sudden death and that reduction in the incidence of late death has been seen at some

centers[48] after instituting a policy of aggressive drug treatment for all patients with frequent or complex ectopy on Holter recordings. Others contend that nonsustained arrhythmias on Holter monitoring are not necessarily good predictors of poor outcome.[137] At Boston Children's Hospital, treatment decisions are based primarily on invasive electrophysiologic testing. Holter recordings are performed at 1–3 year intervals for most postoperative patients as routine surveillance, and those with nonsustained VT are further evaluated with programmed ventricular stimulation at cardiac catheterization. Patients with inducible VT are treated, but the remainder are usually followed closely without therapy if they remain asymptomatic. At present there is no firm agreement on proper management of these patients, although a national protocol for tetralogy patients is currently in progress to clarify the issue.[16]

Treatment of VT in congenital heart disease may involve both correction of residual hemodynamic defects and suppressive drug therapy. In difficult cases, surgical excision of a monomorphic VT focus is feasible and is a particularly attractive option if the patient is returning to the operating room for other hemodynamic reasons. There is no specific antiarrhythmic drug which is likely to be effective in all cases. Class IB agents (phenytoin,[48] mexiletine[107]) are reported to be effective in suppressing ventricular ectopy by Holter criteria, although parallel data with programmed stimulation are incomplete. Beta blockers, procainamide, flecainide, and amiodarone have also been used successfully in some patients, but the final choice remains largely a trial and error process.

Ventricular Tachycardia Associated with Myopathy. The management of ventricular arrhythmia in the setting of cardiomyopathy remains a major therapeutic challenge. The predictive value of Holter monitoring[110] and electrophysiologic study[103] seems reduced for these disorders, and drug suppression of ectopy may often result in worsening of already compromised ventricular function. Thus, therapeutic emphasis must be placed on optimizing hemodynamic variables, along with judicious administration of antiarrhythmic drugs.

Dilated myopathies are the most difficult in this regard. In general, therapy involves drugs that have relatively modest myocardial depression (such as procainamide and mexiletine), while avoiding agents such as disopyramide and sotalol, which have more potent negative inotropic properties. Amiodarone has the attraction of minimal influence on cardiac function and may ultimately be the only drug such patients can tolerate, but it is usually reserved as a second- or third-line agent because of its potential noncardiac toxicities.

Therapeutic response to these drugs can be evaluated with a combination of Holter recording, electrophysiologic testing, and repeated measurements of hemodynamics as part of follow-up electrophysiologic catheterization. Nonpharmacologic management, including implantation of an automatic defibrillator, or even cardiac transplant, may be the only reliable option for some patients who have advanced dilated myopathy with refractory ventricular arrhythmias and marked ventricular dysfunction.

For **hypertrophic myopathy,** the negative inotropic effects of antiarrhythmic drugs are less of an issue, but, unfortunately, ventricular arrhythmias remain as refractory and unpredictable as in any other form of myopathy. The utility of electrophysiologic testing is not well examined for this disorder, although some small series[90] have suggested reasonable reproduction of clinical arrhythmias. Indeed, electrophysiologic testing is often contraindicated in patients with marked subaortic obstruction, given the potential for induction of prolonged ventricular fibrillation, because it is difficult to support circulation with closed chest massage in conditions with severe left-sided obstruction.

At Boston Children's Hospital treatment of ventricular arrhythmias in cases of hypertrophic cardiomyopathy usually involves initial attempts to improve hemodynamics with agents such as verapamil[126] or a beta blocker. If ventricular arrhythmias persist, disopyramide, sotalol, or amiodarone may be tried as second-line therapy, although no controlled studies have yet verified long-term efficacy of any one agent in this condition.

Idiopathic Ventricular Tachycardia. High grade ventricular arrhythmias are seen occasionally in young patients without demonstrable cardiac pathology.[38] Typically the VT is monomorphic and characterized by relatively slow rates (120–180/ min), often appearing during or immediately after exercise and stress. Based on QRS morphology from surface ECG recordings and limited data from intracardiac mapping studies, an origin in the right ventricular outflow tract seems most common. Several reviews of such patients have suggested a relatively benign prognosis for this form of VT,[10] but most also recognize that an occasional patient has a poor outcome.[21] At present, because this condition is not universally benign, detailed diagnostic study appears justified.

The diagnosis of idiopathic VT depends on a complete noninvasive evaluation, as well as cardiac catheterization, with ventricular and coronary angiography and endomyocardial biopsy. At Boston Children's Hospital, if no pathology is detected, asymptomatic patients are not treated. Symptomatic patients are treated, the most successful agents being beta blockers, mexiletine, and even verapamil. This somewhat unusual drug-response profile, as well as atypical findings at electrophysiologic study, may support triggered automaticity as the cellular mechanism for this particular variety of VT.[146]

BRADYCARDIA DUE TO DEPRESSED PACEMAKER FUNCTION

Sinus Bradycardia

Although normal values are well established for resting sinus rates in all age groups, individual variation is so dramatic that it is hazardous to dictate firm cut-off values as positively diagnostic of pathologic bradycardia in children. Much depends on the clinical setting. An awake resting sinus rate of 45/min may be normal for a healthy, fit teenager, but would be strictly abnormal for a similar-aged patient with poor cardiac function.

The electrocardiographic picture for pathologic sinus node behavior is a slow P-wave rate, usually with marked sinus arrhythmia, allowing a variety of escape rhythms from low atrial and junctional foci (Fig. 46). Additionally, the sinus node may display abrupt pauses because of exit block or even complete sinus arrest.

Management of sinus bradycardia depends on the etiology (Table 8). Primary SA-node injury in the setting of organic heart disease, the so-called "sick sinus syndrome," will be discussed separately below. For many of the remaining causes listed in Table 8, bradycardia is seen as a secondary phenomenon which can be corrected eventually by treating the underlying cause or eliminating the offending drug. In the emergency setting, intravenous atropine or isoproterenol can be used to support the rate until the primary pathology is reversed. Alternatively, pacing, using a transesophageal or transvenous lead, can be employed.

Sick Sinus Syndrome

Classically, this disorder results from direct injury to the SA node, and it is an all too frequent problem following surgery for congenital heart disease. No open heart procedure, even simple closure of an atrial septal defect, is without risk for SA-node dysfunction, although complex atrial baffling procedures (such as the Mustard,[35] Senning,[100]

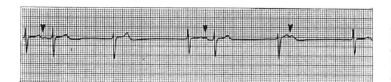

Figure 46. Sinus node dysfunction in a patient 10 years after the Mustard operation. The P waves are slow and irregular (arrows), allowing a slow junctional escape rhythm.

Table 8. Causes of Sinus Bradycardia

Primary SA Node Dysfunction (Sick Sinus Syndrome)
  Certain myopathies and inflammatory diseases
  Following surgery for congenital heart disease
  Complex heterotaxy with "absent SA node"

Secondary SA Node Dysfunction
  Hypothyroidism
  Hypothermia
  Hypoglycemia
  Acidosis and hypoxia
  Malnutrition (including anorexia nervosa)
  Gram-negative sepsis
  CNS injury

Drug-induced
  Digoxin
  Beta blockers
  Verapamil
  Sotalol
  Amiodarone

Autonomic-mediated
  Long Q-T syndrome
  Hypervagotonia
  Pallid breathholding spells

and Fontan[148] operations) seem to result in the highest incidence. This syndrome may also occur in complex anatomic heart disease or myopathy in the absence of surgical trauma.

The electrocardiogram (Fig. 47) shows slow and irregular sinus rates with a variety of escape rhythms, frequently associated with episodic atrial reentry tachycardia (atrial flutter, or fibrillation). The situation may be further complicated by ventricular arrhythmias, which can be conditioned by the low rates and/or may arise because of coexistent pathology in ventricular muscle.

Occasionally, patients with the sick sinus syndrome experience syncope and even sudden death. Surprisingly, the exact mechanism of malignant arrhythmia in this disorder is not clearly established and may include SVT with rapid ventricular response, abrupt bradycardia (as a primary event or following termination of a prolonged tachyarrhythmia), or ventricular tachycardia.

The diagnosis of sick sinus syndrome is usually first suspected on the basis of slow rates on a routine electrocardiogram. Such patients are further evaluated with Holter monitoring in order to examine diurnal heart rate variation, to detect abrupt sinus pause or arrest, and to quantitate the degree of supraventricular or ventricular ectopy. It is often helpful to review serial electrocardiograms and Holter recordings looking for progressive trends in sinus slowing, and electrophysiologic evaluation may be of use occasionally. Techniques measuring sinus-node recovery time (SNRT) and sinoatrial conduction time (SACT) (see pp. 152–153) are fair

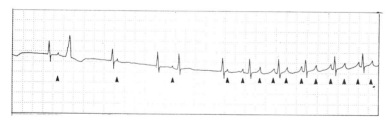

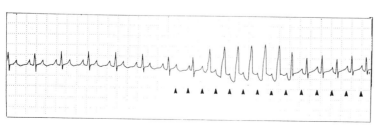

Figure 47. Holter recordings from a patient with the "sick sinus syndrome" 5 years after a Senning operation showing both the "brady" and "tachy" phases. The slow rhythm in the upper strip is abruptly interrupted by a rapid, regular atrial rhythm (arrows), which is atrial muscle reentry or "flutter." This initially conducts 2:1, but on the lower strip it changes to 1:1 conduction; there is transient QRS aberration at the onset of the rapid ventricular response.

indicators of SA-node integrity, but both tests are limited by a high false-negative rate. Grossly abnormal data are valuable, but normal SA-node measurements in young patients are of little consequence if electrocardiographic and Holter data are strongly indicative of nodal dysfunction.

Treatment at Boston Children's Hospital is usually reserved for patients with symptoms or documented tachyarrhythmias. Asymptomatic patients with isolated bradycardia may not require therapy unless there are coexistent hemodynamic problems that could be aggravated by chronotropic incompetence (such as poor ventricular function or valvar regurgitation). Patients requiring therapy who have bradycardia as the primary component of their syndrome are treated with pacemaker insertion. The simple expedient of correcting bradycardia frequently reduces episodes of SVT. If SVT remains an issue, suppressive medical therapy is begun. Of note, it may be hazardous to institute drug treatment with any agent other than digoxin in patients with marked bradycardia unless a pacemaker is already in place[37] because of the risk of further slowing of the SA node or escape foci, although this recommendation is still debated.[92]

An alternate therapy for both the fast and slow components of this disorder is use of an atrial antitachycardia pacemaker.[57] Such devices can detect and interrupt atrial flutter in addition to providing routine-demand atrial pacing and thus may eliminate the need for drug therapy in selected patients.

DISORDERS OF ATRIOVENTRICULAR CONDUCTION

Abnormalities of atrioventricular conduction may involve either the AV node or the proximal His-Purkinje system. They can be subdivided by grades according to the P-QRS relationship on the surface ECG.

First-degree AV Block

In first-degree block, every atrial beat is conducted to the ventricle, although conduction velocity is abnormally slow. This appears on the surface electrocardiogram as a prolonged P-R interval for age (Fig. 48). Although delay in the AV node is the most common cause of first-degree block, His-Purkinje delay may be operative in some cases.

The causes of first-degree block are numerous and include congenital cardiac malformations (atrial septal defects, AV-canal defects, L-looped ventricles), antiarrhythmic medications, myocardial inflammation or myopathy, hypothyroidism, surgical trauma, and high levels of vagal tone. In general, first-degree AV block requires no therapy and is a well-tolerated condition.

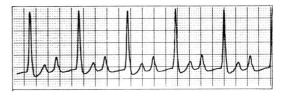

Figure 48. First-degree AV block with a P-R interval of 0.39 msec.

Second-degree AV Block

Second-degree block refers to intermittent failure of conduction for a single atrial impulse and may be subclassified as either the Mobitz I (Wenckebach) or Mobitz II variety. In the former condition there is a gradual but progressive increase in the P-R interval, culminating in a single nonconducted beat, typically recurring in a sequence that can be described by the ratio of P waves to QRS complexes (2:1, every other beat blocked, 3:2, every third beat blocked, etc.). Mobitz I block is usually due to a conduction disorder at the level of the AV node (Fig. 49).

In Mobitz II block there is no premonitory conduction delay, but rather an abrupt nonconducted atrial impulse with equal P-R intervals for the flanking conducted beats (Fig. 50). This disorder usually occurs with disease of the bundle of His and is often associated with a more diffuse disturbance of His-Purkinje conduction; therefore it is rare to observe true Mobitz II block in a patient without some form of bundle branch block on the electrocardiogram.[155]

The distinction between Mobitz I and Mobitz II block is clinically important and can often be made by analyzing the surface electrocardiogram for Wenckebach patterns and the duration of the QRS. In difficult cases, an electrogram of the bundle of His can be recorded to determine the site of the block more precisely.

Mobitz I (Wenckebach) AV Block. Mobitz I block is well tolerated and rarely requires therapy. It may be a normal finding on Holter recordings in many healthy adolescents and young adults during sleep. Etiologies are similar to those associated with first-degree block. Although most patients are asymptomatic, in some there may be progression to higher degrees of block, and in rare instances symptomatic bradycardia may also occur. For acute symptoms, treatment with intravenous atropine or isoproterenol usually provides temporary improvement in conduction, but a pacemaker is the safest long-term therapy in symptomatic patients. For patients in whom the conduction disturbance is only intermittent and appears to be related to excessive vagal tone, therapy with vagolytic agents (such as theophylline)[3] can be used on a trial basis.

Mobitz II AV Block. Second-degree block due to His-Purkinje disease is a less predictable situ-

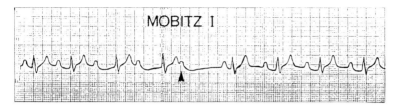

Figure 49. Second-degree AV block of the Mobitz I type, showing gradual and progressive prolongation of the P-R interval before a nonconducted beat (arrow). The subsequent conducted beat has a normal P-R, after which progressive prolongation resumes.

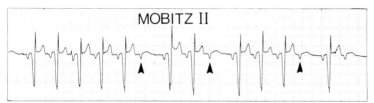

Figure 50. Second-degree AV block of the Mobitz II type, which developed in a patient after aortic valve surgery. The P-R intervals are identical for all conducted beats, and the episodic block (arrows) follows no predictable pattern. The QRS is wide because of coexistent bundle branch block.

ation that usually follows inflammatory or traumatic injury below the level of the AV node. Abrupt progression to complete block may occur in this disorder,[82] thus necessitating a higher level of concern that does Mobitz I block.

Mobitz II block is rare in children. When it occurs as the result of surgical trauma, implantation of a pacemaker has been advised.[37] When observed as an isolated phenomenon in an asymptomatic patient, Mobitz II block can be followed conservatively but carefully.

Third-degree (Complete) AV Block

In third-degree heart block electrical communication between the atria and ventricles is completely interrupted. The atria continue to beat at their own rate, while the slower ventricular rhythm is supplied by escape foci in the AV node or the His-Purkinje system, thereby creating complete dissociation of the P and QRS on the electrocardiogram (Fig. 51). QRS complexes are narrow when the escape rhythm arises above the bifurcation of the common His bundle, but occasionally may be wide if the escape focus arises low in the conducting system or if the patient has concomitant bundle branch block. Complete heart block should not be confused with benign AV dissociation that may be seen with some accelerated junctional or ventricular rhythms.

Third-degree block may be congenital or acquired (Table 9). The prognosis and therapy vary widely depending on etiology.

Congenital Complete AV Block. The most common causes of congenital heart block include anatomic cardiac defects[114] (particularly ventricular inversion or atrioventricular canal defects) and fetal exposure to maternal antibodies related to con-

nective tissue disease (primarily systemic lupus erythematosus).[115] Often, it is first diagnosed in utero when a slow fetal pulse is detected on routine obstetrical evaluation. Fetal echocardiography can be performed to rule out structural cardiac defects and to record an M-mode tracing that views simultaneous atrial and ventricular wall motion (Fig. 52). Third-degree block is readily diagnosed if the faster atrial motion is completely dissociated from the slow ventricular contraction. If block is seen in the absence of structural defects, maternal testing for antinuclear antibody titers should be performed. It is estimated that as many as 60% of mothers will have clinical and/or serologic evidence of connective tissue disease in this setting.[102]

Congenital heart block is usually well tolerated in utero, but there are well described instances of fetal hydrops and even fetal death. Unfortunately, treatment for a distressed fetus is difficult because in utero pacing techniques are not yet perfected.[12] At present, the only safe course for a hydropic infant is early delivery and immediate pacing but this option is frequently limited by fetal lung immaturity.

Fortunately, in most cases the fetus adapts well to slow heart rates and will usually come to term without difficulty. Delivery should be performed at a center with pediatric cardiology back-up, because abrupt extrauterine decompensation may occur occasionally even if the fetus did well in utero. Emergency pacemaker placement will stabilize such infants promptly. For the vast majority of newborns with congenital heart block, the transition to extrauterine life is smooth unless complicated by prematurity, lung disease, or anatomic cardiac defects.

Although the short-term prognosis for most patients with congenital block is generally good, the

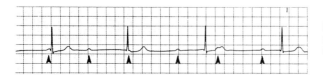

Figure 51. Complete heart block showing nonconducted P waves (arrows) and a junctional escape rhythm at 37 bpm.

Table 9. Causes of Third-degree Atrioventricular Block

Congenital
  Structural heart disease
    L-looped ventricles
    AV canal defects
    ASD and VSD (rare)
    Ebstein's anomaly (rare)
  Maternal lupus antibodies
  Idiopathic
  Kearns-Sayre syndrome
  Myotonic/muscular dystrophy
  Refsum's syndrome

Acquired
  Surgical trauma
  Catheter trauma
  Endocarditis
  Cardiac tumors
  Antiarrhythmic drugs
  Chagas' disease
  Lyme disease
  Diphtheria
  Myopathy

long-term outlook is guarded and many of them ultimately require pacemaker insertion. In a review of 30 years of experience with congenital block in patients with normal cardiac anatomy, 32% of unpaced patients eventually developed symptoms, including 5% who had sudden cardiac arrest.[128] A large international review of this condition[105] found the incidence of early death to be 8% for patients with normal cardiac anatomy, and 28% for those with structural defects. Certainly, all symptomatic patients should be treated promptly with pacing, but pacemaker implant should also be considered in advance of symptoms for any patient thought to be at risk for sudden events. Potential risk factors for poor outcome have been sought in multiple studies and have included: (1) a resting ventricular rate below 55/min for neonates,[114] (2) a resting ventricular rate below 50/min for older patients,[23] (3) a prolonged Q-T interval,[31] (4) a wide QRS escape rhythm,[30] (5) ventricular ectopy,[149] and (6) advanced cardiomegaly and/or ventricular dysfunction.[128]

It remains uncertain which of these factors is the single best predictor of the need for prophylactic pacer insertion, but given the low risk and high reliability of modern pacer technology, the threshold for recommending the procedure should be low. If none of the above factors is present, it appears reasonable to follow the patient conservatively, particularly the very young child in whom small body size may complicate pacemaker implantation.

Acquired Complete AV Block. The most common etiology for acquired AV block in the pediatric age group is direct injury to the conduction tissues during cardiac surgery or catheterization. In about one-third of the cases, traumatic AV block is a transient disturbance which needs only to be treated with temporary pacing until normal conduction returns. If improvement is not observed within 6–10 days, recovery becomes unlikely.

The prognosis for traumatic AV block is poor unless the patient receives a permanent pacemaker. A 50–60% fatality rate was observed[72,96] in follow-up of children with postoperative block in the era before pacemaker therapy was routinely available. At present, there does not appear to be any clinical setting in which pacemaker implant can safely be deferred for persistent third-degree surgical block.[37]

Complete block can also be acquired from inflammatory processes, metabolic disease, neuromuscular disorders,[112] and infectious diseases in the pediatric age group. Unless the block can be reversed by treatment of the underlying cause, pacemaker implant is advisable.

PHARMACOLOGIC THERAPY FOR ARRHYTHMIAS

Antiarrhythmic drugs are commonly classified according to their effects on cardiac cell action potentials, as initially proposed by Vaughan Williams in 1970.[142] In this scheme, the drugs are divided into four major groups:

Class I   Local anesthetic agents that reduce upstroke velocity of phase 0 in atrial, ventricular, and Purkinje cells (sodium channel blockers)

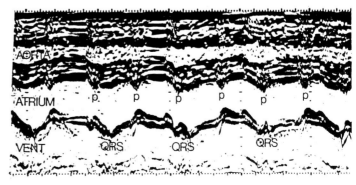

Figure 52. M-mode fetal echocardiogram showing complete dissociation of the atrial wall motion (P) and ventricular motion (QRS) in a fetus with congenital heart block.

Class II Drugs that inhibit sympathetic activity (beta blockers)

Class III Drugs that prolong duration of the action potential without changing phase 0

Class IV Drugs that block the slow inward current (calcium channel blockers)

Class I agents are usually split into subclasses A, B, and C, depending on the degree of modification in the upstroke of phase 0, as well as on their effects on repolarization and conduction velocity.[69] This grouping of agents by in-vitro cellular effect is a useful method for understanding the genesis of electrocardiographic changes, as well as a starting point for matching drug effect with arrhythmia mechanism. However, it cannot be overemphasized that drugs within the same class may not have equivalent action in vivo and can vary widely in terms of bioavailability, efficacy, side effects, and proarrhythmic potential.

The current formulary of antiarrhythmic agents is reviewed briefly here, with particular emphasis on cellular effects and caveats regarding their use in children. Drugs that do not fall into the standard Vaughn Williams classification are discussed as "miscellaneous" agents. Data regarding pediatric dosages, therapeutic serum levels and side effects are presented in the Appendix, p. 760. In depth discussion of these topics is available in several reviews of antiarrhythmic pharmacology in children.[89,106,113]

Class IA Drugs (Quinidine, Procainamide, Disopyramide)

The IA agents cause a moderate depression of phase 0 upstroke, a slowing of repolarization, and a prolongation of conduction time in the fast-response cells of atrial muscle, ventricular muscle, His-Purkinje cells, and accessory pathways.[151] When these cellular events are translated to the intact heart, the major effects are increased duration of the QRS and prolongation of the Q-T interval on the surface electrocardiogram (Fig. 53).

Although IA agents have minimal direct action on slow-response cells of the normal SA and AV nodes, indirect changes may be mediated through the autonomic nervous system. The IA drugs all possess some anticholinergic activity, which may increase the rate of sinus node discharge and enhance AV node conduction.

Class IA agents are used primarily for treatment of reentry tachycardia involving atrial muscle (e.g., atrial fibrillation or flutter), ventricular muscle (ventricular tachycardia), and accessory pathways (e.g., WPW syndrome).

Quinidine is the most commonly used IA drug for oral administration in children. Intravenous quinidine can be associated with marked hypotension and should be avoided. When a parenteral IA drug is required, **procainamide** can be employed. Long-term oral procainamide is often limited by poor absorption in infants and by side-effects (particularly the lupus-like syndrome) in teenagers and young adults. **Disopyramide** is an alternate IA oral agent, but its use must be restricted to patients with good ventricular function because of its negative inotropic properties.

The side effect of all class IA agents that is of the most concern is the small, but real, potential for the development of proarrhythmia, specifically new or worsened ventricular arrhythmias of the torsade de pointes variety. When beginning type IA drugs, hospitalization and monitoring are required.

Class IB Drugs (Lidocaine, Mexiletine, Tocainide, Phenytoin)

The cellular effects of IB agents are subtle. In therapeutic concentrations they cause a trivial decrease in the slope of phase 0 of a normal fast-response action potential, although the effect becomes much more pronounced under conditions of cell damage, acidosis, or hyperkalemia. In both healthy and injured fast-response cells, the duration of the action potential and to an even greater degree the refractory period, is shortened.[130] This effect appears primarily in Purkinje fibers and ventricular myocytes and is much less prominent in atrial tissue. Slow-response cells of the normal SA and AV nodes are not affected by IB agents, and the influence on autonomic tone is negligible. These cellular actions all translate to a surface electrocardiogram that is largely unchanged from the pre-drug state, except perhaps for a slight decrease in the QT interval (Fig. 54).

The IB drugs are used for suppression of most forms of ventricular arrhythmias and are particularly well suited to emergency treatment of arrhythmias that may occur in the setting of abnormal Q-T prolongation. Having minimal effect on atrial cells, they are not very effective for management of supraventricular arrhythmias.

Lidocaine is the prototype IB agent but, owing to rapid hepatic metabolism, it is available only for intravenous use. **Mexiletine** and **tocainide** are structural analogues of lidocaine with prolonged elimination half-life that allows oral administration. **Phenytoin** is a weaker IB agent that can be administered by either route.

Proarrhythmia is less common with these agents than with other class I drugs, but there still are well-documented instances of rhythm degeneration with mexiletine and tocainide, necessitating careful inpatient monitoring and follow-up.

Class IC Drugs (Flecainide, Encainide, Propafenone)

The IC agents cause marked depression of phase 0 upstroke and profound slowing of conduction in

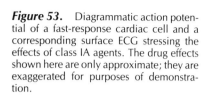
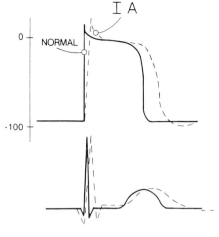

Figure 53. Diagrammatic action potential of a fast-response cardiac cell and a corresponding surface ECG stressing the effects of class IA agents. The drug effects shown here are only approximate; they are exaggerated for purposes of demonstration.

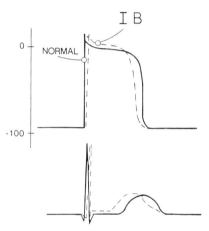

Figure 54. Diagrammatic action potential of a fast-response cardiac cell and a corresponding surface ECG stressing the effects of class IB agents. The drug effects shown here are only approximate; they are exaggerated for purposes of demonstration.

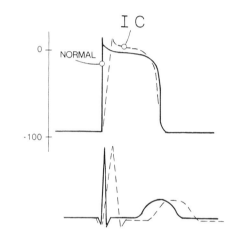

Figure 55. Diagrammatic action potential of a fast-response cardiac cell and a corresponding surface ECG stressing the effects of class IC agents. The drug effects shown here are only approximate; they are exaggerated for purposes of demonstration.

fast-response cells. The influence on repolarization and duration of the action potential are minimal, such that the refractory period for an individual cell is not typically prolonged. However, in the intact heart measured "effective refractory periods" may be increased,[32] particularly in the His-Purkinje system and accessory pathways. Drugs in this class do not appear to affect slow inward calcium currents in vitro or to alter autonomic tone. On the surface electrocardiogram, the most notable change is an increase in QRS duration caused by slowing of intraventricular depolarization. The measured Q-T interval may be prolonged as a consequence of the widened QRS, but the T wave itself is not significantly modified (Fig. 55). Some P-R prolongation may also be seen.

The IC drugs are potent inhibitors of abnormal automaticity and reentry within atrial muscle, ventricular muscle, and accessory pathways, but because of growing evidence for a relatively high proarrhythmic potential,[13] use should be reserved for "life-threatening" arrhythmias that have failed to respond to other treatment modalities.

Flecainide and **encainide** are available for oral use, and both efficacy[135,154] and proarrhythmic potential[34] have been well documented in the pediatric population. **Propafenone** has been used intravenously under an investigational protocol in children,[47] but experience is still limited with oral administration.

Class II Drugs (Propranolol, Nadolol, Atenolol, Esmolol)

The mechanisms by which beta blockade may modify cardiac arrhythmias are complex.[143] The predominant effect is competitive inhibition of catecholamine binding at cardiac receptors, which reduces both normal and abnormal automaticity and slows AV-node conduction. However, direct membrane effects may also occur, including prolonging the duration of the action potential and effective refractory periods, as well as increasing the threshold for ventricular fibrillation. These direct cellular actions are most pronounced during chronic administration of high doses.

Class II agents are used to treat a diverse spectrum of arrhythmias in children. They are often effective in catecholamine-mediated tachycardias from either abnormal automaticity or triggered activity at both the atrial and ventricular levels. They are less useful for reentry tachycardias but often prove effective if they suppress premature beats which serve as the initiating event for the reentry circuit. Additionally, some forms of reentry SVT may be effectively treated by beta blocker therapy if the AV node is a necessary part of the circuit and can be sufficiently slowed to prevent rapid conduction. Finally, beta blockade plays a major role in management of the long Q-T syndrome.

Propranolol is the prototype beta blocker. It is "nonselective" and it affects both B_1 (cardiac) and B_2 (bronchial and blood vessel) receptors. Both oral and intravenous administration is possible. Intravenous administration is more likely to produce acute cardiac side effects (hypotension, bradycardia, AV node block) and should be used only when oral administration is impossible.

Propranolol is usually well tolerated. Important limitations include its B_2 blockade properties, which can aggravate reactive airway disease, and its B_1 blockade, which may further depress ventricular function in patients with poor contractility.

Nadolol is likewise a nonselective beta blocker that differs from propranolol in requiring less frequent dosing, as well as in having reduced penetration across the blood-brain barrier.

Atenolol is designated as a cardioselective beta blocker, although some cross-reactivity with B_2 receptors may still occur at high doses. It has low central nervous system penetration and maintains effectiveness with oral administration only once or twice a day. For most arrhythmias that respond to propranolol, nadolol and atenolol are usually effective, although the long Q-T syndrome may be an exception.[139]

Esmolol is a B_1 selective agent which is unique in its rapid onset and short duration,[97] thus lending itself to emergency management of arrhythmias, as well as to therapeutic trials during electrophysiologic testing. Experience with this drug is still limited in children, but rapid drug elimination (less than 10 min) offers a potentially dramatic advantage over intravenous propranolol.

Class III Drugs (Amiodarone, Sotalol, Bretylium)

Drugs that prolong the action potential plateau without affecting phase 0 (Fig. 56) are grouped in

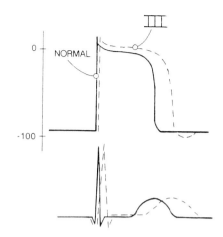

Figure 56. Diagrammatic action potential of a fast-response cardiac cell and a corresponding surface ECG stressing the effects of class III agents. The drug effects here are only approximate; they are exaggerated for purposes of demonstration.

class III. All such agents exhibit mixed electrical properties as well as variable effects on the autonomic nervous system.

Amiodarone is the prototype class III agent and is like no other cardiac drug in terms of its pharmacokinetics, side effects, and potency.[101] It should be reserved for treatment of "life-threatening" rhythm disorders that are refractory to all other forms of treatment.

Amiodarone's electrical effects are felt at all levels of the heart. Most notable is prolongation of action potential duration (and hence refractory period) in all fast response cells of atrial muscle, ventricular muscle, Purkinje fibers, and accessory pathways. Unlike Class I agents, it also has direct effects on the SA and AV nodes, decreasing the rate of automatic discharge in the former and slowing conduction in the latter. Amiodarone also possesses both alpha and beta blocking properties.

Widespread changes occur on the surface electrocardiogram, including sinus slowing, P-R prolongation, a slight increase in QRS width, and Q-T prolongation.

Amiodarone has an elimination half-life longer than one month. Thus, there are steady serum levels with administration only once a day, but treatment responses are delayed and, more importantly, should toxicity develop, drug elimination is very slow.

Like all potent antiarrhythmic agents, new or worsened rhythm disorders may develop during administration of amiodarone requiring inpatient monitoring during the oral loading phase and careful outpatient follow-up. Amiodarone also has multiple noncardiac toxicities. These may include corneal microdeposits, hyper- or hypothyroidism, pulmonary interstitial fibrosis, "adult respiratory distress syndrome" following cardiac surgery, hepatitis, peripheral neuropathy, photosensitive skin rash, and blueish discoloration of the skin. Fortunately, serious side effects have not been common in children,[65] but careful surveillance is still mandatory.

Sotalol remains an investigational antiarrhythmic agent that is currently undergoing clinical trials. It acts primarily as a nonselective beta blocker at low doses, but exhibits class III activity at higher levels. Preliminary data[118] suggest efficacy in treatment of both supraventricular and ventricular arrhythmias in children, although use must be restricted to those with well-preserved ventricular function because of its beta blockade properties.

Bretylium exerts unique antiarrhythmic and autonomic effects.[98] When administered intravenously, bretylium is selectively concentrated at sympathetic nerve terminals, causing an acute release of norepinephrine, gradually followed by block of norepinephrine release. Consequently, there is a biphasic cardiovascular response characterized by initial sinus tachycardia with a rise in blood pressure and occasional transient worsening of arrhythmias, which is then is followed by mild hypotension and delayed onset of class III antiarrhythmic activity.

The most important clinical application of bretylium is for treatment of ventricular fibrillation in cardiac arrest, but it is used occasionally for suppressing ventricular tachycardia when other drugs have failed.

Class IV Drugs

Verapamil is the most commonly used calcium channel antagonist for treatment of cardiac arrhythmias. Enthusiasm for this agent in pediatric practice has become somewhat tempered by the observation of potentially serious side effects in small infants and the introduction of alternate drugs and pacing techniques for SVT management. Nevertheless, it remains a useful treatment option for older children and adults. Verapamil acts predominately on the slow calcium current in cells of the SA and AV nodes, causing a decrease in the rate of phase 4 automaticity, a slowing of phase 0 depolarization, and a prolongation of refractoriness and conduction time. Except for a slight decrease in plateau amplitude, its effect on the normal fast-response action potential is negligible. These actions all translate to a surface electrocardiographic picture of mild sinus slowing and prolongation of the P-R interval, but no noticeable change in the QRS or T wave (Fig. 57). Under pathologic conditions, however, verapamil can affect injured cells of ventricular or atrial tissue that may deviate from their normal fast-response characteristics.[59]

Verapamil is available for both oral and intravenous administration. The most common clinical indication is reentry supraventricular tachycardia

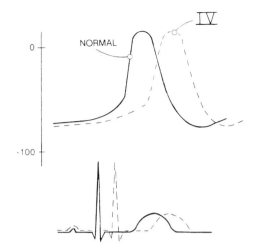

Figure 57. Diagrammatic action potential of a slow-response cardiac cell and a corresponding surface ECG stressing the effects of class IV agents. The drug effects here are only approximate; they are exaggerated for purposes of demonstration.

that involves the SA or AV node as part of the circuit. Thus, SA-node reentry, AV-node reentry, or macroreentry involving an accessory connection (with anterograde conduction over the AV node) may all respond with abrupt termination following an intravenous dose. By contrast, tachycardias arising from atrial muscle (e.g., ectopic atrial tachycardia, atrial flutter) are less likely to respond, although verapamil will slow AV-node conduction to control the ventricular response rate in such disorders.

There are several caveats surrounding the use of this agent. Most relevant to the pediatric population is the observation that neonates may develop marked hypotension and bradycardia following intravenous use.[28] Intravenous verapamil should generally be avoided in the first 6 months of life, particularly now that there are safer alternate techniques for termination of SVT (e.g., esophageal pacing).

A second limitation of verapamil relates to its enhancement of accessory pathway conduction in the WPW syndrome. In the setting of atrial fibrillation or flutter, verapamil may increase the ventricular response rate to dangerous levels in patients with short effective refractory periods and/or multiple accessory pathways.[67] Although verapamil is safe for emergency termination of orthodromic reentry, it should never be given for management of atrial fibrillation or flutter in patients with WPW, nor should it be used for long-term therapy of this syndrome unless comprehensive electrophysiologic testing has confirmed its safety.

Miscellaneous Drugs

The antiarrhythmic actions of **digoxin** are complex; there is a direct effect on the cell membrane, along with a major contribution through the action on the autonomic nervous system.[132] The predominant clinical response to this agent (SA-node slowing and depression of AV-node conduction) appears to be due almost exclusively to enhancement of vagal tone. However, there are measurable direct cellular effects in atrial muscle, ventricular muscle, and specialized conduction tissue (including accessory pathways) which may be best summarized as a mild decrease in the duration of the action potential and shortening of the effective refractory period.[60]

The above actions cause predictable changes on the surface electrocardiogram that involve sinus slowing, P-R prolongation, and a slight shortening of the Q-T interval. Mild depression of the S-T segment and flattening of the T wave may occur also.

As an antiarrhythmic agent, digoxin is used primarily for its effect on atrioventricular conduction. Reentry tachycardias that involve the AV node as part of their circuit may be terminated and/or prevented with this agent, while the ventricular response rate can be controlled in other forms of SVT (e.g., atrial fibrillation), even though digoxin does not exert a significant direct effect on the primary atrial abnormality.

The WPW syndrome is one condition in which digoxin should be used with caution.[125] Because of its potential for shortening refractory periods in accessory pathways, the ventricular response during atrial fibrillation or flutter may be dangerously increased. Although digoxin appears to be safe for acute management of orthodromic reentry in WPW, chronic outpatient administration of this drug seems unwise, because one can never guarantee that a patient's next episode of tachycardia will not be fibrillation or flutter. In rare instances in which digoxin is the only reasonable treatment option, it may be used if electrophysiologic testing has confirmed its safety.

Digoxin intoxication in children usually produces sinus bradycardia, disturbances in AV conduction, nausea, and somnolence. Digoxin toxicity can be managed[70] by withholding the drug, correcting electrolyte abnormalities which can potentiate toxic effects (hypokalemia, hypercalcemia), temporary pacing for high-grade block, and administration of phenytoin for ventricular ectopy. Digoxin is not removed from the circulation by dialysis or cardiopulmonary bypass, but can be rendered inactive by the intravenous administration of digoxin-specific Fab fragments.[131] This antibody therapy should be used promptly for any potentially life-threatening intoxication.

Adenosine is a new and very promising pharmacologic option for abrupt termination of supraventricular tachycardia.[111] This agent is an endogenous nucleoside found in all cells of the body, but when administered as a large rapid bolus, it transiently impairs AV node conduction and slows SA-node automaticity by a direct cellular effect. Adenosine is promptly removed from the circulation by erythrocytes and endothelial cells, resulting in a half-life of less than 10 seconds. It can be used to interrupt narrow QRS reentry tachycardias that involve the AV node as part of the circuit because of its rapid onset of action and absence of lingering side effects.

PACEMAKER THERAPY FOR ARRHYTHMIAS

Until recently, cardiac pacemakers were implanted for the sole purpose of relieving bradyarrhythmias, but generators are now available that are capable of treating both bradycardia and tachycardia, including automatic defibrillation for malignant rhythm disorders. Furthermore, generator sizes have been drastically reduced (Fig. 58) and battery longevity markedly prolonged, such that pacemaker implant is now a generally practical and safe procedure in even the smallest of infants.[92]

The clinical indications for pacemaker insertion have been discussed elsewhere in this chapter. Comments here are restricted to the technical aspects of cardiac pacing.

Permanent Pacing Leads and Implant Techniques

The interface between the pacemaker lead and cardiac tissue is the most crucial component of the pacing system. The lead tip(s) must be positioned in the atrium and/or ventricle such that there is proper recognition of intrinsic electrical activity ("sensing" function), as well as of low energy requirements for pacing ("threshold" or "capture" function).

The leads may be attached to either the epicar-

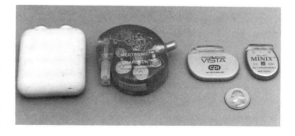

Figure 58. Evolution of the pacemaker generator size in the last three decades. Shown here are some single-chamber units. From left-to-right: 1960s, 1970s, 1980s, 1990. Early mercury-powered batteries lasted 6–18 months. Today's lithium-powered batteries last 5–10 years or more.

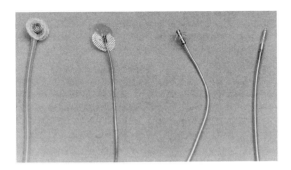

Figure 59. Pacemaker leads. From left-to-right: two types of epicardial leads ("corkscrew" and "fish-hook") and two endocardial leads ("tine-tip" and micro "corkscrew").

dium (via a small thoracotomy or subxyphoid incision) or the endocardium (using a transvenous approach). Although transvenous leads are generally preferred for superior sensing function and less traumatic surgery, the epicardial technique is still used in select pediatric cases, such as: (1) very small infants; (2) patients with right to-left intracardiac mixing who are at risk for systemic embolic events; (3) patients with caval-pulmonary anastomosis (who lack venous connection to the heart); and (4) patients undergoing cardiac surgery in whom the pacemaker is implanted as part of a more complex procedure.

Epicardial leads are fixed to cardiac tissue by direct suturing, or by a "fish-hook" or "corkscrew" at the tip. Endocardial leads may use a screw-tip for "active fixation" or may rely on "passive fixation" of small tines which become entrapped in muscle trabeculae (Fig. 59). Leads are also now available which exude small quantities of steroid to reduce local fibrotic reaction and possibly prolong lead life.

Generators and Pacing Modes

The earliest pacemakers were "asynchronous" units that generated stimuli at a single fixed rate regardless of the patient's underlying cardiac rhythm. "Demand" pacing evolved when generators were equipped with circuitry that sensed na-

tive cardiac activity and temporarily inhibited stimulus output if the intrinsic heart rate exceeded the pacemaker rate. In essence, all modern pacing units operate according to subtle variations on this basic demand theme. They are programmed to recognize spontaneous cardiac events in the atrium and/or ventricle, and respond to the presence or absence of native beats by being **inhibited** or **triggered.**

A shorthand notation involving a 3–5 letter code[5] has been developed to describe various pacing modes. The first letter indicates the chamber paced, the second refers to the chamber sensed, and the third describes the unit's response to a sensed event (Table 10). For example, an AAI pacemaker involves a single atrial lead that can pace the atrium (when needed), sense the atrium (if spontaneous atrial beats are present at rates faster than the set pacemaker rate), and respond to a sensed atrial event by being inhibited (Fig. 60). This type of generator would be suited to a patient with isolated sinus bradycardia and normal AV node conduction. The VDD mode requires both atrial and ventricular wires. It will pace the ventricle only, but senses native electrical activity in both chambers. When a spontaneous atrial signal is recognized, the unit begins to scan for a ventricular event, and if none occurs after a preset time interval (the so-called AV delay), the ventricular wire is triggered to pace (Fig. 61). The DDD mode combines the above functions and is able to pace both atrium and ventricle to prevent bradycardia, while ensuring AV synchrony (Fig. 62). The VVI mode simply paces the ventricles without regard for atrial events (Fig. 63).

The choice of pacing mode is subject to many variables, such as patient size, status of AV conduction, and underlying hemodynamics. Decisions must be made on a case by case basis.

Specialized Functions. Specialized pacing options, most notably rate modulation and antitachycardia functions, are important advances in pacing technology. In the past, generators were simply programmed to a minimum rate for demand pac-

Table 10. Pacemaker Codes

Basic Three-letter Code			Special Function Codes	
I Chamber Paced	**II** Chamber Sensed	**III** Response to Sensed Event	**IV** Other Functions	**V** Antitachy Functions
A–atrium V–ventricle D–dual O–none	A–atrium V–ventricle D–dual O–none	I–inhibited T–triggered D–dual (T&I) O–none	R–rate responsiveness P–simple programmable M–multiprogrammable C–communicating O–none	P–pacing S–shock D–dual (P&S) O–none

Adapted from North American Society of Pacing and Electrophysiology/British Pacemaker and Electrophysiology Group (NASPE/BPEG) Generic (NBG) Pacemaker Code Recommendations, 1987.[5]

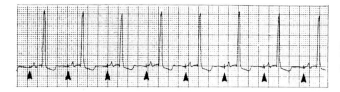

Figure 60. Atrial pacing (arrows) in a patient with sinus bradycardia and intact atrioventricular conduction.

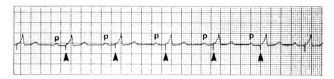

Figure 61. Operation of the VDD mode in a patient with heart block but normal sinus node function. One lead senses atrial activity (P); the generator then waits for a 200-msec time delay and paces the ventricle through a second lead.

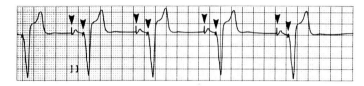

Figure 62. Dual chamber pacing in a patient with sinus bradycardia and complete heart block. Both atrial and ventricular leads pace in this case (arrows).

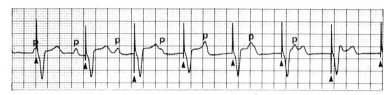

Figure 63. Ventricular pacing (arrows) in the VVI mode. Atrial activity (P) is completely dissociated. Absence of AV synchrony caused no difficulties in this patient with congenital heart block and otherwise normal cardiac anatomy and function.

ing, but this often limited the cardiac output during exercise and stress. Rate modulation restores a chronotropic response. These specialized generators are equipped with sensors that track a physiologic parameter (e.g., skeletal muscle contraction, respiration, venous temperature, etc.) and adjust the pacing rate automatically in an effort to better match metabolic demands. Rate responsiveness is now available for both single and dual chamber generators, and is so designated by addition of a fourth letter (R) to the basic three-letter code.

Antitachycardia pacemakers are becoming increasingly popular as alternatives (or adjuncts) to pharmacologic therapy for both supraventricular and ventricular arrhythmias. There are two general categories of devices: those that sense rapid regular reentrant rhythms and respond with burst pacing (so designated by a fifth code, the letter P) and those that can detect tachycardia and/or fibrillation, and respond with a DC shock (so designated by a fifth code, the letter S). Some newer investigational devices can combine burst pacing with a backup DC shock option.

The burst generator is used exclusively for interruption of reentry SVT, and is now in use for selected pediatric patients.[57] It is not much larger than a single chamber generator, and requires only an atrial lead. The most common application is in the child with postoperative sick sinus syndrome,

where the unit can provide routine atrial demand pacing, along with the automatic capacity to detect and interrupt atrial flutter (Fig. 64).

The automatic implantable cardioverter defibrillator (AICD) is used for life-threatening ventricular arrhythmias that have not responded to conventional pharmacologic therapy.[83] It is a relatively large device (Fig. 65), and requires a thoracotomy for placement of the defibrillating patches which are positioned directly on the epicardial surface. Shocks in the range of 2–20 joules are delivered automatically when malignant arrhythmias are detected. Candidates for this device obviously require careful selection and close follow-up. AICD implant is now being performed in the pediatric population,[91] although the experience is still quite limited.

SURGICAL AND TRANSCATHETER THERAPY FOR ARRHYTHMIAS

Pharmacologic therapy for tachyarrhythmias, while often effective, is strictly palliative and subject to the limitations of side effects. The ability to "cure" arrhythmias by permanently destroying the site of origin has thus captured the attention of cardiologists, particularly in pediatrics, in which projected exposure time to potentially toxic medications spans many decades. Ablation of arrhythmia foci or abnormal pathways was originally re-

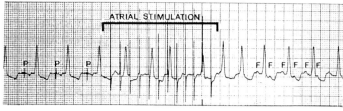

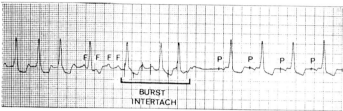

Figure 64. Function of an atrial anti-tachycardia pacer. In the upper strip, the patient is paced (P) in the AAI mode. Burst atrial pacing was then performed as part of an electrophysiology study, and atrial flutter (F) was induced. The generator was able to sense this abnormal rhythm, and in the lower strip automatically responded with 7 beats of burst pacing to terminate the flutter.

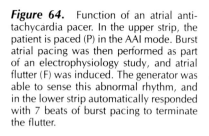

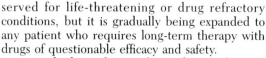

Figure 65. An autonomic implantable cardioverter defibrillator (AICD) showing 2 leads for epicardial sensing and two epicardial patches for delivering shocks. (Photo courtesy of Cardiac Pacemakers, Inc., St. Paul, MN.)

Surgical Techniques

Successful arrhythmia surgery hinges upon accurate mapping of the abnormal focus or pathway. This begins with review of surface electrocardiogram recordings and a preoperative electrophysiologic study in which intracardiac recordings are used to confirm the arrhythmia mechanism and pinpoint the area of interest.

With the heart exposed and beating at surgery, similar mapping is repeated using a handheld electrode (Fig. 66) that is moved over the cardiac surface by the surgeon to record the local electrical signals (Fig. 67), and reconfirm the suspected focus of origin. Additionally, it is often necessary to map the location of normal conduction tissues in the operating room in order to avoid unwanted trauma to these areas during destruction of the pathologic focus. As final confirmation, an "ice map" can be performed by placing a cryoprobe over the suspected focus and cooling the area slightly. If the arrhythmia is eliminated during this temporary cooling, the surgeon may proceed to more definite

served for life-threatening or drug refractory conditions, but it is gradually being expanded to any patient who requires long-term therapy with drugs of questionable efficacy and safety.

Any arrhythmia that involves a discrete focus or abnormal pathway is amenable to these techniques. The largest experience has come from surgical division of accessory pathways in the WPW syndrome,[41] but successful procedures are also possible for ventricular tachycardia,[43] ectopic atrial tachycardia,[53] Mahaim fibers,[68] junctional ectopic tachycardia,[54] AV node reentry,[17] and other arrhythmias.[88]

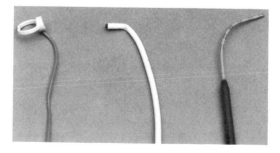

Figure 66. Probes for intraoperative mapping. Shown here are a ring electrode and a handheld probe for single site recording, and a band electrode that can record six simultaneous signals (e.g., along the AV groove for WPW mapping).

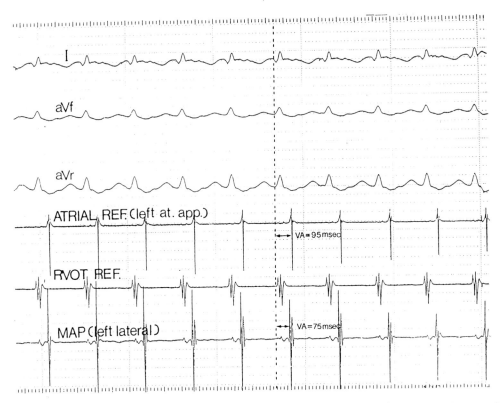

Figure 67. Intraoperative mapping during orthodromic tachycardia in a patient with the WPW syndrome and a left lateral pathway. Shown are three surface ECG recordings, along with signals from two reference electrodes (attached to the right ventricular outflow tract and the left atrial appendage) and the signal from the mapping probe. The V-A interval of 75 msec in the left lateral region was the shortest atrial activation time recorded during the map and corresponded to the atrial insertion site of the abnormal pathway.

destruction of the area with considerable confidence in the map's accuracy.

Several techniques may be employed for destroying the unwanted focus, the most common being direct surgical dissection or local freezing with a cryoprobe. One reported advantage of cryosurgery for WPW is that the heart need not be arrested and cardiopulmonary bypass may not be necessary,[66] but for many arrhythmia foci (e.g., septal accessory pathways in WPW, ectopic atrial foci, ventricular tachycardia) it is still essential to expose the endocardium for both mapping and destruction, and bypass cannot be avoided.

Following surgery, serial electrocardiograms and electrophysiologic studies are performed to confirm successful elimination of the focus or pathway (Fig. 68). Usually this is done just before closing the chest in the operating room and again several days after surgery. By using temporary epicardial pacing wires placed at the time of operation, the need for a second electrophysiologic catheterization can be eliminated. Surgical therapy for pediatric arrhythmias has been highly promising.[46] Success rates of greater than 95% are reported for the WPW syndrome, with very low surgical morbidity and mortality.

Transcatheter Ablation of Arrhythmia Foci

As an alternative to surgery, methods are now being perfected to destroy arrhythmia foci with the tip of specialized catheters at the time of intracardiac electrophysiologic study. Such techniques are logical extensions of catheter mapping technology but are still in their developmental stages both in terms of energy delivery and catheter design.

Potentially, transcatheter ablation may be achieved with several energy forms, including: DC shock,[36] radiofrequency energy,[7] laser,[117] local chemical infusion (e.g., ethanol),[76] and local freezing with a specialized cryocatheter.[55] The first two modalities have received the most attention to date, but the list will likely change and expand.

Most ablation attempts have been performed using electrical shocks delivered through a standard electrode catheter from DC cardioversion equipment. The sudden discharge of DC energy results in an intense electrical arc at the catheter tip which fulgurates local tissue by a combination of heat, light, and barotrauma.[8] The DC shock technique has been used in both adults and children for accessory pathways and ventricular tachycardias, and for the modification or destruction of atrioventricular conduction. An advantage of DC ablation is

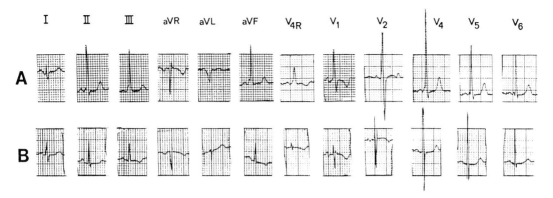

Figure 68.   Preoperative **(A)** and postoperative **(B)** ECG from the patient shown in Figure 67. The delta wave is absent and SVT could no longer be induced following surgical ablation of the left lateral pathway.

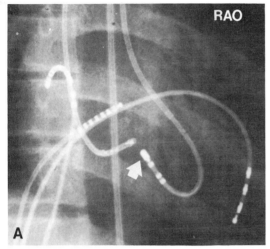

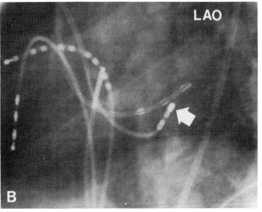

Figure 69.   Catheter positions (RAO and LAO) during successful radiofrequency ablation of a left-sided accessory pathway. The ablation catheter (arrow) has been inserted into the left ventricle, using a retrograde arterial approach, and is positioned behind the mitral valve at the level of the annulus. Radiofrequency discharge through the catheter tip eliminated the abnormal pathway.

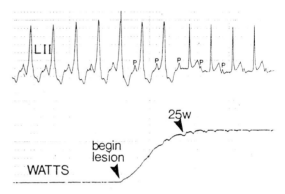

Figure 70.   Recording of sinus rhythm from lead II on the surface ECG of a patient with the WPW syndrome at the time of successful radiofrequency ablation of the accessory pathway. There is an obvious delta wave and a short P-R interval at baseline which disappear within three beats of beginning radiofrequency discharge. Both anterograde and retrograde conduction through the abnormal pathway were completely (and permanently) eliminated.

its relatively large lesion size; however, the energy discharge is somewhat uncontrolled and can create myocardial damage or perforation, as well as precipitate rhythm degeneration. Such procedures are generally performed with surgical backup readily available.

Radiofrequency ablation has recently evolved as a more controlled technique for destroying arrhythmia foci. The energy is generated by a device that is somewhat similar to a surgical electrocautery unit, although the delivered power is less than that used for routine surgical coagulation and does not create a spark or arc within the heart. Instead, tissue around the catheter tip is slowly heated over 20–60 seconds, resulting in local tissue desiccation and coagulation necrosis.[75] The lesion size is somewhat smaller than that achieved with DC ablation, and more exacting electrode placement is required (Fig. 69), but the risk of cardiac perforation and rhythm degeneration appears reduced. Recently, Jackman and coworkers[78] have used this technique in more than 100 adults to ablate accessory pathways with 100% success and no significant morbidity. At Children's Hospital in Boston the same technique has been used successfully for children and young adults (Fig. 70).[119]

Transcatheter ablation is likely to evolve in this decade as a realistic (and possibly preferred) alternative to drug therapy or surgical therapy for many arrhythmias in childhood.

REFERENCES

1. Akhtar M, Tchou PJ, Jazayeri M: Mechanism of clinical tachycardias. Am J Cardiol 61:9A–19A, 1988.
2. Bash SE, Shah JJ, Albers WH, et al: Hypothermia for the treatment of postsurgical greatly accelerated junctional ectopic tachycardia. J Am Coll Cardiol 10:1095–1099, 1987.
3. Benditt DG, Benson DW, Kreitt J, et al: Electrophysiologic effects of theophylline in young patients with recurrent symptomatic bradyarrhythmias. Am J Cardiol 52:1223–1229, 1983.
4. Benson DW, Smith WM, Dunnigan A, et al: Mechanisms of regular wide QRS tachycardia in infants and children. Am J Cardiol 49:1778–1788, 1982.
5. Bernstein AD, Camm AJ, Fletcher RD, et al: The NASPE/BPEG generic pacemaker code for antibradyarrhythmia and adaptive-rate pacing and antitachyarrhythmia events. Pace 10:794–799, 1987.
6. Bhandari AK, Scheinman MM, Morady F, et al: Efficacy of left cardiac sympathectomy in the treatment of patients with the long QT syndrome. Circulation 70:1018–1023, 1984.
7. Borggrefe M, Budde T, Podcyeck A, et al: High frequency alternating current ablation of an accessory pathway in humans. J Am Coll Cardiol 10:576–582, 1987.
8. Boyd EG, Hoet PM: The biophysics of catheter ablation techniques. J Electrophysiol 1:62–77, 1987.
9. Brodsky M, Wu D, Denes P, et al: Arrhythmias documented by 24 hour continuous electrocardiographic monitoring in 50 male medical students without apparent heart disease. Am J Cardiol 39:390–395, 1977.
10. Buxton AE, Waxman HL, Marchlinski FE, et al: Right ventricular tachycardia: clinical and electrophysiologic features. Circulation 68:917–927, 1983.
11. Campbell RM, Dick M, Jenkins JM, et al: Atrial overdrive pacing for conversion of atrial flutter in children. Pediatrics 75:730–736, 1985.
12. Carpenter RJ, Strasburger JF, Garson A, et al: Fetal ventricular pacing for hydrops secondary to complete atrioventricular block. J Am Coll Cardiol 8:1434–1436, 1986.
13. (CAST) The Cardiac Arrhythmia Suppression Trial (CAST) Investigators: Preliminary report: effect of encainide and flecainide on mortality in a randomized trial of arrhythmia suppression after myocardial infarction. N Engl J Med 321:406–412, 1989.
14. Casta A, Wolff GS, Mehta AV, et al: Dual atrioventricular nodal pathways: a benign finding in arrhythmia-free children with heart disease. Am J Cardiol 46:1013–1018, 1980.
15. Chameides L, Truex RC, Vetter V, et al: Association of maternal systemic lupus erythematosus and congenital complete heart block. N Engl J Med 297:1204–1207, 1977.
16. Chandar JS, Wolff GS, Garson A, et al: Ventricular arrhythmias in postoperative tetralogy of Fallot. Am J Cardiol 65:655–661, 1990.
17. Cox JL, Holman WL, Cain ME: Cryosurgical treatment of atrioventricular node reentrant tachycardia. Circulation 76:1329–1336, 1987.
18. Critelli G, Gallagher JJ, Thiene G, et al: The permanent form of junctional reciprocating tachycardia. In Benditt DG, Benson DW (eds): Cardiac Preexcitation Syndromes. Boston, Martinus Nijhoff, 1986, p. 233.
19. Damiano BP, Rosen M: Effects of pacing on triggered activity induced by early after depolarization. Circulation 69:1013–1025, 1984.
20. Deal BJ, Keane JF, Gillette PC, et al: Wolff-Parkinson-White syndrome and supraventricular tachycardia during infancy: management and follow-up. J Am Coll Cardiol 5:130–135, 1985.
21. Deal B, Miller S, Scagliotti D, et al: Ventricular tachycardia in a young population without overt heart disease. Circulation 73:1111–1118, 1986.
22. Deanfield JE, McKenna WJ, Presbitero P, et al: Ventricular arrhythmia in unrepaired and repaired tetralogy of Fallot. Br Heart J 52:77–81, 1984.
23. Dewey RC, Capeless MA, Levy AM: Use of ambulatory electrocardiographic monitoring to identify high-risk patients with congenital complete heart block. N Engl J Med 316:835–839, 1987.
24. Dunnigan A, Benditt DG, Benson DW: Modes of onset of paroxysmal atrial tachycardia in infants and children. Am J Cardiol 57:1280–1287, 1986.
25. Dunnigan A, Benson DW, Benditt DG: Transesophageal study of infant supraventricular tachycardia: electrophysiologic characteristics. Am J Cardiol 52:1002–1006, 1986.
26. Dunnigan A, Pierport ME, Smith SA, et al: Cardiac and skeletal myopathy associated with cardiac dysrhythmias. Am J Cardiol 53:731–737, 1984.
27. Eldar M, Griffin JC, Abbott JA, et al: Permanent cardiac pacing in patients with the long QT syndrome. J Am Coll Cardiol 10:600–607, 1987.
28. Epstein ML, Kiel EA, Victoria BE: Cardiac decompensation following verapamil therapy in infants with supraventricular tachycardia. Pediatrics 75:737–740, 1985.
29. Epstein ML, Stone FM, Benditt DG: Incessant atrial tachycardia in childhood: association with rate-dependent conduction in an accessory atrioventricular pathway. Am J Cardiol 44:498–504, 1979.
30. Esscher E: Congenital complete heart block. Acta Paediatr Scand 70:131–136, 1981.
31. Esscher E, Michaelsson M: QT interval in congenital complete heart block. Pediatr Cardiol 4:121–124, 1983.
32. Estes NA, Garson H, Ruskin JN: Electrophysiologic properties of flecainide acetate. Am J Cardiol 53:26B–29B, 1984.
33. Evans VC, Garson A, Smith RJ, et al: Ethmozine: a promising drug for "automatic" atrial ectopic tachycardia. Am J Cardiol 60:83F–86F, 1987.
34. Fisk FA, Gillette PC, Benson DW, et al: Incidence of death, cardiac arrest, and proarrhythmia in young patients receiving flecainide or encainide (abstract). Circulation 80:II–387, 1989.
35. Flinn CJ, Wolff GS, Dick M, et al: Cardiac rhythm after the Mustard operation for complete transposition of the great arteries. N Engl J Med 310:1635–1638, 1984.
36. Fontaine G, Frank R, Tonet J, et al: Treatment of rhythm disorders by endocardial fulguration. Am J Cardiol 64:83J–86J, 1989.
37. Frye RL, Collins JT, Desanctis RW, et al: Guidelines for permanent cardiac pacemaker implantation. J Am Coll Cardiol 4:434–442, 1984.
38. Fulton DR, Chung KJ, Tabakin BS, et al: Ventricular tachycardia in children without heart disease. Am J Cardiol 55:1328–1331, 1985.
39. Gallagher JJ, Pritchett ELC, Sealy WC, et al: The

preexcitation syndrome. Prog Cardiovasc Dis 20:285–327, 1978.

40. Gallagher JJ, Selle JG, Sealy WC, et al: Surgical interruption of nodoventricular Mahaim fibers with preservation of normal AV conduction (abstract). J Am Coll Cardiol 7:133A, 1986.

41. Gallagher JJ, Selle JG, Svenson RH, et al: Surgical treatment of arrhythmias. Am J Cardiol 61:27A–44A, 1988.

42. Gallagher JJ, Smith WM, Kasell JH, et al: Role of Mahaim fibers in cardiac arrhythmias in man. Circulation 64:176–189, 1981.

43. Garan H, Nguyen K, Mcgovern B, et al: Perioperative and long term results after electrophysiologically directed ventricular surgery for recurrent ventricular tachycardia. J Am Coll Cardiol 8:201–209, 1986.

44. Garson A, Gillette PC: Junctional ectopic tachycardias in children: electrocardiography, electrophysiology, and pharmacologic responses. Am J Cardiol 44:298–302, 1979.

45. Garson A, Gillette P, Titus JL, et al: Surgical treatment of ventricular tachycardia in infants. N Engl J Med 310:1443–1445, 1984.

46. Garson AJ, Moak JP, Friedman RA, et al: Surgical treatment of arrhythmias in children. Cardiol Clin 7:319–329, 1989.

47. Garson A, Moak JP, Smith RT, et al: Usefulness of intravenous propafenone for control of postoperative junctional ectopic tachycardia. Am J Cardiol 59:1422–1424, 1987.

48. Garson A, Randall DC, Gillette PC, et al: Prevention of sudden death after repair of tetralogy of Fallot: treatment of ventricular arrhythmias. J Am Coll Cardiol 6:221–227, 1985.

49. German LD, Gilbert MR, Kasell JH: The role of electrophysiologic studies in preexcitation syndromes. In Benditt DG, Benson DW (eds): Cardiac Preexcitation Syndromes. Boston, Martinus Nijhoff, 1986, p. 346.

50. German LD, Packer DL, Bardy GH, et al: Ventricular tachycardia induced by atrial stimulation in patients without symptomatic cardiac disease. Am J Cardiol 52:1202–1207, 1983.

51. Gikonyo BM, Dunnigan A, Benson DW: Cardiovascular collapse in infants: association with paroxysmal atrial tachycardia. Pediatrics 76:922–926, 1985.

52. Gillette PC: The mechanisms of supraventricular tachycardia in children. Circulation 54:133–139, 1976.

53. Gillette PC, Garson A, Hesslein PS, et al: Successful surgical treatment of atrial, junctional and ventricular tachycardia unassociated with accessory connections in infants and children. Am Heart J 102:984–991, 1981.

54. Gillette PC, Garson A, Porter CJ, et al: Junctional ectopic tachycardia: new proposed treatment by transcatheter His bundle ablation. Am Heart J 106:619–623, 1983.

55. Gillette P, Thompson M, Swindle M, et al: Requirements for transvenous catheter cryoablation of AV conduction (abstract). Circulation 80:II–388, 1989.

56. Gillette PC, Wampler DG, Garson A, et al: Treatment of atrial automatic tachycardia by ablation procedures. J Am Coll Cardiol 6:405–409, 1985.

57. Gillette PC, Wampler DG, Shannon C, et al: Use of cardiac pacing after the Mustard operation for transposition of the great arteries. J Am Coll Cardiol 7:138–141, 1986.

58. Gilmour RF, Heger JJ, Prystowsky EN, et al: Cellular electrophysiologic abnormalities of diseased human ventricular myocardium. Am J Cardiol 51:137–144, 1983.

59. Gilmour RF, Zipes DP: Cellular basis for cardiac arrhythmias. Cardiol Clin 1:3–11, 1983.

60. Gomes JA, Dhatt MS, Akhtar M, et al: Effects of digitalis on myocardial and His Purkinje refractoriness and reentry in man. Am J Cardiol 42:931–937, 1978.

61. Gomes JA, Hariman RJ, King PS, et al: Sustained symptomatic sinus node reentrant tachycardia: incidence, electrophysiologic observations and the effects of antiarrhythmic agents. J Am Coll Cardiol 5:45–57, 1985.

62. Gorgels AP, Vos MA, Brugada P, et al: The clinical relevance of abnormal automaticity and triggered activity. In Brugada P, Wellens HT (eds): Cardiac Arrhythmias: Where to Go from There? Mount Kisco, Futura, 1987.

63. Goy JJ, Fromer M, Schlaepfer J, et al: Clinical efficacy of radiofrequency current in the treatment of patients with atrioventricular nodal reentrant tachycardia. J Am Coll Cardiol 16:418–423, 1990.

64. Grant JW, Serwer GA, Armstrong BE, et al: Junctional tachycardia in infants and children after open heart surgery for congenital heart disease. Am J Cardiol 59:1216–1218, 1987.

65. Guiccione P, Paul T, Garson A: Long-term follow-up of amiodarone therapy in the young. J Am Coll Cardiol 15:1118–1124, 1990.

66. Guiraudon G, Klein GJ, Sharma AD, et al: Surgical treatment of Wolff-Parkinson-White syndrome. The epicardial approach. In Benditt DG, Benson DW (eds): Cardiac Preexcitation Syndromes. Boston, Martinus Nijhoff, 1986, pp. 535–542.

67. Gulamhusein S, Ko P, Carruthers G, et al: Acceleration of the ventricular response during atrial fibrillation in the Wolff-Parkinson-White syndrome after verapamil. Circulation 65:348–354, 1982.

68. Haissaguerre M, Warin JF, LeMetayer P, et al: Catheter ablation of Mahaim fibers with preservation of atrioventricular nodal conduction. Circulation 82:418–427, 1990.

69. Harrison DC: Antiarrhythmic drug classification: new science and preexcitations application. Am J Cardiol 56:185–187, 1985.

70. Hastreiter AR, Van der Horst RL, Chow-Ting E: Digitalis toxicity in infants and children. Pediatr Cardiol 5:131–148, 1984.

71. Henthorn RW, Okumura K, Olshansky B, et al: A fourth criteria for transient entrainment: the electrogram equivalent of progressive fusion. Circulation 77:1003–1012, 1988.

72. Hofschire PJ, Nicoloff DM, Moller JH: Postoperative complete heart block in 64 children treated with and without cardiac pacing. Am J Cardiol 39:559–562, 1977.

73. Holman WL, Hackel DB, Lease JG, et al: Cryosurgical ablation of atrioventricular nodal reentry: histologic localization of the proximal common pathway. Circulation 77:1356–1362, 1988.

74. Horowitz LN, Vetter VL, Harken AH, et al: Electrophysiologic characteristics of sustained ventricular tachycardia occurring after repair of tetralogy of Fallot. Am J Cardiol 46:446–452, 1980.

75. Huang SK: Radio-frequency catheter ablation of cardiac arrhythmias: appraisal of an evolving therapeutic modality. Am Heart J 118:1317–1323, 1989.

76. Inoue H, Waller BF, Zipes DP: Intracoronary ethyl alcohol or phenol injections ablates aconitine-induced ventricular tachycardias in dogs. J Am Coll Cardiol 10:1342–1349, 1987.

77. Jackman WM, Friday KJ, Anderson JC, et al: The long QT syndromes: a critical review, new clinical observations and a unifying hypothesis. Prog Cardiovasc Dis 41:115–172, 1988.

78. Jackman W, Wang X, Moulton K, et al: Role of the coronary sinus in radiofrequency ablation of left free wall accessory AV pathways (abstract). Circulation 82:III–689, 1990.

79. Jacobson JR, Garson A, Gillette PC, et al: Premature ventricular contractions in normal children. J Pediatr 92:36–38, 1978.

80. Josephson ME, Kastor JA: Supraventricular tachycardia: mechanism and management. Ann Intern Med 87:346–358, 1977.
81. Katy NM, Blackstone EH, Kirklin JW, et al: Late survival and symptoms after repair of tetralogy of Fallot. Circulation 65:403–410, 1982.
82. Kelly DT, Brodsky SJ, Krovetz LJ: Mobitz type II atrioventricular block in children. J Pediatr 79:972–976, 1971.
83. Kelly PA, Cannon DS, Garan H, et al: The automatic implantable cardioverter-defibrillator: efficacy, complications and survival in patients with malignant ventricular arrhythmias. J Am Coll Cardiol 11:1278–1286, 1988.
84. Kerr CR, Gallagher JJ, German LD: Changes in ventriculoatrial intervals with bundle branch block aberration during reciprocating tachycardia in patients with accessory atrioventricular pathways. Circulation 66:196–201, 1982.
85. Kimura S, Cameron JS, Kozlousky PL, et al: Delayed afterdepolarizations and triggered activity induced in feline Purkinje fibers by alpha-adrenergic stimulation in the presence of elevated calcium levels. Circulation 70:1074–1082, 1984.
86. Klein GJ, Bashore TM, Sellers TD, et al: Ventricular fibrillation in the Wolff-Parkinson-White syndrome. N Engl J Med 301:1080–1085, 1979.
87. Klein GJ, Guiraudon GM, Kerr CR, et al: "Nodoventricular" accessory pathways: evidence for a distinct accessory atrioventricular pathway with atrioventricular node-like properties. J Am Coll Cardiol 11:1035–1040, 1988.
88. Klein GJ, Guiraudon GM, Sharma AD, et al: Demonstration of macroreentry and feasibility of operative therapy in the common type of atrial flutter. Am J Cardiol 57:587–591, 1986.
89. Klitzner TS, Friedman WF: Cardiac arrhythmias: the role of pharmacologic intervention. Cardiol Clin 7:299–318, 1989.
90. Kowey PR, Eisenberg R, Engle TR: Sustained arrhythmias in hypertrophic obstructive cardiomyopathy. N Engl J Med 310:1566–1569, 1984.
91. Kron J, Oliver RP, Norsted S, et al: The automatic implantable cardioverter-defibrillator (AICD) in young patients (abstract). Circulation 80:II–389, 1989.
92. Kugler JD, Danford DA: Pacemakers in children: an update. Am Heart J 117:665–679, 1989.
93. Levine JH, Michael JR, Guarnieri T: Treatment of multifocal atrial tachycardia with verapamil. N Engl J Med 312:21–25, 1985.
94. Liberthson RR, Colan SD: Multifocal or chaotic atrial rhythm: report of nine infants, delineation, and review of the literature. Pediatr Cardiol 2:179–184, 1982.
95. Liberthson RR, Dinsmore RE, Fallon JT: Aberrant coronary artery origin from the aorta. Circulation 59:748–754, 1979.
96. Lillehei CW, Sellers RD, Bonnabeau RC, et al: Chronic postsurgical complete heart block with particular reference to prognosis, management and a new P wave pacemaker. J Thorac Cardiovasc Surg 46:436–456, 1963.
97. Lowenthal DT, Porter S, Saris SD, et al: Clinical pharmacology, pharmacodynamics and interactions with esmolol. Am J Cardiol 56:14F–17F, 1985.
98. Lucchesi BR: Rationale of therapy in the patient with acute myocardial infarction and life-threatening arrhythmias: a focus on bretylium. Am J Cardiol 54:14A–19A, 1984.
99. Mancini GB, Goldberger AL: Cardioversion of atrial fibrillation: consideration of embolization, anticoagulation prophylactic pacemaker and long term success. Am Heart J 104:617–621, 1982.
100. Martin TC, Smith L, Hernandez A, et al: Dysrhythmias following the Senning operation for dextro-trans-

101. position of the great arteries. J Thorac Cardiovasc Surg 85:928–932, 1983.
101. Mason JW: Amiodarone. N Engl J Med 316:455–466, 1987.
102. McCue CM, Mantakas ME, Tingelstad JB, et al: Congenital heart block in newborns of mothers with connective tissue disease. Circulation 56:82–90, 1977.
103. Meinertz T, Treese N, Kasper W, et al: Determinants of prognosis in idiopathic dilated cardiomyopathy as determined by programmed electrical stimulation. Am J Cardiol 56:337–341, 1985.
104. Merideth J, Mendez C, Mueller WJ, et al: Electrical excitability of atrioventricular nodal cells. Circ Res 23:69–85, 1968.
105. Michaelsson M, Engle MA: Congenital complete heart block: an international study of the maternal history. Cardiovasc Clin 4:85–101, 1972.
106. Moak JP: Pharmacology and electrophysiology of antiarrhythmic drugs. In Gillette PC, Garson A: Pediatric Arrhythmias: Electrophysiology and Pacing. Philadelphia, W.B. Saunders, 1990, pp. 37–115.
107. Moak JP, Smith RT, Garson A: Mexiletine: an effective antiarrhythmic drug for treatment of ventricular arrhythmias in congenital heart disease. J Am Coll Cardiol 10:824–829, 1987.
108. Moe GK, Abildoshov JA: Antiarrhythmic drugs. In Goodman LS, Gilman A (eds): The Pharmacologic Basis of Therapeutics. New York, Macmillan, 1975, p. 688.
109. Morady F, Scheinman MM, Winston SA, et al: Efficacy and safety of transcatheter ablation of posteroseptal accessory pathways. Circulation 72:170–177, 1985.
110. Olshausen KV, Stienen V, Math D, et al: Long term prognostic significance of ventricular arrhythmias in idiopathic dilated cardiomyopathy. Am J Cardiol 61:146–151, 1988.
111. Overholt ED, Rheuban KS, Gutgesell HP, et al: Usefulness of adenosine for arrhythmias in infants and children. Am J Cardiol 61:336–340, 1988.
112. Perloff JK: Neurologic disorders and heart disease. In Braunwald E (ed): Heart Disease. Philadelphia, W.B. Saunders, 1984, pp. 1704–1721.
113. Pickoff AS, Singh S, Gelband H: The medical management of cardiac arrhythmias. In Roberts NK, Gelband H (eds): Cardiac Arrhythmias in the Neonate, Infant and Child. Norwalk, CT. Appleton-Century-Crofts, 1983, pp. 297–340.
114. Pinsky WW, Gillette PC, Garson A, et al: Diagnosis, management and long term results of patients with congenital complete atrioventricular block. Pediatrics 69:728–733, 1982.
115. Rosen KM, Rahimtoola SH, Gunnar RM: Pseudo AV block secondary to premature nonpropagated His bundle depolarization. Circulation 42:367–373, 1970.
116. Rossi P, Massumi A, Gillette PC, et al: Arrhythmogenic right ventricular dysplasia: clinical features, diagnostic techniques, and current management. Am Heart J 103:415–421, 1982.
117. Saksena S: Catheter ablation of tachycardia with laser energy: issues and answers. Pace 12:196–203, 1989.
118. Saul JP, Rhodes LA, Walsh EP: Sotalol: investigational therapy for infants and children with refractory supraventricular and ventricular arrhythmias (abstract). J Am Coll Cardiol 15:176A, 1990.
119. Saul JP, Walsh EP, Langberg JJ, et al: Radiofrequency ablation of accessory atrioventricular pathways: early results in children with refractory SVT (abstract). Circulation 80:III–222, 1990.
120. Scher DL, Arsura EL: Multifocal atrial tachycardia: mechanisms, clinical correlates and treatment. Am Heart J 118:574–580, 1989.
121. Scheinman MM: Catheter ablation for patients with ventricular preexcitation syndromes. In Benditt DG,

Benson DW (eds): Cardiac Preexcitation Syndromes. Boston, Martinus Nijhoff, 1986, p. 493.

122. Scherf L, Neufeld HN: The Preexcitation Syndrome: Facts and Theories. New York, Yorke Medical Books, 1978.

123. Schwartz PJ: Idiopathic long QT syndrome: progress and questions. Am Heart J 109:399–412, 1985.

124. Schwartz PJ, Mallian A: Electrical alternation of the T wave: clinical and experimental evidence of its relationship with the sympathetic nervous system and with the long QT syndrome. Am Heart J 89:45–50, 1975.

125. Sellers TD, Bashore TM, Gallagher JJ: Digitalis in the preexcitation syndrome: analysis during atrial fibrillation. Circulation 56:260–267, 1975.

126. Shaffer EM, Rocchini AP, Spicer RL, et al: Effects of verapamil on left ventricular diastolic filling in children with hypertrophic cardiomyopathy. Am J Cardiol 61:413–417, 1988.

127. Sharma AD, Klein GJ, Guiraudon GM, et al: Atrial fibrillation in patients with Wolff-Parkinson-White syndrome: incidence after surgical ablation of the accessory pathway. Circulation 72:161–169, 1985.

128. Sholler GE, Walsh EP: Congenital complete heart block in patients without anatomic cardiac defects. Am Heart J 118:1193–1198, 1989.

129. Sholler GE, Walsh EP, Mayer JE, et al: Evaluation of a staged treatment protocol for postoperative rapid junctional tachycardia (abstract). Circulation 78:II–597, 1988.

130. Singh BN, Collett JT, Chew CY: New prospectives in the pharmacologic therapy of cardiac arrhythmias. Prog Cardiovasc Dis 22:243–301, 1980.

131. Smith TW, Butler VP, Haber E, et al: Treatment of life threatening digitalis intoxication and digoxin-specific Fab antibody fragments. N Engl J Med 307:1357–1362, 1982.

132. Smith TW, Haber E: Digitalis. N Engl J Med 289:945–951, 1973.

133. Southall DP, Johnson F, Shinebourne EA, et al: 24 hour electrocardiographic study of heart rate and rhythm in population of healthy children. Br Heart J 45:281–291, 1981.

134. Southall DP, Richards J, Mitchell P, et al: Study of cardiac rhythm in healthy newborn infants. Br Heart J 43:14–20, 1980.

135. Strasburger JF, Moak JP, Smith RT, et al: Encainide for refractory supraventricular tachycardia in children. Am J Cardiol 58:49C–55C, 1986.

136. Strasburger JF, Smith RT, Moak JP, et al: Encainide for resistant supraventricular tachycardia in children: follow-up report. Am J Cardiol 62:50L–54L, 1988.

137. Sullivan ID, Presbitero P, Gooch VM, et al: Is ventricular arrhythmia in repaired tetralogy of Fallot an effect of operation or a consequence of the course of the disease? Br Heart J 58:40–47, 1987.

138. Till JA, Rowland E, Shinebourne EA, et al: R-wave synchronized atrial pacing in the management of post surgical His bundle tachycardia (abstract). Circulation 78:II–597, 1988.

139. Trippel DL, Gillette PC: Should atenolol be used in children with long QT syndrome? (abstract) Circulation 80:II–338, 1989.

140. Tzivoni D, Banai S, Schuger C, et al: Treatment of torsade de pointes with magnesium sulfate. Circulation 77:392–397, 1988.

141. Valdes-Dapena M: Are some crib deaths sudden cardiac deaths? J Am Coll Cardiol 5:113B–117B, 1985.

142. Vaughan Williams EM: Classification of antiarrhythmic drugs. In Sandoe E, Flensted-Jansen E, Olesen KH (eds): Symposium on Cardiac Arrhythmias. Sodertalje, Sweden, AB Astra, 1970, pp. 449–472.

143. Venditte FJ, Garan H, Rusbin JN: Electrophysiologic effects of beta blockers in ventricular arrhythmias. Am J Cardiol 60:3D–10D, 1987.

144. Viitasalo MT, Kala R, Eisalo A: Ambulatory electrocardiographic findings in young athletes between 14 and 16 years of age. Eur Heart J 5:2–6, 1984.

145. Waldo AL, Akhtar M, Benditt DG, et al: Appropriate electrophysiologic study and treatment of patients with Wolff-Parkinson-White syndrome. J Am Coll Cardiol 11:1124–1129, 1988.

146. Walsh EP, Rhodes LA, Saul JP: Triggered activity as the possible mechanism for exercise-induced ventricular tachycardia in young patients (abstract). Pace 13:541, 1990.

147. Walsh EP, Rockenmacher S, Keane JF, et al: Late results for patients with tetralogy of Fallot repaired during infancy. Circulation 77:1062–1067, 1988.

148. Weber HS, Hellenbrand WE, Kleinman CS, et al: Predictors of rhythm disturbances and subsequent morbidity after the Fontan operation. Am J Cardiol 64:762–767, 1989.

149. Winkler RB, Freed MD, Nadas AS: Exercise induced ventricular ectopy in children and young adults with complete heart block. Am Heart J 99:87–92, 1980.

150. Wolff L, Parkinson J, White PD: Bundle branch block with short PR interval in healthy young people prone to paroxysmal tachycardia. Am Heart J 5:685–704, 1930.

151. Woosley RL, Funck-Brentano C: Overview of the clinical pharmacology of antiarrhythmic drugs. Am J Cardiol 61:61A–69A, 1988.

152. Wu D, Denes P, Amat-Y-Leon F, et al: Clinical, electrocardiographic and electrophysiologic observations in patients with paroxysmal supraventricular tachycardia. Am J Cardiol 41:1045–1051, 1978.

153. Yeager SB, Hougen TJ, Levy AM: Sudden death in infants with chaotic atrial rhythm. Am J Dis Child 138:689–692, 1984.

154. Zeigler V, Gillette PC, Hammill B, et al: Flecainide for supraventricular tachycardia in children. Am J Cardiol 622:410–430, 1988.

155. Zipes DP: Second-degree atrioventricular block. Circulation 60:465–472, 1979.

156. Zipes DP: Specific arrhythmias: diagnosis and treatment. In Braunwald E (ed): Heart Disease. Philadelphia, W.B. Saunders, 1984, p. 700.

157. Zipes DP, Foster PR, Troup PJ, et al: Atrial induction of ventricular tachycardia: reentry versus triggered automaticity. Am J Cardiol 44:1–8, 1979.

Section IX
CONGENITAL HEART DISEASE

Chapter 28

VENTRICULAR SEPTAL DEFECT

Donald C. Fyler, M.D.

DEFINITION

The term ventricular septal defect describes an opening in the ventricular septum. Ventricular defects may be located anywhere in the ventricular septum, may be single or multiple, and may be of variable size and shape. At Children's Hospital in Boston, **ventricular septal defect** includes patients with isolated or multiple ventricular septal defects and ventricular defects with an associated atrial defect, patent ductus arteriosus, or some valvar abnormalities (Exhibit 1).

PREVALENCE

Sixteen percent of patients seen with heart disease at Children's Hospital in Boston in recent years have had ventricular defects as defined above. The following facts confuse the estimation of the incidence of ventricular septal defect.

1. There can be confusion about which patients should be included in the category ventricular septal defect. If 50% of patients with congenital heart disease have a ventricular opening, which ones should be included under the heading ventricular septal defect? Truncus arteriosus, tricuspid atresia, tetralogy of Fallot, common atrioventricular canal, and others characteristically have ventricular defects. These specific syndromes and other well-recognized complexes are excluded from consideration; those patients who are born with ventricular defects as the dominant lesion or have an associated patent ductus arteriosus or atrial septal defect are included. The definition used here is arbitrary but reflects our local usage.

2. Ventricular septal defect is more common among premature infants and stillborns.[33,46,47]

3. Spontaneous closure of ventricular septal defect occurs in 15–50% of observed cases,[1,2,7,22,47,58] largely in the first 6 months of life. Consequently, the incidence may be underestimated if the list of patients does not include neonates and infants.

4. Case discovery depends on the tools employed. For example, in the past, the diagnosis often was based on presence of a blowing, regurgitant murmur at the left sternal border without other supporting evidence. Errors were introduced because, in the first days of life, a murmur of ventricular septal defect is not yet present while similar murmurs of tricuspid regurgitation and pulmonary stenosis are. The decrease in relative frequency of ventricular septal defects in recent years can be attributed to improved diagnosis (see ch. 18) primarily because of the increased use of echocardiograms.

5. Echocardiographic diagnosis has become available only recently and as yet a detailed prospective study has not been carried out.

6. Because detection of small, isolated ventricular defects is of little practical consequence, the impetus to learn the "true" incidence is not compelling.

It is a tenable hypothesis that in an undetermined but significant number of children, the ventricular septum does not close as expected during the course of fetal and postnatal life but that the open ventricular septum does close later. As a corollary, at any time from the first 2 weeks after conception through adulthood, there are a decreasing number of individuals with an opening in the ventricular septum.

Exhibit 1

Boston Children's Hospital Experience 1973–1987 **Ventricular Septal Defect**			
Associated Defects		Hierarchical listing*	All†
Aortic Stenosis		117	117
Valvar stenosis	40		
Supravalvar stenosis	4		
Subvalvar stenosis	69		
Nonspecific stenosis	22		
Aortic Regurgitation		90	138
Mitral Stenosis		22	30
Valvar stenosis	26		
Supravalvar stenosis	5		
Cor triatriatum	3		
Mitral Regurgitation		72	102
Pulmonary Stenosis		425	533
Valvar stenosis	334		
Subvalvar stenosis	61		
Double-chambered right ventricle	135		
Supravalvar stenosis	37		
Peripheral stenosis	98		
Pulmonary Regurgitation		22	64
Tricuspid Valve		83	189
Valvar regurgitation	180		
Ebstein's disease	4		
Valvar stenosis	7		
Other	20		
Patent Ductus Arteriosus		170	296
Atrial Septal Defect		86	238
Uncomplicated Ventricular Septal Defect		2235	2235
Total		3322	

*Arbitrarily records each patient once according to position in the hierarchial list.
†Lists each time a lesion was found; thus, some patients appear several times.
There were 3322 patients classified as having a ventricular septal defect as the dominant lesion. Almost 54% were first seen in the first year of life, while 76% had been seen by the age of 5 years and 88% by the age of 10 years. Each year during this period, 100–200 new patients were encountered. They were subcategorized by associated cardiac lesions.

Despite the high incidence of spontaneous closure, isolated ventricular septal defect is the most common congenital heart defect encountered after the first weeks of life and remains the most common congenital cardiac defect seen through the first three decades of life (see ch. 18). Depending on the ages of the children examined and the type of examination, figures ranging from 1 to 7 per 1000 live births are given as the incidence of ventricular defects.[33,36,46,47,50]

There is a need to plan diagnostic and therapeutic services for infants with ventricular septal defect. There are 0.35–0.50 infants per 1000 live births who have a ventricular septal defect of sufficient size to require diagnostic or therapeutic intervention[23] (15% of all ventricular defects).[15]

In the late 1970s an epidemic of ventricular septal defect was reported by the Centers for Disease Control.[38,53] Retrospectively, the prevalence of several congenital cardiac lesions rose during this time in response to deliberate attempts to improve case discovery. With improved imaging techniques, the number of patients labeled as having ventricular septal defect has decreased considerably in recent years (see ch. 18).

EMBRYOLOGY

A ventricular septal defect results from a delay in closure of the interventricular septum beyond the first 7 weeks of intrauterine life; the reasons for delayed or incomplete closure are unknown.

Any theory of etiology should consider and explain the following observations. A variety of other cardiac and noncardiac anomalies are associated with ventricular defects, and some chromosomal abnormalities and many syndromes include ventricular defects as a problem. There is some evidence suggesting variation in incidence for certain years[53,61] and different seasons. Geographic differences have been noted but these seem to be related mostly to differences in case finding. Asian populations have a greater incidence of subpulmonary defects.[3,49] The offspring of survivors have a higher incidence of congenital heart disease[71] but the familial incidence of ventricular defect is not as prominent a feature[52] as it is among some other congenital cardiac defects (3% of children of parents with ventricular septal defect also have a ventricular defect).[17] Ventricular defects are distinctly more common among premature infants and those with low birth weights, with reports of incidence as high as 7.06 per 1000 live premature births.[47] Studies of birth order and maternal age show no correlation with the presence of a ventricular septal defect.[62]

ANATOMY

Ventricular defects are classified by their location in the septum (Fig. 1).

A wide variety of terms is used to classify the location of ventricular septal defects. A partial list includes: membranous, high, subaortic, subarterial, subpulmonary, doubly committed, infundibular, supracristal, intracristal, subcristal, trabecular, muscular, posterior, anterior, mid, apical, Swiss cheese, endocardial cushion type, atrioventricular canal type, malalignment, inlet, outlet, hyphenated combinations of the above and others (Fig. 1).[11,18,26,27,41,63] At Children's Hospital in Boston, the following classifications are used:

Membranous Defects

Membranous defects are by far the most common, accounting for fully 75% of ventricular septal

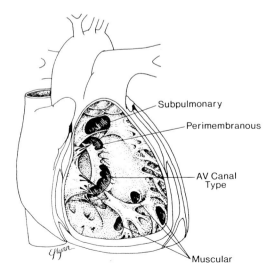

Figure 1. Diagram of types of ventricular septal defects as viewed from the right ventricle.

defects (Exhibit 2). The membranous septum is a small area, immediately adjacent to and under the aortic valve on the left side, contiguous to the septal leaflet of the tricuspid valve on the right side, and overlapping a small segment of the right atrium. Congenital or acquired abnormalities of the aortic valve may be associated with membranous defects. The tricuspid valve may be involved in the formation of a ventricular septal aneurysm and may be damaged by the jet of blood passing through a small membranous defect. Rarely, a defect in the membranous septum opens solely into the right atrium, allowing a left ventricular–right

Exhibit 2

Boston Children's Hospital Experience 1973–1987 **Ventricular Septal Defect Location in Septum**		
Location	Isolated	All
Membranous	872	973
Muscular	122	198
Infundibular	40	58
Endocardial cushion type	14	48
Malalignment	11	26
Multiple	36*	107
Combinations	138†	
Total	1233‡	

*No other categorization was used.

†This figure may not represent multiple ventricular defects because a single defect could be described in different ways on different occasions—multiple ventricular defect can be no higher than 138 or lower than 107.

‡Categorization of location in the septum was not systematically carried out until echocardiographic identification became possible.

The location of the ventricular septal defect in the ventricular septum was not routinely recorded in the earlier years. Of 1233 for whom there was data, 71% of isolated defects were said to be membranous; 79% had a membranous ventricular defect, if those with multiple defects are included.

Spontaneous closure was a feature of membranous and muscular ventricular defects. There were no instances of spontaneous closure among the endocardial cushion, subpulmonary, or malalignment defects. Spontaneous closure of the ventricular defect was noted in 492 patients (20%). The defect was described as closed or the patient was later declared to have a normal heart. This was noted most commonly in the earlier years in patients in whom the diagnosis was based solely on clinical observations, without the backup of echocardiography or cardiac catheterization. Among patients whose diagnosis was documented with catheterization or echocardiography, only 8% were listed as having spontaneous closure, whereas almost 30% of patients diagnosed as having a ventricular septal defect on clinical grounds were later thought to have had spontaneous closure. These data are somewhat misleading because patients diagnosed by echocardiography (mostly in recent years) have offered less opportunity for follow-up than have all others and, of necessity, this group included the sicker patients.

atrial shunt. Because the membranous septum is a small area, most defects extend into the immediately adjacent infundibular region; hence the synonymous term **perimembranous**. There may be **malalignment** of the great arteries and ventricles favoring either the right or left (anterior or posterior) and associated with encroachment of either right or left ventricular outflow. Malalignment defects are characteristic of the tetralogy of Fallot syndrome (see ch. 30).

Muscular Defects

Muscular defects may be located anywhere in the apical, mid, anterior, or posterior muscular septum and are often multiple. Sometimes these defects seem multiple when viewed from the right ventricle (the usual surgical approach) because trabeculations overlie a large defect that is discovered to be single when viewed from the left ventricular side (Fig. 2).

Infundibular (Subpulmonary) Defects

These are located under the pulmonary valve when viewed from the right ventricle, and when viewed from the left ventricle they are immediately beneath the aortic valve. The adjacent aortic valve cusps often prolapse into the ventricular defect with or without aortic regurgitation.

Endocardial Cushion Type of Defects

These are located beneath the tricuspid valve, extending to the tricuspid valve ring, and they occupy the area where an atrioventricularis communis opening would be found. The other stigmata of endocardial cushion defects, leftward-superior axis on the electrocardiogram and atrioventricular valve abnormalities, are not necessarily present.

The incidence of the various types of ventricular defects is reported to be the same in patients with or without coarctation of the aorta but different among patients with D-transposition.[48] Although not studied in detail, this distinction has not been obvious in our experience.

PHYSIOLOGY

The size of the defect and the pulmonary vascular resistance determine the hemodynamics in these patients. Normally, high fetal, pulmonary arteriolar resistance decreases rapidly with the first breath and in the first hours of life; later the decrease is more gradual (see ch. 10) and it stabilizes at adult levels about the age of 3–6 months. After birth, as pulmonary vascular resistance falls, left-to-right shunting through the ventricular defect begins and increases in the first days and weeks of life. Smaller defects allow the right ventricular and pulmonary arterial pressure to fall proportional to the drop in pulmonary resistance. With large defects (greater than 50% of the aortic diameter) there is obligatory equilibration of pressures between the two ventricles. Fortunately, in these infants involution of the fetal pulmonary arteriolar structures is delayed or is reinstated very early[34] (there is considerable individual variation); otherwise, the systemic circulation would bleed into the pulmonary circulation. The larger the ventricular defect and the lower the pulmonary resistance the greater the left-to-right shunt. Up to the point of equalization of the right and left ventricular pressures the size of the shunt is dictated by the size of the hole. When the ventricular pressures are equilibrated, the size of the shunt is determined by the relative levels of the pulmonary arterial and the systemic resistances (Fig. 3).

The bulk of shunting occurs in systole with lesser amounts in diastole. Muscular defects may become smaller in systole, allowing less shunting than expected for the size of the defect.

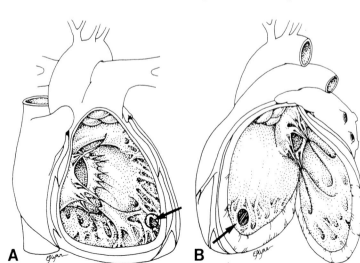

Figure 2. Diagram of apical muscular ventricular septal defect as viewed from the right (**A**) and left (**B**) ventricle. Note that from the right side, shunted blood passes through multiple trabeculations, whereas from the left ventricle a single defect is present. An occluding patch is more readily applied to the left septal wall.

A   B

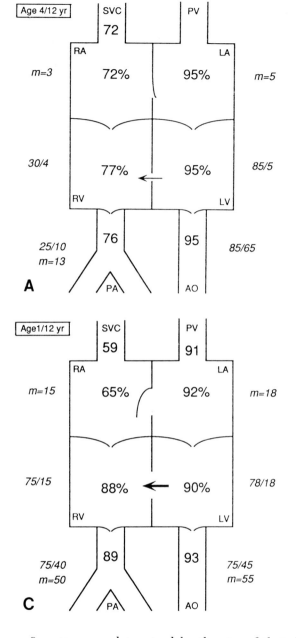

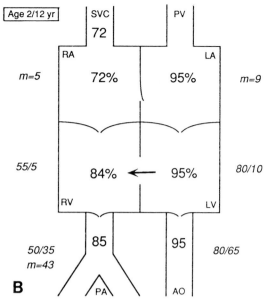

Figure 3. Diagrams of small (A), medium (B), and large (C) ventricular septal defects. **A,** There is no pulmonary hypertension and the left to right shunt is small. **B,** There is significant shunting and some elevation of the right ventricular pressure. **C,** There is equilibration of the right and left ventricular pressures and a very large shunt. Note that the borderline arterial oxygen saturation results from low pulmonary venous oxygen due either to pulmonary overcirculation or pulmonary edema.

Symptoms are determined by the size of the shunt. If the shunt is small, the infant is asymptomatic; if the shunt is large (pulmonary flow greater than or equal to 2.5 times the systemic blood flow), congestive heart failure may appear. With a large defect congestive heart failure can occur within days of birth, but it is usually delayed until the third week of life or, rarely, as late as 6 months after birth with solitary lesions. Other factors that promote the appearance of congestive failure in the first days of life include additional cardiac defects (sometimes unsuspected), intercurrent respiratory infection, anemia, noncardiac congenital anomalies, and prematurity.[47]

Left-to-right shunting increases the amount of blood passing through the right ventricle, pulmonary arteries, left atrium, and left ventricle and, if the defect is large enough, there is also hypertension of the pulmonary artery, right ventricle and left atrium. The abnormalities of chest x-rays, electrocardiograms, angiocardiograms, and echocardiograms are direct functions of these hemodynamic realities.

An additional patent ductus arteriosus increases the amount of left-to-right shunting, but if the combination of a patent ductus arteriosus and a ventricular defect results in equilibration of pressures, the amount shunted depends primarily on the relative pulmonary and systemic resistances, with little relation to the combined size of the defects.

An additional atrial septal defect increases the amount of left-to-right shunting by venting the left atrium, but elevation of right ventricular pressure is still dependent on the size of the ventricular defect and the pulmonary vascular resistance.

Additional valvar abnormalities, such as aortic stenosis, aortic regurgitation, mitral regurgitation, or mitral stenosis, influence the hemodynamics in proportion to the added pressure and volume work demanded.

A large ventricular defect is better tolerated when there is counterbalancing pulmonary stenosis. The relation of the systemic resistance to the resistance provided by pulmonary stenosis determines whether there is right-to-left or left-to-right shunting and how much. Two decades ago, when the repair of ventricular septal defects had a high mortality, surgeons successfully reduced the left-to-right shunting through pulmonary artery banding. Subsequently, there was improvement in congestive heart failure and improved growth in infants formerly in critical trouble with ventricular septal defects.

Elevation of pulmonary vascular resistance by any mechanism reduces left-to-right shunting. Hypoxia (high altitude) increases pulmonary vascular resistance and decreases the amount of left-to-right shunt. At high altitudes children with ventricular defects develop congestive heart failure less commonly than their contemporaries at sea level, and they may develop heart failure on descent to sea level.[67] Similarly, patients with pulmonary arterial hypertension caused by pulmonary venous hypertension have less of a left-to-right shunt. Surgical relief of mitral stenosis in the presence of a large ventricular septal defect can result in a large left-to-right shunt and congestive heart failure even though the patient was cyanotic originally (Fig. 4). As patients with large ventricular defects get older (age 12 months or older), irreversible pulmonary vascular obstructive disease may occur.[12,30,51] The hemodynamic effect is comparable to pulmonary artery banding and may actually help the patient symptomatically by reducing the volume load; however, if the pulmonary vascular disease becomes irreversible, it becomes the overriding determinant of the future of the patient.[29,56,57] Fortunately, normal fetal pulmonary vascular changes usually involute after birth, only rarely persisting and advancing to permanent abnormality after the age of 12 months. During the window of delayed appearance the ventricular defect can be repaired safely, but once irreversible pulmonary vascular disease is established, repair of the defect is not helpful and may be fatal.

CLINICAL MANIFESTATIONS

Discovery

Most infants with ventricular septal defect are asymptomatic because most defects are too small to allow sufficient left-to-right shunting to cause symptoms. Consequently, most ventricular septal defects are discovered through routine auscultation by the pediatrician on discharge from the neonatal nursery or at the first postnatal checkup. Another significant group (20–30% of symptomatic patients) is discovered when some other noncardiac congenital anomaly is observed and a search for additional anomalies leads to discovery of a heart murmur. Larger defects may produce only tachypnea, but among the largest ones, symptoms of gross congestive failure, tachypnea, dyspnea, reduced fluid intake, and poor growth call attention to the underlying abnormality.

The age at which the murmur of ventricular septal defect first appears is not well documented because the scheduling of routine well-baby visits determines when the pediatrician listens for a murmur. This murmur is present in the first week of life unless there is some other cardiac or pulmonary defect that prohibits the normal regression of pulmonary hypertension.

While a small number of infants who are symptomatic because of a ventricular defect are transferred to a cardiac unit in the first week of life, the average age at first cardiac hospitalization is 6 weeks. In general, the sickest babies are the youngest but many who come to the attention of a cardiologist in the first week of life have other major congenital anomalies that prompted the examination for heart disease. Often superimposed respiratory infections precipitate hospitalization (respiratory syncytial virus is common).

Even though only about 15% of all ventricular septal defects are large enough to cause symptoms, this is still the most common form of congenital heart disease requiring hospitalization after the first 2 weeks of life.

Symptoms

Infants with large defects present with symptoms caused by congestive heart failure and superimposed respiratory infections. Tachypnea, with respiratory rates regularly over 60 breaths per minute, is a first symptom, often recognized in retrospect by the mother or grandmother as having been present from birth. Such a baby may grow and develop normally for some time without other symptoms. Those with more severe dyspnea will be unable to nurse normally, resting frequently and requiring more than 20 minutes to ingest an appropriate feeding. Regurgitation is common and vomiting occurs when there is severe congestive failure (see ch. 7). Growth failure is a common problem,[40,50,73] although growth may be satisfactory initially, only later slowing down. In the worst case, the infant never exceeds birth weight because of poor caloric intake and increased oxygen consumption due to excessive work of the heart and lungs.

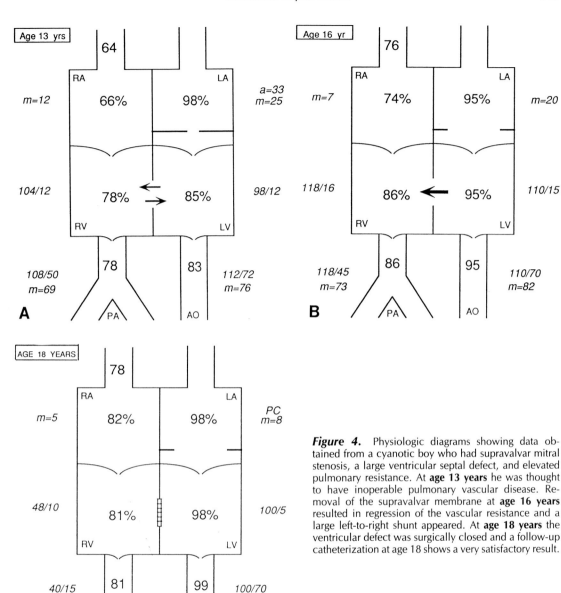

Figure 4. Physiologic diagrams showing data obtained from a cyanotic boy who had supravalvar mitral stenosis, a large ventricular septal defect, and elevated pulmonary resistance. At **age 13 years** he was thought to have inoperable pulmonary vascular disease. Removal of the supravalvar membrane at **age 16 years** resulted in regression of the vascular resistance and a large left-to-right shunt appeared. At **age 18 years** the ventricular defect was surgically closed and a follow-up catheterization at age 18 shows a very satisfactory result.

Older patients seen for the first time may be referred because of arrhythmia, congestive heart failure, hemoptysis, and bacterial endocarditis.[19]

Physical Examination

The sick infant is most often malnourished and scrawny. Often there is tachypnea with respiratory rates ranging upwards of 100 breaths per minute, associated with subcostal, sternal, or suprasternal retractions. The liver is large and the spleen may be palpable. Surprisingly, the peripheral pulses are generally good even when the infant looks quite ill. The heart rate is fast. The cardiac impulse is hyperdynamic.

The systolic murmur of ventricular septal defect is influenced by the size of the defect, the pressure difference between the two ventricles, and the amount of left-to-right shunting. As a rule, ventricular septal defects with solely right-to-left shunting do not produce systolic murmurs. This intuitively unexpected phenomenon results from the fact that right-to-left shunting is comparatively small and not associated with a difference in pressure between the ventricles. It follows that the systolic murmur in patients who are cyanotic with the tetralogy of Fallot syndrome results from pulmonary stenosis, not from the ventricular septal defect. The smaller defects produce the loudest murmurs. These systolic, ejection murmurs peak in midsystole and are usually heard best at the lower left sternal border where there may be a thrill (Fig. 5).

Among patients with larger defects the murmur is pansystolic and of constant intensity, without a midsystolic peak. Thrills are less common. Because of excessive blood flow through the mitral valve, there is usually a loud third heart sound and often an apical diastolic rumble (Fig. 6). On initial examination of these sick infants, the heart rate is so fast that an apical diastolic rumble cannot be heard with certainty. Often a loud gallop can be heard. Only later, with treatment and with a slower heart rate, can the diastolic rumbling murmur be more confidently described. Usually, the second heart sound is narrowly split and the pulmonary component accentuated. The presence of pulmonary rales most often signifies pulmonary infection or atelectasis and not pulmonary edema, although pressure by the enlarged left atrium on the bronchus may be the cause of rales in these children.

Beyond infancy a small ventricular septal defect (a few mm in diameter) produces the characteristic findings of the **Maladie de Roger**. The murmur is loud, commonly grade 5, and is associated with a thrill at the point of maximal intensity. The murmur is maximal at the lower left sternal border but may be heard higher when the defect is subpulmonary. It is heard well at the xiphoid, the cardiac apex, and along the upper left sternal border. With progressively smaller defects the murmur becomes less intense.

Uncomplicated large ventricular septal defects

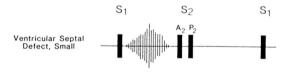

Figure 5. Diagram of auscultatory findings in a child with a small ventricular septal defect. S_1, first heart sound; S_2, second heart sound; A_2, aortic closure; P_2, pulmonary closure. The diamond-shaped murmur suggests a pressure gradient from the left to the right ventricle. Note the similarity to the murmur of pulmonary stenosis. (From Avery ME, First LP (eds): Pediatric Medicine. Baltimore, Williams & Wilkins, 1989, with permission.)

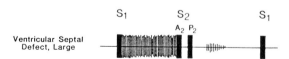

Figure 6. Diagram of auscultatory findings in a child with a large ventricular septal defect. S_1, first heart sound; S_2, second heart sound; A_2, aortic valve closure; P_2, pulmonary valve closure. Note the high frequency, pansystolic murmur that extends from the first to the second heart sound. Note the low-frequency apical diastolic rumble. (From Avery ME, First LP (eds): Pediatric Medicine, Baltimore, Williams & Wilkins, 1989, with permission.)

are seen rarely in older children today. Very large ones may produce little murmur, either because of the large size of the defect or because there is minimal shunting because of pulmonary vascular disease (see p. 449).

The apical, diastolic, rumbling murmur heard in patients with large ventricular septal defects results from excessive blood flow through the mitral valve. The presence of a rumble is a crude indication of the size of the shunt and the defect, although, rarely, it is the result of some anatomic obstruction of the mitral valve.

Electrocardiography

Patients with small ventricular septal defects have normal electrocardiograms. With larger defects the electrocardiogram shows left ventricular hypertrophy of the volume overload type (see ch. 12) and with high right ventricular pressure there is right ventricular hypertrophy as well. There may be left atrial P waves.

Presumably, at birth, the electrocardiogram is normal in all patients because the fetal circulation with ventricular septal defect, large or small, is scarcely different from normal. Therefore it follows that the electrocardiographic abnormalities are acquired after birth. Of course, this is difficult to document because the largest defects produce the least murmurs and are rarely evaluated before symptoms develop, the electrocardiogram having had an opportunity to evolve.

Chest X-ray

The volume overload caused by the left-to-right shunt produces chamber enlargement proportional to the size of the shunt. It is difficult to learn from the x-ray which chambers contribute to the enlargement, with the possible exception of left atrial enlargement as estimated in appropriate views. The best measure of the amount of left-to-right shunting is the presence of increased pulmonary vascularity associated with comparable overall cardiac enlargement. The excessive water in the lungs of patients with large right shunts[66] is not visible, although signs of congestive heart failure, especially as indistinct and increased vascular markings, may be present. Outright pulmonary edema sufficient to cause Kerley B lines is rare.

Echocardiography

Whether directly demonstrable by two-dimensional imaging or detectable by the more sensitive Doppler techniques, especially the most sensitive Doppler color flow mapping, essentially all ventricular septal defects can be identified provided there is sufficient shunting. Because defects with minimal or no shunting are not detected by the Doppler examination, such defects may be overlooked if the size is below the limits of resolution of the imaging device. This is particularly true if there is more than one defect. It has become axiomatic that whenever two ventricular defects are identified, unidentified additional defects are likely to be present. Usually, the septal location of a ventricular defect can be confidently defined. The size of the left-to-right shunt can be estimated by the relative sizes of the chambers and by the Doppler techniques.

Subxiphoid views, especially the short-axis views, are excellent for imaging most ventricular septal defects in infants and small children.[72] However, for accurate localization, a defect should be imaged in at least two planes—a long-axis and short-axis plane of the heart.

Membranous defects are seen well in parasternal short-axis (Fig. 7) and apical four-chamber views. An "aneurysm" (really the septal leaflet of the tricuspid valve) associated with the defect is seen best in these views as well. In the parasternal short-axis view the membranous defect is posterior and rightward, near the crux of the heart. The parasternal short-axis view usually provides the most advantageous orientation for Doppler examination.

Muscular ventricular septal defects should be imaged in a subxiphoid or parasternal short-axis view to determine the location and in an anterior-posterior axis and an apical view to define the position in an apex-to-base direction (Fig. 8). Doppler color flow mapping can be performed in these views as well (see Fig. 6, p. 165). Color flow mapping is essential for identifying muscular defects and for distinguishing defects from intertrabecular spaces.

Atrioventricular canal defects are characterized by a defect at the inlet which borders on the tricuspid valve annulus. Subxiphoid long axis, short axis, and apical four-chamber views usually best

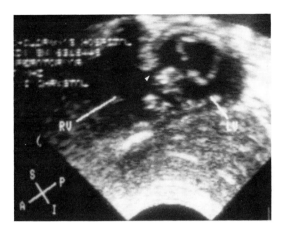

Figure 8. An echocardiogram in subxiphoid short-axis view showing a midmuscular ventricular septal defect (arrow). RV, right ventricle; LV, left ventricle.

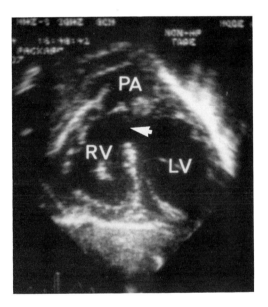

Figure 9. An echocardiogram in subxiphoid oblique view (between the long and short axis) showing a subpulmonary ventricular septal defect. Note that the defect is immediately below the pulmonary valve. PA, pulmonary artery; RV, right ventricle; LV, left ventricle.

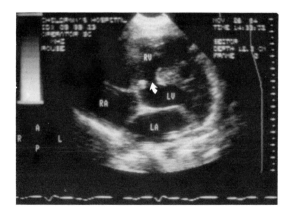

Figure 7. An echocardiogram in parasternal short-axis view showing a membranous ventricular septal defect. Note the rightward and posterior location of the defect, behind the septal leaflet of the tricuspid valve and near the crux of the heart. RV, right ventricle; LV, left ventricle; RA, right atrium; LA, left atrium.

demonstrate these defects. The overlying septal leaflet of the tricuspid valve may obscure the defects, especially in diastole. Doppler color flow mapping may be very helpful in determining their extent.

Subpulmonary defects result from partial or complete absence of the infundibular septum. A subxiphoid view rotated halfway between the long- and short-axis plane demonstrates the subpulmonary defect and its relation to the pulmonary valve (Fig. 9). In the parasternal short-axis view the subpulmonary defect is more anterior and leftward than the membranous defect and is related to the right coronary leaflet of the aortic valve (see p. 451).

Magnetic Resonance Imaging

Magnetic resonance imaging is gradually improving and may be the imaging technique for visualization of ventricular defects in the future.[16]

Cardiac Catheterization

Cardiac catheterization (see ch. 14) is mandatory in the critically ill infant who is a likely candidate for surgery. Confirmation of the clinical diagnosis, quantification of the hemodynamic burden, and exclusion of associated defects are the goals. Nothing is more dangerous to the infant and more embarrassing to the cardiologist and the cardiac surgeon than the discovery of a hidden second problem in the postoperative period when the patient is doing poorly. Because the clinical and echocardiographic features of ventricular septal defect are largely dependent on the amount of left-to-right shunting and because indirect estimations of intracardiac pressures are not sufficiently reliable, cardiac catheterization is required in some patients to measure pulmonary vascular resistance. Electrocardiographic evidence of right ventricular hypertrophy without associated left ventricular hypertrophy in an infant more than 6 months old requires study to evaluate the possibility of pulmonary vascular disease. In practice, an infant older than 6 months who might have pulmonary hypertension is studied, even though asymptomatic.

With the smallest of defects there may be no physiologic abnormalities discovered by conventional oximetry. Somewhat larger defects show evidence of left-to-right shunting in the form of an oxygen increase at the ventricular level (see Fig. 3). With even larger defects the evidence for shunting is greater and there is pulmonary hypertension (see Fig. 3).

Evidence of pressure gradients across the pulmonary outflow tract, in the form of pulmonary stenosis, is noted, as well as evidence of obstruction at the mitral or aortic valve. Retrograde arteriograms are performed routinely in patients with pulmonary hypertension to rule out a patent ductus arteriosus. Aortic and mitral regurgitation are also quantified by angiography.

Angiography. Membranous ventricular defects are seen best with the catheter pointed toward the apex of the left ventricle and the patient in the long axial oblique position, filming at right angles in biplane. The contrast (2.0 ml/kg of body weight) should be delivered as fast as possible. The membranous ventricular defect will show on the lateral film as the dye passes from the left to the right ventricle just beneath the aortic valve (Fig. 10).

Midmuscular and **apical ventricular defects** also

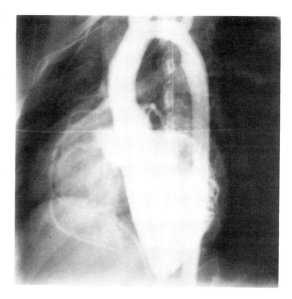

Figure 10. Angiogram showing a membranous ventricular septal defect. The injection is into the left ventricle with the patient in the long axial oblique position. Note passage of the contrast from the left to the right ventricle just beneath the aortic valve. The upper border of the shunted dye represents an aneurysm that may ultimately close the defect.

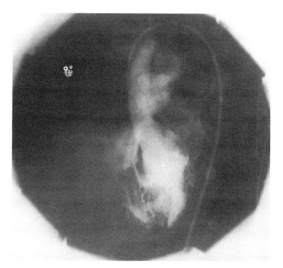

Figure 11. Angiogram showing multiple apical and midmuscular ventricular septal defects. The injection of contrast material is into the left ventricle with the patient in the left anterior oblique position.

are best recorded in the long axial oblique view by the lateral camera (Fig. 11). **Anterior muscular defects** are seen as the dye passes well below the pulmonary valve into the pulmonary artery in the right anterior oblique view. **Posterior muscular defects** are seen best in the hepatoclavicular view.

Subpulmonary defects are best shown in the right anterior oblique view with the passage of dye almost directly into the pulmonary artery (Fig. 12).

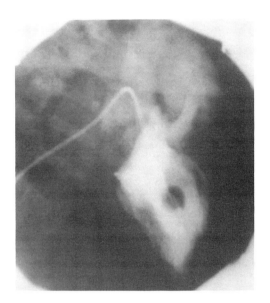

Figure 12. Angiogram showing a subpulmonary ventricular septal defect. The injection of contrast is into the left ventricle with the patient in an anteroposterior position. Dye is seen to pass almost directly into the main pulmonary artery.

An endocardial cushion type of ventricular defect is seen well in the hepatoclavicular view (Fig. 13).

Minor Laboratory Tests

Hemoglobin and hematocrit measurements may be important because any degree of anemia aggravates the symptoms produced by a left-to-right shunt. Evidence of a superimposed infection, as demonstrated by fever or an elevated white count, may reveal the aggravating cause of congestive heart failure in these infants. Positive blood cultures guide antibiotic therapy. Careful plotting of the growth curve is needed to decide about surgery.

MANAGEMENT

Influence of Size of Defect

Small Ventricular Septal Defects. All infants with the murmur of ventricular septal defect should be examined by two-dimensional echocardiography as soon after discovery as is reasonable. Although the diagnosis is most often confirmed, sometimes it is not, and a search for other causes of the murmur is needed.

The majority of ventricular defects are small. The child who has reached the age of 6 months without evidence of congestive heart failure and without evidence of pulmonary hypertension can be managed conservatively. Ventricular defects do not get bigger, only smaller; rarely, however, left-

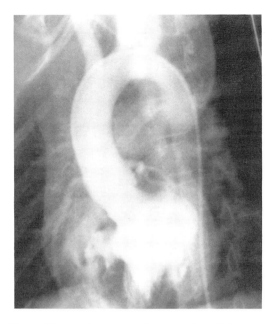

Figure 13. Angiogram showing an endocardial cushion type of ventricular septal defect. The injection of contrast is into the left ventricle with the patient in the hepatoclavicular position. Note the passage of contrast through the mid septum. A midmuscular ventricular defect in the posterior septum might result in the same picture.

to-right shunting is increased by the development of additional lesions causing left ventricular hypertension. After the first year of life, asymptomatic infants known to have small membranous ventricular septal defects should be examined every 2–3 years to watch for the development of aortic regurgitation as well as to document any decrease in size of the defect (see p 449). Prophylactic antibiotics should be used to prevent the possibility of infective endocarditis when oral, dental, or genitourinary surgery is undertaken.

Large Ventricular Septal Defects. Defects large enough to cause **congestive heart failure** are managed first with digoxin and diuretics (see ch. 7).[5,8] Correction of anemia by careful administration of packed red blood cells followed by oral iron therapy may be helpful and afterload reduction may be needed.[6,42] In early infancy, a trial period of anticongestive measures usually is indicated to see if growth failure can be overcome and to allow time for closure. When growth is satisfactory it is our practice at Children's Hospital in Boston to delay surgery; on the other hand, growth failure is *the indication* for ventricular septal defect repair within the first 6 months of life (Fig. 14). Congestive heart failure must be severe enough to impair growth before the risk of corrective surgery in early infancy can be justified. Because of the common association of other congenital anomalies, often it is necessary to exclude or to correct noncardiac problems that may affect growth. Because of the higher mortality in the first 2 months of life, only

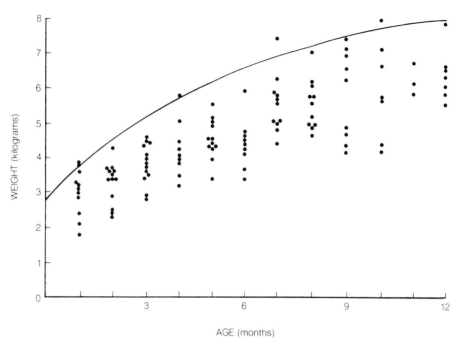

Figure 14.   Age and weight of patients at the time of surgery for primary closure of a ventricular septal defect. The solid line represents the third percentile for normal infants. (Reprinted with permission from the American College of Cardiology, Journal of the American College of Cardiology 3:1269–1276, 1984.)

those infants in this age group who are in desperate difficulty are referred to surgery.

With this management, the mortality among these frequently very sick infants is surprisingly small. Often, it comes down to whether the nurse-mother feeding team can get the infant to grow. When they fail, surgery is undertaken. It follows that the enthusiasm, strength and experience of the nurse and the mother determine when surgery will be needed. Frequent feedings of increased calories per ounce via a nasogastric tube to relieve the stress of nursing may be helpful. Careful attention to superimposed respiratory problems such as aspiration, pneumonia, and atelectasis is desirable. Whether the gain in growth outweights the surgical risk is a question which the cardiologist, nurse-mother feeding team, and the surgeon should face squarely prior to operation. Following surgery, improvement in growth is nearly universal.[73]

Older infants with evidence of **pulmonary hypertension** who otherwise are growing well are studied at cardiac catheterization after the age of 6 months and before the first birthday. An infant with pure right ventricular hypertrophy (as shown on the electrocardiogram), a large defect discerned at echocardiography, and echocardiographic evidence of pulmonary hypertension is a candidate for cardiac catherization even when there are no symptoms. The more convincing the evidence for pulmonary hypertension, the earlier the catheter-

ization is carried out; in any case, cardiac catheterization should be performed before the age of 1 year if there is any question of pulmonary hypertension. Infants with pulmonary arterial pressure greater than 50% of systemic pressure should have surgical correction after the age of 6 months and before the first birthday.

After the first birthday, children with ventricular septal defects producing left-to-right shunts with Qp/Qs in excess of 2:1, regardless of the pulmonary arterial pressure, are candidates for surgical closure.

Generally, the operative technique is transatrial though other approaches are utilized occasionally (e.g., transaortic, transpulmonary, transventricular, and apical left ventricular).[4,45,59,73] Surgical mortality is relatively high (20%) in the first month of life, but is low (2%) after the age of 6 months (Exhibit 3).

Closure of ventricular septal defects using umbrella devices extruded from cardiac catheters is a fascinating technique that holds considerable promise. Ventricular defects adjacent to important structures, such as the aortic valve, cannot be safely closed using this method. Muscular defects, especially the multiple muscular defects, may be specific candidates for their use. The technique involves passing a catheter from the left ventricle through the defect to the right side. The venous end is snared and brought to the outside. The occluding device is passed over the venous end of

Exhibit 3

Boston Children's Hospital Experience
1973–1987

Ventricular Septal Defect
Number of Patients Undergoing Surgical Repair in Three Time Periods
n = 641

Age at Repair	Years			Total	30-Day Mortality
	1973–77	1978–82	1983–87		
0–2 mo	9	8	18	35	20%
3–6 mo	22	51	62	135	4%
7–12 mo	25	51	61	137	3%
1–5 yr	50	59	91	200	1%
6–10 yr	21	20	23	64	0%
11–15 yr	15	5	9	29	0%
16–20 yr	8	8	7	23	4%
21–	3	3	9	15	0%
Total	153	205	280*	638*	3%

*Three patients had faulty data.
A total of 908 (26%) of the children had cardiac surgery, 209 before 1973. Of 765 who had cardiac surgery after 1973, the vast majority (641) had primary repiar of the ventricular septal defect. Sixty-seven children had had a prior pulmonary artery band. Three died during repair and band takedown.

Life table with and without surgery

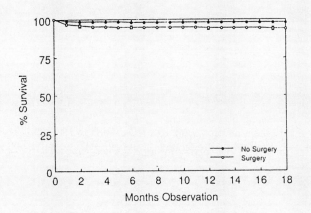

Surgical Repair of Ventricular Septal Defect

Years	No. of Patients	30-Day Mortality	Late Mortality
1973–77	153	5 (3%)	
1978–82	205	6 (3%)	
1983–87	283	8 (3%)	
Total	641	19 (3%)	12 (2%)

The 30-day surgical mortality was remarkably constant for each of the 5-year periods from 1973–1987.

the catheter to the ventricular defect. The device is positioned through manipulation of both the venous and retrograde ends and then released (see ch. 14).[43]

Influence of Type of Defect

Membranous Defects. It is fortunate that the majority of ventricular septal defects are in the membranous location and that these defects are likely to become smaller (±50%). Even large membranous defects have been known to close spontaneously. Because of this tendency toward improvement with time, the struggle with the difficult problem of poor growth is more likely to be rewarding with these than with ventricular defects in other locations. Among those with good growth, expectation of decrease in the amount of left-to-right shunting as the child gets older is justified, even though decrease in shunt size is by no means a certainty.

Because of the proximity of the tricuspid valve,

distortion of valve leaflets after surgical patching of a membranous ventricular defect is nearly universal. With good closure of the defect, right ventricular pressure is normal and functional problems caused by the tricuspid deformity are negligible.

The rare malalignment membranous defect is not thought to close spontaneously or to get smaller. These defects are usually large and associated with pulmonary hypertension; consequently, all should be surgically closed. The vast majority are associated with pulmonary stenosis in the context of cyanotic or acyanotic tetralogy of Fallot and are surgically corrected either electively or because of symptoms (see p. 479).

Muscular Defects. Muscular defects are often small and multiple. Because spontaneous closure of muscular defects is likely, the general plan of management is similar to that for membranous defects. Unfortunately, not all muscular defects decrease in size and surgery may be needed to prevent pulmonary vascular obstructive disease. Watchful waiting is desirable, particularly among those with multiple defects. Usually, **multiple defects** involve the muscular septum, at least in part.[20] Because surgical repair is difficult, spontaneous regression is the most satisfactory outcome. Otherwise, the indications for surgical correction of multiple defects are the same as for membranous defects; however, the operative mortality and the risk of residual defects is greater, hence delay in operative intervention usually is justified. Occasionally a large defect in the apical, trabecular septum requires a left ventricular incision and a left-sided patch. Rarely, some of these patients undergo pulmonary banding to combat congestive heart failure and enhance growth while waiting for the spontaneous decrease in size of the defects. The possibility of closing a muscular defect with a catheter-introduced device is an attractive concept, particularly in a child with a trabeculated, muscular ventricular defect which otherwise would require a left ventricular incision.

Infundibular (Subpulmonary) Defects. Because subpulmonary defects are rarely small and are not known to get smaller, and because aortic regurgitation develops commonly, all patients are referred to the surgeons after the age of 6 months, or earlier if there is growth failure.

Endocardial Cushion Type of Defect. The other stigmata of endocardial cushion defects are not necessarily present (i.e., leftward-superior axis on the electrocardiogram and cleft atrioventricular valves). Because these defects do not regress spontaneously or get smaller and since small defects are uncommon, surgery is almost invariably needed.

COURSE

Children with smaller defects reach adulthood normally without surgery, and although bacterial endocarditis is a risk, it is uncommon in this group of patients. Only a single patient with bacterial endocarditis superimposed on a small ventricular defect has been encountered in the past 15 years at Boston Children's Hospital. The Natural History Study confirms perceived clinical experience. The incidence of bacterial endocarditis was higher among those with large ventricular defects (41.4 per 10,000 person-years of follow-up).[70]

Rarely, the murmur of the small defect becomes so loud that it is distracting to nearby individuals; more often, it becomes less intense as the chest grows. Defects in the membranous area that seem small may be partially occluded by a prolapsed aortic valve and aortic regurgitation may develop. This possibility dictates follow-up of patients with membranous ventricular defects that are clinically small.

Patients with larger defects which have been surgically closed usually do well, regaining their destined position on growth chart if surgery is done early enough and if there are no noncardiac anomalies that inhibit growth (Fig. 14). Even with late surgical correction, the child is not dwarfed but is smaller than the parent or siblings. There are late deaths. The Natural History Study[70] reported 82% survival of patients first identified to have a ventricular defect 25 years earlier. Many of these patients had pulmonary vascular disease when first evaluated. With this problem now controlled, longer survival is anticipated.

Some survivors have a small residual defect (20%)[73] that is the result of an unrecognized second defect or a leak around the patch. Rarely, a second operation is needed and when undertaken does not have the same likelihood of success as an initial operation.

Complete right bundle branch block and bifascicular block are relatively common (30–85%) and occur regardless of whether the ventricular septal defect is patched via a transventricular or atrial approach. The long-range implications of these electrocardiographic abnormalities are not known. Persistent complete heart block occurs in about 5% (0–11%) of patients, the incidence being no higher among infants than older children.[9,32,73] As with all patients who have intraventricular surgery, late ectopy found on a 24-hour Holter monitor or discovered on stress testing is observed in 5% of patients.[70]

Follow-up cardiac catheterization shows a decrease in pulmonary artery pressure (Fig. 15) and resistance.[73] Postoperative tricuspid valve deformity is believed to be common; frequently it may be related to the proximity of the patching material used in repair. Without residual pulmonary hypertension or pulmonary stenosis, tricuspid regurgitation has been an insignificant problem.

At Children's Hospital in Boston there have been no cases of late infective endocarditis in a patient with postoperative ventricular septal defect

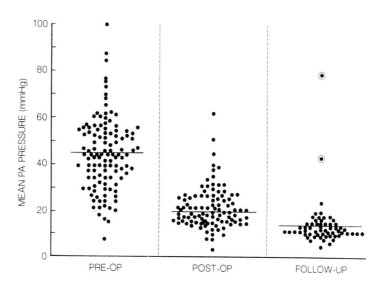

Figure 15. Mean pulmonary artery (PA) pressures measured during the preoperative catheterization, the early postoperative period and the follow-up recatheterization. The circled points represent the two patients with large residual ventricular septal defects who subsequently underwent reoperation. The solid lines represent the median of each group. (Reprinted with permission from the American College of Cardiology, Journal of the American College of Cardiology 3:1269–1276, 1984.)

in whom the defect was successfully closed. The Natural History Study II found a different experience, with bacterial endocarditis as likely to occur among patients managed surgically as among those who were not.[70]

Spontaneous Diminution in Size

For many years it has been known that a ventricular septal defect may close spontaneously and, more often, may become smaller in size.[33] In recent years this phenomenon has been the subject of multiple reports.[1,2,7,22,47,58] The wide variation in reports of diminishing size of defects results from the varying methods of discovery, methods of diagnosis, ages at first discovery and types of ventricular septal defect.

Infundibular (subpulmonary) and endocardial cushion ventricular defects are not known to close. Because these defects often extend into the adjacent muscular septum it is reasonable to postulate that some may get smaller over time, but this remains to be documented. Malalignment defects are not known to get smaller or close. The remarkable constancy in relative size of the ventricular defect in patients with tetralogy of Fallot is an example. One word of caution; the conviction that malalignment defects "never" close has become so ingrained that if a malalignment defect ever did close, it would be reviewed and reclassified as membranous. Indeed, at the present time the definition of malalignment defects includes the fact that they do not close or get smaller, a self-fulfilling prophecy.

Membranous and muscular defects are known to get smaller with time. Upward of 50% of membranous ventricular defects get smaller and some close. Rarely, the decrease in the diameter of the defect may be delayed over years though the most dramatic changes occur in the first 6 months of life.

Usually, the changing anatomy involves the septal leaflet of the tricuspid valve and evolves as an aneurysm, or wind sock, of the membranous ventricular septum,[22,58] sometimes producing a systolic click. Muscular defects commonly close, particularly in small infants. The mechanisms of closure must involve the regular muscular contraction with the attendant changes in size and shape of the defect. Because many of these defects are tiny, the rim of the defect must rub in rhythmic contact.

Given the number of factors involved, the variation in reports of spontaneous closure of ventricular septal defects is understandable. Short of prospective echocardiography of large numbers of unselected newborns, it is unlikely that greater precision will ever be achieved.

The factors considered in a decision to wait for spontaneous diminution in size of a ventricular defect are:

1. The age of the patient. Most of the change in size of the defect occurs before the age of 6 months.
2. The location of the defect. Only membranous and muscular defects are known to get smaller.
3. Surgical mortality. The risk is greater in the first months of life.
4. Multiple defects. The risk of surgery is greater and may require a left ventricular incision.
5. Noncardiac causes of symptoms. Growth failure and respiratory difficulty may be caused by associated anomalies.
6. Adequacy of medical management.

Development of Pulmonary Vascular Disease

In the past pulmonary vascular disease (Eisenmenger's syndrome) appeared with increasing frequency as children survived longer with large ventricular septal defects.[34] About 15% of patients with ventricular defects in the 20-year-old group had pulmonary vascular disease. Although all patients with large ventricular defects had some pulmonary arteriolar abnormality on biopsy,[73] the development of permanent pulmonary vascular disease is very rare before the first birthday; the numbers increase afterward.[51,64] In general, pulmonary vascular disease is more common when the ventricular septal defect is large, multiple, or associated with a patent ductus arteriosus. Nowadays, with early surgery the incidence of pulmonary vascular obstructive disease should approach zero and, for practical purposes, it has. With early surgery the disease has disappeared before the mechanisms which cause it are understood.

With pulmonary hypertension, the second heart sound is accentuated, often palpable, and usually single. In some patients, the murmur of pulmonary regurgitation is recognizable (Fig. 16). The electrocardiogram shows right ventricular hypertrophy. Any degree of left ventricular hypertrophy suggests left-to-right shunting and a potentially operable candidate. Because pulmonary vascular resistance limits the amount of left-to-right shunting, the patient tends to have a smaller heart on the chest x-ray and is much less likely to have congestive heart failure. The pulmonary vasculature is described as "pruned," with prominent central vessels and decreased caliber of the peripheral vessels. Blind evaluation of this feature has convinced us that it is at best a dubious observation, even though postmortem casts of the pulmonary vascular tree show this phenomenon.

Any suggestion of pulmonary hypertension in patients older than 6 months with ventricular septal defect requires cardiac catheterization for evaluation. Careful estimation of the pressures encountered in the right side of the heart, pulmonary arteries, and the left atrium (or as reflected in the pulmonary arterial wedge position) is needed. Measurement of the shunt size should be recorded. The catheterization data should not be confused by general anesthesia or use of agents that might affect the pulmonary circulation. Results suggesting pulmonary vascular disease of any degree should prompt collection of further confirmatory evidence such as the response to pulmonary arterial vasodilators, the most effective one being oxygen.

Urgent surgical intervention should be undertaken to reverse the process if the pulmonary vascular disease is of recent origin. Virtually all children with ventricular septal defect and any evidence of pulmonary vascular disease undergo surgical correction in the first year of life because the appearance of pulmonary vascular disease must have occurred in the recent past. Beyond the age of 6 months the decision to operate depends on whether the vascular change is minimal or advanced, is of recent onset, or shows evidence of reversibility. These decisions cannot be readily tabulated and are associated with significant error. In general, all patients with pulmonary resistance estimated at less than 8 units/m^2 of body surface and all patients under 2 years of age in whom there is any evidence of developing pulmonary vascular disease are referred to the surgeons. Significant left-to-right shunting (Qp/Qs >2:1) is taken as an indication for surgery even in the face of elevated pulmonary vascular resistance. Patients who clearly respond to vasodilator therapy, such as oxygen, are subjected to surgery (although lung biopsies are taken during surgery as a matter of documentation,[56,57] despite known pitfalls[10]). Minimal evaluation of pulmonary vascular resistance may be measured during vigorous exercise.[44] Patients with resistance levels higher than 8 units/m^2, particularly those who have no left-to-right shunt, those with a dominant right-to-left shunt, those older than the age of 2 years, and those who show no response to pulmonary arterial vasodilation are not considered candidates for surgical correction.

The bad outcome for patients with pulmonary vascular disease and ventricular septal defect has been somewhat exaggerated. Many of these patients survive much longer than was formerly thought and are known to be functional, although somewhat limited, into the fourth and fifth decades. Pregnancy poses a prohibitive risk for women with pulmonary vascular disease secondary to congenital heart problems (50% mortality). The tendency to survive pregnancy, even delivery, but then to succumb suddenly within 1–2 weeks seems well established.[54] For this reason, these patients are strongly discouraged from becoming pregnant as a matter of life and death. Contraceptive pills, which might promote pulmonary infarction, and mechanical devices, which promote infection as well as clotting, are also contraindicated. Tubal ligation offers a safe but not always acceptable alternative. Clearly the management of contraception and pregnancy in these young women is a matter of importance.

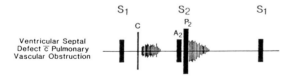

Figure 16. Diagram of auscultatory findings in a child with ventricular septal defect and pulmonary vascular obstructive disease. S_1, first heart sound; S_2, second heart sound; C, click; A_2, aortic valve closure; P_2, pulmonary valve closure. Note the minimal systolic murmur and loud P_2. The high-frequency early diastolic murmur following P_2 results from pulmonary regurgitation. The diastolic murmur and the click are not invariably present. (From Avery ME, First LP (eds): Pediatric Medicine. Baltimore, Williams & Wilkins, 1989, with permission.)

With all this, it is noteworthy that no infant with an isolated ventricular septal defect has developed pulmonary vascular disease at Children's Hospital in Boston in the last 15 years. There have been 2 children with ventricular defect and coarctation who have; in 1 case, mild residual pulmonary vascular disease developed after surgical closure of the ventricular defect and in the other there was severe pulmonary vascular disease and no attempt was made to close the defect (Fig. 17).

Development of Aortic Regurgitation

Prevalence. Aortic regurgitation develops in less than 5% of patients with unspecified types of ventricular septal defect (Exhibit 1).[13] Subpulmonary ventricular defects are much more common in Asiatic populations and are more likely to cause aortic regurgitation. In the United States, where most of the ventricular defects are in the membranous location, the appearance of aortic regurgitation is less likely but it does occur. The relative numbers of membranous versus subpulmonary defects varies considerably among various reports, even excluding the Asian experience, although 25% of the ventricular defects in a large series of patients in the United States who developed aortic regurgitation were subpulmonary.[60]

Anatomy. The ventricular defect is not large and is immediately adjacent to and under the aortic valve. When viewed from the right ventricle, the defect is either subpulmonary or membranous.[65] The adjacent aortic valve cusps (right and/or non-coronary) are variably elongated and prolapsed, sometimes into and sometimes through the ventricular defect into the right ventricle (Fig. 18).

About 10% of patients with ventricular septal defect who are discovered to have aortic regurgitation do not have prolapsed aortic valve cusps but have a bicuspid aortic valve.[35]

The potential relation between patients with aortic regurgitation who have membranous ventricular defects and subpulmonary stenosis and those with tetralogy of Fallot, who have similar anatomy and also acquire aortic regurgitation (see ch. 30), is not clear but, for the most part, those with tetralogy have less severe aortic regurgitation.

Physiology. The left-to-right shunt tends to be small, partly because the ventricular defect is not large and partly because the ventricular defect is obstructed by the aortic cusp. Usually, there is a pressure gradient across the right ventricular outflow tract, sometimes resulting from a prolapsed cusp, but more often the result of mild infundibular obstruction. Pulmonary arterial pressure as high as the systemic pressure is rare and pulmonary vascular disease is unknown.

Clinical Manifestations. A history of congestive heart failure in infancy is rare. Aortic regurgitation is not recognized at birth. The youngest child with the murmur of aortic regurgitation reported in the literature was 6 months old.[28] At Children's Hospital in Boston, the youngest was 18 months old. In our experience, the median age at discovery of aortic regurgitation was 5 years and the latest was 17 years. Discovery is through detection of the

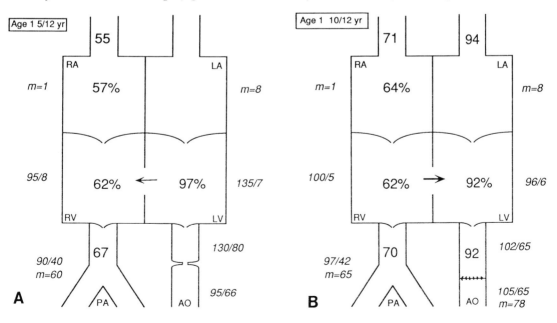

Figure 17. Physiologic diagrams showing the findings in a child with (**A**) ventricular septal defect, coarctation of the aorta, and pulmonary vascular obstructive disease. **B,** After the coarctation was surgically relieved, shunting through the ventricular defect reversed direction. There being no significant left-to-right shunt, no further surgery was undertaken. Ten years later, this girl is an excellent dancer.

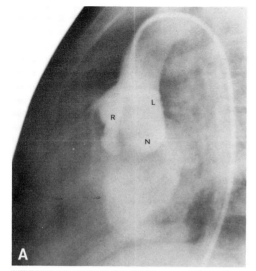

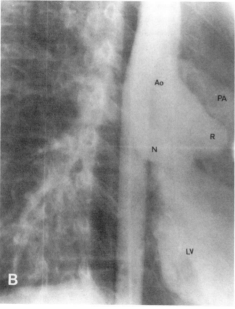

Figure 18. **A,** Aortogram filmed in the lateral position in a patient with subaortic ventricular septal defect and aortic regurgitation. The contrast outlines a prolapsed right and noncoronary cusp. **B,** Aortogram filmed in the right anterior oblique position in a patient with subpulmonary ventricular septal defect and aortic regurgitation. The contrast outlines prolapse of the right and noncoronary cusp. L, left cusp; R, right cusp; N, noncoronary cusp; Ao, aorta; PA, pulmonary artery; LV, left ventricle.

characteristic murmur of aortic regurgitation in a patient who is otherwise thought to have a small ventricular septal defect. In recent years, with routine echocardiography, some patients have been found to have a prolapsed aortic valve without aortic regurgitation, but to date none of these has developed auscultatory evidence of aortic regurgitation.

Management. Because subpulmonary defects frequently are associated with aortic regurgitation and are not known to get smaller or close, surgical repair is undertaken regardless of the size of the defect, to prevent the development of aortic regurgitation.[49] Subpulmonary defects are surgically closed in infancy because of symptoms and after the age of 6 months to prevent aortic regurgitation.

Children with asymptomatic small membranous defects are reviewed yearly to detect those who may develop aortic regurgitation.

Once aortic regurgitation has developed the decision to ask the surgeons to close the ventricular defect or to attempt surgical improvement of aortic valve function, or both, is a matter of some debate. Aortic valvuloplasty[39] is sometimes, but not invariably, successful. Advanced aortic regurgitation requires surgery, sometimes including aortic valve replacement. Closure of the ventricular defect may or may not prevent progression of the regurgitation. Regardless of the type of surgery, it is important to emphasize that no patient with ventricular defect and aortic regurgitation is cured.

Course. The management of these children before and after surgery is still not clearly defined despite claims of success using various techniques. It is expected that systematic evaluation with newer echocardiographic methods[14] will not only improve the surgical outcome but will provide needed information about the natural progress of the disease.

The incidence of infective endocarditis is high, occurring in 16% of the patients (14 episodes in 85 patients).[60] Children with known membranous or subpulmonary defects should be followed systematically to detect this serious complication.

Because aortic regurgitation becomes progressively and even dangerously more severe in about one-third of patients, close observation is required. Other patients are stable for years.

Development of Subaortic Stenosis

Subaortic stenosis associated with a membranous ventricular septal defect most often involves a discrete fibrous or fibromuscular ridge situated at a variable distance beneath the aortic valve.[35,37,68,69] Rarely, the ventricular defect opens into the outflow of the left ventricle, distal to the stenosis.

The substrate for the development of subaortic stenosis must be present at birth whether or not it is associated with a ventricular septal defect; still it is virtually never recognized in the first days of life. It is common among patients with coarctation and ventricular septal defect and for some reason develops following pulmonary artery banding.[21] It may appear also following repair of a ventricular septal defect. Because it is a progressive lesion, surgical relief is usually undertaken relatively early; unequivocal documentation of a subaortic membrane with a gradient of more than 30 mm Hg is sufficient indication for surgical intervention. Long-term follow-up of these infants is mandatory, even though, so far, surgery appears to be largely curative.

A murmur known to be present from birth is unlikely to result from subaortic stenosis, and later the murmur of subaortic stenosis may be indistinguishable from that of a small ventricular defect. Confusion arises when the infant who has a membranous ventricular septal defect subsequently develops subaortic stenosis, sometimes after surgical patching of the ventricular defect.[31] Isolated subaortic stenosis in the older child may be indistinguishable from a small ventricular septal defect by auscultatory, radiologic, and electrocardiographic means; the combination of ventricular defect and subaortic stenosis is an even more formidable diagnostic problem without imaging techniques. In experienced hands, echocardiography reveals a subaortic membrane that may be quite thin and often is difficult to recognize. A Doppler gradient across the left ventricular outflow tract is a clear indication for further anatomic evaluation of this region. Cardiac catheterization is almost never needed in this differential diagnosis but is useful in determining severity. The association of membranous ventricular septal defect, subaortic membrane, and double-chambered right ventricle is sufficiently common to require special consideration when either of these two lesions complicate ventricular septal defect.

At cardiac catheterization in early infancy, this lesion may be unrecognizable either as a pressure gradient or as an anatomic lesion visible on angiography—only to be present later, sometimes after surgical closure of the ventricular defect. The wary clinician will react to electrocardiograms showing left ventricular hypertrophy and strain pattern in an infant who is unexpectedly doing poorly and has a loud murmur following closure of a ventricular septal defect. The association of subaortic stenosis with coarctation of the aorta, interrupted aortic arch, mitral stenosis, and double-chambered right ventricle should raise the possibility of subaortic stenosis whenever these lesions are encountered with a ventricular septal defect.

Surgical resection of the obstructing ring of fibrous tissue is generally curative.

VARIATIONS

Ventricular Septal Defect and Secundum Atrial Septal Defect

The combination of a ventricular septal defect and a secundum atrial defect is difficult to recognize short of 2-D echocardiography or cardiac catheterization. This combination is relatively common (7% of ventricular septal defects) (Exhibit 1). Some-times the distinction between an atrial defect of the secundum type and a dilated, patent foramen ovale is difficult. Some of these patients have a rightward bulging flap of the foramen ovale, left atrial hypertension, and atrial left-to-right shunting. The left-to-right shunt disappears after the excess left atrial flow and pressure are relieved by closure of the ventricular septal defect. In those with a true secundum atrial defect, the left atrial overload resulting from the ventricular septal defect is relieved by the atrial defect and there is no atrial hypertension. Indeed, the one possible observation that points to the diagnosis of atrial defect in the presence of a large ventricular defect is a left atrium which is not large.

If the total left-to-right shunt is large, surgical relief is undertaken. Both the atrial and ventricular septa are inspected and repaired as needed. Surgical mortality for this combination has been reported to be higher than for uncomplicated ventricular septal defect, but this difference has not been detectable in recent years.

The incidence of extracardiac anomalies may be somewhat higher than for isolated ventricular septal defects.[23]

Ventricular Septal Defect and Patent Ductus Arteriosus

This is a recognized subset of the ventricular septal defects (9%). Within the first days of life all infants have a patent ductus arteriosus, but a few infants with ventricular defects have a persistently patent ductus.

Continued patency of the ductus contributes to the equilibration of pressure between the ventricles and may provide additional left-to-right shunting if the pulmonary resistance favors this. When one or the other defect is larger, the hemodynamics reflects the dominant defect. When either or both defects are large the net flow depends on relative pulmonary vs. systemic resistance. The differences in ductal versus ventricular shunting because of arterial-to-arterial shunting through the ductus and shunting from ventricle-to-ventricle through the ventricular septal defect, as well as the differences in shunting in systole and diastole, have an almost unfathomable complexity. Practically, when both defects are large and the amount of left-to-right shunting is determined by the pulmonary resistance, dividing the ductus, even if it is large, may not affect the size of the shunt. With any suggestion that the ventricular defect will turn out to be restrictive, it may be beneficial to divide the ductus. The contrasting possibility of a possibly restrictive ductus requires that both defects be managed simultaneously because of the necessity to control the ductus during pump oxygenator surgery.

Clinical suspicion of this diagnosis depends on discovery of a continuous murmur at the upper left sternal border or at least the characteristic late crescendic systolic murmur (see ch. 33). In general, the auscultatory findings reflect the dominant defect.[24] If the ductus is relatively small, it cannot be recognized by auscultation; the diagnosis will depend on imaging techniques or cardiac catheterization.

Treatment consists of surgical closure of the defects, ideally after the age of two months and before the age of one year. If the infant grows the decision is elective; if not, anticongestive medications in a vigorous attempt to promote growth are indicated. Surgery is indicated in any infant who fails to grow.

Because this combination tends to produce a large left-to-right shunt as well as equilibration of both right- and left-sided pressures, the tendency for the development of pulmonary vascular disease may be greater than with either defect alone. In assessing possible pulmonary vascular disease, closure of the ductus may be desirable to allow more precise assessment of pulmonary vascular disease with cardiac catheterization at a later date.

Ventricular Defects with Pulmonary Stenosis

Ventricular defects associated with pulmonary stenosis occur most commonly in the framework of tetralogy of Fallot. Occasionally patients with valvar pulmonary stenosis and a ventricular defect do not fit the criteria for diagnosis of tetralogy of Fallot and some others have moderator bands associated with the ventricular defect. Still others have the tetralogy of Fallot syndrome with additional moderator bands. All types of outflow obstruction may be progressive.[25,55] Rarely, patients with ventricular septal defect will have varying degrees of peripheral pulmonary stenosis (Exhibit 1).

Those with the anatomy of tetralogy of Fallot most often go on to develop the classical tetralogy of Fallot syndrome and are discussed in that context (see ch. 30).

Acyanotic Tetralogy of Fallot. The characteristic physical findings associated with a small ventricular septal defect (16% in the Boston Children's Hospital experience) are sufficiently similar to those of acyanotic tetralogy of Fallot that confusion between the two diagnoses is perhaps the most common error in pediatric cardiology. Acyanotic tetralogy of Fallot, with or without some left-to-right shunting, sometimes produces a murmur indistinguishable from the murmur of small ventricular septal defect. Whether there are one or two components of the second heart sound is difficult to recognize, especially in the small infant in whom this differentiation most often is necessary. The heart size and pulmonary vascularity on x-ray may be the same in both conditions. The electrocardiogram may not show evidence of an abnormal degree of right ventricular hypertrophy, particularly in small infants. Any electrocardiographic ev-

idence of an abnormal degree of right ventricular hypertrophy is cause for concern when the tentative diagnosis is isolated ventricular defect; if the electrocardiographic interpretation is correct, there is either pulmonary hypertension or pulmonary stenosis. In the past, occasionally, parents of such an infant were advised that their baby had a small ventricular defect that might close and, in any case, would never require surgery, only to have the infant become visibly cyanotic weeks or months later. Echocardiography has largely, but not completely, eliminated this problem. Two-dimensional echocardiographic diagnosis of tetralogy of Fallot requires demonstration of an overriding aorta, but echocardiography is relatively poor in locating the infundibular pulmonary stenosis.

Recognition of a left-to-right shunt by Doppler technique does not help unless some reversal of the shunt is seen. Doppler recognition of a significant pressure gradient across the outflow tract is most helpful, and for this reason, at Boston Children's Hospital, Doppler examination of the outflow tract has become a required part of the examination of any infant with ventricular septal defect. Equalization of pressures between the two ventricles is recognizable and clearly incompatible with the diagnosis of small ventricular septal defect. When the right ventricular pressure is less than that of the left ventricle, the probability of the development of the classical tetralogy of Fallot syndrome is unlikely. Discovery at Doppler examination of a membranous ventricular septal defect with some outflow gradient and without an overriding aorta is not a rare phenomenon. Which one will develop into tetralogy of Fallot is more a matter of experience than an easily defined fact. Therefore, prognostic reservation is justified. Some of these infants develop the tetralogy of Fallot and some lose the flow gradient as the ventricular defect becomes smaller. Predictions are still wrong occasionally.

Cardiac catheterization produces the same dilemma but is used whenever the diagnosis of tetralogy of Fallot seems a reasonable possibility (see ch. 30).

Ventricular Defect and Valvar Pulmonary Stenosis. Infants with ventricular defect and valvar pulmonary stenosis make up about 10% of all ventricular septal defects. The incidence of spontaneous closure of the ventricular septal defect in this group of patients is zero, suggesting either that this is a variant of tetralogy of Fallot or that the hemodynamics prevents closure of the ventricular septal defect. The lack of right aortic arches in this group of patients points to some other embryologic etiology. The point of maximal intensity of the murmur depends on the degree of right ventricular obstruction. With left-to-right shunting the murmur of a ventricular septal defect may be audible at the fourth left intercostal space, while a similarly loud murmur may be audible at the second left intercostal space because of pulmonary stenosis.

Electrocardiograms show more right ventricular hypertrophy than is expected with simple ventricular septal defects. Chest x-rays may not be very helpful. Two-dimensional echocardiograms are particularly insensitive to mild degrees of valvar pulmonary stenosis, although doming of the valve may suggest it and detection of a Doppler gradient may focus attention on the valve. Usually, the ventricular septal defect is in the membranous location but it may be elsewhere. Occasionally at cardiac catheterization, a restrictive ventricular defect is found with right ventricular pressure greater than left ventricular pressure.

Whether treatment is indicated or not depends on the severity of the defects. It may be that neither defect is sufficient to require surgery.

Ventricular Septal Defect with Double-chambered Right Ventricle. Muscle bundles arising from the lower infundibular septal region and traversing and obstructing the right ventricular outflow tract result in a double-chambered right ventricle. This lesion is surprisingly common and yet has received only limited attention in the literature. The ventricular defect is usually membranous and may get smaller or close spontaneously. The muscle bundles tend to become more obstructive with time;[55] hence, surgery is usually required.

Double-chambered right ventricle produces a murmur indistinguishable from that of a small ventricular septal defect. When both lesions coexist, the auscultatory, electrocardiographic, and x-ray features are not sufficiently reliable for a certain diagnosis. The electrocardiographic findings sometimes show significant right ventricular hypertrophy, suggesting right ventricular hypertension. As with acyanotic tetralogy of Fallot, those with more advanced obstruction can be identified by the echocardiographer, particularly with the Doppler technique. A smaller gradient results in less prognostic confidence whether observed by echocardiography or cardiac catheterization. Usually, the diagnosis is recognized at echocardiography and the severity is reasonably documented by Doppler techniques. All patients should undergo cardiac catheterization. The difficulty in recognizing the low-lying obstruction at cardiac catheterization has been known for some years. The casual withdrawal of the catheter from the right ventricular outflow tract may result in the small area of right ventricular hypertension immediately beneath the tricuspid valve being overlooked. A percentage of these patients develop membranous subaortic stenosis as time goes by.[68,69]

Usually, surgical treatment is required because the obstruction is almost invariably progressive. Usually, excision of the muscle bundles requires a right ventricular exposure. The low-lying obstruction, when exposed by a ventricular excision, may be confusing to the inexperienced surgeon. Mistaken patch closure of the outflow tract is rare at the present time.

Ventricular Septal Defect and Mitral Valve Disease

Rarely, a patient with ventricular septal defect also has either mitral stenosis or mitral regurgitation. Increased left atrial pressure and/or volume may be substantial if the atrial septum is intact. In this case, two possible causes of pulmonary vascular abnormality (left-to-right shunting and elevated pulmonary venous pressure) may coexist. Fortunately, the two are not additive. Nonetheless, detailed cardiac catheterization data are mandatory for rational management.

If there is **mitral regurgitation,** the child is managed as other children with a ventricular defect. With adequate growth, observation and perhaps anticongestive medications may be employed. With uncontrolled, poor growth, the ventricular defect should be closed unless it is tiny. Both lesions, mitral regurgitation and a ventricular defect, require an excess volume of blood to be pumped by the left ventricle. Consequently, with closure of the ventricular defect, there may be marked improvement in congestive heart failure. With severe mitral regurgitation and a small or surgically closed ventricular defect, mitral valvuloplasty (particularly if the ventricular defect is of the endocardial cushion type), or even mitral valve replacement, can be remarkably successful. Obviously, surgery of the mitral valve is avoided if at all possible.

When there is more than minimal **mitral stenosis** associated with the ventricular defect, the patient's course usually will be determined by the severity of the mitral stenosis. If the mitral valve is minimally obstructed and there is moderate pulmonary hypertension or less, management is the same as that for the usual ventricular defect. If there is moderate mitral stenosis and the ventricular defect is of some size, there will be systemic levels of pressure in the pulmonary artery. The amount of left-to-right shunting will depend largely on the comparative levels of pulmonary and systemic resistance. Elevated pulmonary resistance may be calculated, and concern about whether this is reversible or not is usual. Fortunately, the two causes of pulmonary vascular resistance are not additive, and for any given level of resistance the outcome (so far as the pulmonary vascular disease is concerned) is likely to be better than that for a patient with a comparable ventricular defect alone.

When there is severe mitral stenosis, the level of pulmonary resistance may become so high that ventricular shunting reverses and the patient becomes cyanotic. The ultimate success of management depends on the success in treating the mitral stenosis. If it can be relieved, the pulmonary vascular resistance will reverse and the problem becomes one of left-to-right shunting (see Fig. 4). If the mitral stenosis cannot be relieved (e.g., because of a hypoplastic valve), the only solution may be atrial septectomy, provided that the ventricular defect is large. With lowering of the left atrial pressure and consequent increased left-to-right shunting, a pulmonary artery band may be needed. Ultimately, a Fontan procedure might be imaginable. This management is, of course, more theory than fact for this rare combination of defects.

REFERENCES

1. Alpert BS, Cook DH, Varghese PJ, et al: Spontaneous closure of small ventricular septal defects: ten year follow-up. Pediatrics 63:204–206, 1979.
2. Anderson RH, Lenox CC, Zuberbuhler JR: Mechanisms of closure of perimembranous ventricular septal defect. Am J Cardiol 52:341–345, 1983.
3. Ando M, Takao A: Racial differences in the morphology of common cardiac anomalies. Japan, Bulletin of the Heart Institute, 1979, p. 47.
4. Arciniegas E, Farooki, ZQ, Hakimi M, et al: Surgical closure of ventricular defect during the first twelve months of life. J Thorac Cardiovasc Surg 80:921–928, 1980.
5. Artman M, Graham TP: Congestive heart failure in infancy: recognition and management. Am Heart J 103:1040–1055, 1982.
6. Beekman RH, Rocchini AP, Rosenthal A: Hemodynamic effects of hydralazine in infants with a large ventricular septal defect. Circulation 65:523–528, 1982.
7. Beerman LB, Park SC, Fischer DR, et al: Ventricular septal defect associated with aneurysm of the membranous septum. J Am Coll Cardiol 5:118–123, 1985.
8. Berman W, Yabek SM, Dillon T, et al: Effects of digoxin in infants with a congested circulatory state due to a ventricular septal defect. N Engl J Med 308:363–366, 1983.
9. Blake RS, Chung EE, Wesley H, et al: Conduction defects, ventricular arrhythmias, and late death after surgical closure of ventricular septal defect. Br Heart J 47:305–315, 1982.
10. Braunlin EA, Moller JH, Patton C, et al: Predictive value of lung biopsy in ventricular septal defect: long-term followup. J Am Coll Cardiol 8:1113–1118, 1986.
11. Capelli H, Andrade JL, Somerville J: Classification of the site of ventricular septal defect by 2-dimensional echocardiography. Am J Cardiol 51:1474–1480, 1983.
12. Collins G, Calder L, Rose V, et al: Ventricular septal defect: clinical and hemodynamic changes in the first five years of life. Am Heart J 84:695–705, 1972.
13. Corone P, Doyon F, Gaudeau S, et al: Natural history of ventricular septal defect: a study involving 790 cases. Circulation 55:908–915, 1977.
14. Craig BG, Smallhorn JF, Burrows P, et al: Cross-sectional echocardiography in the evaluation of aortic valve prolapse associated with ventricular septal defect. Am Heart J 112:800–807, 1986.
15. Dickinson DF, Arnold R, Wilkinson JL: Ventricular septal defect in children born in Liverpool 1960 to 1969. Br Heart J 46:47–54, 1981.
16. Didier D, Higgins CB: Identification and localization of ventricular septal defect by gated magnetic resonance imaging. Am J Cardiol 57:1364–1368, 1986.
17. Driscoll D, Michels V, Gersony WM, et al: Occurrence of congenital heart defects in offspring of patients with ventricular septal defect, aortic stenosis, or pulmonary stenosis: results of the second natural history study of congenital heart defects (abstract). J Am Coll Cardiol 13:136A, 1989.
18. Edwards JE: Congenital malformations of the heart and great vessels. In Gould SE (ed): Pathology of the Heart. Springfield, IL, Charles C Thomas, 1960.
19. Ellis JH, Moodie DS, Sterba R, et al: Ventricular septal defect in the adult: natural history and unnatural history. Am Heart J 114:115–120, 1987.
20. Fellows KE, Westerman GR, Keane JF: Angiography of multiple ventricular septal defects in infancy. Circulation 66:1094–1099, 1982.
21. Freed MD, Rosenthal A, Plauth WH, et al: Development of subaortic stenosis after pulmonary artery banding. Circulation 47(Suppl III):7–10, 1973.
22. Freedom RM, White RD, Pieroni DR, et al: The natural history of the so-called aneurysm of the membranous ventricular septum in childhood. Circulation 49:375–384, 1974.
23. Fyler DC, Buckley LP, Hellenbrand WE, et al: Report of the New England Regional Infant Cardiac Program. Pediatrics 65(Suppl):376–460, 1980.
24. Fyler DC, Gallaher ME, Nadas AS: Auscultation in the evaluation of children with heart disease. Prog Cardiovasc Dis 10:363–384, 1968.
25. Gasul BM, Dillon RF, Vrla V, et al: Ventricular septal defects, their natural transformation into those with infundibular stenosis or into the cyanotic or noncyanotic type of tetralogy of Fallot. JAMA 164:847–853, 1957.
26. Goor DA, Lillehei CW, Rees R, et al: Isolated ventricular septal defect: developmental basis for various types and presentation of classification. Chest 58:468–482, 1970.
27. Hagler DJ: Standardized nomenclature of the ventricular septum and ventricular septal defects, with applications for two-dimensional echocardiography. Mayo Clin Proc 60:741–752, 1985.
28. Halloran KH, Talner NS, Browne MJ: A study of ventricular septal defect associated with aortic insufficiency. Am Heart J 69:320–326, 1965.
29. Haworth SG, Sauer U, Buhlmeyer K, et al: Development of the pulmonary circulation in ventricular septal defect: a quantitative structural study. Am J Cardiol 40:781–788, 1977.
30. Heath D, Edwards JE: The pathology of hypertensive pulmonary vascular disease. Circulation 18:533–547, 1958.
31. Hegesh JT, Marx GR, Allen HD: Development of a subaortic membrane after surgical closure of a membranous defect in an infant. Am Heart J 114:889–902, 1987.
32. Hobbins SM, Izukawa T, Radford DJ, et al: Conduction disturbance after surgical correction of ventricular defect by the atrial approach. Br Heart J 41:289–293, 1979.
33. Hoffman JIE, Rudolph AM: The natural history of ventricular septal defects in infancy. Am J Cardiol 16:634–653, 1965.
34. Hoffman JIE, Rudolph AM, Heymann MA: Pulmonary vascular disease with congenital heart lesions: pathologic features and causes. Circulation 64:873–877, 1981.
35. Keane JF, Plauth WH, Nadas AS: Ventricular septal defect and aortic regurgitation. Circulation 56(Suppl):I-72–I-77, 1977.
36. Keith JD, Rowe RD, Vlad P: Heart Disease in Infancy and Childhood, 3rd ed. New York, Macmillan, 1979, pp. 4–13.
37. Lauer RM, DuShane JW, Edwards JE: Obstruction of

left ventricular outlet in association with ventricular septal defect. Circulation 22:110–125, 1960.

38. Layde PM, Dooley K, Erickson JD, et al: Is there an epidemic of ventricular septal defects in the USA. Lancet 1:407–408, 1980.

39. Leung MP, Beerman LB, Siewers RD, et al: Long-term follow-up after aortic valvuloplasty and defect closure in ventricular septal defect with aortic regurgitation. Am J Cardiol 60:890–894, 1987.

40. Levy RJ, Rosenthal A, Miettinen OS, et al: Determinants of growth in patients with ventricular septal defect. Circulation 57:793–797, 1978.

41. Lincoln C, Jamieson S, Joseph M, et al: Transatrial repair of ventricular septal defects with reference to their anatomic classification. J Thorac Cardiovasc Surg 74:183–190, 1977.

42. Lister G, Hellenbrand WE, Kleinman CS, et al: Physiologic effects of increasing hemoglobin concentration in left-to-right shunting in infants with ventricular septal defects. N Engl J Med 306:502–506, 1982.

43. Lock JE, Keane JF, Fellows KE: Diagnostic and Interventional Cardiac Catheterization in Congenital Heart Disease. Boston, Martinus Nijhoff, 1987.

44. Maron BJ, Redwood DR, Hirshfeld JW, et al: Postoperative assessment of patients with ventricular septal defect and pulmonary hypertension: response to intense upright exercise. Circulation 48:864–874, 1973.

45. McNicholas K, DeLeval M, Stark J, et al: Surgical treatment of ventricular septal defect in infancy. Br Heart J 41:133–138, 1979.

46. Mitchell SC, Korones SB, Berendes HW: Congenital heart disease in 56,109 births. Circulation 43:323–332, 1971.

47. Moe DG, Guntheroth WG: Spontaneous closure of uncomplicated ventricular septal defect. Am J Cardiol 60:674–678, 1987.

48. Moene RJ, Oppenheimer-Dekker A, Bartelings MM, et al: Ventricular septal defect with normally connected and with transposed great arteries. Am J Cardiol 58:627–632, 1986.

49. Momma K, Toyama K, Takao A, et al: Natural history of subarterial infundibular ventricular septal defect. Am Heart J 108:1312–1317, 1984.

50. Nadas AS, Fyler DC: Pediatric Cardiology. Philadelphia, W.B. Saunders, 1972, pp. 348, 360.

51. Nadas AS, Ellison RC, Weidman WH: Pulmonary stenosis, aortic stenosis, ventricular septal defect: clinical course and indirect assessment. Circulation 56:I-1–I-87, 1977.

52. Newman TB: Etiology of ventricular septal defects: an epidemiologic approach. Pediatrics 76:741–749, 1985.

53. Pinkley K, Stoesz PA: Current trends: ventricular septal defect. MMWR 30:609–610, 1981.

54. Pitts JA, Crosby WM, Basta LL: Eisenmenger's syndrome in pregnancy. Am Heart J 93:321–326, 1977.

55. Pongiglione G, Freedom RM, Cook D, et al: Mechanism of acquired outflow tract obstruction in patients with ventricular septal defect: an angiography study. Am J Cardiol 50:776–780, 1982.

56. Rabinovitch M, Haworth SG, Castaneda AR, et al: Lung biopsy in congenital heart disease: morphometric approach to pulmonary vascular disease. Circulation 58:1107–1122, 1978.

57. Rabinovitch M, Keane JF, Norwood WI, et al: Vascular structure in lung tissue obtained at biopsy correlated with pulmonary hemodynamic findings after repair of congenital heart defects. Circulation 69:655–667, 1984.

58. Ramaciotti C, Keren A, Silverman NH: Importance of (perimembranous) ventricular septal aneurysm in the natural history of isolated perimembranous ventricular septal defect. Am J Cardiol 57:268–272, 1986.

59. Richardson JV, Schieken RM, Lauer RM, et al: Repair of large ventricular septal defects in infants and small children. Ann Surg 195:318–322, 1982.

60. Rhodes L, Keane JF, Fellows KE, et al: Long follow-up (to 43 years) of ventricular septal defect with audible aortic regurgitation. Am J Cardiol 66:340–345, 1990.

61. Rothman KJ, Fyler DC: Association of congenital heart defects with season and population density. Teratology 13:29–34, 1976.

62. Rothman KJ, Fyler DC: Sex, birth order, and maternal age characteristics of infants with congenital heart defects. Am J Epidemiol 104:527–534, 1976.

63. Soto B, Becker AE, Moulaert AJ, et al: Classification of ventricular septal defects. Br Heart J 43:332–343, 1980.

64. Van Hare GF, Soffer LJ, Sivakoff MC, et al: Twenty-five-year experience with ventricular septal defect in infants and children. Am Heart J 114:606–614, 1987.

65. Van Praagh R, McNamara JJ: Anatomic types of ventricular septal defect with aortic insufficiency: diagnostic and surgical considerations. Am Heart J 75:604–619, 1968.

66. Vincent RN, Lang P, Elixson EM, et al: Extravascular lung water in children after operative closure of either isolated atrial septal defect or ventricular septal defect. Am J Cardiol 56:536–539, 1985.

67. Vogel JHK, McNamara DG, Blount SG: Role of hypoxia in determining pulmonary vascular resistance in infants with ventricular septal defects. Am J Cardiol 20:346–349, 1967.

68. Vogel M, Freedom RM, Brand A, et al: Ventricular septal defect and subaortic stenosis: an analysis of 41 patients. Am J Cardiol 52:1258–1263, 1983.

69. Vogl M, Smallhorn JF, Freedom RM, et al: An echocardiographic study of the association of ventricular septal defect and right ventricular muscle bundles with a fixed subaortic abnormality. Am J Cardiol 61:857–860, 1988.

70. Weidman W, et al: Natural history study II: followup in patients with ventricular septal defect, aortic stenosis, and pulmonary stenosis. Unpublished data.

71. Whittemore R, Hobbins JC, Engle MA: Pregnancy and its outcome in women with and without surgical treatment of congenital heart disease. Am J Cardiol 50:641–651, 1982.

72. Williams RG, Bierman FZ, Sanders SP: Echocardiographic diagnosis of congenital anomalies. Boston, Little, Brown and Co., 1986.

73. Yeager SB, Freed MD, Keane JF, et al: Primary surgical closure of ventricular septal defect in the first year of life: results in 128 infants. J Am Coll Cardiol 3:1269–1276, 1984.

Chapter 29

PULMONARY STENOSIS

Donald C. Fyler, M.D.

DEFINITION

Obstruction to outflow from the right ventricle, whether within the body of the right ventricle, at the pulmonary valve, or in the pulmonary arteries, is described as pulmonary stenosis. Often these obstructions occur with other major cardiac abnormalities. For the purposes of this discussion, those associated with another cardiac abnormality (except for patent ductus arteriosus, atrial septal defect, and patent foramen ovale) will be excluded; only those with an intact ventricular septum will be considered.

PREVALENCE

There were 1,500 patients (10.7%) seen between 1973 and 1987 at The Children's Hospital in Boston who were described as having pulmonary stenosis or pulmonary regurgitation as isolated defects (Exhibit 1). Pulmonary stenosis with an intact ventricular septum is the second most common congenital cardiac defect (see ch. 18) and, when it is associated with other congenital cardiac lesions, pulmonary stenosis may occur in as many as 50% of all patients with congenital heart disease.

Most authors report that between 7.5 and 12% of their patients have pulmonary stenosis with an intact ventricular septum (see ch. 18).

ANATOMY

Pulmonary valvar stenosis is characterized by fused or absent commissures. In most patients the valve is a mobile, dome-shaped structure with an orifice that may be tiny and sometimes eccentric (Fig. 1). The jet of blood through the valve usually causes poststenotic dilatation, most often involving the main and left main pulmonary arteries, because that is the direction of the jet (Fig. 2). When there is severe valvar stenosis, there is right ventricular hypertrophy, including infundibular muscle, which may contribute to the obstruction.

Exhibit 1

Boston Children's Hospital Experience 1973–1987	
Pulmonary Outflow Problems*	
Basis for Diagnosis n = 1174	
Clinic visit	954
Echocardiography	313
Cardiac catheterization	384
Cardiac surgery	207
Dead	6
Types of Pulmonary Stenosis n = 1174	
Diagnosis	*No. of patients†*
Valvar pulmonary stenosis	1022
Pulmonary regurgitation	150
Peripheral pulmonary stenosis	132
Abnormal pulmonary valve	47
Subvalvar stenosis	38
Excessive moderator bands	18
Maternal rubella	16
Noonan syndrome	8
Williams syndrome	6

*There were 1500 patients with pulmonary outflow problems; 1174 were first seen after January 1973.
†Some patients are listed in more than one category.

Dysplastic valves consisting of thickened, irregular, immobile tissue and a variably small pulmonary valve annulus are much less common.[4]

Obstructive muscle in the outflow tract, perhaps erroneously called "moderator bands," is seen in patients with tetralogy of Fallot and in some patients with membranous ventricular septal defect (see pp. 455, 489). Occasionally, because some of these ventricular defects close spontaneously, patients are discovered to have important muscular obstruction in the outflow of the right ventricle as an apparently isolated lesion. Whether some patients have excessive muscle without ever having had a ventricular defect is not known. These muscular obstructions occur in the region of the mod-

459

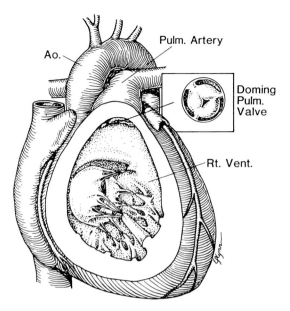

Figure 1. Diagram of a patient with valvar pulmonary stenosis. Note the domed pulmonary valve and poststenotic dilatation.

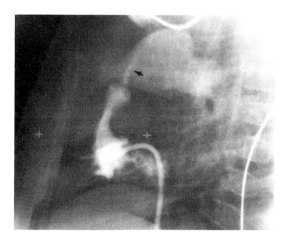

Figure 2. Right ventricular angiogram in a patient with valvar pulmonary stenosis. Note the jet of contrast through the domed valve (arrow) and the poststenotic dilatation.

erator band at the proximal infundibulum and, in some patients, they tend to be progressive.[24,31,33]

Infundibular stenosis of the type associated with the tetralogy of Fallot syndrome is rarely seen as an isolated lesion with an intact ventricular septum. The diagnosis of infundibular pulmonary stenosis with no ventricular septal defect is immediately suspect and the presence of excessive muscle bands is likely.

Peripheral pulmonary stenosis may take several forms. There may be a single obstructive lesion, multiple similar lesions located at approximately the same distance from the pulmonary valve, or symmetrical or asymmetrical pulmonary arterial

hypoplasia (Figs. 3 and 4). Some of these obstructions are centrally located and accessible to the surgeon. Others are located more distally in the lung and are surgically inaccessible. Some involve the main pulmonary artery and the right and left main pulmonary arteries as discrete obstructions (Fig. 3). There may be some proximal dilatation because of hypertension, and distal, poststenotic dilatation because of a jet through the obstructive orifice. Rarely, a pulmonary artery is completely absent.

A particular pattern of right and left main pulmonary artery hypoplasia is seen in patients who are suffering from the maternal rubella syndrome.[30] Diffuse peripheral pulmonary stenosis is part of Alagille syndrome[1] and may be associated with intrabiliary obstruction. Peripheral pulmonary arterial obstruction is seen sometimes in Noonan syndrome,[22] and peripheral as well as main pulmonary artery obstructions are seen in patients with Williams syndrome.[37]

PHYSIOLOGY

To provide an adequate cardiac output, the right ventricular pressure must be elevated sufficiently to overcome the pulmonary stenosis. With exercise the requirement for cardiac output is increased and right ventricular pressure rises proportionately until the capacity of the right ventricular muscle is surpassed.[17] To estimate the severity of the obstruction, it is important to know the amount of blood being pumped across the valve as well as the pressure required. For this reason, estimates of the severity of obstruction require either a reproducible basal state or direct measurement of blood flow. The increase in pressure needed to produce greater cardiac output is predictable, once the pressure gradient in the resting state is known. Consequently, a well-documented pressure gradient, measured with the child in a calm, relaxed state (ideally asleep but not anesthetized), is the ultimate standard for categorizing the severity of pulmonary stenosis (Fig. 5).

The point between the right ventricle and the pulmonary artery at which the pressure drops is the point of anatomic obstruction (Fig. 6).

Chronic elevation of right ventricular pressure results in right ventricular hypertrophy and a less compliant right ventricle. Greater right atrial pressures are required to fill the ventricle, and relative right and left atrial pressures may be reversed, favoring persistent patency of the foramen ovale and right-to-left shunting.

Deformity and malfunctioning of the left ventricle occur in proportion to the right ventricular hypertension and can be demonstrated using sophisticated techniques.[13,32] However, they are of little practical consequence, because they improve with relief of the right ventricular hypertension.

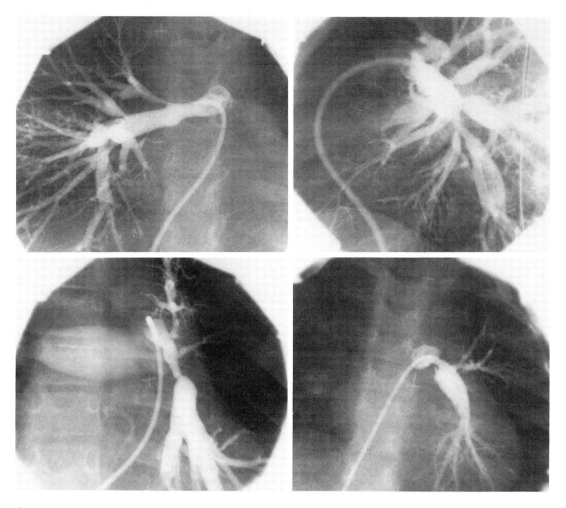

Figure 3. Several angiograms of patients with various forms of peripheral pulmonary stenosis. Note the areas of hypoplasia, branch stenosis, and poststenotic dilatation in obstructed branches.

Figure 4. Pulmonary artery angiogram in a patient with the bilateral peripheral pulmonary artery disease. Note the marked hypoplasia of the pulmonary arteries.

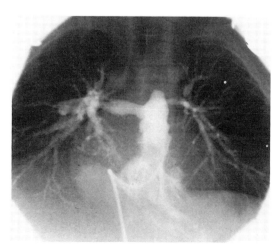

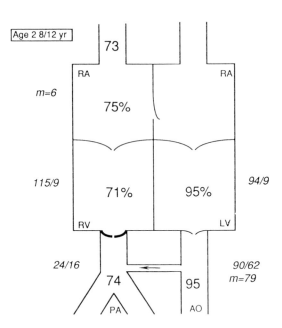

Figure 5. Physiologic diagram of a 2-year-old patient with valvar pulmonary stenosis. Note the normal pulmonary artery pressure with suprasystemic right ventricular pressure.

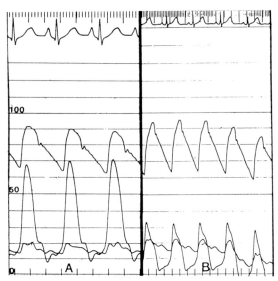

Figure 6. **A,** Simultaneous pressure tracings from the aorta, right ventricle, and pulmonary artery in a patient with valvar pulmonary stenosis. The pressure scale is in mm Hg. Note that the right ventricular systolic pressure is 70, whereas the pulmonary artery systolic pressure is 20 mm Hg. **B,** Following balloon dilatation of the pulmonary valve, the recording speed has been halved and the heart rate is slower. The right ventricular systolic pressure is now 30 mm Hg, while the pulmonary artery systolic pressure is unchanged compared with panel A.

VALVAR PULMONARY STENOSIS

Clinical Manifestations

Characteristically, children with valvar pulmonary stenosis and an intact septum, who are not cyanotic, grow well and are asymptomatic. In Boston Children's Hospital experience, there has been no predilection in either sex.

The cardiac defect is discovered on routine auscultation, usually at birth, although the patient with maximal obstruction may be discovered because of cyanosis. The systolic murmur is loudest at the second left intercostal space; it is ejection in type, the maximal intensity being at mid-systole or later (Fig. 7). The later the peak intensity of the murmur, the greater is the obstruction (Figs. 8 and 9). Often, there is a systolic thrill in the same area. The second heart sound is split, proportionate to the severity of the obstruction (Fig. 10). The greater the obstruction, the longer the right ven-

tricle takes to empty and the wider is the splitting. The second component, the pulmonary component, is decreased in intensity in proportion to the pressure in the pulmonary artery. The lower the pressure, the softer is the second component of the second heart sound and, with maximal obstruction, it may be inaudible. Usually there is an ejection click early in systole; without a click other diagnoses should be considered. The smaller the interval between the first sound and the click, the more severe is pulmonary stenosis (Fig. 11).[11,21]

"A" wave pulsations in the neck veins are not unusual, but clinical right-sided congestive heart failure is rare. When there are prominent "A" waves a fourth heart sound may be audible. A small infant with maximal obstruction may have a minimal murmur, sometimes overlooked, and cyanosis.

Electrocardiography

The electrocardiogram shows right-axis deviation and right ventricular hypertrophy proportion-

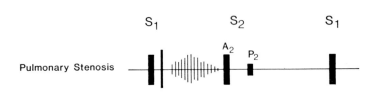

Figure 7. Diagrammatic presentation of the murmur in a patient with valvar pulmonary stenosis. Compare with phonocardiogram in Figure 8. S_1, first sound; S_2, second sound; A_2, aortic component of the second heart sound. (From Avery ME, First LP (eds): Pediatric Medicine. Baltimore, Williams & Wilkins, 1989, with permission.)

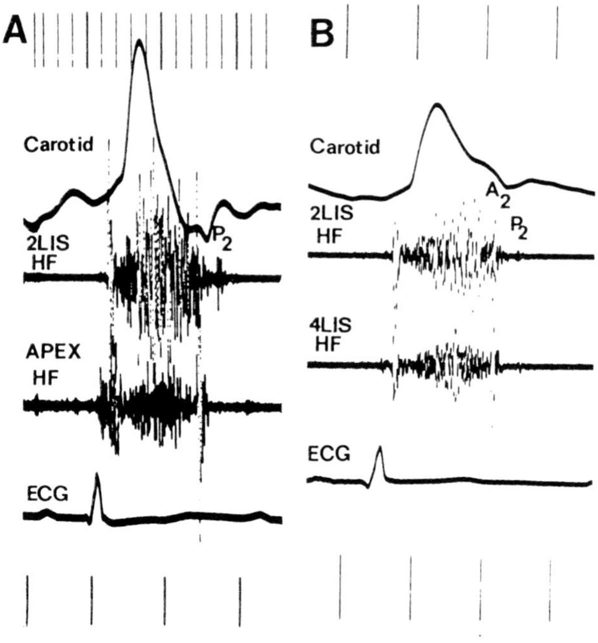

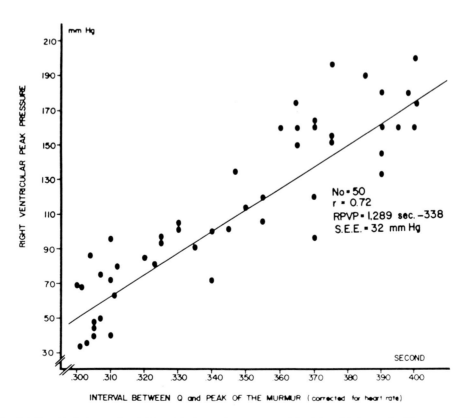

Figure 8. Phonocardiograms from two patients with pulmonic stenosis and intact ventricular septum. **A,** A moderately split second sound with an appreciable pulmonic component, indicating mild stenosis. **B,** Widely split second sound with a low-intensity pulmonic component characteristic of severe stenosis. Note the late apex of the diamond in B. (From Nadas AS, Fyler DC: Pediatric Cardiology, Philadelphia, W.B. Saunders, 1973, with permission.)

Figure 9. Relationship between the right ventricular peak pressure and the interval between the Q wave and the peak intensity of the murmur. (From Gamboa R, et al: Accuracy of the phonocardiogram in assessing severity of aortic and pulmonary stenosis. Circulation 30:35–46, 1964, by permission of the American Heart Association, Inc.)

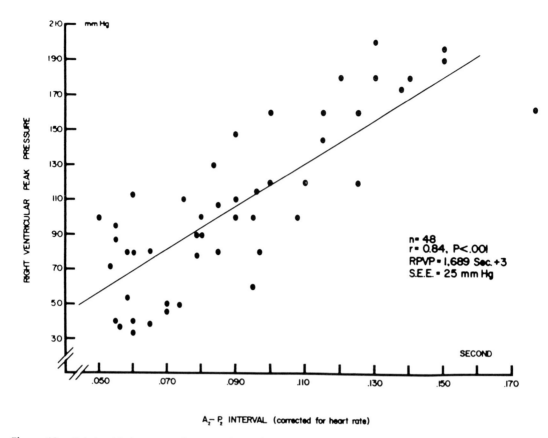

Figure 10. Relationship between right ventricular peak pressure and the amount of splitting of the second heart sound (A₂–P₂ interval). (From Gamboa R, et al: Accuracy of the phonocardiogram in assessing severity of aortic and pulmonary stenosis. Circulation 30:35–46, 1964, by permission of the American Heart Association, Inc.)

ate to the amount of obstruction (Fig. 12). The R-wave in the right chest leads is roughly predictive of the right ventricular pressure. There may be P pulmonale. In infants with maximal obstruction, bordering on pulmonary atresia, the evidence for right ventricular hypertrophy may be less convincing and, rarely, left dominance is observed.

Chest X-ray

Except in cases of maximal obstruction in early infancy, the heart size is normal or only slightly enlarged. Poststenotic dilatation of the main and left main pulmonary artery may be visible. In the cyanotic patient the pulmonary vasculature is decreased. Also, acyanotic children may have decreased pulmonary vascular markings when the pulmonary stenosis is severe enough to limit the upper extremes of pulmonary blood flow during exercise. In these children the average day-to-day blood flow through the lungs is less than normal even though the resting blood flow is normal. Occasionally, in a patient with maximal obstruction, the right ventricle may be grossly dilated (seen as cardiomegaly on the conventional chest x-ray).

Echocardiography

The presence and magnitude of the pressure gradient across the outflow tract usually can be detected and measured by Doppler echocardiography as a maximum instantaneous velocity, which is about 10% greater than the peak-to-peak gradient measured at cardiac catheterization.

The size of the pulmonary valve ring also can be estimated, as well as the size of structures immediately before and after the obstruction. Poststenotic dilatation can be documented. The echocardiographer may have difficulty imaging peripheral pulmonary stenosis, although central obstructions usually are readily seen.

The presence and severity of pulmonary stenosis can be determined by 2-D and Doppler echocardiography. The size of the pulmonary valve annulus and the mobility and consistency of the leaflets can be seen using parasternal long- (Fig. 13) and short-axis views.[36] The leaflets are typically thickened but dome in systole. Dysplastic valves are characterized by markedly thickened and immobile leaflets as well as annular hypoplasia. Doppler echocardiography is quite reliable for estimating the gradient across the pulmonary valve.[19] Multiple trans-

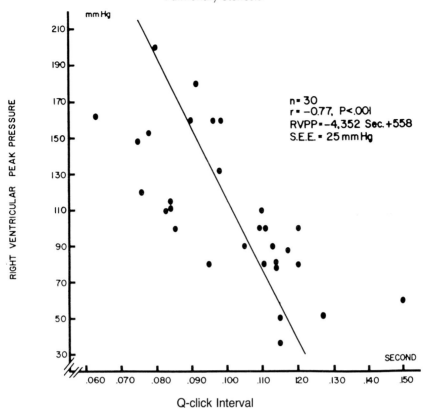

Figure 11. Relationship between right ventricular peak pressure and the Q-X (Q-click) interval in patients with pulmonary valvar stenosis. (From Gamboa R, et al: Accuracy of the phonocardiogram in assessing severity of aortic and pulmonary stenosis. Circulation 30:35–46, 1964, by permission of the American Heart Association, Inc.)

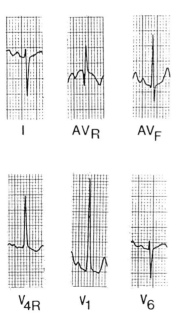

Figure 12. Electrocardiogram in patient with valvar pulmonary stenosis.

ducer locations, including parasternal, para-apical, and subxiphoid, should be used to minimize the likelihood of underestimating the gradient.

Cardiac Catheterization

Although cardiac catheterization is not needed to establish the anatomy or the severity of the pulmonary stenosis, all patients with echocardiographic evidence of significant pulmonary stenosis (a gradient of 40–50 mm Hg) should undergo cardiac catheterization for more precise estimation of the gradient and for balloon dilatation of the pulmonary valve if needed. Balloon valvuloplasty is feasible at any age[28,38] but the procedure is safest and technically simplest in children older than 18 months of age.

A right ventricular angiogram is recorded to document the anatomy. With the patient in the anteroposterior and lateral positions, an injection of 1 ml of contrast agent over 1 second is made into the right ventricle (Fig. 2). Because the catheter tends to recoil into the right atrium, a balloon-tipped angiography catheter is pushed to the apex of the right ventricle while the balloon is inflated. It is important not to inflate the balloon after the catheter has been positioned because of the trabecular nature of this part of the right ventricle.

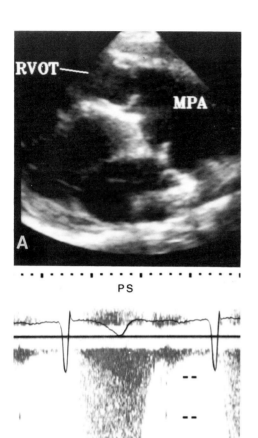

PS

4.3 m/s

B

Figure 13. **A,** Parasternal long-axis view of the right ventricular outflow tract demonstrating a doming pulmonary valve with thickened leaflets. MPA, main pulmonary artery; RVOT, right ventricular outflow tract. **B,** Continuous-wave Doppler recording through the valve. The peak velocity is 4.3 m/sec, indicating a peak pressure gradient of about 75 mm Hg.

The tip may be lodged between trabeculae and, with inflation of the balloon, angiography may cause a myocardial stain.

Management

Patients with mild pulmonary stenosis do not require special concessions. Physical exercise should not be limited and, because of the rarity of infective endocarditis, prophylaxis during dental procedures is not needed (see ch. 26). Almost half

of the children who are diagnosed clinically as having pulmonary stenosis do not need further evaluation (Table 1), although in recent years many now undergo echocardiography.

When more severe forms of pulmonary stenosis are suspected, cardiac catheterization is carried out. At the Children's Hospital in Boston, about one-third of patients with pulmonary stenosis had obstructions severe enough to require balloon valvuloplasty. Since the advent of balloon valvuloplasty,[16,18,29] the shift from cardiac surgery to balloon valvuloplasty has been virtually complete (Exhibit 2). There have been no deaths resulting from surgical or balloon valvuloplasty, and the need for reoperation is uncommon. Balloon valvuloplasty is useful whether there is fusion of commissures or the valve is dysplastic, although the dysplastic valves respond less well.[7,20] Provided the catheter can be advanced though the valve, balloon valvuloplasty has been successful in neonates.[28,38] Technical discussions about using larger balloons[20] or multiple balloons[26] simultaneously are matters of current interest.

Whether to use the transventricular[6] or pulmonary artery approach, and whether to use pump oxygenators or inflow occlusion in the surgical management of pulmonary valvar stenosis are subjects of debate among surgeons.[2,12,23] The differences in outcome are negligible.[6] Which neonates require a supplementary Blalock shunt because of persistent cyanosis[5] may be a moot question now that these babies are managed with balloon valvuloplasty, particularly with the availability of prostaglandins E as an alternate means of maintaining supplementary pulmonary blood supply (Exhibit 2).[9]

Whether the stenosis is relieved by open surgery or by balloon valvuloplasty, there may be residual obstructing muscular hypertrophy in the infundibulum. Immediately following either approach, there may be a residual gradient across the subvalvar area which clears within hours or days. Vis-

Table 1. Pulmonary Stenosis: Progressive Severity of Obstruction

Initial Gradient Between Right Ventricle and Pulmonary Artery (mm Hg)	No. of Patients with Progression of Obstruction Severe Enough to Require Surgery (%)
>25	4
26–49	21
50–79	79
80–	97

From Hayes CJ, Gersony WM, Driscoll DJ, et al., Results of treatment of patients with pulmonary stenosis. In The Report of the Second Natural History Study of Congenital Heart Defects (NHS-2). Circulation, in press, by permission of the American Heart Association, Inc.)

These data are based on a large series of patients followed for an average of 22 years.

Exhibit 2

Boston Children's Hospital Experience 1973–1987 **Procedural Management of Valvar Pulmonary Stenosis** n = 223 procedures						
			Years			
Procedure	1973–77	1978–83	1983	1984	1985	1986	1987
Surgical Procedure	56	65	10	10	3	2	0
Catheterization	0	0	0	7	19	23	28

There were 384 patients who underwent cardiac catheterization and 207 who underwent cardiac surgery. The 214 who had pulmonary valvuloplasty for valvar pulmonary stenosis are shown in this table. Nine patients had more than one intervention. Note the trend toward balloon valvulopasty in recent years.

	Ages at Valvuloplasty		
Procedure	Less than 1 month	1–12 months	Older than 12 months
Surgical Procedure	24	24	98
Catheterization	6	13	58

One 2-day-old infant died following surgical valvotomy and was discovered at postmortem examination to have had aortic stenosis as well. There were no other deaths. Three infants had shunting procedures within a few days of the valvuloplasty.

Surgical Procedures
n = 205

Operative Procedure	No. of procedures*
Valvulopasty	146
Patent ductus ligation	29
Atrial defect closure	45
Subvalvar surgery	21
Pulmonary artery reconstruction	17
Systemic artery–pulmonary artery shunt	5

*Some patients had more than one operative procedure.

ible infundibular hypertrophy may be demonstrable by angiography weeks afterward.

In the past, older patients whose ventricular pressure exceeded 200 mm Hg were at some added risk because the infundibular obstruction did not promptly regress, and deaths were reported. These patients were thought of as having a "suicide" right ventricle, a problem that is no longer encountered, perhaps because now patients are operated on at an early age.

Course

Patients with mild pulmonary stenosis continue to have mild pulmonary stenosis, usually without progression, although occasionally the stenosis has been known to progress.[14]

In patients with moderate or severe pulmonary valvar stenosis, the obstruction has a tendency to progress (Table 1);[14] therefore, these patients are candidates for either surgical or balloon valvuloplasty. Among those who have undergone successful operation, the need for subsequent surgery is extremely rare, and actuarial survival (whether or not surgery is required and without respect to the initial severity) is at least as good as that of the normal population.[14] There is no reason to believe that the outcome after successful balloon valvulo-

plasty will be different. Right ventricular hypertrophy regresses after relief of the obstruction, but it is the author's impression that incomplete right bundle branch block patterns often persist long afterward. Mild exercise limitation is detectable years after surgical valvuloplasty.[8] The incidence of infective endocarditis is negligible (5.6/10,000 patient years) and the incidence of brain abscess is even less (3.3/10,000 patient years).

VARIATIONS

Critical Pulmonary Stenosis in the Neonate

Maximal pulmonary stenosis in a small infant is a life-threatening problem. There are two variations on this theme.

With maximal pulmonary stenosis (near pulmonary atresia), the infant is cyanotic and may have a small right ventricle. Right ventricular pressure equals systemic pressure or is greater.[10] Some infants resemble patients who have pulmonary atresia with an intact septum; in these the electrocardiogram shows left ventricular hypertrophy. With surgical or balloon relief, the cyanosis often does not clear immediately but, rather, improves gradually over the ensuing weeks. Occasionally, because of persisting cyanosis, a systemic artery-pulmonary artery shunting procedure is considered necessary,[5] but for the most part this can be avoided (Fig. 14). Prostaglandins E offer an alternative means of maintaining pulmonary blood flow during this transition period. As with patients who have pulmonary atresia and an intact ventricular septum, the size of the right ventricle[35] and the diameter of the tricuspid orifice provide clues to the likely course after valvuloplasty. It as been a matter of some interest to those of us at Children's Hospital in Boston that any orifice in the valve seems to obviate the need for a shunting operation, whereas atresia of the valve most often requires an arterial shunt for survival (see p. 639). Others have not had similar experience.[5] Usually, the small right ventricle grows in the surviving patients. Whether this improvement is due to closure of the patent foramen ovale (force feeding the ventricle) or to relief from high pressure is not clear.[27]

Other infants, who are not seen until some weeks after birth, have maximal pulmonary stenosis with a considerably enlarged heart on the chest x-ray and severe right ventricular hypertrophy on the electrocardiogram. Often there is no visible cyanosis. At cardiac catheterization there is supraventricular pressure in the right ventricle, elevated right ventricular end-diastolic pressure, and elevated right atrial pressure. These infants usually respond promptly to balloon or surgical valvuloplasty.

Rarely, a child will have persistent cyanosis.

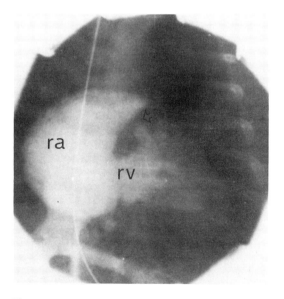

Figure 14. Angiogram of a patient with critical valvar pulmonary stenosis (same patient as in Fig. 13). This angiogram was interpreted as showing pulmonary valvar atresia. At surgery a tiny orifice was found in the pulmonary valve (arrow). After valvotomy she remained cyanotic for 2 months. No further surgery was done until age 5 years when a residual gradient across the valve was removed by balloon dilatation. ra, right atrium; rv, right ventricle.

Whether or not the atrial opening should be closed can be determined by occluding the atrial defect with a balloon; if this is tolerated well, the atrial defect can be closed safely.[3]

Peripheral Pulmonary Stenosis

These children are discovered to have an ejection murmur. If the obstruction is bilateral, the murmur is found to be equally loud all over the chest. The discovery of an ejection murmur of minimal intensity heard equally loud in all parts of the chest is virtually diagnostic of peripheral pulmonary stenosis, and if the electrocardiogram is normal, the severity can be said to be mild. Fortunately, these obstructions do not seem to be progressive and, for clinical purposes, are largely a curiosity. Most patients with peripheral pulmonary stenosis require little or no intervention. Of 132 children at Children's Hospital in Boston who were labeled with this diagnosis, 62 came to cardiac catheterization and 19 were considered candidates for surgery or balloon dilatation (17 had surgical reconstruction, 10 had balloon angioplasty and 8 had both) (Exhibit 1). Balloon dilatation may be the treatment of choice (it is for patients with tetralogy of Fallot who have more severe peripheral pulmonary stenosis), and, for those distal obstructions that are inaccessible to the surgeon, it may be the only possibility.

Infants born of mothers who had **rubella** around the time of conception commonly have a patent ductus arteriosus and a characteristic form of peripheral pulmonary stenosis. There is tapering hypoplasia of the origins of both right and left main pulmonary arteries that is rarely severe enough to require surgery but is typical enough to suggest the possibility of maternal German measles. This, along with the associated problems of deafness, blindness, and mental retardation, has almost completely disappeared since routine immunization against rubella has been adopted.

Asymmetric peripheral pulmonary stenosis is encountered and, rarely, even unilateral **congenital absence of a pulmonary artery** without any other cardiac abnormality (Fig. 15).[25] When there is unilateral peripheral pulmonary stenosis, it is important to remember that the bulk of pulmonary blood flow goes through the unobstructed lung, often at normal pressure. In this case the estimation of relative pulmonary blood flow to each lung can be made with radionucleotide scans. On occasion, angiography reveals that a mild obstruction to one lung is associated with a predominant blood flow to the opposite lung, and the decision to use surgical or balloon angioplasty is self evident. Similarly, a radionucleotide scan can used to assess improvement after angioplasty.

Bands of muscle obstructing the outflow of the right ventricle (**moderator bands**) which are not

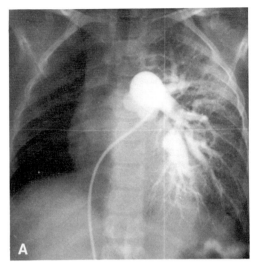

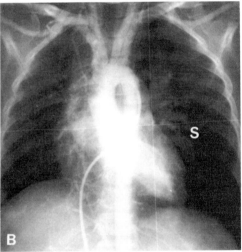

Figure 15. Angiogram of a patient with a congenitally absent right pulmonary artery. **A,** With injection of contrast material in the main pulmonary artery, there is no opacification of the right pulmonary artery. **B,** On the levophase of the same angiogram, there is no other source of perfusion of the right pulmonary artery. At catheterization this man had a normal pulmonary artery pressure. Fifteen years later he is well and vigorously pursuing a career as a cat burglar.

associated with a ventricular septal defect are encountered occasionally (Exhibit 1). Those associated with a ventricular septal defect tend to be progressive and, occasionally, even if the ventricular septal defect closes spontaneously or is surgically patched, the outflow obstruction may still progress (see p. 455).

Noonan syndrome must be considered in an infant with pulmonary stenosis, lymphedema, webbed neck, dysmorphic facies, and hypotonia. The pulmonary valve is dysplastic and variably obstructive. The chromosomes are normal. Older patients may have cardiomyopathy.[22]

Some patients with **Williams syndrome** develop stenoses in the pulmonary arteries. Generally, these are associated with arterial stenoses, such as characteristic supraaortic stenosis, coarctation of the aorta, and renal artery stenoses. These lesions can develop at any time and tend to be progressive. Supravalvar pulmonary stenosis usually is mild. When it is discovered, the possibility of Williams syndrome should be considered.[37]

Pulmonary Regurgitation

Pulmonary regurgitation is a common observation following surgery for tetralogy of Fallot and is seen occasionally following correction of pulmonary stenosis (Exhibit 1). Rarely, it is an isolated congenital abnormality manifested by an early diastolic, decrescendo murmur that is accidentally discovered during routine auscultation. The main pulmonary artery is large, and is sometimes coincidentally recognized on a chest x-ray taken for some other reason. Pulmonary regurgitation has been a benign lesion in the author's experience, despite reports of problems in neonates with this abnormality.[15] Since the advent of Doppler echocardiography, the incidence of isolated pulmonary regurgitation has risen tenfold. Only recently it has been learned that most normal individuals have trivial pulmonary regurgitation that can be detected only by this technique.[34] Hence, there is little relation between the incidence of isolated pulmonary regurgitation recognized by auscultation and that recognized by echocardiography.

REFERENCES

1. Alagille D, Odievre M, Gautier M, et al: Hepatic ductular hypoplasia associated with characteristic facies, vertebral malformations, retarded physical, mental and skeletal development and cardiac murmur. J Pediatr 86:63–71, 1975.
2. Awariefe SO, Clarke DR, Pappas G: Surgical approach to critical pulmonary valve stenosis in infants less than six months of age. J Thorac Cardiovasc Surg 85:375–387, 1983.
3. Bass JL, Fuhrman BP, Lock JE: Balloon occlusion of atrial septal defect to assess right ventricular capability in hypoplastic right heart syndrome. Circulation 68:1081–1086, 1983.
4. Becu L, Somerville J, Gallo A: "Isolated" pulmonary valve stenosis as part of more widespread cardiovascular disease. Br Heart J 38:472–482, 1976.
5. Coles JG, Freedom RM, Olley PM, et al: Surgical management of critical pulmonary stenosis in the neonate. Ann Thorac Surg 38:458–465, 1984.
6. Daskalopoulos DA, Pieroni DR, Gingell RL, et al: Closed transventricular pulmonary valvotomy in infants. J Thorac Cardiovasc Surg 84:187–191, 1982.
7. DiSessa TG, Alpert BS, Chase NA, et al: Balloon valvuloplasty in children with dysplastic pulmonary valves. Am J Cardiol 60:405–407, 1987.
8. Driscoll DJ, Wolfe RR, Gersony WM, et al: Exercise response of patients with pulmonary stenosis. In Report of the Second Natural History Study of Congenital Heart Defects (NHS-2). Circulation (in press).

9. Freed MD, Heymann MA, Lewis AB, et al: Prostaglandin E in infants with ductus arteriosus-dependent congenital heart disease. Circulation 64:899–905, 1981.

10. Freed MD, Rosenthal A, Bernhard WF, et al: Critical pulmonary stenosis with diminutive right ventricle in neonates. Circulation 48:875–881, 1973.

11. Gamboa R, Hugenholtz PG, Nadas AS: Accuracy of the phonocardiogram in assessing severity of aortic and pulmonic stenosis. Circulation 30:35–46, 1964.

12. Griffith BP, Hardesty RL, Siewers RD, et al: Pulmonary valvulotomy alone for pulmonary stenosis: results in children with and without muscular infundibular hypertrophy. J Thorac Cardiovasc Surg 83:577–583, 1982.

13. Harinck E, Becker AE, Gittenberger-DeGroot AC, et al: The left ventricle in congenital isolated pulmonary valve stenosis. Br Heart J 39:429–435, 1977.

14. Hayes CJ, Gersony WM, Driscoll DJ, et al: Results of treatment of patients with pulmonary stenosis. In The Report of the Second Natural History Study of Congenital Heart Defects (NHS-2). Circulation, in press, Nov. 1991.

15. Ito T, Engle MA, Holswade GR: Congenital insufficiency of the pulmonic valve: a rare cause of neonatal heart failure. Pediatrics 28:712–718, 1961.

16. Kan JS, White RF, Mitchell SE, et al: Percutaneous balloon valvulopasty: a new method for treating congenital pulmonary valve stenosis. N Engl J Med 307:540–542, 1982.

17. Krabill KA, Wang Y, Einzig S, et al: Rest and exercise hemodynamics in pulmonary stenosis: comparison of children and adults. Am J Cardiol 56:360–365, 1985.

18. Labibidi Z, Wu J: Percutaneous balloon pulmonary valvulopasty. Am J Cardiol 52:560–562, 1983.

19. Lima CO, Sahn DJ, Valdez-Cruz LM, et al: Noninvasive prediction of transvalvular pressure gradient in patients with pulmonary stenosis by quantitative two-dimensional echocardiographic Doppler studies. Circulation 67:866–871, 1983.

20. Marantz PM, Huhta JC, Mullins CE, et al: Results of balloon valvulopasty in typical and dysplastic pulmonary valve stenosis: Doppler echocardiographic follow-up. J Am Coll Cardiol 12:476–479, 1988.

21. Nadas AS, Fyler DC: Pediatric Cardiology. Philadelphia, W.B. Saunders, 1972, pp. 293–294.

22. Noonan JA, Ehmke DA: Associated non-cardiac malformations in children with congenital heart disease. J Pediatr 63:468–470, 1963.

23. Polansky DB, Clark EB, Doty DB: Pulmonary stenosis in infants and young children. Ann Thorac Surg 39:159–164, 1985.

24. Pongiglione G, Freedom RM, Cook D, et al: Mecha-

nism of acquired right ventricular outflow tract obstruction in patients with ventricular septal defect: an angiocardiographic study. Am J Cardiol 50:776–780, 1982.

25. Pool PE, Vogel JH, Blount SG: Congenital unilateral absence of a pulmonary artery. Am J Cardiol 10:706–732, 1962.

26. Radtke W, Keane JF, Fellows KE, et al: Percutaneous balloon valvotomy of congenital pulmonary stenosis. J Am Coll Cardiol 8:909–915, 1986.

27. Rao PS, Liebman J, Borkat G: Right ventricular growth in a case of pulmonic stenosis with intact ventricular septum and hypoplastic right ventricle. Circulation 53:389–394, 1976.

28. Rey C, Marache P, Francart C, et al: Percutaneous transluminal balloon valvuloplasty of congenital pulmonary valve stenosis, with a special report on infants and neonates. J Am Coll Cardiol 11:815–820, 1988.

29. Rocchini AP, Kveselis DA, Crowley D, et al: Percutaneous balloon valvuloplasty for treatment of congenital pulmonary valvular stenosis in children. J Am Coll Cardiol 3:1005–1012, 1984.

30. Rowe RD: Cardiovascular disease in the rubella syndrome. In Keith JD, Rowe RD, Vlad P (eds): Heart Disease in Infancy and Childhood, 3rd ed. New York, Macmillan, 1979, pp. 3–13.

31. Rowland TW, Rosenthal A, Castaneda AR: Double-chamber right ventricle: experience with 17 cases. Am Heart J 89:455–462, 1975.

32. Sholler GF, Colan SD, Sanders SP: Effect of isolated right ventricular outflow obstruction on left ventricular function in infants. Am J Cardiol 62:778–784, 1988.

33. Simpson WF, Sade RM, Crawford FA, et al: Double-chambered right ventricle. Ann Thorac Surg 44:7–10, 1987.

34. Takao S, Miyatake K. Izumi S, et al: Clinical implications of pulmonary regurgitation in healthy individuals: detection by cross sectional pulsed Doppler echocardiography. Br Heart J 59:542–550, 1988.

35. Trowitzsch E, Colan SD, Sanders SP: Two-dimensional echocardiographic evaluation of the right ventricular size and function in newborns with severe right ventricular outflow tract obstruction. J Am Coll Cardiol 6:388–393, 1985.

36. Weyman AE, Hurwitz RA, Girod DA, et al: Cross-sectional echocardiographic visualization of the stenotic pulmonary valve. Circulation 56:769–774, 1977.

37. Williams JCP, Barrett-Boyes BG, Lowe JB: Supravalvar aortic stenosis. Circulation 24:1311–1318, 1961.

38. Zeevi B, Keane JF, Fellows KE, et al: Balloon dilation of critical pulmonary stenosis in the first week of life. J Am Coll Cardiol 11:821–824, 1988.

Chapter 30

TETRALOGY OF FALLOT

Donald C. Fyler, M.D.

DEFINITION

In 1888 Fallot[10] described a group of patients with infundibular pulmonary stenosis, a ventricular septal defect, dextroposed aorta (overriding aorta), and right ventricular hypertrophy. Although Fallot's name is attached to this syndrome, Stensen[49] earlier reported a patient with the same findings.

PREVALENCE

Except for the first weeks of life, tetralogy of Fallot is the leading form of heart disease that causes cyanosis. Nine percent of infants seen with critical congenital heart disease in the first year of life have the tetralogy of Fallot (0.196–0.258/1000 live births).[16] The overall incidence in the Boston Children's Hospital series of children with congenital heart disease was 8% (see ch. 18). Keith[28] reported 9.7% in his group of patients. Repaired tetralogy of Fallot is a common congenital cardiac lesion in surviving patients (see ch. 18).

EMBRYOLOGY

The relationship between the severity of the subpulmonary stenosis and the degree of overriding of the aorta is the basis for a theory of embryologic development. It is proposed that the fundamental problem is underdevelopment of the pulmonary infundibulum, all other features of the disease being secondary.[52] Whether this "monology" theory is an oversimplification or not, all observers focus on the infundibular anatomy, especially the relationship and abnormalities of the parietal and septal bands, as fundamental to the development of the syndrome of Fallot's tetralogy.

ANATOMY

The ventricular defect is located in the membranous septum, is subaortic (sometimes extending into the subpulmonary region), and is appropriately described as a **malalignment defect,** because the aortic root is overriding. The defect is large and of constant size relative to the size of the child, being large enough to equilibrate the right and left ventricular pressures. These defects, unlike most ventricular septal defects, do not get smaller with time and are not known to close spontaneously (Fig. 1).

In contrast, the degree of outflow obstruction is quite variable, ranging from very slight obstruction, to severe pulmonary stenosis, to complete pulmonary atresia. Classically, there is infundibular hypoplasia and obstruction, without which the diagnosis of tetralogy of Fallot is in doubt. The distinction between excessive moderator bands (see pp. 455, 459) and the infundibular obstruction of tetralogy should be made, because the two syndromes have different prognoses and different courses. At the same time, it must be kept in mind that the two problems may appear together (see p. 489). Additionally, most children with tetralogy of Fallot have hypoplasia of the pulmonary annulus

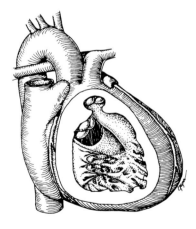

Figure 1. Drawing of the anatomy of tetralogy of Fallot. There is infundibular obstruction, a ventricular septal defect (through which the aortic leaflets can be seen), and a right aortic arch.

which may be severe. Characteristically, over time, obstruction of the pulmonary outflow tract becomes more severe, sometimes progressing to pulmonary atresia. Usually the pulmonary valve is deformed and often it is stenotic, presumably, in part, from hydraulic damage resulting from the jet produced by the underlying subpulmonary stenosis. Occasionally, the pulmonary valve is represented by only nubbins of tissue (see p. 486) (Exhibit 1).

The pulmonary arteries are usually small and often asymmetrically formed, with variable peripheral stenosis. The main pulmonary arteries may be more hypoplastic than the larger distal vessels (which are nonetheless smaller than normal), because distal blood flow may be supplied, in large part, by bronchial or collateral circulation. This is in contrast to patients with valvar pulmonary stenosis who have abnormally large central vessels and smaller distal vessels. The true **bronchial arteries** follow the bronchi and are normal structures, whereas the **collateral vessels** arising from the descending thoracic aorta are bizarre, primitive vessels. These tortuous structures supply sections of lung, sometimes crossing the midline to the opposite side of the chest (Fig. 2). Either bronchial

or collateral vessels may supply the bulk of distal pulmonary blood flow. Peripheral stenoses and areas of hypoplasia of the pulmonary arteries are common. Obstruction at the origin of the left main pulmonary artery, at the point of insertion of the ductus arteriosus, is particularly common. In its extreme form, the left main pulmonary artery is completely occluded. The pulmonary artery immediately distal to the obstruction is small, because it carries very limited blood flow. The principle that pulmonary arterial growth is dependent on the amount of blood flow is further emphasized by the remnants of main pulmonary arteries, or even absence of main pulmonary arteries, sometimes seen when there is pulmonary atresia (Exhibit 1).

Although the main and central pulmonary arteries are usually small or hypoplastic, the ascending aorta is comparatively and absolutely large. The degree to which the aorta overrides the ventricular septum is roughly proportionate to the severity of the right ventricular outflow obstruction. In the extreme form of overriding, both great arteries arise from the right ventricle and the patient is appropriately described as having a **double-outlet right ventricle** (see ch. 41). Between those with

Exhibit 1

Boston Children's Hospital Experience 1973–1987				
Tetralogy of Fallot*				
	Pulmonary Stenosis n = 1071	Absent Pulmonary Valve n = 22	Atrioventricular Canal n = 54	Pulmonary Atresia n = 256
First Seen				
−1972	446	8	8	52
1973–1977	163	2	12	25
1978–1982	209	4	19	55
1983–1987	253	8	15	124

*Patients with dextrocardia and tetralogy of Fallot are excluded.
Among 1403 patients with tetralogy of Fallot, 22 had an absent pulmonary valve, 54 were classified as having tetralogy of Fallot with an atrioventricular canal, and 256 were classified as having pulmonary atresia. Prior to 1973, 514 patients had been seen at Boston Children's Hospital.

Tetralogy of Fallot: Complicating Features			
	Pulmonary Stenosis n = 1071	Absent Pulmonary Valve n = 22	Atrioventricular Canal n = 54
Multiple Ventricular Defects	60	2	3
Abnormal Coronary Anatomy	51	0	3
Pulmonary Artery Stenosis or Hypoplasia*	299	–	12
Atresia of the Left Pulmonary Artery*	21	–	2
Atresia of the Right Pulmonary Artery*	5	–	1

*Some of these pulmonary artery abnormalities are congenital, some are iatrogenic, and some have developed over time. The number of observations are a function of the level of interest in the problem and the period of time that the interest was sustained. Are these data, then, an under-, over-, or precise estimation of reality? The author is not certain.

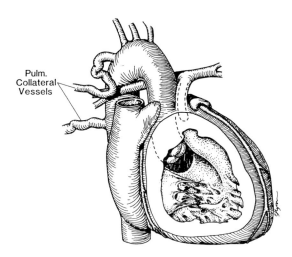

Pulm.
Collateral
Vessels

Figure 2. Drawing of the anatomy of tetralogy of Fallot with pulmonary atresia. There is no outflow from the right ventricle because of pulmonary atresia. The entire right ventricular output passes through the ventricular defect into the left ventricle and aorta. The main pulmonary artery is small (sometimes only a remnant exists). There are bizarre vessels supplying the lung (collaterals) which arise from the descending aorta.

tetralogy of Fallot with mild overriding of the aorta and those with double-outlet right ventricle lie a group of patients who might be categorized as having either one or the other diagnosis.

Among the 18% of children with tetralogy of Fallot who have pulmonary atresia (Exhibit 1), some are born with it whereas others develop atresia as they grow. With pulmonary outflow atresia, the main pulmonary artery varies from normal size, to small, to a string-like remnant of variable length. In the majority (70%) of patients with pulmonary atresia, the pulmonary blood supply is through a duct-like collateral from the undersurface of the aorta at about the point where a ductus arteriosus would be expected. In the remainder (30%),[43] pulmonary blood is provided from the descending aorta via collateral vessels. Rarely, these may be sufficiently large and numerous to cause congestive heart failure in infancy. Patients with pulmonary atresia have small, central pulmonary arteries, occasionally so small that surgical repair is impossible. Others have only limited distribution of true pulmonary vessels, whole lobes or segments of the lungs being unconnected to the pulmonary arterial tree. In these patients the collateral circulation may be required for survival, even if the pulmonary arteries eventually can be connected to the right ventricular outflow. It is rare to find bizarre collateral vessels supplying a major portion of pulmonary blood flow when there is pulmonary stenosis; collaterals are a feature of pulmonary atresia.

The younger the child, the more likely there will be a patent foramen ovale (pentalogy of Fallot)— 40% of the patients overall. In 25% the ascending aorta arches to the right. Five percent of patients have an anomalous coronary artery, arising from the right coronary artery, which supplies the left anterior descending coronary (Exhibit 1). This "conus coronary" passes over the right ventricular outflow, prohibiting an outflow incision and, thereby, greatly influencing the surgical options.

PHYSIOLOGY

In the mildest form of tetralogy of Fallot, the pulmonary stenosis may be so slight, particularly in early infancy, that significant resistance to pulmonary blood flow is nonexistent, and congestive heart failure, because of excessive left-to-right shunting, is the dominant problem (Fig. 3). With more severe stenosis the hemodynamics may be balanced, there being little shunting either to the right or to the left. The balance between the fixed pulmonary outflow obstruction and the relatively variable systemic resistance determines the degree of cyanosis at any given moment. When the outflow obstruction is severe, ultimately an almost inevitable development for most patients, most of the cardiac output passes through the ventricular defect into the aorta. The degree of cyanosis would be intolerable but for other sources of pulmonary blood flow, such as a patent ductus arteriosus, bronchial vessels, or collaterals. In the most extreme form there is complete atresia of the pulmonary outflow tract and the entire cardiac output passes through the ventricular septal defect, right-to-left. In this case the entire pulmonary blood flow is supplied by bronchial or collateral vessels once the ductus arteriosus has closed.

Cyanosis is the clinical manifestation of arterial oxygen unsaturation. Whether cyanosis is visible or not depends on the percent of arterial oxygen saturation and on the hemoglobin concentration. An arterial oxygen saturation of 50% with a hemoglobin of 20 gm results in 10 gm of reduced hemoglobin and visible cyanosis. With a 50% oxygen saturation and 10 gm of hemoglobin, there will be 5 gm of reduced hemoglobin, with barely visible cyanosis. In the second example it follows that only 5 gm of hemoglobin is available for oxygen delivery, the practical equivalent of severe anemia.

When the right-sided outflow obstruction and the systemic resistance balance each other, the potential for abrupt increases in right-to-left shunting exists through constriction of the muscular right ventricular outflow tract or reduction in the prevailing systemic resistance with exercise. Both of these effects may occur in an excited infant with tetralogy of Fallot and result in the sudden appearance of marked cyanosis and the other features of a cyanotic spell (see ch. 8).[19]

With chronic cyanosis, erythropoietin, the mediator to the production of hemoglobin, is pro-

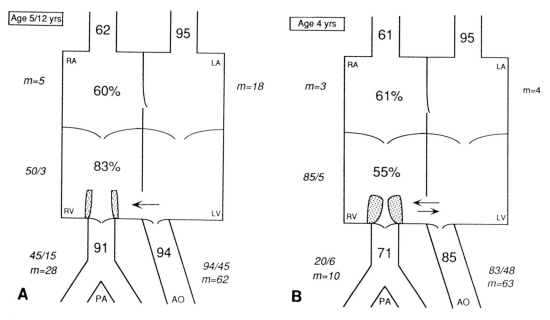

Figure 3. Diagram of the circulation in an acyanotic patient with ventricular septal defect and pulmonary stenosis (A) who progresses to the physiology of tetralogy of Fallot (B). RA, right atrium; LA, left atrium; RV, right ventricle; LV, left ventricle; PA, pulmonary artery; AO, aorta; large bold numbers, oxygen % saturation; italics, pressure in mmHg.

duced by the kidneys, and, available iron stores being sufficient, it stimulates the hematocrit to rise proportionate to the degree of oxygen unsaturation. This response occurs in a muted form in the first months of life because of limited iron stores, but later, with normal dietary intake of iron, the hematocrit becomes a direct reflection of the average arterial oxygen saturation.

CLINICAL MANIFESTATIONS

The child with tetralogy of Fallot is discovered to have a murmur at birth. This murmur emanates from the obstructing right ventricular infundibulum, not from the ventricular septal defect. Although this murmur may sound like the murmur of ventricular septal defect, a ventricular defect murmur is almost never audible within the first hours of life, because left-to-right shunting is required to produce such a murmur. This is unlikely because, in the first days of life, there is residual elevation of pulmonary resistance left over from fetal life.

Cyanosis at birth is not common unless there is pulmonary atresia, and even with pulmonary atresia, cyanosis may not be visible if there is extensive collateral circulation. When there are extensive collaterals, cyanosis may go unrecognized for some time. With closure of the ductus arteriosus in the first days of life, cyanosis becomes more marked.

The symptoms in an infant with tetralogy of Fallot depend on whether there is excessive left-to-

right shunting and congestive heart failure or excessive right-to-left shunting and cyanosis. Many babies are either asymptomatic or have only mild cyanosis. Because pulmonary stenosis is progressive, congestive failure is a feature of early infancy. This improves later and is finally replaced by cyanosis. Twenty-five percent of infants are cyanotic at birth, whereas 75% have become recognizably cyanotic by 1 year of age.[55] Growth may be limited by either congestive heart failure or cyanosis.

Cyanotic spells (hypoxic spells) are characteristic of young children with tetralogy of Fallot. In a typical cyanotic spell, the infant or child becomes distressed, most often in the morning, not necessarily because of external stimuli. With crying, the child becomes unconsolable, hyperpneic, and increasingly blue. Mothers of "spelling" infants discover that holding the baby upright on the shoulder with the baby's knees tucked firmly against the belly may relieve the symptoms. Otherwise, the distress becomes more marked, there is increasing hyperpnea, finally unconsciousness and, rarely, convulsions. Spells are self-aggravating; the more upset the baby becomes, the more profound the hypoxemia, the more noticeable the discomfort, and the more upset the infant becomes. "Spells" are not common in neonates and are noted mostly in infants and toddlers. After the age of 4 or 5 years, spells are again uncommon but not unknown. The most surprising spells occur in infants who, either because of low hemoglobin or high resting arterial oxygen content, or both, are not visibly cyanotic. Sometimes these babies pass through the sequence of symptoms to unconsciousness before it is realized that hypoxemia is the problem. Usually after being calmed, the infant sleeps and, on awakening, is his or her usual self. Anything that distresses the baby may precipitate a cyanotic spell. Thus, the strange surroundings, giving injections, or taking blood samples may be life-threatening. It is not surprising, therefore, that the first spell sometimes occurs when the child is first admitted to the hospital to be evaluated for heart disease. Cardiac catheterization is particularly dangerous because the symptoms of a spell are modified by premedication, the knee-chest position is impossible, and unconsciousness can be attributed to drugs rather than to profound hypoxemia.

Because of the profound hypoxemia, cyanotic spells may produce brain injury ranging from reduced intelligence quotients to hemiparesis, to severe neurologic sequelae and death. For this reason, any infant with the anatomy of tetralogy of Fallot, whether cyanotic or not, who has temper tantrums, holds its breath, or has unusual fussy episodes is viewed with alarm. Similarly, any infant with the anatomy of tetralogy of Fallot in whom there is marked variation of oxygen saturation is viewed with concern. A child who, while undergoing cardiac catheterization, has excessive variation in arterial oxygen saturation, is a potential candidate for a cyanotic spell.

Whether a child with tetralogy of Fallot and congestive heart failure due to a left-to-left shunt can have cyanotic spells is a question that arises regularly. Clearly, this depends on the degree and certainty of the diagnosis of congestive failure. With debatable evidence of congestive heart failure, cyanotic spells are a possible problem, but with outright congestive failure and increased pulmonary blood flow, spells are unknown. Some months after a first bout of congestive failure and, with an intervening period of time during which the infundibular stenosis becomes more severe, the possibility of a cyanotic spell is greater.

In an older child with unrepaired tetralogy of Fallot, exercise produces increasing cyanosis through decreased systemic resistance, and rest may be required to overcome discomfort. The older child discovers that the discomfort associated with arterial oxygen unsaturation during excitement or exercise is relieved by a squatting position, sitting on the heels with the chin on the knees. A particularly articulate patient, in describing her spells, talked of terrifying air hunger and the miraculous relief from pressing her legs firmly against her chest. She made a sharp distinction between simply squatting, her preferred sitting position, and firm pressure of her legs against her chest to relieve the discomfort brought on by exercise. Whether the age distribution of spells and squatting is related to more dynamic infundibular obstruction in the younger child, is due to societal

pressures, or occurs simply because there are few unrepaired older children with tetralogy of Fallot, is not known. Still, the impression remains that older age groups have less trouble with spells and squatting. The mechanism of relief is not well understood, but the rapid rise in arterial oxygen saturation with squatting can be easily documented (see Fig. 2, p. 75). When the legs are pressed against the chest, there is increased peripheral resistance and decreased venous return from the legs. In effect, a significant part of the venous return is removed, the need for cardiac output is decreased, and the patient becomes pinker.

It is not necessary to have infundibular pulmonary stenosis to have spells. Although patients with pulmonary atresia have fewer spells because their pulmonary blood supply is not affected by infundibular muscle, an excessive drop in systemic resistance with vigorous activity can result in sufficient reduction of an already limited pulmonary blood flow to cause a spell.

Physical Examination

Clubbing of the fingers and toes, recognizable in older infants and children, is a manifestation of chronic cyanosis (see Fig. 1, p. 103).

Growth is limited in severely cyanotic patients, but in the 1990s this is rarely an important issue because of early surgical intervention.

Without pulmonary atresia, there is a loud, systolic ejection murmur that is heard well at the lower left sternal border, but is usually transmitted upward along the entire left sternal border and toward the suprasternal notch. The second heart sound is single, composed only of the aortic component, and may be accentuated because of the proximity of the anteriorly displaced, (dextroposed) ascending aorta (Fig. 4). With pulmonary atresia, the continuous murmurs of collateral circulation may be audible, particularly over the back; indeed, in a neonate with cyanosis and continuous murmurs, tetralogy of Fallot with pulmonary atresia is the most prominent diagnostic possibility.

Electrocardiography

The electrocardiogram shows right-axis deviation and right ventricular hypertrophy. Without these findings, the diagnosis of tetralogy, with or without pulmonary atresia, is in doubt. When there is minimal pulmonary stenosis with substantial left-to-right shunting, the electrocardiogram may show combined ventricular hypertrophy. A leftward, superior axis suggests tetralogy of Fallot with an atrioventricular canal defect.

Chest X-ray

Classically, the chest x-ray shows the heart size to be normal with decreased pulmonary vascularity. Generally, the main pulmonary artery segment

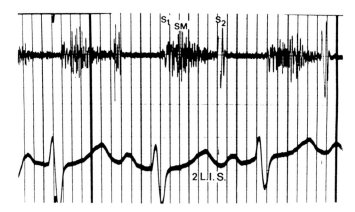

Figure 4. Phonocardiogram of a patient with tetralogy of Fallot. Note the stenotic murmur with a loud single second sound. 2 L.I.S, second left interspace; S_1, first heart sound; SM, systolic murmur; S_2, second heart sound.

is deficient. Given excessive left-to-right shunting, the pulmonary vasculature may be increased and the heart enlarged and indistinguishable from the features seen in an infant with a ventricular septal defect. With pulmonary atresia and excessive collateral circulation, the heart may be somewhat larger than normal but the main pulmonary artery segment is usually absent. Absence of the main pulmonary artery segment gives the heart the appearance of a shoe and has earned the name *coeur en sabot*. Usually, when the aorta arches to the right, it is readily seen on the plain chest film. Unusual vascular patterns on the chest film sometimes are recognized as collateral circulation.

Echocardiography

On echocardiography it is possible to demonstrate the ventricular septal defect, typically conoventricular with anterior deviation of the infundibular septum. The aortic root is large and variably overriding (Fig. 5). The pulmonary outflow narrowing is usually readily visualized and obstruction can be documented by Doppler techniques. It is now possible for echocardiographers to identify additional ventricular septal defects in other parts of the ventricular septum with color Doppler techniques, and the coronary artery anatomy can often be seen sufficiently well to recognize abnormal conal branches in the right ventricular outflow tract at the point where surgical incision may be required. Proximal peripheral pulmonary stenoses and relative hypoplasia of central pulmonary vessels can be visualized. There are not yet sufficient data to recommend that surgical correction of tetralogy of Fallot be carried out with anatomic diagnostic information based solely on echocardiography, but it does seem likely that this will be the case in the foreseeable future.

Subxiphoid and parasternal views most clearly demonstrate the ventricular septal defect, the overriding aorta, and the right ventricular outflow tract obstruction. The branch pulmonary arteries are usually seen in parasternal and suprasternal short-axis views. The anatomy of the left coronary

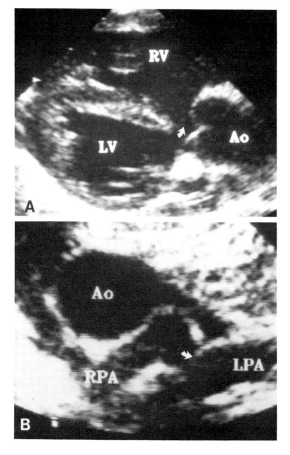

Figure 5. **A,** Echocardiogram in the parasternal long-axis view showing the ventricular septum through the malalignment ventricular defect (arrow). **B,** Echocardiogram in the short-axis view in a patient with tetralogy of Fallot and pulmonary atresia. The pulmonary artery bifurcation is seen. There is discrete left pulmonary artery stenosis (arrow). RV, right ventricle; Ao, aorta; LV, left ventricle; LPA, left pulmonary artery; RPA, right pulmonary artery.

artery can be seen in a parasternal short-axis view or a long-axis view angled toward the left shoulder.

Unfortunately, as patients grow older and bigger, echocardiographic definition diminishes and angiocardiography becomes mandatory.

Cardiac Catheterization

With a reliable echocardiographic diagnosis of tetralogy of Fallot, there is little or no need for cardiac catheterization and angiography if a shunting operation is planned. When a reparative operation is to be undertaken, angiography is required to clarify the following issues (Exhibit 1):

1. Are there additional ventricular septal defects (5%)?

2. Is there a coronary artery crossing the right ventricular outflow tract (5%)?

3. Is there peripheral pulmonary stenosis (28%)?

If present, any of these abnormalities may be a problem in the repair or in the postoperative period. Although most of these details can be ascertained by echocardiography with relatively high reliability, the high price for a missed diagnosis dictates the necessity for cardiac catheterization before surgery.

Stenosis of the left pulmonary artery is best demonstrated angiographically in a slightly left anterior oblique position with the child sitting up (see Fig. 11, ch. 14) (Fig. 6). The coronary anatomy is usually well demonstrated in the left axial oblique position during left ventricular injection of the contrast. Any question that a conus coronary artery crosses the right ventricular outflow tract at the

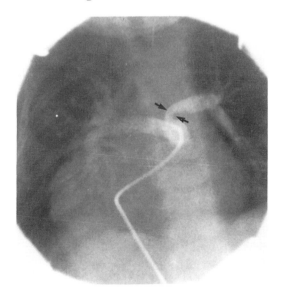

Figure 6. Angiocardiogram in a patient with tetralogy of Fallot showing stenosis at the origin of the left main pulmonary artery (arrows).

point of intended incision requires further evaluation (usually including an aortic root injection if not a direct coronary angiogram) to be confident of the anatomy preoperatively (Fig. 7). The source of blood flow to the left anterior descending coronary should be identified also. Perhaps a conduit repair will be the only possibility. Additional ventricular septal defects, apical and midmuscular defects, are demonstrated with left ventricular angiography in the left anterior oblique position (Fig. 8). Anterior muscular defects are seen in the corresponding right anterior oblique view.

A right ventricular angiogram usually is made to demonstrate the basic anatomy of tetralogy of Fallot.

MANAGEMENT

Cyanotic Spells

A cyanotic spell is cause for concern. Initially, having the mother simply comfort the infant, who is in knee-chest position, is effective treatment. All unpleasant treatments are likely to aggravate cyanotic spells. So, injections, finger pricks, intravenous therapy, or restraints are likely to make the situation worse. The point at which simply comforting the infant should be abandoned and more aggressive treatment undertaken is a matter of experience and judgment, and knowledge of the child. It is a matter of interest that mothers report recurring spells at home managed with success, only to find that the first spell in the hospital is a panicky episode ending up with the infant sedated, intubated, on intravenous feeding, and curarized. On awakening, such an infant usually has another spell upon realizing the strange surroundings. This form of treatment leads to surgery on that admission, but is sometimes unavoidable.

Useful treatment for cyanotic spells includes morphine, an almost specific drug for this problem, and propranolol. Morphine suppresses the sensation of suffocation and relieves fear, whereas propranolol relaxes infundibular spasm, sometimes with dramatically beneficial effect on arterial oxygen saturation. Former concerns that propranolol compromises later surgery seem unfounded. Any drug that increases peripheral resistance (i.e., neosynephrine) may be helpful. It may be that the improvement with the knee-chest position and squatting is owing as much to the increase in peripheral resistance as to anything else. Usually, oxygen is used but it has little demonstrable effect. Within minutes of onset, a severe spell results in metabolic acidosis, which can be controlled with intravenous sodium bicarbonate in repeated doses if the spell continues. Finally, and fortunately rarely, a patient may respond so poorly to everything else that surgery must be carried out as an emergency. In this situation, an emergency sys-

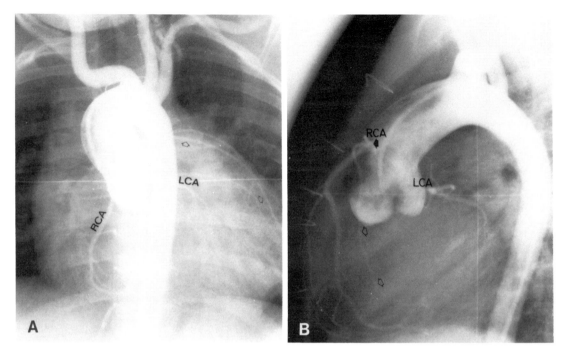

Figure 7. Angiocardiogram in a patient with tetralogy of Fallot with injection of contrast material into the aortic root, showing that the blood supply to the left anterior descending coronary artery (arrows) comes from the right coronary. Comparing the anteroposterior view (**A**) and the lateral view (**B**) of the angiogram, it becomes obvious that the supply to the left anterior descending coronary crosses the right ventricular outflow tract.

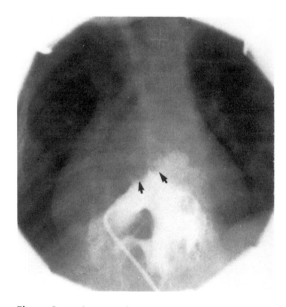

Figure 8. Left ventricular angiogram in a patient with tetralogy of Fallot taken from the left anterior oblique position. Note the large malalignment ventricular septal defect and the additional defect, or defects, toward the apex. The arrows indicate the aortic valve.

temic arterial–pulmonary artery shunt procedure may not only be lifesaving but may help to avoid brain damage.

In general, aggressive treatment commits the patient to surgery during that hospitalization, because the treatment itself will aggravate the child, causing more spells. To put this another way, there is nothing more likely to provoke a cyanotic spell than for the child to find himself tied down, being intravenously fed and jabbed by needles. Often the child simply goes from a spell to surgery, even though the spell has been controlled.

Nowadays, having recognized the presence of heart disease because of a murmur, and having diagnosed tetralogy of Fallot by echocardiographic techniques, the slightest spell is taken as reason to proceed to surgery. Difficulty in recognizing a spell occurs mainly when the patient has been sedated either for a prior spell or, more likely, for cardiac catheterization or echocardiography. Spells in patients who have been sedated are particularly dangerous, because the physician feels secure that a spell is not likely because of the sedation. Increasing cyanosis, appearance of hyperpnea, widely fluctuating arterial saturation, very low arterial saturation, acidosis, or unexplained prolonged unconsciousness are all signals to the careful observer that the child, even though not awake, may be having a spell.

The use of vasodilators must be avoided in patients with tetralogy of Fallot; dropping the systemic resistance and systemic blood pressure is likely to cause a spell.

Fortunately, functioning shunt operations prevent spells almost entirely.

Timing of Cardiac Catheterization

At Boston Children's Hospital, an asymptomatic, cyanotic infant who is growing and gaining undergoes cardiac catheterization electively early in infancy to clarify the coronary anatomy, to rule out the possibility of additional ventricular defects, and to measure possible peripheral pulmonary stenosis. In general, it is preferable to perform catheterization earlier rather than later, to avoid cyanotic spells in the laboratory. Nonetheless, children who have had spells are studied at cardiac catheterization, but with considerable caution.

Surgery

With few exceptions, symptomatic infants are referred to surgery for repair (Exhibits 2 and 3).[5,20] With no symptoms and with no technical problems anticipated, elective repair is carried out by the first birthday. In recent years, the average age at repair has gradually become younger (Exhibits 2 and 3). At present, it cannot be documented that reparative surgery at 6 months of age has a different risk than later repair. Repair consists of a right ventricular incision, a patch to close the ventricular defect, and most often a transannular outflow patch.

Not all agree with this plan. The points of discussion include the timing of repair as well as the type of surgery. Some believe that reparative surgery should be delayed until the child is older, even to the point of supporting the child's growth and easing spells with a shunt procedure in early infancy.[30,42] Modified Blalock procedures have been in favor in recent years.[26] Whether to try to avoid transannular patches on the theory that a competent pulmonary valve is needed to ensure a long life or to sacrifice pulmonary valve function to provide a wide open outflow tract is still under discussion.[35]

If possible, surgery for the asymptomatic child who has a "conus coronary" crossing the right ventricular outflow tract is delayed until the age of 3–4 years, because a conduit may be required between the right ventricle and the main pulmonary artery to get around the anomalous coronary. The bigger the child, the larger the conduit that can be used, and the longer it is likely to last. By the age of 4 years, a conduit large enough to last 5–10 years can be inserted. When surgery is required because of symptoms, the choices lie between a systemic artery–pulmonary artery shunt or repair using a conduit. The argument for a shunting operation is that it is easier, faster, and less traumatic. The argument for repair is that the circulation is made normal sooner and replacement of the conduit later is acceptable, because the shunting operation also presupposes a second operation. Rarely, the outflow can be enlarged by tunneling under the anomalous coronary.

Generally, additional ventricular septal defects

Exhibit 2

Boston Children's Hospital Experience 1973–1987

Tetralogy of Fallot with Pulmonary Stenosis: Interventions

Type of Operation	No. of Patients
Surgical Repair	601
Arterial-Pulmonary Shunt	18
Conduit Repair	19
Pulmonary Artery Reconstruction	93
Balloon Pulmonary Arterioplasty	32
Coil Embolization	4
Pulmonary Valve Replacement	6

Tetralogy of Fallot: Reparative Surgery % of 30-Day Mortality

Year	Pulmonary Stenosis n = 496		Absent Pulmonary Valve n = 14		Atrioventricular Canal n = 26	
	n	% mortality	n	% mortality	n	% mortality
1973–77	131	7			7	29
1978–82	177	5	14	38	11	9
1983–87	188	6			8	13

located in the muscular septum will close spontaneously or are so small that specific surgery is not needed. This is not invariably true; the discovery of a second, large, unrepaired ventricular defect in the intensive care unit requires a second, unexpected operation.

COURSE

Progression

Tetralogy of Fallot is a progressive disease. With time, patients with acyanotic tetralogy of Fallot become cyanotic and cyanotic patients become more cyanotic. In part, this is because infundibular stenosis becomes more severe with time, and in part because the hematocrit level gradually rises over time, increasing the absolute amount of reduced hemoglobin and, thus, visible cyanosis. Progression is most noticeable (and dangerous) in the first 6 months of life, when cyanotic spells may appear without warning.

Suprasystemic Right Ventricular Pressure

Rarely, the ventricular defect may become partially occluded by tricuspid valve tissue.[9,12] When this occurs in the presence of severe pulmonary stenosis, the right ventricular pressure may become suprasystemic. It is not known why these patients have a high mortality with surgery, but the dangers have been rediscovered repeatedly.[13]

Aortic Regurgitation

Over time an increasing percentage of patients with uncorrected tetralogy of Fallot develop aortic regurgitation.[4] It is presumed that the greater than normal blood flow through the aortic valve accounts for dilatation of the valve ring and valvar incompetence. According to this theory, the more severe the pulmonary stenosis, the more likely there will be aortic regurgitation. This seems to be true, because aortic regurgitation is most commonly associated with pulmonary atresia. Because these patients are the ones who are likely to have diastolic murmurs arising from bronchial or collateral circulation, special vigilance is required to recognize this problem.

In a patient with infective endocarditis, suspicion that the aortic valve is the site of the vegetations is warranted, because a regurgitant aortic valve is a favorite location for endocarditis. On a few occasions aortic regurgitation has been severe enough to be a management problem. Presumably with early repair this complication is avoided.

Left Pulmonary Artery Stenosis or Atresia

In most patients stenosis at the origin of the left pulmonary artery can be managed during surgical repair (Fig. 6). Some have residual obstruction that often can be satisfactorily relieved with balloon dilatation (Exhibit 3). In the extreme form there is atresia, the patient obtaining his entire oxygen uptake from the right lung. This is a special problem, because repair with circulation to only one lung may result in some degree of pulmonary hypertension. Because of the problem of pulmonary regurgitation in the presence of pulmonary hypertension, an artificial pulmonary valve is required in the repair of this form of tetralogy of Fallot. It is the author's impression that the number of children with this problem has decreased since early intervention has come into vogue and, indeed, the condition has been rarely seen at birth. Perhaps this is another feature of this disease that develops with time.

Pulmonary Vascular Obstructive Disease

Pulmonary vascular disease is seen in adults with long-standing, large aortopulmonary shunts (i.e., Waterston or Potts procedures) and, rarely, in patients with Blalock-Taussig shunts or with excessive collateral circulation. In part, this problem has led to diminished use of the large vessel, side-to-side shunts, such as Waterston or Potts operations. The use of coils to occlude large collaterals may have a beneficial effect on preventing pulmonary vascular obstructive disease, which is now so rare as to be a curiosity.

Arrhythmias

As the survivors with repaired or palliated tetralogy of Fallot grow older, increasing numbers are found to have ventricular ectopy.[54] Also, the older the child is at the time of repair,[7,29] the more likely it is that ectopy will occur. It has been related to late sudden death.[18] Whether this is specific to tetralogy of Fallot repair or is a problem with all intracardiac surgery is not clear, but the thought that it may be an inherent feature of intracardiac surgery is inescapable.

Holter monitoring of survivors at regular intervals to find patients at risk is mandatory, and exercise testing of survivors uncovers additional cases.[17] Treatment is directed at the identified rhythm disturbance. Unifocal ventricular ectopic beats, multifocal ventricular ectopy, and runs of ventricular tachycardia should evoke different treatments (see ch. 27). When needed, antiarrhythmic medication is usually successful in suppressing rhythm problems, although, rarely, surgical excision of a focus has been used.[21] Based on the presently available data, and contrary to some recommendations,[18] prophylactic medication for all of these patients based on the likelihood of developing ectopy does not seem justified.

Exhibit 3

Boston Children's Hospital Experience 1973–1987 **Pulmonary Artery Obstruction** n = 299*		
	Management	
Pathology	*Surgery†*	*Catheterization*
Right Pulmonary Artery Stenosis	43	Right Pulmonary Arterioplasty 42
Right Pulmonary Artery Hypoplasia	40	–
Right Pulmonary Artery Absence	4	–
Left Pulmonary Artery Stenosis	71	Left Pulmonary Arterioplasty 41
Left Pulmonary Artery Hypoplasia	56	–
Left Pulmonary Artery Absent	20	–
Nonspecific‡ Peripheral Pulmonary Stenosis	132	Peripheral Pulmonary Arterioplasty 65
Nonspecific‡ Peripheral Pulmonary Hypoplasia	51	–

*Patients with pulmonary atresia excluded.
†Patients with either balloon and/or surgical arterioplasty were counted once. There is considerable overlap. No attempt was made to relate the development of peripheral pulmonary stenosis to prior shunt surgery.
‡Side not indicated.

Tetralogy of Fallot with Pulmonary Stenosis: Surgical Procedures*

	Age at operation			
	< 1 Year		*> 1 Year*	
Year	Shunt	Repair	Shunt	Repair
1973–77	3	38	3	176
1978–82	5	73	3	117
1983–87	3	101	1	106

*Excludes atrioventricular canal, absent pulmonary valve, and pulmonary atresia. There were 182 patients with prior shunts from the era preceding 1973, or who had shunt surgery elsewhere. 40 patients had more than one operation.

Tetralogy of Fallot with Pulmonary Stenosis n = 1071

Complication	*No. of Patients*	*%*
Infective Endocarditis	20	2
Aortic Regurgitation	50	5
Gall Stones	3	1
Brain Abscess	6	1
Cerebral Vascular Accident	5	1
Other Central Nervous System Problem	11	1
Scoliosis	41	4
Pulmonary Vascular Obstructive Disease	28	3

Myocardial Dysfunction

Separate from the acute myocardial infarction that can occur with surgical damage to an anomalous coronary artery supplying the left anterior descending coronary, is the late myocardial dysfunction that may occur in some patients after surgical repair. Measurements of myocardial function suggest that this is less common when repair is accomplished at an earlier age[2,3] and when there are no residual defects, particularly residual ventricular septal defects.[45] As a corollary, patients who have repeated surgical procedures often have myocardial dysfunction. Ventricular ectopy and sudden death are also related to myocardial dysfunction.[27] Although much is to be learned about this topic, with modern management, including early repair, the number of patients with myocardial problems seems to be diminishing.

Reoperation

Eighteen percent of the patents at Children's Hospital in Boston have required reoperation because of significant residual ventricular defects, residual outflow obstruction, obstructed conduits, or pulmonary artery distortion. Conduits have a limited life (estimated 10 years) (see p. 740) and require regular replacement.[51]

Late Death

Late death following repair of tetralogy of Fallot occurs in 2–7% of patients, varying with the duration of follow-up.[15] Most observers have attributed these deaths to ventricular arrhythmias.[6,7,56]

Brain Abscess

Any patient with right-to-left shunting is at risk for brain abscess. Sudden onset of unusual headache, the first appearance of a seizure, or other neurologic signs should raise this question. Generally, computed tomography of the brain identifies or eliminates the possibility. With the appearance of central nervous system signs or symptoms in a child with tetralogy of Fallot, brain abscess is *the* diagnosis to be excluded (see ch. 9) (Exhibit 3).

Cerebrovascular Accident

Sometimes, cerebrovascular accidents are preceded by a typical cyanotic spell and, on other occasions, they appear without warning in the unrepaired child. In small infants anemia is found more often than polycythemia, suggesting that the hypoxemia is the underlying cause. In older, unrepaired patients, polycythemia can always be incriminated, although limited oxygen delivery to the brain seems the most likely cause. Again, brain abscess must be excluded (see ch. 9) (Exhibit 3).

Depressed Intelligence Quotient

Chronic cyanosis is associated with a lower than predicted intelligence quotient, even long after the cyanosis has been corrected by surgery (see ch. 9).[36]

Scoliosis

Chronic cyanosis is associated with scoliosis, particularly in females, and is a particular problem for patients with tetralogy of Fallot.[44] Whether this will be a diminishing problem now that these children are aggressively repaired in early childhood is not known. In any case, a growing child with chronic cyanosis should be examined on a regular basis for this complication (see ch. 8, Exhibit 1).

Gout

Gout is reported to occur in older patients who are cyanotic and polycythemic.[47]

Gallstones

The surgical removal of pigment gallstones in symptomatic adolescents and young adults with chronic cyanosis has been required several times in Boston Children's Hospital's series of patients.

Infective Endocarditis

Twenty patients with tetralogy of Fallot have had infective endocarditis in the past 15 years. Mostly, the vegetations are located on the aortic valve (see ch. 26).

Polycythemia

Children with chronic cyanosis experience a rising hematocrit level during adolescence and, in some, this polycythemia becomes sufficiently severe to result in prohibitively high blood viscosity. The more viscous blood is difficult to pump, oxygen delivery to the tissues is diminished, and symptoms appear. Red cell pheresis may be helpful (see ch. 8).

Complete Heart Block

The incidence of postoperative complete heart block has been stable at about 1% for the past 15 years.

Pulmonary Atresia and Ventricular Septal Defect

The combination of pulmonary atresia (acquired postnatally or congenital) and a ventricular septal defect has, in the past, been described as a pseudotruncus or a truncus arteriosus type IV. It is now considered to be an extreme variation of the tetralogy of Fallot syndrome and is referred to as tetralogy of Fallot with pulmonary atresia.

Definition

This combination of anomalies resembles the tetralogy of Fallot in all respects, with the additional feature of pulmonary atresia. The nature of the outflow obstruction varies somewhat, but literally no blood passes directly from the right ventricle to the pulmonary artery.

Prevalence

Among infants with congenital heart disease who are seen in the first year of life, 22% of those with tetralogy of Fallot had pulmonary atresia.[16] There are two sources of error in this number. First, with the passage of time additional patients develop complete outflow obstruction; second, some patients with the tetralogy of Fallot syndrome may not be critically ill in the first year of life and so may not appear in this series. At Boston Children's Hospital over the past 15 years, 18% of patients with tetralogy of Fallot had pulmonary atresia (see ch. 18).

Anatomy (Fig. 2)

The anatomy of the outflow obstruction varies somewhat. Complete occlusion may be at the infundibular or valvar level. The central pulmonary arteries may be string-like over short distances and there may be no connection between the right and left main pulmonary arteries. Rarely, at the other extreme, the pulmonary arteries may be near normal in size.

The ventricular septal defect is the typical membranous malalignment type characteristic of tetralogy of Fallot. There may be additional ventricular defects located elsewhere in the septum, but there is a malalignment defect of the size usually found in all patients with tetralogy of Fallot. Pulmonary atresia with a ventricular septal defect that is not of the tetralogy of Fallot type probably exists, but for practical purposes, the vast majority of patients with pulmonary atresia and a ventricular septal defect have variations of the tetralogy theme.

The aorta arches to the right in 25% of patients.[28]

The pulmonary circulation is supplied through a ductus arteriosus, bronchial circulation, and, in some patients (30%), by bizarre collateral vessels arising from the descending aorta.[22,31,46] These vessels arise distal to the ductus arteriosus and may be multiple. Occasionally the tortuous course extends upward into the neck before returning to the pulmonary circulation. On other occasions the collateral vessel may arise from branches of the aorta, even from the arterial vessels in the neck. These structures do not respect right- or left-sidedness; a collateral vessel may arise from one side and supply blood to either the right or left lung or both. Collateral vessels connect to the pulmonary arteries, most often feeding the pulmonary circulation through the hilar pulmonary arteries. Almost invariably there is obstruction within the collateral vessels, with the result that the central pulmonary arteries are only rarely exposed to the systemic pressure.[23]

Distal to the entry point of the collateral circulation, the pulmonary arteries are larger than the central pulmonary arteries because the distal vessels carry more blood.

Embryology

Early in normal embryologic life, the pulmonary circulation is supplied by vessels arising from the descending aorta. These vessels later disappear as blood flow is established from the heart to the main pulmonary artery. When there is pulmonary atresia, these peculiar collateral vessels arising from the descending aorta may persist.

When normal blood flow from the right ventricle to the pulmonary artery has been established, the collaterals usually regress. Subsequent development of pulmonary atresia leaves the patient with the sole pulmonary blood supply being through the ductus arteriosus and bronchial circulations. Consequently, there are two kinds of pulmonary atresia in tetralogy of Fallot at birth: (1) those with persistent primitive vessels supplying the lung and (2) those with the pulmonary arteries supplied by bronchial vessels and, rarely, a persistent patent ductus arteriosus. Additionally, pulmonary atresia may develop after birth in a patient with otherwise typical tetralogy of Fallot. This has occurred often enough in the author's experience to indicate that many patients with tetralogy of Fallot, who survive long enough, may develop pulmonary atresia.

The relative distribution of the pulmonary arteries and the collateral vessels is unpredictable.[50] Some areas of the lung are supplied only by collateral circulation; others have both forms of blood supply, and some areas are supplied by pulmonary arteries connected to other parts of the lung that derive blood flow from collateral circulation. Thus, it is possible for blood to flow from the right pulmonary artery toward the left pulmonary artery because of excessive collaterals into the right pulmonary vessels.

Physiology

As in most patients, all systemic venous blood is returned to the right atrium. From here some passes right-to-left through the usually patent foramen ovale, whereas the remainder enters the right ventricle and passes through the ventricular septal defect into the aorta. The entire cardiac output, including that destined for the pulmonary circulation and that destined for the systemic circulation, passes through the aortic valve. The aortic valve is, of necessity, larger than normal and, as a consequence, is sometimes somewhat incompetent (14%). The pulmonary blood flow enters the lung via the ductus arteriosus. When the ductus closes, as scheduled, the patient has immediate problems with hypoxemia unless there is sufficient bronchial or collateral circulation to provide enough pulmonary blood flow to survive.

Pressure within the collateral vessels is equal to that in the aorta up to the point of obstruction, usually close to the native pulmonary artery. Only rarely does the tortuosity or the obstruction allow passage of a cardiac catheter through to the pulmonary artery. When the pulmonary artery pressures have been measured (usually through a surgical arterial pulmonary shunt), the pulmonary artery pressure is normal or below normal. Pulmonary venous wedge measurements confirm this observation. Rarely, there is pulmonary hypertension because of excessive flow, often to an isolated area of the lung.

Clinical Manifestations

These patients are cyanotic at birth. The degree of cyanosis depends on the patency of the ductus arteriosus and the extent of the collateral and bronchial blood supply. There is no systolic murmur. Continuous murmurs arising from the collateral circulation may be heard anywhere over the chest. The second heart sound is single. A systolic click originating from the large aorta may be audible.

If the collateral circulation is greatly excessive (a rare event occurring exclusively in early infancy), there may be congestive heart failure and no visible cyanosis.

Electrocardiography. The electrocardiogram shows right-axis deviation and right ventricular hypertrophy.

Chest X-ray. The chest x-ray shows a variable heart size, often a boot-shaped heart because of the absent main pulmonary segment, and sometimes an irregular pattern of pulmonary vasculature, suggesting bronchial or collateral vessels. A right aortic arch may be recognized.

Echocardiography. On echocardiographic examination, the malaligned ventricular septal defect can be recognized, as well as the small and abnormal pulmonary arteries. Absence of blood flow across the pulmonary valve can be established. The extent of the atretic segment can be seen in parasternal short-axis view. The branch pulmonary arteries are best examined in a high parasternal or suprasternal view. The branch pulmonary arteries should be imaged carefully, seeking and measuring narrowed segments. Collateral vessels can often be seen arising from the descending aorta with Doppler color-flow mapping. The side of the aortic arch (right or left) should be determined (see ch. 13), because this might influence the type of shunt that will be created.

Cardiac Catheterization. Cardiac catheterization is required for all infants who have pulmonary atresia in the context of tetralogy of Fallot and is carried out once the echocardiographic diagnosis is made. An exception is the markedly cyanotic newborn who urgently needs a shunting operation. In addition to the usual data required in the management of patients with tetralogy of Fallot (i.e., determination of possible additional ventricular septal defects, evaluation of coronary anatomy, and evaluation for stenosis of the left pulmonary artery), the patient with pulmonary atresia requires careful angiographic documentation of the pulmonary circulation in all lobes of the lungs. Are the pulmonary arteries present and of sufficient size to be used in the repair? How are the pul-

monary arteries perfused? Is there a patent ductus arteriosus? Do abnormal collateral vessels supply some areas of the lungs? Are these areas of the lungs solely supplied by collateral vessels which might become infarcted if a collateral were occluded? What happens to the arterial oxygen saturation if a collateral vessel is occluded with an inflated balloon?

Detailed angiographic delineation of the precise circulation to each lobe and each segment of the lung is needed to plan a repair. Sometimes all the required information cannot be obtained at a single catheterization because the circulation is too complicated; in others, there having been no previous surgery, there is no way to get useful opacification of the pulmonary arteries. Injection of contrast material into each of the individual collaterals is mandatory, in part to see the anatomy of the collateral and in part to see the pulmonary artery anatomy in as much detail as possible. It may be necessary to resort to pulmonary vein wedge injections to backfill the pulmonary arteries, including puncture of the atrial septum to gain access to the left atrium and pulmonary veins. Often it is necessary to repeat the catheterization once the right ventricular outflow is opened to the pulmonary artery, or an arterial-pulmonary shunt has been put in place, so that a catheter can be introduced into the pulmonary circulation for appropriate angiography.

With large collateral vessels supplying the pulmonary circulation, the possibility of occluding collateral vessels with coils extruded from a catheter should be considered. If there are demonstrable pulmonary arterial vessels supplying the same area as the collateral vessels, and if, on balloon occlusion of the collateral vessel, the arterial oxygen saturation does not fall to dangerous levels, coils can be safely placed in that vessel. This maneuver is rarely considered unless surgical provision for increased pulmonary blood flow is planned for the near future.

Magnetic Resonance Imaging. Magnetic resonance imaging allows identification of the pulmonary arteries and measurement of their size.[32] Whether this is practical enough to be useful in the management of these patients remains to be seen.

Management (Exhibit 4)

The goal, if possible, is to establish continuity between the right ventricle and the pulmonary arteries, to close the ventricular septal defect, and to eliminate excessive collateral circulation. Because the main pulmonary arteries tend to be small, often the first step is to increase blood flow to the central vessels to distend them and to stimulate growth. It is presumed that the earlier in life an increase in flow is established, the greater will be the later improvement in the capacity of the

Exhibit 4

Boston Children's Hospital Experience 1973–87

Pulmonary Atresia and Ventricular Septal Defect: Surgical Procedures*

Year of Operation	Age at Operation			
	< 1 Year		> 1 Year	
	Shunt	Repair	Shunt	Repair
1973–77	6	0	8	14
1978–82	12	6	25	32
1983–87	26	28	15	60

*Some patients had a preceding shunt operation. Many were performed elsewhere or in the time period preceding 1973. In each 5-year period, an increasing percentage of patients are being repaired.

Tetralogy of Fallot with Pulmonary Atresia
n = 256

Complication	No. of Patients	%
Infective Endocarditis	7	3
Aortic Regurgitation	37	14
Gall Stones	0	
Brain Abscess	2	1
Cerebral Vascular Accident	1	
Other Central Nervous System Problem	0	
Scoliosis	3	1
Pulmonary Vascular Obstructive Disease	12	5

Note that aortic regurgitation is three times more common among patients with pulmonary atresia than among those without pulmonary atresia, giving support to the theory that dilatation of the aortic annulus is the cause. Compare with Exhibit 1.

Tetralogy of Fallot with Pulmonary Atresia: Interventions

Type of Operation	No. of Patients
Surgical Repair	136
Arterial-Pulmonary Shunt	82
Conduit Repair	106
Pulmonary Artery Reconstruction	50
Balloon Pulmonary Arterioplasty	38
Coil Embolization	34
Pulmonary Valve Replacement	1

pulmonary arteries. Sometimes opening and enlarging the pulmonary annulus and main pulmonary artery with a transannular patch is possible. A conduit from the right ventricle to the pulmonary arteries may be used as well, and, as a less desirable alternative, an arterial-pulmonary shunt may be undertaken. If relatively free access from the right ventricle to the pulmonary arteries is established, allowing unobstructed blood flow, the blood may shunt left-to-right through the ventricular septal defect and the patient may require a trial of closure of the ventricular defect. If this is poorly tolerated, the ventricular septal patch may later be fenestrated.

Theoretically, a right ventricle-to-main pulmonary artery connection could be established, but when the pulmonary artery is hypoplastic or absent, a conduit may be necessary to make the connection. Whether to use a modified Blalock shunt or a small conduit from the right ventricle to the main pulmonary artery in a small symptomatic infant is a matter of debate.[38] At Children's Hospital in Boston, we favor the use of a conduit, where possible, believing that the earlier in life normal or nearly normal hemodynamics are established, the better. Which method is used should be determined by the preference of the surgeon and the difficulties with later management of residual pulmonary artery obstructions.

In the presence of excessive aortopulmonary collaterals, any open heart operation is complicated by excessive pulmonary blood flow via collateral circulation during use of a pump oxygenator. Occlusion of collateral vessels, either by permanent obstruction with coils (see p. 217) or temporarily with balloons, may be helpful.

Coil Embolization of Aortopulmonary Collaterals. Collateral vessels may arise from head and neck arteries, the abdominal aorta, or coronary arteries, as well as from the descending thoracic aorta. Their courses within the thorax are erratic, often crossing the midline. This unpredictable anatomy may make intraoperative recognition difficult; besides, vessels that arise from the descending aorta usually need to be approached from a posterior thoracotomy incision. As a result, most aortopulmonary collateral vessels are not closed at the time of reparative surgery and require a second incision.

In recent years, catheter techniques[14,37] have been used to close most aortopulmonary collateral vessels and reduce the number of operations required. Angiograms can be used to evaluate the result quite precisely. Success rates are high, morbidity low, and recanalization rare.

Technique. Precise angiographic definition is mandatory to identify the optimal coil size and location. Because the course of the vessel is often tortuous, multiple views and selective injections are needed. Coils are chosen to be 10–30% larger than the diameter of the vessel to be closed: smaller coils are nonocclusive, and larger coils may extrude into the aorta (see p. 217). Frequently multiple coils are needed, with the larger coils used as a framework and smaller coils added subsequently to get complete occlusion.

Peripheral Pulmonary Stenosis. Even though central pulmonary blood flow has been improved, the residual pulmonary arteries may be so obstructive or distorted that further surgery or balloon dilatation is needed. Balloon dilatation of pulmonary arterial obstruction can be remarkably helpful (see p. 210).

Unifocalization. In principle, surgical interconnection of adjacent collateral vessels and pulmonary arterial blood vessels (unifocalization),[39] providing blood flow from the right ventricle, is highly desirable and often possible, at least in part.

The theory of isolating the section of the descending aorta from which the collateral circulation arises, and connecting this localized segment to the right ventricle via a conduit, should provide separation of the pulmonary and systemic circulations. A bypass graft around the isolated section of the aorta is necessary to reconstitute the descending aorta. Such a plan results in the requirement for systemic pressure in the right ventricle to overcome the obstructions within the collateral vessels. It is hard to be optimistic about the potential of this approach.

Course

The precise proportion of patients who begin life with tetralogy of Fallot and later develop pulmonary atresia is not known, but it is not rare. Because the entire pulmonary and systemic blood flow must pass through the aortic valve, the aortic annulus is dilated and aortic regurgitation is more common in those patients than in the patient with tetralogy of Fallot and pulmonary stenosis (Exhibit 4).

The course for an unrepaired patient with pulmonary atresia and ventricular septal defect is one of chronic cyanosis and its problems. Patients with limited pulmonary circulation may die in infancy, whereas others with greater pulmonary blood flow may survive into the third or fourth decade without surgical assistance, albeit with all the problems of chronic hypoxia. In general, patients with congestive heart failure early in life have less congestive trouble later and more difficulty with cyanosis. Those with anatomy nearest to that of the tetralogy of Fallot are repaired as are other patients with tetralogy of Fallot and have the same expectations for the future. In some patients the excessive collateral vessels may be inoperable; other patients are marginally improved with shunts and conduits; and in still others closure of the ventricular septal defect may provide a pulmonary circulation adequate for a reasonable life.

So far as is presently known, a child who has been repaired, who has no residual ventricular defect, who has no residual obstruction in the right heart or in the pulmonary arteries, and who has reasonably normal distribution of pulmonary blood flow has the same potential for survival as the other patients with repaired tetralogy of Fallot. Exercise tolerance tests will uncover some limitation in most survivors,[1] and patients with a conduit face the necessity for later conduit replacement.[25,34]

For patients with bizarre collateral circulation

and borderline pulmonary arteries there are additional problems. It must be understood that the attempt to provide near normal circulation requires determination and persistence. Repeated diagnostic catheterizations, interventional catheterizations, and surgical procedures are necessary. Each intervention must be followed by evaluation with appropriate techniques, including echocardiography, cardiac catheterization, and nuclear scans to evaluate pulmonary blood flow. Sometimes, instead of improving pulmonary blood flow, one lobe of lung may be completely disconnected or occluded. Pulmonary infarction occurs.

While the principles that should guide management of patients of this type are not yet firmly established, it is the author's belief that they should include the following:

1. The earlier in life the pulmonary circulation begins to receive increased flow, the larger the ultimate capacity of the pulmonary arterial circulation will become.

2. A central pulmonary artery 2 mm in diameter will still be 2 mm in diameter 10 years later if no attempt is made to improve flow through the structure.

3. The sooner the source of pulmonary blood flow is from the right ventricle, the better.

4. In general, a repair of tetralogy of Fallot with a single functional lung is undesirable and is often associated with pulmonary hypertension. Assuming adequate circulation, approximately 1½ lungs or ¾ of the usual available lung space (right and left) will provide a reasonable probability of a normal life.

5. All bizarre collateral vessels should be removed if adequate alternative flow to that area of lung can be identified.

It must be emphasized that one cannot generalize in detail. The management of these patients requires individual, tailor-made decisions by experienced cardiologists and surgeons.

Hemoptysis

Occasionally, patients with excessive collateral circulation will suffer hemoptysis. This relatively uncommon problem has been managed conservatively with success. The possibility of identifying the bleeding vessel and plugging it with a coil has been raised, but as yet has not been needed (see p. 217).

TETRALOGY OF FALLOT WITH ABSENT PULMONARY VALVE

Definition

Rarely, in patients with the tetralogy of Fallot syndrome the pulmonary valve leaflets are absent, and pulmonary regurgitation dominates the clinical picture.

Prevalence

This is an uncommon combination of anomalies. Twenty-two patients who had tetralogy of Fallot with an absent pulmonary valve were seen at Children's Hospital in Boston in the 15 years between 1973 and 1987 (Exhibit 1).

Anatomy

The pulmonary valve leaflets are represented by nubbins of tissue (Fig. 9), whereas all other intracardiac structures resemble those of the tetralogy of Fallot. There is the usual malalignment ventricular septal defect, infundibular pulmonary stenosis, and overriding of the aorta. However, the pulmonary arteries are very different from those in the usual tetralogy of Fallot. There is aneurysmal dilatation of the main, right main, and/or left main pulmonary arteries. While, at first, this appears to be simply dilatation secondary to pulmonary regurgitation, in at least some of these patients, the pulmonary vessels are inherently abnormal to several generations of pulmonary artery branches (Fig. 10).[40,41] These tortuous and dilated vessels may obstruct the airways with resulting pockets of emphysema and atelectasis. Other children, despite central aneurysmal dilatation, have no peripheral vessel tortuosity or, at least, it is so mild that after corrective surgery for the tetralogy of Fallot there is no recognizable residual pulmonary abnormality. In this condition there is usually no demonstrable ductus arteriosus,[8,11]

Physiology

The murmur of pulmonary regurgitation is audible at birth and, presumably, has been present long before birth; the right ventricle and central pulmonary vessels are large because of it. The pulmonary stenosis is rarely severe, perhaps because severe pulmonary stenosis prohibits severe pulmonary regurgitation, or perhaps simply because the right ventricle and its outflow must dilate to accommodate the regurgitated volume. So, these children are rarely more than slightly cyanotic and cyanotic spells are unlikely.

There is long-standing discussion about whether these children suffer congestive heart failure or not. Physiologic measurements do not support clinical findings that suggest the presence of congestive heart failure.

Clinical Manifestations

At birth a systolic-diastolic, to-and-fro, saw-like murmur is audible, and if a very large main, right main, or left main pulmonary artery is visible on the plain chest x-ray, the diagnosis is usually established. These infants are not more than slightly cyanotic and are not sick initially. Some will develop respiratory distress that is clinically indistinguishable from congestive heart failure.

Electrocardiography. The electrocardiogram shows right ventricular hypertrophy.

Chest X-ray. Often the plain chest x-ray demonstrates the aneurysmal dilatation of the central pulmonary arteries (Fig. 11), although occasionally the enlarged vessel is camouflaged by other structures.

Echocardiography. The features of tetralogy of Fallot with the addition of aneurysmal enlargement of the central pulmonary arteries can be demonstrated. Pulmonary regurgitation can be documented using Doppler techniques.

Cardiac Catheterization. The main purpose of cardiac catheterization is to delineate the pulmonary artery anatomy. Abnormal branching and distribution of pulmonary arteries may be found, and decisions about surgical intervention will be possible.

Management

There are two groups of patients:

1. Those who do not have trouble in infancy are similar to those with ordinary tetralogy of Fallot; these children actually do better than patients with the usual tetralogy of Fallot. Unlike the average child with the tetralogy, cyanosis does not worsen with time. These children are rarely cyanotic enough to have spells and squatting.

2. The other group has serious respiratory difficulty early in infancy, and early deaths are common. Some of these babies have compression of the tracheobronchial tree that sometimes can be relieved by surgically plicating the pulmonary artery or fixing the position of the vessels so that airway compromise is lessened.[24,48] Others have

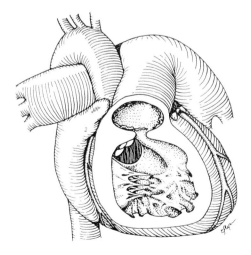

Figure 9. Drawing showing absence of the pulmonary valve. Note the lumpy bits of tissue at the usual site of the pulmonary valve, the greatly enlarged main, right main, and left main pulmonary arteries. The infundibular stenosis and ventricular septal defect are characteristics of tetralogy of Fallot.

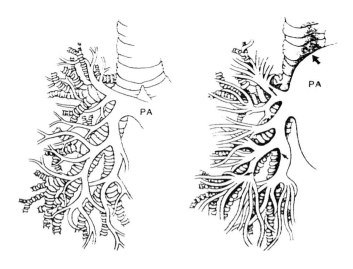

Figure 10. Drawing of a bizarre pulmonary vascular pattern found in some patients with tetralogy of Fallot and absent pulmonary valve. Arrow indicates point of compression of the right main stem bronchus by the enlarged pulmonary artery. (From Rabinovitch M, Grady S, David I: Am J Cardiol 50:804–813, 1982,[40] with permission.)

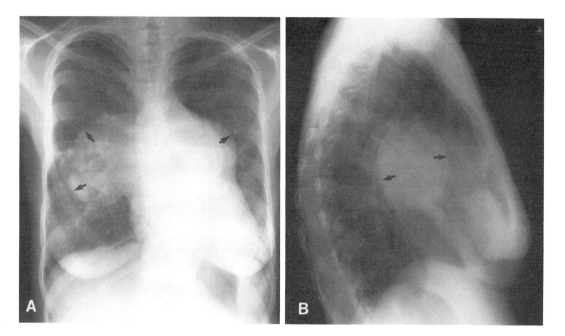

Figure 11. Anteroposterior and lateral chest x-rays of an asymptomatic mother (who has three children) with tetralogy of Fallot and absent pulmonary valve. There is gross enlargement of the main, right main, and left main pulmonary arteries (arrows). (Courtesy of the Grenada Heart Association.)

widespread abnormalities of the tracheobronchial tree for which no surgical procedure is possible (Fig. 9).

Surgical correction of the first group proceeds as for tetralogy of Fallot,[33] with the exception that the surgery is delayed until the child is older so that an artificial valve can be inserted. In general, most surgical groups are using artificial pulmonary valves or homografts in these repairs, although the requirement for this is not well demonstrated.

The second group presents a much more difficult problem. Therapy centers around providing the best possible pulmonary function. Survival is the goal (Exhibit 2).[11]

Course

It is expected that the survivors of surgical repair will have the same life expectancy as any other patient with repaired tetralogy of Fallot.

TETRALOGY OF FALLOT AND COMMON ATRIOVENTRICULAR CANAL

The combination of tetralogy of Fallot and common atrioventricular canal is a rare problem; 54 were seen at Boston Children's Hospital during the recent 15-year period (Exhibit 1).

Anatomy

Virtually all the variations of the anatomy of the tetralogy of Fallot and the anatomy of endocardial cushion defects are encountered in combination (see pp. 471, 577).

Physiology

The physiology is essentially that of tetralogy of Fallot, except that there may be incompetence of the atrioventricular valve as well. Progressive outflow obstruction and cyanotic spells are seen.

Clinical Manifestations

The history is that of tetralogy of Fallot. There may be a greater incidence of the Down syndrome. The auscultatory findings are similar to those of tetralogy of Fallot. The electrocardiogram usually shows the leftward-superior axis characteristic of atrioventricular canal defects. On chest x-ray the findings are similar to those of tetralogy of Fallot.

Echocardiography. The diagnosis is established by echocardiography, the presence of both lesions being demonstrable (see p. 584) (see ch. 36). The common atrioventricular valve virtually always has a true floating and undivided superior leaflet.

Cardiac Catheterization. The combination is sufficiently rare and the possibilities for complications sufficiently great that, except for those being considered for a shunting operation, cardiac catheterization is carried out. The distribution of the coronaries, possible additional ventricular defects, and distortion or obstruction in the pulmonary arteries are evaluated, and it is determined whether either ventricle is hypoplastic.

Management

Management consists of maintaining a level of arterial oxygen sufficient to provide reasonable growth and prevent cyanotic spells. Repair is scheduled for about 1 year of age, or earlier if there are severe symptoms.[53] Occasionally, a very small infant may undergo a shunting procedure because of cyanosis and poor growth.

Course

Survival with surgery (shunting with later repair or primary repair alone) is poorer than it is for either lesion alone (Exhibit 2).

OBSTRUCTING MUSCLE BUNDLES IN THE INFUNDIBULUM

Large muscle bundles (moderator bands) obstructing the outflow of the right ventricle are found in 5% of patients with tetralogy of Fallot (Fig. 12). These structures are identical to those described as causing double-chambered right ven-

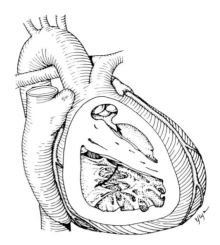

Figure 12. Drawing of the cardiac anatomy in a patient with tetralogy of Fallot with obstructive moderator bands. Compare with Figure 1. The arrow indicates the means of egress from the body of the right ventricle to the pulmonary outflow under the obstructive muscle tissue.

tricle (see ch. 29). It is important to recognize this abnormality so that the muscle can be severed or removed to prevent residual obstruction. As with any patient with double-chambered right ventricle, when there has been incomplete removal, the muscular obstruction can recur. The distinction between double-chambered right ventricle as an isolated entity and tetralogy of Fallot depends on the difference between a malalignment ventricular defect and a membranous ventricular defect (see ch. 41). Patients with no ventricular defect or a spontaneously closed defect are readily classified as having double-chambered right ventricle. When there is a double-chambered right ventricle alone, the main pulmonary artery is normal in size, whereas in patients with tetralogy of Fallot, the main pulmonary artery is almost always smaller than normal. When the two defects occur together, the features of tetralogy of Fallot are present in addition to the features of double-chambered right ventricle. The surgeon will need to relieve the obstruction caused by the moderator bands, as well as to repair the usual features of the tetralogy of Fallot syndrome.

REFERENCES

1. Barber G, Danielson GK, Puga FJ, et al: Pulmonary atresia with ventricular septal defect; preoperative and postoperative responses to exercise. J Am Coll Cardiol 7:630–638, 1986.
2. Borow KM, Green LH, Castaneda AR, et al: Left ventricular function after repair of tetralogy of Fallot and its relationship to age at surgery. Circulation 61:1150–1158, 1980.
3. Borow KM, Keane JF, Castaneda AR, et al: Systemic ventricular function in patients with tetralogy of Fallot,

ventricular defect and transposition of the great arteries repaired in infancy. Circulation 64:878–885, 1981.

4. Capelli H, Ross D, Somerville J: Aortic regurgitation in tetralogy of Fallot and pulmonary atresia. Am J Cardiol 49:1979–1983, 1982.

5. Castaneda AR, Freed MD, Williams RG, et al: Repair of tetralogy of Fallot in infancy: early and late results. J Thorac Cardiovasc Surg 74:372–381, 1977.

6. Chen DG, Moller JH: Comparison of late clinical status between patients with different hemodynamic findings after repair of tetralogy of Fallot. Am Heart J 113:767–772, 1987.

7. Deanfield JE, McKenna WJ, Hallidie-Smith KA: Detection of late arrhythmia and conduction disturbance after correction of tetralogy of Fallot. Br Heart J 44:248–253, 1980.

8. Emmanouilides GC, Thanopoulos B, Siassi B, et al: "Agenesis" of ductus arteriosus associated with the syndrome of tetralogy of Fallot and absent pulmonary valve. Am J Cardiol 37:403–409, 1976.

9. Faggian G, Frescura C, Thiene G, et al: Accessory tricuspid valve tissue causing obstruction of the ventricular septal defect in tetralogy of Fallot. Br Heart J 49:324–327, 1983.

10. Fallot A: Contribution a l'anatomie pathologique de la maladie bleue (cyanose cardiaque). Marseille Med 25:77, 138, 207, 270, 341, 403, 1988.

11. Fischer DR, Neches WH, Beerman LB, et al: Tetralogy of Fallot with absent pulmonic valve: analysis of 17 patients. Am J Cardiol 53:1433–1441, 1984.

12. Fisher EA, Thanopoulos BD, Eckner FAO, et al: Pulmonary atresia with obstructed ventricular septal defect: spectrum of echocardiographic findings. J Am Coll Cardiol 11:386–395, 1988.

13. Flanagan MF, Foran RB, Van Praagh P, et al: Tetralogy of Fallot with obstruction of the ventricular septal defect: spectrum of echocardiographic findings. J Am Coll Cardiol 11:386–395, 1988.

14. Fuhrman B, Bass JL, Castaneda-Zuniga W, et al: Coil embolization of congenital thoracic vascular anomalies in infants and children. Circulation 70:285–289, 1984.

15. Fuster V, McGoon DC, Kennedy MA, et al: Long-term evaluation (2–22 years) of open heart surgery for tetralogy of Fallot. Am J Cardiol 46:635–642, 1980.

16. Fyler DC: Report of the New England Regional Infant Cardiac Program. Pediatrics 65(Suppl):375–461, 1980.

17. Garson A, Gillette PC, Gutgesell HP, et al: Stress-induced ventricular arrhythmia after repair of tetralogy of Fallot. Am J Cardiol 46:1006–1012, 1980.

18. Garson A, Randall DC, Gillette PC, et al: Prevention of sudden death after repair of tetralogy of Fallot: treatment of ventricular arrhythmias. J Am Coll Cardiol 6:221–227, 1985.

19. Guntheroth WG, Morgen BC, Mullins GL: Physiologic studies of paroxysmal hyperpnea in cyanotic congenital heart disease. Circulation 31:66–76, 1965.

20. Gustafson RA, Murray GF, Warden HE, et al: Early repair of tetralogy of Fallot. Ann Thorac Surg 45:235–241, 1988.

21. Harken AH, Horowitz LN, Josephson ME: Surgical correction of recurrent sustained ventricular tachycardia following complete repair of tetralogy of Fallot. J Thorac Cardiovasc Surg 80:779–781, 1980.

22. Haworth SG: Collateral arteries in pulmonary atresia with ventricular septal defect: a precarious blood supply. Br Heart J 44:5–13, 1980.

23. Haworth SG, Macartney FJ: Growth and development of pulmonary circulation in pulmonary atresia with ventricular septal defect and major aortopulmonary collateral arteries. Br Heart J 44:14–24, 1980.

24. Ilbawi MN, Fedorchik J, Muster AJ, et al: Surgical approach to severely symptomatic newborn infants with tetralogy of Fallot and absent pulmonary valve. J Thorac Cardiovasc Surg 91:584–589, 1986.

25. Jonas RA, Freed MD, et al: Long-term follow-up of patients with synthetic right heart conduits. Circulation 72(Suppl II):77–83, 1985.

26. Karpawich PP, Bush CP, Antillon JR, et al: Modified Blalock-Taussig shunt in infants and young children. J Thorac Cardiovasc Surg 89:275–279, 1985.

27. Kavey RW, Thomas FD, Byrum CJ, et al: Ventricular arrhythmias and biventricular dysfunction after repair of tetralogy of Fallot. J Am Coll Cardiol 4:126–131, 1984.

28. Keith J, Vlad P, Rowe RD: Heart disease in Infancy and Childhood, 3rd ed. New York, Macmillan, 1979, pp. 3–13; 475.

29. Kobayashi J, Hirose H, Nakano S, et al: Ambulatory electrocardiographic study of the frequency and cause of ventricular arrhythmia after correction of tetralogy of Fallot. Am J Cardiol 54:1310–1313, 1984.

30. Lamberti JJ, Carlisle J, Waldman JD, et al: Systemic-pulmonary shunts in infants and children. J Thorac Cardiovasc Surg 88:76–81, 1984.

31. Liao PK, Edwards WK, Julsrud PR, et al: Pulmonary blood supply in patients with pulmonary atresia and ventricular septal defect. J Am Coll Cardiol 6:1343–1350, 1985.

32. Lois JF, Gomes AS, Brown K, et al: Magnetic resonance imaging of the thoracic aorta. Am J Cardiol 60:358–362, 1987.

33. McCaughan, BC, Danielson GK, Driscoll DJ, et al: Tetralogy of Fallot with absent pulmonary valve. J Thorac Cardiovasc Surg 89:280–287, 1985.

34. McGoon DC, Danielson GK, Puga FJ, et al: Results after extracardiac conduit repair for congenital cardiac defects. Am J Cardiol 49:1741–1749, 1982.

35. Misbach GA, Turley K, Ebert PA: Pulmonary valve replacement for regurgitation after repair of tetralogy of Fallot. Ann Thorac Surg 36:684–691, 1983.

36. Newburger JW, Silbert AR, Buckley LP, et al: Cognitive function and duration of hypoxemia in children with transposition of the great arteries. N Engl J Med 310:1495–1499, 1984.

37. Perry SB, Radtke W, Fellows KE, et al: Coil embolization of aorto-pulmonary collaterals and shunts in patients with congenital heart disease. J Am Coll Cardiol 13:100–108, 1989.

38. Piehler JM, Danielson GK, McGoon DC, et al: Management of pulmonary atresia with ventricular septal defect and hypoplastic pulmonary arteries by right ventricular outflow construction. J Thorac Cardiovasc Surg 80:552–565, 1980.

39. Puga FJ, Leone FE, Julsrud PR, et al: Complete repair of pulmonary atresia, ventricular septal defect, and severe peripheral arborization abnormalities of the central pulmonary arteries. J Thorac Cardiovasc Surg 98:1018–1029, 1989.

40. Rabinovitch M, Grady S, David I, et al: Compression of intrapulmonary bronchi by abnormally branching pulmonary arteries associated with absent pulmonary valves. Am J Cardiol 50:804–813, 1982.

41. Rabinovitch M, Herrera-DeLeon V, Castaneda AR, et al: Growth and development of the pulmonary vascular bed in patients with tetralogy of Fallot with or without pulmonary atresia. Circulation 64:1234–1249, 1981.

42. Rittenhouse EA, Mansfield PB, Hall DG, et al: Tetralogy of Fallot: selective staged management. J Thorac Cardiovasc Surg 89:772–779, 1985.

43. Rome J: Personal communication.

44. Roth A, Rosenthal A, Hall JE, et al: Scoliosis in congenital heart disease. Clin Orthop Rel Res 93:95–102, 1973.

45. Sandor GGS, Patterson MWH, Tipple M, et al: Left ventricular systolic and diastolic function after total correction of tetralogy of Fallot. Am J Cardiol 60:1148–1151, 1987.

46. Shem-Tov A, Dicker D, Blieden LC, et al: The pulmonary circulation and its systemic arterial supply in pulmonary atresia. Clin Cardiol 5:489–492, 1982.

47. Somerville J: Gout in cyanotic congenital heart disease. Br Heart J 23:31–34, 1961.

48. Stellin G, Jonas RA, Goh TH, et al: Surgical treatment of absent pulmonary valve syndrome in infants: relief of bronchial obstruction. Ann Thorac Surg 36:468–475, 1983.

49. Stensen N: Quoted by Goldstein HI: Bull Hist Med 29:526, 1948.

50. Thiene G, Frescura C, Borolotti U, et al: The systemic pulmonary circulation in pulmonary atresia with ventricular septal defect: concept of reciprocal development of the fourth and sixth aortic arches. Am Heart J 101:339–344, 1981.

51. Uretzky G, Puga FJ, Danielson GK, et al: Reoperation after correction of tetralogy of Fallot. Circulation 66:202–206, 1982.

52. Van Praagh R, Van Praagh S, Nebesar RA, et al: Tetralogy of Fallot: underdevelopment of the pulmonary infundibulum and its sequelae. Am J Cardiol 26:25–28, 1970.

53. Vargas FJ, Coto EO, Mayer JE, et al: Complete atrioventricular canal and tetralogy of Fallot: surgical considerations. Ann Thorac Surg 42:258–263, 1986.

54. Walsh EP, Rochenmacher S, Keane JF, et al: Late results in patients with tetralogy of Fallot repaired during infancy. Circulation 77:1062–1067, 1988.

55. Wood P: Diseases of the Heart and Circulation, 3rd ed. London, Eyre and Spottiswoode, 1968.

56. Zhao H-X, Miller DC, Reitz BA, et al: Surgical repair of tetralogy of Fallot: long-term follow-up with particular emphasis on late death and reoperation. J Thorac Cardiovasc Surg 89:204–220, 1985.

Chapter 31

AORTIC OUTFLOW ABNORMALITIES

Donald C. Fyler, M.D.

VALVAR AORTIC STENOSIS

Definition

Obstruction to outflow from the left ventricle by an abnormal aortic valve is described as valvar aortic stenosis.

Prevalence

Valvar aortic stenosis is one of the most common congenital cardiac defects. It is rare in infancy (0.04–0.34 per 1000 live births); it ranks 16th among infants with critical heart disease (2%) (see ch. 18). However, in progressively older age groups, patients with aortic stenosis make up an increasing percentage of congenital heart disease. By the third decade, it is second only to ventricular septal defect (see ch. 18). Among men of draft age at the time of World War I, the incidence was 0.11%.[73] Often, aortic stenosis is not recognized in early infancy; however, when it is discovered, it is frequently shown to be based on a congenitally bicuspid valve. Because of the high incidence of congenital abnormality of the leaflets, it is thought of as a congenital abnormality. Still, there are instances of stenosis of a three-leafed valve that could be examples of an acquired disease.

Pathology

In a patient with valvar aortic stenosis, the periphery of each commissure may be fused, the valve ring may be hypoplastic, and the leaflets may be thickened and deformed. The orifice of the valve is small and may be eccentric.[21] In the young infant with critical aortic stenosis, the aortic valve may, at times, be a nodular, gelatinous mass scarcely resembling a valve. The valve is commonly bicuspid;[42] rarely, it is unicuspid. Even the tricuspid valves may have asymmetric leaflets, one leaflet being of different size in comparison to the others. Often, the ascending aorta is dilated because of the jet produced by left ventricular ejection.

Combinations of more than one type of obstruc-

tion in the left ventricular outflow tract are common (Exhibit 1).

In the later stages of the disease, there may be calcification of the valve (rare before the age of 20 years), and, finally, the myocardium may show evidence of fibrotic scarring after prolonged exposure to elevated left ventricular pressure.

Pathogenesis. In formulating a theory of the pathogenesis of congenital valvar aortic stenosis, the following observations must be reconciled:

1. Aortic stenosis tends to be a progressive disease. Although there are few infants with valvar aortic stenosis, in each older age group there are greater numbers of patients affected, so much so that among the group with congenital heart disease older than 30 years of age, valvar aortic stenosis shares the lead with ventricular septal defects. This trend may be exaggerated by the loss of patients with other kinds of congenital heart disease. Still, the difference is convincing (see ch. 18). With serial observations, the severity of valvar obstruction has been documented to get worse.[68]

2. Many patients with aortic stenosis have bicuspid valves. Bicuspid aortic valve is a common anomaly that has an incidence in the order of 10–20 times that of aortic stenosis (see p. 510). The majority of patients with coarctation of the aorta have a bicommissural aortic valve, yet only a few develop valvar stenosis. A bicuspid valve is very common in the younger age groups with aortic stenosis, but is less common in the very old.[59]

3. Aortic stenosis is sometimes familial.

4. Among 1000 patients with rheumatic fever, only two developed aortic stenosis after 20 years of follow-up.[10]

As a working hypothesis, it is proposed that there may be a genetic factor that predisposes to the combination of bicuspid aortic valve and aortic stenosis, but that a bicuspid aortic valve by itself does not necessarily predispose to aortic stenosis. Aortic stenosis is a progressive lesion; **aortic stenosis begets aortic stenosis.** Rheumatic fever is not a factor in the pathogenesis of valvar aortic stenosis, at least

493

Exhibit 1

Boston Children's Hospital Experience 1973–87 **Aortic Outflow Abnormalities**					
Type of Aortic Stenosis	Valvar Aortic Stenosis	Supravalvar Aortic Stenosis	Subvalvar Aortic Stenosis	Aortic Regurgitation*	Bicuspid Valve
Valvar Aortic Stenosis n = 835	835	1	79	454	338 (40%)
Supravalvar Stenosis n = 63	–	63	17	26	9 (14%)
Subvalvar Stenosis n = 75	–	–	75	44	3 (4%)
Aortic Regurgitation n = 87	–	–	–	87	24 (24%)

*Includes preoperative and postoperative aortic regurgitation.

The patients were arbitrarily divided into groups with mutually exclusive primary problems and then examined for associated left ventricular outflow lesions. Aortic regurgitation was common, whereas pure aortic regurgitation was rare. Because of the methods of data collection, the numbers of patients with bicuspid valves may be underestimated. Still, the trends are apparent.

	Male (%)	Female (%)
Valvar Aortic Stenosis	75	25
Subaortic Stenosis	65	35
Supravalvar Aortic Stenosis	59	41
Aortic Regurgitation	54	46
Bicuspid Aortic Valve	70	30

Age When First Seen 1973–87

Primary Diagnosis	Age*						Total
	0–2 months n (%)	3–12 months n (%)	1–5 years n (%)	6–9 years n (%)	10–19 years n (%)	20– years n (%)	
Valvar Aortic Stenosis	69 (8)	61 (7)	142 (17)	218 (26)	309 (37)	33 (4)	832
Aortic Regurgitation	0	6 (7)	3 (3)	24 (28)	38 (44)	15 (17)	86
Subvalvar Aortic Stenosis	3 (4)	7 (9)	17 (23)	26 (35)	20 (27)	1 (1)	74
Supravavar Aortic Stenosis	1 (2)	11 (17)	17 (27)	14 (22)	16 (25)	4 (6)	63

*Age could not be calculated for five patients because of faulty data.

in the young. Aortic stenosis in the aged is unrelated to congenital aortic stenosis and has a different pathogenesis.

Physiology

The degree of obstruction is best expressed in terms of the pressure loss across the valve in systole (Fig. 1). This is a mathematical relationship involving the ventricular pressure required to deliver the cardiac output at the required perfusion pressure (see ch. 14).[30] With exercise, anemia, hyperthyroidism, or any other cause for increased cardiac output, the left ventricular pressure needed to produce increased output is proportionately higher.

During cardiac catheterization, the usual method of measurement involves recording the pressure while the catheter crosses the valve, or, alternatively, when recordings of left ventricular pressure and ascending aortic pressure can be made simultaneously. If the peak systolic pressure distal to the valve is measured at some remote site (i.e., the radial artery), an error due to the standing wave effect is introduced, and if the distal pressure is measured by a different technique (pressure cuff), further error is introduced. Theoretically, in severe stenosis, the pressure gradient could be affected by the catheter within the valve, but aortic stenosis that severe is rarely encountered except possibly in very small infants who are seriously ill.

Measurement of the maximal instantaneous gradient using echo-Doppler techniques produces a

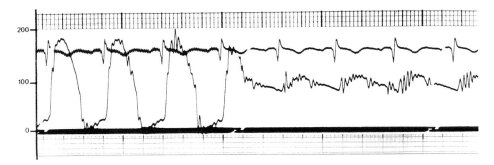

Figure 1. Pressure gradient observed in a patient with valvar aortic stenosis as the catheter is withdrawn from the left ventricle to the aorta. Note the change in systemic pressure.

somewhat different gradient for several reasons.[18,54] Echocardiography relies on the determination of the maximal velocity of the jet of blood passing through the orifice of the valve during systole and, by itself, gives a result that is different from the peak systolic pressure gradient measured with a cardiac catheter. An eccentric jet may cause an error in the echocardiographic estimation. Additionally, the patient is more often awake during an echocardiographic examination and, therefore, may have some anxiety. Fortunately, the differences between the two techniques are usually not great; when echocardiographic measurements and catheterization measurements are made simultaneously, the correlation is much improved. The echocardiographic gradient is useful in following the course of the disease, but not for therapeutic decisions. This is a point of little consequence now that virtually all patients undergo cardiac catheterization for balloon valvuloplasty, and pressure gradients are measured directly prior to that procedure.

The systemic arterial pressure is characterized by a smaller than normal pulse pressure. The small pulse of aortic stenosis (pulsus parvus) has stimulated many attempts to determine the severity of the aortic stenosis from the arterial pressure wave. Although this idea is solidly based in science and may be useful, to a degree, in adults, it is not reliable in children.

Left ventricular hypertrophy interferes with the pumping function of the ventricle. Wall-stress abnormalities and diastolic filling problems should be documented and may be useful measures in following the course of this disease (see ch. 15).[23,47] With extreme left ventricular hypertrophy, fibrosis may be so extensive that there is involvement of the papillary muscles, tethering the mitral valve. Mitral regurgitation is the result. Endocardial fibroelastosis is common in critically ill infants but rare in older patients.

Clinical Manifestations[68]

The usual child with valvar aortic stenosis is a male (75%), is asymptomatic, and is growing and developing normally (Exhibit 1). He is discovered to have a heart murmur during a routine physical examination. Discovery of unexpected aortic stenosis in teenagers is common enough that the required examination of students participating in sports uncovers a few new patients each year (Exhibit 1).

Less commonly, a child will complain of typical angina pectoris with exercise. In the toddler and small child, this symptom is not well articulated, yet sometimes a child is observed who suddenly stops and clutches the anterior chest during exercise. Fainting is another ominous finding in these children; nevertheless, exercise intolerance is not a common symptom.

On physical examination, the child is well developed and well nourished. The peripheral pulses may be small and the measured pulse pressure is less than normal. Often there is a systolic thrill in the suprasternal notch and, with more severe stenosis, a thrill may be felt at the second right intercostal space. On auscultation, a systolic click usually precedes the crescendo-decrescendo systolic murmur. The murmur is loudest at the second right interspace and is typically stenotic. It transmits well into the neck (Fig. 2).

Because ventricular systole is prolonged proportionate to the severity of aortic stenosis, the

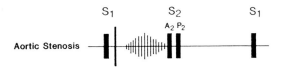

Figure 2. Diagram of the ejection murmur of valvar aortic stenosis. Note the early systolic click characteristic of valvar aortic stenosis. The crescendo-decrescendo murmur reaches peak intensity in mid systole.

aortic component at the second heart sound is delayed, producing a narrowly split second heart sound, sometimes with the aortic closure appearing after pulmonary closure (reverse splitting). Verification of this phenomenon requires phonocardiography.

Because aortic regurgitation is commonly associated with aortic stenosis, there may be an early diastolic regurgitant murmur as well (Fig. 3).

Electrocardiography. Usually, when there is mild aortic stenosis, the electrocardiogram is normal. With greater obstruction there may be increased left-sided R wave voltage, and with severe obstruction there are changes in the S-T segment and T wave in the left precordial leads (strain pattern). However, there is not a strict correlation between these electrocardiographic findings and the measured severity of the obstruction. The electrocardiogram tends to reflect the average pressure gradient during the child's daily life and the amount of myocardial injury that has occurred over the years. Therefore, there is some variation between the observations recorded on the electrocardiogram and the resting observations made during cardiac catheterization or echocardiography. Despite this, on the average, the electrocardiogram provides a reflection of the severity of the stenosis (Fig. 4).

Chest X-ray. The chest x-ray provides little useful information. The heart (except in small infants in congestive heart failure) is rarely more than slightly enlarged and is often normal. Occasionally, the ascending aorta is dilated because of poststenotic dilatation.

Echocardiography. The number of aortic leaflets, the size of the ascending aorta, and the maximal instantaneous pressure gradient across the valve can be determined. Evaluation of ventricular function by volume measurements and by contraction indices gives clues to the functional status of the myocardium (see ch. 15).[19]

The morphology of the aortic valve is best determined from parasternal long- and short-axis views (Fig. 5). The thickness of the leaflets and

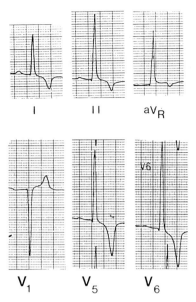

Figure 4. Electrocardiogram in an outstanding athlete with valvar aortic stenosis. Besides voltage evidence of left ventricular hypertrophy, there are S-T and T-wave abnormalities particularly noticeable in V_6 and aV_F. He dropped dead during a squash match a few months after this electrocardiogram was taken. He had been warned that competitive sports might be fatal.

systolic doming are detected in the long-axis views. The commissural anatomy is best determined from the short-axis view, primarily in systole when the valve opens.[12] In diastole most aortic valves appear to be trileaflet. If a commissure is present, the valve leaflets separate all the way to the valve annulus, but, if commissural fusion is present, separation is incomplete and a raphe can be seen connecting the more peripheral aspects of the adjacent leaflets.

The commissure between the right and left coronary leaflets and the commissure between the right coronary and noncoronary leaflets are the common sites of fusion. The commissure between the left coronary and noncoronary leaflets is almost never involved (one case in the files of Children's Hospital in Boston).

The function of the valve should be assessed using Doppler examination. Regurgitation is seen best in apical or parasternal long-axis views, using Doppler color-flow mapping or pulsed Doppler examination. At best, quantification of the regurgitation is approximate, but it should be based on the diameter of the flow jet at the level of the valve seen by Doppler color-flow mapping, the size of the left ventricle, and the Doppler flow pattern in the descending aorta (see p. 178). Stenosis of the valve can be evaluated using pulsed or continuous-wave Doppler examination, with the transducer located in the apex, the right sternal border, or

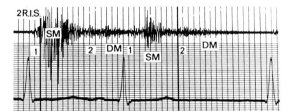

Figure 3. Phonocardiogram of the murmurs present in a patient with valvar aortic stenosis and aortic regurgitation. Note the diamond-shaped systolic murmur peaking in early to mid systole and the high-frequency, lower intensity murmur throughout diastole. 2RIS, second right intercostal space; SM, systolic murmur; DM, diastolic murmur; 1, first heart sound, 2, second heart sound.

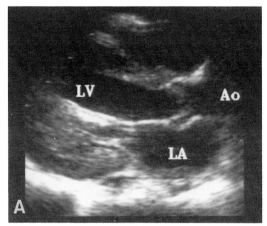

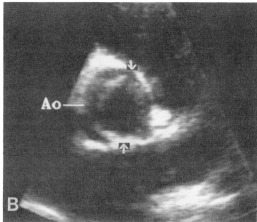

Figure 5. Parasternal views in a patient with a bicommissural aortic valve. **A,** Long-axis view demonstrating doming and mild thickening of the valve leaflets. **B,** Short-axis view demonstrating the two commissures (arrows) that open completely to the valve annulus. Ao, ascending aorta, LA, left atrium; LV, left ventricle.

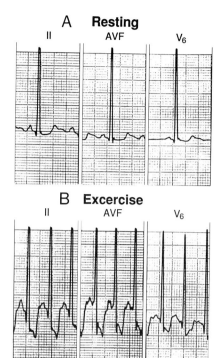

Figure 6. Electrocardiograms recorded before and during treadmill exercise. Note the normal T waves at rest, which become inverted with exercise. Depression of the S-T segment also appears.

the suprasternal notch. The results may be more reliable if the patient is sedated.[49]

Stress Testing. Maximal exercise testing can be a useful procedure.[4,35,44] Because the endpoints of angina, syncope, or changes in the S-T segment and T wave are positive outcomes, exercise testing in patients who already have these changes does not add useful information. In the asymptomatic child with normal, borderline, or suspicious findings, a stress test may result in changes in the S-T segment and T wave. This finding suggests that a significant degree of obstruction is present (Fig. 6).

Cardiac Catheterization. Today, cardiac catheterization is rarely undertaken to determine the severity of aortic stenosis; rather, it is used to dilate the valvar obstruction. Once the clinician has reached the conclusion that sufficient aortic stenosis is present to require dilatation, catheteriza-

tion is undertaken. The indications for cardiac catheterization include the following:[63]

1. Fainting. A fainting episode in a patient who has aortic stenosis, regardless of all else, requires mandatory cardiac catheterization. Clearly, if the echo-Doppler estimation of the pressure gradient suggests mild obstruction, a search for other causes of syncope is needed; but none being found, fainting, in the presence of aortic stenosis, is a signal for further study and probable therapy. Episodes of feeling dizzy or faint without actual syncope are also encountered and these require careful evaluation in making a decision.

2. Angina. Anginal pain that is convincing has the same significance as syncope.

3. Changes in the S-T segment and T wave. The appearance of these changes, either on routine follow-up electrocardiograms or during stress tests, requires cardiac catheterization.

4. An echocardiographic pressure gradient of 60 mm Hg or more is an indication for cardiac catheterization and probable dilatation of the valve.

5. Given a lesser echo-Doppler gradient in an asymptomatic child who has no changes in the S-T segment and T wave, the decision to catheterize is based on the amount of left ventricular hypertrophy, the intensity of the murmur, and the clinician's estimate of the child's physical activity (a

couch-potato is one type, whereas a weight-lifting, backyard athlete is another).

6. Ectopy. Because ventricular ectopy further complicates the delivery of cardiac output through an obstructive valve, and may otherwise be a signal of left ventricular impairment, the tendency to intervene is increased when ectopy is present.

The pressure gradient across the valve is a precise measure of the degree of obstruction, provided the cardiac output is not depressed. The measured gradient determines whether a balloon angioplasty can be carried out (Fig. 7).

The aortic valve and the supravalvar region are well demonstrated with the angiographic catheter above, not touching, the aortic valve. Because the aortic valve often overlies the spine and the descending aorta, rotation of the patient in either direction improves visualization. Usually, filming in biplane in the right and left anterior oblique views, while injecting 1.0–1.5 ml of contrast material per kg of body weight, not only results in good visualization of the aortic valve but gives evidence of the degree of aortic regurgitation as well. This technique also gives a good view of a subaortic membrane.

Management

Except for infants in congestive heart failure where the issue is survival (see p. 501), the main consideration in managing a child or young adult with valvar aortic stenosis is the preservation of left ventricular muscle function. At some point in the natural course of this disease, there will be evidence of left ventricular muscle dysfunction. The plan of management is to relieve valvar obstruction before permanent muscle damage occurs.

Episodes of fainting, anginal pain, ventricular rhythm disturbance, echocardiographic evidence of left ventricular dysfunction, or electrocardiographic evidence of changes in the S-T segment and T wave (at rest or on exercise) suggest the need for intervention, beginning with cardiac catheterization. If there is a pressure gradient of 50 mm Hg or more across the aortic valve, in the absence of aortic regurgitation, balloon valvuloplasty is undertaken (see ch. 14) (Exhibit 2). Because the best residual pressure gradient that can be expected is between 25 and 30 mm Hg, an initial gradient between 30 and 50 mm Hg scarcely justifies balloon valvuloplasty. The largest patients may require simultaneous inflation of two balloons to get the desired result.[5,31,67]

The complications of balloon valvuloplasty are associated with insertion of larger catheters into arterial vessels. Deaths have occurred only in infants with critical aortic stenosis.[69]

Pediatricians and internists have a different view of the indications for intervention in patients with aortic stenosis. A 20-year-old with aortic stenosis is managed in Children's Hospital in Boston with one form of treatment, whereas the same patient would be managed in our associated adult hospitals in a different manner. Physicians concerned with adults are primarily influenced by symptoms and much less by ventricular function. Hence, the average patient subjected to valvuloplasty in a pediatric hospital would be treated more conservatively by our friends in internal medicine. This is not a matter of criticism; rather it is a matter of fact, which is recognized, considered, and debated by all concerned.

There has been insufficient experience with bal-

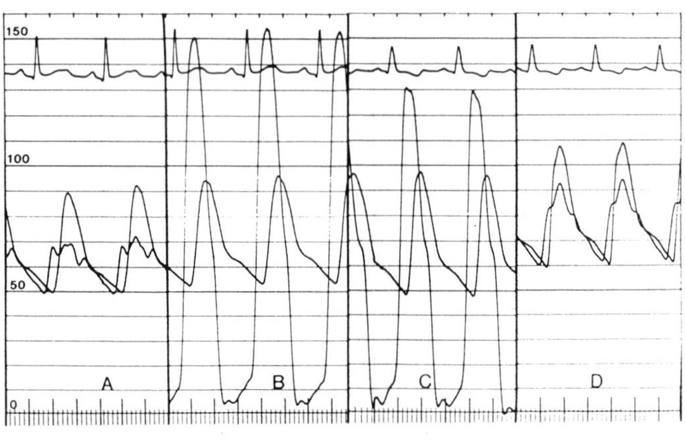

Figure 7. Pressure recordings in a patient with valvar aortic stenosis. The numerical scale on the left is in mm Hg. **A,** Comparison of the pressure recorded from the ascending aorta with that in the femoral artery. Note that the pressure tracing is delayed in the femoral artery and is 20 mm Hg higher in the femoral artery than in the ascending aorta. This is an example of the standing wave effect (see ch. 14). **B,** Comparison of the femoral artery pressure with the left ventricular pressure. Note that the gradient of pressure across the valve measures 55 mm Hg but underestimates the true gradient by 20 mm Hg. **C,** Comparison of the femoral artery pressure and the left ventricular pressure following balloon dilatation of the aortic valve. Note that the pressure gradient is now smaller, the arterial pulse pressure is greater, and the electrocardiogram now shows bundle branch block, a transitory phenomen. **D,** Comparison of the ascending aorta and femoral artery pressures after ballooning the aortic valve. Note that the pulse contour of the ascending aorta has changed; the pulse pressure is greater and the pressures are higher than in panel A.

Exhibit 2

Boston Children's Hospital Experience
1973–1987
Valvar Aortic Stenosis: Valvuloplasty

Year of Procedure	Age at Procedure*						
	0–2 months	3–12 months	1–5 years	5–9 years	10–19 years	20– years	Total
Surgery							
1973–77	6	2	3	3	25	7	46
1978–82	11	4	4	6	17	10	52
1983–1987	11	0	1	0	11	5	28
Catheterization							
1983–87	10	7	13	10	22	6	68
Total	38	13	21	19	75	28	194

*Note that 25% of these aortic valvuloplasties took place in the first year of life.

Method	Year of Procedure							Total	Mortality (%)
	1973–77	1978–82	1983	1984	1985	1986	1987		
Surgery*	46 (4)	52 (5)	8 (2)	8	4	6	2 (1)	126 (12)	10%
Catheterization	0	0	0	1	11	33 (2)	23 (1)	68 (3)	4%

*Numbers in parentheses are the number of patients who died in association with valvuloplasty. All deaths occurred in critically ill infants.

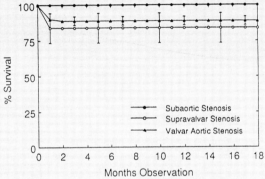

Actuarial survival curves for patients who underwent aortic outflow surgery for otherwise uncomplicated aortic outflow disease.

Infective Endocarditis Associated with Aortic Outflow Abnormalities*

	Primary Diagnosis	Infective Endocarditis	Secondary Diagnosis	Infective Endocarditis
Valvar Aortic Stenosis	835	25 (3%)	642	10 (2%)
Supravalvar Stenosis	75	0 (0)	351	10 (3%)
Subvalvar Stenosis	63	2 (3%)	140	1 (1%)
Aortic Regurgitation	87	6 (8%)	547	41 (7%)
Bicuspid Aortic Valve	71	0	737	20 (4%)

*All but two patients with endocarditis and a primary diagnosis of aortic outflow disease had primary or associated aortic regurgitation; all but 12 of the patients with a secondary diagnosis of aortic outflow disease and infective endocarditis had associated aortic regurgitation.

Aortic Valve Replacement*

Original Lesion	Boston Children's Hospital	Late Replacement Elsewhere	Total
Valvar Aortic Stenosis	46	8	54
Subaortic Stenosis	1	0	1
Supravalvar Stenosis	7	0	7
Aortic Regurgitation	14	1	15
Total	68	9	77

*The majority of these operations were performed because of aortic regurgitation, often acquired or aggravated by prior valvoplasty. At least three had a preceding Konno procedure. Because this is a pediatric population that is growing older, some patients had valve replacement elsewhere, and it is likely that additional adult patients have had valve replacement elsewhere.

loon valvuloplasty to prove that the results are as good as those following surgical valvuloplasty. They seem to be. Still, surgical valvuloplasty[2,36] is a valuable option even if there has been preceding unsuccessful balloon valvuloplasty.

With balloon procedures, the number of valve cusps does not influence the relief of valvar obstruction, but it does seem to predict complicating aortic regurgitation.[63] That all types of valvar stenosis respond at least somewhat to balloon valvuloplasty seems established. Intuitively, the number of times balloon valvuloplasty can be repeated may be unlimited, whereas surgical valvuloplasty, involving reopening of scars, is unlikely to be accepted as a repetitive solution.

Aortic valve replacement is required when the previously mentioned indications for intervention are present and, in addition when: (1) the aortic valve is grossly deformed, especially if it is calcified—a phenomenon that occurs as early as 20 years of age, or (2) there is enough aortic regurgitation that it is as much the cause of the patient's problems as the associated stenosis (or to put it another way, when attempts to relieve the stenosis with valvuloplasty will only make matters worse).

Patients who have aortic stenosis require prophylaxis against infective endocarditis,[27] because aortic valvar abnormalities are particularly prone to this complication.[14]

Course

The natural course of mild aortic stenosis is relatively benign, although the number of late deaths is greater than that expected for the normal population.[40] Although fewer of these patients progress to the need for intervention than do those with more severe stenosis, progression to more severe stenosis does occur and must be kept in mind.

Those with moderate or severe stenosis are much more likely to develop, increasing obstruction with time. Although this is not universally true, it is, nonetheless, sufficiently likely that patients must be managed with this thought in mind. Therefore, these patients should be followed closely, watching for changes in serial observations that suggest a need for valvuloplasty. The recurrence or new appearance of symptoms is rare; still, symptoms suggesting angina or syncope should be taken seriously, as they usually indicate the need for interventional treatment.

Exercise intolerance is not a common symptom and is rarely a factor in deciding management questions. In contrast, stress tests do uncover patients who are prone to changes in the S-T segment and T wave during maximal exercise, an observation that should be taken seriously.

Rhythm abnormalities, at rest or on exercise, are encountered and are taken as a sign of ventricular dysfunction. Rarely, arrhythmia influences the decision to intervene, but it is almost never the sole reason.

Abnormalities in ventricular function tests, volume measurements, shortening fractions, and other indices (see ch. 15) should be taken seriously, particularly if a pattern of deterioration is documented in the course of follow-up.

The appearance of changes in the left-sided S-T segments and T waves, whether occurring spontaneously or during maximal exercise testing, requires serious consideration, because sudden death occurs primarily among patients who have these abnormalities.[20,46]

Unfortunately, it remains to be shown that valvuloplasty influences the incidence of late sudden death.[40] For the present, optimists (like the author) assume that the number of late sudden deaths would be greater without their ministrations.

To control the problems associated with aortic stenosis, the following steps should be taken:

1. The average patient with valvar aortic stenosis should be seen at least annually to have an electrocardiographic tracing. Follow-up is a lifetime commitment and, for most patients, requires visits to the cardiologist when there are, in fact, no symptoms or limitations.

2. Holter monitoring should be carried out at 5-year intervals, or more often if there is any suggestion of rhythm problems.

3. In the absence of ST-T changes and with more than minimal obstruction by echocardiography, maximal exercise tolerance testing should be carried out at 2-year intervals.

4. Echocardiographic evaluation of the severity of stenosis and ventricular function should be recorded at 2-year intervals.

Infective endocarditis is a serious threat, occurring 27.1 times per 10,000 patient-years.[27] There were 16 instances of infective endocarditis with aortic valve disease at Children's Hospital in Boston in a 15-year period (Exhibit 2).

Sudden death hangs over the head of all patients with aortic stenosis, but it is mainly a threat to those with symptoms, especially those with abnormalities in the S-T segment and T wave.[28,32,46]

Vigorous exercise, particularly in competitive sports, is associated with sudden death. Because of this, vigorous physical activity should be prohibited for those with more than mild obstruction, particularly if there is any evidence of changes in the S-T segment and T wave, whether or not valvuloplasty has been carried out. This can be a particularly difficult problem, because many of these children are well-developed, physically able boys, who sometimes are excellent athletes. Anyone with a known gradient of more than 40 mm Hg or changes in the S-T segment and T wave should be prohibited from participating in vigorously competitive sports. For some, in the interest of the child's self-image, some sports, such as baseball and other less violent activities, are permitted. Occasionally, simply prohibiting varsity sports suffices. The best outcome results when the parents redesign the child's physical activities and promote a less vigorous style of life while the boy is still prepubertal. This is easier said than done, and when siblings are athletically inclined, especially older siblings, compromises are the only recourse, and sooner or later a rebellious teenager will drop dead (Fig. 6).

Avoiding the problem of sudden death while maintaining a healthy psychological outlook is the goal. Obtaining the best compromise with the individual patient is a matter of understanding the family, the child, and the physiology of the cardiac problem.

A second surgical valvotomy can be successful,[26] but repeated operations carry little promise in the long run. Whether repeated balloon valvuloplasty will be successful and how many times it can be done before valve replacement is necessary remains to be seen.

Artificial Valves

Because of the difficulty in obtaining a good surgical result in second or third attempts at valvuloplasty, valve replacement is commonly used to obtain a reasonable physiologic result. The patient who is in need of an operative procedure and in whom valvuloplasty is unlikely to help is a candidate for valve replacement (see ch. 54).[8] Excessive aortic regurgitation is a common reason. With prolonged follow-up, as many as 25% of patients who have undergone surgical valvuloplasty have ended up with an artificial valve (Exhibit 2).[40] Although an artificial valve has a finite useful expectancy, the newer valves are much improved. Complications are not common and the need to replace the valve is less than in former years. In any case, valve function is usually excellent and the requirement for anticoagulation is manageable.

It is obvious that the treatment of aortic stenosis is palliative.[33,57] No surgical or catheterization procedure cures these patients. The goal is simply to maintain reasonable well-being for as long as possible.

INFANT AORTIC STENOSIS

Infants with critical valvar aortic stenosis constitute a special group with maximal aortic valve obstruction. A murmur may have been noticed at birth and, indeed, the diagnosis of aortic stenosis may have been made. Congestive failure develops in the first weeks of life and, very rapidly, a life-threatening situation evolves.

The valves in these babies are notable, sometimes appearing as gelatinous blobs of tissue unrecognizable as leaflets. The left ventricle may be quite small, and for some infants it is too small to be compatible with life. A newborn ventricle that can accommodate a maximal volume of 20 ml is borderline in its ability to support life. Because of left ventricular failure and gross elevation of left atrial pressures, the foramen ovale becomes incompetent, and atrial left-to-right shunting adds to the problems, further aggravating congestive heart failure (Fig. 8). Shunting right to left through the ductus arteriosus may be helpful in this situation, because it supplies some cardiac output that does not have to pass through the aortic valve. Indeed, in the most critical situation there is pulmonary hypertension, and the administration of prostaglandin E1 to open the ductus, thereby adding to the cardiac output, may be lifesaving.[37]

On physical examination the infant is in congestive heart failure, sometimes in shock, and is ashen and pulseless. The electrocardiogram shows right or left ventricular hypertrophy with changes in the S-T segment and T wave. The chest x-ray shows an enlarged heart with pulmonary edema. On echocardiography, the diagnosis is established.

Diagnostic cardiac catheterization in these small infants is not difficult, but balloon valvuloplasty can be a problem because the catheters are relatively large, and induced aortic regurgitation is significant (see ch. 14).[63] Still, the loss of life associated with balloon valvuloplasty does not yet approach the risk associated with surgery in these small babies and, therefore, it is the treatment of choice at the present time (Exhibit 2) (see p. 499).[45,60,75]

As an alternative treatment, surgical valvotomy can be carried out at an acceptable mortality with

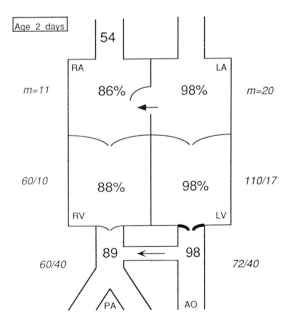

Figure 8. Hemodynamic data from a very ill infant with valvar aortic stenosis. Note that left ventricular failure has caused elevation of left atrial pressure, forcing open the foramen ovale and allowing a large left-to-right shunt, which adds a further hemodynamic burden for the heart and lungs.

good results.[40,50,56] In either of these interventions, it should be kept in mind that a small increase in the valvar orifice will provide considerable benefit, because the pressure required to produce an output follows an exponential function of the radius of the orifice. Widely opening the valve may carry more danger than benefit.

If the infant responds well, the congestive heart failure is controlled, the pulses return, and the infant grows. With close follow-up over the course of the next few months, it is often gratifying to see the child become a nearly normal infant, despite the fact that usually there is clear evidence of residual aortic stenosis.

The mortality, regardless of the kind of treatment, is high compared with that for other children with aortic stenosis, and it remains high with later interventions. It is clear that the more severe the aortic stenosis, the more troubles the child will have with the first intervention and subsequently (Exhibit 2).[40,56]

It is of interest that at surgery some years later, these valves have been noted to be no longer gelatinous, and sometimes they have acquired the appearance of three-leafed aortic valves.[39]

SUBAORTIC STENOSIS

Definition

Obstruction to outflow from the left ventricle beneath the aortic valve is called subaortic stenosis.

Prevalence

Subaortic stenosis is rarely recognized in the newborn period but is common in infancy and childhood. It may be associated with other defects such as ventricular septal defect,[17,24] coarctation of the aorta, interrupted aortic arch (see ch. 34), double-chambered right ventricle,[29] and atrioventricular canal.[6] Isolated subaortic stenosis is not uncommon, comprising 0.5% of the series at Children's Hospital in Boston, but the anomaly is more frequently associated with other defects (Exhibit 3).

Pathology

There are four types of subvalvar aortic stenosis.

Discrete Type. The most common form of subaortic stenosis is a discrete, thin, fibromuscular ridge located beneath the aortic valve, sometimes so close to the valve that the obstructing tissue is difficult to distinguish from the valve itself (Fig. 9). The term membranous subaortic stenosis is occasionally used; this can be misleading because the obstructing tissue usually has some thickness. The opening may be eccentric. Often there is deformity of the, usually tricuspid, aortic valve caused by the jet of blood passing through the subvalvar obstruc-

Exhibit 3

Boston Children's Hospital Experience 1973–1987	
Subvalvar Aortic Stenosis: Associated Cardiac Defects	
Associated Cardiac Defect	No. of Patients
Coarctation of the Aorta	113
Ventricular Septal Defect	96
Double-Outlet Right Ventricle	58
D-Transposition of the Great Arteries	49
Endocardial Cushion Defects	44
Others	170
Total	530
Supravalvar Aortic Stenosis: Associated Problems	
Associated Problems	No. of Patients
Williams' Syndrome	23
Systemic Hypertension	2
Coarctation of the Aorta	8
Pulmonary Stenosis	20
None Described	10
Total	63

tion, with resulting aortic regurgitation. Older patients appear to have greater degrees of aortic incompetence than do younger patients (a point that is yet to be firmly established). Downstream cardiac defects that obstruct blood flow, such as interrupted aortic arch or severe coarctation, are common and sometimes are associated with a membranous ventricular septal defect and/or a mitral valve deformity.[64] The subvalvar obstruction is almost never discovered at birth, and in the newborn period it is often overlooked by physiologic and imaging studies. It seems likely that the development of subaortic stenosis is predestined and that the patients in whom this lesion is likely to develop could be identified at birth if we knew how to do it. Subaortic stenosis may be overlooked at a cardiac catheterization, which is undertaken to study another defect, and is only discovered later (Fig. 10).[6,16]

Tunnel Type. The rarer fibromuscular tunnel seems to be a part of the same pathologic process, but it has greater length, often affecting 1 cm or more of the outflow tract. Because of its length, or perhaps contributing to it, the anterior leaflet of the mitral valve is often involved, a feature of some significance at the time of surgical correction.

Hypertrophic Subaortic Stenosis. Cardiomyopathy of the idiopathic hypertrophic variety often produces clinically important subaortic obstruction due solely to muscle (see ch. 24).

Obstructive Bulboventricular Foramen. When the aorta arises from a hypoplastic ventricle, as in tricuspid atresia with transposition of the great arteries or in the most common form of single ventricle, the only communication between the aorta

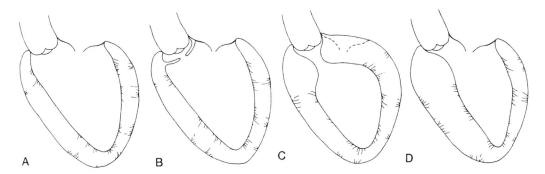

Figure 9. Drawings illustrating three types of subaortic stenosis: **A,** normal; **B,** membranous; **C,** fibromuscular tunnel; **D,** hypertrophic cardiomyopathy with subaortic obstruction. See Figure 11 for two additional forms of left ventricular outflow obstruction. See Figure 5, ch. 42 for an example of an obstructed outflow to the aorta at the bulboventricular foramen (physiologically subaortic stenosis) in a patient with a single left ventricle.

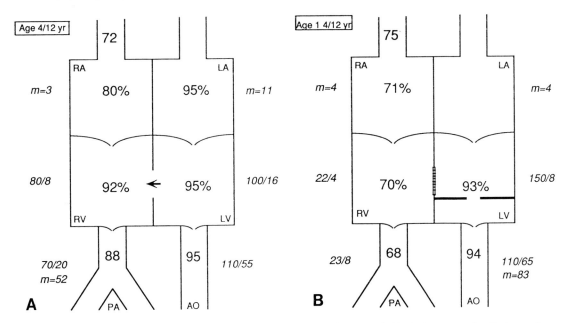

Figure 10. Physiologic diagrams of two cardiac catheterizations in the same child. **A,** Age 4 months. **B,** A year later. Because there was no gradient across the left ventricular outflow, the presence of subaortic stenosis was not suspected at the first study. Whether subaortic stenosis was masked by the ventricular defect on the first study or whether it developed is a matter of speculation.

and the ventricle may be a ventricular septal defect (bulboventricular foramen), which may be small and tends to become smaller (see ch. 42). The functional effect is that of subaortic stenosis in the context of a complex cardiac lesion.

Accessory Endocardial Cushion Tissue. Rarely, bits of tissue presumed to be derived from the embryologic endocardial cushions may obstruct the left ventricular outflow tract. These bits of tissue may be attached to a pedicle or act as a sail or sheet across the outflow tract, moving with cardiac contraction and the flow of blood (Fig. 11).[1,3]

Pathogenesis

The association of subaortic stenosis with anomalies of the aortic arch has led to the theory that chronic limitation of left ventricular outflow leads to aortic arch anomalies. An alternate theory might be that low flow in the aorta and obstructions within the aorta are the cause for subaortic stenosis. Although neither theory is generally accepted, the association among left ventricular anomalies, subaortic obstruction, and aortic arch anomalies is well documented.[21,64]

Physiology

The physiologic abnormalities are comparable to those seen in valvar aortic stenosis, except that subaortic stenosis is almost never severe enough to cause congestive heart failure in infancy, at least as an isolated lesion. The associated aortic regur-

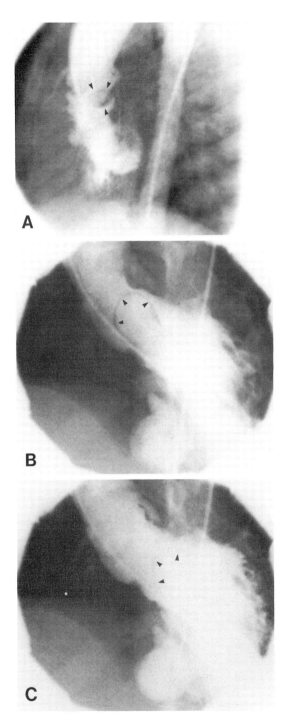

Figure 11. Left ventricular angiograms in two babies with obstructing tissue in the left ventricular outflow tract. In each case the obstructing material was mobile. **A,** The rounded object under the valve was surgically removed with great difficulty through the valve, with resulting aortic regurgitation. **B** and **C,** Systolic and diastolic views of a sail-like membrane flopping back and forth in the left ventricle. This material was surgically removed without difficulty or residual problem.

gitation is rarely severe. A practical, yet difficult, physiologic problem is the absence of a gradient across the subaortic stenosis when the ductus arteriosus supplies the distal systemic circulation. In this framework, subaortic stenosis may be severe without a significant gradient, making the assessment of its severity guesswork, particularly if the infant has congestive heart failure. Unfortunately, this problem arises in the sickest patients, in whom ligation of the ductus may result in the sudden discovery of subaortic stenosis.

Clinical Manifestations

Isolated subaortic stenosis produces a stenotic systolic murmur that is indistinguishable from that of valvar aortic stenosis or smaller ventricular septal defects. Usually, the murmur is heard best over the base of the heart, but it may be heard maximally at the third left intercostal space. Usually there is no systolic click; some patients have an early diastolic blowing murmur of aortic regurgitation. The peripheral pulses are rarely thought of as small, and congestive heart failure resulting from isolated subaortic stenosis is virtually nonexistent.

Electrocardiography. The electrocardiogram shows left ventricular hypertrophy in proportion to the degree of obstruction. Mild obstruction produces no abnormality, whereas severe obstruction results in left ventricular hypertrophy with changes in the S-T segment and T wave.

Chest X-ray. The isolated form of subaortic stenosis is not characterized by cardiac enlargement or enlargement of the ascending aorta. Finding an abnormality on the chest x-ray is unusual unless there are associated defects.

Echocardiography. Echocardiography is an excellent method for recognition and evaluation of subaortic stenosis (Fig. 12). The area of obstruction is usually well visualized, and a Doppler gradient can be measured.[71] The turbulence produced by the jet of blood sometimes causes early closure of the aortic valve.[61] The presence of other anomalies can be investigated (see Fig. 11, ch. 13).

Cardiac Catheterization. Cardiac catheterization provides the most reliable documentation of the pressure gradient across the outflow tract of the left ventricle (Fig. 13). The location and length of the obstruction can be demonstrated by angiography, and evaluation of associated defects can be accomplished. As a practical matter, whether to refer the patient for surgery, based on echocardiographic evidence alone, or to confirm the echocardiographic data with cardiac catheterization must be decided. At Boston Children's Hospital few patients undergo surgery without catheterization.

Management

Discrete subaortic stenosis of the fibromuscular (membranous) type is usually a progressive dis-

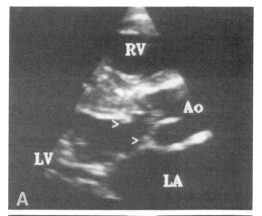

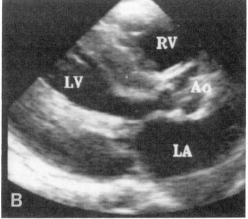

Figure 12. **A,** Parasternal long-axis view of the outflow tract of the left ventricle in a patient with discrete membranous subaortic stenosis. The arrows indicate the membrane. **B,** Parasternal long-axis view of the left ventricular outflow tract in a patient with tunnel subaortic stenosis. The area of obstruction is apparent. RV, right ventricle; LV, left ventricle; Ao, aorta; LA, left atrium.

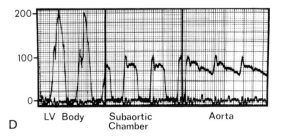

Figure 13. Pressure recording during withdrawal of a catheter from the left ventricle to the aorta in a patient with subaortic stenosis. Note that as the catheter passes the obstructed area the left ventricular pressure falls; only when it is withdrawn across the aortic valve does a typical arterial pressure contour appear. Sometimes, the space between the subvalvar obstruction and the aortic valve is so small that this type of tracing cannot be recorded.

ease.[13,53,62,66,74] Hence, planning is not so much a matter of whether intervention should be done, but rather when it should be undertaken. Balloon dilatation of a subaortic membrane[22,45] has been used, but complete surgical excision of the collar of tissue seems more likely to prevent recurrence. Generally, with complete surgical excision of the obstructing tissue there is no mortality and little likelihood of recurrence.[13,53] Because the disease is known to progress and because surgery is so successful, it is the policy at Children's Hospital in Boston to refer these individuals to our surgeons almost as soon as the diagnosis is certain. A directly measured pressure gradient in excess of 30 mm Hg is sufficient to recommend surgical removal of the obstruction. The surgical approach is through the aortic root, with excision of the fibromuscular tissue under direct vision.

When there is obstructive endocardial cushion tissue, the decision to refer the patient for surgery is based primarily on the anatomy. Often the pieces of tissue are flopping around in the left ventricular outflow region in a manner that cries out for surgical removal to prevent some from getting loose. (To the present time, none has come loose.) During surgical removal the surgeon must be careful not to injure the mitral valve[3] and may discover an underlying subaortic membrane.[1]

The tunnel type of subaortic stenosis is a more formidable problem. Surgical excision of the outflow muscle amounts to resection of a wedge of tissue from the septal side of the obstructing tunnel. A Konno procedure may be helpful.[43,51] Others have replaced the aortic root with a homograft.[65] Surgery is less often as effective as it is for other types of subaortic stenosis; it is rarely curative and may be hazardous to the mitral valve on the one hand and the conduction system on the other.[52] Rarely, the mitral valve must be replaced. If the anatomy seems to be dominantly muscle, the postoperative use of beta-blockers is probably indicated.

Course

Subaortic stenosis tends to become more severe with time, except for the rare obstructions caused by endocardial cushion tissue. Surgical excision of a discrete membrane or excision of aberrant endocardial cushion tissue seems curative, although earlier follow-up studies have indicated substantial recurrence.[38] The tunnel type is rarely completely relieved, often requiring repeated operations, and is obviously a lesion that needs a new idea. The ingenious valved conduit from the left ventricle to the descending aorta turned out to be a disappointment.

SUPRAVALVAR AORTIC STENOSIS

Definition

Supravalvar aortic stenosis denotes obstructive constriction of the ascending aorta above the aortic valve. This anomaly is commonly associated with elfin facies (Williams' syndrome)[7,72] and other areas of vascular stenosis, such as peripheral pulmonary stenosis, coarctation, or renal artery stenosis.

Prevalence

Supravalvar aortic stenosis is a rare anomaly that is sometimes familial. There have been 63 patients with this diagnosis listed in the files of Children's Hospital in Boston over the past 15 years. Of these, a third had Williams' syndrome (Exhibit 3).

Pathology

The obstructing ring, sometimes asymmetric, is situated above the aortic valve and the sinuses of Valsalva. The edge of the obstructing tissue may impinge upon a sinus of Valsalva, compromising flow to the coronary ostia. Occasionally the coronary occlusion is complete, a leaflet of the distorted aortic valve adhering to the obstructing collar of tissue. When the aortic lumen is compromised, there is proportionate left ventricular hypertension and hypertrophy. The obstruction may be localized, virtually membranous, or may extend diffusely into the ascending aorta (Fig. 14). The aortic cusps are thickened and distorted, sometimes adherent to the aortic wall, but although aortic regurgitation is common, it is rarely severe.

Some patients have other vascular obstructions. Peripheral pulmonary stenosis with hypoplasia of the pulmonary arteries occurs in 30%, coarctation of the aorta in 15%, renal artery stenosis in 5%; obstructions may also occur in branches of the

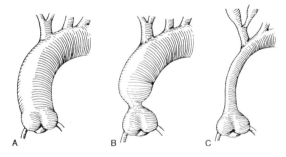

Figure 14. The anatomic types of supravalvar aortic stenosis: **A,** normal; **B** and **C,** two forms of supravalvar stenosis. The difference between these two forms is in the length of the obstruction, which sometimes involves virtually all of the ascending aorta. Note the obstructions in the innominate and common carotid arteries as they arise from the aortic arch. Other obstructions, such as coarctation of the aorta, renal artery stenosis, and pulmonary artery stenosis, are found in some patients.

aorta. Abdominal coarctation of the aorta has been described[48] and may lead to renal vascular involvement. These obstructions in the aorta can be acquired and are often progressive. Indeed, all of these peripheral phenomena may be seen in the absence of supravalvar stenosis and are sometimes readily recognized as part of Williams' syndrome. Severe mitral regurgitation has been described also in a patient with Williams' syndrome.[48]

Physiology

The physiology is comparable to that of valvar aortic stenosis except that coronary blood flow may be under increased pressure and coronary ostia may be obstructed (Fig. 15). In any case, the demands of a hypertrophied ventricle, with or without coronary ostial obstruction, are likely to result in a mismatch of myocardial demand and perfusion.

Hypercalcemia is seen in patients with Williams' syndrome in early infancy.[9]

Clinical Manifestations

Patients with Williams' syndrome have typical elfin facies, dental problems, and mental retardation (see Fig. 12, ch. 5). Patients in whom this diagnosis is suspected should be evaluated for possible supravalvar aortic stenosis. Otherwise, supravalvar stenosis is discovered in these patients because of a basilar murmur, sometimes associated with a thrill. There may be a family history of supravalvar aortic stenosis. These children tend to grow poorly; they may have exercise intolerance and, occasionally, angina with effort. Syncope has been reported.

On physical examination, other than evidence of Williams' syndrome, patients have a systolic murmur over the base of the heart, radiating into the neck. There may be hypertension if coarctation of the aorta or renal artery stenosis is present. Murmurs suggesting peripheral pulmonary stenosis may be audible, as may the murmur of minimal aortic insufficiency.

Electrocardiography. If the obstruction in the ascending aorta is severe, there will be left ventricular hypertrophy.

Chest X-ray. The heart may be somewhat enlarged, but a chest x-ray is rarely helpful in this diagnosis.

Echocardiography. The diagnosis becomes evident at echocardiography. The anatomy of the aortic valve leaflets, the sinuses of Valsalva, and the supravalvar obstructing collar can be visualized and Doppler estimations of the pressure gradient across the obstructed area measured.[70] The supravalvar narrowing is most readily imaged in a parasternal long-axis view (Fig. 16), the appearance of the lesion being generally much less impressive than the measured gradient. Wall thickening at the site of

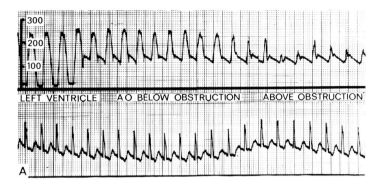

Figure 15. Pressure tracing recorded in a patient with supravalvar aortic stenosis during withdrawal of a catheter from the left ventricle to the ascending aorta. Note that there is no change in systemic pressure as the catheter passes the valve and an arterial pressure trace appears. Further withdrawal shows a drop from a higher to a lower arterial pressure.

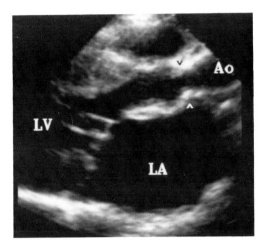

Figure 16. Parasternal long-axis view of the left ventricle illustrating supravalvar aortic stenosis. The supravalvar ridge and proximal ascending aorta are narrowed (arrow) and the vessel wall appears thickened. Ao, Aorta; LA, Left atrium; LV, Left ventricle.

obstruction is generally apparent. The aortic valve leaflets may appear thickened and may move abnormally despite absence of commissural fusion.

The aortic arch and brachiocephalic vessels should be imaged, because coarctation and stenosis of the brachiocephalic arteries commonly accompany supravalvar aortic stenosis. Occasionally, the origin of a coronary artery is stenosed. However, this is rarely detectable by echocardiography.

Doppler examination should be performed from the apex and the suprasternal notch, using continuous-wave Doppler.

Magnetic Resonance Imaging. This technique of imaging arterial structures that may be remote from the echocardiographic beam may be valuable in assessing these children.[11]

Cardiac Catheterization. Generally, cardiac catheterization is undertaken in these patients, not because the echocardiographic diagnosis is doubted, but to evaluate other possible problems. The renal arteries, the site of usual coarctation, the possibility of stenosis of branches of the aortic arch,

and evidences of pulmonary stenosis and coronary obstruction are evaluated.

Management

With sufficient obstruction, symptoms, or a gradient of pressure greater than 50 mm Hg, patch angioplasty of the ascending aorta is undertaken and usually relieves the obstruction.[41]

Course

Further obstruction may develop even though there has been successful surgical relief of the supravalvar obstruction. Coarctation of the aorta, renal artery stenosis, or obstructions of the branches of the aortic arch may develop or recur. Each new problem is evaluated on its own merits and managed independently.[25]

AORTIC REGURGITATION

Definition

The reflux of blood from the ascending aorta into the left ventricle during diastole is described as aortic regurgitation or aortic insufficiency.

Prevalence

Aortic regurgitation is found in association with almost all known pediatric cardiac problems. At Children's Hospital in Boston, it was mentioned as a complicating feature of pediatric heart disease in more than 1,100 patients; in 250 of these, the diagnosis was made by echocardiography alone. Less than 5% of them had rheumatic heart disease and only about a third had isolated aortic valve abnormalities (Exhibit 4).

Exclusive of those diagnosed by echocardiography alone, it was a primary lesion in only 87 patients; 35 children had rheumatic aortic regurgitation.

Pathology

There is no specific pathology for aortic regurgitation because there are multiple causes. There

Exhibit 4

Boston Children's Hospital Experience 1973–1987	
Aortic Regurgitation Associated with Other Congenital Heart Defects*	
Category of Congenital Heart Disease	No. of Patients
Aortic Stenosis	556
Ventricular Septal Defect	129
Coarctation of the Aorta	85
Tetralogy of Fallot	79
Truncus Arteriosus	53
D-Transposition of the Great Arteries	52
Malposition	20
Double-Outlet Right Ventricle	16
Endocardial Cushion Defects	14
Mitral Valve Disease	13
Single Ventricle	10
Other	89
Total	1116

*Categorical diagnoses are mutually exclusive. When the diagnoses based only on echocardiography are excluded (250 cases), the distribution of associated categories of congenital heart disease is unchanged.

Association of Bicuspid Aortic Valve with Other Congenital Defects*

Associated Cardiac Defect	Total Patients	Bicuspid Aortic Valve (%)	Keith[42]
Aortic Stenosis	835	338 (40%)	19%
Aortic Regurgitation Pure	87	27 (31%)	—
Aortic Regurgitation Associated with Other Defects	1116	334 (30%)	—
Coarctation of Aorta	820	85 (10%)	29%
Ventricular Defect	3322	58 (2%)	13%
Endocardial Cushion	717	7 (9%)	8%

*Because bicuspid aortic valve is not a lesion with hemodynamic effects, reporting may be less than complete. The percentages presented should be considered as minimum figures.

may be dilatation of the valve ring, as seen in patients with tetralogy of Fallot (see ch. 30) or Marfan syndrome. There may be a primarily abnormal valve, as in valvar aortic stenosis, or an incompetent valve resulting from valvuloplasty for aortic stenosis (see p. 500). There may be deformity of the valve from a jet caused by subaortic stenosis (see p. 503). There may be adherence of the valve leaflet because of supravalvar aortic stenosis (see p. 506). There may be prolapse of the aortic valve leaflets associated with a ventricular septal defect (see ch. 28). The primary pathology may be rheumatic (see ch. 22). Aortic regurgitation is often found with bicuspid aortic valves (see p. 510) (Exhibit 4).[55,59]

Physiology

Whether the minimal aortic regurgitation found so frequently by echocardiographers has a specific pathologic meaning or is a normal variant, the amount of leak found by this technique is often tiny.[15] Whether these valves are sites for endocarditis is not yet known.

When there is aortic regurgitation, the amount

of blood that is refluxed must be pumped forward in addition to that supplying the appropriate cardiac output. The left ventricular volume is thereby enlarged in direct proportion to the amount of regurgitated blood. With increased amounts of regurgitation, the left ventricular volume increases, ultimately resulting in a huge heart. The runoff from the aorta to the left ventricle results in a wide pulse pressure, the systolic pressure becoming higher as the diastolic becomes lower with increasing regurgitation.

Ultimately, over many years, increasing aortic regurgitation leads to congestive heart failure, which presages death, usually within 12–24 months.

Clinical Manifestations

A high-frequency, early diastolic blowing murmur, usually best heard along the left sternal border, is virtually diagnostic of aortic regurgitation (Figs. 17 and 18). The frequency of the murmur (the blowing quality) is higher with aortic regurgitation than it is with pulmonary regurgitation. This murmur is quite difficult to discover, let alone distinguish, when there are continuous murmurs

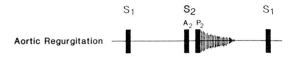

Figure 17. Schematic drawing of the murmur of aortic regurgitation. Note the decrescendo, early diastolic murmur that begins after the second heart sound. S1, first heart sound; S2 second heart sound composed of A2 (aortic closure) and P2 (pulmonary closure).

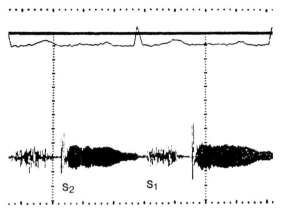

Figure 18. Phonocardiogram in a patient who suddenly developed a loud, high-frequency murmur of aortic regurgitation because of a perforation in an aortic valve leaflet.

from other causes such as patent ductus arteriosus, collateral circulation, shunt operations, and other lesions. The murmur is heard well in a small child lying down, but among teenagers, it is easier to hear with the patient sitting up and leaning forward. It is easier to hear with the diaphragm of the stethoscope pressed firmly against the chest at the left sternal border, usually at the third left interspace.

In the past, the discovery of isolated aortic regurgitation was synonymous with the diagnosis of rheumatic heart disease; this is no longer the case. Still, this possibility should be considered for each patient with isolated aortic regurgitation, and any history or family history suggesting rheumatic fever should be carefully reviewed.

With increasing degrees of aortic regurgitation, the peripheral pulses become more prominent as the pulse pressure increases. Prominent peripheral pulses result in those interesting signs of physical diagnosis—Corrigan pulse, Duroziez's sign, Quincke's sign, and pistol shots. Generally, with routine observation of the carotid pulsations, the pediatrician sees the wide pulse pressure before he or she feels it. Confirmation of the wide pulse pressure by blood pressure measurement documents the somewhat elevated systolic pressure and low diastolic pressure.

The cardiac impulse is depressed downward and toward the left, sometimes reaching the anterior axillary line at the sixth interspace. The hyperactive impulse conveys the impression of forceful ejection of large amounts of blood.

Electrocardiography. With increasing left ventricular volume overload, there is increased left ventricular voltage on the electrocardiogram and, in the extreme form, there may be depression of the S-T segment and T-wave inversion.

Chest X-ray. The heart size is directly proportional to the amount of aortic regurgitation, or it may be grossly enlarged through the dilatation of congestive heart failure superimposed on a large regurgitated volume (Fig. 19).

Echocardiography. The regurgitant flow across the aortic valve is readily detected by color Doppler interrogation. Indeed, this technique is so sensitive that reports of aortic regurgitation without an audible murmur are common. Perhaps, some aortic regurgitation is normal but, in any case, ac-

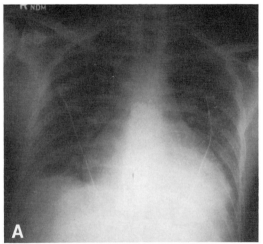

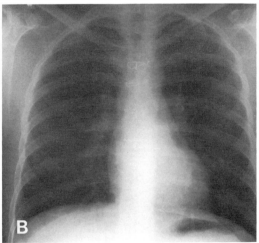

Figure 19. Preoperative (**A**) and postoperative (**B**) chest x-rays in a patient who had valve replacement for severe aortic regurgitation. Note the postoperative decrease in heart size.

commodation to this extension of our diagnostic ability is as yet incomplete (see Fig. 5B, ch. 13).

Cardiac Catheterization. Cardiac catheterization is not needed in the evaluation of a patient with aortic regurgitation. However, because most of these children have other defects, cardiac catheterization is often used to discover and evaluate the presence and relative difficulty posed by each lesion. Evaluation of the degree of aortic regurgitation during cardiac catheterization is accomplished by the injection of contrast material above the aortic valve (the catheter not in contact with the valve) and observing the amount that enters the ventricle.

Management

Any patient with known aortic regurgitation who has syncope or anginal chest pain, or who has developed congestive heart failure is a candidate for surgery. A patient in whom there is progressive enlargement of the left ventricle on serial observation of chest x-rays or echocardiograms is considered for aortic valve replacement. A patient who develops depression of the S-T segment, or T-wave inversion, either spontaneously or on exercise, is viewed as a potential surgical candidate, because it is believed that these changes reflect myocardial damage. The combination of dysrhythmia and changes in the S-T segment and T wave is taken as even stronger evidence of progressive myocardial deterioration.

Whenever possible, the surgeons undertake valvuloplasty, which is sometimes dramatically successful, particularly for perforated leaflets or prolapsed valves. But, unfortunately, most often damaged valves require valve replacement.

Course

Moderate or severe aortic regurgitation from any cause tends to be progressive, although occasionally patients will live for many years without change. Minimal aortic regurgitation is most often a stable problem except, possibly, in patients with rheumatic disease. A regurgitant aortic valve is particularly prone to infective endocarditis. Perhaps more than any others with cardiac lesions, these patients need to have good dental hygiene and must pay strict attention to the use of prophylactic antibiotics during dental surgery.

BICUSPID AORTIC VALVE

Definition

Congenital bicuspid aortic valve is characterized by two leaflets, often with a rudimentary third leaflet.

Prevalence

Bicuspid aortic valves without aortic stenosis or aortic regurgitation are said to be present in between 0.9 and 2.0% of the population.[34,42,58] Many bicuspid aortic valves are associated with other cardiac defects (e.g., valvar aortic stenosis, aortic regurgitation, coarctation of the aorta, ventricular defect, and others) (Exhibit 4).[42]

Clinical Manifestations

Bicuspid aortic valve is more common in males (Exhibit 1).

The diagnosis is suggested by an early systolic click that does not vary with respiration. The additional presence of the murmur of aortic regurgitation or aortic stenosis at the second right interspace should raise the question of a bicuspid aortic valve.

Electrocardiography. No specific electrocardiographic changes are associated with bicuspid aortic valve.

Chest X-ray. There are no specific findings of bicuspid aortic valve on the routine chest x-ray.

Echocardiography. Echocardiographic examination of the entire valve will reveal whether or not it is bicommissural (Fig. 5) (see ch. 13).

A practical question is whether to get an echocardiogram when there is an early systolic click. At Boston Children's Hospital, we do not believe that every person who has a systolic click, whether early, mid, or late in systole, should have echocardiography. When the click is associated with a murmur of aortic stenosis or a murmur of aortic regurgitation, we believe that an echocardiogram is an appropriate test.

Management

It is conventional wisdom that a bicuspid aortic valve is prone to infective endocarditis. Surely this is correct when there is associated aortic regurgitation, however mild, or if there is aortic stenosis. That a bicuspid valve without functional abnormality (i.e., not producing turbulence) has a high probability to serve as a nidus for infective endocarditis remains to be shown. It seems unlikely. Still, we do recommend the use of prophylactic antibiotics for all patients with repaired coarctation of the aorta when oral surgical procedures are to be undertaken because of the high incidence of bicuspid aortic valve, as well as the frequent residual coarctation murmur and the commonly associated mitral valve abnormalities.

Prophylactic antibiotics to prevent infective endocarditis are recommended when a patient has a bicuspid aortic valve with an associated murmur of aortic stenosis or aortic regurgitation.

Course

Concern that all bicuspid aortic valves will eventually cause late aortic stenosis is based on the fact that many older individuals with aortic stenosis have bicuspid valves. In fact, there is no documentation for this conviction and older individuals with normally functioning bicuspid aortic valves have been reported.

REFERENCES

1. Alboliras ET, Tajik JA, Puga FJ, et al: Accessory mitral valve tissue in association with discrete subaortic stenosis: a two-dimensional echocardiographic diagnosis. Echocardiography 2:191–195, 1985.
2. Ankeney JL, Tzeng TS, Liebman J: Surgical therapy for congenital aortic valvular stenosis: a 23 year experience. Cardiovasc Surg 85:41–48, 1983.
3. Ascuitto RJ, Ross-Ascuitto NT, Kopf GS, et al: Accessory mitral valve tissue causing left ventricular outflow obstruction (two-dimensional echocardiographic diagnosis and surgical approach). Ann Thorac Surg 42:581–584, 1986.
4. Barton CW, Katz B, Schork MA, et al: Value of treadmill exercise test in pre- and postoperative children with valvular aortic stenosis. Clin Cardiol 6:473–477, 1983.
5. Beekman RH, Rocchini AP, Crowley DC, et al: Comparison of single and double balloon valvuloplasty in children with aortic stenosis. J Am Coll Cardiol 12:480–485, 1988.
6. Ben-Shacher G, Moller JH, Castaneda-Zuniga W, et al: Signs of membranous subaortic stenosis appearing after correction of persistent common atrioventricular canal. Am J Cardiol 48:340–344, 1981.
7. Beuren AJ, Apitz J, Harmjanz D: Supravalvular aortic stenosis in association with mental retardation and a certain facial appearance. Circulation 26:1235, 1962.
8. Bissett III GS, Meyer RA, Hirschfield SS, et al: Aortic valve replacement in childhood: evaluation of left ventricular function by electrocardiography, echocardiography and graded exercise testing. Am J Cardiol 52:568–572, 1983.
9. Black JA, Bonham-Carter RE: Association between aortic stenosis and facies of severe infantile hypercalcemia. Lancet 2:745–748, 1963.
10. Bland EF, Jones TD: Rheumatic fever and rheumatic heart disease: a twenty-year report on 1000 patients followed since childhood. Circulation 4:836–843, 1951.
11. Boxer RA, Fishman MC, LaCorte MA, et al: Diagnosis and postoperative evaluation of supravalvar aortic stenosis by magnetic resonance imaging. Am J Cardiol 58:367–368, 1986.
12. Brandenberg RO, Tajik AJ, Edwards WD, et al: Accuracy of 2-D echocardiographic diagnosis of congenitally bicuspid aortic valve. Am J Cardiol 51:1469–1473, 1983.
13. Brown J, Stevens L, Lynch L, et al: Surgery for discrete subvalvular aortic stenosis: actuarial survival, hemodynamic results, and acquired aortic regurgitation. Ann Thorac Surg 40:151–155, 1985.
14. Campbell M: The natural history of congenital aortic stenosis. Br Heart J 30:514–526, 1968.
15. Choong CY, Abascal VM, Weyman J, et al: Prevalence of valvular regurgitation by Doppler echocardiography in patients with structurally normal hearts by two-dimensional echocardiography. Am Heart J 117:636–639, 1989.
16. Christy C, Noonan JA, O'Connor WN: Discrete subvalvar aortic stenosis after tetralogy of Fallot repair. Br Heart J 49:510–512, 1983.
17. Chung KJ, Fulton DR, Kreidberg MB, et al: Combined discrete subaortic stenosis and ventricular septal defect in infants and children. Am J Cardiol 53:1429–1432, 1984.
18. Currie PJ, Hagler DJ, Seward JB, et al: Instantaneous pressure gradient: a simultaneous Doppler and dual catheter correlative study. J Am Coll Cardiol 7:800–806, 1986.
19. Donner R, Black I, Spann JF, et al: Improved prediction of peak left ventricular pressure by echocardiograph with aortic stenosis. J Am Coll Cardiol 3:349–355, 1984.
20. Doyle E, Arumugham P, Lara E, et al: Sudden death in young patients with aortic stenosis. Pediatrics 53:481–489, 1974.
21. Edwards JE: Pathology of left ventricular outflow tract obstruction. Circulation 31:586–599, 1965.
22. Feldman T, Chiu YC, Carroll JD: Catheter balloon dilatation for discrete subaortic stenosis in the adult. Am J Cardiol 60:403–404, 1987.
23. Fifer MA, Borow KM, Colan SD, et al: Early diastolic left ventricular function in children and adults with aortic stenosis. J Am Coll Cardiol 5:1147–1154, 1985.
24. Fisher DJ, Snider AR, Silverman NH, et al: Ventricular septal defect with silent discrete subaortic stenosis. Pediatr Cardiol 2:265–269, 1982.
25. Flaker G, Teske D, Kilman J, et al: Supravalvar aortic stenosis: a 20-year clinical perspective and experience with patch aortoplasty. Am J Cardiol 51:256–260, 1983.
26. Fulton DR, Hougen TJ, Keane JF, et al: Repeat aortic valvotomy in children. Am Heart J 106:60–63, 1983.
27. Gersony WM, Hayes CJ, Driscoll DJ, et al: Bacterial endocarditis in patients with aortic stenosis, pulmonary stenosis, or ventricular septal defect. The Report of the Second Natural History Study of Congenital Heart Defects. Circulation. In press.
28. Glew RH, Varghese PJ, Krovetz LJ, et al: Sudden death in congenital aortic stenosis: a review of eight cases with an evaluation of premonitory clinical features. Am Heart J 78:615–625, 1969.
29. Golan M, Hegesh J, Massini C, et al: Double-outlet right ventricle associated with discrete subaortic stenosis. Pediatr Cardiol 5:157–158, 1984.
30. Gorlin R, Gorlin SG: Hydraulic formula for calculation of area of stenotic mitral valve, other valves and central circulatory shunts. Am Heart J 41:1–29, 1951.
31. Helgason H, Keane JF, Fellows KE, et al: Balloon dilation of the aortic valve: studies in normal lambs and in children with aortic stenosis. J Am Coll Cardiol 9:816–822, 1987.
32. Hossack KF, Neutze JM, Lowe JB et al: Congenital valvar aortic stenosis: natural history and assessment or operation. Br Heart J 43:561–573, 1980.
33. Hsieh K-S, Keane JF, Nadas A, et al: Long-term follow-up of valvotomy before 1968 for congenital aortic stenosis. Am J Cardiol 58:330–341, 1986.
34. Hurst JW: The Heart. New York, McGraw-Hill, 1985, p. 642.
35. James FW, Schwartz DC, Kaplan S, et al: Exercise electrocardiogram blood pressure and working capacity in young patients with valvular or discrete subvalvular aortic stenosis. Am J Cardiol 50:769–774, 1982.
36. Jonas RA, Castaneda AR, Freed MD: Normothermic caval inflow occlusion: application to congenital heart surgery. J Thorac Cardiovasc Surg 89:780–786, 1985.
37. Jonas RA, Lang P, Mayer JE, et al: Importance of prostaglandin E1 in resuscitation of the neonate with critical

aortic stenosis. J Thorac Cardiovasc Surg 89:314–315, 1985.

38. Jones M, Garnhart GR, Morrow AG: Late results after operations for left ventricular outflow tract obstruction. Am J Cardiol 50:569–578, 1982.

39. Keane JF, Bernhard W, Nadas AS: Aortic stenosis surgery in infancy. Circulation 52:1138–1143, 1975.

40. Keane JF, Driscoll D, Gersony W: Results of treatment of patients with aortic stenosis. The Report of the Second Natural History Study of Congenital Heart Defects. Circulation 1990, in press.

41. Keane JF, Fellows KE, LaFarge CG, et al: The surgical management of discrete and diffuse supravalve aortic stenosis. Circulation 54:112–117, 1976.

42. Keith JD: Bicuspid aortic valve. In Keith JD, Rowe RD, Vlad P (eds): Heart Disease in Infancy and Childhood, 3rd ed. New York, Macmillan, 1979, pp. 728–735.

43. Konno S, Imai Y, Iida Y, et al: New method for prosthetic valve replacement in congenital aortic stenosis associated with hypoplasia of the aortic valve ring. J Thorac Cardiovasc Surg 10:909–917, 1975.

44. Kveselis DA, Rocchini AP, Rosenthal A, et al: Hemodynamic determinants of exercise induced ST-segment depression in children with valvar aortic stenosis. Am J Cardiol 55:1133–1139, 1985.

45. Lababidi Z, Weinhaus L, Stoeckle H, et al: Transluminal balloon dilatation for discrete subaortic stenosis. Am J Cardiol 59:423–425, 1987.

46. Lambert EC, Menor VA, Wagner HR, et al: Sudden unexpected death from cardiovascular disease in children: a cooperative international study. Am J Cardiol 34:89–96, 1974.

47. Lavine SJ, Follansbee WP, Shreiner DP, et al: Left ventricular diastolic filling in valvular aortic stenosis. Am J Cardiol 57:1349–1355, 1986.

48. Maisuls H, Alday LE, Thuer O: Cardiovascular findings in the Williams-Beuren syndrome. Am Heart J 114:897–899, 1987.

49. Martin GR, Soifer SJ, Silverman NH, et al: Effects of activity on ascending aortic velocity in children with valvar aortic stenosis. Am J Cardiol 59:1386–1390, 1987.

50. Messina LM, Turley K, Stanger P, et al: Successful aortic valvotomy for severe congenital valvular aortic stenosis in the newborn infant. J Thorac Cardiovasc Surg 88:92–96, 1984.

51. Misbach GA, Turley K, Ullyot DJ, et al: Left ventricular outflow enlargement by the Konno procedure. J Thorac Cardiovasc Surg 84:696–703, 1982.

52. Moses RD, Barnhart GR, Jones M: The late prognosis after localized resection for fixed (discrete and tunnel) left ventricular outflow tract obstruction. J Thorac Cardiovasc Surg 87:410–420, 1984.

53. Newfeld EA, Muster AJ, Paul MH, et al: Discrete subvalvular aortic stenosis in childhood. Am J Cardiol 38:53–61, 1976.

54. Oh JK, Taliercio CP, Holmes DR, et al: Prediction of the severity of aortic stenosis by Doppler aortic valve area determination: prospective Doppler-catheterization correlation in 100 patients. J Am Coll Cardiol 11:1227–34, 1988.

55. Olson LJ, Subramanian R, Edwards WD, et al: Surgical pathology of pure aortic insufficiency: a study of 225 cases. Mayo Clin Proc 59:835–41, 1984.

56. Pelech AN, Dyck JD, Trusler GA, et al: Critical aortic stenosis: survival and management. J Thorac Cardiovasc Surg 94:510–517, 1987.

57. Presbitero P, Somerville J, Revel-Chion R, et al: Open aortic valvotomy for congenital aortic stenosis: late results. Br Heart J 47:26–34, 1982.

58. Roberts WC: The congenitally bicuspid valve: a study of 85 autopsy cases. Am J Cardiol 49:151, 1970.

59. Roberts WC, Morrow AG, McIntosh CC, et al: Congenitally bicuspid aortic valve causing severe, rare aortic regurgitation without superimposed infective endocarditis: analysis of 13 patients requiring aortic valve replacement. Am J Cardiol 47:206–209, 1981.

60. Rupprath G, Neuhaus KL: Percutaneous balloon valvuloplasty for aortic stenosis in infancy. Am J Cardiol 55:1855–1856, 1985.

61. Sabbah HN, Stein PD: Mechanism of early systolic closure of the aortic valve in discrete membranous subaortic stenosis. Circulation 65:399–402, 1982.

62. Shem-Tov A, Schneeweiss A, Motro M, et al: Clinical presentation and natural history of mild discrete subaortic stenosis: follow-up of 1–17 years. Circulation 66:509–512, 1982.

63. Sholler GF, Keane JF, Perry SB, et al: Balloon dilation of congenital aortic valve stenosis. Results and influence of technological features on outcome. Circulation 78:351–360, 1988.

64. Shone JD, Sellers RD, Anderson RC, et al: The developmental complex of "parachute mitral valve," supravalvular ring of left atrium, subaortic stenosis, and coarctation of aorta. Am J Cardiol 11:714–725, 1963.

65. Somerville J, Ross D: Homograft replacement of aortic root with reimplantation of coronary arteries: results after one to five years. Br Heart J 47:473–482, 1982.

66. Somerville J, Stone S, Ross D: Fate of patients with fixed subaortic stenosis after surgical removal. Br Heart J 43:629–647, 1980.

67. Vogel M, Benson LN, Burrows P, et al: Balloon dilatation of congenital aortic valve stenosis in infants and children: short-term and intermediate results. Br Heart J 62:148–53, 1989.

68. Wagner HR, Ellison RC, Keane JF, et al: Clinical course in aortic stenosis. Report from the Joint Study of the Natural History of Congenital Heart Defects. Circulation 56:I–47–55, 1977.

69. Waller BF, Girod DA, Dillon JC: Transverse aortic wall tears in infants after balloon angioplasty for aortic valve stenosis: relation of aortic wall damage to diameter of inflated angioplasty balloon and aortic lumen in 7 necropsy cases. J Am Coll Cardiol 4:12135–1241, 1984.

70. Weyman AE, Caldwell RL, Hurwitz RA, et al: Cross-sectional echocardiographic characterization of aortic obstruction. I. Supravalvar aortic stenosis and aortic hypoplasia. Circulation 57:491–497, 1978.

71. Wilcox WD, Seward JB, Hagler DJ, et al: Discrete subaortic stenosis: two-dimensional echocardiographic features with angiographic and surgical correlation. Mayo Clin Proc 55:425–433, 1980.

72. Williams JCP, Barrett-Boyes BG, Lowe JB: Supravalvar aortic stenosis. Circulation 24:1311–1318, 1961.

73. Wooley CF, Boudovlas H: From irritable heart to mitral valve prolapse: World War I—the US experience and the prevalence of apical systolic murmurs and mitral regurgitation in drafted men compared with present day mitral valve prolapse studies. Am J Cardiol 81:895–899, 1988.

74. Wright GB, Keane JF, Nadas AS, et al: Fixed subaortic stenosis in the young: medical and surgical course in 83 patients. Am J Cardiol 52:830–835, 1983.

75. Zeevi B, Keane JF, Castaneda AR, et al: Neonatal critical valvar aortic stenosis. Circulation 80:831–839, 1989.

Chapter 32

ATRIAL SEPTAL DEFECT SECUNDUM

Donald C. Fyler, M.D.

DEFINITION

Any opening in the atrial septum, other than a competent foramen ovale, is described as an atrial septal defect. Those that involve tissue derived from the endocardial cushions (ostium primum defects) are discussed in the chapter on Endocardial Cushion Defects (see ch. 36). "Secundum" atrial septal defects include those with an incompletely formed or fenestrated septum primum covering the fossa ovalis. Defects involving the embryologic sinus venosus (sinoseptal defects) include (1) sinus venosus defects at the orifice of the superior vena cava, (2) partially or completely unroofed coronary sinus, and (3) sinus venosus defects in the region of the inferior vena cava. Sinoseptal defects often include, apparent or real, anomalous entry of the right pulmonary veins into the right superior vena cava or the right atrium (Exhibit 1).

Partial anomalous pulmonary veins entering the systemic venous circulation have many of the physiologic characteristics of an atrial defect and usually are associated with a defect in the atrial septum. For these reasons partial anomalous pulmonary veins will be discussed with the secundum and sinoseptal defects in this chapter.

PREVALENCE

The incidence of atrial septal defect is difficult to determine. The murmurs produced are not readily noticed and therefore are easily overlooked; consequently, many are not discovered until the person is well beyond the pediatric age group. Atrial defects are first recognized in all age groups, including octogenarians.[42]

Isolated atrial defects, including those with partial anomalous pulmonary venous return, accounted for 6% of Boston Children's Hospital patients with heart disease and comprise the fifth most common category of cardiac defects (see Table 2, ch. 18).[17] Between 33 and 50% of children with congenital heart disease have an atrial defect as

Exhibit 1

Boston Children's Hospital Experience 1973–1987 **Atrial Septal Defect n = 891**	
Primary Classification	*Number*
Atrial septal defect	769
Sinus venosus defect (SVC type)	70
Partial anomalous pulmonary veins	78
Scimitar syndrome	6
Unroofed coronary sinus	3

Average Age When First Seen

Date	Age first seen, years	Age at operation, years
1973–1977	6	7
1978–1982	4	5
1983–1987	3	5

Listed under other primary diagnoses were 89 patients with pulmonary stenosis and atrial defect and 17 with ventricular defect and atrial defect who underwent operation for atrial septal defect only. There were 65 patients with patent foramen ovale and no other defect (see ch. 18), 7 patients with scimitar syndrome (see ch. 37), and 4 patients with unroofed coronary sinus (see ch. 37).

part of their cardiac problem. Among the patients seen at The Hospital for Sick Children in Toronto, 11%, or about 1 child per 1550 live births, had an atrial defect.[30] Atrial defects are discovered less commonly in young infants but still occur in as many as 2.9% of infants thought to be critically ill with heart disease (0.3–0.07 per 1000 live births) (see Table 1, ch. 18).

The prevalence of atrial septal defect increases progressively in populations living at higher altitudes.[38]

ANATOMY

Atrial defects may be single or multiple and can be located anywhere in the atrial septum. The defects range from millimeters in diameter to virtual absence of the septum (Fig. 1).

Secundum atrial defects are located in the area of the fossa ovalis and within the substance of the septum primum. They represent persistent foramina secunda, often resulting from failure of the septum primum to cover the fossa ovalis as it evolves from the sinus venous tissue at the junction of the inferior vena cava and grows upward to cover the fossa ovalis. The septum primum is the valve of the foramen ovale during fetal life, becoming part of the atrial septum postnatally.

A **sinoseptal defect** is an opening between the sinus venosus component of the right atrium and the left atrium (Fig. 2). The term **sinus venosus defect** is used loosely to describe the most common sinoseptal defect located at the entry of the superior vena cava into the right atrium. An opening in the lower part of the atrial septum between the entry of the inferior vena cava and the left atrium is called an **inferior vena caval type of sinus venosus defect**. A communication between the left atrium and the coronary sinus is called an **unroofed coronary sinus**.

The most common **sinus venosus defects** are located near the entry of the superior vena cava into the right atrium. The right upper pulmonary veins normally enter the left atrium at about this point, and when there is a sinus venosus defect, these veins may appear to be anomalously entering the right atrium. While there is anomalous drainage of right pulmonary veins into the superior vena cava

and right atrium in this condition, the actual connection of the pulmonary veins is normal. Although true abnormal connection of one or more of the right pulmonary veins to the right superior vena cava does exist, the incidence of this malformation is probably overestimated.[56]

The **inferior vena caval type of sinoseptal defect** is rare. It involves an opening into the lower right atrium at the orifice of the inferior vena cava. Because it lies between the right-sided pulmonary veins and the inferior vena cava, the pulmonary veins appear to enter anomalously into the right atrium.[56] True anomalous connection of the right pulmonary veins with the inferior vena cava occurs only in the scimitar syndrome.

An **unroofed coronary sinus** involves an anomalous communication between the coronary sinus and the left atrium.[19] Sometimes there is entry of a left superior vena cava into the coronary sinus and the left atrium through the unroofed area.[44] In any case the unroofed coronary sinus allows blood to pass from left atrium, to the coronary sinus, to the right atrium—in effect, a left-to-right shunt. If the coronary sinus is completely absent, the left superior vena cava will appear to be connected to the left atrium. If the atrial septum is intact, the orifice of the coronary sinus may appear to be a "posterior" atrial septal defect (Raghib syndrome).[44] Physiologically it functions as an atrial septal defect, but anatomically it represents the orifice of the unroofed coronary sinus. If there is a left superior vena cava, the patient is cyanotic. Often the left superior vena cava does not communicate with the right vena cava because of absence of the innominate vein, an important consideration in contemplating surgical repair.

Usually, **partial anomalous pulmonary veins** returning to the systemic venous circulation occur with atrial septal defects; however, rarely, they may occur with an intact atrial septum. A number of anatomic variations of partial anomalous veins have been described. The most common entry is into the superior vena cava or the right atrium.

The **scimitar syndrome**[11,28,40,41] is associated with anomalous entry of all or some of the right pulmonary veins into the inferior vena cava, hypoplasia of the right lung, often, an atrial defect, and left-to-right shunting. Parts of the right lung may be supplied by anomalous arterial blood vessels arising from the descending aorta.

The term **single atrium** or **common atrium** refers to virtual absence of all the components of the atrial septum and, as such, includes that part of the septum derived from the endocardial cushions. This is discussed in chapter 36, Endocardial Cushion Defects.

PHYSIOLOGY

The amount of shunting through a large atrial defect is determined by the relative right and left

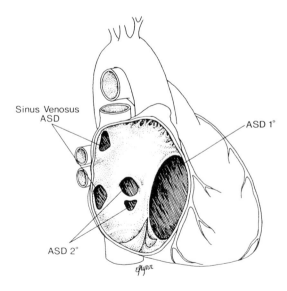

Figure 1. Diagram of the atrial septum showing several types of atrial septal defects. An ostium primum defect (ASD1) is located immediately adjacent to the mitral and tricuspid valves. Ostium secundum defects (ASD2) are located near the fossa ovalis in the center of the septum. Sinus venosus defects are located in the area derived from the embryologic sinus venosus (see Fig. 2).

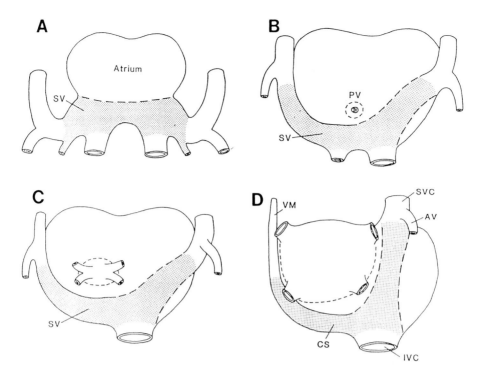

Figure 2. Embryologic evolution of the sinus venosus as viewed from the back of the heart. The coronary sinus, parts of a left superior vena cava, the points of entry of the superior and inferior venae cavae, as well as the parts of the right atrium nearest to the entry of the right pulmonary veins, are derived from the sinus venosus. Defects in the region of the sinus venosus that allow communication between the right and left atria include: unroofed coronary sinus, scimitar syndrome, and superior or inferior vena caval–sinus venosus defects. (From Van Mierop L: Isomerism of the cardiac atria in the asplenia syndrome. Lab Invest 11:1303–1315, 1962, © U.S.–Canadian Academy of Pathology, Inc., with permission.)

ventricular compliance. Early in infancy, the right ventricle is less compliant than later and left-to-right shunting is minimal, becoming greater as the right ventricle becomes more compliant with age. Years later, with normally decreasing left ventricular compliance with age (a thicker left ventricle), there is a further increase in the left-to-right shunt. Therefore, it is a tenable hypothesis that atrial defects are associated with increasing left-to-right shunting as the patient gets older. Perhaps this hypothesis explains the clinical course of individuals who appear in adulthood with pulmonary vascular obstructive disease or congestive heart failure and an atrial defect but no history of congenital heart disease in childhood.

The left-to-right shunt is phasic, varying with systole and diastole. Usually, with sensitive techniques, a small right-to-left shunt arising from the inferior cava can be detected. Perhaps this accounts for the slightly lower than normal, average arterial oxygen saturation found in these patients.[43]

Although most infants with an atrial septal defect are asymptomatic, rarely some develop congestive heart failure and growth failure. It is the author's opinion that, most often, these atypical infants have large left-to-right shunts in early infancy because there are additional defects. Specifically, left-sided problems, such as ventricular septal defect, patent

ductus arteriosus, myocardial dysfunction, an anatomically small left ventricle or systemic hypertension, may be associated with early symptoms. The high incidence of associated extracardiac anomalies[20] may also account for the growth failure in some of these children. Surprisingly, a number of these infants in early difficulty undergo spontaneous closure of the defect,[14,22,34] suggesting that many of these "defects" are actually dilated patent foramina ovale that became incompetent because of elevated left atrial pressure for whatever reason. Later, with resolution of the underlying left-sided problem, the foramen ovale closes.

Older patients may develop pulmonary vascular disease. In general, this unfortunate occurrence is rare before the age of 20 years and can be expected to occur in 5–10% of adults with atrial septal defect who have not undergone surgical repair.[2,57] Improvement in the reliability of this statistic is unlikely because most atrial defects are now being surgically closed on discovery, thus preventing the development of pulmonary vascular disease.

Whether patients with partial anomalous pulmonary venous return, in the absence of an atrial defect, ever develop pulmonary vascular disease is not known. The life expectancy of patients with partial anomalous pulmonary venous return, without an atrial defect, may be equivalent to normal life expectancy.

CLINICAL MANIFESTATIONS

The age at which an atrial septal defect is first discovered has been steadily decreasing. In the last 5 years, at Children's Hospital in Boston, the average age at which atrial defects were discovered was 3 years (Exhibit 1). Still, children with this congenital anomaly are not discovered at birth, often not recognized in infancy, and sometimes are found to have congenital heart disease many years after birth. The lack of symptoms and the lack of a readily audible murmur may account for the delay in discovering these patients.

Generally, the cardiac problem is uncovered during routine examination of an otherwise well child. Discovery at the first preschool examination is common.

The vast majority of children with an atrial septal defect of the secundum variety are asymptomatic. A few small infants and many older adults present with congestive heart failure.

Atrial septal defects of the secundum type occur more commonly among females (56%) who are often described as gracile, tall, thin.

Physical Examination

The cardiac impulse is hyperactive when the shunt is large and there may be left chest prominence. The systolic murmur rarely is loud; it resembles that of mild pulmonary stenosis, and, in fact, arises from the usually trivial pressure gradient across the pulmonary valve. A loud systolic murmur results from a bigger pressure gradient and implies some degree of pulmonary stenosis. Rarely, there may be no systolic murmur and, even less frequently, there may be no auscultatory abnormality at all (silent atrial defect).[50]

The first heart sound is accentuated in proportion to the size of the shunt. The second heart sound is widely split, 0.05 sec or greater, the splitting varying little with respiration. This is in contrast to normal children in whom splitting of the second heart sound clearly varies with respiration. The wide split is easily appreciated, but the lack of variation with respiration maybe more difficult to hear because small children are rarely able to control respiratory depth and rate on request. In this case, changing the patient's position from lying to sitting or standing may elicit convincing evidence of lack of variation. The wide split results from delayed emptying of the overloaded right ventricle; the fixed split is the consequence of unlimited communication between the two atria, allowing for equalization of the influence of respiratory variation on the right and left ventricular output. When the shunt is large there may be a diastolic rumble at the lower left sternal border which seems to arise early in diastole, primarily because the murmur arises from the tricuspid valve and, secondarily, because the second part of the second heart sound is delayed (Fig. 3). These auscultatory findings are virtually diagnostic of atrial septal defect.

Electrocardiography

The electrocardiogram usually shows incomplete right bundle branch block, which is a normal finding in the age group when atrial defects are usually first discovered. Rarely, there is right ventricular hypertrophy. Later in life, in those with pulmonary vascular obstructive disease, the evidence for right ventricular hypertrophy may be more convincing. Right ventricular hypertrophy in the presence of an atrial septal defect may be found also if there is more than minimal pulmonary stenosis, a not unusual concomitant.

Chest X-ray

On chest x-ray, the heart size is enlarged proportionate to the amount of shunting. With a shunt of average size (2:1 QP/QS), the heart size may be normal, with the only abnormal finding being an increase in the pulmonary vascularity. It is curious that the superior vena cava rarely is seen to the right of the spine on the plain chest film in patients with atrial septal defect.

Echocardiography

The echocardiographic diagnosis of atrial septal defect has evolved to the point where it can be made with virtual certainty. The echocardiographer looks for an opening in the atrial septum and, to be confident that this is more than a patent foramen ovale, looks for abnormalities resulting from left-to-right shunting. There may be increased right ventricular volume,[16] an enlarged main pulmonary artery,[16] abnormal respiratory variation in right ventricular dimensions,[36] and abnormal motion of the ventricular septum.[12] The presence of an atrial septal aneurysm should raise the probability of an atrial defect.[25] In any case, the diagnosis of atrial septal defect without evidence of right ventricular overload is suspect. The pattern of Doppler flow velocity across the atrial septum may provide a useful measure of the shunt size.[35]

Atrial septal defects are best visualized using a subxiphoid view because the echo beam is perpendicular to the atrial septum (Fig. 4). Even the thin fossa ovalis is visible when approached in this manner.[3,49] False dropout of the mid portion of the atrial septum is common in apical views because the echo beam is parallel to the thin septum primum. Other helpful views include the parasternal short-axis view and the right sternal border view.[54]

Atrial Septal Defect
2°

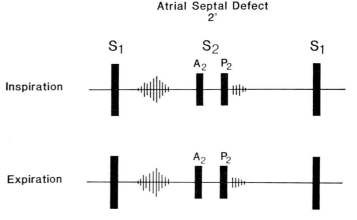

Figure 3. Auscultatory findings resulting from an atrial septal defect. S_1 = first heart sound, S_2 = second heart sound, A_2 = aortic valve closure, P_2 = pulmonic valve closure. The second heart sound is widely split and does not vary with respiration. There is a minimal systolic murmur of the ejection type. Often there is an early diastolic rumble that arises from excess flow across the tricuspid valve and seems to occur early in diastole, in part, because of the widely split second heart sound.

Doppler color flow mapping is especially useful in detecting shunt flow across an atrial defect (see Fig. 6, p. 165).[53] This helps to distinguish between false dropout and real defects. Also, the Doppler examination indicates the direction of flow across the defect.

Supporting evidence for a shunt should always

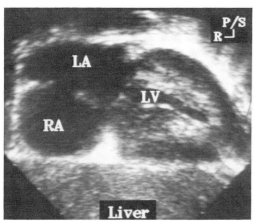

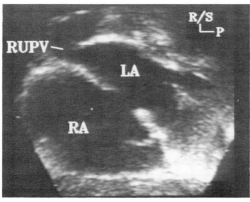

Figure 4. Subxiphoid long-axis (**above**) and short-axis (**below**) views in a child with a typical secundum atrial septal defect. LA, left atrium; LV, left ventricle; P, posterior; R, right; RA, right atrium; RUPV, right upper pulmonary vein; S, superior.

be sought when the diagnosis of an atrial septal defect is entertained. Dilatation of the right ventricle indicates volume loading due to the left-to-right shunt. Reversed septal motion on the M-mode echocardiogram is another manifestation of right ventricular dilatation. The pulmonary artery is often dilated as well. If there is no supporting evidence for increased right heart volume, the diagnosis of atrial septal defect is suspect and confirmation by another means is required.

Transesophageal echocardiography is an excellent means of imaging the atrial septum in older patients.[26] This new window affords excellent imaging of the atrial septum even in large adults with poor transthoracic echocardiographic windows (Fig. 5). Most systems make Doppler color flow mapping available with the transesophageal transducer as well.

The flow velocity across the defect measured by pulsed Doppler examination has been reported to correlate with the shunt volume,[35] but we have not found this parameter particularly useful. For example, in patients with elevated left atrial pres-

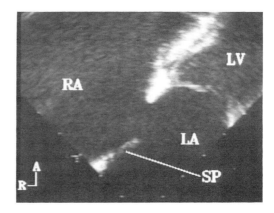

Figure 5. Transesophageal image of a secundum atrial septal defect in a 17-year-old girl. The thin septum primum (SP) could not be imaged using transthoracic windows, leading to overestimation of the size of the defect. Correct determination of the size of the defect is important for deciding if device closure is possible. A, anterior; LA, left atrium; LV, left ventricle; R, right; RA, right atrium.

sure, the velocity of flow across a patent foramen ovale may be quite high despite a trivial shunt volume.

Cardiac Catheterization

Usually, cardiac catheterization is not required for the preoperative diagnosis of atrial septal defect of the secundum type.[18] Occasionally, questions of pulmonary vascular obstructive disease arise and suggestions of associated defects are raised that lead to cardiac catheterization, but, for the usual patient with secundum atrial septal defect, cardiac catheterization is not needed.

At cardiac catheterization, the diagnosis of atrial septal defect is based largely on detection of an atrial left-to-right shunt, because no satisfactory angiographic method of visualization of the defect itself is available. An increase in oxygen saturation of 10% or more from the superior vena cava to the right atrium, if reproducible, and the persistence of the high level of oxygen saturation throughout the lesser circulation, is diagnostic. The normal variability of atrial oxygen saturations can be surmounted by repeated sampling. For reproducibility, there should be careful positioning of the catheter tip; it should face toward the right lateral atrial wall, halfway between the orifices of the superior and inferior venae cavae. Comparison is made with the midsuperior vena caval sample, because this has the more predictable systemic venous saturation. The variability of inferior vena caval samples is such that in our laboratory at Children's Hospital in Boston, these measurements are ignored as unreliable. The inferior vena caval variation results from streaming of lower body (low saturation) and renal (high saturation) blood, the variation of random samples being as much as 20%.

Injection of contrast material into the right-sided circulation shows contrast returning to the right atrium after passage through the lungs, most convincing if the hepatic veins are opacified.

MANAGEMENT

Surgery

For practical purposes, patients with atrial septal defects are referred to the surgeon for closure once the diagnosis is certain. Quibbling about cardiac surgery based on the size of the shunt places more reliance on the data than is justified. Given the proved presence of an atrial defect with left-to-right shunting in a child more than 3 years old, closure is reasonable. To be detected, a left-to-right shunt must allow a ratio of at least 1.5:1 QP/QS; hence, documenting the presence of a shunt is sufficient evidence to proceed. In first year or so of life, there is some merit in delaying until it is certain that the defect will not close spontaneously.

After the age of 3 years, further delay is scarcely justified.[14,22,34]

The primary indication for closing an atrial defect is to prevent pulmonary vascular obstructive disease. Prevention of late rhythm problems and late development of congestive heart failure might also be considered but, in fact, the defect could be closed later if these problems developed. Today the risk of cardiac surgery for atrial septal defect of the secundum variety is virtually zero. Of 430 patients operated on at The Children's Hospital in Boston, there was no mortality except for one very sick small infant who underwent ligation of a patent ductus arteriosus (Exhibit 2). The likelihood of incomplete closure at surgery is rare. Late complications after surgery are rare and are primarily problems with atrial rhythm. Opposing this experience is the devastating problem of pulmonary vascular obstruction in the 5–10% of patients[51,57] who develop this disease. Pulmonary vascular obstructive disease is almost uniformly fatal within a few years and, by itself, is sufficient reason to consider surgical repair of all atrial defects.

Exhibit 2

Boston Children's Hospital Experience 1973–1987	
Basis for Atrial Defect Surgery*	
Clinical evaluation only	273
Echocardiography	61
Cardiac catheterization	176
Echocardiogram and cardiac catheterization	6

*Comment: 20 patients had other surgery, mostly for ligation of a patent ductus arteriosus. The former practice of referring patients for surgery based solely on clinical observations has been supplanted in recent years by echocardiography. Cardiac catheterization for patients with atrial septal defect is now very unusual.

Complications

Rhythm Problems
Sixty-four patients had rhythm abnormalities; 34 were first noted after cardiac surgery and 30 were noted either before surgery or the child did not have cardiac surgery. Five have pacemakers: 2 because of complete heart block and 3 because of the sick sinus syndrome. All of these had had prior cardiac surgery. Three had their first onset of rhythm problem more than 15 years ago.

Deaths
There were 15 deaths. Two died from pulmonary vascular obstructive disease and nine deaths were associated with extracardiac anomalies. There were four deaths in patients who had had cardiac surgery: one after pneumonectomy for scimitar syndrome (age 6 mos.), two after ligation of patent ductus arteriosus (ages 10 days and 6 mos.), and one 10 years after pericardiectomy for constrictive pericarditis and atrial defect closure (age, 26 years). There were no deaths associated with atrial septal defect repair.

Catheter Closure of Atrial Septal Defects

Double-umbrella devices (Fig. 6) that are inserted with a cardiac catheter are now used to close many atrial defects. The smaller and more centrally located defects are particularly suited to this approach. The obvious difficulties of proximity of the atrioventricular valves and other structures, such as the orifices of the venae cavae, are apparent and, as yet, systems for delivering devices big enough to close large defects are not available. The desirability of avoiding intrathoracic dissection and opening the heart is obvious.

Technique. A most important step in transcatheter closure of atrial defects is accurate assessment of the number, size, and location of the defects. Those larger than 25 mm in diameter, multiple defects including those outside the fossa ovalis, sinus venosus defects extending into the venae cavae, and defects with tissue rims less than 3–6 mm from the tricuspid valves or right pulmonary veins are avoided. For patients with suitably located defects, the size is determined by inflating a balloon and measuring the stretched diameter. An umbrella is chosen which is 80% larger than the stretched diameter of the defect. The distal arms of the umbrella are opened in the left atrium and pulled slowly but firmly to bow the septum rightward. Then, the right-sided arms are opened and the umbrella is advanced to a neutral position. The proper location is confirmed and the umbrella released. Patients are monitored overnight, discharged the next day, and maintained on antibiotic prophylaxis for 6–9 months.

Results. By the end of 1989, more than 50 atrial defects had been closed in children and young adults[32] without mortality or significant complica-

tion at Children's Hospital in Boston (see p. 219). Closure has been complete in most, although one boy had multiple defects.

COURSE

The natural course of atrial septal defect, except for the largest openings and those associated with other cardiac defects, is relatively benign.[10] Many patients have lived into the fourth, fifth, sixth, and seventh decades with atrial defects of some size before they develop symptoms.[42] Late symptoms are those of atrial fibrillation, congestive heart failure and, less often, those of pulmonary vascular obstructive disease.

Follow-up of Patients after Surgery

Rarely, an incompletely patched atrial defect or a second unrecognized defect is encountered, but, for the most part, atrial defect surgery is remarkably successful. Late appearance of pulmonary vascular disease or congestive heart failure after closure of the defect is virtually unknown.

Among patients who have undergone operation in the past, the right ventricular volume has remained increased for some years despite closure of the defect.[37] It is suggested that earlier surgery might eliminate this result.

Atrial arrhythmias are the most common late problems following closure.

Atrial Arrhythmias

Unrepaired atrial defects are associated with atrial dysrhythmia, particularly in older patients.[7,24] Atrial fibrillation and atrial flutter are not common complications of atrial septal defect in children but are seen often in adult patients. Preoperative electrophysiologic measurements in patients of all ages detect conduction abnormalities in as many as 40% of patients.[6,29] Following surgery, some of the electrophysiologic aberrations improve; others do not.[45] The prevalence of significant arrhythmia is higher after surgery, occurring in from 7–20% of repaired patients (Exhibit 2).[5,6,8] A small number (0.5–2%)[5,6] may need pacemakers because of the sick sinus syndrome or even surgically induced complete heart block (Exhibit 2). Postoperative abnormalities are more likely if suturing involves the region of the sinus node or if cannulation of the superior vena cava is needed.[4,13] Postoperative rhythm abnormalities also are associated with repair of partial anomalous pulmonary veins.[5]

Pulmonary Vascular Obstruction

Pulmonary vascular disease occurs in about 5–10% of patients with untreated atrial defects,[51,57] predominantly in females. Usually it occurs after the age of 20 years, although rare cases in early childhood have been recorded.[27]

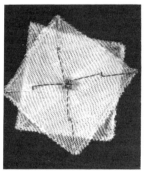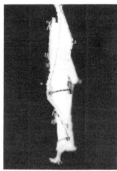

Figure 6. A clamshell device (33 mm) used to close an atrial septal defect. The two umbrellas are covered with thrombin-soaked cloth to provide a surface for growth of endothelium. The device is extruded from the catheter tip placed in the left atrium. After the umbrella springs open, the catheter is pulled back to the atrial septum. With the first umbrella opened and applied firmly to the septum, the catheter is pulled back further and the second cloth-covered umbrella opens to cover the right side of the septum. With satisfactory position, the device is released.

It is interesting that individuals who develop pulmonary vascular obstructive disease with atrial septal defects seldom report cardiovascular problems earlier in life and often are not known to have heart disease. Patients who have symptoms as children are less likely to get pulmonary vascular disease.[27] Whether it is the increase in shunt size over many years or the development of thromboses in the pulmonary artery, usually in adults,[47] that ultimately causes pulmonary vascular obstructive disease, the conclusion that all atrial defects of detectable size should be surgically closed to prevent its development seems inescapable. At Children's Hospital in Boston, two patients have been seen who, elsewhere, were not considered candidates for surgery because of a small atrial septal defect. Each had undergone cardiac catheterization and was found to have a small left-to-right shunt; years later, both succumbed to pulmonary vascular disease (Fig. 7).

Whether the defect should be closed after pulmonary vascular obstructive disease has developed is debatable. Little is accomplished by closing the atrial defect to prevent left-to-right shunting when, in truth, there is minimal left-to-right shunt and the opening provides some cardiac output (albeit unsaturated blood) when a patient is under stress. Closure of the defect may remove this tenuous safeguard.

In deciding which patients who have atrial septal defects and evidence of pulmonary vascular ob-

structive disease should undergo closure of the defect, detailed hemodynamics are required. As with any other patient with evidence of pulmonary vascular disease, every effort should be made to find reversible causes of the increased resistance. Any evidence that the pulmonary hypertensive vascular abnormality is a consequence of high altitude, upper airway obstruction, or sleep apnea should be investigated with care, because these problems are reversible. Otherwise, closure is recommended if there is a significant left-to-right shunt (greater than 1.5:1 QP/QS) and minimal right-to-left shunting or pulmonary resistance of less than 8 units. Even after having survived surgery, these patients face significant mortality in the ensuing years (Exhibit 2).[15]

VARIATIONS

Symptomatic Infants

There are a few infants, often with congestive heart failure, who have relatively large atrial septal defects[14,22,34] and in whom further evaluation uncovers no other abnormality. Because surgery carries some risk and spontaneous closure is known to occur in infants, conservative treatment is the first choice in management. Infants who recover spontaneously subsequently seem normal. The explanation of these observations is elusive. It is believed that there may have been left ventricular

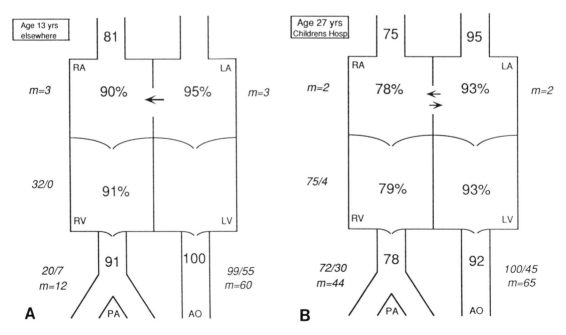

Figure 7. Catheterization data derived from two studies of the same patient. The data obtained at age 13 (**A**) were interpreted as compatible with a small atrial defect of insufficient size to require closure. Some years later she had developed pulmonary vascular obstructive disease (**B**) and was no longer shunting enough to recommend surgery. Death occurred 5 years later. RA, right atrium; LA, left atrium; RV, right ventricle; LV, left ventricle; PA, pulmonary artery; AO, aorta; large bold numbers, oxygen % saturation; Italics, pressure in mmHg.

myocardial disease or hypoplasia of the left ventricle to account for the apparent improvement without anatomic abnormality. There may never have been a true atrial defect, the foramen ovale having become incompetent with elevated left atrial pressure and closed spontaneously with improvement of the left-sided disease. The possibility that the septum primum is incomplete at birth and continues to evolve after birth would also account for a demonstrable left-to-right shunt that later disappears.

Occasionally, when there is congestive heart failure and poor growth, it is recommended that the atrial defect be surgically closed. It must be remembered that the surgical risk in this group of patients is greater than for older children with atrial septal defect.

Patent Foramen Ovale

At birth, all babies have a patent foramen ovale. Rarely, absence of the foramen ovale is encountered and often it is associated with major left-sided cardiac abnormalities.

Normally, the flap of the foramen ovale closes after birth because of the relatively higher pressure in the left atrium; the defect becomes anatomically closed later. Cardiac defects that favor a higher right versus left atrial pressure are associated with persistent patency. Any abnormality that causes right ventricular hypertension (i.e., valvar pulmonary stenosis) is likely to be associated with an open foramen ovale and a possible right-to-left shunt. Any defect associated with higher left than right atrial pressure, (i.e., ventricular septal defect or patent ductus arteriosus) is likely to be associated with a closed foramen ovale. In the majority of children and adults the foramen is closed; however, it is open in 34% of patients in groups aged 1–9, 10–19, and 20–29 years. For older patients, a persistent foramen is less likely (20% over the age of 80 years).[23]

In early infancy, whenever there is severely elevated left atrial pressure and volume, the foramen may be stretched open and the flap inverted into the right atrium, allowing important left-to-right shunting. The atrial shunt is reversed once the left-sided disease has been controlled (see ch. 24).

With increasing use of 2-D echocardiography, otherwise normal patients with a patent foramen ovale are being identified. Paradoxical embolus, rarely reported in all age groups, is a risk, but considering the number of people with a patent foramen, it is not justifiable to close patent formina ovale to prevent this problem in the absence of evidence of embolization.

Sinoseptal Defects

Superior Vena Caval Sinus Venosus Defect. These defects, usually called "sinus venosus atrial septal defects," are not large and shunting usually does not often exceed 2:1 QP/QS. Sinus venosus defects are the second most common atrial defect, constituting about a quarter of all atrial defects not derived from the endocardial cushions. All are referred for surgical closure. For the future, closure with catheter extruded devices is under consideration but seems unlikely because of the proximity of the superior vena cava. Whether the incidence of pulmonary vascular disease is the same as for other atrial defects is unknown; it may be less because these defects are not huge. The incidence of rhythm problems is known to be higher in the postoperative patient.[5]

Unroofed Coronary Sinus. This diagnosis can best be made by sophisticated echocardiography. Surgical repair is tailored to the anatomy present. In principle, the left superior vena cava, if present,[44] is redirected to the right atrial side either through ligation, if an adequate innominate vein is present, or with a baffle or tunnel in the atrium.[46] The left-to-right shunt is removed by a patch or baffle, or through closure of the orifice of the coronary sinus. Whether the coronary venous blood flow drains into the left atrium or is redirected to the right is of little practical consequence.

Inferior Vena Caval Sinoseptal Defect. The rare sinoseptal defects that are adjacent to the orifice of the inferior vena cava most often seem to be associated with partial anomalous veins to the right atrium. Because the defect lies between the orifice of the inferior vena cava and the orifice of the right pulmonary veins, the suggestion that the pulmonary veins enter abnormally may be more apparent than real.[56] A single patch appropriately applied will close the defect with the veins on the correct side, the patch assuming the normal position of the atrial septum.

Partial Anomalous Venous Return. Partial anomalous pulmonary veins are a relatively common anomaly (1/200 autopsies),[30] often complicating other cardiac abnormalities. Most often there is an associated atrial defect and the hemodynamics are those of an atrial defect. In the absence of an atrial defect, the second sound may be well split but is not fixed relative to respiration. As an isolated defect, partial anomalous pulmonary veins only rarely cause symptoms.

A variety of anomalies of pulmonary venous return have been described (Fig. 8). Anomalous entry of the right upper and middle pulmonary veins into the superior vena cava is associated with sinus venosus atrial defects. Entry of right-sided pulmonary veins into the inferior vena cava is part of the scimitar syndrome. Entry of the left upper pulmonary veins into the left vertical vein is, in many ways, comparable to the anatomy found in some patients with total anomalous pulmonary venous return. Rarely, the left lower pulmonary veins drain into the coronary sinus.[33]

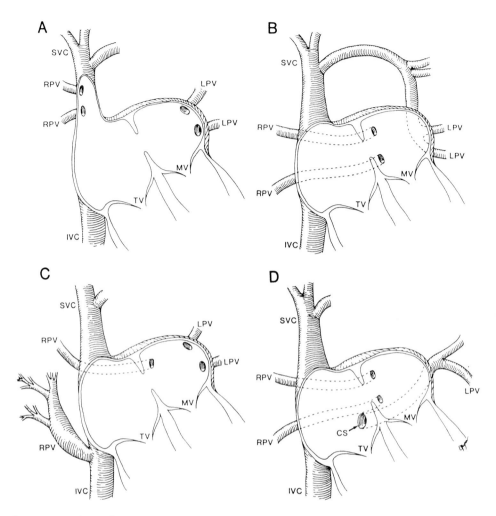

Figure 8. Diagram of several connections of anomalous pulmonary veins to the systemic venous circulation. **A,** Drainage of the right upper veins to the superior vena cava. **B,** Drainage of left pulmonary veins via connections to the innominate veins. **C,** Drainage of lower right-sided veins into the inferior vena cava (scimitar syndrome). **D,** Drainage of left pulmonary veins into the coronary sinus. SVC, superior vena cava; IVC, inferior vena cava; RPV, right pulmonary vein; LPV, left pulmonary vein; MV, mitral valve; TV, tricuspid valve; CS, coronary sinus.

For the most part, these partially anomalous veins can be corrected, but the surgical difficulty, the likelihood of success, and the probable benefits should be weighed carefully before proceeding. Abnormal entry of a single small pulmonary vein does not require surgical intervention. Most have associated atrial defects that should be closed, and the decision is easy. The anomalous veins pose the practical problem of what to do when the chest has been opened to repair an atrial defect. Small pulmonary veins entering the left superior vena cava have been ligated without a problem. Pulmonary veins entering the inferior vena cava and those entering the superior vena cava can be redirected to the left atrium. Management of the left-sided anomalous pulmonary veins is more problematic but they can be corrected by direct connection to the left atrium. In each case, tailoring the response to the anatomy is required.

Scimitar Syndrome. Anomalous entry of the right pulmonary veins, in part or totally, into the inferior vena cava (often associated with hypoplasia of the right lung, sometimes with mesocardia or dextrocardia, atrial defect, and anomalous arterial supply to the right lung from the descending aorta) is called the **scimitar syndrome**.[11,28,31,40,41] Usually, this relatively rare problem is readily recognized on the plain chest x-ray because there is hypoplasia of the right lung, the heart shadow is shifted to the right, and the visible right pulmonary veins (the scimitar) curve toward the inferior vena cava (Fig. 9). Sometimes, the physiologic advantage of surgical correction is not obvious because the amount of blood shunting through the small right lung may be small. Recurrent pulmonary infections, an obvious concern, have not been a problem but pulmonary vascular disease[27] has been reported in infants as an unexplained complication.

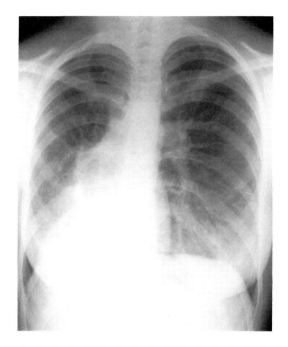

Figure 9. X-ray of an asymptomatic patient with scimitar syndrome. Note the hypoplasia of the right lung and the corresponding increase in size of the left lung. The right diaphragm is high and the anomalous pulmonary vein (scimitar) is visible above the diaphragm.

Uncomplicated Atrial Defect with Cyanosis

Rarely, patients with atrial septal defect or patent foramen ovale, without other cardiac abnormality, are cyanotic, particularly on exercise.[9,21,39,52,55] This is considered to be an extreme version of the small right-to-left shunt measurable in all patients with an atrial septal defect and perhaps is aggravated by an unusually large eustachian valve often found in these people. Closing the defect is curative.

Lutembacher's Syndrome

Wherever there is rheumatic fever, some patients will be identified who have an atrial septal defect and rheumatic mitral valve dysfunction. The combination of mitral stenosis and an atrial defect is called Lutembacher's syndrome.[1] With the near disappearance of rheumatic fever, the association of an atrial defect and rheumatic mitral stenosis is now rare in the United States. At Children's Hospital in Boston, only one patient was found among 882 individuals with atrial septal defect and in that one the diagnosis was questionable.

Mitral Valve Prolapse

Mitral valve prolapse (see pp. 614–616) is a curious but common finding, without known practical consequence, among patients with atrial septal defect. That mitral valve prolapse is caused in part by the atrial defect itself is suggested by improvement in the degree of prolapse after repair of the atrial defect.[48]

REFERENCES

1. Bashi VV, Ravikumar E, Jairaj PS, et al: Coexistent mitral valve disease with left-to-right shunt at the atrial level: clinical profile, hemodynamics, and surgical considerations in 67 consecutive patients. Am Heart J 114:1406–1414, 1987.
2. Besterman E: Atrial septal defect with pulmonary hypertension. Br Heart J 23:587–598, 1961.
3. Bierman FZ, Williams RG: Subxiphoid two-dimensional imaging of the interatrial septum in infants and neonates with congenital heart disease. Circulation 60:80–90, 1979.
4. Bink-Boelkens ME, Meuzelaar KJ, Eygelaar A: Arrhythmias after repair of secundum atrial septal defect: the influence of surgical modification. Am Heart J 115:629–633, 1988.
5. Bink-Boelkens ME, Velvis H, Homan van der Heide JJ, et al: Dysrhythmias after atrial surgery in children. Am Heart J 106:125–130, 1983.
6. Bolens M, Friedli B: Sinus node function and conduction system before and after surgery for secundum atrial septal defect: an electrophysiologic study. Am J Cardiol 53:1415–1420, 1984.
7. Brandenburg RO, Holmes DR Jr, Brandenburg, RO Jr, et al: Clinical follow-up study of paroxysmal supraventicular tachyarrhythmias after operative repair of a secundum type atrial septal defect in adults. Am J Cardiol 51:273–276, 1983.
8. Bricker JT, Gillette PC, Cooley DA, et al: Dysrhythmias after repair of atrial septal defect. Texas Heart Inst J 13:203–208, 1986.
9. Burton DA, Chin A, Weinberg PM, et al: Identification of cor triatriatum dexter by two-dimensional echocardiography. Am J Cardiol 60:409–410, 1987.
10. Campbell M: Natural history of atrial septal defect. Br Heart J 32:820–826, 1970.
11. Canter CE, Martin TC, Spray TL, et al: Scimitar syndrome: a report of nine cases. Am J Cardiol 58:652–654, 1986.
12. Chazal RA, Armstrong WF, Dillon JC, et al: Diastolic ventricular septal motion in atrial septal defect: analysis of M-mode echocardiograms in 31 patients. Am J Cardiol 52:1088–1090, 1983.
13. Clark EB, Kugler JD: Preoperative secundum atrial septal defect with coexisting sinus node and atrioventricular node dysfunction. Circulation 65:976–980, 1982.
14. Cockerham JT, Martin TC, Gutierrez FR, et al: Spontaneous closure of secundum atrial septal defect in infants and young children. Am J Cardiol 52:1267–1271, 1983.
15. Dalen JE, Haynes FW, Dexter L: Life expectancy with atrial septal defect: influence of complicating pulmonary vascular disease. JAMA 200:442–446, 1967.
16. Denef B, Dumoulin M, Van Der Hauwaert LG: Usefulness of echocardiographic assessment of right ventricular and pulmonary trunk size for estimating magnitude of left-to-right shunt in children with atrial septal defect. Am J Cardiol 55:1571–1574, 1985.
17. Ferencz C, Rubin JD, McCarter RJ, et al: Congenital heart disease: prevalence at birth. The Baltimore-Washington Infant Study. Am J Epidemiol 121:31–36, 1985.
18. Freed MD, Nadas AS, Norwood WI, et al: Is routine preoperative cardiac catheterization necessary before

repair of secundum and sinus venosus atrial septal defects? J Am Coll Cardiol 4:333–336, 1984.

19. Freedom RM, Culham JAG, Rowe RD: Left atrial to coronary sinus fenestration (partially unroofed coronary sinus): morphological and angiographic observations. Br Heart J 46:63–68, 1981.

20. Fyler DC, Buckley LP, Hellenbrand WE, et al: Report of the New England Regional Infant Cardiac Program. Pediatrics 65(Suppl):376–460, 1980.

21. Gallaher ME, Sperling DR, Gwinn JL, et al: Functional drainage of the inferior vena cava into the left atrium—three cases. Am J Cardiol 12:561–566, 1963.

22. Ghisla RP, Hannon DW, Meyer RA, et al: Spontaneous closure of isolated secundum atrial septal defects in infants: an echocardiographic study. Am Heart J 109:1327–1333, 1985.

23. Hagen PT, Scholz DG, Edwards WD: Incidence and size of patent foramen ovale during the first 10 decades of life: an autopsy of 965 normal hearts. Mayo Clin Proc 59:17–20, 1984.

24. Hamilton WT, Haffajee CI, Dalen JE, et al: Atrial septal defect secundum: clinical profile with physiologic correlates in children and adults. In Roberts WC (ed): Adult Congenital Heart Disease. Philadelphia, F.A. Davis, 1979.

25. Hanley PC, Tajik AJ, Hynes JK, et al: Diagnosis and classification of atrial aneurysm by 2-dimensional echocardiography: report of 80 consecutive cases. J Am Coll Cardiol 6:1370–1382, 1985.

26. Hanrath P, Schluter M, Langenstein BA, et al: Detection of ostium secundum atrial septal defects by transesophageal cross-sectional echocardiography. Br Heart J 49:350–358, 1983.

27. Haworth SG: Pulmonary vascular disease in secundum atrial septal defect in childhood. Am J Cardiol 51:265–272, 1983.

28. Haworth SG, Sauer U, Buhlmeyer K: Pulmonary hypertension in Scimitar syndrome in infancy. Br Heart J 50:182–189, 1981.

29. Karpawich PP, Antillon JR, Cappola PR, et al: Pre- and postoperative electrophysiologic assessment of children with secundum atrial septal defect. Am J Cardiol 55:519–521, 1985.

30. Keith JD, Rowe RD, Vlad P: Heart Disease in Infancy and Childhood, 3rd ed. New York, Macmillan, 1979, pp. 380–404.

31. Kieley B, Filler J, Stone S, et al: Syndrome of anomalous venous drainage of the right lung to the inferior vena cava: a review of 67 reported cases and three new cases in children. Am J Cardiol 20:102–116, 1967.

32. Lock JE, Keane JF, Fellows KE: Diagnostic and Interventional Catheterization in Congenital Heart Disease. Boston, Martinus Nijhoff, 1987.

33. Lucas RV: Anomalous venous connections, pulmonary and systemic. In Adams FH, Emmanouilides GC (eds): Heart Disease in Infants, Children, and Adolescents. Baltimore, Williams & Wilkins, 1983, pp. 458–490.

34. Mahoney LT, Truesdell SC, Krzmarzick TR, et al: Atrial septal defects that present in infancy. Am J Dis Child 140:1115–1118, 1986.

35. Marx GR, Allen HD, Goldberg SJ, et al: Transatrial septal velocity measurement by Doppler echocardiography in atrial septal defect: correlation with QP/QS ratio. Am J Cardiol 55:1162–1167, 1985.

36. Mauran P, Fouron JC, Carceller AM, et al: Value of respiratory variations of right ventricular dimension in the identification of small atrial septal defects (secundum type) not requiring surgery: an echocardiographic study. Am Heart J 112:548–552, 1986.

37. Meyer RA, Korfhagen JC, Covitz W, et al: Long-term follow-up study after closure of secundum atrial septal defect in children: an echocardiographic study. Am J Cardiol 50:143–148, 1982.

38. Miao C, Zuberbuhler JS, Zuberbuhler JR: Prevalence of congenital cardiac anomalies at high altitude. J Am Coll Cardiol 12:224–228, 1988.

39. Morishita Y, Yamashita M, Yamada K, et al: Cyanosis in atrial septal defect due to persistent eustachian valve. J Thorac 40:614–616, 1985.

40. Neill CA, Ferencz C, Sabiston DC, et al: The familial occurrence of hypoplastic right lung with systemic arterial supply and venous drainage "scimitar syndrome." Bull Johns Hopkins Hosp 107:1–21, 1960.

41. Oakley D, Naik D, Verel D, et al: Scimitar vein syndrome: report of nine new cases. Am Heart J 107:596–598, 1984.

42. Paolillo V, Dawkins KD, Miller GAH: Atrial septal defect in patients over the age of 50. Int J Cardiol 9:139–147, 1985.

43. Parisi LF, Nadas AS: Natural history of atrial septal defects. In Kidd BSL, Keith JK (eds): The Natural History and Progress in Treatment of Congenital Heart Defects. Springfield, IL, Charles C Thomas, 1971.

44. Raghib G, Ruttenberg HD, Anderson RC, et al: Termination of left superior vena cava in left atrium, atrial septal defect, and absence of coronary sinus. Circulation 31:906–918, 1965.

45. Ruschhaupt DG, Khoury L, Thilenius OG, et al: Electophysiologic abnormalities of children with ostium secundum atrial septal defect. Am J Cardiol 53:1643–1646, 1984.

46. Sand ME, McGrath LB, Pacifico AD, et al: Repair of left superior vena cava entering the left atrium. Ann Thorac Surg 42:560–564, 1986.

47. Schamroth CL, Sareli P, Pocock WA, et al: Pulmonary arterial thrombosis in secundum atrial septal defect. Am J Cardiol 60:1152–1156, 1987.

48. Schreiber TL, Feigenbaum H, Weyman AE: Effect of atrial septal defect repair on left ventricular geometry and degree of mitral valve prolapse. Circulation 61:888–896, 1980.

49. Shub C, Dimopoulos IN, Seward JB, et al: Sensitivity of two-dimensional echocardiography in the direct visualization of atrial septal defect utilizing the subcostal approach: experience with 154 patients. J Am Coll Cardiol 2:127–135, 1983.

50. Shub C, Tajik AJ, Seward JB: Clinically "silent" atrial septal defect: diagnosis by two-dimensional and Doppler echocardiography. Am Heart J 110:665–667, 1988.

51. Steele PM, Fuster V, Cohen M, et al: Isolated atrial septal defect with pulmonary vascular obstructive disease: long-term follow-up and prediction of outcome after surgical correction. Circulation 76:1037–1042, 1987.

52. Strunk BL, Cheitlin MD, Stulbarg MS, et al: Right-to-left shunting through a patent foramen ovale despite normal intracardiac pressures. Am J Cardiol 60:413–414, 1987.

53. Suzuki Y, Kambara H, Kadota K, et al: Detection of intracardiac shunt flow in atrial septal defect using a real-time two-dimensional color-coded Doppler flow imaging system and comparison with contrast two-dimensional echocardiography. Am J Cardiol 56:347–350, 1985.

54. Tei C, Tanaka H, Yoshimura H, et al: Real-time cross-sectional echocardiographic evaluation of the interatrial septum by right atrium–interatrial septum–left atrium direction of the sound beam. Circulation 60:539–546, 1979.

55. Thomas JD, Tabakin BS, Ittleman FP: Atrial septal defect with right to left shunt despite normal pulmonary artery pressure. J Am Coll Cardiol 9:221–224, 1987.

56. Van Praagh S, Kakou-Guikahue M, Kim H-S, et al: Atrial situs in patients with viseral heterotaxy and congenital heart disease: conclusions based on findings in 104 postmortem cases. Coeur 19:484–452, 1988.

57. Zaver AG, Nadas AS: Atrial septal defect—secundum type. Circulation 32(Suppl III):III-24–III-32, 1965.

Chapter 33

PATENT DUCTUS ARTERIOSUS

Donald C. Fyler, M.D.

DEFINITION

Functional patency of the ductus arteriosus is abnormal if it persists more than a few hours after birth. Persistent, sometimes intermittent, patency for up to 10 days after birth is encountered in patients with circulatory or ventilatory abnormalities, and among premature infants the ductus may remain open for longer periods before closing. For the purposes of this section, persistent patency of the ductus beyond a few days will be considered abnormal.

PREVALENCE

A patent ductus arteriosus was the fifth or sixth most common congenital cardiac defect in most surveys (see ch. 18), although there was as much as a tenfold difference in estimated numbers per thousand live births (0.06 per 1,000 to 0.77 per 1,000). At the Children's Hospital in Boston in the past 15 years, among all age groups, patent ductus arteriosus has been the sixth most common defect. Studies of infants carried out in recent years found fewer patients with patent ductus arteriosus than were found in previous studies. Perhaps the ductus arteriosus, in premature infants at least, is becoming the concern of another specialty—neonatology.

Not only does patency of the ductus arteriosus persist longer among premature infants, but prematurity accounts for some of the patent ductus arteriosus seen long after infancy. Children born of mothers who have had rubella around the time of conception have a high incidence of patent ductus. Maternal rubella is thought to be the cause of its seasonal incidence, which was noted before immunization was widely introduced.[33] Children born at high altitudes more often have a persistently patent ductus than those born at sea level.[1,23] The number increases as the altitude increases, suggesting that patency is a direct function of ambient oxygen.[23]

ANATOMY

The ductus arteriosus is derived from the left sixth embryologic arch and connects the origin of the left main pulmonary artery to the aorta, just below the left subclavian artery. During fetal life, the ductus is as large, or larger, than the ascending aorta and carries outflow from the right ventricle to the descending aorta (Fig. 1). Within hours of birth, the ductus closes, usually at the pulmonary end, often leaving behind a remnant on the aorta, a ductus diverticulum. Occasionally, a diverticulum persists at the point of origin from the pulmonary artery as well. With a right aortic arch the ductus is usually left sided, although rarely it arises in mirror image, entering the right pulmonary artery. Bilateral ductus are rare. When the right ventricular outflow is occluded, as in pulmonary atresia, the ductus must shunt left-to-right during fetal life, supplying blood to the developing lung. In this case, the ductus is small because the flow it carries is a small fraction of that normally passing right-to-left to the aorta in the fetus. In patients with tetralogy of Fallot, the ductus is often absent.

The ductus closes through muscular constriction a few hours after birth. Later there is obliteration of the lumen, initially by a pile up of endothelium and, finally, by complete occlusion through thrombosis, the ductus withering to a fibrous strand. The histopathology of a persistently patent ductus is different from that found in a normal ductus not yet closed, suggesting that persistent patency is usually a primary anomaly and not a secondary effect.[15,16] On histologic examination, the ductus is notably edematous, friable, and lacerated after the use of prostaglandins.[4,17]

It is proposed that strands of ductal muscle sometimes snare the descending aorta causing coarctation,[32,36] or ensnare the proximal pulmonary artery, producing stenosis at the origin of the left pulmonary artery. That constriction of the aorta is associated with a right-to-left shunting duct, whereas constriction of the pulmonary artery is associated

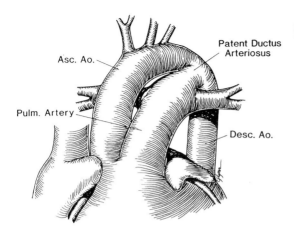

Figure 1. Anatomic drawing of a large persistent patent ductus arteriosus.

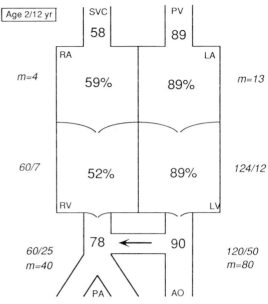

Figure 2. Diagram of the hemodynamics in a patient with a patent ductus arteriosus and moderate pulmonary hypertension. Note the low pulmonary venous oxygen that results from a combination of excess pulmonary flow, congestive heart failure, and pulmonary infection. Note also the wide pulmonary arterial and aortic pulse pressures.

with a left-to-right shunt (i.e., in patients with tetralogy of Fallot) is an intriguing curiosity.

In premature infants, the process of ductal closure is the same but is delayed, sometimes for weeks. The baby is born too soon; ductal closure occurs on schedule. However, not all close. The incidence of persistent patency of the ductus well past infancy in patients who were premature is greater than it is in the normal population.

PHYSIOLOGY

With the first respiratory gasps after birth, pulmonary arteriolar resistance falls abruptly; the ductus arteriosus reverses its flow and begins to shunt from left to right. Normally, the ductus begins to close with the first gasping respiration, and in a matter of hours the ductus may be functionally closed. If the ductus remains widely patent, there is equilibration of the aortic and pulmonary arterial pressures. In this situation, the pulmonary resistance falls, causing increasing left-to-right shunting and congestive failure. If the ductus is large and there is continued elevation of pulmonary resistance, it may become irreversible, although pulmonary vascular disease is rare before the first birthday.

When there is a persistently large runoff from the aorta to the pulmonary artery, there is excessive blood flow to the lungs, left atrium, left ventricle, and ascending aorta (Fig. 2), with enlargement of these structures in proportion to the size of the left-to-right shunt. The volume overload within the thorax is great enough that blood transfusion after ductal ligation is rarely needed. The larger the runoff, the greater is the arterial pulse pressure, and the more striking the peripheral pulsations. When there is a large volume overload, the flap covering the foramen ovale may become incompetent, allowing additional left-to-right shunting and further volume overload.

The mechanism of ductal closure is a complex interaction of the level of arterial oxygen, circulating prostaglandins, genetic predetermination, and unknown factors.[26] Low oxygen tension is a factor in maintaining ductal patency in the fetus, and the sharp increase in arterial oxygen saturation with the first breath is thought to be the initiating step in ductal closure. On the other hand, high ambient oxygen does not help to close a persistently patent ductus, although the increased incidence of patent ductus in infants born at high altitudes is thought to be the result of low ambient oxygen.[1,23]

Prostaglandin E1 is a powerful ductal dilator.[27] Prostaglandins may be required to maintain ductal patency in utero, but some other arachidonic derivative may be involved as a counterbalancing effect to cause closure.[26] The reciprocal relation between the effects of oxygen and prostaglandins varies with maturity. Oxygen is more effective in promoting ductal closure in the mature infant and less in the immature. Prostaglandin E1 is more effective in promoting ductal patency in the premature infant and less effective in the mature.

Indomethacin given to the baby, or corticosteroids given to the mother,[14] will promote ductal closure. In the natural course of events, the ductus regularly and inappropriately closes in the first days of life even though the baby depends on left-to-right (pulmonary atresia) or right-to-left shunting (interrupted aortic arch) to survive.

How maternal rubella interrupts the sequence of closure is not known but probably it has a direct effect on the ductal tissue itself, since adjacent structures (the origins of the right and left pulmonary arteries) are also affected.

CLINICAL MANIFESTATIONS

Patency of the ductus arteriosus in a full-term or older infant or child (largely females 2:1) produces symptoms and signs proportionate to the amount of blood passing into the pulmonary circulation. When the ductal shunt is small, the only abnormality may be the presence of a murmur. When the ductus is large, symptoms of congestive heart failure or pulmonary hypertension may be present and the murmur may not be typical.

Most children are discovered to have a murmur within days or weeks of birth (Exhibit 1). The murmur is not characteristically continuous in the early weeks of life, but it is recognized as a systolic murmur. If the ductus is large, symptoms of congestive heart failure (tachypnea, dyspnea, intercostal or subcostal retractions, hepatomegaly, or growth failure) may signal the cardiac problem. These children are not cyanotic unless there is pulmonary edema.

Classically, in the older child, there is a crescendo systolic murmur, peaking in intensity at aortic closure, and continuing into diastole as a high-frequency, decrescendo diastolic murmur (Figs. 3 and 4). Usually, although not invariably, the diastolic component of the murmur extends the entire length of diastole. Often there are coarse sounds (clicks or "shaking dice" noises) during systole which contribute to the typical machinery sound. The murmur is loudest at the second left intercostal space; maximal intensity anywhere else should raise concern about the diagnosis of a patent ductus arteriosus. In the small infant it is uncommon to hear the diastolic component of the murmur even if the ductus is large. In older infants with a large ductus and equilibration of aortic and pulmonary pressures, there may be only a systolic murmur, usually recognizable because of its location, its crescendo quality, and the clicks. When the ductus is large there is often an apical diastolic rumble (because of excessive mitral valve flow) that is hard to differentiate from the transmitted sounds of the loud continuous murmur.

The presence of a continuous murmur of crescendo-decrescendo quality, loudest at the time of the second sound, with systolic clicks, and located in the second right intercostal space, should be interpreted as resulting from a patent ductus arteriosus. Among other causes of these findings, the most common is an aortopulmonary window; but, even here, the size of the window is usually so big that a continuous murmur is unusual. Other problems that could more or less mimic these findings include:

1. A **venous hum** is usually louder when the patient is sitting rather than lying down and it may be louder to the right of the sternum. Hums have an evanescent quality, changing with respiration as well as position.

2. A **fistula between a coronary artery and a cardiac chamber** may produce a continuous murmur of crescendo-decrescendo quality which is usually not loudest at the second right intercostal space. The murmur may be louder in systole or diastole depending on the hemodynamics (see ch. 50).

3. A **ruptured sinus of Valsalva** also produces a continuous murmur, not previously heard, which most often is not loudest at the second right interspace.

4. **Tetralogy of Fallot with pulmonary atresia and collateral circulation** produces continuous murmurs which are heard all over the front and back of the chest, and if there are sufficient collaterals the patient may not be visibly cyanotic.

Usually, all of these possibilities are readily eliminated by cardiac auscultation.

In patients with a patent ductus arteriosus, heart failure is a feature of early infancy and is rare after the age of 6 months.

The peripheral arterial pulsations depend on the size of the ductus and the size of the shunt. The larger the ductus and the larger the left-to-right shunt, the more prominent are the peripheral arterial pulsations.

Electrocardiography

The electrocardiogram is normal when there is a small ductus; it shows left ventricular hypertrophy with a somewhat larger ductus, and shows combined ventricular hypertrophy with a large ductus and pulmonary hypertension. When pulmonary vascular disease dominates the clinical picture there may be only right ventricular hypertrophy. Because the presence of a continuous murmur and significant right ventricular hypertrophy are contradictory observations, careful investigation of patients with this combination of findings is required.

Chest X-Ray

The aorta, left ventricle, left atrium, pulmonary vessels, and main pulmonary arteries are enlarged in proportion to the amount of left-to-right shunt and may appropriately affect the cardiac silhouette on the plain chest film.

Echocardiography

The relative enlargement of the various cardiac chambers is recognizable. Patency of the ductus may be visualized and, with Doppler scanning, the

Exhibit 1

Boston Children's Hospital Experience 1973–1987
Patent Ductus Arteriosus
There were 866 patients with a primary diagnosis of patent ductus arteriosus seen between 1973 and 1987; 92 were first seen before 1973. 478 underwent surgical closure in this time period, usually by ligation, and in 38 the ductus was closed using an umbrella device. There were 19 recurrences; 7 occurred after catheter closure and 12 after surgical ligation. Some had had surgery elsewhere. In 64 the ductus closed spontaneously. The incidence of noncardiac medical problems was high: more than 228 had some respiratory problem and 281 had noncardiac anomalies; 169 were considered to have a specific syndrome; 14 patients had pulmonary vascular obstructive disease; and 4 patients had infective endocarditis.

Age on First Admission

Age at First Admission	1973–77	1978–82	1983–87	Total
0–1 month	80	126	135	341
2–12 months	44	64	61	169
1–5 years	45	55	50	150
6–10 years	25	14	22	61
11– years	15	13	25	53

Repair of Patent Ductus Arteriosus

Age at Ductal Ligation	1973–77		1978–82		1983–87*	
	No.	Mortality	No.	Mortality	No.	Mortality
0–2 months	50	14%	113	11%	56	4%
2–6 months	12	8%	15	16%	10	0
6–12 months	11	0	14	0	10	0
1–5 years	41	0	49	0	26	0
6– years	33	0	21	0	17	0

*During this period, 38 of these children had ductus closures using umbrella devices (see pp. 207, 218). Three later had ductus surgery.

Deaths

	Age in Months		
Risk Factors*	0–1 (n = 53)	2–12 (n = 23)	12– (n = 6)
Syndrome	13	7	0
Noncardiac anomalies	29	17	2
Respiratory distress or prematurity	28	16	2
Cardiac surgery	21	20	0
None listed	19	1	6†

*None of the risk factors listed (except for surgery) is a mandatory entry in the computer system. Birth weight is not recorded. Hence, the emphasis on prematurity and respiratory disease in this table is probably underestimated.

†Of these, 1 had pulmonary vascular obstructive disease (age 28 years), 1 had a diaphragmatic hernia (age 1 year), 1 had a respiratory anomaly (age 3 years), and in 3 the cause of death was unexplained (ages 3, 7, 9).

left-to-right shunt may be quantified. The size of the ductus, the size of the pulmonary arteries, and the position of the ventricular septum may give information about the level of pulmonary artery pressure. Although there is usually a gradient of pressure observed between the aorta and pulmo-nary artery, absence of a gradient may be taken as evidence of pulmonary hypertension at the systemic level. In upward of 60% of patients, some incompetence of the foramen ovale, allowing left-to-right shunting, may be discovered using Doppler techniques (Fig. 5).[41]

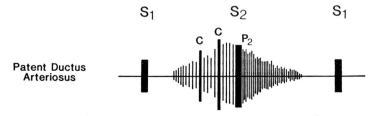

Figure 3. Diagram of the machinery murmur of patent ductus arteriosus. Typically the murmur is maximally loud at the time of the second heart sound. Clicking noises in systole contribute to the machinery sound.

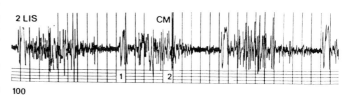

Figure 4. Phonocardiogram of the murmur of a ductus arteriosus with simultaneous recordings of aortic (Ao) and pulmonary artery (PA) pressure. The murmur is continuous at the second left interspace. Note the late systolic crescendo, with the apex of the murmur coinciding with the second sound and with the peak of aortic systolic pressure. It is at this point in the cycle that the pressure difference, the gradient, between the aorta and the pulmonary artery is maximal. (From Nadas AS, Fyler DC: Pediatric Cardiology. Philadelphia, W.B. Saunders Co., 1973, with permission.)

The ductus is best imaged in a high, left, parasternal, parasagittal plane view. The ductus connects with the distal main pulmonary artery just superior to the left pulmonary artery. In this view the ductus is seen in its long axis, and both aortic and pulmonary ends can be imaged. Doppler color flow mapping in the same view demonstrates the flow through the ductus. Continuous-wave Doppler color examination is useful for estimating the pulmonary artery pressure by indicating the difference between aortic and pulmonary artery pressure.

Cardiac Catheterization

Cardiac catheterization is rarely needed for the diagnosis of a patent ductus arteriosus; it is reserved for evaluation of confusing findings or when there is suspicion that additional defects may be present. This was true before the advent of echocardiography, and now the need for diagnostic cardiac catheterization has been virtually eliminated.

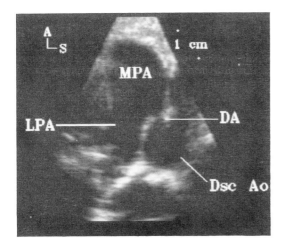

Figure 5. Echocardiogram showing a patent ductus arteriosus. A, anterior; S, superior; MPA, main pulmonary artery; LPA, left main pulmonary artery; Dsc Ao, descending aorta; DA, ductus arteriosus.

MANAGEMENT

Interrupting the left-to-right shunt is the goal of management of an uncomplicated patent ductus arteriosus. The reasons for intervention include elimination of congestive heart failure and promotion of growth in the small infant, prevention of infective endocarditis, and prevention of pulmonary vascular disease. For practical purposes every isolated patent ductus arteriosus without associated problems should be closed. Age and size are not a consideration in surgical management, even in the smallest babies. If the patient has failed to thrive or has overt congestive heart failure the ductus should be interrupted. Legitimate reservations arise when the ductus is small and of little physiologic consequence; then the only question remaining concerns the prevention of infective endocarditis.

Surgical ligation or division of the ductus is a time-honored and proven form of management with minimal risk, well-defined results, and minimal complications (Exhibit 1). This standard of care has been challenged in recent years by inventive techniques of ductal occlusion using devices extruded from cardiac catheters (Exhibit 1) (see ch. 14). The attraction of an ambulatory procedure that occludes the ductus without the problems of thoracic surgery is obvious.[40] Besides, if this approach fails, the surgical option can still be exercised. Unresolved problems concern the potential for harm. The numbers of times that a device becomes loose in the circulation, the cost in terms of X-radiation, and the problems associated with arterial introduction of very large catheters are being studied. For the present, in older infants and children, at the Children's Hospital in Boston all but the largest ductus arteriosus are electively closed using occluding devices. The size of the devices available limits their use to children older than 18 months.

Catheter closure of patent ductus arteriosus was first shown to be practical by Porstman[28] more than 20 years ago. Present-day technique utilizes a single venous catheter and an ingenious double umbrella device proposed by Rashkind.[3,29,30,31] Under general anesthesia, the tip of a No. 7 French sheath is positioned at the aortic end of the ductus, and a device that opens like an umbrella is extruded from the catheter. The open umbrella is pulled against the aortic wall; then the rest of the device, another umbrella in reversed orientation, is allowed to open. If this can be appropriately seated, as proved by angiography, the device is released. The arms of the umbrellas are covered with cloth that has been soaked in a thrombolytic solution before its use. The use of heparin is avoided in these procedures (see Fig. 28, ch. 14).

After the placement of several hundred devices by cardiologists in several institutions, the following statements can be made:

1. The ductus must be small enough to hold the device. Ductus large enough to allow the largest devices to pass through have been encountered, and retrieval of the device by catheter or surgical techniques has usually been considered necessary.

2. Although most ductus are occluded, some still allow a small left-to-right shunt. A residual shunt in a patient who was subjected to the procedure only to prevent later infective endocarditis should, perhaps, indicate failure, although subsequent surgery is still possible. Whether a persistent shunt detected only by echocardiography poses a risk of infective endocarditis is not known. There are limited data concerning the presence of residual shunting after surgery; some patients have a shunt following ligation.

3. Ambulatory cardiac catheterization is not always possible because of excessive bleeding (large catheters must be used).

4. Catheter closure may not be possible because arterial vessels are compromised and require heparin or streptokinase therapy.

None of these difficulties is crippling; most seem to be the technical difficulties of a new procedure and are probably surmountable.

COURSE

Given the ease with which a patent ductus is closed, the natural history of untreated patent ductus arteriosus is unlikely ever to be documented. Based on the admittedly poor, retrospective data available in 1967, Campbell[5] noted that after a heavy mortality in infancy, the main features are spontaneous ductal closure, bacterial endocarditis, late congestive heart failure, and the development of pulmonary vascular disease. Ignoring the infants, now recognized as the sickest patients, he estimated 20% mortality by the age of 20 years, 42% by the age of 45 years, and 60% mortality by the age of 60 years. He noted 0.6% per annum spontaneous closure. Persistent patency of the ductus arteriosus among adults is associated with significant mortality, with or without surgery.[11]

An infant with congestive heart failure caused by a patent ductus arteriosus may be helped with anticongestive medications, but the sure way to improve the symptoms and, above all, to help the baby grow, is to interrupt the left-to-right shunt. Unfortunately, catheter devices suitable for use in infants are not yet available. Congestive heart failure first appearing after the age of 6 months is rare.

The management of a patent ductus arteriosus in a premature infant will be discussed later.

An untreated large patent ductus arteriosus may cause **pulmonary vascular obstructive disease,** occasionally as early as 10 months of age and commonly by the age of two years. If the infant has not been seen in early infancy the first examination may not reveal a characteristic murmur; the peripheral pulses may not be bounding; the heart may not be very large. The electrocardiogram may show pure right ventricular hypertrophy. On chest x-ray a large main pulmonary artery may be visible (Fig. 6). Echocardiograms, even if not clearly documenting the diagnosis, will cause sufficient concern to require cardiac catheterization, the most reliable way to assess the degree of pulmonary resistance and provide the information needed to decide whether surgery is possible. When repeated observations within a single cardiac catheterization show pulmonary resistance measurements over 8.0 units, or when there is a dominant right-to-left shunt, surgery should be avoided. Efforts should be made to influence the pulmonary arteriolar resistance using high concentrations of ambient oxygen or other substances known to affect pulmonary resistance (Fig. 7). Well-documented and significant variation in pulmonary arteriolar resistance

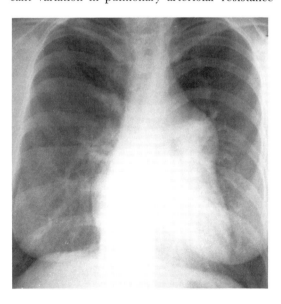

Figure 6. Chest x-ray in a young woman with a large patent ductus arteriosus and advanced pulmonary vascular disease. This patient died within a year after this picture was taken. Note the very large main pulmonary artery and the near normal size of the heart.

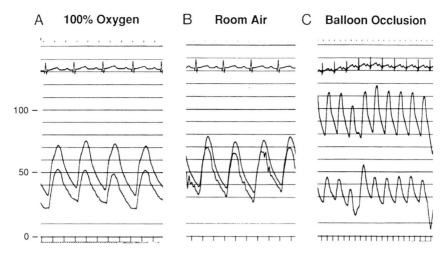

Figure 7. Pulmonary and aortic pressure tracings in a 3-year-old child with a large patent ductus arteriosus and elevated pulmonary vascular resistance. **A,** Breathing 100% oxygen. The pulmonary artery pressure is lower at the time the left-to-right shunt was very large. **B,** Breathing room air. The pressures are virtually identical at the time the left-to-right shunt was minimal and estimated pulmonary vascular resistance was prohibitively high. **C,** With the ductus occluded by a balloon. Note the wide separation of pressures. The ductus was later divided and the child is well without evidence of heart disease.

may tip the balance toward surgery, particularly if the patient is an infant or toddler, because these babies could not have had pulmonary vascular disease for long. As a corollary, pulmonary vascular disease known to be present for several years is taken as a contraindication to surgery even if the resistance data are suggestively favorable. Temporary balloon occlusion of the ductus may provide further indication of the likely success of ductal closure.

Without surgery, survival with pulmonary vascular disease is a matter of some years, possibly decades. Polycythemia may be quite marked despite minimal, if any, blueness of the lips and fingernails, because the ductus directs the right-to-left shunt into the descending aorta, causing greater stimulation of the kidneys to produce erythropoietin and hemoglobin than is suspected from the degree of upper body cyanosis.

An untreated patent ductus arteriosus is a favored site for **infective endocarditis.** The chance of developing endocarditis is estimated at 0.45% per year.[5] Ligation or division of the ductus eliminates this possibility.

Ductal ligation has been followed by later appearance of a left-to-right shunt either because of an incomplete ligation or **recanalization.**[8] Double ligation may be helpful but does not eliminate the possibility of recanalization. Dividing the ductus and oversewing the stumps is not associated with recanalization. The difficulties and dangers of division, although small, are nonetheless sufficient that many surgeons favor ligation in most circumstances.

Generally, late **spontaneous closure** of a persistently patent ductus arteriosus is observed in infants with a small ductus. It is difficult to document this clinical observation with certainty because the ductus is small and documentation has been largely dependent on auscultation. There were 64 patients labeled as having spontaneous closure of a persistently patent ductus in the files of Children's Hospital in Boston between 1973 and 1987 (Exhibit 1).

Occasionally, a child is referred with the late discovery of a typical ductus arteriosus murmur. Some of these children are found to have an intermittently audible murmur and can be shown to have an **intermittently closed ductus arteriosus.**[7] The oldest patient encountered with these findings was a 15-year-old girl followed for years by a reliable pediatrician, who first noticed the murmur when she was 14 years old. Subsequently the murmur was heard variably and, finally, the ductus was occluded with a Rashkind device. Variability of ductal patency has been documented occasionally by echocardiography.[9,12,37,39]

VARIATIONS

Ductus Arteriosus in Premature Infants

Natural closure of the ductus arteriosus is programmed to occur within a few minutes to a few hours after delivery, following normal gestation. With survival after incomplete gestation, the timing of ductal closure may be delayed in proportion to prematurity. In a premature infant, a patent ductus arteriosus, with or without the respiratory distress syndrome, may add significant morbidity and mortality.[20]

Prevalence. Of 1,700 infants weighing less than

1,750 gm at birth, 20.5% had a patent ductus arteriosus;[14] 42% of these weighed less than 1000 gm and 7% weighed more than 1500 gm.[10] Among 146 older infants with patent ductus arteriosus, 19% weighed less than 2 kg at birth and 17% were born after less than 34 weeks of gestation.

Anatomy. The gross and histopathologic anatomy of a premature ductus arteriosus is indistinguishable from that of the normal patent ductus arteriosus.[18]

Physiology. The level of pulmonary resistance in premature infants is less than it is in full-term babies.[21] This, coupled with persistent patency of the ductus, favors the early appearance of left-to-right shunt, which may be excessive. The presence of respiratory distress promotes continued patency of the ductus because of hypoxemia, and this aggravates respiratory difficulty either because of congestive heart failure or because of the excessive pulmonary blood volume associated with the shunt, which compromises the intrathoracic volume available for respiration. Pulmonary venous oxygen desaturation and pulmonary hypertension were constant features of premature infants who underwent cardiac catheterization in the early days of studying this problem.

Clinical Manifestations. Although prominence of the peripheral pulses is a good indication that the ductus is large enough to cause problems, the murmur in premature infants is usually atypical, rarely being more than a systolic murmur, and not necessarily crescendo. Indeed, any systolic murmur in a very small premature baby should be considered indicative of a patent ductus arteriosus until proved otherwise.[10] Rarely, a premature infant may have a known patent ductus with no audible murmur. Whether this indicates a very large ductus or equal resistance to flow in both the pulmonary and systemic circuits is a matter of opinion. The author favors the latter explanation.

Electrocardiography. The electrocardiogram shows tachycardia, right axis deviation, and right ventricular hypertrophy that is rarely in excess of that normally expected for the age.

Chest X-ray. The chest x-ray is dominated by signs of the respiratory distress syndrome. There is commonly enough gross pulmonary opacity to obscure the cardiac shadow completely.

Echocardiography. Not only does echocardiography confirm the presence of an open ductus arteriosus, but it provides excellent information on which to base the estimation of the size of the shunt, the level of pulmonary pressure, and the response to indomethacin.[34,35]

Cardiac Catheterization. Cardiac catheterization is not used for this condition.

Management. The controversy about the relative merits of indomethacin or surgery[24] to close a patent ductus arteriosus in the management of respiratory distress in premature infants provoked a multicenter study. The National Collaborative Study on Patent Ductus Arteriosus in Prematures[14] recommended the following treatment regimen for babies with hemodynamically significant patent ductus (diagnosed by clinical means and confirmed by echocardiography):

1. There should be 48 hours of conventional management (respiratory assistance and anticongestants).

2. If no closure occurs, indomethacin (0.2 mg/kg, first dose) is administered intravenously, to be followed by two further doses at 12-hour intervals. For babies less than 48 hours old, on account of their poor renal function, the subsequent second and third doses should be 0.1 mg/kg. Infants older than 48 hours receive 0.2 mg/kg for the second and third doses.

With this management schema, about 80% of the ductus will close or become hemodynamically insignificant and remain so. For babies in whom this plan is not effective, surgery (with risk of less than 3%) is recommended.[38]

Possible adverse effects of indomethacin are under investigation.[2] Indomethacin used to treat premature labor has been shown to constrict the fetal ductus.[25]

Course. In the National Collaborative Study, the overall mortality rate by the age of 1 year was approximately 20%, principally owing to pulmonary insufficiency, intracranial hemorrhage, necrotizing enterocolitis, and sepsis. It is unlikely that the ductus played the dominant role in the ultimate outcome for these babies; severe untoward events and death were caused mostly by prematurity and the respiratory distress syndrome. It must be remembered also that at 1 year of age 65–70% of the original group were alive without major handicaps.

Even with the best of management, some premature infants will succumb. The mortality associated with ductus ligation is significant; all of the early and late deaths encountered among patients with surgically managed patent ductus arteriosus at the Children's Hospital in Boston in the past 15 years were among premature infants (Exhibit 1).

The surviving small premature babies require continued observation for some months because ductus may remain patent or reopen later, whether they are treated medically or surgically.[6,8]

Aneurysm of the Ductus Arteriosus

Aneurysm of the closed ductus arteriosus is a variation of the normal ductus diverticulum (the remnant of the ductus at the point of attachment to the aorta). When the diverticulum is large, it is described as an aneurysm. Rarely, the aneurysmal diverticulum may cause obstruction of the aorta,[22] develop clots, obstruct the pulmonary artery,[13,19] be a source of emboli, become infected, or rupture.

Maternal Rubella

The dreadful consequences of maternal rubella about the time of conception are nearly a thing of the past. These variously blind, deaf, retarded infants, who often have a patent ductus arteriosus, are seen nowadays only in populations that are not immunized.

In this disease, the ductus arteriosus may be large, sometimes large enough to cause congestive heart failure, although most often congestive heart failure, if present, can be readily controlled with medication. Although there is concern that poor growth is secondary to heart failure, ligation of the ductus does not necessarily correct the problem. Pulmonary vascular disease is not common, probably because of the frequent association of peripheral pulmonary stenosis. The combination of patent ductus arteriosus and characteristic peripheral pulmonary stenosis suggests the possibility of maternal rubella, even if other stigmata are absent.

The clinical picture is often dominated by defects of the central nervous system. Whenever it seems possible that ductal shunting is contributing to the patient's symptoms, the ductus should be closed. On the other hand, routine ductal closure for a bedridden child seems scarcely needed on physiologic grounds and infective endocarditis is sufficiently rare, especially in early infancy, that delay to learn how the other medical problems will evolve is, perhaps, wise.

REFERENCES

1. Alzamora V, Rotta A, Battilana G, et al: On the possible influence of great altitudes on the determination of certain cardiovascular anomalies. Pediatrics 12:259–262, 1953.
2. Appleton RS, Graham TP, Cotton RB, et al: Decreased early diastolic function after indomethacin administration in premature infants. J Pediatr 112:447–451, 1988.
3. Benson LN, Dyck J, Hecht B: Technique for closure of the small patent ductus arteriosus using the Rashkind occluder. Cathet Cardiovasc Diagn 14:82–84, 1988.
4. Calder AL, Kirker JA, Neutze JM, et al: Pathology of the ductus arteriosus treated with prostaglandins: comparison with untreated. Pediatr Cardiol 5:85–92, 1984.
5. Campbell M: Natural history of persistent ductus arteriosus. Br Heart J 30:4–12, 1968.
6. Clyman RJ, Campbell DC, Heymann MA et al: Persistent responsiveness of the neonatal ductus arteriosus in immature lambs: a possible cause for reopening of patent ductus arteriosus after indomethacin-induced closure. Circulation 71:141–145, 1985.
7. Cokkinos DV, Leachman RD, Lufschanowski R: Intermittent disappearance of a patent ductus arteriosius murmur: report of a case and review of the literature. Texas Heart Inst J 9:57–60, 1982.
8. Daniels SR, Reller MD, Kaplan S: Recurrence of patency of the ductus arteriosus after surgical ligation in premature infants. Pediatrics 73:56–58, 1984.
9. Dubrow IW, Fisher E, Hastreiter A: Intermittent functional closure of a patent ductus arteriosus in a 10 month old infant: hemodynamic documentation. Chest 68:110–112, 1975.
10. Ellison RC, Peckham GJ, Lang P, et al: Evaluation of the preterm infant for patent ductus arteriosus. Pediatrics 71:364–372, 1983.
11. Fisher RG, Moodie DS, Sterba R et al: Patent ductus arteriosus in adults—long-term follow-up: nonsurgical versus surgical treatment. J Am Coll Cardiol 8:280–284, 1986.
12. Friedberg DZ, Rajpal RS, Litwin SB, et al: Persistent reactivity of patent ductus with a review of the mechanism of spontaneous closure. Am J Dis Child 135:472–473, 1981.
13. Fripp RR, Whitman V, Waldhausen JA, et al: Ductus arteriosus aneurysm presenting as pulmonary artery obstruction: diagnosis and management. J Am Coll Cardiol 6:234–236, 1985.
14. Gersony WM, Peckham GJ, Ellison RC, et al: Effects of indomethacin in premature infants with patent ductus arteriosus: results of a national collaborative study. J Pediatr 102:895–906, 1983.
15. Gittenberger-de Groot AC: Persistent ductus arteriosus: most probably a primary congenital malformation. Br Heart J 39:610–618, 1977.
16. Gittenberger-de Groot AC, Strengers JLM, Mentink M, et al: Histologic studies on normal and persistent ductus arteriosus in the dog. J Am Coll Cardiol 6:394–404, 1985.
17. Gittenberger de-Groot AC, Strengers JLM: Histopathology of the arterial duct (ductus arteriosus) with and without treatment with prostaglandin E1. Int J Cardiol 19:153–166, 1988.
18. Gittenberger-deGroot AC, van Ertbruggen I, Moulaert AJMG: The ductus arteriosus in the preterm infant: histologic and clinical observations. J Pediatr 96:88–93, 1980.
19. Jesseph JM, Mahony L, Girod DA, et al: Ductus arteriosus aneurysm in infancy. Ann Thorac Surg 40:620–622, 1985.
20. Jones RWA, Pickering D: Persistent ductus arteriosus complicating the respiratory distress syndrome. Arch Dis Child 52:274–281, 1977.
21. Levin DL, Rudolph AM, Heymann MA, et al: Morphological development of the pulmonary vascular bed in fetal lambs. Circulation 53:144–151, 1976.
22. McFaul RC, Keane JF, Norwicki ER, et al: Aortic thrombosis in the neonate. J Thorac Cardiovasc Surg 81:334–337, 1981.
23. Miao C, Zuberbuhler JA, and Zuberbuhler JR: Prevalence of congenital cardiac anomalies at high altitude. J Am Coll Cardiol 12:224–228, 1988.
24. Mikhail M, Lee W, Toews W, et al: Surgical and medical experience with 734 premature infants with patent ductus arteriosus. J Thorac Cardiovasc Surg 83:349–357, 1982.
25. Moise KJ, Huhta JC, Sharif DS, et al: Indomethacin in the treatment of premature labor: effects on the fetal ductus arteriosus. N Engl J Med 319:327–331, 1988.
26. Olley PM, Coceani F: Lipid mediators in the control of the ductus arteriosus. Am Rev Respir Dis 136:218–219, 1987.
27. Olley PM, Coceani F, Bodach E: E type prostaglandins: a new emergency therapy for certain cyanotic congenital heart malformations. Circulation 53:728–731, 1976.
28. Porstmann W, Wierny L, Warnke H, et al: Catheter closure of patent ductus arteriosus, 62 cases treated without thoracotomy. Radiol Clin North Am 9:203–218, 1971.
29. Rashkind WJ: Transcatheter treatment of congenital heart disease. Circulation 67:711–716, 1983.
30. Rashkind WJ, Cuaso CC: Transcatheter closure of pat-

ent ductus arteriosus: successful use in a 3.5 kilogram infant. Pediatr Cardiol 1:3–7, 1979.

31. Rashkind WJ, Mullins CE, Hellenbrand WE, et al: Nonsurgical closure of patent ductus arteriosus: clinical application of the Rashkind PDA occluder system. Circulation 75:583–592, 1987.

32. Rudolph AM, Heymann MA, Spitznas U: Hemodynamic considerations in the development of narrowing of the aorta. Am J Cardiol 30:514–525, 1972.

33. Rutstein DD, Nickerson RJ, Heald FP: Seasonal incidence of patent ductus arteriosus and maternal rubella. Am J Dis Child 84:119–213, 1952.

34. Smallhorn JP, Gow R, Olley PM, et al: Combined noninvasive assessment of the patent ductus arteriosus in the preterm infant before and after indomethacin treatment. Am J Cardiol 54:1300–1304, 1984.

35. Swensson RE, Valdes-Cruz LM, Sahn DJ, et al: Realtime Doppler color flow mapping for detection of patent ductus arteriosus. J Am Coll Cardiol 8:1105–1112, 1986.

36. Talner NS, Berman MA: Postnatal development of obstruction in coarctation of the aorta, role of the ductus arteriosus. Pediatrics 56:562–569, 1975.

37. Thapar MK, Rao PS, Rogers JH Jr, et al: Changing murmur of patent ductus arteriosus. Pediatrics 92:939–941, 1978.

38. Wagner HR, Ellison RC, Zierler S, et al: Surgical closure of patent ductus arteriosus in 268 preterm infants. J Thorac Cardiovasc Surg 87:870–875, 1984.

39. Weber JW, Stocker F, Gurtner HP: Ungewohlniche variationen des links-rechts shunts durch einen ductus Botalli. Z Kreislauf 60:533–544, 1971.

40. Wessel DL, Keane JF, Parnes I, et al: Outpatient closure of the patent ductus arteriosus. Circulation 77:1068–1071, 1988.

41. Zhou T-F, and Guntheroth WG: Valve-incompetent foramen ovale in premature infants with ductus arteriosus: Doppler echocardiographic study. J Am Coll Cardiol 10:193–199, 1987.

Chapter 34

COARCTATION OF THE AORTA

Donald C. Fyler, M.D.

DEFINITION

Coarctation of the aorta is an obstruction in the descending aorta located almost invariably at the insertion of the ductus arteriosus.

PREVALENCE

Nine percent of all children with congenital cardiac defects have some degree of coarctation of the aorta (see Exhibit 1). When coarctation is the dominant lesion, it ranks as the fourth most common cardiac defect causing symptoms in infancy (between 0.20 and 0.62 patients per 1000 live births) (see ch. 18, Fig. 1) and accounts for 7.5% of critically ill infants with heart disease. At the Children's Hospital in Boston it is the seventh most common cardiac defect and coarctation repair is the fifth most common cardiac operation (see ch. 18).

EMBRYOLOGY

It has been suggested that less than normal blood flow through the aortic arch during fetal life may result in hypoplasia of the arch and, thereby, promote the likelihood that coarctation will develop.[49] Thus, patients with aortic stenosis would tend to have coarctation of the aorta. However, the patients with the largest isthmic flow, albeit retrograde, are the ones with the hypoplastic left heart syndrome who have a high incidence of coarctation.

It has been proposed that aberrant ductal tissue, lassoing the aorta in a juxtaductal position, constricts the aorta during ductal closure. The posterior shelf at the point of coarctation supports this view (Fig. 1).[73] This hypothesis allows for the possibility that not only is the ductus itself relaxed by prostaglandins, but strands of ductal tissue around the aorta, causing coarctation, may also be relaxed, relieving the coarctation, a phenomenon suspected but difficult to prove.

The rarity of coarctation of the aorta in association with pulmonary stenosis or pulmonary atresia, and the common left pulmonary artery stenosis associated with pulmonary outflow obstruction, suggests that patients with an embryologic left-to-right shunting ductus arteriosus are at risk for lassoing of the left main pulmonary at the insertion of the ductus, whereas those with a right-to-left shunting ductus are more prone to develop coarctation of the aorta.

Whatever theory is employed, coarctation of the aorta, including interruption of the aortic arch, is often associated with other cardiac anomalies (Exhibit 1). Bicuspid aortic valve and minor mitral valve deformities are common.[21,74] Less common are subaortic stenosis, parachute mitral valve or supravalvar mitral stenosis, as in Shone's syndrome.[66] That a particular genetic substrate is required is indicated by the presence of these associated cardiac anomalies, the rarity of coarctation in patients with Down's syndrome (see ch. 18), the predominance of males, and the association with Turner's syndrome.[39]

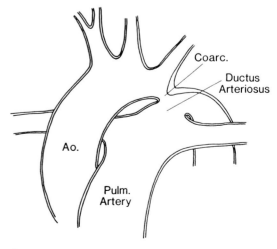

Figure 1. Diagram of coarctation of the aorta.

Exhibit 1

Boston Children's Hospital Experience 1973–1987
Cardiac Problems Associated with Coarctation of the Aorta
n = 1270*

Associated Cardiac Problems	Classified under Coarctation						Other Classification	
	Uncomplicated (n = 539)		Ventricular Defect (n = 217)		Interrupted Aortic Arch (n = 70)		Complex Cardiac Anomalies (n = 444)	
	No.	%	No.	%	No.	%	No.	%
Aortic stenosis	88	(16)	42	(19)	31	(44)	107	(24)
Valvar	76	(14)	24	(11)	10	(14)	52	(12)
Subvalvar	24	(4)	25	(12)	28	(40)	66	(15)
Aortic regurgitation	61	(11)	16	(7)	10	(14)	45	(10)
Mitral stenosis	28	(5)	33	(15)	2	(3)	65	(15)
Mitral regurgitation	57	(11)	25	(12)	8	(11)	66	(15)
Atrial defect or patent foramen ovale	61	(11)	87	(40)	48	(69)	267	(60)
None	197	(37)	—		—		—	

*9% of children with congenital heart disease.

In addition to 826 children classified as having coarctation of the aorta or interrupted aortic arch as the primary diagnosis, there were 444 individuals who had coarctation in association with other, more complex cardiac problems. 227 patients were first seen before 1973 and, as might be predicted, were mainly children with the least complicated problems and therefore most likely to survive. Only three children from the prior era survived with a repaired interrupted aortic arch.

Coarctation of the Aorta with Other Complex Cardiac Defects
n = 444

	No.	%
Hypoplastic left ventricle	116	26
D-transposition of the great arteries	64	14
Single ventricle	39	9
Double-outlet right ventricle	37	8
Endocardial cushion defect	36	8
Malposition	24	5
Tricuspid atresia	18	4
Truncus arteriosus	14	3
Tetralogy of Fallot	0	0
Pulmonary atresia with intact ventricular septum	0	0
Other	96	23
Total	444	100%

The vast majority of patients with coarctation of the aorta have other cardiac defects, often multiple lesions. Not shown in this table are the very common bicuspid aortic valves and the minor abnormalities of the mitral valve found in patients with coarctation of the aorta. Note the high incidence of aortic stenosis in the patients with interrupted aortic arch. Coarctation is ony rarely associated with pulmonary stenosis or pulmonary atresia.

ANATOMY

There has been some confusion regarding the classification and description of coarctation of the aorta over the years. Misleading age-related terms such as *infantile*, *adult*, *preductal*, and *postductal* coarctation were in common use. Then data were presented indicating that most coarctations that are present at birth and, in the past, would have been called *infantile*, evolved with growth and age into the *adult* form,[22] a suspected but unsupported observation until that time.

Almost without exception, the obstructing indentation of the aorta is located opposite the entry of the ductus arteriosus (juxtaductal). The infolding of the aortic wall is asymmetric, being most marked in the wall opposite the entry of the ductus. Often there is tapered hypoplasia of the aortic arch, which reaches its narrowest point at the coarctation itself. The degree of hypoplasia may be severe, but the narrowest point is at the entry of the ductus arteriosus (Fig. 1). The coarctation may be immediately above or below the origin of the left subclavian artery. Rarely it is associated with an aberrant right subclavian artery arising distal to the coarctation and, very rarely, both right and left subclavian arteries arise below the coarctation, the only vessels above the coarctation being the carotid arteries.

The normal aortic arch tapers, reaching its narrowest diameter at the aortic isthmus just above the ductus arteriosus. In the fetus, the blood supply below this point is supplied by the right ventricle via the ductus arteriosus; the blood above is supplied by flow from the left ventricle via the ascending aorta. For fetal survival, it is not required that blood pass either way through the aorta at the isthmus and, in fact, the blood flow at this point is small enough so that, normally, the aortic diameter here is the narrowest in the thoracic aorta.[59] With growth, this normal, narrow point disappears and, similarly, the abnormal hypoplasia of the arch associated with coarctation improves with time.

Coarctation of the aorta commonly becomes more obstructive as the child grows. The gradually accumulating intimal proliferation is balanced by compensatory recruitment of collateral circulation, including the intercostal, internal mammary, and spinal vessels. Thus, because of extensive collateral circulation, it is possible to have severe obstruction of the aorta with only a small difference in blood pressure between the arms and the legs. The collateral vessels become larger and more tortuous with time, the intercostals ultimately eroding the undersurface of the ribs (rib notching). The interconnecting arteries of the collateral circulation are present at birth, enlarging to accommodate the need for increased flow as needed.

Almost any cardiac defect may be associated with coarctation of the aorta. An exception to this rule is the rare association of pulmonary atresia, pulmonary stenosis, or tetralogy of Fallot with coarctation of the aorta (Exhibit 1).

Distortion or kinking of the aorta at the usual site of coarctation, without the usual anatomy of coarctation and without demonstrable obstruction, is sometimes called **pseudocoarctation**. This is a misleading term because the aorta is abnormal, not obstructed.

PHYSIOLOGY

The physiologic effects of coarctation of the aorta are a direct function of the difference in blood pressure between the upper and lower body. In theory, this difference could be large but in the average patient it is not often more than 30 or 40 mm Hg. This can be accounted for by the fact that collateral blood vessels circumvent the coarctation and also that only part of the cardiac output must pass the obstructed area. Although collateral vessels tend to reduce the resting pressure gradient across the coarctation, with exercise the upper body pressures may rise to high levels.[44] There is little reason to believe that the pressure in the arm rises to unexpectedly high levels, the pressures observed being those required to provide adequate blood pressure and flow to the lower part of the body. The mechanisms by which this is regulated include the baroreceptors, the renin-angiotensin system, and circulating catecholamines.[3,7,28,58]

Coarctation affects the heart by causing left ventricular hypertension and hypertrophy, the patient presenting with hypertensive heart disease.

CLINICAL MANIFESTATIONS

The majority of patients with coarctation of the aorta, usually males (56%), are asymptomatic older children, adolescents, or adults. They tend to have simple, relatively uncomplicated coarctations, discovered on routine examination of the blood pressure; in searching for the cause of hypertension, the coarctation of the aorta is uncovered. Others are found when femoral or dorsalis pedis pulses are weak or absent. A few, perhaps, are found when chest x-rays taken for noncardiac reasons show rib notching, an indented aorta, or cardiomegaly. Some are discovered because of the presence of murmurs (Exhibit 1).

Twenty to thirty percent of patients with uncomplicated coarctation of the aorta are first referred to the Boston Children's Hospital before the age of 6 months, usually because of congestive heart failure. This is in contrast to all other patients with coarctation of the aorta. With interrupted aortic arch, 70–90% are first seen in the neonatal period.

Children who have coarctation of the aorta that has not caused symptoms grow normally unless there is some added cardiac or noncardiac anomaly. Although there are reports that lower torso growth is affected in some patients, in our experience at Boston Children's Hospital this observation is overworked, particularly because this anomaly is more common in males where broad shoulders and narrow hips are common.

The femoral pulses are absent or weak and delayed compared with brachial pulses. Because the left subclavian artery may arise above, at, or below the coarctation and the right subclavian artery occasionally arises below, comparisons of the right and left brachial and femoral pulses are important.

Repeated measurements of systolic pressures higher in the arm than in the leg are sufficient to indicate the possibility of coarctation of the aorta, and repeated differences of 20 mm Hg or more represent significant obstruction. Normally the systolic pressure in the femoral artery is as many as 20 mm Hg higher than in the arm; therefore, discovery of a femoral pressure even a few mm Hg lower than that in the arms is suspicious. Generally, the diastolic pressures in the arms and in the legs are the same, although in some adults and even in older children, diastolic pressure gradients are reported. When the pressures are measured directly, there is damping of the lower body pressure curves compared with those for the upper body (Fig. 2). Diastolic hypertension in the lower extremities, despite a systolic pressure gradient, suggests hypertension of some other cause (i.e., abdominal coarctation with involvement of the renal arteries).

With direct measurement of the intra-arterial pressures at cardiac catheterization, the pressure differences usually are not as marked as those noted in a clinical situation, although simultaneous measurements of the cuff and intra-arterial pressures compare favorably. The reason for the difference is that many intra-arterial measurements with the patient sedated and lying on the catheterization table are being compared with a few cuff measurements in an awake, apprehensive patient who only recently climbed onto the examination table.

A systolic ejection murmur of low intensity is

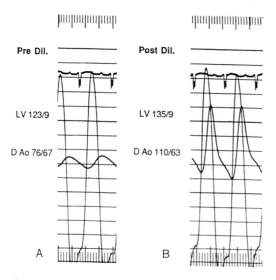

Figure 2. **A,** Simultaneous recording of descending aorta pressure (D Ao) and left ventricular pressure (LV) in a patient with a residual coarctation of the aorta. Note the damped aortic tracing showing a small pulse pressure and a systolic gradient of 47 mm Hg between the left ventricle and the aorta. **B,** A similar recording following balloon dilatation of the coarctation. Note that a gradient of 15 mm Hg remains. The aortic systolic pressure is now higher and is no longer damped.

audible over the base of the heart and also heard well in the axilla and the left interscapular region. Usually, the murmur is loudest over the back. Because auscultatory identification of systole and diastole is made by listening to the heart sounds and the origin of the murmur is downstream, diastole has begun for the heart before the systolic pulse in the descending aorta has ended. Consequently, the murmur appears to extend into diastole (Fig. 3). Usually, there is a systolic click, which can be attributed to a bicuspid aortic valve. In the older child, adolescent, or adult, collateral circulation may be sufficiently developed that continuous murmurs are audible over the intercostal arteries. In a more advanced form these are sometimes palpable and even visible.

Because of the association of mitral valve abnormalities, careful auscultation at the cardiac apex for the apical systolic murmur of mitral regurgitation and the diastolic murmur of mitral stenosis should be undertaken. In more than 25% of patients with otherwise uncomplicated coarctations, there is a minimal apical diastolic rumble or blowing pansystolic murmur, which suggests a minor mitral valve abnormality. The murmurs of associated aortic stenosis or aortic regurgitation may be encountered. Often the question of aortic stenosis is raised because the murmur of coarctation is a stenotic murmur heard well anteriorly. Generally, however, because the murmur of coarctation is not loudest to the right of the sternum or the suprasternal notch and is at least as loud over the back as it is anteriorly, the distinction between the murmur of coarctation and that of aortic stenosis is not difficult.

Electrocardiography

The asymptomatic child or adult with coarctation of the aorta may show left ventricular hypertrophy in proportion to the degree of upper body hypertension. Left-sided changes in the S-T segment and T wave are not part of the clinical picture of coarctation of the aorta and raise the possibility of an additional cardiac defect.

Chest X-ray

On chest x-ray the asymptomatic older child may show a prominent aortic knob, an indentation of the left border of the descending aorta at the usual site of coarctation and, during barium swallow, an opposing indentation on the esophagus. Rib notching is rarely seen before the age of 10 years.

Echocardiography

In infants the aortic isthmus and proximal descending aorta can be imaged routinely, using either a high, left, parasternal, parasagittal plane view (Fig. 4) or a suprasternal notch view.[32,69,70]

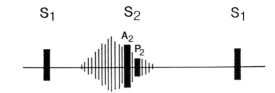

Figure 3. Diagram of the murmur of coarctation of the aorta. Usually, the murmur is heard best over the left interscapular area. In relation to the heart sounds, the murmur extends into diastole.

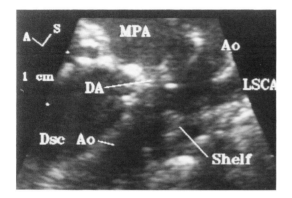

Figure 4. High left parasternal, parasagittal plane view in an infant with a discrete coarctation. Note the "shelf" (Shelf) opposite the ductal remnant (DA). A, anterior; Ao, aorta; Dsc Ao, descending aorta; LSCA, left subclavian artery; MPA, main pulmonary artery; S, superior.

Simple coarctation almost always occurs just distal to the left subclavian artery, at the site of insertion of the ductus arteriosus. The characteristic feature is indentation of the posterior and lateral aspects of the aorta by a wedge-shaped "shelf" of tissue. If the images are not of excellent quality, the thin lip of the shelf may not be detected, leading to underestimation of the severity of the narrowing. Often, Doppler color flow mapping is useful for defining the width of the flow jet. The segment of aorta distal to the coarctation usually is dilated.

Because there is often associated hypoplasia of the aortic arch, the transverse aortic arch should be imaged and measured using a suprasternal notch view. A diameter of less than 4 mm is associated with persistence of a pressure gradient, despite adequate repair of the discrete coarctation.

The branching pattern of the aortic arch should be determined using suprasternal notch views.

The gradient across the coarcted segment can be determined using continuous-wave Doppler cardiography from the suprasternal notch.[46] A small, nonimaging transducer is best because it can be inserted deeper into the suprasternal notch without producing discomfort. The transducer should be directed inferiorly and posteriorly and adjusted until a well-defined, negative flow signal is obtained. High-velocity, continuous flow is usually recorded (Fig. 5). The velocity proximal to the coarctation should be recorded with pulsed Doppler echocardiography, using the two-dimensional image to locate the sample volume proximal to the narrowing. This allows the proximal velocity to be taken into account when calculating the pressure drop across the narrowing. Otherwise, the drop in pressure is likely to be overestimated.

Indirect Doppler evidence for coarctation can be obtained by recording the flow pattern in the descending aorta at the diaphragm.[60,65] Normally, there is anterograde flow during systole, with a rapid upstroke and downstroke, followed by a small, retrograde flow signal early in diastole and minimal flow late in diastole. In contrast, if a coarctation is present, the upstroke velocity is reduced and there is a continuous, anterograde flow throughout the cardiac cycle (Fig. 6).

In older patients, the ability to image the aortic isthmus and proximal descending aorta is variable. The same views are used but the results are less predictable. The flow pattern in the descending aorta may provide evidence that a coarctation is present or absent. If adequate images cannot be obtained with echocardiography, magnetic resonance imaging should be employed.

Cardiac Catheterization

There is no need for diagnostic cardiac catheterization in a child with clinically uncomplicated coarctation of the aorta unless there is reason to suspect some additional problem that might be clarified.

Magnetic Resonance Imaging

This new technique demonstrates coarctation of the aorta clearly (see ch. 11).[10]

MANAGEMENT

Indications for Intervention

An uncomplicated coarctation with a consistent systolic blood pressure gradient between the arms and legs of more than 20 mm Hg is an indication for surgical correction. Generally, in the absence of congestive heart failure, surgery can be scheduled at the convenience of the family and the surgeon. Sometimes there is concern that the collateral circulation is insufficient to safely cross-clamp the aorta during repair. Cross-clamping of the aorta may result in spinal cord damage when there is inadequate collateral circulation.[8] Paralysis of the lower limbs occurs in about 0.4% of coarctation surgery[12] and can be related to absence of upper

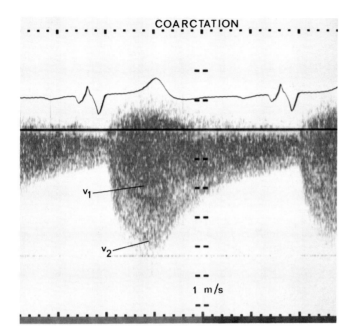

Figure 5. Continuous-wave Doppler tracing from the suprasternal notch in a patient with coarctation. The peak velocity in the coarctation is indicated by the outer envelope (v_2) and the velocity proximal to the coarctation by the dark band within the tracing (v_1).

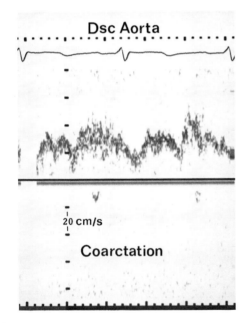

Figure 6. Doppler tracing from the descending aorta at the diaphragm in a patient with coarctation. Note the delayed upstroke and the continuous flow throughout the cardiac cycle.

arm hypertension or to the presence of femoral pulses, in effect, to a mild coarctation with limited collateral circulation. A small gradient may signify a minimal obstruction but could result from a more severe coarctation with good collateral circulation. Confusion about these possibilities can be resolved with imaging techniques (e.g., magnetic resonance imaging or echocardiography); rarely, retrograde aortic pressure measurements and angiography are required. When there is doubt, surgery is postponed.

It is important to recognize that reduction in the average diameter of the descending aorta to less than one-third of normal is needed to produce any systolic pressure gradient at all. With imaging techniques, a gradient of 20 mm Hg almost invariably looks like a severe coarctation.

Surgery

Surgical repair of coarctation of the aorta is accomplished by resection and end-to-end anastomosis,[18,20,30] or by using the left subclavian artery as a patch in a plasty operation,[13,78] or by using an artificial patch.[17,80] Very rarely a bypass graft is needed.[34] The technique of choice varies from institution to institution and is a matter of current debate.[5,82] At Boston Children's Hospital the surgeons individualize each case. Survival is good (Exhibit 2).

In the postoperative period there may be persistent, paradoxical hypertension and abdominal pain which, at times, can be very severe. Systolic blood pressures in the arms and legs are the same, but are inordinately high. The abdominal pain is attributed to mesenteric arteritis. These problems are thought to be related to: (1) the differential arm and leg resistance prevailing before surgery and persisting postoperatively.[28] (On histologic examination, the appearance of vessels above and below the coarctation is different, the coronaries being abnormal[62] and the upper aorta having a thicker and stiffer wall.)[64] (2) A disordered renin-angiotensin system,[53,58] (3) a disordered baroreceptor re-

Exhibit 2

	Boston Children's Hospital Experience 1983–1987							
	Surgical Experience with Coarctation of the Aorta or Interrupted Aortic Arch							
	Uncomplicated		Ventricular Defect		Interrupted Aortic Arch		Complicated*	
Age	No.	% 30-day Mortality	No.	% 30-day Mortality	No.	% 30-day Mortality	No.	% 30-day Mortality
Less than 2 months	17	(0)	28	(7)	27	(11)	89	(26)
More than 2 months	85	(0)	35	(0)	8	(13)	56	(13)
Total	102	(0)	63	(3)	35	(11)	145	(21)

*Includes some with interrupted aortic arch.
The initial mortality with surgical management of coarctation of the aorta is a direct reflection of the complexity of the associated defects and the age of the baby. These recent data suggest that surgical repair of uncomplicated coarctation of the aorta has virtually no mortality.

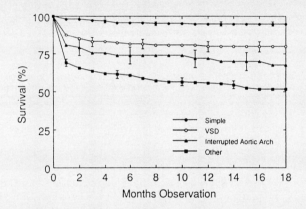

The survival curves for 401 patients with simple coarctation of the aorta, 185 patients with coarctation, and a ventricular defect, 67 patients with interrupted aortic arch and 390 patients with other forms of complex heart disease associated with coarctation of the aorta are shown in this life table. Patients first seen before 1973 are excluded. Compare with above table showing 30-day mortality for the most recent group of patients.

sponse,[3] or (4) abnormal levels of circulating norepinephrine.[7] Drugs to reduce the blood pressure, such as propranolol,[28] nitroprusside, or captopril, have proved useful in managing this problem.

Balloon Angioplasty

An unresolved issue is the role of balloon angioplasty. An unrepaired aortic coarctation can be dilated with good initial relief of the gradient (Fig. 2) and minimal short-term complications.[6,38,71] In general, however, the gradient relief is less than that obtained at surgery. Successful procedures succeed by tearing the vascular intima and part or all of the media.[43] This may result in the development of aneurysms, both in experimental animals and in children.[11] For these reasons, at Boston Children's Hospital we do not use balloon dilatation routinely in the management of an unrepaired aortic coarctation. However, there is no doubt that

balloon dilatation can be a useful procedure in a very sick infant or child with complex cardiac anomalies who faces high risk with standard surgical management.

With few exceptions, vascular access is obtained percutaneously via the femoral arteries. Biplane angiography is used to outline the severity and dimensions of the coarctation and the diameter of the aorta above and below the obstruction. A balloon 2.5–3 times the diameter of the narrowing is used first; in more than 50% of the cases larger balloons are required when no improvement is seen on the initial postdilatation angiogram. To prevent injury to the "normal" aorta, long (> 3 cm) balloons and those more than 50% larger than the unaffected aorta are avoided.

Recent reports have noted some long-lasting gradient relief,[2,38,50] but, nonetheless, the recurrence rate is high. The absence of angiographically visible tears in the vessel following dilatation of neonatal coarctations and the "soft" nature of the lesions (a waist is rarely seen in the balloon) suggest that dilatation may stretch ductal tissue, which subsequently contracts again.

In the limited experience of Boston Children's Hospital, complications have not occurred in neonates, children, or young adults following dilatation of native coarctation.

COURSE

Natural History

Coarctation of the aorta is a progressive anomaly. With time and growth the obstruction tends to become more severe and the collateral circulation more extensive. This must be factored into any plan of management. Because of the compensatory development of collateral circulation, there may be little change in relative arm and leg blood pressures while the actual point of coarctation becomes more obstructive.

There is little reliable information about the long-range natural history of unrepaired coarctation of the aorta and little likelihood there will be any additional information in the future because, nowadays, virtually all patients with coarctation of the aorta undergo surgical repair. Only a rare patient in the hinterlands, underdeveloped countries, or royal families escapes surgery. The following bits and pieces constitute the present extent of our knowledge of the natural history of this lesion:

1. Adults seen at autopsy (a less than precise way to determine natural history) who had unrepaired coarctation of the aorta died at a younger age than would otherwise be expected.[14,56]

2. Adults, often young adults, with coarctation suffer hypertensive heart disease, degenerative heart disease, and congestive heart failure.[29]

3. Individuals with long-standing coarctation of the aorta have a greater tendency to have atherosclerotic disease, myocardial infarction, and cerebral vascular accidents.[42,45]

4. Spontaneous rupture and dissection of the aorta occur in patients with coarctation.[72]

5. Infants with symptomatic coarctation of the aorta have a high mortality without surgery.[27]

6. Rupture of the central nervous system (berry aneurysms) is a risk for patients with coarctation of the aorta.[29]

Postoperative Course

It is important to recognize that surgery for coarctation of the aorta is palliative.[79] Not only is the area of repair enclosed in scar tissue and the repaired aorta less resilient, even obstructive, but if surgery is performed in the first years of life, recoarctation is possible. Postoperatively, patients have residual hypertension, earlier atherosclerosis,

subarachnoid hemorrhage, and premature cardiovascular problems.[29,45] Myocardial function is abnormal even years after surgery.[15] Many patients $(27-85\%)$[21,74] have bicuspid aortic valves and are prone to aortic valve dysfunction and infective endocarditis. These considerations account for the increased life insurance rates paid by patients with "repaired" coarctation.[75] It appears that the late complications are fewer if the surgery is performed earlier, but early surgery increases the chance of recoarctation.[9] At Boston Children's Hospital the incidence of reoperation is about the same regardless of the technique used in the initial operation,[82] although this issue is under debate.

Persistent or recurrent hypertension, despite an apparently good repair of the coarctation, is a well-recognized problem. Exercise studies of patients who have had repair of coarctation show a higher rise in systolic pressure in the arm than expected, particularly with maximal treadmill exercise.[26] This occurs even in patients with no evidence of narrowing at the operative site. Arm exercise does not cause the same elevation.[44] These data suggest that the scarred area of the coarctation repair is obstructive to the high flow required by the lower body during leg exercise, despite the absence of a measurable gradient at rest or even visible obstruction on angiography.[67]

There are four possible results from these exercise studies:

1. If there is equal hypertension in the arms and legs before and after exercise the patient has systemic hypertension and should be so managed.

2. With no gradient at rest and one that develops on exercise, no therapy is needed because on a daily basis the child suffers little added work.

3. If there is a minor gradient at rest that dramatically worsens on exercise, antihypertensive drugs should be used.

4. If there is a resting gradient, balloon dilatation should be used.

Postoperative Balloon Angioplasty[1,19]

In the postoperative patient, balloon angioplasty is safer and produces a more satisfactory result because the scarring around the repaired coarctation provides safety and allows use of larger balloons. Even patients with repaired interrupted aortic arches and the reconstructed arches of the hypoplastic left heart syndrome may benefit from this technique.

The procedure is similar to that outlined for the unrepaired aortic coarctation. Initially, balloon size is chosen to be 2.5–3 times the size of the obstruction, but the final balloon size is frequently larger (on average, nearly 4 times the narrowest diameter). As with unrepaired coarctations, the use of a Y adaptor (to allow frequent measurement of gradients and angiographic diameters) is very helpful in deciding when a large enough balloon has been used.

Among 25 patients with obstructions following end-to-end coarctation repair, 34 patients with obstructions following other forms of coarctation repair, 10 patients with narrowings after repair of interrupted aortic arch, and 6 patients with obstructions after palliation for the hypoplastic left heart syndrome, gradient reduction (50% or more) was achieved in 80% of patients.[43] Failures have occurred in long-segment stenosis, whereas discrete lesions appear to be dilatable regardless of the underlying anatomy, type of surgical repair,[61] or patient's age (Fig. 7).

One death occurred among the first 52 patients, a 3-month-old with a postoperative coarctation and severe congestive heart failure who bled into the retroperitoneum (see ch. 14) As of January 1990, 114 procedures (102 patients) have been accomplished (see ch. 14) with no further mortality.

Other complications have included temporary and permanent loss of the femoral pulse.

At present, given the documented early appearance of atherosclerotic heart disease in patients with unrepaired coarctations and in those who were first repaired at an older age, the value of relieving the obstructed aorta as early as possible seems inescapable, particularly now that operative mortalities have improved. Although at the Boston Children's Hospital we are not ready to recommend surgery for every infant less than 2 months old, surgery in the first year of life in an asymptomatic infant with coarctation of the aorta may be the best management. Early surgery and later balloon dilatation or reoperation may be double jeopardy but, in our opinion, the dangers of this plan are outweighed by the incidence of late complications with a single, late operation. The fewer years one lives with an obstructed aorta, the fewer problems occur later.

COARCTATION OF THE AORTA WITH INTACT VENTRICULAR SEPTUM IN INFANTS

Definition

Coarctation of the aorta in infants is almost invariably discovered because of congestive heart failure or while investigating other symptoms of cardiac origin. These sick babies are classified into four groups: (1) those with intact ventricular septum, (2) those with a ventricular septal defect, (3) those with an interrupted aortic arch, and (4) those with other more complex cardiac defects (see Exhibit 1). In each of these groups the infant may have additional atrial defects, a persistently patent ductus arteriosus, or abnormalities of the mitral or aortic valve.

Anatomy

The anatomy of coarctation of the aorta in symptomatic infants is similar to that seen in older patients (see p. 536), except that in infants the obstruction is more severe and develops more suddenly.

Physiology

An infant with severe coarctation of the aorta may present with symptoms of advanced congestive heart failure, having been well days before. Even before the advent of prostaglandins E, such an infant could look well 24 hours after the first hospitalization, having been vigorously treated with digoxin, diuretics, oxygen, and morphine. The mechanisms of this rapidly changing course are not clearly understood. The left ventricle is normally under stress at birth (see ch. 7) and with the added burden of a severe coarctation it may fail. Left ventricular failure results in left atrial hypertension, persistence or resumption of fetal pulmonary hypertension, and right-to-left shunting through the ductus arteriosus. Because of elevated left atrial pressures, the foramen ovale may be sprung open, allowing left-to-right shunting (Fig. 8) and further aggravating the situation by increasing pulmonary and left atrial blood flow. With the spontaneous closure of the ductus arteriosus, the left ventricle assumes the added load of lower body perfusion. These increasing burdens can lead to more congestive heart failure and more pulmonary hypertension. The infant becomes acutely, seriously, and even critically ill. Reopening the ductus

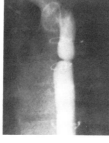 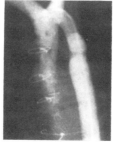 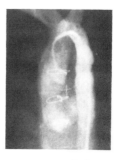

Figure 7.　Three aortograms of a patient with recurrent coarctation of the aorta. Left, before, ballooning; middle, after using a 10-mm balloon; right, after using a 12-mm balloon. PSEG, peak systolic gradient; Coa. Diam., internal diameter at point of obstruction.

Coa. Diam.	4 mm	7.5 mm	9.0 mm
Balloon		10 mm	12 mm
PSEG	31 mmHg		6 mmHg

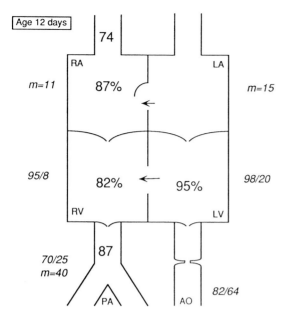

Figure 8. Physiologic diagram of a child with a coarctation of the aorta. This infant was very ill with gross congestive heart failure. Note the elevation of atrial pressures, the incompetent foramen ovale with a large left-to-right shunt, and pulmonary hypertension approaching systemic levels. This child responded well to anticongestive medications and was discharged without surgery.

with prostaglandins E (possibly also relieving the coarctation through relaxation of ductal tissue which was lassoing the aorta) and supporting the left ventricle with anticongestive measures may reduce left atrial pressure, reduce left-to-right shunting, and produce remarkable improvement in a baby's condition in a matter of hours.

Clinical Manifestations

It is a matter of interest that asymptomatic patients with coarctation of the aorta are rarely referred to pediatric cardiologists in infancy. Perhaps this is because of the difficulty of examining the femoral pulses in normal newborns, because the infants are asymptomatic, or because most coarctations develop after birth and are not recognizable in the first days after birth. The fact remains that pediatric cardiologists see very few asymptomatic infants because of a suspected diagnosis of coarctation of the aorta.

Coarctation of the aorta is rarely noted at birth unless there is an associated cardiac anomaly that produces cyanosis or a loud murmur. In retrospect, some infants are tachypneic from birth. Many develop congestive failure as early as the third or fourth day of life, and 60% of babies with congestive heart failure are hospitalized before the fourteenth day of life.[27]

The babies, most often males, may be tachypneic, "shocky," and dangerously ill. There are no palpable pulses. There may be gross evidence of congestive heart failure, pulmonary rales, hepatomegaly, and intercostal retractions. Auscultation is difficult because of tachycardia and respiratory noise. With response to medications the murmur of coarctation may become discernible and evidence of mitral or aortic valve involvement may be discovered. With improvement in the infant's condition, upper body hypertension appears and the difference in arm and leg blood pressures becomes more obvious. With the use of prostaglandins E to improve the infant's condition, the femoral pulses may become palpable.

Electrocardiography

The electrocardiogram of an infant with coarctation of the aorta, as an isolated lesion, shows right ventricular hypertrophy in the first months of life, and only later (usually after the age of 6 months) does left ventricular hypertrophy appear. If left ventricular hypertrophy is found in the first weeks of life, the diagnosis of uncomplicated coarctation of the aorta must be questioned. Right ventricular hypertrophy noted after the age of 6 months suggests that another defect is present, usually one producing pulmonary hypertension.

Chest X-ray

There is cardiomegaly and evidence of congestive failure, and, if there is left-to-right shunting, there is increased pulmonary vascularity.

Echocardiography

The coarctation is visualized and the pressure gradient is recorded. The diameter and tapering of the aortic arch are measured. The condition of the ductus arteriosus is described. The presence of a ventricular septal defect is excluded, the atrial defect or the foramen ovale is described, and the amount of left-to-right atrial shunting is estimated. The aortic valve is examined to discover whether it is bicuspid and stenotic and, if stenotic, the pressure gradient is estimated. Mitral valve abnormalities are looked for and, if present, estimations of the degree of stenosis or regurgitation are made.

Cardiac Catheterization

The sicker the infant and the more complicated the anatomy, the more necessary cardiac catheterization becomes. The purpose of cardiac catheterization is not only to confirm the anatomy, which, usually, has already been established by echocardiography, but to measure the physiologic consequences. Precise measurements of pulmonary artery pressure, left atrial pressure, and gradients across the valves are obtained.

Angiographic demonstration of coarctation is rarely necessary because other techniques provide information adequate for planning surgical repair. Under unusual circumstances or when the coarctation is part of a complex group of anomalies, it may be expedient or necessary to visualize a coarctation. This can be done with a left ventricular injection of contrast material while filming in the left axial oblique projection. Injection of the contrast into the aortic arch will show the aorta in better definition with balloon occlusion of the aorta below the coarctation while injecting a small amount of contrast (0.5 ml/kg) (Fig. 9).

Balloon dilatation of unrepaired coarctation at cardiac catheterization is undertaken in the unusual situation in which the surgical approach to the coarctation will carry increased risk (see p. 213).

Management

Any infant with an uncomplicated coarctation of the aorta who has congestive heart failure is a candidate for interventional relief. Those who respond well to medications can be followed along, but the price paid is some months or years of anticongestive medications and systemic hypertension. At the Boston Children's Hospital we favor surgery, at least until more experience with balloon angioplasty can be documented. With surgery the initial mortality is acceptable (Exhibit 2) and the late risk of recurrence is now between 9 and 24% in young infants.

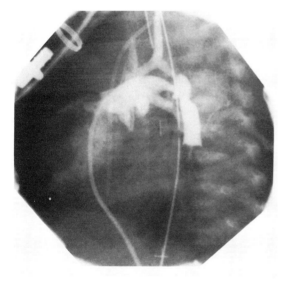

Figure 9. Lateral view of an aortic angiogram in a small infant. A balloon angiographic catheter has been passed through the ductus arteriosus into the descending aorta. With the balloon inflated, a small amount of contrast material, injected through the proximal orifices, backfills the ductus, the main pulmonary artery, a coarctation, and a tiny transverse aortic arch. (From Keane J, McFaul R, Fellows K, et al: Balloon occlusion angiography in infancy: methods, uses, and limitations. Am J Cardiol 56:495–497, 1985, with permission.)

There is little difference in the outcome following various surgical techniques for coarctation repair. All may be associated with inadequate relief of the coarctation or with later recoarctation. Often, the left subclavian artery is sacrificed in the repair, resulting in permanent diminution of the pulse in the left arm. The conclusion that these operations try to provide adequate lower body circulation while sacrificing some circulation to the left arm is correct. Problems caused by diminished circulation to the left arm are rare.

Course

Often, there is a residual coarctation on late follow-up. Among infants whose coarctations were repaired before the age of 4 months, 9% with uncomplicated coarctation of the aorta, 12% of those with a ventricular defect, and 24% of those with an interrupted aortic arch required reoperation or balloon angioplasty. The younger the child is at the time of original repair, the greater is the likelihood of a residual coarctation. This may be caused by incomplete repair of particularly difficult original anatomy or by recoarctation due to either limited growth at the anastomotic site or progressive obstruction.[47] Formerly, these recoarctations were managed with reoperation,[4,54] but in recent years balloon angioplasty has become the preferred treatment (see p. 213).[43] Any residual gradient of more than 25 mm Hg measured at rest should suggest this therapy. The long-range results of balloon angioplasty are not known but initial results are promising; the possibility of subsequent surgical correction and even further ballooning is not excluded.

COARCTATION OF THE AORTA WITH VENTRICULAR SEPTAL DEFECT

Definition

The baby who has coarctation of the aorta and a ventricular septal defect is included in this arbitrary classification.

Prevalence

Forty percent of infants with coarctation of the aorta also have a ventricular septal defect, representing the largest group presenting with symptoms in infancy.[27] Asymptomatic infants with coarctation of the aorta and ventricular defect are rare.

Anatomy

When there is a ventricular defect, tubular hypoplasia of the aortic arch is more common and more severe. Usually, the anatomy of the arch is intermediate between the anatomy in babies with an intact ventricular septum and that in babies with an interrupted aortic arch.

The ventricular defect or defects may be located anywhere in the ventricular septum.[48] Multiple defects are common.[23] Mitral and aortic valve abnormalities are common (Exhibit 1) but rarely cause significant clinical problems.

Physiology

Asymptomatic coarctation of the aorta with a ventricular defect is rare because any ventricular defect carries a larger left-to-right shunt when there is coarctation of the aorta. The size of the shunt is proportionate to the severity of the coarctation as well as to the size of the defect.

When there is a ventricular defect, the usual infant with coarctation of the aorta becomes sick at an earlier age than does the infant with coarctation alone. There is greater left-to-right shunting through the ventricular defect than can be inferred by the size of the defect because of the elevated systemic resistance imposed by the coarctation. Again, closure of the ductus arteriosus may cause a sudden deterioration in the patient. This usually occurs in the second week of life and improves with the reopening of the ductus when prostaglandins are administered. Why apparent closure of the ductus arteriosus in these patients is delayed until the second week of life is unknown. Possibly, the ductus closes on schedule in the first days of life and it simply takes some days for clinical congestive heart failure to develop or perhaps the ductus reopens with the onset of congestion.

With associated abnormalities of the aortic and mitral valves sometimes contributing significantly to the cardiac work load, it is not surprising that some infants with coarctation and a ventricular defect are desperately ill. The common finding of hypoplasia of the isthmus of the aortic arch usually contributes little to the physiologic state of these infants but becomes an important issue for the surgeon when it is time for repair.

Clinical Manifestations

Often, these babies are not recognized as having heart disease in the newborn nursery, there being no murmur and the femoral pulses seeming adequate. Within days the infant becomes ill, some as early as the third day of life, most between 7 and 10 days, and a few somewhat later. Often, the infant is suddenly, surprisingly, ill with gross congestive failure.

On physical examination the infant may be ashen, the peripheral pulses may be absent, and the liver enlarged. There are tachypnea and costal retraction. A systolic murmur is audible despite tachycardia and a gallop rhythm.

Electrocardiography

The electrocardiogram shows right ventricular hypertrophy, sometimes of abnormal degree for age. A leftward-superior QRS axis requires explanation, and left ventricular hypertrophy suggests some other diagnosis, although a large ventricular defect and a minor coarctation could be associated with this finding.

Chest X-ray

On chest x-ray the heart is large with increased pulmonary vascular markings. Sometimes pulmonary edema is evident.

Echocardiography

The anatomy is demonstrated; the severity of the coarctation is assessed; the degree of hypoplasia of the arch is measured; the location and size of the ventricular defects are noted; the function of the aortic and mitral valves is assessed; and the status of the ductus is noted.

Cardiac Catheterization

Having established the diagnosis, the decision to proceed to coarctectomy or to gain further information by cardiac catheterization can be troublesome. Any suggestion that additional surgery in the postoperative period will be needed (i.e., pulmonary artery banding or patching the ventricular defect) requires preoperative cardiac catheterization. Although postoperative cardiac catheterization of patients in the intensive care unit is undertaken with little reservation, it is desirable to avoid this complication.

Cardiac catheterization confirms the anatomy as described by the echocardiographers. It is particularly useful in locating additional ventricular septal defects, documenting severity of obstructions at the aortic and mitral valves, and providing a sharp image of the anatomy of the arch. The techniques used have been described (see ch. 14).

Management

Treatment with anticongestive measures is begun and prostaglandins E are administered. This, with digoxin and diuretics, allows the infant to recover and stabilize while the detailed anatomy is documented and an operation is arranged.

Virtually all infants with coarctation and a ventricular defect who are in congestive heart failure require surgery or balloon aortoplasty in the neonatal period. Theoretically, either relieving the coarctation or repairing the ventricular septal defect will improve the baby's condition. In fact, coarctation surgery, which does not require an oxygenator or hypothermic arrest, is the least complicated answer. Repair of the ventricular septal defect can be done a few days later if it is established that the infant is doing poorly. Many times the ventricular defect becomes smaller or closes spontaneously. It is possible to repair the ventricular septal defect and the coarctation through a single anterior chest incision in a small baby, but the added technical difficulty usually makes this plan unattractive. An alternative is to repair the coarctation and band the pulmonary artery to reduce left-to-right shunting.[31,35] In the view of our surgeons at Boston Children's Hospital, and others,[37] the distortion of the pulmonary arteries caused by banding is an unnecessary complication not always completely amenable to later procedures.

Formerly, the mortality associated with managing these infants was poor but it has improved greatly in recent years (Exhibit 2).

Course

Survival and growth are the immediate goals in managing symptomatic infants with coarctation of the aorta. Remaining problems usually can be dealt with later. Subaortic stenosis (often progressive) and obstruction at, above, or below the mitral valve can be troublesome.

COARCTATION OF THE AORTA WITH MITRAL VALVE ABNORMALITIES

Prevalence

Mitral valve abnormality associated with coarctation of the aorta is common (as many as 25% of the patients) (Exhibit 1). Mitral regurgitation or mitral stenosis that contributes significantly to the patient's course is rare (about 2% of patients with coarctation).[25] Mitral regurgitation with coarctation of the aorta is associated with a variety of abnormalities, including endocardial cushion defects, single ventricle, L-transposition and ventricular septal defect. Whether there is a ventricular defect or not, and even if there are other major cardiac anomalies, mitral regurgitation occurs in about 10% of patients with coarctation (Exhibit 1). In contrast, mitral stenosis associated with coarctation is notably more common among patients with ventricular septal defect.

Anatomy

The regurgitant abnormalities of the mitral valve include perforation of the leaflets and chordal abnormality, including rupture. Mitral stenosis may occur with an obstructing supravalvar ring, with insertion of all the chordae at a single point (**parachute valve**), or simply with hypoplasia of the valve and valve ring.

Physiology

Because the afterload adversely affects adaptation to mitral regurgitation, otherwise tolerable degrees of mitral regurgitation may be intolerable when there is coarctation of the aorta. The relative severity of the two lesions determines the clinical course.

When there is a ventricular septal defect, the physiologic effect of mitral stenosis is accentuated by left-to-right shunting, the flow across the obstructing mitral valve being greater than normal. Closure of the ventricular defect may reduce the gradient across the mitral valve. When there is severe mitral stenosis and elevated pulmonary venous pressure, there will be pulmonary hypertension which, in the presence of a ventricular defect, may be confusing. Whether the pulmonary vascular disease is caused by pulmonary venous hypertension or by the left-to-right shunt is a critical decision, because the first is reversible and the second may become irreversible with time (see ch. 28).

Clinical Manifestations

The clinical picture is an amalgam of the clinical features of coarctation of the aorta and the clinical features of mitral regurgitation or mitral stenosis as isolated lesions. In addition to the findings of coarctation of the aorta, there is an apical systolic murmur that transmits well to the axilla when there is mitral regurgitation and an apical diastolic rumble when there is mitral stenosis.

Electrocardiography

With mitral regurgitation and coarctation of the aorta, there may be left ventricular hypertrophy if either lesion or the combination is severe. When there is mitral stenosis, there may be right ventricular hypertrophy if there is pulmonary hypertension.

Chest X-ray

With severe mitral regurgitation, the heart may be very large, with demonstrable left atrial enlargement because, in general, the heart size is proportionate to the degree of mitral regurgitation. With mitral stenosis and a ventricular defect, the heart may be large because of left-to-right shunting, but with severe mitral obstruction the heart may be smaller because pulmonary vascular disease limits the shunting.

Echocardiography

With mitral regurgitation the left ventricle and left atrium are readily demonstrated to be enlarged proportionate to the regurgitant flow. The regurtitant mitral flow can be quantified. With mitral stenosis the valvar abnormality may be visible. The single insertion of the papillary muscles may be seen if there is a parachute valve. Hypoplasia of the valve and valve ring may be similarly demonstrated. Using Doppler techniques, a diastolic gradient across the valve can be measured. The coarctation may be directly visible in smaller children.

Cardiac Catheterization

The use of cardiac catheterization to evaluate these patients can be questioned because, usually, the details required for surgical planning are shown by echocardiography. Cardiac catheterization is carried out when there are other major cardiac anomalies or in any child in whom an operation for mitral regurgitation or mitral stenosis is contemplated. Whenever mitral valve replacement is under consideration, catheterization is used to document the physiologic status.

Management

Once it is decided that the patient has coarctation of the aorta and either mitral regurgitation or mitral stenosis, relief of the coarctation is undertaken. If significant mitral regurgitation remains, the child is managed as any other with mitral regurgitation. Valvoplasty is preferred but valve replacement may be required (10 cases in 15 years at Children's Hospital in Boston). A relatively large prosthetic valve can be accommodated because the valve ring is dilated if there is sufficient regurgitation to require valve replacement.

Mitral stenosis is a different problem. The valve ring may be small, is never large, and valve replacement in an infant is difficult. Sometimes, a barely adequate valve is all that can be inserted. The only reasonable choice may be to provide improved but incomplete relief with an obstructive artificial valve. The small, scarred valve ring seems to grow, at least in some patients with artificial valves, but repeated valve replacement may be required every few years.

Course

While mitral regurgitation or mitral stenosis is often discovered in early infancy, fortunately, mitral valve surgery is rarely required in the first year of life. Either lesion, particularly mitral regurgitation, may become progressively more severe with time.

COARCTATION OF THE AORTA WITH AORTIC STENOSIS

Definition

Aortic stenosis associated with coarctation of the aorta may be valvar or subvalvar and often is associated with ventricular septal defect and/or mitral valve abnormality. This discussion will be confined to those patients with aortic stenosis and coarctation with an intact ventricular septum.

Prevalence

Five percent of infants critically ill with coarctation of the aorta have aortic stenosis.[27] In 21% of the patients with coarctation of the aorta (excluding those with complex cardiac defects), an aortic valve abnormality other than bicuspid valve is found, but only 2% of these are sufficiently severe to require aortic valve surgery.

Anatomy

The aortic outflow obstruction associated with coarctation of the aorta may be valvar, it may be subvalvar, and, in the case of Williams' syndrome, it may be supravalvar. Subvalvar obstruction is more common when there is an interrupted aortic arch (Exhibit 1).

Physiology

While aortic stenosis and coarctation present the problem of two obstructions in series, the higher coronary perfusion pressure may permit more severe aortic stenosis than might have otherwise been anticipated.

Clinical Manifestations

These patients are discovered early in infancy, some because of the development of congestive heart failure and others because of the discovery of a loud murmur of aortic stenosis. Unlike uncomplicated coarctation of the aorta, there is a loud systolic murmur, sometimes with a thrill, at the base of the heart and along the left sternal border. There may be a click and there may be the murmur of aortic regurgitation. The difference in pulse pressure between the arms and the legs is sometimes less easily determined because the pulse pressure is generally lower when there is aortic stenosis. Measurements of blood pressures in the arms and legs will establish the presence of coarctation of the aorta.

Electrocardiography

If either of the obstructive lesions or both are severe, there will be left ventricular hypertrophy. Left ventricular strain pattern is characteristic of the most severe combinations.

Chest X-ray

The heart is not more than slightly enlarged unless there has been congestive failure or there are other associated defects. The features of either aortic stenosis or coarctation may be visible.

Echocardiography

The aortic outflow obstruction can be recognized, and its anatomy and function evaluated. The coarctation can be visualized.

Cardiac Catheterization

With clinical evidence of more than minimal valvar aortic stenosis, cardiac catheterization is undertaken either before or after repair of the coarctation, with a plan of carrying out balloon dilatation of the aortic valve.

Management

It is rare that both lesions are severe. If balloon dilatation of an obstructive aortic valve is to be carried out, coarctation must allow passage of a catheter appropriately large in diameter. If the coarctation is severe, surgical relief of the coarctation is undertaken, and, at a preplanned later time, cardiac catheterization is scheduled for possible balloon dilatation of the aortic valve.

Course

The combination of coarctation and aortic stenosis, which produces symptoms in infants, is dangerous and requires prompt attention. The mortality is high, although recent experience has been better. Older children who are asymptomatic do better.

COARCTATION OF THE AORTA AND COMPLEX HEART DISEASE

Coarctation of the aorta can be associated with any congenital cardiac defect. An exception may be tetralogy of Fallot, which is almost never associated with coarctation of the aorta (Exhibit 1). All infants with coarctation and complex heart disease are discovered in early infancy and most are critically ill. The coarctation is discovered by noting differences in arm and leg pulses or blood pressures, or during study by echocardiography or cardiac catheterization undertaken because of other more obvious cardiac problems.

Management consists of devising the best plan for the problems presented. With more than mild coarctation, coarctectomy is usually undertaken first; then the patient is reevaluated and remaining problems managed as seems indicated. The only occasion where this might be an error is when there is a patient who has diminished pulmonary blood flow and is dependent on the systemic resistance to provide what pulmonary flow there is. Sudden diminution of systemic resistance by removal of a coarctation may result in cyanosis. Fortunately, this is extremely rare and, if thought of prior to surgery, is avoidable. As might be expected, survival with those complex problems is poor and with every increase in complexity survival is even poorer (Exhibit 2).

INTERRUPTED AORTIC ARCH

Definition

Interruption of the aortic arch describes a point of atresia or absence of a segment of the aortic arch.

Prevalence

Twelve percent of infants with coarctation seen in New England had complete interruption of the aortic arch.[27] This amounted to 1.3% of all infants critically ill with heart disease or to a prevalence of 0.019/1000 live births. At the Boston Children's Hospital, interrupted aortic arch accounts for 5% of all patients with aortic obstruction (Exhibit 1).

Embryology

At least some interruptions represent an extreme form of coarctation of the aorta that has progressed to atresia. Those with absence of segments of the arch likely represent involution of the anlage of various parts of the arch. The association with other cardiac defects suggests some other embryologic background, the disordered circulation perhaps causing the interruption.[77] The association with an aberrant subclavian artery, the DiGeorge syndrome, and truncus arteriosus has led to the thought that Type B interruptions are different from Type A and possibly are related to developmental errors of the neural crest.[36,76]

Anatomy

The aortic arch may be interrupted or atretic in three subtypes, depending on whether the arch is interrupted distal to the left subclavian artery (**Type A**), between the left subclavian artery and the left carotid artery (**Type B**), or between the innominate and left carotid arteries (**Type C**) (Fig. 10). In each case, there is a ventricular septal defect; aortic valve deformity is common (60%), and often there is mitral valve deformity (10%). There may be complete absence of aortic arch continuity or external continuity without an internal lumen.[16] Type B is more common than Type A, accounting for as many as two-thirds in some reports.[52,55] Type C is rare. The ventricular septal defect is often subpulmonary in location but may be located anywhere in the septum. However, the septum may be intact, especially in those with Type A interruption. A bicuspid aortic valve is common (50–80%); an anomalous subclavian artery is particularly common when there is Type B interruption and the DiGeorge syndrome is reported in as many as 48% of patients.[76] It is our experience at

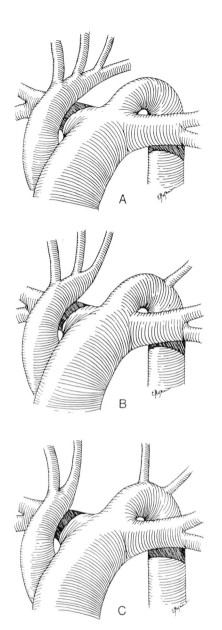

Figure 10. Types of interrupted aortic arch. Type A may be an extreme variation of coarctation of the aorta. Type B is the most common variety of interrupted aortic arch. Type C is a rare anomaly.

Boston Children's Hospital that these patients are likely to have abnormal serum calcium determinations and that less than the usual amount of thymic tissue is found at surgery, although beyond this there has been little problem attributable to the DiGeorge syndrome. Almost any cardiac anomaly may occur with interrupted aortic arch (Exhibit 3). Of particular interest is the association with aortopulmonary window and truncus arteriosus, both lesions also known to be associated with the DiGeorge syndrome.

Physiology

Other major deformities of the heart commonly associated with interruption of the arch may dominate the physiologic picture. At Boston Children's Hospital we tend to divide the case material: those with ventricular defect, patent ductus arteriosus, and valve deformity are classified as relatively uncomplicated and all others are considered under other headings (Exhibit 1).

Regardless of associated defects, the ductus arteriosus is required to supply blood to the lower half of the body. Alternate connections from the upper to the lower body are encountered rarely, but for practical purposes the ductus arteriosus supplies the lower body in the majority of infants. Spontaneous closure of the ductus arteriosus threatens the babies' immediate survival; without circulation to the lower body there is marked metabolic acidosis and circulatory collapse. Average survival is only a matter of days following birth. Presumably, the difference between the infants with coarctation of the aorta who appear in congestive failure in the second week of life and those with interruption of the aorta who appear ill in the first days of life is related to the presence and size of the orifice connecting the upper and lower aorta. Clearly, any opening at the point of obstruction makes an appreciable difference, because the ductus arteriosus likely closes at the same time whether there is coarctation or interruption of the aorta. Often, the use of prostaglandins E to open the ductus helps dramatically in either case (Fig. 11).[41]

Because only a fraction of the cardiac output passes through the aortic valve and systemic pressure is, in large part, supplied by the ductus arteriosus, subaortic stenosis, even if moderately severe, may cause no pressure gradient and consequently go unrecognized (Fig. 12).

Clinical Manifestations

These infants become desperately ill in the first days of life whether they have other major cardiac defects or not. Only those with a reliable blood supply to the lower body (i.e., persistent patent ductus arteriosus) survive longer than a few weeks. The infants are "shocky," tachypneic, and may appear terminally ill. Often, there is a systolic murmur. The peripheral pulses may be weak or absent, sometimes waxing and waning, and only with the improvement following administration of prostaglandins E does the difference between the arm and leg pulses becomes noticeable. The femoral pulses are usually absent or markedly diminished but may vary in intensity from time to time, depending on whether the ductus is open or closed. The child may be cyanotic or not, depending on the associated cardiac defects.

Exhibit 3

	Boston Children's Hospital Experience 1973–1987 Interrupted Aortic Arch: Associated Problems*	
Associated Problem	Uncomplicated n = 56	Complicated n = 74
Asplenia	0	4
Single ventricle	0	16
Hypoplastic left ventricle	0	10
Tricuspid atresia	0	12
Double-outlet right ventricle	0	8
D-transposition of the great arteries	0	8
L-transposition of the great arteries	0	21
Total anomalous pulmonary veins	0	0
Endocardial cushion defect	0	11
Pulmonary atresia with intact septum	0	0
Tetralogy of Fallot	0	0
Aortic valvar stenosis	30	31
Subaortic stenosis	23	26
Aortic regurgitation	9	10
Mitral valve abnormality	6	14
Pulmonary valve abnormality	5	22
Tricuspid valve abnormality	10	22

*Some patients had more than one associated anomaly.

Electrocardiography

The electrocardiogram shows right ventricular hypertrophy in the uncomplicated cases and reflects the abnormal cardiac pathology in others.

Chest X-ray

The chest x-ray shows cardiomegaly, often marked, and often with increased pulmonary vascularity, although this may not be obvious in the early newborn period.

Minor Laboratory Tests

Metabolic acidosis, sometimes quite marked, correlates directly with the state of the patient. The sicker the child appears, the more marked is the acidosis.

Echocardiography

Generally, the diagnosis in all its details is made by echocardiography. Initially, recognition of ductal dependence leads to treatment with prostaglandins E,[41] and later, with a more stable patient, the anatomic details are documented. The likely associated cardiac abnormalities should be kept in mind and the patient evaluated for each as the examination proceeds (Exhibits 1 and 3).[57]

The majority of infants with interrupted aortic arch have a conoventricular septal defect with deviation of the hypoplastic infundibular septum toward the aorta (Fig. 13). The ventricular septal defect is seen best in subxiphoid and parasternal views.[57] The left ventricular outflow tract should be evaluated in parasternal long-axis and apical two-chamber views because of the high incidence of outflow tract obstruction. The minimal diameter

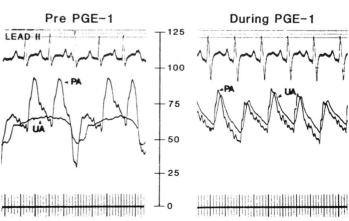

Figure 11. Pressure tracings before and after administration of prostaglandins E in a patient with interrupted aortic arch. Note the nonpulsatile tracing from the umbilical artery (the pressure variation is coincident with mechanical ventilation) and the appearance of pulatile flow after administration of prostaglandins E.

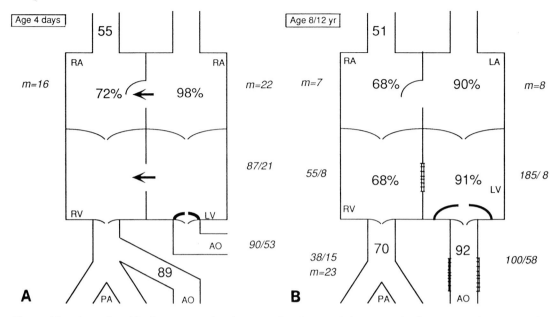

Figure 12. This 4-day-old infant was moribund on arrival and responded to prostaglandins E. **A,** Catheterization data at age 4 days, using 100% oxygen, showed equal pressures above and below a type B interrupted aortic arch. On angiography, there was moderately severe subaortic stenosis, which became clinically manifest after the ventricular defect was patched and a conduit placed between the ascending and descending aorta. **B,** Same patient 8 months later. Severe subaortic stenosis is evident now that the entire cardiac output passes through the aortic valve.

of the outflow tract should be measured from the parasternal long-axis view. A diameter as small as 4 mm may not be associated with significant subaortic stenosis after repair. Doppler evaluation of the outflow tract is best carried out using apical, right sternal border and suprasternal notch views. Absence of a detectable gradient does not exclude obstruction, however.

The ascending aorta is imaged and the diameter measured in a parasternal long axis view. A high, left parasternal, parasagittal plane view (Fig. 14), as used for coarctation, is the best view for demonstrating the arch interruption.[32,57,68] The ascending aorta ends in the brachiocephalic arteries without a posteriorly coursing transverse arch. The main pulmonary artery continues into the descending aorta through the ductus arteriosus. The dis-

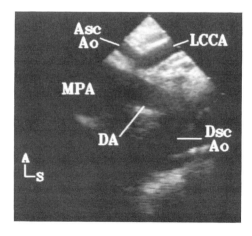

Figure 13. Echocardiogram in a parasternal long-axis view illustrating a conoventricular septal defect with hypoplasia and posterior deviation of the infundibular septum (arrow) toward the aorta. Note the hypoplasia of the left ventricular outflow tract. LA, left atrium; LV, left ventricle; AO, aorta; RV, right ventricle.

Figure 14. Echocardiogram in a high left parasternal, parasagittal plane view showing the ascending aorta separated from the proximal descending aorta, which is supplied by the ductus arteriosus. Asc Ao, ascending aorta; DA, ductus arteriosus; Dsc Ao, descending aorta; MPA, main pulmonary artery; LCCA, left common carotid.

tance between the distal ascending aorta and the proximal descending aorta can be seen in this view.

An aberrant right subclavian artery is common with interrupted aortic arch and can be diagnosed using suprasternal notch views. First, no right subclavian artery can be seen arising from the right brachiocephalic artery when scanning superiorly and rightward. Second, the right subclavian artery can be seen arising from the right side of the proximal descending aorta, adjacent to the origin of the left subclavian artery. The retroesophageal portion of the right subclavian artery cannot be imaged because of the intervening trachea.

Cardiac Catheterization

Given the anatomic diagnosis supplied by echocardiography, it may be useful to the surgeon to record the aortic arch anatomy in greater detail prior to repair. Echocardiographic indications of mitral or aortic valve abnormalities should be pursued and measured in terms of physiologic impairment. The angiographic views used for evaluation of coarctation of the aorta are also valuable for evaluation of interruption of the aortic arch (Fig. 15), except that retrograde examination of the aortic arch is, of course, not possible. Any suggestion that there may be other intracardiac anomalies should be pursued.

Management

Infants suspected of having interrupted aortic arch should be treated promptly with prostaglandins E, a response in the patient's condition confirming the impression of ductal dependence (Fig. 11). An emergency echocardiogram should be obtained and plans for surgery, with or without car-

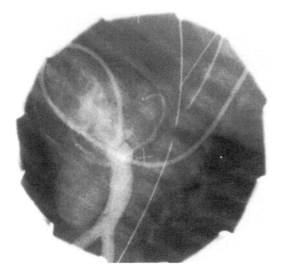

Figure 15. Anteroposterior view of a left ventricular angiogram showing a type B interrupted aortic arch. This picture is characteristic.

diac catheterization, decided. Once the metabolic acidosis has been reasonably controlled, surgical correction should be undertaken.

Generally, in all types, the aortic arch structures can be mobilized and a primary anastomosis of the upper and lower segments of the arch carried out, but artificial conduits or homografts may be unavoidable. Depending on associated intracardiac problems, repair of a ventricular septal defect or placement of a pulmonary artery band may be undertaken. If there is a truncus arteriosus, repair of the truncus as well as the interrupted aortic arch is undertaken. In principle, in so far as is feasible, all abnormalities should be repaired in one operation, although often a second operation must be contemplated because of the intracardiac anatomy.

In the last 10 years there has been steady improvement in the survival of these babies,[24,51,52,55,63,81] the probability of surviving the initial hospitalization being as high as 90% (Exhibit 2).

Course

Without surgery, uncomplicated interrupted aortic arch is a uniformly fatal illness, death occurring within days of birth. Additional intracardiac anomalies add to the problem.

Having survived initial surgery, there are many difficulties to be surmounted. In the immediate postoperative period residual lesions may become evident. When recovery is delayed, an unexplained murmur suggests an additional defect. It is a matter of some interest that subaortic stenosis (40% of patients) is not recognized at birth yet may become obvious days or weeks later. Anatomically it is dissimilar to membranous subaortic stenosis (see ch. 54), the obstructive ridge being thicker and the valve ring, smaller. Postoperative echocardiography and, often, cardiac catheterization are needed, sometimes within days of surgery, to suggest a confident management plan. With significant aortic stenosis, a residual area of obstruction in the aortic arch, or a residual ventricular septal defect, appropriate measures are taken.

There is little information about long-range survival. A number of patients succumb in the late management of other cardiac or noncardiac defects (Exhibit 2). The ultimate survivors are a tribute to the persistence of all concerned.

ATYPICAL COARCTATIONS OF THE AORTA

Rarely, coarctation of the aorta is atypically located in the abdominal aorta, sometimes involving the renal arteries and sometimes the thoracic aorta. Some of these obstructions are acquired, and often the presenting problem is hypertension, occasionally with congestive heart failure. There is a pred-

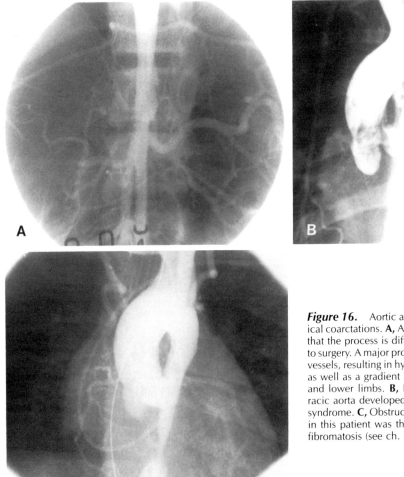

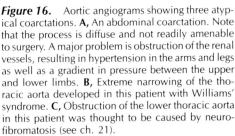

Figure 16. Aortic angiograms showing three atypical coarctations. **A,** An abdominal coarctation. Note that the process is diffuse and not readily amenable to surgery. A major problem is obstruction of the renal vessels, resulting in hypertension in the arms and legs as well as a gradient in pressure between the upper and lower limbs. **B,** Extreme narrowing of the thoracic aorta developed in this patient with Williams' syndrome. **C,** Obstruction of the lower thoracic aorta in this patient was thought to be caused by neurofibromatosis (see ch. 21).

ilection for females. The similarities of the obstructions among patients with **Takayasu's disease,**[33] **abdominal coarctation of the aorta,**[40] or **neurofibromatosis** (see ch. 21), and the aortic obstructions acquired by patients with **Williams' syndrome** are apparent (see ch. 31) (Fig. 16). At times, the distinction among these diagnoses is arbitrary. Treatment must be individualized and is dependent on the location of the obstruction. Renal vascular surgery may be required (see ch. 21). Progression of the obstruction may or may not arrest spontaneously.

REFERENCES

1. Allen HD, Marx GR, Ovitt TW, et al: Balloon dilatation angioplasty for coarctation of the aorta. Am J Cardiol 57:828–832, 1986.
2. Attia IM, Lababidi ZA: Early results of balloon angioplasty of native coarctation in young adults. Am J Cardiol 61:930–932, 1988.
3. Beekman RH, Katz BP, Moorehead-Steffens C, et al: Altered baroreceptor function in children with systolic hypertension after coarctation repair. Am J Cardiol 52:112–116, 1983.
4. Beekman RH, Rocchini AP, Behrendt DM, et al. Reoperation for coarctation of the aorta. Am J Cardiol 48:1108–1114, 1981.
5. Beekman RH, Rocchini AP, Behrendt DM, et al: Long-term outcome after repair of coarctation in infancy: subclavian angioplasty does not reduce the need for reoperation. J Am Coll Cardiol 8:1406–1411, 1986.
6. Beekman RH, Rocchini AP, Dick M, et al: Percutaneous balloon angioplasty for native coarctation of the aorta. J Am Coll Cardiol 10:1078–1084, 1987.
7. Benedict CR, Grahame-Smith DG, Fisher A: Changes in plasma catecholamines and dopamine beta-hydroxylase after corrective surgery for coarctation of the aorta. Circulation 57:598–602, 1978.
8. Berendes JN, Bredee JJ, Schipperheyn JJ, et al: Mechanism of spinal cord injury after cross-clamping of the descending thoracic aorta. Circulation 66(Suppl I):112–116, 1982.
9. Bergdahl L, Bjork VO, Jonasson R: Surgical correction of coarctation of the aorta: influence of age on late results. J Thorac Cardiovasc Surg 85:532–536, 1983.
10. Boxer RA, LaCorte MA, Singh S, et al: Nuclear mag-

netic resonance imaging in evaluation and follow-up of children treated for coarctation of the aorta. J Am Coll Cardiol 7:1095–1098, 1986.

11. Brandt B, Marvin WJ, Rose EF, et al: Surgical treatment of coarctation of the aorta after balloon angioplasty. J Thorac Cardiovasc Surg 94:715–719, 1987.

12. Brewer LA, Fosburg RG, Mulder GA, et al: Spinal cord complications following surgery for coarctation of the aorta. J Thorac Cardiovasc Surg 64:368–379, 1972.

13. Campbell DB, Waldhausen JA, Pierce WS, et al: Should elective repair of coarctation of the aorta be done in infancy? J Thorac Cardiovasc Surg 88:929–938, 1984.

14. Campbell M: natural history of coarctation of the aorta. Br Heart J 32:633–640, 1970.

15. Carpenter MA, Dammann JF, Watson DD, et al: Left ventricular hyperkinesia at rest and during exercise in normotensive patients 2 to 27 years after coarctation repair. J Am Coll Cardiol 6:879–886, 1985.

16. Celoria GC, Patton RB: Congenital absence of the aortic arch. Am Heart J 58:407–413, 1959.

17. Clarkson PM, Brandt PWT, Barratt-Boyes BG, et al: Prosthetic repair of coarctation of the aorta with particular reference to dacron onlay patch grafts and late aneurysm formation. Am J Cardiol 56:342–346, 1985.

18. Cobanoglu A, Teply TF, Grunkemeier GL, et al: Coarctation of the aorta in patients younger than 3 months. J Thorac Cardiovasc Surg 89:128–135, 1985.

19. Cooper RS, Ritter RS, Golinko RJ: Ballon dilatation angioplasty: nonsurgical management of coarctation of the aorta. Circulation 70:903–907, 1984.

20. Crafoord C, Nylin G: Congenital coarctation of the aorta and its surgical treatment. J Thorac Surg 14:347–361, 1945.

21. Edwards JE, Carey LS, Neufeld HN, et al: Congenital Heart Disease, Vol. 2. Philadelphia, W.B. Saunders, 1965, pp. 667–704.

22. Elzinga NJ, Gittenberger-de Groot AC: Localised coarctation of the aorta; an age dependent spectrum. Br Heart J 49:317–323, 1983.

23. Fellows KE, Westerman GR, Keane JF: Angiography of multiple ventricular septal defects in infancy. Circulation 66:1094–1099, 1982.

24. Fowler B, Lucas SK, Razook JD, et al: Interruption of the aortic arch: experience in 17 infants. Ann Thorac Surg 37:25–32, 1984.

25. Freed MD, Keane JF, Van Praagh R, et al: Coarctation of the aorta with congenital mitral regurgitation. Circulation 49:1175–1184, 1974.

26. Freed MD, Rocchini A, Rosenthal A, et al: Exercise induced hypertension after surgical repair of coarctation of the aorta. Am J Cardiol 43:253–258, 1979.

27. Fyler DC, Buckley LP, Hellenbrand WE, et al: Report of the New England Regional Infant Cardiac Program. Pediatrics 65:376–461, 1980.

28. Gidding SS, Rocchini AP, Beekman R, et al: Therapeutic effect of propranolol on paradoxical hypertension after repair of coarctation of the aorta. N Engl J Med 312:1224–1228, 1985.

29. Glancy DL, Morrow AG, Simon AL, et al: Juxtaductal aortic coarctation: analysis of 84 patients studied hemodynamically, angiographically, and morphologically after age 1 year. Am J Cardiol 51:537–551, 1983.

30. Gross RE: Coarctation of the aorta: surgical treatment of 100 cases. Circulation 1:41–55, 1950.

31. Hammon Jr. JW, Graham Jr. TP, Boucek MM, et al: Operative repair of coarctation of the aorta in infancy: results with and without ventricular septal defect. Am J Cardiol 55:1555–1559, 1985.

32. Huhta JC, Gutgesell HP, Latson LA, et al: Two-dimensional echocardiographic assessment of the aorta in infants and children with congenital heart disease. Circulation 70:417–424, 1984.

33. Ishikawa K: Survival and morbidity after diagnosis of occlusive thromboaortopathy (Takayasu's disease). Am J Cardiol 47:1026–1032, 1981.

34. Jacob T, Cobanoglu A, Starr A: Late results of ascending aorta–descending aorta bypass graft for recurrent coarctation of the aorta. J Thorac Cardiovasc Surg 95:782–787, 1988.

35. Kamau P, Miles V, Toews W, et al.: Surgical repair of coarctation of the aorta in infants less than 6 months of age; including the question of pulmonary artery banding. J Thorac Cardiovasc Surg 81:171–179, 1981.

36. Kirby ML, Gale TF, Stewart DE: Neural crest cells contribute to normal aortopulmonary septation. Science 220:1059–1061, 1983.

37. Kopf GS, Hellenbrand W, Kleinman C, et al: Repair of aortic coarctation in the first three months of life: immediate and long term results. Ann Thorac Surg 41:425–430, 1986.

38. Lababidi ZA, Daskalopoulos DA, Stoeckle H: Transluminal balloon coarctation angioplasty: experience with 27 patients. Am J Cardiol 54:1288–1291, 1984.

39. Lacro RV, Jones KL, Benirschke K: Coarctation of the aorta in Turner syndrome: a pathologic study of fetuses with nuchal cystic hygromas, hydrops fetalis, and female genitalia. Pediatrics 81:445–451, 1988.

40. Lande A: Takayasu's and congenital coarctation of the descending thoracic and abdominal aorta: a critical review. Am J Roentgenol 127:227–233, 1976.

41. Lang P, Freed M, Rosenthal A, et al: The use of prostaglandin E1 in an infant with interruption of the aortic arch. J Pediatr 91:805–807, 1977.

42. Liberthson RR, Pennington G, Jacobs ML, et al: Coarctation of the aorta: review of 234 patients and clarification of management problems. Am J Cardiol 43:835–840, 1979.

43. Lock JE, Bass JL, Amplatz K, et al: Balloon dilation angioplasty of coarctation in infants and children. Circulation 68:109–116, 1983.

44. Markel H, Rocchini AP, Beekman RH, et al: Exercise-induced hypertension after repair of coarctation of the aorta: arm versus leg exercise. J Am Coll Card 8:165–171, 1986.

45. Maron BJ, Humphries JON, Rowe RD, et al: Prognosis of surgically corrected coarctation of the aorta: a 20-year postoperative appraisal. Circulation 47:119–126, 1973.

46. Marx GR, and Allen HD: Accuracy and pitfalls of Doppler evaluation of the pressure gradient in aortic coarctation. J Am Coll Cardiol 7:1379–1385, 1986.

47. Metsdorff MT, Cobanoglu A, Grunkemeier GL, et al: Influence of age at operation on late results with subclavian flap aortoplasty. J Thorac Cardiovasc Surg 89:235–241, 1985.

48. Moene RJ, Gitterberger-de Groot, Oppenheimer-Dekker, et al: Anatomic characteristics of ventricular septal defect associated with coarctation of the aorta. Am J Cardiol 59:952–955, 1987.

49. Morrow WR, Huhta JC, Murphy DJ, et al: Quantitative morphology of the aortic arch in neonatal circulation. J Am Coll Cardiol 8:616–620, 1986.

50. Morrow WR, Vick GW, Nihill MR, et al: Balloon dilation of unoperated coarctation of the aorta: short and intermediate term results. J Am Coll Cardiol 11:133–138, 1988.

51. Moulton AL, Bowman FO Jr: Primary definitive repair of type B interrupted aortic arch, ventricular septal defect and patent ductus arteriosus. J Thorac Cardiovasc Surg 85:501–510, 1981.

52. Norwood WJ, Lang P, Castenada AR, et al: Reparative

operations for interrupted aortic arch with ventricular septal defect. J Thorac Cardiovasc Surg 86:832–837, 1983.

53. Parker FB Jr, Streeten DHP, Phil D, et al: Preoperative and postoperative renin levels in coarctation of the aorta. Circulation 66:513–514, 1982.

54. Pollack P, Freed MD, Castenada AR, et al: Reoperation for isthmic coarctation of the aorta: follow-up of 26 patients. Am J Cardiol 51:1690–1694, 1983.

55. Reardon MJ, Hallman GL, Cooley DA: Interrupted aortic arch: brief review and summary of an 18-year experience. J Texas Heart Inst 11:250–259, 1984.

56. Reifenstein GH, Levine SA, Gross RE: Coarctation of the aorta; a review of the 104 autopsied cases of the "adult type" 2 years of age or older. Am Heart J 33:146–168, 1947.

57. Riggs TW, Berry TE, Aziz KU, et al: Two-dimensional echocardiographic features of interruption of the aortic arch. Am J Cardiol 55:1385–1390, 1982.

58. Rocchini AP, Rosenthal A, Barger AC, et al: Pathogenesis of paradoxical hypertension after coarctation resection. Circulation 54:382–387, 1976.

59. Rudolph AM, Heymann MA, Spitznas U: Hemodynamic considerations in the development of narrowing of the aorta. Am J Cardiol 30:514–525, 1972.

60. Sanders SP, MacPherson D, Yeager SB: Temporal flow velocity profile in the descending aorta in coarctation. J Am Coll Cardiol 7:603–609, 1986.

61. Saul JP, Keane JF, Fellows KE, et al: Balloon dilation angioplasty of postoperative aortic obstructions. Am J Cardiol 59:943–948, 1987.

62. Schneeweiss A, Sherf L, Lehrer E, et al: Segmental study of the terminal coronary vessels in coarctation of the aorta: a natural model for study of the effect of coronary hypertension on human coronary circulation. Am J Cardiol 49:1996–2002, 1982.

63. Schumacher G, Schreiber R, Meisner H, et al: Interrupted aortic arch: Natural history and operative results. Pediatr Cardiol 7:89–93, 1986.

64. Sehested J, Baandrup U, Mikkelsen E: Different reactivity and structure of the prestenotic and poststenotic aorta in human coarctation. Circulation 65:1060–1065, 1982.

65. Shaddy RE, Snider AR, Silverman NH, et al: Pulsed Doppler findings in patients with coarctation of the aorta. Circulation 73:82–88, 1986.

66. Shone JD, Sellers RD, Anderson RC, et al: The developmental complex of "parachute mitral valve," supravalvar ring of left atrium, subaortic stenosis and coarctation of aorta. Am J Cardiol 11:714–725, 1963.

67. Simsolo R, Grunfeld B, Gimenez M, et al: Long-term systemic hypertension in children after successful repair of coarctation of the aorta. Am Heart J 115:1268–1973, 1988.

68. Smallhorn JF, Anderson RH, Macartney FJ: Cross-sectional echocardiographic recognition of interruption of aortic arch between the left carotid and subclavian arteries. Br Heart J 48:229–235, 1982.

69. Smallhorn JF, Huhta JC, Adams PA, et al: Cross-sectional echocardiographic assessment of coarctation in the sick neonate and infant. Br Heart J 50:349–361, 1983.

70. Snider AR, Silverman NH: Suprasternal notch echocardiography: a two-dimensional technique for evaluating congenital heart disease. Circulation 63:165–173, 1981.

71. Sperling DR, Dorsey TJ, Rowen M, et al: Percutaneous transluminal angioplasty of congenital coarctation of the aorta. Am J Cardiol 51:562–564, 1983.

72. Strauss RG, McAdams AJ: Dissecting aneurysm in childhood. J Pediatr 76:578–584, 1970.

73. Talner NS, Berman MA: Postnatal development of obstruction in coarctation of the aorta: role of the ductus arteriosus. Pediatrics 56:562–569, 1975.

74. Tawes RL, Berry CL, Aberdeen E: Congenital bicuspid aortic valves associated with coarctation of the aorta in children. Br Heart J 31:127–128, 1969.

75. Truesdell SC, Skorton DJ, Lauer RM: Life insurance for children with cardiovascular disease. Pediatrics 77:687–691, 1986.

76. Van Mierop LHS, Kutsche L: Interruption of the aortic arch and coarctation of the aorta: pathogenetic relations. Am J Cardiol 54:829–834, 1984.

77. Van Praagh R, Bernhard WF, Rosenthal A, et al: Interrupted aortic arch: surgical treatment. Am J Cardiol 27:200–211, 1971.

78. Waldhausen JA, Nahrwold DL: Repair of coarctation of the aorta with subclavian flap. J Thorac Cardiovasc Surg 51:532–533, 1966.

79. Wallentin I, Hanson E, Erikson BO: Non-invasive evaluation of the long-term results of coarctectomy in childhood. Clin Physiol 8:121–128, 1988.

80. Yee ES, Soifer SJ, Turley K, et al: Infant coarctation: a spectrum in clinical presentation and treatment. Ann Thorac Surg 42:488–493, 1986.

81. Zahka KC, Roland JMA, Cutilletta AF, et al: Management of aortic arch interruption with prostaglandin E1 infusion and microporous expanded polytetrafluoroethylene grafts. Am J Cardiol 46:1001–1005, 1980.

82. Zeimer G, Jonas RA, Perry SB, et al: Surgery for coarctation in the neonate. Circulation 74 (Suppl I):I-25–31, 1986.

Chapter 35

D-TRANSPOSITION OF THE GREAT ARTERIES

Donald C. Fyler, M.D.

DEFINITION

D-transposition of the great arteries describes reversal of the anatomic relation of the great arteries. Normally, the aorta is posterior and medial, and the pulmonary artery, anterior and leftward; in a transposition, each vessel assumes the position of the other. Normally, the aorta relates directly to the left ventricle and the pulmonary artery to the right ventricle; when there is transposition, the ventriculoarterial relationships are reversed. The vast majority of patients with transposition of the great arteries are readily characterized using these descriptions. Confusion is possible in the rare case when the two are in conflict, e.g., when the pulmonary artery arises from left ventricle and the relation of the great arteries to each other is otherwise not that of the usual transposition, but for practical purposes this difficulty with definition can be ignored.

Only patients who meet the above definitions of transposition and have undergone normal D-looping (see ch. 2) are considered in this chapter. Patients with L-looping and transposition are discussed elsewhere (see ch. 49). Those with tricuspid or mitral atresia and those with single ventricle or in the context of heterotaxy are discussed under the appropriate heading.

In half of the infants with D-transposition of the great arteries, there is an intact ventricular septum (Exhibit 1); in the rest there is a ventricular septal defect. Some of the ventricular defects are tiny, "virtually intact ventricular septum"; others are large and may or may not be associated with pulmonary stenosis or pulmonary atresia. Other possible associated cardiac anomalies are coarctation of the aorta, pulmonary stenosis, or mitral valve disease (Exhibit 1).

Problems of Classification

There is a spectrum ranging from double-outlet right ventricle (two great arteries arising from the right ventricle) to transposition with ventricular defect. There is another spectrum ranging from patients with transposition and some ventricular hypoplasia to patients with single ventricle. In each case the point of demarcation is indistinct and there are patients in between who might be classified differently by two observers or even by one observer on two different occasions. Because ventricular defects are more common in newborns and tend to get smaller, or even close, the incidence of ventricular defects or "virtually intact ventricular septum" varies with age. As a corollary, the earlier cardiac surgery is undertaken, the more ventricular defects there are to cause difficulties.

Pressure gradients across the left ventricular outflow tract are common and are sufficient to prompt comment in more than 50% of patients. Who among these should be classified as having pulmonary stenosis sufficient to be of concern is a judgmental matter. Measured gradients may overestimate the degree of anatomic obstruction because of the increased flow across the pulmonary valve in these children.

PREVALENCE

D-transposition of the great arteries is the second most common congenital cardiac defect encountered in early infancy and is the leading reason for transfer to a cardiac unit in the first two weeks of life. The number of children born each year with D-transposition (0.218–0.442/1000 live births) is remarkably constant (see ch. 18). The lack of variation in discovery, compared to other congenital cardiac defects, may be related to the ease of recognition of D-transposition because of cyanosis at birth (see ch. 18).

EMBRYOLOGY

It is obvious that the mechanism for division of the truncus arteriosus into two arteries is flawed

Exhibit 1

Boston Children's Hospital Experience 1973–87	
Diagnostic Groups	
Transposition Associated with	*No. of Patients*
Intact Ventricular Septum	362
Virtually Intact Ventricular Septum	78
Ventricular Septal Defect	222
Ventricular Defect and Pulmonary Stenosis	93
Total	755

There were 300 children with transposition of the great arteries who at some time were thought to have a ventricular septal defect; 78 of these were considered insignificant (virtually intact septum). The number of children with ventricular defect or virtually intact ventricular septum varies with age because in many of the small infants the defect closes spontaneously or decreases in size.

Cardiac Problems Associated with Transposition:
Percent of Each Diagnostic Group

	Diagnostic Group			
Problem	*Intact Ventricular Septum n = 362*	*Virtually Intact Ventricular Septum n = 78*	*Ventricular Septal Defect n = 222*	*Ventricular Defect, Pulmonary Stenosis n = 93*
Overriding Tricuspid Valve n = 33	0	1	11	9
Hypoplastic Right Ventricle n = 45	1	1	16	9
Tricuspid valve abnormality n = 224	20	27	45	33
Myocardial Problems n = 90	11	14	12	12
Coarctation of Aorta n = 64	4	9	18	4
Pulmonary Vascular Disease n = 63	1	8	7	2
Pulmonary Atresia n = 34	1	2	2	29
Pulmonary Stenosis n = 396	46	51	49	88
Infective Endocarditis n = 5	0	1	1	2

The recorded incidence of pulmonary vascular obstructive disease represents those who had a palliative Mustard operation because of pulmonary vascular obstructive disease and those who were discovered to have pulmonary hypertension postoperatively. Pulmonary vascular obstruction in patients with pulmonary stenosis was postoperative. Many patients had more than one additional cardiac problem.

in patients with transposition of the great arteries, but the reasons for this are not known. Shaher[69] discussed a number of proposed theories.

Transposition of the great arteries is unlike most of the other congenital cardiac defects. There is no obvious genetic component; the author has yet to see two children in the same family with this diagnosis. It is associated with fewer extracardiac anomalies than are most other congenital cardiac defects, perhaps fewer than the general population. Furthermore, transposition of the great arteries is specifically uncommon among premature infants and those with low birth weights.[23] There is evidence of a higher incidence in rural population,[66] with advanced maternal age, and with higher birth order.[67]

ANATOMY

In D-transposition of the great arteries, the aorta arises from the right ventricle, being most often positioned directly in front in a lateral view, and slightly to the right of the pulmonary artery in the anteroposterior view (Fig. 1). A small percentage of patients have the aorta positioned somewhat leftward. The pulmonary artery arises behind the aorta from the left ventricle, a position that allows straight line ejection from the left ventricle into the right pulmonary artery and probably accounts for the large right pulmonary artery and the somewhat increased flow to the right lung in these patients.[54] There is a subaortic conus as well as pulmonary and mitral valvar fibrous continuity.

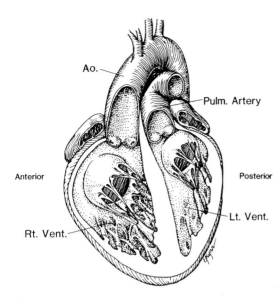

Figure 1. Transposition of the great arteries, lateral view. The aorta arises anteriorly from the right ventricle; the pulmonary artery arises posteriorly from the left ventricle. As diagrammed, there is no communication shown between the pulmonary and systemic circulations, a situation not compatible with life. For survival there must be communication between the two circuits, usually as a patent ductus arteriosus, ventricular defect, or atrial opening.

Because most of these infants are discovered at birth or shortly afterward, the foramen ovale and ductus arteriosus are patent at the time of first encounter.

Among infants with an **intact ventricular septum**, functional obstruction to outflow from the left ventricle (dynamic pulmonary stenosis) is common. This obstruction appears to be caused by bowing of the ventricular septum to the left, because of greater right ventricular pressure; the resulting proximity of the mitral valve and septum causes obstruction. These dynamic, outflow pressure gradients disappear with anatomic correction. Rarely, a patient may have anatomic subvalvar stenosis, a particularly difficult management problem.[33] Valvar stenosis is equally rare. Natural atrial septal septal defects are uncommon but a persistent large ductus arteriosus may be encountered occasionally.

Ventricular defects are present at birth in 50% of the infants with D-transposition of the great arteries, but spontaneous closure in the first year reduces the number of children with ventricular septal defects by one-third. Ventricular defects may be located anywhere in the ventricular septum. However, there is some difference of opinion about whether the relative frequency of the different types of ventricular septal defects is similar to that seen in patients who do not have transposition.[52] At Boston Children's Hospital we have not noticed a distribution convincingly different from that in infants without transposition.[63] The terms

"subpulmonary" and "subaortic" ventricular defects are confusing when the great arteries are transposed; the terms "infundibular" and "perimembranous" are preferred in this setting. Among the children with transposition of the great arteries and ventricular septal defect, additional cardiac anomalies are more common than among those with transposition of the great arteries and intact ventricular septum. Thus, pulmonary stenosis, pulmonary atresia, an overriding or straddling atrioventricular valve, coarctation of the aorta, and interruption of the aortic arch are more likely to be encountered when there is a ventricular septal defect. (Exhibit 1). Right ventricular outflow obstruction is rare.[51]

The coronary anatomy in transposition of the great vessels has been a matter of recent study (see ch. 54),[26,48,72] since the location of the coronaries influences the success of the arterial switching operations. A simple rule that accounts for virtually all variations is that the coronaries arise from the sinuses of Valsalva, which face the pulmonary artery, and the follow the shortest route to their ultimate destination.[25] Only a small number pose a problem in arterial switching surgery.

Minor abnormalities of the tricuspid[16,32] and mitral valves[50] are frequent but are rarely functionally important—mainly when the tricuspid valve serves the systemic ventricle after a Senning or Mustard operation.

Infants with a ventricular septal defect of the endocardial cushion type may have an overriding or straddling tricuspid valve. When the septal cordal attachments extend into the left ventricle, the valve is said to be **straddling.** When the valve allows direct flow into the left ventricle without straddling cordae, it is described as **overriding.** The implications for surgical correction are vitally important. In either case, with an overriding or straddling tricuspid valve, some right atrial blood is ejected into the left ventricle. When this happens, the right ventricle receives less than the usual amount of blood and is correspondingly hypoplastic.

PHYSIOLOGY

With transposition of the great arteries the systemic venous blood passes through the right heart to the aorta, while the pulmonary venous blood passes through the left heart, returning to the lungs. Survival is dependent on the amount of communication between these two parallel circulations. Those with an **intact ventricular septum** survive because of flow through the ductus arteriosus into the pulmonary circuit, returning from the pulmonary circuit via left atrial-to-right atrial shunting through a dilated foramen ovale (Fig. 2). For the required atrial shunt to occur, the flap of the fo-

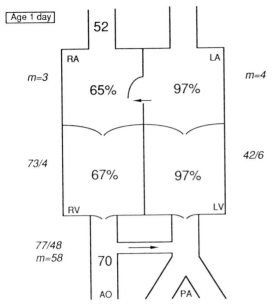

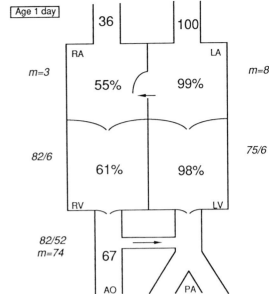

Figure 2. Hemodynamic diagram of the circulation with transposition of the great arteries with intact ventricular septum. This infant survives because of flow through the ductus arteriosus to the lungs and return of equal flow from the left atrium to the right through a "sprung" foramen ovale. It is believed that, at birth, an excess of blood is supplied to the pulmonary circuit by the patent ductus arteriosus, thereby raising the left atrial pressure sufficiently to force open the foramen ovale, and thereby allowing compensatory pulmonary-to-systemic flow. RA, right atrium; RV, right ventricle; AO, aorta; LA, left atrium; LV, left ventricle; PA, pulmonary artery; italics, pressure in mmHg; %, percent oxygen saturation.

Figure 3. Hemodynamic diagram of a newborn infant with transposition of the great vessels and intact ventricular septum who has received prostaglandins E. The pulmonary blood flow is excessive, the left atrial pressure is higher than the right, and there is pulmonary hypertension. Compare with Figure 4.

ramen ovale must become incompetent. At birth the pulmonary circuit is overloaded to the point that elevation of left atrial pressure causes bulging of the atrial septum toward the right, allowing decompression through an incompetent foramen ovale. It is apparent that the amounts of blood flowing into and out of the pulmonary circulation must be equal, or piling up of blood in one circuit or the other would be rapidly fatal. Increasing the ductal left-to-right shunt, as with infusion of prostaglandins E,[22,39] increases the flow into the lung, which must in turn be compensated for by increased flow toward the right atrium and systemic circuit via the foramen ovale. If the incompetent foramen ovale cannot accommodate the increased blood flow, the pulmonary circuit will be overloaded (Fig. 3). At best, a patent foramen ovale and a patent ductus arteriosus allow for marginal survival. Enlarging the atrial opening by balloon atrial septostomy or creation of an atrial defect by surgery allows for increased mixing between the two circulations with improved arterial oxygenation and survival. Administering oxygen has little effect on the amount of shunting into and out of

the pulmonary circuit and, therefore little effect on the systemic arterial oxygen saturation.

Rarely, a patient is born with a **large atrial defect** which allows equal shunting in both directions with good survival. These patients can be recognized because of the equilibration of atrial pressures and the lack of other shunts.

Infants with **ventricular defects** have greater opportunity for mixing and therefore better arterial oxygenation. The ventricular septal defect allows shunting toward the pulmonary circuit, the return to the systemic circuit being via the foramen ovale or the ventricular septal defect if it is large (Fig. 4). Again the left atrial pressure is higher than right atrial pressure, fostering an incompetent foramen ovale. Ventricular septal defects may close spontaneously, leaving the patient with the difficult problem of survival by means of bidirectional shunting through an incompetent foramen ovale (the patent ductus arteriosus by this time having closed). A large ventricular septal defect provides good mixing at the ventricular level, but the unimpeded pulmonary blood flow may result in a relatively pink patient in congestive heart failure.

Obstruction to the pulmonary blood flow by **pulmonary stenosis** will modify the balance between resistance to blood flow to the lungs and blood flow to the aorta. Among infants with an intact ventricular septum, the outflow of the left ventricle is commonly obstructed by dynamic subpulmonary

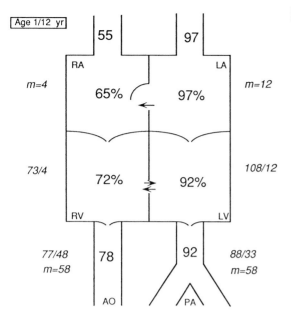

Figure 4. Hemodynamic diagram of a patient with transposition of the great arteries and ventricular septal defect. Note that blood flows toward the lungs via the ventricular defect and from the lungs via both a "sprung" foramen ovale and the ventricular defect. The arterial oxygen saturation (78%) is compatible with growth.

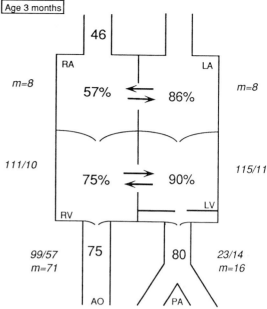

Figure 5. Hemodynamic diagram of a patient with transposition of the great arteries, ventricular septal defect, and subpulmonary stenosis. The balance of the circulation is similar to that shown in Figure 4; however, there is normal pulmonary arterial pressure. The pulmonary stenosis prohibits excess pulmonary blood flow; therefore, left atrial pressures are lower.

stenosis. In large part, these usually mild obstructions are a reversible phenomenon resulting from the leftward position of the ventricular septum due to right ventricular hypertrophy.[14] Close apposition of the septum to the mitral valve accentuates the problem.[71] In any case, the obstruction is rarely severe and, fortunately, tends to involute following arterial switching surgery. Valvar pulmonary stenosis is rare.

In contrast, anatomic pulmonary stenosis, usually subvalvar, is more commonly present when there is a ventricular defect (Fig. 5) (see p. 571). The restriction of pulmonary blood flow coupled with a large ventricular defect provides hemodynamics that are more likely to result not only in a lack of symptoms but also in good growth. Consequently, these babies first come to the cardiologist at a somewhat older age than most of the babies with transposition of the great arteries.

The great difficulty with the hemodynamics in patients with transposition of the great arteries is that surgical approaches to an individual lesion may irretrievably upset the precarious balance of circulation between the systemic and pulmonary circuits. Thus, the patient with transposition of the great arteries and intact ventricular septum in congestive heart failure because of a large patent ductus arteriosus does poorly with division of the ductus. Similarly, correction of an interrupted aortic arch or coarctation of the aorta may upset the balance of circulation between the two circuits if the

intercircuit communications are marginal in the first place. In contrast, an overriding or straddling atrioventricular valve improves mixing and, despite an anatomic deformity difficult or impossible to repair, allows infants to do better than the usual baby with transposition of the great arteries.

The left ventricle pumps at the systemic pressures for the months preceding birth, but the absolute pressures achieved are less than is required of the systemic ventricle after birth. If the ventricular septum is intact, the level of left ventricular pressure required to overcome pulmonary resistance decreases within hours of birth and is less than half of the right ventricular pressure by the end of the first week. Because an arterial switching operation requires the left ventricle to supply blood at systemic pressure immediately following surgery, the practical question is, "How long can the left ventricle function at a low, postnatal, pulmonary pressure and still be able to provide systemic blood pressure after switching?" The interval is not known. Unquestionably, there is considerable variation, depending on the age, the rate of fall of the pulmonary vascular resistance, the size of the ductus arteriosus, and how long it remains open. A switching procedure can be performed safely through the first weeks of life,[11,12,58] but how much longer it is safe cannot be defined precisely; it probably varies. The loss of hypertrophy occurs in days; as a corollary, a pulmonary artery band results in the return of adequate muscle to handle the systemic circulation within days or weeks—at least in small infants.[38]

The left ventricle of infants with a large ventricular septal defect functions at systemic pressure, and so long as the pressure remains at systemic levels an arterial switching operation is possible. Infants with a smaller ventricular defect, as well as those with defects that become smaller over time, have a variable safe time during which a switching procedure can be carried out.

Pulmonary vascular disease is more frequent and occurs earlier in patients with transposition of the great arteries, whether or not there is a ventricular septal defect. Although very early pulmonary vascular disease in an infant with an intact ventricular septum and transposition may have occurred because of a large ventricular septal defect that later closed, it is clear that infants with an intact ventricular septum can get pulmonary vascular disease. Those with a ventricular septal defect are likely to get pulmonary vascular disease earlier than their counterparts without transposition.[30,57] The additional feature that promotes earlier pulmonary vascular disease when there is transposition is elusive. An obvious suggestion is that disorders of oxygen, carbon dioxide, and pH in the pulmonary artery blood may play a role, since these measurements are more extreme in the infant with transposition.[62]

CLINICAL MANIFESTATIONS

The infants are predominantly males (64%) and have normal birth weights. The impression that these infants are larger than normal relates partly to comparisons with other children who have congenital heart disease and, more likely, to the fact that prematurity and low birth weight are not common among babies with transposition.[23]

Cyanosis in the first days of life suggests the possibility of transposition of the great arteries and, if the ventricular septum is intact, the infant may be severely cyanotic within hours of birth. When there is transposition with a large ventricular septal defect, cyanosis is less and may not be noticed in the first months.

Associated with cyanosis there is usually tachypnea. The infant is "happily tachypneic," breathing 60 times per minute or more with a shallow, fluttering of the chest, often without retractions or any suggestion that the infant feels dyspnea. The infant sometimes requires a long time to feed, starting to nurse vigorously, then slowing to rest and try again. Currently, most infants with transposition of the great arteries and intact ventricular septum are recognized, because of cyanosis, in the first days of life.[23]

Infants with small ventricular septal defects may get little additional mixing (virtually intact ventricular septum) and may follow a course comparable to that of infants with no ventricular defect. With a somewhat larger defect, recognition of cyanosis may be delayed and the problem with tachypnea less noticeable. With a large ventricular septal defect, cyanosis may not be noticed and the infant may progress from tachypnea, to dyspnea, to outright congestive failure over days or weeks, in a manner similar to that of infants with ventricular defect without transposition. Infants with a straddling tricuspid valve are likely to follow this course. An infant with a ventricular defect and coarctation of the aorta or an interrupted aortic arch may have gross congestive failure within days of birth.

Physical Examination

Usually, the newborn infant is visibly cyanotic and comfortably tachypneic with a respiratory rate of 60 breaths per minute or more. Except for tachypnea, there is no evidence of congestive heart failure. The cyanosis does not vary with crying or with the administration of oxygen. Systolic murmurs are not a prominent feature in these patients unless there is a pressure gradient across the left ventricular outflow tract. Usually, there is considerable discussion about whether the second heart sound is split or not. Given the rapidity of the heart rate, these discussions are rarely more than roundsmanship. After the first two weeks of life, growth failure may be evident.

When there is a ventricular septal defect, a murmur is present within a few days after birth and, when first examined, the infant often shows signs of congestive failure. There may be tachypnea with intercostal and subcostal retractions and inability to nurse successfully.

It is worthwhile to check the hemoglobin and hematocrit levels in these babies, because a relatively low level may contribute to congestive heart failure (see ch. 7). The comparison of arterial oxygen pO_2, content, or percent of saturation, before and after the administration of 100% oxygen, is sometimes a useful test. When the child has marked cyanosis, there is little increase when oxygen is administered.

Electrocardiography

In most newborns with transposition of the great arteries, the electrocardiogram is within normal limits; later, there is right ventricular hypertrophy. Among infants with an overriding or straddling tricuspid valve, there is left dominance and often a leftward superior axis because of the small right ventricle (Fig. 6).

Chest X-Ray

The chest x-ray is virtually normal in infants presenting with cyanosis within a few days of birth.

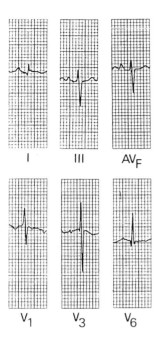

Figure 6. Electrocardiogram of a patient with a straddling tricuspid valve. Often when there is an overriding or straddling tricuspid valve, there is hypoplasia of the right ventricle and excessive blood flow through the left ventricle compared with the right. The electrocardiogram may show a leftward-superior axis and left ventricular hypertrophy.

In those with a large ventricular septal defect who present with symptoms of congestion, there is cardiomegaly, increased pulmonary vascularity, and evidence of congestive heart failure. A right aortic arch is found in 1% of patients with an intact ventricular septum, 3% of patient with a ventricular septal defect, and in 10% of patients with ventricular septal defect and pulmonary stenosis or atresia.

Echocardiography

The diagnosis can be readily made by echocardiography. The discovery of a posterior great artery, arising from the left ventricle, which branches into a right and left pulmonary artery establishes the diagnosis. An anterior aorta arising from the right ventricle provides further confirmation. Left-to-right shunting or bidirectional shunting through a foramen ovale is demonstrable by Doppler technique, with shunting into the pulmonary circuit identifiable at the ventricular or ductal level. The central coronary arteries should be examined in multiple views. Usually, the number and location of vessels can be satisfactorily established as well as the proximal branching pattern.[61] The location of the site and number of ventricular septal defects should be recorded and the degree and nature of left ventricular outflow obstruction evaluated.[13] The presence and degree of mitral or tricuspid deformity must be documented.

Subxiphoid views are the most helpful in making the diagnosis of D-transposition of the great arteries. In a long-axis view the pulmonary root, identified by its bifurcation, can be seen aligned with the posterior left ventricle (Fig. 7A). Further anterior angulation in the long axis sweep displays the anterior aorta to the right and aligned with the right ventricle. Turning into a short-axis or parasagittal plane displays the aorta, including the arch and brachiocephalic vessels (Fig. 7B). Leftward angulation shows the posterior pulmonary artery related to the left ventricle.

The interatrial septum is seen best in subxiphoid long- and short-axis views (Fig. 8). The direction of flow across the septum can be determined using pulsed Doppler technique or Doppler color flow mapping.

Multiple views are required to demonstrate the coronary artery anatomy. The main right and left

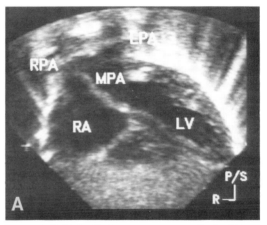

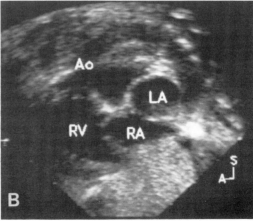

Figure 7. D-transposition of the great arteries seen in: **A,** Subxiphoid long-axis view showing the bifurcating pulmonary artery aligned with the left ventricle. **B,** Subxiphoid short-axis view demonstrating the aorta, including the arch and brachiocephalic vessels, aligned with the right ventricle. RPA, right pulmonary artery; MPA, main pulmonary artery; RA, right atrium; LV, left ventricle; Ao, aorta.

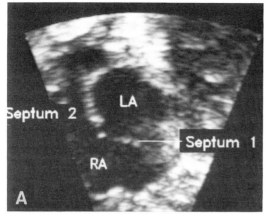

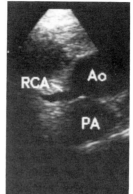 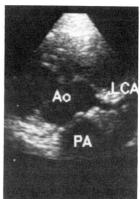

Figure 9. Parasternal short-axis views showing the origin of the left and right coronary arteries from the aorta in a patient with D-transposition of the great arteries. Ao, aorta; RCA, right coronary artery; LCA, left coronary artery; PA, pulmonary artery.

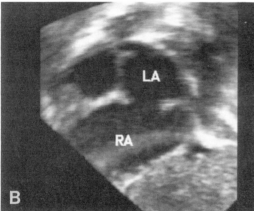

Figure 8. Subxiphoid long-axis view of the interatrial septum in an infant with D-transposition of the great arteries. **A,** Before septostomy. Note the thin septum primum bulging into the right atrium. **B,** After septostomy. Note the remnants of septum primum around the defect. LA, left atrium; RA, right atrium.

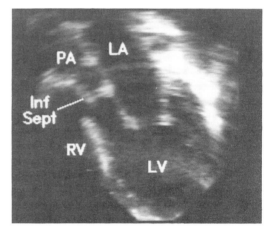

Figure 10. Left ventricular outflow tract in a patient with D-transposition of the great arteries, a posterior malalignment ventricular septal defect, and subpulmonary stenosis due to posterior malalignment of the infundibular septum. PA, pulmonary artery; LA, left atrium; LV, left ventricle; RV, right ventricle.

coronary arteries can be demonstrated in a parasternal short-axis view with clockwise rotation for the left coronary artery and counterclockwise rotation for the right coronary artery (Fig. 9). Usually, the bifurcation of the left coronary artery can be seen well in a parasternal long-axis view, angled to the left. Often an apical or subxiphoid four-chamber view is useful for demonstrating a coronary artery passing posterior to the pulmonary root in cases of single right coronary artery or origin of the left circumflex coronary artery from the right coronary artery.

The size, location, and number of ventricular septal defects should be addressed using subxiphoid, apical, and parasternal views. Doppler color flow mapping is indispensable for detecting multiple defects. Flow mapping, performed in subxiphoid and parasternal short-axis views, is excellent for detecting membranous and atrioventricular canal defects. Scanning with color flow mapping in parasternal short axis, with attention

directed toward the left and anterior aspect of the septum, is the best approach for detecting anterior muscular defects. Posterior and apical muscular defects can be seen best by scanning with color flow mapping in apical four-chamber views.

The left ventricular outflow tract should be examined carefully in parasternal long- and short-axis views, the apical long-axis view and the subxiphoid long-axis view to exclude obstruction (Fig. 10). The morphology of the pulmonary valve should be determined in a parasternal short-axis view. Possible mechanisms of left ventricular outflow obstruction in D-transposition of the great arteries include posterior malalignment of the infundibular septum, posterior bowing of the muscular septum ("dynamic" subpulmonary stenosis), valvar stenosis, subvalvar membrane, accessory atrioventricular valve tissue, and a hypertrophied muscle of Moullaert. Pulsed or continuous-wave Doppler technique can be used from apical long-axis or subxiphoid short-axis views to estimate the outflow tract gradient.

Occasionally in the presence of a basal ventricular septal defect the atrioventricular valve attachments may interfere with repair of the defect. Usually, abnormal attachments of the tricuspid valve to the infundibular septum can be seen in the subxiphoid short-axis views (Fig. 11). Abnormal attachments of the mitral valve can be seen in parasternal short-axis, subxiphoid short-axis, and apical views.

Cardiac Catheterization

Little information is needed in addition to that furnished by echocardiography. The purpose of cardiac catheterization is to perform balloon septostomy and to confirm the coronary anatomy prior to an arterial switching procedure. Occasionally, useful physiologic information about left ventricular outflow obstruction and about the number and location of ventricular septal defects can be added.

The presence, number, and location of any ventricular defects are confirmed by right or left ventricular angiography.

The coronary anatomy is shown either by aortic root angiography with injection just above the aortic valve (1.0 ml/kg contrast) or by injection in the right ventricle (1.5–2.0 ml/kg contrast), with the patient positioned in the long axial oblique and right anterior oblique or with the baby placed in a "laid back," "Mercedes-Benz," anteroposterior-caudal position (Fig. 12).[44] Coronary aortography

is enhanced by balloon occlusion of the aorta distal to the point of injection. The variations of coronary anatomy in patients with D-transposition of the great vessels are discussed further in the Chapter on Surgery (see ch. 54).

Balloon atrial septostomy, introduced by Rashkind and Miller,[64] remains the standard method of creating an atrial septal defect in the newborn. Although intracardiac complications occurred occasionally during the early years, with the advent of biplane fluoroscopy these have virtually disappeared. As experience has accumulated, limitations have become evident. The duration of septal patency is temporary in some infants, and septosomy is not effective in the majority when carried out in infants more than two months of age. Nonetheless, balloon septostomy remains the procedure of choice in the newborn baby with D-transposition whether or not there is a ventricular septal defect.

In recent years we at Children's Hospital in Boston have used, almost exclusively, the Miller™ septostomy catheter (American Edwards Laboratories) introduced through a diaphragm via a 7-French sheath, using a percutaneous umbilical or femoral venous entry site. Usually, the balloon is inflated with 4 ml of dilute contrast material in the left atrium, provided that cavity is large enough to accept this inflated size. Then the balloon is jerked rapidly across the septum; this is repeated at least once. The size of the defect is then estimated and hemodynamic parameters are remeasured.

In an emergency situation balloon septostomy has been safely and adequately accomplished in our intensive care unit, using echocardiography to guide the catheter. In our own experience with newborns in recent years, balloon septosomy has been carried out without intracardiac complications, and has provided an adequate opening in the majority.

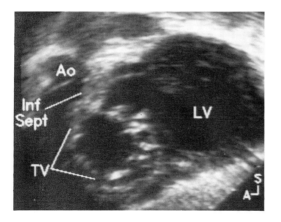

Figure 11. Subxiphoid short-axis view in a patient with D-transposition of the great arteries and an anterior malalignment ventricular septal defect, showing attachments of the tricuspid valve to the infundibular septum. Ao, aorta; TV, tricuspid valve; LV, left ventricle.

MANAGEMENT

Successful management of infants with D-transposition of the great arteries requires the close coordination of the referring hospital, the transport service and the receiving center. If managed suboptimally, brain injury if not death may be the result. It is the author's impression, based on regional autopsy statistics, that a small number of infants with transposition may die within hours of birth before transport can be arranged.

Increasing numbers of babies with transposition are discovered by fetal echocardiography. This is particularly fortunate because the infant can be transported in a personal incubator to the receiving center for scheduled birth and management of the cardiac problem. All concerned can be notified well in advance.

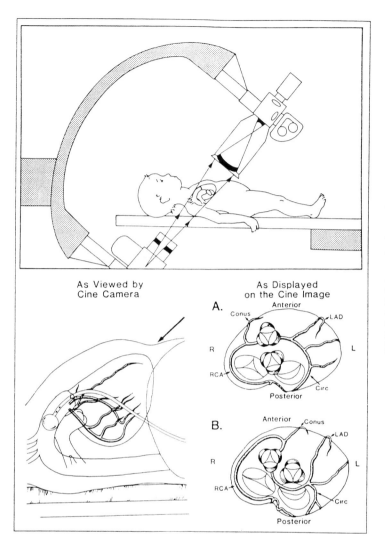

As Viewed by Cine Camera

As Displayed on the Cine Image

A.

Anterior
Conus
LAD
R
L
RCA
Circ
Posterior

B.

Anterior
Conus
LAD
R
L
RCA
Circ
Posterior

Figure 12. The "laid back" view to assess the coronary anatomy in transposition of the great arteries. **A,** Shows the anterior-posterior position of the C-arm with maximal caudal angulation. **B,** Shows the cine image of anterior-posterior great vessels (upper diagram) and side-by-side vessels (lower diagram). **C,** A lateral diagram to show the camera's view of the heart and, particularly, the great vessels and the coronary anatomy. (From Mandell VS, Lock JE, Mayer JE: Am J Cardiol 65: 1379–1383, 1990,[44] with permission.)

The infant who has D-transposition of the great arteries should be transported to the nearest cardiac surgical center as soon as the diagnosis is recognized. Whether balloon septostomy is performed prior to transport depends on the facilities available locally. Prostaglandin E1[22,39] is administered to the baby, who is severely cyanotic, and as soon as it is established that the prostaglandin is well tolerated, the patient is moved. Occasionally prostaglandin will greatly increase the pulmonary blood flow and pulmonary congestion because of an inadequate atrial opening, an observation that suggests that, given a choice, balloon atrial septostomy may be a more desirable first treatment than prostaglandins. Patients receiving prostaglandins should be intubated prior to transport because of the possibility of apnea.

Those with a ventricular septal defect and congestive heart failure should receive anticongestive medications. Surgery is not as urgent for these babies and, as long as the left ventricular pressure is at systemic levels, delay is possible. Unfortunately,

the ventricular defect may get smaller, with a resulting drop in left ventricular pressure. Usually, the infant should not be allowed to function at half systemic pressure in the left ventricle for much more than 2 weeks before arterial switching surgery is carried out. Whenever there is any doubt about how long the left ventricle will remain suitable for switching, surgery should not be delayed. The very few infants whose coronary artery anatomy is unfavorable for arterial switching can have an atrial inversion procedure.

At Children's Hospital in Boston, the plan for infants with transposition of the great arteries and an intact ventricular septum is to carry out an arterial switching procedure as early as possible if there is favorable coronary anatomy and if there are relatively normal semilunar valves. Prior to surgery, cardiac catheterization and balloon atrial septostomy are undertaken to provide some leeway in planning surgery. With all these intravenous manipulations, it must be remembered that these babies are at significant risk from a bolus of medication or air passing from the systemic venous circulation directly to the systemic arterial circulation, with the possibility of brain injury.

In the infant with D-transposition of the great arteries, a large ventricular septal defect and no pulmonary stenosis, elective repair is made by closing the ventricular septal defect and switching the great arteries at about 2 months of age. Earlier surgery may be required if there is doubt about the adequacy of the ventricular septal defect to ensure a left ventricular pressure at systemic levels, and a second preoperative cardiac catheterization may be required to measure the left ventricular pressure.

Surgery

Creation of an atrial septal defect, by the Blalock-Hanlon or open technique, provides improved mixing of the pulmonary and systemic circuits and, thereby, improvement in survival for patients with transposition of the great arteries. These operations have been largely replaced by catheter septostomy techniques in neonates with D-transposition of the great arteries.

A **pulmonary artery banding** procedure, used routinely in the past for D-transposition of the great arteries with a large ventricular septal defect, is now rarely needed because the ventricular septal defects are primarily repaired. This technique is still useful, however, for the patient who has multiple ventricular septal defects. The complications of banding procedures must be considered in these decisions (see ch. 54).

Among the atrial inversion operations, the **Mustard procedure**[53] (Fig. 13) represented a major milestone in managing children with D-transposition of the great arteries. It provided great improvement in survival and in the quality of life for

these infants. The pulmonary venous blood is baffled to the tricuspid valve and the systemic venous blood to the mitral valve and pulmonary circuit. The Mustard procedure accomplishes this baffling using prosthetic material or pericardium. The **Senning procedure,**[68] actually introduced earlier with only limited success, was modified and reintroduced as a means of reducing the complications of the Mustard procedure. The Senning procedure accomplishes similar baffling but uses native structures. There is little difference between the results of the two approaches,[46] the mortality for each being less than 5%. Both procedures are accomplished with reasonable risk in small infants.[17,77]

An **arterial switching procedure** was first successfully performed by Jatene.[36] Transposing the coronary arteries as well as the great arteries, a most difficult problem, was finally accomplished (Fig. 13). Initially, this procedure was available only for older infants who survived with a ventricular septal defect and systemic pressure in the left ventricle.[3,5,37,85] Later,[35,70,86] pulmonary artery banding was used to "prepare" the left ventricle, which had functioned at low pressure, for systemic work. In recent years, arterial switching in the newborn, taking advantage of the naturally "prepared" left ventricle in the neonate with an intact ventricular septum, became a reality and pulmonary artery banding was no longer needed.[11,47,83] At the present time, the preferred management at Children's Hospital in Boston is an arterial switching procedure performed in the first 2 weeks of life in patients with an intact ventricular septum; arterial switching may be delayed for 2–3 months when there is a good-sized ventricular septal defect, but success depends on the left ventricle having been exposed to systemic or near systemic pressure for the preceding 2 or 3 weeks. Present-day mortality is acceptable (Exhibit 2), whether there is a ventricular septal defect or not.[12,19,34,58,75]

The problems with arterial switching operations include limitation of coronary flow,[83] acquired stenosis at the site of anastomosis of the great vessels,[87] aortic regurgitation, and problems with an inadequately prepared left ventricle.

Surgeons **patch the ventricular defect** on the right side of the septum to avoid the conduction bundle. If the repair is to be an atrial inversion procedure, repair of the ventricular defect through the tricuspid valve may damage the valve that is to become the systemic atrioventricular valve. Tricuspid incompetence of any degree is poorly tolerated. Repair through a right ventricular incision is even more damaging, because the right ventricle will become the systemic pump. For this reason the author believes an arterial switching procedure is desirable if there is a ventricular defect, despite comparable survival with atrial inversion surgery.[75] Also, an arterial switching operation is more likely to be successful if there is right ventricular hypo-

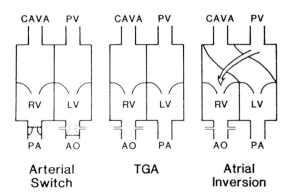

Figure 13. Diagrammatic comparison of atrial inversion in transposition of the great arteries, unrepaired patient with transposition, and arterial switching surgery. Note that atrial inversion requires long atrial suture lines and results in the right ventricle being the systemic pump. Note the necessity to move the coronary arteries with arterial switching surgery; the left ventricle becomes the systemic pump.

Exhibit 2

Boston Children's Hospital Experience 1973–1987
The number of ventricular defects which were surgically closed in less than half of the total cases. Spontaneous closure and decreasing size of ventricular defects account for most of this apparent descrepancy. Patients who were ineligible for ventricular surgery and those who have not yet been operated upon account for some more. The number of children who have pacemakers and the number who have had tricuspid valve replacement, as well as the number with myocardial problems (prior table), influenced the decision to begin arterial switching surgery for transposition of the great arteries.

Surgical Repair of Transposition of the Great Arteries with Intact Ventricular Septum

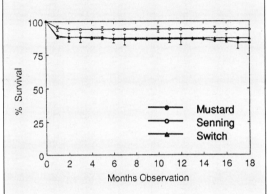

Mustard's procedure (75) was the main operative procedure from 1973–77. Senning's operation (140) was used from 1978–83. Jatene's switching procedure (101) was used from 1983–87. Since this time the mortality with arterial switching surgery has improved further.

Surgical Repair of Transposition of the Great Arteries with Ventricular Septal Defect

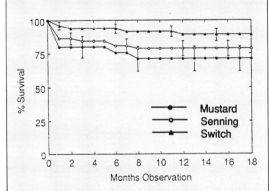

D-transposition of great arteries with ventricular septal defect and no pulmonary stenosis. See prior life table for the time periods when these operations were in use. Mustard's operation (26); Senning's operation (65). The clear advantage of the switching procedure for transposition of the great arteries and a ventricular defect (49) can be seen.

plasia. With an unacceptably small right ventricle, a two-ventricle repair may be out of the question; a Fontan procedure may be the only option.

Surgery for those with large ventricular defects or large patent ductus arteriosus must be carried out in the first 2 to 3 months of life if pulmonary vascular obstructive disease is to be avoided.[63] When there is a ventricular septal defect, it is difficult to close the defect without some damage to either the ventricular muscle or the tricuspid valve; this may contribute to failure of the right ventricle as the systemic pump in patients with atrial inversion surgery.

Relief of subpulmonary stenosis is difficult in the patient with transposition of the great arteries. Both the Senning and Mustard procedures result in the right ventricle remaining the systemic ventricle, the left ventricle functioning under low pressure as the pulmonary ventricle. Subpulmonary stenosis caused by leftward deviation of the ventricular septum with apposition to the mitral valve leaflets is not relieved by atrial switching operations and may require further surgery.[33]

Rastelli proposed a method of patching the ventricular septal defect so that the left ventricular outflow passes through the ventricular defect into the aorta.[65,80] A conduit is placed from the right ventricle to the main pulmonary artery. This approach requires a sizable ventricular septal defect, appropriately located so that a patch can be placed that will redirect the left ventricular flow into the aorta. Sometimes the ventricular defect can be enlarged so that a Rastelli operation becomes possible. This procedure offers a reasonable solution for the patient with transposition and ventricular septal defect in whom arterial switching is not possible because of fixed pulmonary stenosis or unusual coronary patterns. The inherent problems with conduits (see ch. 54) are surmountable.

Conversion from an atrial inversion to an arterial switch is a new idea presently being tested. With the success of arterial switching, it was only a matter of time before patients in difficulty after a Mustard or Senning procedure could be considered to be candidates for conversion to a systemic left ventricle.[49] For this conversion, a pulmonary artery band is applied first to prepare the left ventricle for later systemic work. This, when used in a sick patient who needs relief because of a failing right ventricle, only makes the patient sicker. Fortunately, the time required to prepare the left ventricle is relatively short (2–3 weeks in an infant): then takedown of the original atrial baffling procedure, creation of an atrial septum, removal of the pulmonary artery band, and arterial switching can be performed. It is likely that different periods of time, depending on the patient's age, are required to ready the left ventricle for systemic pressure work.

Finally, patients in whom the intraventricular

anatomy is unfavorable (i.e., multiple ventricular septal defects, hypoplastic right ventricle, or straddling atrioventricular valve) may be amenable to variations on the **Fontan principle** (see ch. 54).

In some children with transposition of the great arteries, a ventricular defect and severe pulmonary vascular disease, **palliative atrial inversion operations** without closure of the ventricular defect, provide surprising improvement.[18,42] The practical effect of this manuever is to give the patient the equivalent of a ventricular defect and pulmonary vascular disease—a status associated with less cyanosis. The results with this operation have been gratifying. It is presumed that arterial switching operations will be equally effective, but it is anticipated that there may be less need for palliative surgery in the future.

It is apparent that there are, in the 1990s, a variety of operative procedures available. Given a choice between the right or left ventricle as the systemic pump, the left ventricle is selected when possible. At the same time, on certain occasions, the right ventricle is a more desirable pumping chamber (e.g., when there must be a left ventricular incision to repair multiple, apical ventricular defects). If the left ventricle has obstructed outflow, a Rastelli procedure can be considered. Hypoplasia of the right ventricle may require a Fontan procedure. For success, the anatomy must be known in minute detail and, after surgery, the team must be prepared for cardiac catheterization and possible reoperation in the postoperative period when progress is not as expected.

COURSE

Survival with D-transposition of the great arteries without surgery is unlikely. Virtually all children with an intact ventricular septum succumb in the first year and most of those with D-transposition and a ventricular septal defect succumb within the first 2 years.[41] Only occasionally does a patient with D-transposition, ventricular defect, and pulmonary stenosis survive to later years. Even fewer patients have survived with an intact septum and a large natural atrial septal defect.

Late follow-up of Mustard and Senning procedures is now proceeding.[9,24,43,76] Although survival generally, is good, the following problems have been recognized.[6,28]

Rhythm Problems

Because of the extensive atrial suturing required in Senning or Mustard surgery, late supraventricular rhythm problems are common. Indeed, it can be suggested that all patients with an atrial inversion operation will have rhythm problems 15 years later. Attempts to avoid the sinus node artery and various other technical maneuvers are not particularly successful. Twenty five percent of patients will have some disorder of native pacemakers or atrial conduction.[9,10,20,21,31,79] By 1987, 19 patients at Children's Hospital in Boston have required permanent pacemakers because of the sick sinus syndrome (Exhibit 3). Later sudden death, with or without pacemaker implantation, occurs at a rate of about 1% of patients per year.

Tricuspid Incompetence

Damage to the tricuspid valve, while acceptable in repair of ventricular septal defect in children without transposition, is unacceptable in patients with transposition of the great arteries following atrial inversion surgery. The reported success of Senning and Mustard repair associated with ventricular septal defect patching is related, in part, to the care in preserving tricuspid valve function.[63]

Right (Systemic) Ventricular Failure

For reasons that are being debated, there is a variable incidence of right ventricular failure following Senning's and Mustard's procedures.[1,4,8,27,29,60,73,74] Congestive heart failure develops in a significant number of patients; in some this is directly related to tricuspid incompetence. Myocardial dysfunction is encountered whether or not there has been prior surgery for a ventricular defect. Because this phenomenon was recognized first in patients who had had repair some years ago and therefore were older at the time of repair, it is possible that exposure to a long period of cyanosis may have impaired ventricular function. The high incidence of damage to the central nervous system with prolonged cyanosis[55] raises the possibility that myocardial function may be similarly lost. In any case, it is not yet known whether arterial switching operations will be associated with the same late incidence of myocardial dysfunction.

Complete Heart Block

A small number of patients have or develop complete heart block and require a permanent pacemaker.

Growth

Following Mustard or Senning surgery, growth is improved and, if the surgery is done early, growth is near normal.[40] Following an arterial switching operation, growth is also normal.[83]

Injury to the Central Nervous System

There is significant risk of injury to the central nervous system in infants with transposition. This may occur spontaneously, in association with cardiac catheterization (Fig. 14), or while awaiting surgical repair (see ch. 9). The longer the exposure

Exhibit 3

	Diagnostic Groups			
Operation	Intact ventricular septum n = 345	Virtually intact ventricular septum n = 78	Ventricular septal defect n = 202	Ventricular defect, pulmonary stenosis n = 92
Pulmonary Artery Band n = 62	1	0	28	0
Coarctation Repair n = 31	2	3	10	3
Pulmonary Outflow Surgery n = 82	8	0	9	39
Arterial-Pulmonary Shunt n = 95	6	1	12	5
Mustard Operation n = 172	27	38	18	13
Senning Operation n = 257	42	38	34	15
Arterial Switch n = 167	29	21	25	0
Rastelli Operation n = 46	0	0	2	46
Ventricular Defect Closure n = 190	0	0	74	43
Fontan Operation n = 12	0	0	3	5
Pacemaker n = 19	2	5	2	3
Tricuspid Valve Replacement n = 11	1	1	4	1

Boston Children's Hospital Experience 1973–1987

Surgical Operations: Percent of Each Diagnostic Group*

*Note: Many patients had more than one operation.

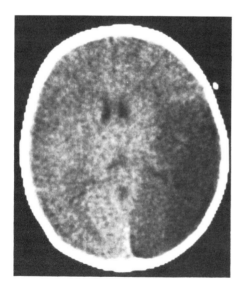

Figure 14. A CT scan of the brain of a child with transposition of the great arteries showing an area of presumed embolic damage suffered during cardiac catheterization. The precise cause is unknown.

to the circulatory abnormality of transposition, the more likely there will be injury to the central nervous system. As many as 10% of patients have had overt signs of brain injury in the past. Studies of late neurologic development show a depressed intelligence quotient and delayed motor function;[56] the later reparative surgery was carried out, the poorer the result on pyschomotor testing. Some of the neurologic problems have been attributed to the surgical techniques, in particular, deep hypothermic cardiac arrest, a technique that is particularly useful in the newborn period. How much the hypothermic circulatory arrest, whether rapidly with core cooling, external cooling, or deep or not so deep hypothermia, may contribute to injury to the central nervous system is not known. This problem is made even more difficult by the remarkable recovery of small infants from major central nervous system injury. Despite gross injury, only minor symptoms may be noted and later evidence of impairment may be minimal.

Coronary Abnormalities

Because the Jatene procedure requires transposing the coronary arteries in the newborn period, it is of obvious interest whether there is myocardial injury at the time of surgery and whether late coronary function is adequate. There may be evidence of myocardial abnormality in the immediate postoperative period following arterial switching. There are enzyme abnormalities, electrocardiographic abnormalities, and abnormalities seen on thallium or pyrophosphate scans. When these tests are repeated later, the abnormalities usually have disappeared and evidence of injury is rarely detectable. The conclusion that the neonatal myocardium repairs itself in a manner different from that of adults seems likely, at least in our present state of knowledge.

Course Following Arterial Switching

The follow-up after an arterial switching operation has been too short to be confident of the final outcome. Follow-up of possible postoperative coronary insufficiency is under way. So far it appears that myocardial function is good[7,15,59] and rhythm problems and late deaths are uncommon.[2,45,78,82] Iatrogenic supravalvar stenosis, either aortic or pulmonary, is rare but can be managed by balloon dilatation.

VARIATIONS

Transposition of the Great Arteries with Intact Ventricular Septum and Pulmonary Stenosis

As many of 30% of patients with D-transposition of the great arteries and intact ventricular septum have a significant pressure gradient across the left ventricular outflow tract. Most of these have bulging of the ventricular septum toward the left, approximating the mitral valve and producing dynamic obstruction. This type of obstruction resolves following switching surgery.[14] A small number have an anatomic obstruction composed of fibrous tissue along the ventricular septum, with or without abnormal mitral valve attachments. Rarely there is valvar obstruction. Attempts at surgical correction of nonvalvar left ventricular outflow obstruction have met with variable success.[33,84]

At the present time, a patient with transposition of the great arteries and intact septum, with systemic or near systemic pressure in the left ventricle from demonstrable anatomic obstruction in the outflow tract, is viewed with concern. Deciding whether an arterial switching procedure will be tolerated is difficult. Those in whom the obstruction is not surgically remediable are managed with a Senning procedure and an attempt to resect the outflow obstruction. In our small group of patients of this type, all have survived and are well, but none has had complete relief of the left ventricular hypertension.

Transposition and Coarctation of the Aorta

Coarctation of the aorta or interrupted aortic arch is rarely seen in patients with transposition of the great arteries. When present, there is usually a ventricular septal defect as well.[81] Whereas, formerly, this combination of lesions most often proved fatal, in recent years survival has improved. Much of this can be attributed to earlier, more precise diagnosis as well as carefully staged procedures, first correcting the coarctation and later performing transposition repair. Occasionally, all abnormalities can be corrected in a single procedure from the midline.

Transposition of the Great Arteries with Ventricular Defect and Pulmonary Stenosis

This variation accounts for roughly 10% of the cases of transposition of the great arteries (Exhibit 1).[23,75]

The anatomic variations in this group of patients are numerous. Ventricular septal defects may occur anywhere within the ventricular septum and pulmonary stenosis is also variable, ranging from pulmonary atresia (Fig. 15), posterior displacement of the septum, abnormal mitral valve attachments, and subvalvar and valvar stenosis.

These patients are discovered with cyanosis during the first days of life; the more severe the pul-

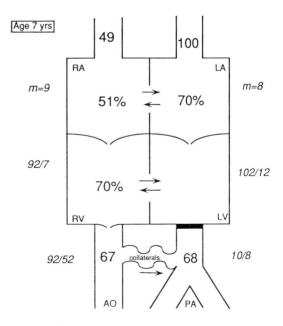

Figure 15. A hemodynamic diagram of a patient with transposition of the great arteries, ventricular defect, and pulmonary atresia. Note that the only blood supply to the lungs is via major collaterals arising from the descending aorta. Compare with a similar situation encountered in patients with tetralogy of Fallot and pulmonary atresia (see ch. 30).

monary stenosis and the smaller the ventricular septal defect, the earlier the patients are seen.

The diagnosis is made by echocardiography and confirmed by cardiac catheterization.

A management plan tailored to each child is required. Is it possible to consider a Rastelli procedure? Is it possible that the best approach would be a Senning operation plus an attempt to relieve pulmonary stenosis? Perhaps an arterial-pulmonary shunting procedure and later a Fontan operation can be considered. Excision of a subpulmonary diaphragm and closure of the ventricular defect has been successful.

Because the most common difficulty in early infancy is marked cyanosis, a shunting procedure may be needed. This takes the form of a modified Blalock operation, an atrial defect being created (balloon or surgical septectomy) at the same time if mixing is thought likely to be marginal. Those with a more balanced combination may do well for months with no surgical interference, the infant having no significant congestive heart failure and tolerable cyanosis (Fig. 15). Those with lesser degrees of pulmonary stenosis may have congestive heart failure as the dominant symptom. With a small or closing ventricular septal defect, the infant will follow the course of patients with transposition of the great arteries with intact ventricular septum and pulmonary stenosis.

With an appropriately located ventricular septal defect in an older child, a Rastelli procedure can be considered. In this operation the ventricular defect is patched in such a way that the left ventricular outflow passes through the ventricular defect to the aorta. The pulmonary artery is disconnected from the left ventricle and connected via a conduit to the right ventricle, resulting in "complete" correction. The ventricular defect must be large enough to carry the systemic output; if it is not, it is sometimes possible to enlarge the ventricular opening. An inappropriately located ventricular defect (i.e., muscular or endocardial cushion defect) prohibits the possibility of a Rastelli operation. Among those with pulmonary atresia, treatment consists of a shunting procedure, usually a modified Blalock operation, and, depending on the adequacy of mixing, the creation of an atrial septal defect as well. Later, a Rastelli procedure is undertaken.

Usually, arterial switching operations are not possible because of the pulmonary stenosis, but they have been successful when pulmonary stenosis can be surgically relieved with a competent valve remaining.

Atrial inversion, closing the ventricular defect, and resection of pulmonary stenosis are possible, although complete relief of the stenosis usually is not possible.

Those with pulmonary atresia may require attention to relieve excessive collateral circulation.

Overriding Tricuspid Valve

An overriding or straddling tricuspid valve is a difficult complication of D-transposition of the great arteries (Fig. 16). The right ventricle is likely to be small in proportion to the degree of straddling. Severe hypoplasia dictates future therapy. Because there is good mixing, these infants often have minimal cyanosis.

If the chordae of the tricuspid valve are inserted on the ventricular septum, repair with an arterial switch may be possible. If the ventricular septal defect can be closed without major disruption of the tricuspid valve, all is likely to be well. If the right ventricle is small, arterial switching is the reparative surgery of choice, because the hypoplastic right ventricle may well manage as a pulmonary circuit pump while it would be ineffective as a systemic ventricle. Other complicating features, such as difficult coronary anatomy, unfavorable location of the ventricular septal defect or some other lesion, are likely to result in prohibitive risk.

If the tricuspid chordae insert on the left ventricular side of the septum the tricuspid valve might be damaged in the repair of the ventricular defect. Clearly, the patient with a diminutive right ventricle is unlikely to survive a Senning procedure, particularly if tricuspid valve function is compromised in the process.

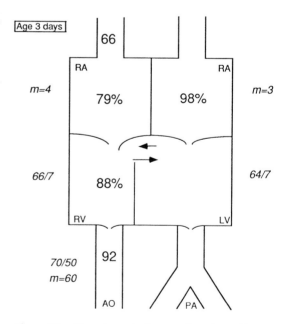

Figure 16. Hemodynamic diagram of a patient with transposition of the great arteries, ventricular septal defect, and straddling tricuspid valve. The direct communication of the right atrium to the pulmonary ventricle (anatomic left ventricle) improves mixing of the pulmonary and systemic circulations. The arterial saturation is better than that in the usual patient with transposition of the great arteries despite an added major and surgically uncorrectable problem.

If the right ventricle is prohibitively small, a Fontan operation or one of the Fontan variants may be the only reasonable plan.

REFERENCES

1. Alpert BS, Bloom, KR, Olley PM, et al: Echocardiographic evaluation of right ventricular function in complete transposition of the great arteries: angiographic correlates. Am J Cardiol 44:270–75, 1979.
2. Arensman FW, Bostock J, Radley-Smith R, et al: Cardiac rhythm and conduction before and after anatomic correction of transposition of the great arteries. Am J Cardiol 52:836–839, 1983.
3. Arensman FW, Sievers H, Lange PE, et al: Assessment of coronary and aortic anastomoses after anatomic correction of transposition of the great arteries. J Thorac Cardiovasc Surg 90:597–604, 1985.
4. Benson LN, Bonet J, McLaughlin P, et al: Assessment of right ventricular function during supine bicycle exercise after Mustard's operation. Circulation 65:1052–1059, 1982.
5. Bical O, Hazan E, Lecompte Y, et al: Anatomic correction of transposition of the great arteries associated with ventricular septal defect: midterm results in 50 patients. Circulation 70:891–897, 1984.
6. Bink-Boelkens MThE, Bergstra A, Cromme-Dijkhuis AH, et al: The asymptomatic child a long time after the Mustard operation for transposition of the great arteries. Ann Thorac Surg 47:45–50, 1989.
7. Borow KM, Arensman FW, Webb C, et al: Assessment of left ventricular contractile state after anatomic correction of transposition of the great arteries. Circulation 69:106–112, 1984.
8. Borow KM, Keane JF, Castaneda AR, et al: Systemic ventricular function in patients with tetralogy of Fallot, ventricular defect and transposition of the great arteries repaired in infancy. Circulation 64:878–885, 1981.
9. Butto F, Dunnigan A, Overholt ED, et al: Transesophageal study of recurrent atrial tachycardia after atrial baffle procedures for complete transposition of the great arteries. Am J Cardiol 57:1356–1362, 1986.
10. Byrum CJ, Bove EL, Sondheimer HM, et al: Hemodynamic and electrophysiologic results of the Senning procedure for transposition of the great arteries. Am J Cardiol 58:138–142, 1986.
11. Castaneda AR, Norwood WI, Jonas RA, et al: Transposition of the great arteries and intact ventricular septum: anatomical repair in the neonate. Ann Thoracic Surg 5:438–443, 1984.
12. Castaneda AR, Trusler GA, Paul MH, et al: The early results of treatment of simple transposition in the current era. J Thorac Cardiovasc Surg 95:14–27, 1988.
13. Chin AJ, Yeager SB, Sanders SP, et al: Accuracy of prospective two-dimensional echocardiographic evaluation of left ventricular outflow tract in complete transposition of the great arteries. Am J Cardiol 55:759–764, 1985.
14. Chiu I, Anderson RH, Macartney FJ, et al: Morphologic features of an intact ventricular septum susceptible to subpulmonary obstruction in complete transposition. Am J Cardiol 53:1633–1638, 1984.
15. Colan SD, Trowitzsch E, Wernovsky G, et al: Myocardial performance after arterial switch operation for transposition of the great arteries with intact ventricular septum. Circulation 78:132–141, 1988.
16. Deal BJ, Chin AJ, Sanders SP, et al: Subxiphoid two-dimensional echocardiographic identification of tricuspid valve abnormalities in transposition of the great arteries with ventricular septal defect. Am J Cardiol 55:1146–1151, 1985.
17. DeLeon VH, Hougen TJ, Norwood WI, et al: Results of the Senning operation for transposition of the great arteries with intact ventricular septum in neonates. Circulation 70:21–25, 1984.
18. Dhasmana JP, Stark J, deLeval M, et al: Long-term results of the "palliative" Mustard operation. J Am Coll Card 6:1138–1141, 1985.
19. Di Donato RM, Wernovsky G, Walsh EP et al: Results of the arterial switch operation for transposition of the great arteries with ventricular septal defect: surgical considerations and midterm follow-up data. Circulation 80:1689–1705, 1989.
20. Duster MC, Bink-Boelkens MThE, Wampler D, et al: Long-term follow-up of dysrhythmias following the Mustard procedure. Am Heart J 109:1323–1326, 1985.
21. Flinn CJ, Wolff GS, Dick M, et al: Cardiac rhythm after the Mustard operation for complete transposition of the great arteries. N Engl J Med 310:1635–1638, 1984.
22. Freed MD, Heymann MA, Lewis AB, et al: Prostaglandin E1 in infants with ductus arteriosus-dependent congenital heart disease. Circulation 64:899–905, 1981.
23. Fyler DC, Buckley LP, Hellenbrand WE, et al: Report of the New England Regional Infant Cardiac Program. Pediatrics 65(Suppl):376–460, 1980.
24. George BL, Laks H, Klitzner TS, et al: Results of the Senning procedure in infants with simple and complex transposition of the great arteries. Am J Cardiol 59:426–430, 1987.
25. Gittenberger-de Groot AC, Sauer U, Oppenheimer-Dekker A, et al: Coronary arterial anatomy in transposition of the great arteries: a morphologic study. Pediatr Cardiol 4:(Suppl)15–24, 1983.
26. Gittenberger-de Groot AC, Sauer U, Quaegebeur J: Aortic intramural coronary artery in three hearts with transposition of the great arteries. J Thorac Cardiovasc Surg 91:566–571, 1986.
27. Graham TP Jr, Atwood GF, Boucek RJ, et al: Abnormalities of right ventricular function following Mustard's operation for transposition of the great arteries. Circulation 52:678–684, 1975.
28. Hagler DJ, Ritter DG, Mair DD, et al: Clinical, angiographic, and hemodynamic assessment of late results after Mustard operation. Circulation 57:1214–1220, 1978.
29. Hagler DJ, Ritter DG, Mair DD, et al: Right and left ventricular function after the Mustard procedure in transposition of the great arteries. Am J Cardiol 44:276–283, 1979.
30. Haworth SG, Radley-Smith R, Yacoub M: Lung biopsy findings in transposition of the great arteries with ventricular septal defect: potentially reversible pulmonary vascular disease is not always synonymous with operability. J Am Coll Cardiol 9:327–333, 1987.
31. Hayes CJ, Gersony WM: Arrythmias after the Mustard operation for transposition of the great arteries: a long-term study. J Am Coll Cardiol 7:133–137, 1986.
32. Huhta JC, Edwards WD, Danielson GK, et al: Abnormalities of the tricuspid valve in complete transposition of the great arteries with ventricular septal defect. J Thorac Cardiovasc Surg 83:569–576, 1982.
33. Idriss FS, DeLeon SY, Nikaidoh H, et al: Resection of left ventricular outflow obstruction in D-transposition of the great arteries. J Thorac Cardiovasc Surg 74:343–351, 1977.
34. Idriss FS, Ilbawi MN, DeLeon SY, et al: Arterial switch in simple and complex transposition of the great arteries. J Thorac Cardiovasc Surg 95:29–36, 1988.

35. Ilbawi MN, Idriss FS, DeLeon SY, et al: Preparation of the left ventricle for anatomical correction in patients with simple transposition of the great arteries. J Thorac Cardiovasc Surg 94:87–94, 1987.

36. Jatene AD, Fontes VF, Paulista PP, et al: Anatomic correction of transposition of the great vessels. J Thorac Cardiovasc Surg 72:364–370, 1976.

37. Jatene AD, Fontes VF, Souza LCB, et al: Anatomic correction of transposition of the great arteries. J Thorac Cardiovasc Surg 83:20–26, 1982.

38. Jonas RA, Giglia TM, Sanders SP, et al: Rapid two-stage arterial switch for transposition of the great arteries and intact ventricular septum beyond the neonatal period. Circulation 80:I023–I208, 1989.

39. Lang P, Freed MD, Bierman FZ, et al: Use of Prostaglandin E1 in infants with d-transposition of the great arteries and intact ventricular septum. Am J Cardiol 44:76–81, 1979.

40. Levy RJ, Rosenthal A, Castaneda AR, et al: Growth after surgical repair of simple d-transposition of the great arteries. Ann Thorac Surg 25:225–230, 1978.

41. Liebman J, Cullum L, Belloc NB: Natural history of transposition of the great arteries: anatomy and birth and death characteristics. Circulation 40:237, 1969.

42. Lindesmith GG, Stanton RE, Lurie PR, et al: An assessment of Mustard's operation as a palliative procedure for transposition of the great vessels. Ann Thorac Surg 19:514–520, 1975.

43. Mahony L, Turley K, Ebert P, et al: Long-term results after atrial repair of transposition for the great arteries in early infancy. Circulation 66:253–258, 1982.

44. Mandell VS, Lock JE, Mayer JE, et al: The "laid-back" aortogram: an improved angiographic view for demonstration of coronary arteries in transposition of the great arteries. Am J Cardiol 65:1379–1383, 1990.

45. Martin RP, Radley-Smith R, Yacoub MH: Arrhythmias before and after anatomic correction of transposition of the great arteries. J Am Coll Cardiol 10:200–204, 1987.

46. Marx GR, Hougen TJ, Norwood WI, et al: Transposition of the great arteries with intact ventricular septum: results of Mustard and Senning operations in 123 consecutive patients. J Am Coll Cardiol 1:476–483, 1983.

47. Mavroudis C: Anatomical repair of transposition of the great arteries with intact ventricular septum in the neonate: guidelines to avoid complications. Ann Thorac Surg 43:495–501, 1987.

48. Mayer JE, Sanders SP, Jonas RA, et al: Coronary artery pattern and outcome of the arterial switch operation for transposition of the great arteries (abstract). Circulation 1989.

49. Mee RBB: Severe right ventricular failure after Mustard or Senning operation: two-stage repair—pulmonary artery banding and switch. J Thorac Cardiovasc Surg 92:385–390, 1986.

50. Moene RJ, Oppenheimer-Dekker A: Congenital mitral valve anomalies in transposition of the great arteries. Am J Cardiol 49:1972–1978, 1982.

51. Moene RJ, Oppenheimer-Dekker A, Bartelings MM: Anatomic obstruction of the right ventricular outflow tract in transposition of the great arteries. Am J Cardiol 51:1701–1704, 1983.

52. Moene RJ, Oppenheimer-Dekker A, Wenink ACG, et al: Morphology of ventricular septal defect in complete transposition of the great arteries. Am J Cardiol 55:1566–1570, 1985.

53. Mustard WT: Successful two stage correction of transposition of the great vessels. Surgery 55:469–472, 1964.

54. Muster AJ, Paul MH, Van Grondelle A, et al: Asymmetric distribution of the pulmonary blood flow between the right and left lungs in d-transposition of the great arteries. Am J Cardiol 38:352–361, 1976.

55. Newburger JW, Silbert AR, Buckley LP, et al: Cognitive function and age at repair of transposition of the great arteries in children. N Engl J Med 310:1495–1499, 1984.

56. Newburger JW, Tucker AD, Silbert AR, et al: Motor function and timing of surgery in transposition of the great arteries, intact ventricular septum (abstract). Pediatr Cardiol 4:317, 1983.

57. Newfeld EA, Paul MH, Muster AJ, et al: Pulmonary vascular disease in complete transposition of the great arteries: a study of 200 patients. Am J Cardiol 34:75–82, 1974.

58. Norwood WI, Dobell AR, Freed MD, et al: Intermediate results of the arterial switch repair: a 20-institution study. J Thorac Cardiovasc Surg 96:854–863, 1988.

59. Okuda H, Nakazawa M, Imai Y, et al: Comparison of ventricular function after Senning and Jatene procedures for complete transposition of the great arteries. Am J Cardiol 55:530–534, 1985.

60. Parrish MD, Graham TP Jr, Vender HW, et al: Radionuclide angiographic evaluation of right and left ventricular function during exercise after repair of transposition of the great arteries: comparison with normal subjects and patients with congenitally corrected transposition. Circulation 67:178–183, 1983.

61. Pasquini L, Sanders SP, Parness IA, et al: Diagnosis of coronary artery anatomy by two-dimensional echocardiography in patients with transposition of the great arteries. Circulation 75:557–564, 1987.

62. Paul MH: Complete transposition of the great arteries. In Adams FH, Emmanouilides GC, Riemenschneider TA (eds): Moss' Heart Disease in Infants, Children, and Adolescents. Baltimore, Williams & Wilkins, 1968, pp. 371–423.

63. Penskoske PA, Westerman GR, Marx GR, et al: Transposition of the great arteries and ventricular septal defect: results with the Senning operation and closure of the ventricular septal defect in infants. Ann Thorac Surg 36:281–288, 1983.

64. Rashkind WJ, Miller WW: Creation of an atrial septal defect without thoracotomy: a palliative approach to complete transposition of the great arteries. JAMA 96:991–992, 1966.

65. Rastelli GC, Wallace RB, Ongley PA: Complete repair of transposition of the great arteries with pulmonary stenosis: a review and report of a case corrected by using a new surgical technique. Circulation 39:83–95, 1969.

66. Rothman KJ, Fyler DC: Association of congenital heart defects with season and population density. Teratology 13:29–34, 1976.

67. Rothman KJ, Fyler DC: Sex, birth order and maternal age characteristics of infants with congenital heart defects. Am J Epidemiol 104:527–534, 1976.

68. Senning A: Surgical correction of transposition of the great vessels. Surgery 45:966–980, 1959.

69. Shaher R: Complete Transposition of the Great Arteries. New York, Academic Press, 1973, pp. 83–120.

70. Sievers HH, Lange PE, Arensman FW, et al: Influence of two-stage anatomic correction on size and distensibility of the anatomic pulmonary/functional aortic root in patients with simple transposition of the great arteries. Circulation 70:202–208, 1984.

71. Silove ED, Taylor JFN: Angiographic and anatomical features of subvalvar left ventricular outflow obstruction in transposition of the great arteries: the possible role of the anterior mitral valve leaflet. Pediatr Radiol 1:87–93, 1973.

72. Smith A, Arnold R, Wilkinson JL, et al: An anatomical study of the patterns of the coronary arteries and sinus

nodal artery in complete transposition. Int J Cardiol 12:295–304, 1986.

73. Trowitzsch E, Colan SD, Sanders SP: Global and regional right ventricular function in normal infants and infants with transposition of the great arteries after Senning operation. Circulation 72:1003–1014, 1985.

74. Trowitzsch E, Colan SD, Sanders SP: Two-dimensional echocardiographic estimation of right ventricular area change and ejection fraction in infants with systemic right ventricle (transposition of the great arteries or hypoplastic left heart syndrome). Am J Cardiol 55:1153–1157, 1985.

75. Trusler GA, Castaneda AR, Rosenthal A, et al: Current results of management in transposition of the great arteries, with special emphasis on patients with associated ventricular septal defect. J Am Coll Cardiol 10:1061–1071, 1987.

76. Turina M, Siebenmann R, Nussbaumer P, et al: Long-term outlook after a trial correction of transposition of the great arteries. J Thorac Cardiovasc Surg 95:828–835, 1988.

77. Turley K, Hanley FL, Verrier ED, et al: The Mustard procedure in infants (less than 100 days of age): ten-year followup. J Thorac Cardiovasc Surg 96:849–853, 1988.

78. Vetter VL, Tanner CS: Electrophysiologic consequences of the arterial switch repair of d-transposition of the great arteries. J Am Coll Cardiol 12:229–237, 1988.

79. Vetter VL, Tanner CS, Horowitz LN: Electrophysiologic consequences of the Mustard repair of d-transposition of the great arteries. J Am Coll Cardiol 10:1265–1273, 1987.

80. Villagra F, Quero-Jimenez M, Maitre-Azcarate MJ, et al: Transposition of the great arteries with ventricular septal defects: surgical considerations concerning the Rastelli operation. J Thorac Cardiovasc Surg 88:1004–1011, 1984.

81. Vogel M, Freedom RM, Smallhorn JF, et al: Complete transposition of the great arteries and coarctation of the aorta. Am J Cardiol 53:1627, 1984.

82. Walsh EP, Wernovsky G, Keane JF, et al: Prospective evaluation of arrhythmias after arterial switch operation for transposition of the great arteries (abstract). Circulation 76(Suppl):IV-549, 1987.

83. Wernovsky G, Hougen TJ, Walsh EP, et al: Midterm results after the arterial switch operation for transposition of the great arteries with intact ventricular septum: clinical, hemodynamic, echocardiographic, and electrophysiologic data. Circulation 77:1333–1334, 1988.

84. Wernovsky G, Jonas RA, Colan SD et al: Results of the arterial switch operation in patients with abnormalities of the mitral valve or left ventricular outflow tract. J Thorac Cardiovasc Surg 95:828–835, 1988.

85. Yacoub MH: The case for anatomic correction of transposition of the great arteries. J Thorac Cardiovasc Surg 78:3–6, 1979.

86. Yacoub M, Bernhard A, Lange P, et al: Clinical and hemodynamic results of the two-stage anatomic correction of simple transposition of the great arteries. Circulation 62(Suppl):190–196, 1980.

87. Yacoub MH, Bernhard A, Radley-Smith R, et al: Supravalvular pulmonary stenosis after anatomic correction of transposition of the great arteries: causes and prevention. Circulation 66(Suppl):193–197, 1982.

Chapter 36

ENDOCARDIAL CUSHION DEFECTS

Donald C. Fyler, M.D.

DEFINITION

Abnormalities of the structures derived from the embryologic endocardial cushions are called endocardial cushion defects. These include a variety of anomalies of the atrial and ventricular septa and the adjacent parts of the mitral and tricuspid valves.

EMBRYOLOGY

The primitive atrioventricular canal connects the atria to the left ventricle. The endocardial cushions make up the circumference of the canal and divide naturally into superior, inferior, right, and left lateral cushions. These ridges of mesenchymal tissue contribute to the adjacent parts of the atrial septum, the ventricular septum, the septal leaflet of the tricuspid valve, and the anterior leaflet of the mitral valve. A flaw in this development results in an endocardial cushion defect.

It has been proposed that in patients with atrioventricular canal defects or ostium primum defects, the main deficiency is in the ventricular septum, the usual amount of atrial septum being largely present, but the atrioventricular valves are located lower on the septum.[17] Thus, with an ostium primum defect there is less than the usual amount of ventricular septum with near normal amounts of atrial septum, and the position of the atrioventricular valves is lower than normal.

ANATOMY

The anatomic categorization of the endocardial cushion defects has been a controversial topic for some time. To start with, the implication that these defects are derived from the embryologic endocardial cushions is not entirely correct.[39] To discuss the many points of classification that have been raised is beyond the scope of this book.[1,4,28,29,32,38] The discussion that follows presents the anatomy

as discussed in the day-to-day work of the cardiologists at Children's Hospital in Boston, where complete agreement on any topic is unknown.

Endocardial cushion defects (also known as common atrioventricular canals, common atrioventricular orifices, or atrioventricular septal defects) involve the septal portions of the mitral and tricuspid valves and the adjacent ventricular and atrial septa. The degree of abnormality of the septa is variable; at worst, virtually the entire atrial and ventricular septa may be absent. Or there may be a defect confined to one septum or the other. Thus, there may be a very large ventricular defect and no atrial defect, or the reverse. When there is deficiency of both the atrial and ventricular septa, the mitral and tricuspid valves cannot attach normally. Their anterior leaflets may form a single sail-like structure, which is part of a surprisingly competent valve extending across the septal orifice. When there is dominantly an atrial defect (ostium primum defect), the mitral valve is usually cleft and is often incompetent, sometimes allowing gross regurgitation. Rarely, the atrioventricular valve deformity is the sole abnormality, there being little or no septal defect. The variations in these deformities provide the basis for the many terms used in classification: **complete common, partial, transitional, intermediate, type A, type B, type C, left-sided, right-sided,** and **balanced** atrioventricular canals.

The **ventricular defect** can be very large, extending well beyond the part of the septum that is derived from endocardial cushion tissue. Usually, the ventricular opening is large and extends into the adjacent atrial septum as well (Fig. 1), although rarely there may be a large typical ventricular defect with only a minimal atrial opening and, very rarely, no atrial defect at all.[33] An isolated ventricular defect without an atrial opening, usually without atrioventricular valvar deformity, may be located immediately adjacent to the anterior leaflet of the mitral valve and under the septal leaflet of the tricuspid valve, and is described as a ventric-

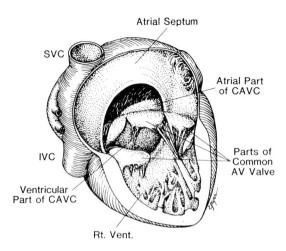

Figure 1. Drawing of a common atrioventricular canal. Note the extension of valvar tissue across the defect. Note that the defect extends as one common orifice from the mid-atrial septum to the mid-ventricular septum. There is considerable variation in the size of the orifice and in the relative involvement of the atrial and ventricular septums. IVC, inferior vena cava; SVC, superior vena cava; CAVC, common atrioventricular canal.

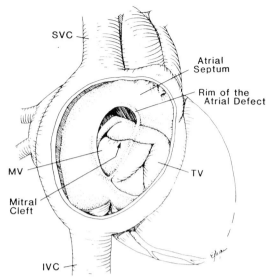

Figure 2. Drawing of an atrial septal defect of the ostium primum type. Note that the defect extends to the valve insertions on each side and that there is a cleft in the mitral valve. SVC, superior vena cava; IVC, inferior vena cava; MV, mitral valve; TV, tricuspid valve.

ular defect of the endocardial cushion type (see p. 438).

The **atrial defects** are equally variable, ranging from a small septal opening to complete absence of the atrial septum (including the entire atrial septum well beyond the territory of the cushions) (i.e., common atrium, single atrium). An isolated atrial defect with little or no ventricular opening is described as an ostium primum defect (Fig. 2). The terms partial, incomplete, transitional, and intermediate describe endocardial cushion defects that range between an ostium primum defect and a persistent, complete common atrioventricular canal.

The **atrioventricular valves** are almost invariably involved in these anomalies. With an ostium primum defect, there is almost always a cleft of the anterior leaflet of the mitral valve (Fig. 3), often, but not necessarily, associated with mitral regurgitation. Occasionally a mitral valve has a double orifice (Fig. 3).[38] There may be varying degrees of mitral regurgitation and, occasionally, mitral regurgitation is the dominant lesion, a small associated atrial septal opening being of little physiologic consequence. With persistence of the common atrioventricular canal, the anterior leaflet of the atrioventricular valve is shared between the right and left ventricles, forming a sail-like structure. This leaflet extends across the septum and poses a significant problem when the atrioventricular canal defect is to be repaired. The relationships of the leaflets to the crest of the ventricular septum have been used as a surgical classification of atrioventricular canal defects.[32]

The tricuspid valve may **override** the ventricular septum or it may **straddle** the septum, with insertion of the chordae in the opposite ventricle. The distinction between overriding and straddling is determined by the insertion of the chordae. If insertion is on the appropriate side of the septum, or on the septal crest the term *overriding* is used. If insertion is across the septum in the opposing ventricle, the term *straddling* is used. The implications for surgical repair are obvious. When either the overriding or straddling is significant, the blood from one atrium is distributed to both ventricles, the proportions being dependent on the degree of displacement of the valve. The underlying right ventricle will be hypoplastic in proportion to the limitation of blood flow that results from the diversion of flow to the other ventricle. Marked hypoplasia of a ventricle may prohibit any possibility of a two-ventricle repair.[12]

Some patients with a common atrioventricular canal defect have a single left ventricular papillary muscle (or two immediately adjacent papillary muscles) which, when a repair has been undertaken, leaves one papillary muscle in the left ventricle. The functional result amounts to a parachute mitral valve, obstructing left ventricular inflow.[10,30,36,38]

The chordae may be relatively short, the atrioventricular valve displaced, and the geometry of the left ventricle distorted. Which deformity is the basic one and which is the natural consequence of the other is a personal conclusion.

Atrioventricular canal defects may be associated with pulmonary stenosis; many of these cases are

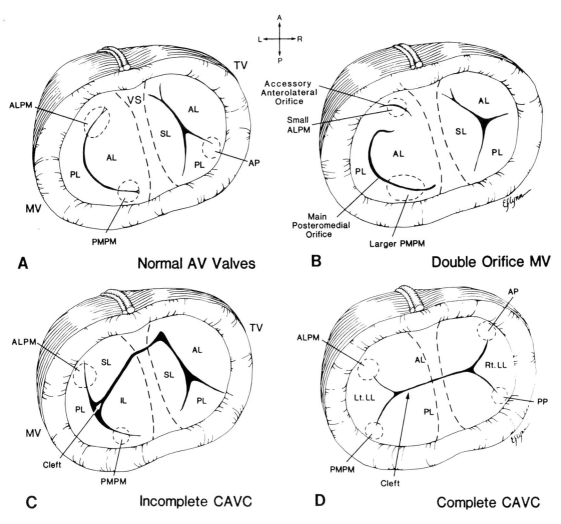

Figure 3. Views of the atrioventricular valves from above in patients with endocardial cushion defects compared with those in normal patients. **A,** Normal. **B,** Double-orifice mitral valve. Note that there is a papillary muscle associated with each orifice. **C,** Ostium primum defect (incomplete complete atrioventricular canal) showing a cleft mitral valve. **D,** Common atrioventricular canal. Note the valve tissue extending across the defect. PMPM, posterior medial papillary muscle; MV, mitral valve; ALPM, anterolateral papillary muscle; TV, tricuspid valve; AL, anterior leaflet; PL, posterior leaflet; SL, superior leaflet (mitral side) or septal leaflet (tricuspid side); IL, inferior leaflet; Rt.LL, right lateral leaflet; Lt.LL, left lateral leaflet; VS, ventricular septum; CAVC, complete atrioventricular canal.

variants of the tetralogy of Fallot syndrome (see p. 488). In other instances, valvar pulmonary stenosis or peripheral pulmonary stenosis may be associated with the ventricular defect.

However one chooses to think about these questions, it is obvious that the surgeon must be familiar with the anatomy and its variations and must have a philosophy of management that has proved successful, regardless of the nomenclature and the embryologic theories.

A common atrioventricular canal defect is present in half of patients with Down syndrome and congenital heart disease (Exhibit 1). In patients who do not have Down syndrome, the ventricles

are sometimes asymmetric and one of the ventricles is hypoplastic; however, in children with Down syndrome, ventricular hypoplasia is less common. Sometimes the ventricles may assume a superior-inferior relationship, with the outflow to both great vessels via the right ventricle (double-outlet right ventricle, see ch. 41).

Almost any known congenital cardiac defect may be associated with an endocardial cushion defect unless the child has Down syndrome. Additional cardiac defects, such as coarctation of the aorta or D-transposition of the great arteries, are rare in children with Down syndrome[13] and are common in other children with endocardial cushion defects (Exhibit 1).

Exhibit 1

<table>
<tr><td colspan="3" align="center">Boston Children's Hospital Experience
1973–87</td></tr>
<tr><td colspan="3" align="center">Number of Patients with Endocardial Cushion Defects By Year First Seen</td></tr>
<tr><td align="center">Year</td><td align="center">With Down
Syndrome</td><td align="center">Without Down
Syndrome</td></tr>
<tr><td align="center">–1973</td><td align="center">10</td><td align="center">100</td></tr>
<tr><td align="center">1973–1977</td><td align="center">54</td><td align="center">64</td></tr>
<tr><td align="center">1978–1982</td><td align="center">110</td><td align="center">87</td></tr>
<tr><td align="center">1983–1987</td><td align="center">153</td><td align="center">139</td></tr>
<tr><td align="center">Total</td><td align="center">327</td><td align="center">390</td></tr>
</table>

There were 717 patients whose primary cardiac diagnosis was an endocardial cushion defect (327 had Down syndrome and 390 did not). An additional 427 patients were categorized under some other heading who had endocardial cushion defects as well (49 had Down syndrome and 378 did not).

Note the 10-fold difference between the numbers of patients with and without Down syndrome before 1973, and the increasing numbers of patients with Down syndrome subsequently.

Types of Endocardial Cushion Defects

<table>
<tr><td align="center">Type</td><td align="center">With Down
Syndrome
n = 327</td><td align="center">Without Down
Syndrome
n = 390</td></tr>
<tr><td>Ostium Primum Defect</td><td align="center">51</td><td align="center">158</td></tr>
<tr><td>Common Atrioventricular Canal</td><td align="center">262</td><td align="center">119</td></tr>
<tr><td>Isolated Valvar Deformity</td><td align="center">4</td><td align="center">13</td></tr>
<tr><td>First Seen Before 1973</td><td align="center">10</td><td align="center">100</td></tr>
</table>

Although atrioventricular canal is more common in patients with Down syndrome, ostium primum defects are more common in those who do not have Down syndrome. The data prior to 1973 are shown separately because of the small numbers of patients with Down syndrome seen at that time.

Primary Diagnosis of Patients with Endocardial Cushion Defect as a Secondary Diagnosis
1983–1987

<table>
<tr><td align="center">Primary
Diagnosis</td><td align="center">With Down
Syndrome
n = 33</td><td align="center">Without Down
Syndrome
n = 223</td></tr>
<tr><td>Coarctation of Aorta</td><td align="center">0</td><td align="center">2</td></tr>
<tr><td>Ventricular Septal Defect</td><td align="center">9</td><td align="center">17</td></tr>
<tr><td>Aortic Valve Abnormality</td><td align="center">0</td><td align="center">4</td></tr>
<tr><td>Single Ventricle</td><td align="center">0</td><td align="center">7</td></tr>
<tr><td>Malposition</td><td align="center">0</td><td align="center">97</td></tr>
<tr><td>Hypoplastic Left Heart</td><td align="center">0</td><td align="center">10</td></tr>
<tr><td>Double-Outlet Right Ventricle</td><td align="center">1</td><td align="center">16</td></tr>
<tr><td>D-Transposition of Great Arteries</td><td align="center">0</td><td align="center">16</td></tr>
<tr><td>Tetralogy of Fallot</td><td align="center">18</td><td align="center">15</td></tr>
<tr><td>Atrial Septal Defect</td><td align="center">1</td><td align="center">5</td></tr>
<tr><td>Other</td><td align="center">4</td><td align="center">34</td></tr>
</table>

Note that other than endocardial cushion defects, Down syndrome is associated with ventricular septal defect and tetralogy of Fallot.

PHYSIOLOGY

The physiologic consequences of endocardial cushion defects are those expected of ventricular or atrial defects or both, with the added possibility of atrioventricular valvar regurgitation. A cleft valve is not necessarily incompetent and a common atrioventricular canal, despite the extensive atrioventricular valve deformity, tends to have little or no regurgitation. However, every possible variation in the size of the defect, the location of the defect, and the degree of atrioventricular valvar incompetence is seen.

When there is mitral regurgitation through a cleft, the presence of an atrial defect may result in reflux of the blood from the left ventricle to the right atrium. Consequently, the left atrium is not enlarged, despite significant regurgitation and obvious enlargement of the left ventricle.

With valvar overriding there is greater mixing of the pulmonary and systemic venous return, depending on the degree of override, and when one ventricle is very small the degree of mixing is equivalent to that of a single ventricle.

When there is a large ventricular opening, the risk of pulmonary vascular disease is high. In this case there is equilibration of right and left ventricular pressures and, unless there is pulmonary stenosis, there is obligatory pulmonary hypertension from birth. The development of pulmonary vascular disease is age-related and, with a large ventricular component, it occurs at least as early as it does with any other large ventricular defect.

There has been debate about the development of pulmonary vascular disease in patients with persistent atrioventricular canal defects who have Down syndrome. Most agree that the average pulmonary resistance in patients with Down syndrome is higher than it is in comparable children of the same age who do not have the Down syndrome. Some have interpreted this to be irreversible pulmonary vascular obstructive disease of the type seen with large ventricular defects, but appearing earlier because of the genetic abnormality.[6,37] Histopathologic examination does not bear out this hypothesis.[14] The author is persuaded that the equally well-established ventilatory problems in children with Down syndrome are a contributing cause for pulmonary hypertension. Respiratory problems such as upper airway obstruction, central hypoventilation, or chronic respiratory disease, in varying combinations, are particularly common in children with Down syndrome and are associated with reversible pulmonary hypertension.[15] The presence of obligatory pulmonary hypertension because of a large ventricular septal defect and a variable left-to-right shunt further impinges on the borderline ventilatory capability. The result is elevation of pulmonary resistance to levels tending to limit left-to-right shunting. This is partly relieved by improved ventilation and oxygenation. However, relaxation of the pulmonary vascularity does not always occur in minutes; sometimes it requires days of improved oxygenation. Whether irreversible pulmonary vascular disease is more common in children with Down syndrome than in children who do not have Down syndrome remains to be established. In the author's experience it is not—at least in the first years of life.

CLINICAL MANIFESTATIONS

Discovery

Endocardial cushion defects are features of several syndromes which are readily recognized. Fully 30% of patients with Down syndrome have congenital heart disease, more than half of which are forms of atrioventricular canal abnormality (see p. 46). Common atrium is a characteristic lesion in patients with the Ellis Van Creveld syndrome, and many patients with asplenia (Ivemark's syndrome) have common atrioventricular canals (see p. 590). The diagnosis of any one of these syndromes should raise the question of an endocardial cushion defect.

In the absence of a recognizable syndrome, the cardiac lesion is often discovered in early infancy because of a readily audible murmur, although oc-

casionally a baby with Down syndrome has no audible murmur, presumably because of pulmonary hypertension (Fig. 4). Such infants have been overlooked as having important heart disease. Consequently, all newborn infants with Down syndrome should have an electrocardiogram, as a screening tool, to discover the presence of heart disease. The presence of a leftward-superior QRS axis suggests the possibility of an endocardial cushion defect even if there is no murmur.

Ostium Primum Defects

History. Infants discovered through routine screening methods to have an ostium primum type of atrial septal defect are largely asymptomatic. Rarely, a child with an ostium primum defect will have symptoms of congestive heart failure with tachypnea and growth failure. Usually this is a consequence of mitral regurgitation aggravating the left-to-right shunt.

Physical Examination. Generally, children with atrial septal defects of the ostium primum type grow well and have no signs of congestive heart failure. The cardiac impulse may be hyperactive if the shunt is large and particularly if there is mitral

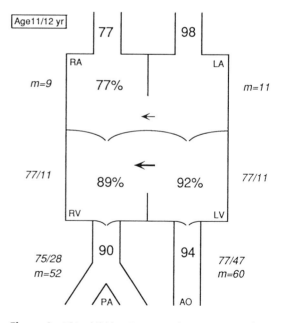

Figure 4. This child has Down syndrome. Because there were no abnormal findings on repeated physical examination, she was thought to have no heart disease until an electrocardiogram was taken at 11 months of age. There was a leftward superior axis (see Fig. 3). When examined by a cardiologist there was no abnormality on auscultation. Subsequently, the diagnosis of a very large common atrioventricular canal was made by echocardiography. The infant survived surgery and is now well. Italics, mm Hg; %, percent oxygen saturation; RA, right atrium; RV, right ventricle; LV, left ventricle; LA, left atrium; AO, aorta; PA, pulmonary artery.

regurgitation. The second heart sound is well split and does not vary with respiration. There is a systolic murmur at the upper left sternal border which is stenotic in character and usually is not loud. With a large shunt there may be a rumbling murmur in early to mid diastole at the lower left sternal border. A systolic murmur of mitral regurgitation may be audible at the cardiac apex, although often, in some of these patients, the murmur of mitral regurgitation is heard equally well at the lower left sternal border.

Electrocardiography. The electrocardiogram has a leftward, superior axis usually ranging between −30 degrees and −90 degrees (Fig. 5). Incomplete right bundle branch block is usually present and if there is significant mitral regurgitation, there may be left ventricular hypertrophy.

Chest X-ray. Depending on the size of the left-to-right shunt and the amount of mitral regurgitation, the heart may be enlarged and the pulmonary vasculature engorged. The left atrium is not enlarged because it is decompressed by the septal defect; in effect, the left ventricular regurgitant flow passes directly into the right atrium. There may be enlargement of the heart out of proportion to the degree of pulmonary vascular engorgement if mitral regurgitation is a prominent feature.

Echocardiography. The two-dimensional technique demonstrates the atrial defect, and the left-to-right shunt can be recognized with Doppler examination. The presence of a mitral valve cleft and mitral regurgitation are readily appreciated. The diagnostic precision of echocardiography in conjunction with the other clinical findings is accurate enough to avoid the need for diagnostic cardiac catheterization in most of these patients.[24]

The primum atrial septal defect can be imaged using apical, parasternal, and subxiphoid views.[18,22] The defect is in the atrioventricular canal portion of the atrial septum, adjacent to the atrioventricular valves. The inlet into the atrioventricular valves is common and resembles a complete common atrioventricular canal defect. The attachments of the valve leaflets to the crest of the ventricular septum separate the outlet into the two valve orifices and close the potential ventricular septal defect. The apical four-chamber view shows all of these features. The morphology of the mitral valve is seen best in subxiphoid and parasternal short-axis views (Fig. 6). The number and spacing of the left ventricular papillary muscles, the cleft in the anterior mitral leaflet, and the attachments of the valve to the septum can be seen in a short-axis view. Doppler color flow mapping from an apical view is excellent for the detection and quantification of atrioventricular valve regurgitation.

Cardiac Catheterization. Given a confident diagnosis by echocardiography, there is little need for cardiac catheterization. However, in the child

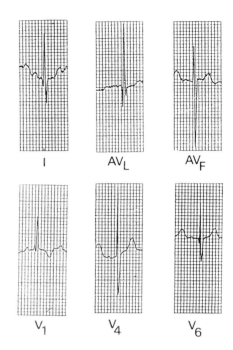

Figure 5. This electrocardiogram is typical of the endocardial cushion defects. Note that the QRS axis is leftward and superior.

with severe mitral regurgitation it may be useful to use cardiac catheterization to evaluate the physiology before going on to surgery and possible valve replacement. Patients with atypical echocardiographic findings or observations inconsistent with the other clinical findings should undergo diagnostic catheterization.

Management. Surgical repair of an ostium primum defect is associated with low mortality and good results and, were it not for the commonly associated mitral valve problems, all ostium primum defects could be closed in infancy. Because of the potential for mitral valvuloplasty and even valve replacement arising as an issue in the course of the operation, caution about scheduling these children for surgery is needed. Fortunately, repair of double-orifice mitral valves,[2,23] and most regurgitant valves, is possible.[7,8] As the years go by fewer mitral valve replacements seem to be needed and it is possible that this issue is disappearing. In the meantime, there being little added risk in waiting, it seems wisest to delay surgery until it is possible to replace the valve if it is needed.[34]

The results of surgical repair of ostium primum defects are excellent (Exhibit 2).[19,20,25,27,31,35]

Course. It is impossible to close an ostium primum atrial defect, tinker with a regurgitant mitral valve, and leave the patient with a normal heart. Some incompetence of the mitral valve is expected and, therefore, a residual murmur is common. In some situations mitral regurgitation is self-aggravating and becomes more pronounced with the

Exhibit 2

Boston Children's Hospital Experience
1973–1987

**Endocardial Cushion Defects
Surgical Procedures
1973–1987**

Surgical Procedure	Primary Diagnosis		Secondary Diagnosis	
	With Down Syndrome n = 258	Without Down Syndrome n = 272	With Down Syndrome n = 26	Without Down Syndrome n = 143
Atrioventricular Canal Repair	208	70	12	15
Ostium Primum Repair	34	167	1	14
Mitral Valve Replacement	20	35	4	11
Fontan's Procedure	0	2	0	45
Ventricular Defect Repair	32	29	14	45
Atrial Defect Repair	25	28	2	51

Many patients had more than one procedure. Note the number of patients who had a mitral valve replacement.

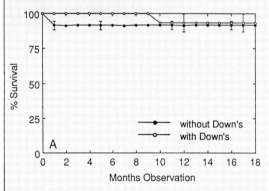

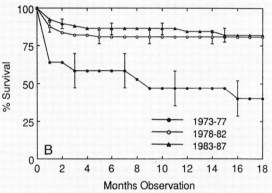

Life table comparing survival of 30 patients with Down syndrome and 103 patients without Down syndrome whose first surgery was repair of ostium primum defect.

Life table comparing survival of patients who had atrioventricular canal repair in three different time periods. 1973–77, 20 patients; 1978–1982, 98 patients; 1983–1987, 142 patients.

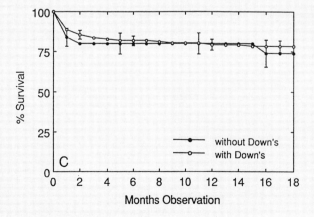

Life table comparing survival of 201 patients with Down syndrome and 59 patients without Down syndrome whose first surgery was repair of common atrial ventricular canal.

passage of time. Fortunately, this is not common. Thus far, follow-up of repaired patients suggests an uncomplicated future for most of them.

Atrioventricular Canal

History. The majority (69%) of children with common atrioventricular canal defects have Down syndrome (Exhibit 1). With recognition that the patient has Down syndrome (see ch. 18), the possibility of congenital heart disease must be considered and, when heart disease is found, there is a 50% chance that the child has a persistent common atrioventricular canal. While, occasionally, a baby with Down syndrome who has no auscultatory findings has an atrioventricular canal defect, the majority with this defect have easily recognized auscultatory findings suggesting congenital heart disease (usually a systolic murmur). Congestive heart failure and failure to grow adequately are common presenting problems.

Physical Examination. Besides the possible evidences of congestive heart failure, there may be a hyperactive cardiac impulse. Most patients have a systolic murmur that is loudest at the lower left sternal border and sometimes is heard well toward the apex. Third heart sounds, gallop rhythms, and apical diastolic rumbling murmurs are often encountered. The second (pulmonary) component of the second heart sound is usually accentuated.

Electrocardiography. The electrocardiogram has a superior, frequently "northwest" axis, often being between $-150°$ and $-90°$ in the frontal plane. Evidence of right, or both right and left, ventricular hypertrophy is present (Fig. 5). Rarely, a patient with severe right ventricular hypertrophy

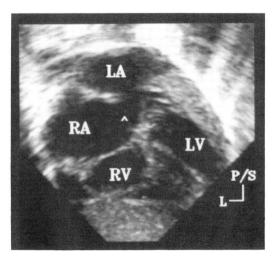

Figure 6. Subxiphoid four-chamber view in a patient with primum atrial septal defect (arrow). Note the attachments of the atrioventricular valve onto the crest of the ventricular septum that close the potential ventricular defect. L, left; LA, left atrium, LV, left ventricle; P, posterior; RA; right atrium; RV, right ventricle; S, superior.

will not have the characteristic leftward-superior axis, but will have right-axis deviation instead.

Chest X-ray. The heart size is enlarged and the pulmonary vascularity is engorged in proportion to the amount of left-to-right shunting. Usually, the left atrium is not enlarged despite evidence of a large shunt.

Echocardiography. Echocardiography has been an invaluable tool in delineating atrioventricular canal defects. Documentation of the size of the ventricular septal defect, the size and shape of the atrial defect, and the relative and absolute sizes of the ventricles, as well as evaluation of the components of the atrioventricular valve, is possible using sophisticated 2-dimensional and Doppler echocardiography. The degree of atrioventricular regurgitation, the number and location of the papillary muscles, and the presence of associated defects are recorded.

The subxiphoid view demonstrates the primum atrial septal defect, the common atrioventricular valve, and the ventricular septal defect component. The alignment of the common valve vis-à-vis the ventricular septum and the left papillary muscle architecture is well seen in the short-axis view. The apical four-chamber view demonstrates the size of the ventricular septal defect and is an excellent view for a Doppler examination of the valves. The apical and parasternal long-axis views can demonstrate abnormal valve attachment that produces subaortic stenosis.

Cardiac Catheterization. Virtually all patients with an echocardiographic diagnosis of an atrioventricular canal defect should undergo cardiac catheterization to evaluate pulmonary hypertension and pulmonary resistance. Additional ventricular defects can be excluded and the relative size of the ventricles documented.

With the patient in the hepatoclavicular position, a pigtail or balloon angiographic catheter is placed in the left ventricle, either across the atrioventricular valve or retrograde across the aortic valve. An angiogram is recorded following an injection of contrast of 1.5–2.0 ml/kg of body weight. This view will not only outline a complete atrioventricular canal and additional ventricular septal defects, but is as good a view as any for determining the degree of mitral regurgitation. Occasionally, a catheter course across the mitral valve, or the rapid injection of contrast medium, may artifically induce mitral valve leakage. When mitral regurgitation is observed, the angiogram may be repeated with the injection at a lower flow rate (and perhaps with retrograde passage of the catheter) to reduce the chances of catheter-induced valvar regurgitation. The angiogram is used primarily to rule out associated muscular ventricular septal defects and to check further on ventricular size.

An aortogram is recorded to discover a patent ductus arteriosus, a common finding in patients with Down syndrome and a common atrioventricular canal.

Management. In the past, children with common atrioventricular canal underwent banding of the main pulmonary artery in early infancy to control congestive heart failure, promote growth, and prevent the development of pulmonary vascular disease. It was planned, at a later date, to remove the band and repair the intracardiac anatomy. The initial mortality with this approach was high,[3,16] and later repair was complicated by the prior operation.[26] Consequently, complete repair in infancy, early enough to prevent pulmonary vascular disease and to promote growth, became the treatment of choice.[9]

Given two ventricles of suitable size, judged adequate to support normal circulation, and no additional defects, surgical correction is undertaken. The defect between the ventricles and atria is patched with one or two patches[5] and the available valve tissue is fashioned into functioning mitral and tricuspid valves. Clearly, the surgeon strives for a functioning mitral valve, because dysfunction on the left side is a major deficit, whereas right-sided atrioventricular valve (tricuspid) dysfunction is much better tolerated. Ideally, surgery is carried

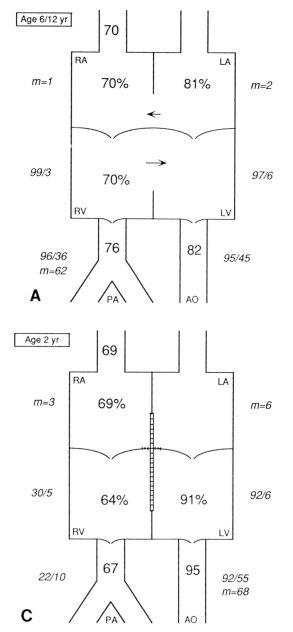

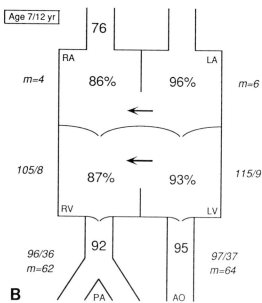

Figure 7. **A,** This infant has Down syndrome and a common atrioventricular canal. At catheterization at age 6 months there was pulmonary hypertension at systemic levels and relatively little left-to-right shunt. As a consequence, the calculated pulmonary resistance was high. **B,** The child was placed on 100% oxygen and showed a marked increase in the pulmonary blood flow because of a large increase in the left-to-right shunt. He underwent uneventful surgical repair and was brought back for follow-up cardiac catheterization (**C**) because of a residual murmur. He was found to have a small muscular ventricular septal defect that had been overlooked. There was no evidence of residual elevation of pulmonary resistance. Abbrevations, see Figure 4.

out sometime after the first months of life and before the child develops pulmonary vascular disease. After the first birthday the chance of developing irreversible pulmonary vascular disease increases as the months go by. The infant who is less than 1 year old but who appears to have prohibitive pulmonary vascular disease is repaired on discovery (Fig. 7). Further evaluation, including a trial of chronic oxygen therapy, may be indicated, and even lung biopsy may be helpful. Rarely, patients, with or without Down syndrome, have irreversible pulmonary vascular disease even before the first birthday; others may have some permanent elevation of pulmonary resistance that will add to the risk of the operation. Nevertheless, operative deaths attributed to pulmonary vascular disease are rare and, after surgical repair, the development of pulmonary vascular disease in survivors is not common. In older children, with or without the Down syndrome, the usual criteria for decisions about surgery for a ventricular septal defect are applied.

Overall the mortality of surgery for atrioventricular canal defects is acceptable (Exhibit 2). The factors influencing the outcome are: (1) the atrioventricular anatomy, (2) ventricular hypoplasia, (3) malalignment of the atrioventricular valve and the ventricles, (4) double-orifice mitral valve,[23] (5) single left-sided papillary muscles, and (6) additional muscular defects.[11,12,21,40] There is essentially no difference in survival between patients with and without the Down syndrome (Exhibit 2). Surgical mortality is influenced by the associated cardiac defects (Exhibit 2). Postoperative disruption of the repair is a dramatic event sometimes confused with overwhelming sepsis, because there may be high fever and marked leukocytosis in a patient who suddenly becomes extremely ill. Fortunately, this has become less common as experience has accumulated.

Course. Among children sick with untreated atrioventricular canal defects, the mortality in the first year of life is as much as 50%.[16] Irreversible pulmonary vascular disease becomes increasingly common in the surviving child with an unrepaired common atrioventricular canal defect.

REFERENCES

1. Anderson RH, Zuberbuhler JR, Penkoske PA, et al: Of clefts, commissures, and things. J Thorac Cardiovasc Surg 90:605–610, 1985.
2. Bano-Rodrigo A, Van Praagh S, Trowitzsch E, et al: Double-orifice mitral valve: a study of 27 postmortem cases with developmental, diagnostic and surgical considerations. Am J Cardiol 61:152–160, 1988.
3. Bender HW, Hammon JW, Hubbard SC, et al: Repair of atrioventricular canal malformation in the first year of life. J Thorac Cardiovasc Surg 84:515–522, 1982.
4. Bharati S, Kirklin JW, McAllister HA Jr, et al: The surgical anatomy of common atrioventricular orifice associated with tetralogy of Fallot, double outlet right ventricle, and complete regular transposition. Circulation 61:1142–1149, 1980.
5. Bove EF, Sondheimer HM, Kavey R-EW, et al: Results with the two-patch technique for repair of complete atrioventricular septal defect. Ann Thorac Surg 38:157–161, 1984.
6. Bull C, Rigby ML, Shinebourne EA: Should management of complete atrioventricular canal defect be influenced by coexistent Down syndrome? Lancet 1:1147–1149, 1985.
7. Carpentier A: Surgical anatomy and management of the mitral component of the atrioventricular canal defects. In Anderson RH, Shinebourne EA (eds): Pediatric Cardiology. London, Churchill Livingstone, 1979, pp. 477–490.
8. Carpentier A: Congenital malformations of the mitral valve. In Stark J, de Leval M (eds): Surgery for Congenital Heart Defects. London, Grune & Stratton, 1983, pp. 467–482.
9. Castaneda AR, Mayer JE, Jonas RA: Repair of complete atrioventricular canal in infancy. World J Surg 9:590–597, 1985.
10. Chin AJ, Bierman FZ, Sanders SP, et al: Subxyphoid 2-dimensional echocardiographic identification of left ventricular papillary muscle anomalies in complete common atrioventricular canal. Am J Cardiol 51:1695–1699, 1983.
11. Chin AJ, Keane JF, Norwood WI, et al: Repair of complete common atrioventricular canal in infancy. J Thorac Cardiovasc Surg 84:437–445, 1982.
12. Clapp SK, Perry BL, Farooki ZQ, et al: Surgical and medical results of complete atrioventricular canal: a ten year review. Am J Cardiol 59:454–458, 1987.
13. De Biase L, Di Ciommo V, Ballerini L, et al: Prevalence of left-sided obstructive lesions in patients with atrioventricular canal without Down's syndrome. J Thorac Cardiovasc Surg 91:467–472, 1986.
14. Fried R, Fyler D, Reid L: Pulmonary artery hypertension (PAH) in infants with atrioventricular canal (AVC) and Down's syndrome (DS) (abstract). Circulation 1984.
15. Fujii AM, Rabinovitch M, Keane JF, et al: Radionuclide angiocardiographic assessment of pulmonary vascular reactivity in patients with left to right shunt and pulmonary hypertension. Am J Cardiol 49:356–361, 1982.
16. Fyler DC, Buckley LP, Hellenbrand WE, et al: Report of the New England Regional Infant Cardiac Program. Pediatrics 65(Suppl):375–461, 1980.
17. Gutgesell HP, Huhta JC: Cardiac septation in atrioventricular canal defect. J Am Coll Cardiol 8:1421–1424, 1986.
18. Hagler DJ, Tajik AJ, Seward JB, et al: Real-time wide-angle sector echocardiography: atrioventricular canal defects. Circulation 59:140–150, 1979.
19. Houyel L, Petit J, Langlois J et al: Mid-term follow-up of patients operated upon for incomplete persistent atrioventricular canal: a series of 128 cases. Arch Mal Coeur 81:501–505, 1988.
20. King RM, Puga FJ, Danielson GK, et al: Prognostic factors and surgical treatment of partial atrioventricular canal. Circulation 74(Suppl I):I-42–I-46, 1986.
21. Lacour-Gayet F, Planche C, Langlois J, et al: Surgical repair of complete atrioventricular canal, regular and irregular forms, in 75 patients. Arch Mal Coeur 79:708–716, 1986.
22. Lange DJ, Sahn DJ, Allen HD, et al: Subxiphoid cross-sectional echocardiography in infants and children with congenital heart disease. Circulation 59:513–524, 1979.
23. Lee C-N, Danielson GK, Schaff HV, et al: Surgical treatment of double-orifice mitral valve in atrioventricular canal defects. J Thorac Cardiovasc Surg 90:700–705, 1985.

24. Lipshultz SE, Sanders SP, Mayer JE, et al: Are routine preoperative cardiac catheterization and angiography necessary before repair of ostium primum atrial septal defect? J Am Coll Cardiol 11:373–378, 1988.

25. Losay J, Rosenthal A, Castaneda AR, et al: Repair of atrial septal defect primum. J Thorac Cardiovasc Surg 75:248–254, 1978.

26. Mavroudis C, Weinstein G, Turley K, et al: Surgical management of complete atrioventricular canal. J Thorac Cardiovasc Surg 83:670–679, 1982.

27. Pan-Chih, Chen-Chun: Surgical treatment of atrioventricular canal malformations. Ann Thorac Surg 43:150–154, 1987.

28. Penkoske PA, Neches WH, Anderson RH, et al: Further observations on the morphology of atrioventricular septal defects. J Thorac Cardiovasc Surg 90:611–622, 1985.

29. Piccoli GP, Gerlis LM, Wilkinson JL, et al: Morphology and classification of atrioventricular defects. Br Heart J 42:621–632, 1979.

30. Piccoli GP, Siew Y-H, Wilkinson JL, et al: Left-sided obstructive lesions in atrioventricular septal defects. J Thorac Cardiovasc Surg 83:453–460, 1982.

31. Portman MA, Beder SD, Ankeney JL, et al: A 20-year review of ostium primum defect repair in children. Am Heart J 110:1054–1058, 1985.

32. Rastelli GC, Kirklin JW, Titus JL: Anatomic observations on the complete form of persistent common atrioventricular canal with special reference to atrioventricular valves. Mayo Clin Proc 41:296–308, 1966.

33. Rowley KM, Kopf GS, Hellenbrand W, et al: Atrioventricular canal with intact atrial septum. Am Heart J 115:902–906, 1988.

34. Spevak PJ, Freed MD, Castaneda AR, et al: Valve replacement in children less than 5 years of age. J Am Coll Cardiol 8:901–908, 1986.

35. Stewart S, Alexson C, Manning J: Partial atrioventricular canal defect: the early and late results of operation. Ann Thorac Surg 43:527–529, 1987.

36. Tandon R, Moller JH, Edwards JE: Single papillary muscle of the left ventricle associated with persistent common atrioventricular canal: variant of parachute mitral valve. Pediatr Cardiol 7:111–114, 1986.

37. Thieren M, Stijns-Cailteux M, Tremouroux-Wattiez M, et al: Congenital heart disease and pulmonary obstructive vascular disease in Down's syndrome: report of 142 children with trisomy 21. Arch Mal Coeur 81:655–661, 1988.

38. Van Praagh S, Antoniadis S, Otero-Coto E, et al: Common atrioventricular canal with and without conotruncal malformations: an antomic study of 251 postmortem cases. In Nora JJ, Takao A (eds): Congenital Heart Disease: Causes and Processes. Mt. Kisco, New York, Futura, 1984, p. 599.

39. Wenink ACG (ed): The Ventricular Septum of the Heart. The Hague, Martinus Nijhoff, 1981, pp. 131–138.

40. Williams WH, Guyton RA, Michalik RE, et al: Individualized surgical management of complete atrioventricular canal. J Thorac Cardiovasc Surg 83:670–679, 1982.

Chapter 37

CARDIAC MALPOSITIONS WITH SPECIAL EMPHASIS ON VISCERAL HETEROTAXY (ASPLENIA AND POLYSPLENIA SYNDROMES)

Stella Van Praagh, M.D., Francesco Santini, M.D., and Stephen P. Sanders, M.D.

Abnormal sidedness of the heart, lungs, or abdominal viscera is usually readily recognized and is an important clue for the pediatrician and the cardiologist because this finding is associated with a high incidence of complex cardiac anomalies.

Prior to the introduction of modern two-dimensional echocardiography, accurate diagnosis was difficult and involved multiple cardiac catheterizations and repeated angiocardiograms. At present, detailed diagnosis of all of the cardiac malformations is usually achieved by echocardiography or magnetic resonance imaging.

DEFINITION

The term **cardiac malposition** indicates that the heart is abnormally located within the chest (dextrocardia, mesocardia) or is abnormally located relative to the situs of the abdominal contents (levocardia with abdominal visceral heterotaxy). The heart can also be displaced outside of the thorax (ectopia cordis).

CLASSIFICATION

Dextrocardia indicates that the heart is located in the right chest. Patients with dextrocardia may be divided into those with normally located abdominal viscera (visceroatrial situs solitus), those with inversely located atria and abdominal viscera (visceroatrial situs inversus), and those with visceral heterotaxy (inconsistent visceroatrial situs).

Mesocardia indicates that the heart is displaced toward the right though not completely into the right chest.

Levocardia describes a heart that is located in the left chest, levocardia with normally located abdominal viscera being normal. The abnormal possibilities include levocardia with visceroatrial situs inversus and levocardia with visceral heterotaxy (isolated levocardia).

It is important to recognize that cardiac malposition does not imply anything specific about the various cardiac segments or the connections and alignments between these segments (see ch. 4). Segmental analysis of the heart can be achieved with the use of the same criteria in levocardia, mesocardia, or dextrocardia. Accurate diagnosis requires the identification of the situs of the various cardiac segments and the description of the associated defects.

PREVALENCE

Because the infant mortality in patients with cardiac malposition is high, the incidence of these lesions is best determined in the neonatal period. Four percent of 2251 consecutive infants born with congenital heart disease were found to have cardiac malposition (0.103 per 1000 live births).[16] In a recent 15-year period there were 335 patients with cardiac malpositions seen at The Children's Hospital in Boston, of whom 260 were seen for the first time (Exhibit 1).

PATHOLOGY

The heart may be misplaced into the right chest because of hypoplasia of the right lung or by virtue of an associated anomaly such as diaphragmatic hernia. Cardiac malposition also occurs with defects or deformities of the anterior chest wall, i.e., the Cantrell syndrome,[7] complete thoracic ectopia cordis, or Siamese twins. In all those cases the

Exhibit 1

	Boston Children's Hospital Experience 1973–1987		
	Patients with Viscero-Cardiac Malposition		
Clinical Diagnosis	No. of Patients	Known Dead	% Mortality
Ectopia cordis	7	5	71
Asplenia	71	37	52
Polysplenia	38	14	37
Dextrocardia			
Situs inversus totalis	2	0	0
Extrinsic dextrocardia	12	6	50
Intrinsic dextrocardia	205	51	25
Totals	335	113	34

Intrinsic dextrocardia includes 7 patients with scimitar syndrome (see p. 522). There were 10 instances (20 individuals) of Siamese twins not included in the above table.

cardiac malposition is secondary to noncardiac malformations. Primary cardiac malposition (usually dextrocardia) represents a disturbance in the direction of cardiac looping or the lateralization of the thoracic viscera (see ch. 4).

Any arrangement of cardiac segments and virtually any combination of cardiac defects may be encountered in patients with cardiac malposition.

PHYSIOLOGY

The hemodynamics associated with cardiac malpositions range from normal to those incompatible with life and are a direct consequence of the intracardiac defects.

Clinical Manifestations

The discovery of patients with cardiac malposition is usually made when a chest x-ray is taken, or because of symptoms of cyanosis or congestive heart failure, or because of the presence of noncardiac anomalies. Dextrocardia or abnormal location of the abdominal viscera is recognized and the patient is referred to a cardiologist. The cardiologist needs not to be unduly concerned about the malposition, as it has little to do with the ultimate outcome. He should concentrate on a systematic segment-by-segment analysis of the heart, using echocardiography and angiocardiography, as the only way to arrive at details needed to plan surgical treatment. Dogged pursuit of the anatomic minutia is the prerequisite to successful management. There are no specific clinical findings and symptoms for cardiac malposition since they depend on the associated cardiac malformations.

SPECIFIC ENTITIES

Visceral Heterotaxy (the Asplenia and Polysplenia Syndromes)

In visceral heterotaxy, not only the heart but several of the abdominal viscera may be malpositioned. This term derives from the Greek words "heteros," meaning other, and "taxis," meaning order or arrangement, i.e., "other than normal arrangement."

Patients with visceral heterotaxy show a high incidence of cardiac malformations. A recent study[47] of 109 postmortem cases from the Cardiac Registry of The Children's Hospital in Boston provided important new data that help in the understanding and management of these patients. Hence, this group of patients is presented in detail.

The fundamental characteristics of visceral heterotaxy are an abnormal symmetry of certain viscera and veins (lungs, liver, venae cavae) and situs discordance between various organ systems, as well as between the various segments of the heart.

The spleen is almost always affected in patients with visceral heterotaxy although the reason for this is not understood. The spleen may be absent (asplenia). It may be composed of a cluster of small splenuli, a large spleen and several small ones, or it may be multilobed (polysplenia). It may also be of normal size but abnormally located in the right upper quadrant of the abdomen (single, right-sided spleen), while the heart is left-sided and the lungs are solitus inversus or symmetrical.[46,47] Rarely, it may be of normal size and normally located.[43]

Although the cardiac malformations in heterotaxic individuals show considerable variability, there is also definite syndromic clustering that often corresponds to the type of splenic malformation present. This association between the cardiac malformations and the status of the spleen, first described by Polhemus in 1952[32] and further elaborated upon by Ivemark in 1955,[20] is responsible for the terms "asplenia" and "polysplenia syndrome." Ivemark also observed and emphasized the association between malformations of the conotruncus and the atrioventricular canal in patients with asplenia. Because the atrioventricular canal and the conotruncus undergo division at about the same time that the splenic primordia appear (30–32 days of gestation), he postulated that it was possible for the same teratogenic factor to adversely affect the formation of the spleen and the division of the atrioventricular canal and the conotruncus. The recent identification of the iv locus on chromosome 12 of the iv/iv mice,[6] which are known to exhibit a high frequency of visceral heterotaxy with cardiac malformations similar to those observed in humans,[24] and the occurrence of heterotaxy with asplenia or polysplenia in more than one member of the same family[2,32] favors a genetic etiology of the heterotaxy syndromes.

Although the presence of visceral heterotaxy—at least in animals—and the absence or multiplicity of the spleen has been known since the time of Aristotle,[1,5] detailed accounts of abnormalities of the visceral situs began to appear in the German literature in 1745 when Troschel described the existence of partial situs inversus.[39] Eighty-one years later, in 1826, G. Martin[27] (a medical student from L'Ecole-Pratique et des Hopitaux Civils de Paris) described the first known case of asplenia with congenital heart disease and visceral heterotaxy in man. Since that time, numerous publications have been devoted to this fascinating disturbance in the lateralization of the abdominal and thoracic viscera, which is associated with a wide variety of cardiac malformations, many of them lethal. The realization that, as a rule, patients with asplenia have bilaterally trilobed lungs and bilaterally eparterial bronchi justified the terms "double rightness"[33] and "right pulmonary isomerism."[5] The observation of bilateral superior venae cavae entering the ipsilateral atrium, bilateral systemic venous connections from below (inferior vena cava and hepatic veins), and totally anomalous pulmonary venous connections to a systemic vein in the majority of patients with asplenia, led to the conclusion that the left atrium was absent; hence the term "right atrial isomerism" appeared appropriate.[40]

The high frequency of bilaterally bilobed lungs and bilateral hyparterial bronchi in patients with polysplenia appeared to justify the term "left lung isomerism." The frequent absence of the hepatic segment of the inferior vena cava and the "ipsilateral" drainage of the pulmonary veins in several cases of polysplenia, in addition to the tendency of the right atrial appendage to resemble the left atrial appendage, formed the basis of the concept of "bilateral" left-sidedness.[29]

In recent years, new impetus has been given to the concept of right and left atrial isomerism by several investigators who have concluded that the atrial situs in visceral heterotaxy is indeterminate and should be diagnosed as right or left atrial isomerism on the basis of the shape of the atrial appendages.[8,15,19,26] Although the proponents of this approach did not really believe that heterotaxic patients have two anatomic right atria or two anatomic left atria,[15,26] the effect of this terminology has been the abandonment of any effort to identify the atrial situs (solitus or inversus) in heterotaxic patients. In order to clarify this question and to decide if, in fact, it is possible to diagnose the atrial situs in heterotaxic patients with accuracy, the authors undertook the study of 109 heart specimens from patients with visceral heterotaxy and congenital heart disease. This chapter will include the data and the conclusions of this study.[47]

Prevalence

Heterotaxy affects 0.8% of patients with congenital heart disease seen at Boston Children's Hospital in a 15-year-period (1973–1987). While, in the past, heterotaxic patients with congenital heart disease were of interest mainly to the pathologist, at present an increasing number of these patients survive, requiring medical and surgical treatment. During a 1-year period (June 1, 1989 to May 31, 1990), 43 patients with visceral heterotaxy underwent echocardiographic examination and cardiac catheterization at this hospital, 14 (38%) of whom were seriously ill infants less than 6 weeks old.

Pathology

Spleen. The most consistent abnormality involved the spleen. Of the 109 cases of visceral heterotaxy with congenital heart disease seen at autopsy, 58 (53%) had asplenia, 46 (42%) had polysplenia, and 5 (5%) had a single, normal-sized spleen that was abnormally located in the upper right side of the abdomen, while the heart was in the left side of the chest and the situs of the lungs was solitus, inversus or symmetrical. The multiple spleens were right-sided in 29 of the 46 patients with polysplenia and left-sided in the remaining 17 patients. It is interesting that right-sided polysplenia was almost twice as frequent as left-sided polysplenia in this postmortem series.

The authors are aware of the existence of living patients who have a normal, left-sided spleen (diagnosed by splenic scan) and cardiac defects similar to those seen in patients with visceral heterotaxy. Those patients were not included in our study, which was limited to postmortem cases. There are also patients who have visceral heterotaxy but no heart defect and, for this reason, are not included in this chapter.

Lungs. The lungs were abnormally symmetrical. The most common pattern in the asplenia group was bilaterally trilobed lungs with eparterial bronchi; in the polysplenia group, bilaterally bilobed lungs with hyparterial bronchi were most common (Fig. 1 and Table 1).

Liver. The liver was abnormally symmetrical in 76% of the patients with asplenia, 67% of those with polysplenia, and 20% of those with a right-sided, single spleen (Table 1). Absence of the gallbladder or extrahepatic biliary atresia has been found in several patients with visceral heterotaxy and polysplenia, usually without significant heart defects.[9]

Mesentery. Mesenteric abnormalities, such as a common mesentery, abnormal mesenteric attachments, and malrotation or malposition of the intestines, are frequent findings with visceral heterotaxy.[42] The mesenteric abnormalities are responsible for the intestinal obstruction observed in heterotaxic patients, usually those with polysplenia.

Systemic Veins. The systemic venous connections are summarized in Table 2.

Inferior Vena Cava. The inferior vena cava was intact in all patients with asplenia and in all patients with a right-sided, single spleen (Table 2) (Fig. 2). In one patient with aspenia the inferior vena cava was small and connected with a dilated azygos vein. During cardiac catheterization, the catheter preferentially entered the dilated azygos vein and gave the false impression of an interrupted inferior vena cava. The potential for this venous pattern should be kept in mind if a patient who otherwise has the characteristic features of the asplenia syndrome seems to have interruption of the inferior vena cava and azygos continuation.

The inferior vena cava was interrupted (i.e., the renal-to-suprahepatic segment of the inferior vena cava was absent and a dilated azygos vein continued from the renal veins to the superior vena cava) in 80% of the patients with polysplenia (Table 2). In one of these, the right-sided, interrupted inferior vena cava had bilateral azygos extensions to the ipsilateral superior venae cavae (Fig. 3).

Hepatic Veins. All the hepatic veins connected with the inferior vena cava in 72% of the patients with asplenia. In the remaining 28%, the hepatic vein draining the lobe of the liver on the side opposite to the inferior vena cava connected with the atrial segment separately from the inferior vena cava. In one of these latter cases, the hepatic vein connected with an intact coronary sinus, while the coronary sinus was completely unroofed in the others. The point of connection of the hepatic vein was similar externally in both circumstances, suggesting that the apparent connection of a hepatic vein with the left atrium or the left atrial portion

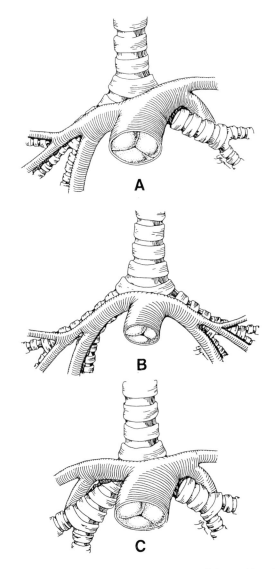

Figure 1. Diagrammatic representation of the positional relationship between the mainstem bronchi and the right and left pulmonary arteries (anterior view). **A**, Normal relationship. The left mainstem bronchus is longer than the right, and the left pulmonary artery (1st and 2nd branches) courses over it to enter the left lung (hyparterial bronchus). The right mainstem bronchus is shorter and its branch for the right upper lobe is over the second branch of the right pulmonary artery (eparterial bronchus). **B**, Bilateral eparterial bronchi that usually occur in asplenic patients. **C**, Bilateral hyparterial bronchi found as a rule in polysplenic patients. In our series, the eparterial or hyparterial position of the bronchi did not appear to be influenced by the size of the pulmonary arteries.

of a common atrium is actually a connection with the unroofed coronary sinus. An example of left polysplenia and identical systemic venous connections (a right-sided inferior vena cava and a left-sided hepatic vein entering a normal coronary sinus) is shown in Figure 4. The hepatic veins con-

Table 1. Lung Lobation, Bronchial Pattern, and Liver Situs in Visceral Heterotaxy with Congenital Heart Disease*

	N = 109 Postmortem Cases					
	Asplenia (n = 58)		Single right spleen (n = 5)		Polysplenia (n = 46)	
	No.	%	No.	%	No.	%
Lung Lobation						
Solitus	1	2	2	40	5	12
Inversus	1	2	1	20	4	9
Bilateral trilobed	45	81	2	40	3	7
Bilateral bilobed	1	2			31	72
Bilateral multilobed	6	11				
Bilateral unilobed	1	2				
Unknown	3				3	
Bronchial Pattern						
Solitus	1	2	1	20	3	9
Inversus	1	2			3	9
Bilateral eparterial	40	95	4	80	4	12
Bilateral hyparterial					22	68
Unknown	16				14	
Liver Situs						
Solitus	7	13			11	26
Inversus	6	11	4	80	3	7
Symmetrical	42	76	1	20	29	67
Unknown	3				3	

*All percentages calculated on the basis of known cases; unknowns excluded for the purposes of percentage computations.

Table 2. Systemic Venous Connections in Visceral Heterotaxy with Congenital Heart Disease

	N = 109 Postmortem Cases					
	Asplenia n = 58		Single right spleen n = 5		Polysplenia n = 46	
Type of Systemic Venous Connection	No.	%	No.	%	No.	%
Continuous (not interrupted) IVC	58	100	5	100	9	20
Continuous IVC and contralateral hepatic vein	16*	28			1*	2
Interrupted IVC					37	80
Interrupted IVC and bilateral hepatic veins					2†	4
Bilateral SVCs	41	71	2	40	23	50
Absent coronary sinus septum	55	95	4	80	12	26

IVC, inferior vena cava; RA, right atrium; SVC, superior vena cava.

*In 1 of the 16 cases of asplenia and in the single case of polysplenia, the hepatic vein contralateral to the IVC drained directly into a normal (not unroofed) coronary sinus and indirectly into the RA.

†In 1 of these 2 cases, the coronary sinus septum was partly present, making possible atrial identification. In the other case, the larger of the two hepatic veins was on the same side with the solitus liver and it was interpreted as draining into the anatomic right atrium.

nected with the inferior vena cava in all 5 patients with a right-sided, single spleen. In the patients with polysplenia, if the inferior vena cava was intact, both right and left hepatic veins joined the inferior vena cava in all except 1 case. In this case a hepatic vein drained into a normal coronary sinus and, indirectly, into the right atrium (Fig. 4). Among patients with interruption of the inferior vena cava, the hepatic veins connected with the anatomically right atrium as a single trunk in all except 2 cases. In another series of patients, sep-

arate connections of the right and left hepatic veins was more common.[26]

Coronary Sinus Septum. The coronary sinus septum was absent in 95% of patients with asplenia, 80% with a single, right-sided spleen, and 26% with polysplenia (Table 2).

Superior Vena Cava. The superior vena cava was present bilaterally in 71% of the patients with asplenia, 40% of patients with a single, right-sided spleen and 50% of patients with polysplenia (Table 2). The coronary sinus septum was absent in all

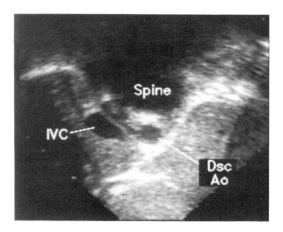

Figure 2. Echocardiogram in the subxiphoid transverse view showing the aorta and inferior vena cava on the same side (right) of the spine in a patient with asplenia. IVC, inferior vena cava; Dsc Ao, descending aorta.

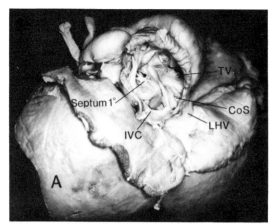

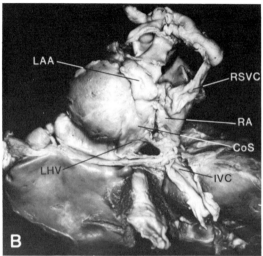

Figure 4. Heart and liver of a 2-day-old white male infant with visceral heterotaxy, left polysplenia, tetralogy of Fallot, and tracheal agenesis. **A**, Internal view of the right atrium (RA). The septum primum (septum 1°) has several small fenestrations. The entry of the inferior vena cava (IVC) into the RA is indicated (arrow). The left hepatic vein (LHV) also enters the RA at the site of the coronary sinus orifice (CoS). **B**, Posterior view of the heart and posteroinferior view of the liver. The left hepatic vein (LHV) enters the coronary sinus area (CoS) of the RA immediately below the left atrial appendage (LAA). If the CoS septum is absent, the LHV would give the false impression of connecting directly with the left atrium. TV, tricuspid valve. (Modified from Van Praagh S, Kakou-Guikahue M, Kim HS, et al.,[46] with permission.)

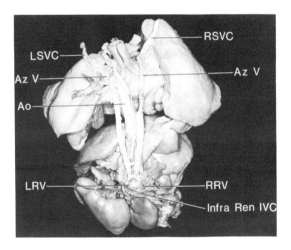

Figure 3. Posterior view of the heart, lungs, liver, and kidneys of a 6½-month-old boy with visceral heterotaxy and left-sided polysplenia. There is interruption of the right-sided inferior vena cava, with bilateral azygos veins (AZV) connecting with bilateral superior venae cavae. The right superior vena cava (RSVC) entered the right atrium directly. The left superior vena cava (LSVC) continued into the coronary sinus, which drained normally into the morphologically right atrium. All the pulmonary veins also drained into the right-sided morphologically right atrium. Multiple fenestrations in the septum primum and a moderate-sized membranous ventricular septal defect allowed blood to enter the morphologically left atrium and left ventricle. There was no deficiency of the atrioventricular canal septum, the atrioventricular valves were normal, and the great arteries were normally related to the ventricles. The segmental combination of this heart was: solitus atria, D-loop ventricles, and normally related great arteries. Ao, aorta; LRV, left renal vein; RRV, right renal vein; Infra Ren IVC, infrarenal inferior vena cava.

patients with asplenia who had bilateral superior venae cavae but in only about half of polysplenic patients.

Bilateral Superior Venae Cavae. The high incidence of bilateral superior venae cavae in the patients with absence of the coronary sinus septum indicates that the distal portion of the left horn of the sinus venosus (or the right horn in situs inversus) is present in the majority of these patients. Consequently, the apparent absence of the coronary sinus (the usual derivative of the left horn of the sinus venosus) seems unlikely. It seems more likely that the deep fold that normally develops in embryos older than 25 somites, and separates the left horn of the sinus venosus from the left atrium,[40] failed to form. This makes the coronary sinus inapparent, because it becomes incorporated into the left atrial portion of the common atrium.[46] When, in addition, the common pulmonary vein fails to develop from the back of the common atrium, and the septum primum and secundum are absent, the only component of the left atrium present is its appendage. This type of common atrium is formed primarily from the two horns of the sinus venosus and, in this sense, could be viewed as "bilaterally right atria." Nonetheless, even this type of common atrium, which occurred in the asplenia cases with totally anomalous pulmonary venous connection to a systemic vein, is not composed of two right atria. It is composed of the right atrium, the unroofed coronary sinus, and the left atrial appendage.

When both atria receive systemic veins (e.g., bilateral superior venae cavae, bilateral hepatic veins, or an inferior vena cava to one atrium and hepatic vein to the other), the true abnormality is not bilaterally right atria but, rather, unroofing of the coronary sinus. Because the coronary sinus is located in the posteroinferior wall of the left atrium, any systemic vein that connects with the coronary sinus will drain into the left atrium when the coronary sinus is unroofed. This is true for all patients with or without visceral heterotaxy, because all the systemic veins connect directly only with the sinus venosus (Fig. 5). The proximity of the left atrium to the coronary sinus (the left horn of the sinus venosus) is shown in Figure 5 and is responsible for the apparent "direct" connection of

any of the systemic veins with the left atrium when the coronary sinus is unroofed.

Pulmonary Veins. The pulmonary venous connections are summarized in Table 3.

Anomalous connections of all the pulmonary veins to a systemic vein occurred in 64% of the patients with asplenia, 60% of those with a right-sided, single spleen, and in only 1 (2%) with polysplenia (Figs. 6–8).

In all of the polysplenic patients with partial or total anomalous pulmonary venous return to the right atrium, the connection of the pulmonary veins appears normal externally. That is, the veins connected with the superior part of the posterior atrial wall between the superior venae cavae when present bilaterally (Fig. 6C), or to the left of a right superior vena cava in situs solitus, or to the right of a left superior vena cava in situs inversus (Fig. 8C). The anomalous pulmonary venous return appeared to be due to abnormal "shifting" of the atrial septum toward the anatomically left atrium rather than to an abnormal connection of the pulmonary veins with the right atrium.[11,29,46,47]

Usually, absence or hypoplasia of the septum secundum appeared to be responsible for the abnormal position and attachments of the septum primum. The abnormal attachments of the septum primum to the free wall of the left atrium, and to the left of half or all of the orifices of the pulmonary veins, were usually associated with stenosis or obliteration of the foramen ovale (Figs. 6A and 8A). In addition, the upper border of the septum primum (i.e., the valve of the foramen ovale) could be viewed from the anatomically right atrium (Figs. 6A, 7A, and 8A).

Depending on the extent of displacement of the septum primum, the two right pulmonary veins, or all four pulmonary veins, drained into the an-

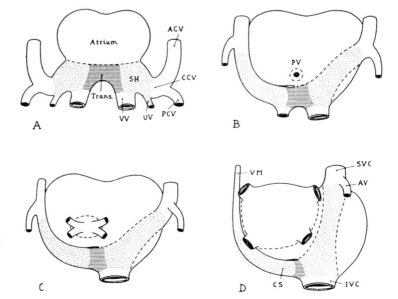

Figure 5. Posterior view (diagrammatic) of the sinus venosus in embryos of various ages: **A**, 3 mm crown-rump length; **B**, 5 mm; **C**, 12 mm; **D**, newborn. ACV, anterior cardinal vein; AV, azygous vein; CCV, common cardinal vein; CS, coronary sinus; IVC, inferior vena cava; PCV, posterior cardinal vein; PV, pulmonary vein; SH, sinus horn; SVC, superior vena cava; trans., transverse portion of sinus venosus; UV, umbilical vein; VM, vein of Marshall; VV, vitelline vein. (From Van Mierop LHS, Wigleworth FW: Isomerism of the cardiac atria in the asplenia syndrome. Lab Invest 11:1303–1315, 1962, © U.S.–Canadian Academy of Pathology, with permission.)

Table 3.   Pulmonary Venous Connections in Visceral Heterotaxy with Congenital Heart Disease

N = 109 Postmortem Cases

Type of Pulmonary Venous Connection	Asplenia n = 58		Single Right Spleen n = 5		Polysplenia n = 46	
	No.	%	No.	%	No.	%
Normal to LA	6		2	40	15	
Normal to CA	2				13	
To LA with single orifice	12	21				
Totals	20	34			28	61
All PVs to RA with abnormal attachments of septum 1°	1	2			10	22
To ipsilateral atrium					7	15
To a systemic vein	37	64	3	60	1	2

CA, common atrium; LA, left atrium; PV, pulmonary vein; RA, right atrium; septum 1°, septum primum.

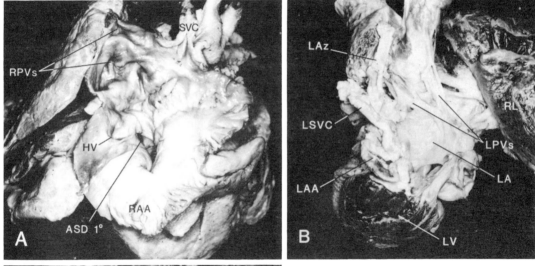

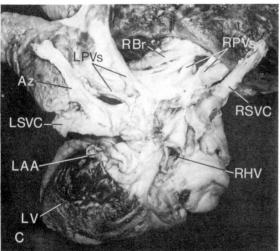

Figure 6. The heart and lungs of a 13-week-old girl with visceral heterotaxy, right polysplenia, and ipsilateral pulmonary veins. **A**, Interior view of the anatomically right atrium, which is right-sided. ASD 1° indicates an atrial septal defect of the ostium primum type. Note the large atrial appendage (RAA), with only its apex simulating the left atrial appendage. The white arrow is through the restrictive foramen ovale. The septum primum is seen well from the right atrial aspect. The septum primum attachments are to the left of the right pulmonary veins (RPVs). The confluence of the hepatic veins (HV) enters the morphologically right atrium. **B**, The interior of the morphologically left atrium (LA). The left superior vena cava (LSVC) receives the azygos extension of the interrupted inferior vena cava and enters the LA directly because of absence of the coronary sinus septum. The left atrial appendage (LAA) is long, narrow, posteriorly placed, and considerably smaller than the RAA of this heart. The valve of the foramen ovale (septum primum) is not seen from the LA aspect. The left pulmonary veins (LPVs) enter the LA. **C**, Posterior view of the heart. The right and left PVs connect with the atrial portion of the heart as in normal hearts, i.e., superiorly and between the entry of the two SVCs. Hence, the ipsilateral pulmonary venous drainage is not due to an anomalous pulmonary venous connection but to the malposition of the septum primum. Az, azygos vein; LAz, left azygos; LV, left ventricle. RBr, right bronchus; RHV, right hepatic venous confluence. RL, right lung. (Modified from Van Praagh S, Kakou-Guikahue M, Kim HS, et al.,[46] with permission.)

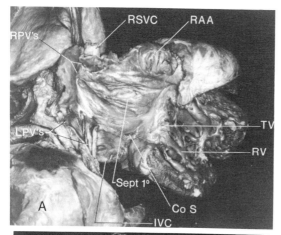

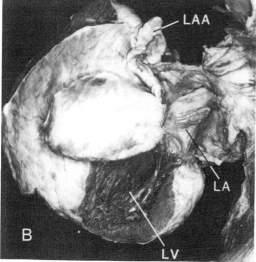

Figure 7. Totally anomalous pulmonary venous return to the right atrium in a 7-year-old girl with visceral heterotaxy, right-sided polysplenia, solitus atria, normally positioned ventricles (D-loop), and normally related great arteries. **A,** Interior view of the right atrium and right ventricle (RV). The septum primum (1°) is to the left of the right and left pulmonary veins (RPVs and LPVs), and its attachments can be seen from the right atrial side of the septum. The right superior vena cava (RSVC), the inferior vena cava (IVC), and the coronary sinus (CoS) connect normally with the RA. The right atrial appendage (RAA) is opened and partly amputated. The tricuspid valve (TV) attaches normally on the hypertrophied RV. **B,** Interior of the very small left atrium (LA) and the left ventricular inflow (LV). The appendage of the left atrium (LAA) is long and narrow. (Modified form Van Praagh S, Kreutzer J, Alday L, et al.,[47] with permission.)

atomically right atrium. In such cases, the anatomically right atrium contained half or all of the common pulmonary vein component that is usually incorporated into the left atrium. The anatomically left atrium was represented by a small chamber that connected with the left atrial appendage and the mitral valve or the mitral component of a common atrioventricular valve, and it received either

only the left or none of the pulmonary veins (Figs. 6B, 7B, and 8B). In some rare cases a persistent superior vena cava, associated with an unroofed coronary sinus, drained into the small left atrium.

Therefore, ipsilateral drainage of the pulmonary veins does not indicate bilaterally left atria but, rather, incorporation of part of the left atrium into the right atrium due to malposition of the septum primum.

This realization has significant therapeutic repercussions. Surgical correction of this type of partial or total anomalous pulmonary venous return can be achieved by resecting the malpositioned atrial septum and placing a new atrial septum in such a position that all the pulmonary veins will be incorporated into the new left atrium. One such patient had only a small additional ventricular septal defect which could be closed easily (Fig. 8C). Of the 18 patients (17 with polysplenia and 1 with asplenia) with either ipsilateral pulmonary venous drainage or with all the pulmonary veins draining into the anatomically right atrium, 11 had normally related great arteries and anatomy suitable for complete surgical repair.

Atrial Septum and Atrioventricular Canal Septum. The incidence of a deficiency, absence, or malattachment of the septum primum in the various heterotaxic groups is presented in Table 4. The same table includes the incidence of deficiency or absence of the atrioventricular canal septum.

Atrial Situs. In patients with visceral heterotaxy the atrial situs is often difficult to determine on the basis of septal morphology[25] because the atrial septum is usually very deficient or absent. Consequently, the term "situs ambiguus" was coined to describe patients with unclear situs[41] and should be used when the atrial situs cannot be diagnosed with certainty. The diagnosis of atrial situs in visceral heterotaxy is considered important for at least two reasons. First, it may lead to enhanced understanding of the etiology of visceral heterotaxy by demonstrating the high incidence of atrial situs inversus in these patients. Second, it makes possible the determination of atrioventricular situs concordance or discordance, which is essential for the more complete understanding of the internal organization of these hearts, and it can be predictive of the course of the conduction system. Review of specimens in this series has shown that atrial situs can be determined in the majority of patients with visceral heterotaxy on the basis of the following considerations.

It is generally accepted that the atrium into which the right horn of the sinus venosus is incorporated is the morphologically right atrium.[23,40] The right horn of the sinus venosus includes the orifices of the inferior and superior venae cavae and the smooth atrial wall between them. The coronary sinus, which represents the reduced left horn of the sinus venosus (Fig. 5), normally opens

Figure 8.   The heart of a $12\frac{7}{12}$-year-old boy with visceral heterotaxy, right polysplenia, inversus atria and ventricles, total anomalous pulmonary venous return to the left-sided right atrium, and double-outlet right ventricle with only sub-pulmonary conus. **A**, Interior of the left-sided right atrium. The foramen ovale is restrictive and its valve, i.e., septum 1°, is seen from the right atrial side. **B**, Interior of right-sided left atrium (LA). Note the long and narrow left atrial appendage (LAA) contrasting with the very large RAA. S 1° is not seen from the LA side. **C**, Posterior view of the same heart. The position of the LPVs and RPVs to the right of the left-sided SVC and HV is normal in viscer-oatrial situs inversus. The left bronchus (LBr) passes under the left pulmonary artery (LPA), i.e., the left bronchus is hyparterial. Ao, aorta; LV, left ventricle; ASD 1°, atrial septal defect of the os-tium primum type; CAVV, common atrioventric-ular valve; CoS, coronary sinus; CT, crista ter-minalis; HV(L), hepatic vein, left-sided; LPVs, left pulmonary veins; RA, right atrium; RPVs, right pulmonary veins; S 1°, septum primum with at-tachments to the right of RPVs; SVC(L), superior vena cava, left-sided. (From Van Praagh S, Kakou-Guikahue M, Kim HS, et al.,[46] with per-mission.)

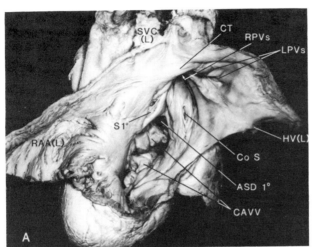

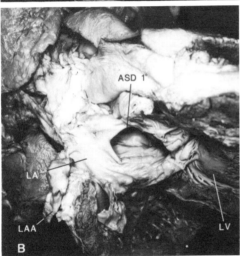

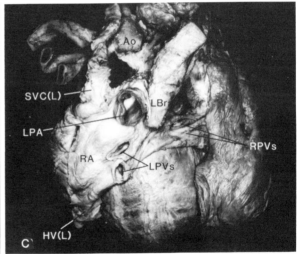

into the sinus venosus component of the morpho-logically right atrium. Hence, the atrium that re-ceives the superior and inferior venae cavae and the orifice of the coronary sinus is the anatomically right atrium.

It is also well documented that some or all of the pulmonary veins may drain into the right atrium because of malposition of the septum pri-mum (see p. 595). Therefore, when all of the sys-temic veins and some or all of the pulmonary veins drain into one atrium, which is not a common atrium because another small atrium is present, this large atrium contains the morphologically right atrium.

Until recently, it was thought that the unin-terrupted inferior vena cava always connected directly with the right atrium and could be used as a marker for atrial situs identification.[46] However, the au-thors are now aware of a case in which a nonin-terrupted, left-sided, and small inferior vena cava connected with a normally roofed coronary sinus and indirectly with the right atrium.[47] This inferior vena cava received only one hepatic vein. All the other hepatic veins formed a larger confluence that entered the right atrium directly. It could be pos-sible then, in rare cases, for the inferior vena cava to drain into the left atrium via an unroofed cor-onary sinus, leading to an erroneous diagnosis of the atrial situs. In these cases, the size and position of the atrial appendages and the connections of the pulmonary veins help to determine the atrial situs. The above-mentioned embryologic and pathologic findings were used to identify the atrial situs in the 109 patients in this series.

Anatomically Right Atrium. The anatomically right atrium was considered to be the atrium that received (1) all the systemic veins while a separate atrium received all of the pulmonary veins; (2) all

Table 4. Atrial Septa, Atrioventricular Canal, and Ventricular Size in Visceral Heterotaxy with Congenital Heart Disease

	Aspelenia n = 58		Single Right Spleen n = 5		Polysplenia n = 46	
N = 109 Postmortem Cases	No.	%	No.	%	No.	%
Atrial Septa						
Septum primum present with normal attachments	10	19	3	60	8	19
Septum primum displaced toward the morphologically LA	1	2			15	35
Septum primum resected or artifacted	4*				3*	
Absent septum primum, septum secundum and AVC septum	31	57			13	30
Septum primum present with uncommitted attachment	12	22	2	40	7	16
Atrioventricular Canal						
Complete CAVC with CAVV	40	69	2	40	15	33
Incomplete CAVC (ASD primum or common atrium with cleft MV)					10	22
Incomplete CAVC with MAt	2	3	1	20	2	4
Incomplete CAVC with straddling TV and MS					1	2
CAVC with single RV	8	14				
Incomplete CAVC with tricuspid atresia	4	7	1	20	2	4
Intact AVC septum with 2 AVV	4	7	1	20	16	35
Ventricles						
Both ventricles well developed	26	45	2	40	29	63
LV hypoplasia	16	28	2	40	11	24
RV hypoplasia	6	10	1	20	5	11
LV absent	8	14				
RV absent	2	3			1	2

*Surgically or postmortem artifacted cases excluded for the purpose of percentage computations.

ASD, atrial septal defect; AVC, atrioventricular canal; AVV, atrioventricular valve; CAVC, common atrioventricular canal; CAVV, common atrioventricular valve; LA, left atrium; LV, left ventricle; MAt, mitral atresia; MS, mitral stenosis; MV, mitral valve; RV, right ventricle; TV, tricuspid valve.

of the systemic veins and some or all of the pulmonary veins without being a common atrium; and (3) the orifice of a normal coronary sinus. A fourth criterion for identifying the right atrium, based on the review of the specimens in this series, was the size and position of the atrial appendages. Although the shape of the atrial appendages may be similar in many cases of visceral heterotaxy, the right atrial appendage is usually the larger and is more anteriorly placed (Fig. 4B, 6A&B, 7A&B, 8A&B, 9, 10A&B).

Anatomically Left Atrium. The anatomically left atrium was the atrium which received (1) half or all of the pulmonary veins and none of the systemic veins (except for a persistent superior vena cava associated with an unroofed coronary sinus in cases with bilateral superior venae cavae); or (2) none of the pulmonary veins and none of the systemic veins. A third criterion for identification of the left atrium, based on review of the specimens of this series, was the size and position of its appendage, which is usually smaller and more posteriorly lo-

cated than the right atrial appendage (Figs. 4B, 6A&B, 7A&B, 8A&B, 9, 10A&B).

Using criteria 1–3 for the right atrium and 1 and 2 for the left atrium (i.e., the systemic and pulmonary venous connections), it was possible to diagnose the atrial situs in all of the patients with polysplenia (100%), in 21 of those with asplenia (36%), and in 1 patient with a single, right-sided spleen (20%). When the size and position of the atrial appendages were also taken into consideration, it was possible to diagnose the atrial situs in 47 of those with asplenia (81%) and in all of those with a right-sided, single spleen. In the remaining 11 cases of asplenia (19%), the inferior vena cava was contralateral to the larger and more anterior appendage. In these cases, it could not be ascertained whether the inferior vena cava was connected to the left atrium via an unroofed coronary sinus, or whether the inferior vena cava connected directly with the morphologically right atrium that had the smaller atrial appendage. Consequently,

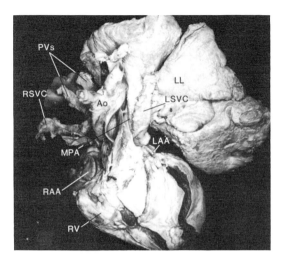

Figure 9. The heart and left lung of a 3²⁄₁₂-year-old girl with visceral heterotaxy, asplenia, double-outlet right ventricle with a bilateral conus, and severe subpulmonary stenosis. The right superior vena cava (RSVC), which receives all the pulmonary veins (PVs), enters the right-sided anatomically right atrium with the larger right atrial appendage (RAA). The left superior vena cava enters the left-sided anatomically left atrium with the smaller left atrial appendage (LAA). The morphologically right ventricle (RV) is to the right of the morphologically left ventricle (D-loop). The ascending aorta (Ao) is to the right and anterior to the hypoplastic main pulmonary artery (MPA). The left lung (LL) is trilobed. (Modified from Van Praagh S, Kreutzer J, Alday L, et al.,[47] with permission.)

the diagnosis of atrial situs ambiguus seemed to be justified.

The presently used methods of echocardiography do not always allow accurate evaluation of the size and position of the appendages. Hence, the diagnosis of the atrial situs is not always possible during life. For these patients, one should use the term "atrial situs ambiguus." It is hoped that the use of other methods, such as magnetic resonance imaging, will provide the means for accurate evaluation of the size and position of the appendages and will make possible the diagnosis of atrial situs in most living patients with visceral heterotaxy.

In this postmortem series, the incidence of atrial situs inversus, determined with the above-outlined criteria, was highest in patients with a single, right-sided spleen (60%). Next in frequency of situs inversus were the asplenias (31%), and last, the polysplenias (22%) (Table 5). There was no significant difference in the distribution of atrial situs between the right and left polysplenic groups. This high incidence of atrial situs inversus in all the heterotaxic patients is noteworthy, and it may provide an important clue in the understanding of the etiology of abnormal visceral lateralization.

Atrioventricular Valves. A common atrioventricular valve (Fig. 11) was present in 69% of the patients with asplenia. The single atrioventricular

valve that was present in each of the 8 cases of asplenia with a single right ventricle (14%) could represent either a common atrioventricular valve entering the single right ventricle or a tricuspid valve with atresia and absence of the mitral valve (Fig. 12). Both atrioventricular valves were normal in 7% of asplenic patients. The distribution of atrioventricular valve abnormalities (Table 4) was similar in the patients with a single, right-sided spleen.

Atrioventricular valve anomalies were present in 65% of patients with polysplenia. A common atrioventricular valve was also the most common anomaly in polysplenia, occurring in 33% of patients. Next most common was a cleft mitral valve with an intact ventricular septum, which occurred in 22%. Two separate and patent atrioventricular valves were present in 35% of patients with polysplenia (Table 4).

The frequent occurrence of partial and complete common atrioventricular canal was noted previously by Ivemark.[20] In his series of heterotaxic patients there appeared to be a linkage between atrioventricular canal defects and malformations of the conotruncus. This linkage was also present in our asplenic patients and in our patients with a single, right-sided spleen. A similar linkage did not appear to exist in polysplenic patients. Despite the high incidence of atrioventricular canal defects, conal development was normal in all except 5 polysplenic patients (Table 5).

Ventricles. Ventricular looping did not differ as strikingly between patients with asplenia and polysplenia as did other aspects of cardiac development. A ventricular D-loop was present in 62% of patients with asplenia and 70% of patients with polysplenia, while in the remainder a ventricular L-loop was present. A ventricular D-loop was present in all 5 patients (100%) with a single, right-sided spleen (Table 5).

The incidence of ventricular inversion (L-loop ventricles) was almost identical with the incidence of dextrocardia in both the asplenias and the polysplenias. The presence of dextrocardia appeared to correlate better with the presence of ventricular inversion than with the presence of atrial inversion in the polysplenic group. Both dextrocardia and ventricular inversion appeared to occur often in patients with visceral heterotaxy (Table 5).

The ventricular development in all three groups is summarized in Table 4. There was a high incidence of left ventricular underdevelopment in all the heterotaxic patients (Table 4). In 8 cases of asplenia (14%), only the right ventricle could be identified (Fig. 12). The authors suspect that the right ventricular predominance in many of the heterotaxic patients is related to the hemodynamic effect of the cardiac malformations present.

Ventricular Outflow Tract Obstruction. The pulmonary outflow tract was obstructed in all patients with a single, right-sided spleen and in all

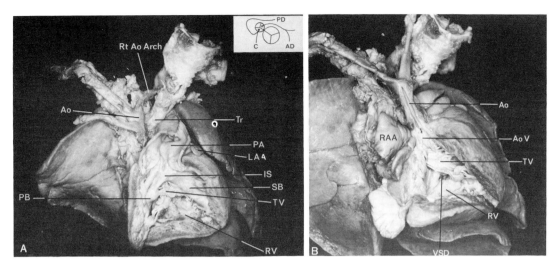

Figure 10. The heart and lungs of a 3-day-old girl with visceral heterotaxy and multiple, right-sided spleens. There was a right aortic arch with a left ductus arteriosus and an aberrant left subclavian. A right superior vena cava and the hepatic venous confluence entered the morphologically right atrium. The inferior vena cava was interrupted and continued into a left azygos, which joined the left superior vena cava and entered the morphologically left atrium (unroofed coronary sinus). All the pulmonary veins entered the morphologically right atrium. **A,** Opened right ventricle (RV) showing the well-developed subpulmonary conus under a normal pulmonary artery (PA). The infundibular septum (IS) and the septal band (SB) are well developed and normally positioned. The small left atrial appendage (LAA) is seen to the left of the PA. **B,** Opened RV showing the severe subaortic stenosis caused by the position of the aortic valve (AoV) between the redundant tricuspid valve component (TV) of the common atrioventricular valve and the infundibular septum (not seen in this view). The AoV and the ascending aorta (Ao) are very underdeveloped. The large right atrial appendage (RAA) is seen to the right of the Ao. The ventricular component of the atrioventricular septal defect is partly seen (VSD). This case is an example of double-outlet right ventricle with solitus atria, normally positioned ventricles (D-loop), and normal conus (i.e., only subpulmonary conus). The normalcy of the ventricular loop and the conus are reflected in the normal origin and distribution of the coronary arteries (see insert in A). AD, anterior descending coronary; C, conus coronary; PB, parietal band; PD, posterior descending coronary; Tr, trachea. (Modified from Van Praagh S, Antoniadis S, Otero-Coto E, et al.,[44] with permission.)

except 2 patients with asplenia. One of the 2 patients without pulmonary outflow obstruction had aortic atresia, which is very rare, and the other had a double-outlet right ventricle.[14,44,45] The pulmonary obstruction was subvalvar in 96% of the patients with asplenia and was often associated with valvar stenosis or atresia (Table 5). The high incidence of pulmonary outflow tract obstruction has been reported in several series of patients with asplenia.[34]

The picture was much less uniform among polysplenic patients. Both outflow tracts were unobstructed in 35% of patients. Subpulmonary stenosis was seen in 43%, and subaortic stenosis in 22% (Table 5).

Ventriculoarterial Alignment. The ventriculoarterial alignments are detailed in Table 5. Asplenic and polysplenic patients diverged widely with respect to ventriculoarterial alignment. In nearly all of the patients with asplenia, the alignment was double-outlet right ventricle (82%) or transposition (9%). Normally related great arteries were present in only 9% of patients. In contrast, the great arteries were normally related in 61% of polysplenic patients. Double-outlet right ventricle was present in 17 patients (37%) with polysplenia, but all except

4 of these patients had only subpulmonary conus without subaortic conus (Fig. 10). Consequently, as a rule, in most of the patients who had polysplenia with a double-outlet right ventricle, the conotruncus was reminiscent of normally related great arteries (subpulmonary conus without subaortic conus). The absence of subaortic conus in cases of double-outlet right ventricle appeared to be responsible for the subaortic stenosis which was present. The aortic valve had descended to the level of the tricuspid valve and was "squeezed" between the tricuspid valve and the conal septum (Fig. 10B). Transposition of the great arteries was present in only one case (2%) of polysplenia. In this single case of polysplenia and transposition of the great arteries, the conus was absent bilaterally, resulting in direct fibrous continuity between both semilunar valves and the anterior leaflet of the common atrioventricular valve.

Segmental Combinations. There was great diversity of segmental combinations in patients with asplenia and polysplenia, reflecting the inconsistency of the situs of the various cardiac segments, which is the hallmark of visceral heterotaxy. The presence of atrioventricular discordance without transposition of the great arteries in 11% of the

Table 5. Heart Position, Cardiac Segments, and Outflow Obstructions in Visceral Heterotaxy with Congenital Heart Disease

N = 109 Postmortem Cases

		Asplenia n = 58		Single Right Spleen n = 5		Polysplenia n = 46	
		No.	%	No.	%	No.	%
Levocardia		37	64	5	100	31	67
Dextrocardia		21	36			15	33
Atrial situs	Solitus	29	50	2	40	36	78
	Inversus	18	31	3	60	10	22
	Ambiguus	11	19				
Ventricular loop	D-	36	62	5	100	32	70
	L-	22	38			14	30
Type of conus	SubPA	5	9	1	20	41	89
	SubAo	5	9				
	Bilat	48	82	4	80	5*	11
Ventriculo-arterial relationship	Normal	5	9			28	61
	DORV	48	82	5	100	17	37
	TGA	5	9			1	2
AV discordance with NRGA						5	11
Outflow obstruction or atresia	None	1	2			16	35
	SubPA	56†	96	5†	100	20†	43
	SubAo	1‡	2			10	22

*In 1 case there was TGA with bilaterally absent conus, resulting in fibrous continuity of the aortic and pulmonary valves with the anterior leaflet of the common AV valve. The other 4 patients had DORV.

†In 21 cases of asplenia (36%), 3 cases of right-sided single spleen (60%), and 2 cases of polysplenia (4%) there was pulmonary atresia.

‡A very rare case of aortic atresia.

AV, atrioventricular; Bilat, bilateral; DORV, double-outlet right ventricle; NRGA, normally related great arteries; SubAo, subaortic; SubPA, subpulmonary; TGA, transposition of the great arteries

patients with polysplenia is noteworthy and reflects one of the most specific characteristics of this group, i.e., absence of subaortic conus (Table 5). Atrioventricular discordance with normally related great arteries results in transposition physiology and can be repaired with the left ventricle as the systemic ventricle by performing an atrial switch operation.[31]

Linkages Between Anomalies. Despite the considerable variation of the situs of the different cardiac segments and the variability of the segmental combinations seen in heterotaxic individuals, several definite linkages between the heart defects were observed.

1. All patients with an unroofed coronary sinus, regardless of the status of the spleen, also had complete or partial common atrioventricular canal. The reverse was true in the groups with asplenia and right-sided, single spleen, but not in patients with polysplenia.

2. All patients who had asplenia or a single, right-sided spleen with an abnormal atrioventricular canal also had an abnormal conus (bilateral or subaortic). The reverse was not always true, and the polysplenic patients did not show this linkage at all.

3. All patients with asplenia, single, right-sided spleen, and polysplenia with totally anomalous pulmonary venous connection to a systemic vein had

an abnormal conus (bilateral or subaortic). The reverse was not always true.

4. Polysplenia was characterized by the absence of subaortic conus even in cases of transposition, double-outlet right ventricle or atrioventricular discordance. Only 4 of the 46 polysplenic patients with double-outlet right ventricle had bilateral conus. The single patient with transposition of the great arteries had bilaterally deficient conus.

In patients with visceral heterotaxy, the association of heart defects makes it possible to suspect asplenia or polysplenia.

Associated Anatomic Findings in Asplenia

Asplenia should be suspected when the following defects coexist: (1) an intact inferior vena cava, (2) an unroofed coronary sinus, (3) totally anomalous pulmonary venous connection to a systemic vein, (4) a common atrioventricular canal, (5) double-outlet right ventricle or transposition with bilateral or subaortic conus, and (6) pulmonary stenosis or atresia.

In a few instances, the same defects may exist in patients with a right-sided, single spleen.

Associated Anatomic Findings in Polysplenia

Polysplenia (right- or left-sided) should be suspected when the following defects coexist: (1) an interrupted inferior vena cava, (2) totally or par-

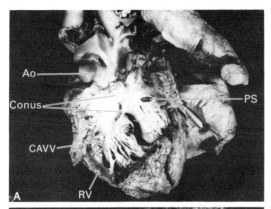

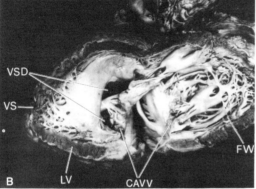

Figure 11. The heart and left lung of a 4⁹/₁₂-year-old girl with visceral heterotaxy and asplenia. The heart was in the left chest. The inferior vena cava was left-sided below the liver but switched to the right at the level of the liver and entered the right-sided atrium, which had the larger and more anterior appendage. All the pulmonary veins entered the common atrium to the left of the subdividing atrial strand (inferior limbic band) through a common orifice. The ventricles were normally located (D-loop) and both great arteries emerged from the morphologically right ventricle (double-outlet right ventricle). Hence, the segmental combination was: solitus atria (S), D-loop ventricles (D), and D-malposed aorta. **A,** Opened right ventricle (RV) showing a well-developed subaortic conus (conus) and a defect within the conal septum representing the site of the severe subpulmonary stenosis (PS). The tricuspid component of the common atrioventricular valve (CAVV) and the right ventricular aorta (Ao) are well seen. **B,** Opened left ventricle (LV) showing the characteristic left ventricular septal surface (VS), the fine trabeculation of the free wall (FW), and the mitral component of the CAVV. VSD, ventricular septal defect. (Modified from Van Praagh S, Antoniadis S, Otero-Coto E, et al.,⁴⁴ with permission.)

Clinical Manifestations

Physical Examination. Because nearly all patients with asplenia or a single, right-sided spleen

tially anomalous pulmonary venous drainage to the right atrium, (3) complete or partial common atrioventricular canal, and (4) normally related great arteries or double-outlet right ventricle without subaortic conus.

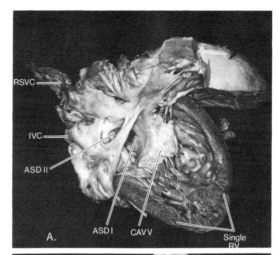

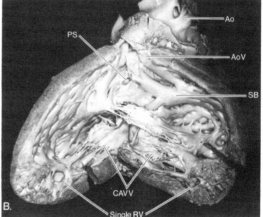

Figure 12. The heart of a 3³/₁₂-year-old boy with visceral heterotaxy and asplenia. **A,** Inferior view of the right-sided morphologically right atrium and the inflow of the morphologically single right ventricle (RV). The RA receives the right superior vena cava (RSVC) and the inferior vena cava (IVC). There is a large secundum type of atrial septal defect (ASD II) superior and posterior to the inferior limbic band; a primum type of atrial septal defect (ASD I) is located in front of and below the inferior limbic band. There was totally anomalous pulmonary venous connection to the junction of the RSVC with the RA. The coronary sinus septum was absent and the left superior vena cava appeared to join the left atrium "directly." The common atrioventricular valve (CAVV) underlies both the right- and left-sided atrium. **B,** Anterior view of the opened single RV. The septal band (SB), moderator band, and anterior papillary muscle group are left-sided, indicating that this is a right-handed (D-loop) RV. Double-outlet right ventricle is present with a bilateral conus (subaortic and subpulmonary) separating both semilunar valves from the CAVV. The aortic valve (AoV) lies anteriorly, superiorly, and somewhat to the left of the stenotic pulmonary valve. The subvalvar pulmonary stenosis (PS) mimics a defect within the conal septum. A left ventricular cavity could not be identified, although its microscopic existence cannot be precluded. Ao, aorta. (Modified from Van Praagh S, Davidoff A, Chin A, et al.,⁴⁵ with permission.)

also have pulmonary stenosis or atresia with a large ventricular septal defect or single ventricle, cyanosis is almost universal. Large aortopulmonary collateral vessels are rare in heterotaxic patients with pulmonary atresia. Therefore, if the ductus is allowed to constrict, profound cyanosis will develop, with metabolic acidosis and circulatory collapse. A harsh systolic murmur is usually indicative of pulmonary stenosis, whereas the absence of a murmur, or a continuous murmur, is more consistent with pulmonary atresia. If atrioventricular valve regurgitation is present it may be difficult to distinguish this murmur from that due to pulmonary stenosis. The liver may be palpable across the abdomen if the two lobes are symmetrical. As previously reported,[34] there was a predominance of males in the group with asplenia and in those with a single, right-sided spleen (Table 6).

In contrast, the clinical findings in polysplenia are highly variable because of the variability of the associated heart defects. In general, infants with polysplenia tend to be less seriously ill than infants with asplenia because of the rarity of pulmonary atresia and totally anomalous pulmonary venous connection to a systemic vein in the former patients. This is reflected in the age range and median age at death (Table 6).

Electrocardiography. The electrocardiogram was often helpful in determining atrial situs on the basis of the frontal plane axis of the P wave. In 42 of the patients with asplenia, one or more 12-lead electrocardiograms were examined for atrial situs (Fig. 13). In 13 of 14 (92%) patients with the anatomic diagnosis of situs inversus, the P-wave axis was greater than 90 degrees, indicating atrial inversion. Also, the P-wave axis correctly indicated atrial situs solitus in 24 of the 28 (86%) patients who had atrial situs solitus at necropsy.

The P-wave axis of the patients with polysplenia was unreliable for determining atrial situs because ectopic rhythms were common. The atrial pacemaker appeared to vary from one examination to the next in many patients.

As noted by other investigators,[49] conduction disturbances and other rhythm disorders occurred frequently in patients with polysplenia. Complete heart block was present in 22%, nodal rhythm in 9%, and coronary sinus rhythm in 7% of our patients for whom an electrocardiogram was available. In some patients the rhythm disorders followed cardiac catheterization or noncardiac surgery (gastrostomy). In at least 2 of the 19 patients with rhythm disorders, fetal bradycardia was observed. This was subsequently determined to be an inherent atrial bradycardia rather than a sign of fetal distress. The diagnosis of the heterotaxy syndrome by fetal echocardiogram in such circumstances should suggest a rhythm disturbance (heart block or atrial bradycardia) as the cause of the bradycardia rather than fetal distress and, thus, prevent an unnecessary cesarean section.

All the patients with asplenia or a single, right-sided spleen had normal sinus rhythm.

Chest X-ray. In the asplenia syndrome the heart size is usually normal or small and the lungs, oligemic. Cardiac enlargement usually indicates atrioventricular valve regurgitation. Symmetry of the liver and ectopic location of the stomach bubble may be noted as well. An overpenetrated frontal view is useful for determining the bronchial anatomy, usually bilaterally eparterial bronchi. Pulmonary venous congestion with hazy lung fields and indistinct vessel outlines may develop in infants with obstructed totally anomalous pulmonary venous connection, especially after the ductus is opened with prostaglandin E1.

Radiographic findings in patients with polysplenia depend on the heart defect(s) present. On the lateral chest radiograph, the inferior vena cava shadow is absent in patients with an interrupted inferior vena cava and azygos extension. An overpenetrated frontal view is useful for determining the bronchial anatomy, usually bilaterally hyparterial bronchi.

Echocardiography. Discovering the variable, and often complex, anatomy seen in the heterotaxy syndrome is a major undertaking. An organized, segmental approach is essential in such patients. The examiner must develop and consciously go through a check list of anatomic structures to be sure that all have been examined. Given a compulsive echocardiographer and a comprehensive check list, most, if not all, pertinent anatomy can be determined using echocardiography.

The inferior vena cava, hepatic veins and their atrial connection(s), as well as the abdominal aorta, are best seen using subxiphoid views.[18] The superior vena cava on either side can be imaged using suprasternal notch or high, left or right parasternal views.[19,38] The superior caval termination of an azy-

Table 6.   Age at Death and Male/Female Ratio in Patients with Heterotaxy and Congenital Heart Disease

	Single Right Spleen n = 5	Asplenia n = 58	Polysplenia* n = 46
Age range	1 d – 22 m	5' – 14 2/12 yr	10 h – 25 yr
Median age at death	6 d	14 d	11.5 m
Male/female ratio	4	1.5	0.9

*Sex and age known in 44 of the 46 patients.
Accent ('), minutes; h, hours; d, days; m, months; yr, years.

Asplenia

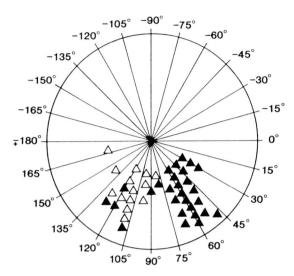

Figure 13. The P-wave axis in the electrocardiogram in 42 patients with asplenia compared with the anatomic diagnosis of atrial situs solitus (closed triangles) or atrial situs inversus (open triangles). Of the 28 patients with atrial situs solitus, 24 (86%) had the expected P axis between 30° and 90°. Of the 14 patients with atrial situs inversus, 13 (92%) had the expected P axis between 90° and 150°. (From Van Praagh S, Kreutzer J, Alday L, et al.,[47] with permission.)

gos vein can also be seen using a right or left, high parasternal, parasagittal view. The coronary sinus is seen well in an apical four-chamber view, angled posteriorly.[37] When dilated, the coronary sinus can also be seen from subxiphoid and parasternal long-axis views.

Normally connecting pulmonary veins can be seen from a number of views, including apical four-chamber, subxiphoid long- and short-axis, and suprasternal short-axis views. Subxiphoid views are especially good for pulmonary veins connecting below the diaphragm.[10] Pulmonary veins connecting anomalously to the innominate vein or the superior vena cava can usually be imaged using suprasternal notch or high parasternal views.[38] Whatever the connection, the individual pulmonary veins can be seen best from suprasternal or high sternal border views. Doppler color flow mapping is extremely useful for detecting flow in the pulmonary veins and for identifying individual veins.

The atria and atrial septum are best examined using subxiphoid and apical views.[3,36] The atrial appendages can be seen in subxiphoid and parasternal short-axis views. The extent of deficiency of the atrial septum can be determined using apical views.

The atrioventricular valves are best examined from subxiphoid long- and short-axis and apical four-chamber views. Doppler color flow mapping and pulsed Doppler mapping are useful for de-

tecting and grading regurgitation. Straddling and abnormal attachments of the valves are best appreciated in subxiphoid or parasternal short-axis and apical four-chamber views.[35]

Ventricular size and morphology should be evaluated in at least two orthogonal views, including one short-axis view. Ventricular volume can be measured using one of the algorithms described elsewhere (see ch. 15). The method for determining the identity of the ventricles and the direction of looping has been described elsewhere (see ch. 4). The ventricular septum should also be examined in at least two views, including subxiphoid or parasternal short-axis and apical four-chamber views.[4] Doppler color flow mapping has proved to be reliable for detecting ventricular septal defects if the septum is scanned in several views.[30]

Outflow tract obstruction should be evaluated using 2-D imaging and Doppler flow velocity measurement. Usually subxiphoid or apical views provide a suitable window for Doppler interrogation of the outflow tracts.

The main pulmonary artery and its branches can usually be seen using high parasternal or suprasternal notch views. They should all be measured. Stenosis of the proximal left pulmonary artery at its junction with the ductus arteriosus is common. The side to which the aorta arches can be determined from the orientation of the transducer when the arch is imaged and from the branching pattern. If aortic outflow tract obstruction is present, coarctation should be suspected. A ductus arteriosus can usually be imaged from a high, left parasternal, parasagittal view.

Cardiac Catheterization. Cardiac catheterization may not be necessary for selected, sick infants with critical pulmonary outflow obstruction, with or without anomalous pulmonary venous connection. If the echocardiogram clearly delineates the pulmonary venous anatomy, atrioventricular valve function, pulmonary artery anatomy, source(s) of pulmonary blood flow and the anatomy of the aortic arch, creation of an aortopulmonary shunt and repair of totally anomalous venous connection may be safely undertaken on the basis of the echocardiographic diagnosis.

Because many of these patients who survive beyond the first year of life are candidates for a modified Fontan procedure,[21] it is essential that the pulmonary artery pressure be measured and that the pulmonary vascular resistance be calculated. When possible, the pulmonary artery pressure should be measured directly. In exceptional cases where the pulmonary artery cannot be entered for technical reasons or because the source of pulmonary blood flow might be compromised by placing a catheter across it, pulmonary venous wedge pressure may be substituted. Pulmonary blood flow and vascular resistance should be calculated using measured oxygen consumption.

The ventricular end-diastolic pressure has been considered an important factor in predicting the outcome of a Fontan type of repair.[13] This can be measured easily at catheterization.

Angiographic assessment of the pulmonary artery anatomy is essential. Stenosis of one or more branches of the pulmonary artery appears to be a significant risk factor for morbidity and mortality after a Fontan type of operation.

Ventricular angiography provides additional information about atrioventricular valve function, ventricular size and function, and about the size, location, and number of ventricular septal defects.

In patients with severe pulmonary stenosis or atresia, a descending aortogram is useful to detect and define aortopulmonary collaterals. A characteristic angiocardiographic finding indicative of asplenia is the juxtaposition of the inferior vena cava and the descending aorta.[12] This is due to the more medial position of the liver which shifts the position of the inferior vena cava closer to the descending aorta.

Laboratory Tests. The presence of Howell-Jolly bodies in the blood smear is indicative of asplenia or a very small hypofunctioning spleen. A splenic scan is very helpful in diagnosing the presence and position of the spleen. It can also demonstrate the presence of multiple spleens. A small, hypofunctioning spleen may not be detected by a splenic scan. Because patients with a small, hypofunctioning spleen need antibiotic prophylaxis as much as asplenic patients do, this misdiagnosis does not create any therapeutic disadvantage.

Diagnosis of Asplenia

The diagnosis of visceral heterotaxy with asplenia can be established during life on the basis of: (1) Howell-Jolly bodies in the blood smear, (2) bilateral eparterial bronchi in the air bronchogram of the chest x-ray, (3) the juxtaposition of the inferior vena cava and the descending aorta, (4) the constellation of the congenital heart defects described above, and (5) the absence of normal uptake on the splenic scan (using heat-damaged red blood cells).

Diagnosis of Polysplenia

The diagnosis of polysplenia can be established during life on the basis of: (1) an interrupted inferior vena cava with unilateral (left or right) or bilateral azygos extension to the ipsilateral superior vena cava, (2) bilateral hyparterial bronchi in the air bronchogram of the chest x-ray, (3) some or all of the characteristic heart defects described above, (4) ectopic atrial pacemakers in the electrocardiogram, and (5) the presence of multiple spleens or a multilobe spleen on the splenic scan.

Noncardiac Anomalies in Visceral Heterotaxy

In reviewing the medical records and the autopsy reports of the 109 patients in this series, the following additional noncardiac anomalies were found.

Five patients (4 with asplenia and 1 with polysplenia) had multiple, severe or lethal anomalies involving many organ systems. These included tracheal agenesis with bronchoesophageal fistula (2 patients), facial dysmorphism (all 5), microphthalmia (3 patients), microcephaly (2 patients), low set ears and a short or webbed neck (3 patients), cleft palate (3 patients) and micrognathia (1 patient). All 5 had central nervous system anomalies, including hydrocephalus (1 patient), encephalocele or meningocele (2 patients), syringomyelia (1 patient), and intraventricular or subarachnoid hemorrhage (1 patient). Similarly, all 5 had skeletal malformations and abnormal kidneys. Three of the 5 were male and all had cryptorchidism. All 5 patients died in the first week of life (age range: 42 hours to 7 days).

These 5 patients appear to represent the result of a more extensive teratogenic mechanism than the one resulting in visceral heterotaxy and congenital heart disease alone. Of interest, 3 of the 5 infants had tetralogy of Fallot instead of the rather complex malformations usually seen in heterotaxy with asplenia.

The remaining 104 (95%) patients seldom had malformations other than the ones expected for heterotaxic individuals. Cryptorchidism was an exception. Six of the 35 males with asplenia (17%) had cryptorchidism, which was bilateral in 4. Five of the 20 polysplenic males (25%) had cryptorchidism, and in all 5 it was bilateral. This frequency of cryptorchidism greatly exceeds the incidence of this anomaly in otherwise normal newborns (3.4%).[17] Also the incidence of bilateral cryptorchidism in the affected males with visceral heterotaxy was much higher (66–100%) than the incidence reported in male infants with cryptorchidism alone (30%).[17]

Management

The presence of a symmetrical liver or a right-sided stomach and dextrocardia in the chest x-ray should alert the clinician to the presence of visceral heterotaxy. When the diagnosis of asplenia is established on the basis of the findings in the blood smear, the air bronchogram, the liver and spleen scan, and the characteristic constellation of the cardiac defects, antibiotic prophylaxis should be given. The recommended regimen for infants and young children is amoxicillin, 125 mg twice daily; for older children and adults, penicillin G, 200,000 units twice daily. Penicillin prophylaxis should continue for life, since fatal septicemia may develop in these patients following a mild upper respiratory infection.[48]

Surgical treatment of the congenital heart defects depends on the nature of the defects. In the asplenic patients with pulmonary atresia, an aortopulmonary or cavopulmonary shunt should not be performed if the pulmonary venous return is abnormal and obstructed. In those cases, the establishment of a normal and nonobstructed pulmonary venous connection should precede the shunt procedure. In some rare cases of asplenia with pulmonary atresia, there may be adequate systemic collaterals, making survival into adulthood possible[43] without any surgical treatment. When the common atrioventricular valve becomes severely regurgitant, cardiac transplantation is a possible, but not an easily achieved, therapeutic option.[28]

Thoracophagus Twins

Siamese twins joined at the thorax may share vascular and cardiac structures; this usually creates an insurmountable surgical problem. If separation of the heart, liver, and bowel seems possible, surgical separation, often with the view of producing one survivor, can be undertaken.

Ectopia Cordis

Rarely, an infant is born with the heart outside of the thorax, usually through a cleft in the sternum (complete thoracic ectopia cordis). The most frequent cardiac malformation is tetralogy of Fallot. The chest cavity is disproportionately small, a feature that may pose great difficulties in surgical repair.

Cantrell's Syndrome

This condition is thoracoabdominal ectopia cordis. It is characterized by midline defects involving the lower part of the sternum and the abdominal epigastrium, with a deficiency in the diaphragm and the diaphragmatic pericardium and, possibly, an omphalocele. Curiously, there is sometimes a peculiar diverticulum from the left ventricle projecting into the epigastric region.

Complete Situs Inversus

When all of the viscera are inverted, situs inversus totalis is said to be present. Although some of these children may have congenital heart disease, there also may be no cardiac anomaly. Situs inversus totalis without heart disease is seldom seen in a hospital population. Hence its prevalence is not known.

Kartagener's Syndrome

A syndrome of situs inversus totalis with sinusitis and bronchiectasis has been described.[22] These patients have disordered cilia, which account for the bronchiectasis and the male infertility seen in this syndrome. Similar cilial abnormality is reputed to be present in some patients without complete situs inversus.

Dextrocardia with Visceroatrial Situs Solitus

Extrinsic Causes

The heart may be displaced into the right chest because of hypoplasia of the right lung (for example, in the scimitar syndrome, see ch. 32), or because of a congenital diaphragmatic hernia, allowing abdominal contents to enter the left side of the chest. In this situation the heart may be normal, although cardiac anomalies are common.

Intrinsic Causes

The heart may occupy the right chest cavity or assume a mesocardial position because of intrinsic reasons related to the process of ventricular looping or visceral lateralization. Intracardiac defects are almost invariably present (Exhibit 1).

Because these patients (the largest group of malpositions, see Exhibit 1) can have almost any cardiac anomaly or combination of anomalies, detailed discussion of the clinical features is scarcely fruitful. As indicated earlier, once malposition has been recognized, the cardiologist begins a systematic evaluation of the segmental relationships and connections of the chambers. That having been done, superimposed anatomic abnormalities can be identified and quantified and a treatment plan outlined.

REFERENCES

1. Aristotle: Historia Animalium. Book II. Translated by A.L. Peck, Loeb Classical Library, Cambridge, MA, Harvard University Press, 1965, p. 132 (507a, 20).
2. Arnold GL, Bixler D, Girod D: Probable autosomal recessive inheritance of polysplenia, situs inversus and cardiac defects in an Amish family. Am J Med Genet 16:35–42, 1983.
3. Bierman FZ, Williams RG: Subxiphoid two-dimensional imaging of the interatrial septum in infants and neonates with congenital heart disease. Circulation 60:80–90, 1979.
4. Bierman FZ, Fellows K, Williams RG: Prospective identification of ventricular septal defects in infancy using subxiphoid two-dimensional echocardiography. Circulation 62:807–817, 1980.
5. Brandt HM, Liebow AA: Right pulmonary isomerism associated with venous, splenic, and other anomalies. Lab Invest 7:469–504, 1958.
6. Brueckner M, D'Eustachio P, Horwich AL: Linkage mapping of mouse gene, iv, that controls left-right symmetry of the heart and viscera. Proc Natl Acad Sci USA 86:5035–5038, 1989.
7. Cantrell JR, Haller JA, Ravitch MM: A syndrome of congenital defects involving the abdominal wall, sternum, diaphragm, pericardium and heart. Surg Gynecol Obstet 197:602–614, 1958.
8. Caruso G, Becker AE: How to determine atrial situs? Considerations initiated by 3 cases of absent spleen with a discordant anatomy between bronchi and atria. Br Heart J 41:559–567, 1979.

9. Chandra RS: Biliary atresia and other structural anomalies in the congenital polysplenia syndrome. J Pediatr 85:649–655, 1974.

10. Cooper MJ, Teitel DF, Silverman NH, et al: Study of the infradiaphragmatic total anomalous pulmonary venous connection with cross-sectional and pulsed Doppler echocardiography. Circulation 70:412–416, 1984.

11. Edwards JE: Pathologic and developmental considerations in anomalous pulmonary venous connection. Mayo Clin Proc 28:441–452, 1953.

12. Elliott LP, Cramer GG, Amplatz K: The anomalous relationship of the inferior vena cava and abdominal aorta as a specific angiocardiographic sign in asplenia. Radiology 87:859–863, 1966.

13. Fontan F, De Ville C, Quagebeur J, et al: Repair of tricuspid atresia in 100 patients. J Thorac Cardiovasc Surg 85:647–660, 1983.

14. Freedom RM: Aortic valve and arch anomalies in the congenital asplenia syndrome. Case report, literature review and re-examination of the embryology of the congenital asplenia syndrome. Johns Hopkins Med J 135:124–135, 1974.

15. Freedom RM, Culham JAG, Moes CAF: Asplenia and polysplenia (a consideration of syndromes characterized by right or left atrial isomerism). In Angiocardiography of Congenital Heart Disease. New York, Macmillan, 1984, pp. 643–654.

16. Fyler DC, Buckley LP, Hellenbrand WE, et al: Report of the New England Regional Infant Cardiac Program. Pediatrics 65:375–461, 1980.

17. Gonzales R, Michael A: Disorders and anomalies of the scrotal contents. In Behrman RE, Vaughn VC, Nelson WL (eds): Nelson's Textbook of Pediatrics, 13th ed. Philadelphia, W.B. Saunders, 1987, pp. 1163–1165.

18. Huhta JC, Smallhorn JF, Macartney FJ: Two-dimensional echocardiographic diagnosis of situs. Br Heart J 48:97–108, 1982.

19. Huhta JC, Smallhorn JF, Macartney FJ, et al: Cross-sectional echocardiographic diagnosis of systemic venous return. Br Heart J 48:388–403, 1982.

20. Ivemark BI: Implications of agenesis of the spleen on the pathogenesis of conotruncus anomalies in childhood. Acta Paediatr Scand [Suppl] 44:1–116, 1955.

21. Jonas RA, Castaneda AR: Modified Fontan procedure: atrial baffle and systemic venous-to-pulmonary artery anastomotic techniques. J Cardiac Surg 3:91–96, 1988.

22. Kartagener M: Zur pathogenese der bronchiektasien, bronchietagien bei situs viscerum inversus. Beitr Klin Tuberk 83:489, 1933.

23. Langman J: Medical Embryology, Human Development: Normal and Abnormal. Baltimore, Williams & Wilkins, 1963, p. 180.

24. Layton WM: Heart malformations in mice homozygous for a gene causing situs inversus. In Rosenquist G, Bersma D (eds): Morphogenesis and Malformation of the Cardiovascular System. New York, Alan R. Liss, 1978, pp. 277–293.

25. Lev M: Pathologic diagnosis of positional variations in cardiac chambers in congenital heart disease. Lab Invest 3:71–82, 1954.

26. Macartney FJ, Zuberbuhler JR, Anderson RH: Morphological considerations pertaining to recognition of atrial isomerism. Br Heart J 44:657–667, 1980.

27. Martin G: Observations d'une deviation organique de l'estomac, d'une anomalie dans la situation, dans la configuration du coeur et des vaisseaux qui en partnet or qui s'y rendent. Bulletin de la Societe Anatomique de Paris 3:39–43, 1826.

28. Mayer JE, Perry S, O'Brien P, et al: Orthoptic heart transplantation for complex congenital heart disease. J Thorac Cardiovasc Surg 99:484–492, 1990.

29. Moller JH, Hakib A, Anderson RC: Congenital cardiac disease associated with polysplenia. Circulation 36:789–799, 1967.

30. Ortiz E, Robinson PJ, Beanfield JE, et al: Localization of ventricular septal defects by simultaneous display of superimposed color Doppler and cross-sectional echocardiographic images. Br Heart J 54:53–60, 1985.

31. Pasquini L, Sanders SP, Parness I, et al: Echocardiographic and anatomic findings in atrioventricular discordance with ventriculoarterial concordance. Am J Cardiol 62:1256–1262, 1988.

32. Polhemus D, Schafer WB: Congenital absence of the spleen: syndrome with atrioventricularis and situs inversus. Pediatrics 9:696–708, 1952.

33. Putschar WGJ, Manion WC: Congenital absence of the spleen and associated anomalies. Am J Clin Pathol 26:429–470, 1956.

34. Rose V, Izukawa T, Moes CAF: Syndromes of asplenia and polysplenia. Br Heart J 37:840–852, 1975.

35. Sanders SP: Straddling atrioventricular valves. In Giuliani ER (ed): Two-dimensional real-time imaging of the heart. Boston, Martinus Nijhoff, 1985, pp. 367–371.

36. Shub C, Dimopoulos IN, Seward JB, et al: Sensitivity of two-dimensional echocardiography in the direct visualization of atrial septal defect utilizing the subcostal approach: experience with 154 patients. J Am Coll Cardiol 2:127–135, 1983.

37. Silverman NH, Schiller NB: Apex echocardiography: a two-dimensional technique for evaluating congenital heart disease. Circulation 57:503–511, 1978.

38. Snider AR, Silverman NH: Suprasternal notch echocardiography: a two-dimensional technique for evaluating congenital heart disease. Circulation 63:165–173, 1981.

39. Troschel: quoted by Schelenz K: Ein neuer Beitrag zur Kenntnis des Situs viscerum inversus partialis. Berl Klin Wchnshr 461:188, 840, 1909.

40. Van Mierop LHS, Wiglesworth FW: Isomerism of the cardiac atria in the asplenia syndrome. Lab Invest 11:1303–1315, 1962.

41. Van Mierop LHS, Eisen S, Schiebler GL: The radiographic appearance of the tracheobronchial tree as indicator of visceral situs. Am J Cardiol 26:432–435, 1970.

42. Van Mierop LHS, Gessner IH, Schiebler GL: Asplenia and polysplenia syndromes. Birth Defects 8:36–44, 1972.

43. Van Praagh S: Unpublished data.

44. Van Praagh S, Antoniadis S, Otero-Coto E, et al: Common atrioventricular canal with and without conotruncal malformations: an anatomic study of 251 postmortem cases. In Nora JJ, Takao A (eds): Congenital Heart Disease: Causes and Processes. Mount Kisco, New York, Futura, 1984, pp. 599–639.

45. Van Praagh S, Davidoff A, Chin A, et al: Double outlet right ventricle: anatomic types and developmental implications based on a study of 101 autopsied cases. Coeur 13:389–439, 1982.

46. Van Praagh S, Kakou-Guikahue M, Kim HS, et al: Atrial situs in patients with visceral heterotaxy and congenital heart disease: conclusions based on findings in 104 postmortem cases. Coeur 19:484–502, 1988.

47. Van Praagh S, Kreutzer J, Alday L, et al: Systemic and pulmonary venous connections in visceral heterotaxy, with emphasis on the diagnosis of atrial situs: a study of 109 postmortem cases. In Clark E, Takao A (eds): Developmental Cardiology: Morphogenesis and Function. Mt. Kisco, NY, Futura, 1990, pp. 671–721.

48. Waldman JD, Rosenthal A, Smith AL, et al: Sepsis and congenital asplenia. J Pediatr 90:555–559, 1977.

49. Wren C, Macartney FJ, Deanfield JE: Cardiac rhythm in atrial isomerism. Am J Cardiol 59:1156–1158, 1987.

Chapter 38

MITRAL VALVE AND LEFT ATRIAL LESIONS

Donald C. Fyler, M.D.

MITRAL VALVE DISEASE

Prevalence

Mitral valve lesions are commonly associated with other congenital and acquired cardiac defects; isolated mitral valve lesions are rare in pediatric populations (Exhibit 1). Rheumatic mitral disease, the most important cardiac problem in children worldwide, is now rare in the United States (see chs. 18 and 22).

Pathology

Any part of the mitral valve apparatus may be congenitally abnormal. The leaflets may be deformed, myxomatous, adherent to adjacent structures, thickened, constricted, or cleft.[15] The commissures may be partially fused or absent; there may be additional orifices. The annulus may be dilated[7] or hypoplastic.[43] The chordae tendineae may be fused (arcade)[5] or shortened and their attachments abnormally located.[43] The papillary muscles may be single or adjacent (parachute valve).[49] Fibrous rings and membranes above the valve are encountered.[49] Prolapse of the leaflets is common, depending somewhat on the criteria used to decide how much prolapse is normal and how much is abnormal.

Acquired problems include the dilatation of the valve ring secondary to ventricular dilatation of any cause or due to inadequate tethering of the valve leaflets because of papillary muscle disease, as is seen in patients with anomalous origin of a coronary artery (see p. 715) and myocarditis (see p. 330). Also, surgery for aortic outflow problems may damage the mitral valve.

Rheumatic mitral valve disease has a characteristic histopathology, the presence of Aschoff nodules being virtually diagnostic (see p. 307).

Physiology

Deformity of the mitral valve produces mitral regurgitation, mitral stenosis, or both. If one imag-

ines absence of the leaflets with an enlarged annulus as characteristic of severe mitral regurgitation, it is obvious that there can be no associated mitral stenosis when there is maximal regurgitation. Similarly, maximal mitral stenosis allows for little mitral regurgitation. If there is a combination of mitral stenosis and regurgitation, the additional amount of regurgitant blood must, in combination with the cardiac output, pass through the stenotic valve. In effect, mitral regurgitation will aggravate the obstruction. The physiologic and clinical features of these two physiologic problems will be discussed separately.

Mitral Regurgitation

When there is mitral regurgitation, each beat contributes to forward stroke volume and, simultaneously, some blood is pumped into the left atrium. The amount of blood regurgitated may be as much as twice the cardiac output. Except in extreme situations, mitral regurgitation is surprisingly well tolerated (better when it develops gradually than when it occurs suddenly). When the left atrium is compliant and is exposed gradually to an increasing left atrial volume, a giant-sized left atrium under low pressure may develop. Acute dilatation of the left atrium can be associated with atrial hypertension (the left atrial wall being relatively noncompliant), and symptoms resulting from pulmonary venous hypertension may ensue. Rarely, with high levels of atrial pressure, pulmonary edema may be experienced. With prolonged elevation of atrial pressure, pulmonary arterial vasoconstriction and pulmonary hypertension may result.

When the left atrium becomes maximally dilated, atrial fibrillation may appear. The sizes of the ventricle and the left atrium are proportionate to the degree of mitral regurgitation and are not necessarily a measure of left ventricular dysfunction. With free mitral regurgitation and a dilated left ventricle, there is decreased left ventricular wall tension, which explains the time-honored clin-

Exhibit 1

Boston Children's Hospital Experience 1973–1987 **Left Atrial and Mitral Valve Problems**		
Left Atrial Problems	Primary Diagnosis	Secondary Diagnosis
Mitral regurgitation		
Congenital	221	1066
Rheumatic	—	58
Mitral stenosis		
Congenital	31	321
Rheumatic	—	43
Supravalvar ring	4	21
Cor triatriatum	10	15
Pulmonary venous stenosis	13	145*
Mitral valve prolapse	367	337

*These patients had suggested diagnoses of obstruction of atrial baffles (atrial inversion operations), obstructed anastomoses after surgery for total anomalous pulmonary veins, and pulmonary venous stenosis. Without a case by case review, it is not possible to distinguish confidently the ones with acquired pulmonary venous stenosis.

Distribution of Left Atrial and Mitral Valve Problems Among Other Primary Cardiac Defects

Primary Diagnosis	Mitral Stenosis n = 321	Supravalvar Stenosis n = 21	Cor Triatriatum n = 15	Mitral Regurgitation n = 1066
Coarctation of the aorta	70	3	5	99
Hypoplastic left heart	89	2	0	14
Endocardial cushion	33	1	2	354
Ventricular defect	26	3	4	113
Aortic outflow problems	24	1	0	164
Double-outlet right ventricle	17	1	0	16
Malposition	14	0	1	42
Single ventricle	15	1	0	40
D-Transposition of great arteries	9	2	1	75
Tetralogy of Fallot	5	3	0	65
L-Transposition of great arteries	1	0	1	26
Tricuspid atresia	1	0	0	39
Other	17	4	1	19

ical observation that relatively severe mitral regurgitation can be well tolerated over long periods of time.[3]

Clinical Manifestations. Minor degrees of mitral regurgitation produce no symptoms. With increased amounts of regurgitation, fatigue may be reported but, except for complaints of being tired, patients with advanced degrees of regurgitation may be surprisingly well. If there is pulmonary venous hypertension, there may be tachypnea or dyspnea, but this is not common. In a child with advanced mitral regurgitation, growth may be limited.

On physical examination, the cardiac pulsations may be visibly and palpably hyperactive, the apex being displaced leftward and posterior in advanced disease. There is no thrill. It is an old observation that apical thrills are almost invariably diastolic and that the systolic murmur of mitral regurgitation is almost never associated with a thrill. The murmur has a blowing quality and is of higher frequency than most left sternal border murmurs of congen-

ital heart disease, but, except for location, it is indistinguishable from the murmur of an unrestricted ventricular septal defect (Fig. 1). Usually, the murmur of mitral regurgitation is well heard outside the anterior axillary line and into the axilla; the murmur of ventricular defect is heard best at the left lower sternal border. Occasionally, with severe mitral regurgitation, the murmur is maximal at the posterior axillary line. A minimal apical mid-diastolic rumble is common; presumably it is due to greatly increased blood flow across the mitral orifice, albeit a dilated orifice.

Electrocardiography. With advanced degrees of mitral regurgitation, there is left ventricular hypertrophy and P-mitrale. It is unusual to find right ventricular hypertrophy caused by pulmonary hypertension secondary to severe mitral regurgitation.

Chest X-ray. The heart is enlarged proportionate to the enlarged left atrium and enlarged left ventricle. The overall size may be huge (Fig. 2).

Echocardiography. The enlarged left atrium and

S_1 S_2 S_1

Figure 1. Diagram of the auscultatory findings in mitral regurgitation. The murmur is of high frequency, begins with the first heart sound, and is holosystolic.

Mitral Regurgitation

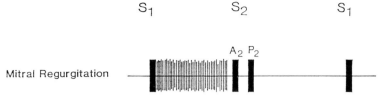

A_2 P_2

left ventricle are readily demonstrated. A Doppler estimation of the regurgitant and forward flows across the mitral valve provides a measure of the severity. Sometimes specific abnormalities of the mitral valve leaflets can be imaged, i.e., a flail or a cleft leaflet.

Cardiac Catheterization. Evaluation of isolated mitral regurgitation does not require cardiac catheterization, although most pediatric patients with mitral regurgitation undergo catheterization to sort out the influence of the various associated defects.

When angiographic documentation is desirable, the patient is best examined in the left anterior oblique view, with contrast injected into the left ventricle. It is best if the catheter has been passed through the aortic valve to avoid inducing or aggravating regurgitation by holding the mitral valve open with a catheter. In general, the selection of angiographic position is more often decided by the associated defects than by the mitral incompetence because mitral regurgitation can be evaluated in most angiographic views, so long as the left atrium and left ventricle do not overlie each other.

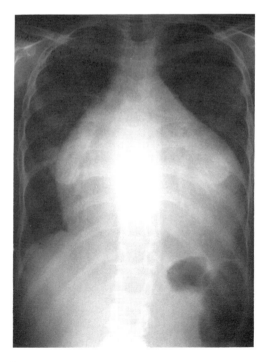

Figure 2. The chest x-ray of an adolescent terminally ill with chronic rheumatic mitral regurgitation.

Management. Because there is a tendency for increasing mitral regurgitation as the child becomes older, patients with minimal mitral regurgitation should be seen regularly. Often there is little change as the years go by and the main medical influence on the disease is the prevention of infective endocarditis, a regurgitant mitral valve being a particularly favored site.

When there are symptoms, anticongestive medications may be helpful, afterload reduction being remarkably successful in some patients. Afterload reduction not only reduces the work of the heart, but it decreases the amount of regurgitation into the left atrium in that the comparative resistance between the left atrium and the systemic circulation has been favorably changed.[35] With continued symptoms or growth limitation, consideration should be given to mitral valve surgery. If valvuloplasty is possible, it is the desirable answer;[4,38,50,52] if not, valve replacement is undertaken.[1] Usually, because of dilatation of the valve ring, a large-sized prosthesis (satisfactory for some years) is possible, even in infants. Bioprostheses have been shown to calcify within a few years. Consequently, mechanical valves, usually requiring chronic anticoagulation,[40,45,46,51] are used (see p. 741).

Course. Except for the milder forms, mitral regurgitation tends to get worse over the years. This is surely the case in patients with rheumatic heart disease and apparently in patients with congenital mitral disease as well. This is thought to be caused by progressive relaxation and dilatation of the valve ring, as well as progressive leaflet deformity (probably because of hemodynamic trauma).

Mitral Stenosis

Mitral stenosis limits blood flow into the left ventricle during diastole. To pump the pulmonary venous return, the left atrial pressure must rise in proportion to the severity of the mitral stenosis. Normally, there is no pressure difference between the left atrium and the left ventricle during diastole, even during exercise. Any pressure gradient suggests obstruction, the degree of obstruction being crudely proportional to the gradient. Left atrial hypertension is transmitted to the pulmonary veins and the pulmonary capillaries where, if oncotic pressure is exceeded, pulmonary edema develops. Thus, the maximal imaginable pressure in the left atrium may be as high as 30–40 mm Hg in the worst case, and at that level it is associated with dyspnea.

According to Gorlin's formula (see p. 197),[21] small changes in flow across the obstructed valve affect the gradient exponentially. Because diastole is proportionately shortened with increases in heart rate, the available time for mitral flow per minute is shortened, and therefore, the necessary pressure gradient is higher. Consequently, patients comfortable at rest may experience dyspnea and pulmonary edema with an increase in activity.

The flow across the mitral valve occurs throughout diastole and is increased in presystole with atrial contraction. Because atrial contraction provides 15–20% of mitral flow, the reduction in flow accompanying the onset of atrial fibrillation may result in the sudden appearance of symptoms.

Elevated pulmonary venous pressure causes reflex pulmonary arteriolar vasoconstriction and pulmonary hypertension. In a small infant this can occur because of persistence of fetal vascularity; in older children it develops over time, reflecting chronic elevation of pulmonary venous pressure. Unlike the pulmonary vascular disease associated with left-to-right shunts, this pulmonary arteriolar vasoconstriction resolves once the pulmonary venous pressure is reduced to normal. With advanced mitral stenosis, pulmonary hypertension may rise to systemic levels. At the same time, the resistance to pulmonary flow posed by the arterioles protects the capillaries from excessive pressure and the development of pulmonary edema. With chronic and progressive obstruction, as in rheumatic heart disease, maximal mitral obstruction is accompanied by severe left atrial hypertension, severe pulmonary hypertension, right ventricular hypertension, and secondary tricuspid valve regurgitation. In the author's experience this secondary tricuspid regurgitation is more common among patients with rheumatic fever than among those with congenital mitral obstruction, possibly because of direct rheumatic involvement of the tricuspid valve.

The severity of mitral stenosis is best expressed by the estimated valve area or, almost as precise, the diastolic gradient across the mitral valve. It must be remembered that the gradient across the valve may not be the sole cause of left atrial hypertension. Elevated left ventricular end-diastolic pressures associated with mitral stenosis and a limited cardiac output form a particularly ominous combination that is not completely relieved with mitral valve surgery. The possibility for increased postoperative cardiac output may be unmanageable for a damaged left ventricle. This is a more than an academic consideration, because the majority of children with congenital mitral stenosis also have other cardiac anomalies and other cardiac operations.

Clinical Manifestations. The first symptom of mitral stenosis in older children is dyspnea and, in infants, tachypnea, but any symptoms are unusual except in advanced cases. Relatively severe mitral stenosis at birth may be surprisingly well tolerated because of secondary persistent pulmonary hypertension. Poor growth is unusual even with maximal obstruction. In everyday practice, the usual patient with mitral stenosis has some associated anomaly that attracts attention through symptoms, a murmur, or gross limitation.

On physical examination, there is a diastolic rumble. It is present in all patients with rheumatic mitral stenosis, but is not invariably present in patients with congenital mitral stenosis. Minimally, the murmur is mid-diastolic or presystolic and, in its characteristic form, it begins in mid-diastole and is accentuated in presystole (Fig. 3). Although an opening snap is rarely noted in congenital mitral stenosis, it is almost invariably present in patients with rheumatic disease. Whether this is related to the difficulty of examining infants with a faster heart rate as opposed to older children with rheumatic heart disease or whether this is inherent in the valve anatomy is not clear. The first heart sound is accentuated in either form. Mitral stenosis may produce an apical diastolic thrill in patients with rheumatic or congenital heart disease. With secondary pulmonary hypertension, there is accentuation of the second heart sound, and sometimes early in diastole the murmur of pulmonary regurgitation (Graham Steell murmur) can be heard.

Electrocardiography. With minimal stenosis the electrocardiogram is normal, but with increasing degrees of mitral stenosis there is increasing evidence of right ventricular hypertrophy and P-mitrale. Extreme obstruction may result in remarkable electrocardiograms (Fig. 4).

Chest X-ray. Although the cardiac silhouette may be enlarged, the enlargement does not approach that seen in patients with mitral regurgitation. The left atrial enlargement is modest in comparison to that seen in mitral regurgitation, but it is detectable as a double density and by elevation of the left main bronchus, and there may be posterior displacement of the esophagus. In severe obstruction there is redistribution of the pulmonary blood flow; when the patient is in the upright position, the apical regions are better perfused than they are in normal individuals.

Echocardiography. Demonstration of limited motion of the mitral valve, abnormal tethering of the mitral valve leaflets, presence of a single papillary muscle, a small valve orifice, and Doppler demonstration of a pressure gradient across the valve are helpful observations in the diagnosis and quantification of mitral stenosis.

Cardiac Catheterization. When considering surgical intervention for mitral stenosis, cardiac catheterization is required. Although echocardiography is helpful in the diagnosis, quantification, and follow-up, the precision of cardiac catheterization is necessary before undertaking surgery. Direct measurement of left atrial and left ventricular

Figure 3. Diagram of the auscultatory findings in pure mitral stenosis. The murmur begins in mid-diastole, becoming increasing louder in a crescentic fashion and ending in a loud first heart sound. This murmur is often mistaken for a systolic murmur and may be associated with a thrill. When it is not loud, it is heard best, sharply localized, at the apex, with the patient in the left lateral decubitus position.

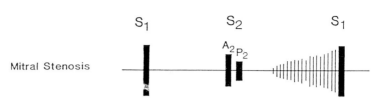

Figure 4. Electrocardiogram in a 6-year-old boy with severe mitral stenosis. There is marked right ventricular hypertrophy. All complexes in this illustration are at half standard. As an infant, he had repair of coarctation of the aorta and, later, his mitral valve was replaced with a small prosthetic valve. It was insufficient to relieve his pulmonary hypertension and episodes of pulmonary edema.

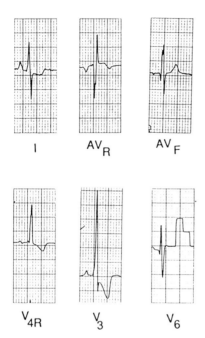

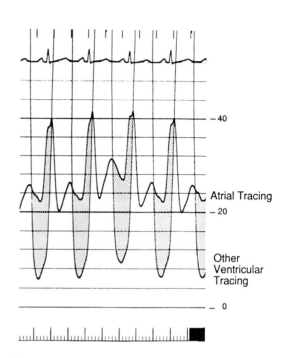

Figure 5. Left ventricular and left atrial pressure tracings recorded at the same attenuation in a 3-month-old baby with severe mitral stenosis. Note the pressure gradient between the left atrium and the left ventricle in diastole.

diastolic pressures, as well as the best available estimation of blood flow across the valve, is needed. Puncture of the atrial septum to gain access to the left atrium is undertaken, even though the targeted left atrium may not be particularly large. Generally, good quality pressure tracings of the left atrium and left ventricle, which can be overlaid for precise comparison, are obtained (Fig. 5).

Usually, angiography with left atrial injection not only confirms the echocardiographic findings but provides further confidence in deciding on a plan of surgical management. A contrast agent with as low osmolality as is available should be selected when high left atrial pressures are discovered.

Any suggestion that the patient has a supravalvar membrane or cor triatriatum (sometimes confused with valvar mitral stenosis) must be diligently pursued because those lesions are readily corrected.

Management. Surgical management of congenital mitral stenosis is less than satisfactory in many patients because valvuloplasty rarely produces sufficient benefit, and valve replacement, even if possible, is not desirable in small children. Additional cardiac defects are common. The mortality is high.[8] Often, the valve ring is small and valve replacement results in some residual obstruction that is likely to become worse as the child grows. Later, as the child grows, upgrading to a larger valve is difficult and sometimes impossible. Various solutions, none completely satisfactory, have been suggested. Excising the mitral valve and inserting a prosthesis above the valve ring have been tried, as has the insertion of a conduit from the left atrium to the left ventricle.[9,25,26,33,34]

For these reasons, surgery for congenital mitral stenosis is delayed until the child is larger, if possible, and it is avoided in infancy. Only when it is certain that there is no alternative to valve replacement is surgery undertaken, even though it is anticipated that valvuloplasty might offer a possible solution.

Correction of associated defects that cause increased mitral valve flow, such as a patent ductus arteriosus or ventricular septal defect, may reduce the transvalvar gradient enough to relieve symptoms.

Rheumatic mitral stenosis is a different problem and, in pure form, is amenable to balloon valvuloplasty[31] or, if necessary, to the full variety of surgical possibilities.

Course. Characteristically, congenital mitral stenosis does not tend to get worse with growth, the valve orifice increasing in proportion to the child's growth. Often, there is concern about pulmonary hypertension that is associated with mitral stenosis. In general, it is reversible with correction of the stenosis, despite years of obstruction, even dating from birth (see p. 441, ch. 28). For this reason, only symptoms of tachypnea or evidence of pulmonary edema are indications for intervention in children with congenital mitral stenosis.

Mitral Valve Prolapse

Mitral valve prolapse is a poorly-defined, controversial condition of uncertain consequence and unclear etiology.[12,28]

Definition. When the mitral valve leaflets billow excessively into the left atrium during systole, mitral valve prolapse is said to be present. By itself, mitral valve prolapse is not abnormal.[41]

Prevalence. The prevalence of mitral valve prolapse is reported to be 4–21% in the general population.[29] The wide variation in prevalence is accounted for by variation in the definition of what constitutes mitral valve prolapse, but whatever definition is used, there are millions of people whose mitral valves billow excessively.

Often there seems to be a genetic component with age-related expression. It is rare in infants and increasingly common with advancing age through childhood; it is more common in women, although among children only slightly more females than males are affected. Because mitral valve prolapse is so common, it is associated with many medical (Exhibit 2) and nonmedical problems, including psychiatric disturbances,[10] sudden otherwise unexplained death,[36] rheumatic fever,[54] atrial septal defect,[30] Marfan's syndrome,[20] (see p. 50), and all other problems known to mankind.

Pathology. Based on the limited pathologic material available, there is excessive mitral valve tissue and the chordae tendineae are lengthened. Myxomatous changes in the valve and laxity of the valve structures are described. The similarity to the cardiac pathology in Marfan's syndrome has prompted the suggestion that mitral valve prolapse is a variant of Marfan's.[20]

Exhibit 2

Boston Children's Hospital Experience 1973–1987 Cardiac Diagnoses Associated with Mitral Valve Prolapse*	
Diagnosis	Number
Mitral valve prolapse alone	367
Mitral regurgitation	68
Atrial septal defect	44
Aortic valve problems	36
Arrhythmia	24
Ventricular septal defect	22
Pulmonary stenosis	18
Extracardiac anomaly	17
Tetralogy of Fallot	12
Endocardial cushion defect	9
Transposition of the great arteries	5
Cardiomyopathy	5
Rheumatic heart disease	4
Other	73
Total	704

*There were 704 patients with mitral valve prolapse. Mitral valve prolapse was associated with most forms of congenital heart disease.

Two children had mitral valve replacement, one as part of surgery for an atrial septal defect of the primum type and a cleft mitral valve. Later, the mitral valve was replaced. The other had mitral valve replacement as treatment for cardiomyopathy. Two children had mitral valvoplasty: one had had the aortic valve replaced for severe aortic stenosis; the other had mitral valvoplasty as part of the treatment for an anomalous left coronary artery arising from the left pulmonary artery.

Six children had infective endocarditis: one with Lennox-Gasteau syndrome had extreme mitral valve prolapse with mitral regurgitation. The other diagnoses included tricuspid atresia, tetralogy of Fallot, ventricular defect, pulmonary atresia with intact ventricular septum, and rheumatic heart disease. It is not known whether the endocarditis was located on the mitral valve in any of these children.

There were 24 children whose primary complaint was a rhythm abnormality but who were also found to have mitral valve prolapse.

Of 65 individuals with Marfan's syndrome; 35 had some form of congenital heart disease; of these, 17 had mitral valve prolapse. Thirty had no other cardiac problem; of these, 16 had mitral valve prolapse. So, of 65 with Marfan's syndrome, 33 children are listed as having mitral valve prolapse.

Most authors imply that inherent changes in the valve lead to prolapse and, ultimately, to mitral regurgitation, occasionally of severe degree.[30] Less often, the obvious fact that mitral regurgitation has multiple causes, some of which cause mitral valve prolapse, is emphasized.[22] Regardless of the theory selected, the amount of mitral regurgitation is the main determinant of the outcome.[14]

Mitral valve prolapse occurs in some patients with an atrial septal defect of the secundum variety. This seems to be a reversible phenomenon, perhaps related to the disproportionately enlarged right ventricle, because the prolapse may improve after surgical closure of the atrial defect.[47]

Physiology. The characteristic midsystolic click moves toward the first heart sound with maneuvers that decrease the volume in the left ventricle (Valsalva, standing erect), and the midsystolic click moves toward the second heart sound with maneuvers that increase the size of the left ventricle (squatting, handgrip). The physiologic effects of mitral regurgitation are similar to those seen in patients with mitral insufficiency of all other causes (see p. 609).

Clinical Manifestations. Many patients with mitral valve prolapse have no symptoms and no abnormality on physical examination.[44]

There is an association between mitral valve prolapse and pseudocardiac complaints, such as twinges of chest pain, feeling faint, sensations of heart pounding, panic reaction, and fatigue. The similarity to "neurocirculatory asthenia" is striking. For the most part, individuals who select themselves for echocardiographic examination are likely to have neurocirculatory asthenia, but they have no more frequent prolapse than carefully selected controls.[13] Others are referred because the pediatrician heard a peculiar squeak or honk during routine auscultation, but most are referred because the pediatrician heard a click. The auditory acuity and evidence of careful auscultation by some of our referring doctors are reassuring.

On physical examination there is a tendency toward a thin, gracile habitus. The anteroposterior diameter of the chest is less than expected for the size of the child and chest deformity, such as pectus excavatum or scoliosis, is common.

To suspect the diagnosis there must be a midsystolic click, which may vary in intensity (Fig. 6). It becomes more readily audible and constant with the patient standing or with the Valsalva maneuver. Sometimes there is a late systolic murmur of mitral regurgitation (also uncovered occasionally when the patient is in the upright position or by the Valsalva maneuver) and, in advanced forms, there may be the typical pansystolic, high-frequency murmur of fullblown mitral regurgitation at the apex. It is the author's opinion that when there is mitral regurgitation the child should be thought of as having **mitral regurgitation, and all that implies,** rather than a **prolapsed mitral valve.**

Electrocardiography. It has been stated that the electrocardiogram may show abnormalities of the S-T segments and T waves in some patients with mitral valve prolapse. In the author's experience, this is not common and, in the view of some,[13] it is not any more likely in these patients than in controls. Occasionally, these patients have ectopy and, rarely, paroxysmal supraventricular tachycardia. Whether this occurs more frequently than would be found in suitable controls remains to be established.

Chest X-ray. The chest x-ray is difficult to discuss because it is rarely needed and, therefore, seldom seen. In patients with the straight back syndrome, pectus excavatum, or scoliosis, the proximity of the ausculting chest piece to the heart, when placed on the anterior chest, produces impressive sounds and suggests either that the heart is compressed or simply that the sounds are heard better in these individuals. The truth may also be that mitral valve prolapse and chest deformities are found in the same people for genetic reasons.

Echocardiography. Echocardiography is the main method for the diagnosis of mitral valve prolapse. Prolapse of the posterior leaflet above the plane of the mitral valve annulus must be demonstrable in the parasternal long-axis view.[28] Because 13% of otherwise normal children have this finding,[55] we at the Children's Hospital in Boston require that the billowing above the ring be "excessive."

The parasternal long-axis view is the primary

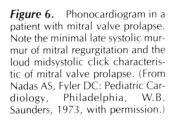

Figure 6. Phonocardiogram in a patient with mitral valve prolapse. Note the minimal late systolic murmur of mitral regurgitation and the loud midsystolic click characteristic of mitral valve prolapse. (From Nadas AS, Fyler DC: Pediatric Cardiology, Philadelphia, W.B. Saunders, 1973, with permission.)

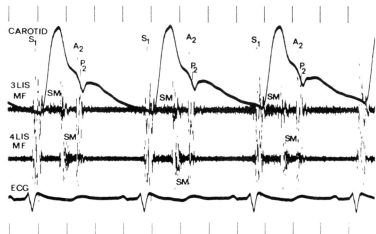

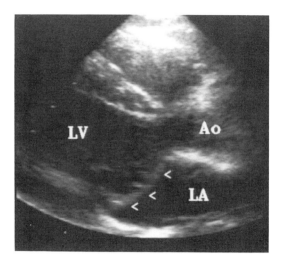

Figure 7. Echocardiogram in the parasternal long-axis view showing prolapse (arrows) of the mitral valve. LV, left ventricle; LA, left atrium; Ao, aorta.

view used (Fig. 7). Although the apical four-chamber view is useful to confirm the findings of other views, a false-positive diagnosis is more likely if this is the only view used.[28] The typical appearance in real time is a biphasic motion of the mitral leaflets in systole. The first phase is the normal closing motion of the valve with apposition of the leaflets. Later in systole, prolapse of the leaflets is seen as a second motion, when the leaflets bulge into the left atrium. Most reports recommend that the leaflets must extend at least 2–3 mm posterior to the plane of the mitral annulus. Careful inspection of the valve leaflets often indicates thickening and redundancy. The chordae tendineae are often elongated and may fold anteriorly in systole as the left ventricle shortens. This finding has been called **anterior prolapse** or **pseudosystolic anterior motion of the mitral valve**. In advanced cases thickening of the leaflets may be so marked that detection of valve-associated masses (vegetations) is difficult.

M-mode echocardiography may be used for detection of mitral valve prolapse but is less sensitive.[28] Prolapse may involve only a portion of a leaflet. Because M-mode echocardiography images only a small part of the valve at a time and one has no global view of the valve to ensure that it is imaged in its entirety, the prolapsing part may be overlooked.

Patients with mitral valve prolapse should have a careful Doppler examination of the valve as well. Doppler color flow mapping is optimal but a systematic interrogation of the atrial side of the valve, using pulsed Doppler cardiography, will also detect regurgitation. Typically, the regurgitation begins after the onset of left ventricular ejection and coincident with the second or prolapsing motion of the mitral valve. Doppler interrogation should

be performed in parasternal long-axis and apical two- and four-chamber views. How much Doppler regurgitation is normal is presently being determined (see p. 177).

Many patients have minor posterior bowing of the mitral leaflets during systole, which is probably a normal variation. Clear biphasic motion of the valve on real time imaging or marked posterior bulging of the valve leaflets (> 4 mm) is required to make the diagnosis. It is easy to fall into the trap of overdiagnosing mitral valve prolapse, especially in the current medicolegal environment. However, the harm done by overzealous interpretation of echocardiograms clearly outweighs any potential benefit.

If the patient being examined has the stigmata of Marfan's syndrome, or has marked mitral prolapse, or prolapse of the tricuspid valve as well, the aortic root should be measured carefully and evidence of aortic regurgitation should be sought.

The premise that mitral valve prolapse is a clinical diagnosis based on symptoms, electrocardiograms, and auscultation, or that the diagnosis can be made in the absence of prolapse revealed on echocardiography, is unacceptable.[27,41] If the echocardiogram shows no prolapse, there is no prolapse, and if the echocardiogram shows prolapse, there is prolapse, regardless of all else. In the author's view, by no means the view of all my associates, the echocardiographers bear the burden of overdiagnosis and underdiagnosis.

The practical clinical question is whether all patients with a midsystolic click should have an echocardiogram. With no other reason but to establish that a midsystolic click results from mitral valve prolapse, the author believes that a routine echocardiogram is overkill, particularly since nothing would be done because of it. If one wants to confirm mitral valve prolapse as part of establishing the diagnosis of Marfan's syndrome, that is a different matter. It follows that the diagnosis of mitral regurgitation is based on auscultation, not on echocardiography. Thus, a patient with mitral valve prolapse who has a mitral valve leak shown at echocardiography, but no systolic murmur, is thought of as being at miniscule risk for infective endocarditis.

Cardiac Catheterization. Cardiac catheterization is not indicated in patients with mitral valve prolapse if there is no evidence of another cardiac lesion.

Management. The symptoms associated with mitral valve prolapse improve when the patients are reassured that no problem exists, but they become permanently embedded when the diagnosis of mitral valve prolapse is solemnly pronounced. Reassurance is of little help when the adolescent has been told that her heart is abnormal. The author is concerned that there has been more harm than benefit caused by the diagnosis of mitral valve prolapse.

Whether or not to recommend the use of prophylactic antibiotics for all patients with mitral valve prolapse is a dilemma for the cardiologist. An unequivocal statement is required; hedging or beating about the bush because of concerns about medicolegal fears is to be deplored. Clearly, the problem is so common that somewhere, someday, infective endocarditis will develop in a patient with mitral valve prolapse and no mitral regurgitation. The cost of counteracting this eventuality with routine prophylactic antibiotics (a less then certain measure) would be astronomical in view of the numbers of people who would require treatment to prevent one case.[6,11] Therefore, at Children's Hospital in Boston, we do not recommend antibiotic prophylaxis during oral surgery if there is only a click and no audible murmur of mitral regurgitation.

The management of mitral regurgitation is discussed elsewhere (see p. 611).

Course. The evidence that mitral valve prolapse may sometimes be progressive is convincing. One should keep this thought in mind when following patients with known prolapse, because mitral regurgitation may be the end result.

LEFT ATRIAL PROBLEMS

Cor Triatriatum

Definition. When a membranous diaphragm divides the left atrium into two chambers, the proximal chamber accepting the pulmonary veins and the distal chamber communicating with the mitral valve and left atrial appendage, cor triatriatum is said to be present.

Prevalence. Cor triatriatum is an extremely rare lesion, occurring 25 times in approximately 14,000 cardiac patients (Exhibit 1) and in 5 of 2251 infants with heart disease. This calculates to 1 per 700 children, or 1 per 450 infants with heart disease, or an incidence of 0.0046/1000 live births.

Pathology. Normally, during cardiogenesis, the common pulmonary vein is absorbed into, and becomes part of, the left atrium. Incomplete absorption, leaving obstructing tissue at the line of connection between the left atrium and the common pulmonary vein, results in cor triatriatum. The degree of obstruction is variable, ranging from being barely detectable to being severe. Often the dividing tissue in the left atrium is a flexible diaphragm, sometimes bulging downward, like a windsock, into the region of the mitral valve. The foramen ovale and the left atrial appendage communicate with the distal left atrium and provide a means to distinguish between cor triatriatum and obstructing supravalvar rings. Atrial defects may communicate between the right atrium and either the proximal or distal left atrial chamber. Cor triatriatum may be associated with a variety of other cardiac lesions (Exhibit 1), although 40% of the time it is a pure and uncomplicated problem. Sometimes one or two, right or left, pulmonary veins are anomalously located and may enter the systemic venous circulation by various routes.[18,24]

Physiology. The physiologic abnormalities associated with cor triatriatum are a direct function of the size of the orifice between the pulmonary venous chamber and the left atrium. When there is sufficient obstruction to raise the pulmonary venous pressure, there is pulmonary hypertension that may reach or exceed systemic levels. With elevated right heart pressure, right-to-left shunting through a foramen ovale may result in cyanosis. In this case, as with mitral stenosis, the cardiac output may be limited and may not increase with exercise. Pulmonary edema is often a clinical problem. In most regards, the clinical picture and course of patients with cor triatriatum are comparable to those for infants with mitral stenosis.

When there are anomalous pulmonary veins, there is differential pulmonary vascular pathology. In the part of the lungs communicating with a severely obstructing membrane there is reflex pulmonary vascular change. The pulmonary vein draining into the systemic venous circulation, offering less resistance, may carry a large part of the total pulmonary flow. However, when there is anomalous pulmonary venous drainage of a single lobe, there is persistence of the fetal vascular muscle and pulmonary hypertension. If there is more than one anomalous pulmonary vein, it is possible that the available vascular space of one lung can manage nearly the entire cardiac output without pulmonary hypertension. In this case there would be greatly different blood flow in the two lungs, drained by the two different routes.

Clinical Manifestations. Many patients with cor triatriatum develop symptoms early in infancy, although some other asymptomatic forms of heart disease are discovered during echocardiographic studies. Uncomplicated cor triatriatum was first discovered in one of our patients at the age of 47 years. When there is mild obstruction there are no symptoms and, if this is an isolated lesion, there is no reason to suspect disease. With severe obstruction there may be pulmonary edema, pulmonary hypertension, and respiratory symptoms, such as tachypnea or dyspnea, early in infancy. Cor triatriatum should be suspected whenever there is unexplained pulmonary edema.

On physical examination there is often little to discern. The second heart sound is accentuated, specifically the pulmonary component of the second heart sound. With pulmonary hypertension, there may be a diastolic murmur of pulmonary regurgitation. Usually, there is no diastolic rumbling murmur at the apex. Why there is a diastolic rumble with valvar mitral stenosis and usually not in patients with cor triatriatum is a matter of some interest. Perhaps the lack of muscular contraction of the common pulmonary venous segment accounts for the lack of a presystolic murmur. Possibly the major reason diastolic murmurs are not heard is that this disease is dominantly a lesion of early infancy when the heart rate is fast and auscultation is not easy.

Electrocardiography. There is right ventricular hypertrophy and P-pulmonale in patients who are symptomatic with cor triatriatum.

Chest X-ray. There is evidence of pulmonary edema and Kerley B lines are present when the degree of obstruction is severe. Usually, the heart is not enlarged.

Echocardiography. The membrane transecting the left atrium can be visualized on 2-D echocardiography. Documentation that the pulmonary venous segment accepts the pulmonary veins, while the distal segment is associated with the foramen ovale and the left atrial appendage makes the diagnosis. The entry point of each of the pulmonary veins should be identified because of the tendency for anomalous drainage in these patients. The need to understand the pulmonary venous anatomy prior to repair is self-evident.

Usually, the distinction between cor triatriatum and a supravalvar obstructing ring is readily apparent. In cor triatriatum, although the membrane may balloon into the mitral valve, the left atrial appendage communicates with the distal compartment, as does the foramen ovale. With a supra-

valvar ring, the left atrial appendage and foramen ovale are proximal to the stenosing structures.

The obstructing membrane can be imaged in subxiphoid or apical chamber views (Fig. 8). Doppler color flow mapping is useful for detecting the orifice in the membrane and for aligning the pulsed or continuous-wave Doppler cursor with the stenotic jet. As for atrioventricular valve stenosis, an average gradient can be calculated from the Doppler tracing by averaging the velocity over the cardiac cycle, using a digitizing tablet and computer. If tricuspid regurgitation is present, the right ventricular pressure can be estimated from the velocity of the regurgitant jet. Otherwise, the right ventricular pressure can be grossly estimated from the orientation of the ventricular septum.

The pulmonary veins should be examined from a suprasternal or parasternal short-axis view to exclude any partially anomalous connection. The usual accessory drainage sites, such as the left innominate vein, the coronary sinus, and the right superior vena cava, should be examined with Doppler color flow mapping as well.

Cardiac Catheterization. Virtually all patients with cor triatriatum come to cardiac catheterization because the diagnosis is sufficiently rare that direct physiologic measurements are usually recorded (Fig. 9). Evaluation of cor triatriatum usually re-

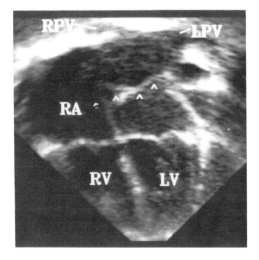

Figure 8. Apical four-chamber view in a patient with cor triatriatum demonstrating the left atrial membrane (arrows). Note the orifice of the left atrial appendage on the side of the membrane closer to the mitral valve and the orifice of a pulmonary vein on the opposite side of the membrane. LV, left ventricle; LPV, left pulmonary vein; RA, right atrium; RPV, right pulmonary vein; RV, right ventricle.

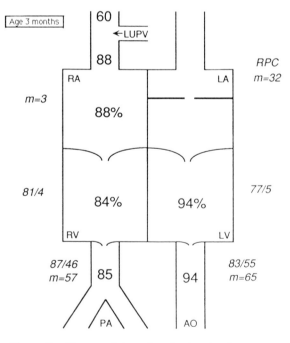

Figure 9. Diagram of the catheterization data from a patient with cor triatriatum and a single left upper pulmonary vein entering the right superior vena cava. Because of pulmonary hypertension, the left-to-right shunt through the left upper lobe is large. One year after surgical excision of the membrane and redirection of the anomalous pulmonary vein, cardiac catheterization showed normal right pressures and no evidence of shunting.

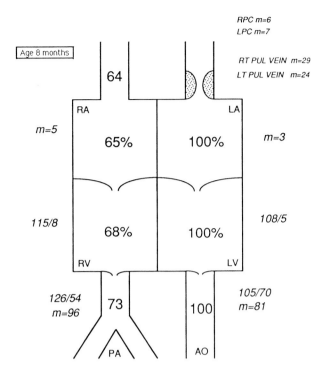

RPC m=6
LPC m=7

Age 8 months

RT PUL VEIN m=29
LT PUL VEIN m=24

64

RA   LA

m=5   65%   100%   m=3

115/8   68%   100%   108/5

RV   LV

126/54   73   100   105/70
m=96   m=81

PA   AO

Figure 10. Catheterization data from a patient with pulmonary venous stenosis. This toddler developed respiratory symptoms that ultimately led to cardiac catheterization and the data presented. Note the suprasystemic pulmonary artery pressure, the elevated pulmonary vein pressures and the repeatedly normal pulmonary artery wedge pressures. All pulmonary veins that could be entered were obstructed and in some cases nearly atretic. Balloon dilatation was transitorily helpful; the infant succumbed some weeks later. (Patient of Dr. D. Tuuri.)

quires a transseptal catheterization to obtain the best data.[48]

Management. The obstructing membrane of cor triatriatum should be resected if the infant is symptomatic.[42] Asymptomatic patients without significant obstruction are managed expectantly. Often a membrane of cor triatriatum is removed when surgical procedures are being carried out for other cardiac defects. Ordinarily, removal of the obstructing membrane is curative.[32,37]

Supravalvar Mitral Membrane

A supravalvar mitral membrane is situated immediately above the mitral valve leaflets and is distinguished from cor triatriatum because the left atrial appendage communicates with the proximal part of the atrium. It is a rare anomaly, occurring about as frequently as cor triatriatum, but it is almost always associated with other cardiac defects, i.e., Shone's syndrome.[49]

The clinical features are those of the associated defects, except in the rare case of an isolated membrane severe enough to cause pulmonary venous hypertension and dyspnea.

The diagnosis can often be recognized by echocardiography. It is necessary to separate the image of the supravalvar membrane from that of the mitral valve leaflets.[19] Sometimes a thin membrane is adherent to the leaflets and is difficult to distinguish. Apical two- and four-chamber views and the parasternal long-axis view are most useful for imaging the membrane. Usually the membrane is at

the annulus of the valve but occasionally it may attach to the leaflet slightly below the annulus. In all patients with evidence of mitral stenosis, a supravalvar membrane should be considered because it is usually a curable lesion,[53] whereas most forms of mitral stenosis are not.

If it is part of a complex of other congenital defects that are being repaired, the membrane should be inspected and removed if possible, even if it is not known to be causing trouble. If it is an isolated lesion causing symptoms or proved obstruction, surgery should be undertaken with the likely expectation of benefit if not cure.

Pulmonary Venous Stenosis

Stenosis of normally positioned pulmonary veins is a rare problem that may occur as an isolated phenomenon or in association with other defects, usually postoperatively.

The stenosis is usually at the junction of the pulmonary vein and the left atrium. Later, the vein itself may become involved, becoming hypoplastic and even atretic.[2,23] Subsequently, other veins may become involved. This disease should not be confused with the obstructions that occur at baffle sites in Senning operations or at the anastomotic site of repaired total anomalous pulmonary veins. At the same time, these operations have preceded the development of individual pulmonary vein obstruction.

Although only one or two veins may be affected, the problem is often progressive, the stenoses becoming more severe and sometimes spreading to affect all the pulmonary veins. Based on presently available information, it is possible that most of these patients have an acquired problem. Some most certainly do, and in others there is no way to be confident. Good documentation of the absence of pulmonary vein disease in patients who subsequently develop pulmonary vein stenosis has been recorded.

With progression of involvement of a single vein and later involvement of other veins, the hemodynamics may be confusing. A single obstructed vein may or may not have an elevated pulmonary arteriolar wedge pressure. When there is involvement of more than one vein, there may be pulmonary hypertension simply because of obstruction of some veins results in excessive blood flow in others.

Clinical Manifestations. Clinically, the symptoms of pulmonary venous hypertension are dyspnea and tachypnea. There is nothing that points to this diagnosis on physical examination other than evidence of pulmonary edema. The electrocardiogram shows right ventricular hypertrophy. The chest x-ray may show pulmonary edema, sometimes asymmetric, and Kerley B lines.

On echocardiography, examination of the extraparenchymal pulmonary veins may show turbulence at the point of entry of the veins into the left atrium.

At cardiac catheterization there is right ventricular and pulmonary hypertension and, usually, elevated pulmonary arteriolar wedge pressure, although this is not necessarily found (Fig. 10). Right-to-left shunting through a foramen ovale and arterial oxygen unsaturation because of pulmonary edema may be seen.

Naturally occurring venous stenosis is usually a fatal disease. Surgical attempts to relieve pulmonary venous obstruction have rarely been successful. Similarly, dilating veins with balloon catheters has been unsuccessful.[16] Although insertion of a stent in a pulmonary vein may be worth trying in this almost universally fatal disease, one has little confidence in its success.

REFERENCES

1. Almeida RS, Elliott MJ, Robinson PJ, et al: Surgery for congenital abnormalities of the mitral valve at the Hospital for Sick Children, London, from 1969–1983. J Cardiovasc Surg 29:95-99, 1988.
2. Bini RM, Cleveland D, Cebailos R, et al: Congenital pulmonary venous stenosis. Am J Cardiol 54:369–375, 1984.
3. Braunwald E: Mitral regurgitation: physiologic, clinical and surgical considerations. N Engl J Med 281:425–433, 1969.
4. Carpentier A: Congenital malformations of the mitral valve. In Stark J, de Leval M (eds): Surgery for Congenital Heart Defects. London, Grune & Stratton, 1983, pp. 467–482.
5. Castaneda AR, Anderson RG, Edwards JE: Congenital mitral stenosis resulting from anomalous arcade and obstructing papillary muscles: report of correction by use of a ball valve prosthesis. Am J Card 24:237–240, 1969.
6. Clemens JD, Horwitz RI, Jaffe CC, et al: A controlled evaluation of the risk of bacterial endocarditis in persons with mitral-valve prolapse. N Engl J Med 307:776–781, 1982.
7. Coles JG, Williams WG, Watanabe T, et al: Surgical experience with reparative techniques in patients with congenital mitral valvular anomalies. Circulation 76(Suppl III):117–122, 1987.
8. Collins-Nakai RL, Rosenthal A, Castaneda AR, et al: Congenital mitral stenosis: a review of 20 years experience. Circulation 56:1039–1047, 1977.
9. Corno A, Giannico S, Leibovich S, et al: The hypoplastic mitral valve. When should a left atrial-left ventricular extracardiac valved conduit be used? J Thorac Cardiovasc Surg 91:848–851, 1986.
10. Crowe RR, Pauls DL, Slyman DJ, et al: A family study of anxiety neurosis: morbidity risk in families of patients with and without mitral valve prolapse. Arch Gen Psychiatry 37:77–79, 1980.
11. Danchin N, Briancon S, Mathieu P, et al: Mitral valve prolapse as a risk factor for infective endocarditis. Lancet 1:743–745, 1989.
12. Devereux RD (ed): Diagnosis and prognosis of mitral-valve prolapse. N Engl J Med 320:1077–1079, 1989.
13. Devereux RB, Kramer-Fox R, Brown WT, et al: Relation between clinical features of the mitral valve prolapse syndrome and echocardiographically documented mitral valve prolapse. J Am Coll Cardiol 8:763–772, 1986.
14. Devereux RB, Kramer-Fox R, Shear MK, et al: Diagnosis and classification of severity of mitral valve prolapse: methodologic, biologic and prognostic considerations. Am Heart J 113:1265–1280, 1987.
15. Di Segni E, Bass JL, Lucas RV, et al: Isolated cleft mitral valve: a variety of congenital mitral regurgitation identified by 2-dimensional echocardiography. Am J Cardiol 51:927–931, 1983.
16. Driscoll DJ, Hesslein PS, Mullins CE: Congenital stenosis of individual pulmonary veins: clinical spectrum and unsuccessful treatment by transvenous balloon dilation. Am J Cardiol 49:1767–1772, 1982.
17. Geggel RL, Fried R, Tuuri DT, et al: Congenital pulmonary vein stenosis: structural changes in a patient with normal pulmonary artery wedge pressure. J Am Coll Cardiol 3:193–199, 1984.
18. Geggel RL, Fulton DR, Chernoff HL, et al: Cor triatriatum associated with partial anomalous pulmonary venous connection to the coronary sinus: echocardiographic and angiocardiographic features. Pediatr Cardiol 8:279–283, 1987.
19. Glaser J, Yakirevich V, Vidne BA: Preoperative echographic diagnosis of supravalvular stenosing ring of the left atrium. Am Heart J 108:169–171, 1984.
20. Glesby MJ, Pyeritz RE: Association of mitral valve prolapse and systemic abnormalities of connective tissue: a phenotypic continuum. JAMA 262:523–528, 1989.
21. Gorlin R, Gorlin SG: Hydraulic formula for calculation of area of stenotic mitral valves, other cardiac valves and central circulatory shunts. Am Heart J 41:1, 1951.
22. Jeresaty RM: Mitral Valve Prolapse. New York, Raven Press, 1979.
23. Kingston HM, Patel RG, Watson GH: Unilateral absence or extreme hypoplasia of pulmonary veins. Br Heart J 49:148–153, 1983.
24. Kirk AJB, Pollock JCS: Concomitant cor triatriatum and coronary sinus total anomalous pulmonary venous connection. Ann Thorac Surg 44:203–204, 1987.

25. Laks H, Hellenbrand WE, Kleinman C, et al: Left atrial-left ventricular conduit for relief of congenital mitral stenosis in infancy. J Thorac Cardiovasc Surg 80:782–787, 1980.

26. Lansing AM, Elbl F, Solinger RE, et al: Left atrial-left ventricular bypass for congenital mitral stenosis. Surg 35:667–669, 1983.

27. Levine RA, Stathogiannis E, Newell JB, et al: Reconsideration of echocardiographic standards for mitral valve prolapse: lack of association between leaflet displacement isolated to the apical four chamber view and independent echocardiographic evidence of abnormality. J Am Coll Cardiol 11:1010–1019, 1988.

28. Levine RA, Weyman AE: Mitral valve prolapse: a disease in search of, or created by, its definition. Echocardiography 1:3–14, 1984.

29. Levy D, Savage D: Prevalence of mitral valve prolapse. Am Heart J 113:1281–1290, 1987.

30. Liberthson RR, Boucher CA, Fallon JT, et al: Severe mitral regurgitation: a common occurrence in the aging patient with secundum atrial septal defect. Clin Cardiol 4:229–232, 1981.

31. Lock JE, Khalilullah M, Shrivastava S, et al: Percutaneous catheter commissurotomy in rheumatic mitral stenosis. N Engl J Med 313:1515–1518, 1985.

32. Marin-Garcia J, Tandon R, Lucas RV, et al: Cor triatriatum: study of 20 cases. Am J Cardiol 35:59–66, 1975.

33. Mazzera E, Corno A, Di Donato R, et al: Surgical bypass of the systemic atrioventricular valve in children by means of a valved conduit. J Thorac Cardiovasc Surg 96:321–325, 1988.

34. Midgley FM, Perry LW, Potter BM: Conduit bypass of mitral valve: a palliative approach to congenital mitral stenosis. Am J Cardiol 56:493–494, 1985.

35. Nakano H, Ueda K, Saito A: Acute hemodynamic effects of nitroprusside in children with isolated mitral regurgitation. Am J Cardiol 56:351–355, 1985.

36. Nishimura RA, McGoon MD, Shub C, et al: Echocardiographic documented mitral-valve prolapse: long-term follow up of 237 patients. N Engl J Med 313:1305–1309, 1985.

37. Oglietti J, Cooley DA, Izquierdo JP, et al: Cor triatriatum: operative results in 25 patients. Ann Thorac Surg 35:415–420, 1983.

38. Okita Y, Shigehito M, Kusuhara K, et al: Early and late results of reconstructive operation for congenital mitral regurgitation in pediatric age group. J Thorac Cardiovasc Surg 96:294–298, 1988.

39. Pacifico AP, Mandke NV, McGrath LB, et al: Repair of congenital pulmonary venous stenosis with living autologous atrial tissue. J Thorac Cardiovasc Surg 89:604–609, 1985.

40. Pass HI, Sade RM, Crawford FA, et al: Cardiac valve prostheses in children without anticoagulation. J Thorac Cardiovasc Surg 87:832–835, 1984.

41. Perloff JK, Child JS, Edwards JE: New guidelines for the clinical diagnosis of mitral valve prolapse. Am J Cardiol 57:1124–1129, 1986.

42. Richardson JV, Doty DB, Sievers RD, et al: Cor triatriatum (subdivided left atrium). J Thorac Cardiovasc Surg 81:232–238, 1981.

43. Ruckmann RN, Van Praagh R: Anatomic types of congenital mitral stenosis: report of 49 autopsy cases with consideration of diagnostic and surgical implications. Am J Cardiol 42:592–601, 1978.

44. Savage DD, Garrison RJ, Devereux RB, et al: Mitral valve prolapse in the general population, epidemiologic features: the Framingham study. Am Heart J 106:571–575, 1983.

45. Schaff HV, Danielson GK, DiDonato RM, et al: Late results after Starr-Edwards valve replacement in children. J Thorac Cardiovasc Surg 88:583–589, 1984.

46. Schaffer MS, Clarke DR, Campbell DN, et al: The St. Jude Medical cardiac valve in infants and children: role of anticoagulant therapy. J Am Coll Cardiol 9:235–239, 1987.

47. Schreiber TL, Feigenbaum H, Weyman AE: Effect of atrial septal defect repair on left ventricular geometry and degree of mitral valve prolapse. Circulation 61:888–896, 1980.

48. Shaffer EM, Rocchini AP, Dick M, et al: Transseptal left heart catheterization as an aid in the diagnosis of cor triatriatum. Pediatr Cardiol 8:123–125, 1987.

49. Shone JD, Sellers RD, Anderson RC, et al: The developmental complex of "parachute mitral valve," supravalvar ring of the left atrium, subaortic stenosis and coarctation of the aorta. Am J Cardiol 11:714–725, 1963.

50. Spencer FC, Colvin SB, Culliford AT, et al: Experiences with the Carpentier techniques of mitral valve reconstruction in 103 patients (1980–1985). J Thorac Cardiovasc Surg 90:341–350, 1985.

51. Spevak PJ, Freed MD, Castaneda AR, et al: Valve replacement in children less than 5 years of age. J Am Coll Cardiol 8:901–908, 1986.

52. Stellin G, Bortolotti U, Mazzucco A, et al: Repair of congenitally malformed mitral valve in children. J Thorac Cardiovasc Surg 95:480–485, 1988.

53. Sullivan ID, Robinson PJ, de Leval M, et al: Membranous supravalvular mitral stenosis: a treatable form of congenital heart disease. J Am Coll Cardiol 8:159–164, 1986.

54. Tomaru T, Uchida Y, Mohri N, et al: Post-inflammatory mitral and aortic valve prolapse: a clinical and pathological study. Circulation 76:68–76, 1987.

55. Warth DC, King ME, Cohen JM, et al: Prevalence of mitral valve prolapse in normal children. J Am Coll Cardiol 5:1173–1177, 1985.

Chapter 39

HYPOPLASTIC LEFT HEART SYNDROME, MITRAL ATRESIA, AND AORTIC ATRESIA

Peter Lang, M.D., and Donald C. Fyler, M.D.

HYPOPLASTIC LEFT HEART SYNDROME

Definition

The term **hypoplastic left heart syndrome** describes a diminutive left ventricle with underdevelopment of the mitral and aortic valves.[24] Because of its small size, the left ventricle is incapable of supporting the systemic circulation.

Some patients have mitral or aortic stenosis, or both, but most have aortic or mitral atresia, or both. A small number of patients with mitral atresia and, rarely, some with aortic atresia have a nearly normal-sized left ventricle. These cases are not properly examples of the hypoplastic left heart syndrome. Similarly, cases of mitral atresia with a double-outlet right ventricle are not examples of the hypoplastic left heart syndrome, nor are those rare instances of mitral atresia with inverse ventricles.

Prevalence

The reported prevalence of hypoplastic left heart syndrome varies between 0.05 and 0.25 per 1,000 live births (see ch. 18). It is the 13th most common defect in the Boston Children's Hospital series, accounting for 1.5% of patients of all ages with heart disease (see ch. 18).

Anatomy

The left ventricle is small, often tiny (Fig. 1). Usually the aortic valve is atretic and hypoplastic, although some babies have severe stenosis. Similarly, the mitral valve may be hypoplastic, severely stenotic, or atretic. The ascending aorta is hypoplastic; above an atretic aortic valve, the diameter of the aorta may be as little as 2 mm, very small but sufficient to supply adequate coronary circulation in a retrograde fashion. Untreated infants show no coarctation of the aorta at autopsy, but coarctation is a common problem among surgically managed survivors, suggesting that the tendency

to develop coarctation is inherent in this anomaly.[16,34] The left atrium is small, reflecting the limited blood flow *in utero*. The atrial septum is thickened; the foramen ovale may be small and, occasionally, may be closed. A patent ductus arteriosus is required for survival.

Recently, anomalies of the brain have been reported to be associated with the hypoplastic left heart syndrome.[13]

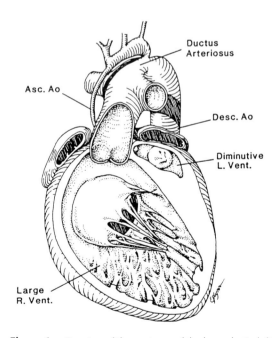

Figure 1. Drawing of the anatomy of the hypoplastic left heart syndrome. Note the tiny ascending aorta that supplies the coronary circulation in a retrograde direction. No blood passes through the diminutive left ventricle. The left atrium empties through an incompetent foramen ovale into the right atrium, where all systemic and pulmonary venous blood becomes mixed. The ductus arteriosus supplies the entire circulation to the body and the lungs.

Physiology

Overview. With an atretic aortic valve, survival beyond birth is dependent on persistent patency of the ductus arteriosus to maintain systemic circulation. There have been occasional reports of "long-term" survival of children with hypoplastic left heart syndrome because of prolonged patency of the ductus arteriosus. The oldest child reported to date survived for 7 years.[10]

Of necessity, the right ventricle supplies both the pulmonary and the systemic circulations via the ductus arteriosus, the coronary arteries and brachiocephalic vessels being supplied in retrograde fashion. The relative flow to the pulmonary and systemic circuits depends on the relative resistances of the two vascular beds. One of the major influences on total pulmonary resistance is the size of the interatrial orifice. A restrictive atrial defect tends to raise left atrial pressure and pulmonary resistance, limiting pulmonary blood flow, whereas a nonrestrictive opening does not.

There is a direct relationship between the amount of pulmonary blood flow and the systemic arterial oxygen saturation. The greater the pulmonary blood flow, the greater the quantity of oxygenated pulmonary venous blood that will return to the heart and mix with the systemic venous return (Fig. 2).

It is interesting to speculate that patients with completely unrestricted pulmonary blood flow are likely to succumb to severe congestive heart failure secondary to right ventricular volume overload, whereas those individuals with some resistance to pulmonary blood flow may survive. Nonetheless, life for more than a few weeks is precluded.

Transitional Circulation. In the hypoplastic left heart syndrome, as in most forms of congenital heart disease, the intrauterine circulation is adequate to meet the needs of the developing fetus. It is noteworthy that this most lethal congenital heart defect supports normal intrauterine growth.

In utero, all circulation, with the exception of the small amount of pulmonary venous return, passes through the right side of the heart. Streams of superior and inferior vena caval blood return to the right atrium and join the pulmonary venous return (5–10% of the cardiac output). The complete admixture of all venous return (that from the placenta as well as the fetus) results in blood flow with identical oxygen saturation to all parts of the fetus. The right atrial return then crosses the tricuspid valve to the right ventricle. The lack of a left ventricular contribution to cardiac output results in a modest right ventricular volume overload.

At this point in the circulation, certain physiologic questions emerge, even *in utero*. The relative flow to the pulmonary or systemic circulation is largely dependent on the relative resistance of the pulmonary and systemic vascular beds. Of equal

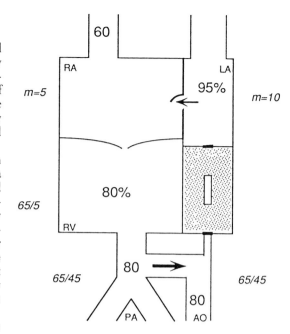

Figure 2. Diagram showing "ideal" preoperative physiology. Low systemic vascular resistance and high pulmonary vascular resistance result in a Q_p/Q_s of approximately 1.

importance is the status of the pulmonary venous return. There is growing evidence that the development of the interatrial septum is abnormal[35] (and even of primary etiologic significance) in the hypoplastic left heart syndrome. In the face of mitral valve atresia, or even severe mitral valve stenosis, an obstructive interatrial septum can result in left atrial hypertension. Even though pulmonary blood flow is low *in utero*, altered intrauterine pulmonary blood flow and pressure might be the best explanation for the abnormal muscularization of the pulmonary veins in these patients. Similarly, the abnormal atrial septal thickness may be caused by left atrial hypertension *in utero*.

There is less speculation about the circulation beyond the ductus arteriosus. It is common to see a posterior aortic ridge of tissue opposite the site of the ductus; systemic blood flow bifurcates at this point. In cases of aortic valve atresia, in which the sole source of systemic blood flow is from the ductus arteriosus, the aortic arch becomes progressively smaller between the ductus and the coronary arteries. Sometimes the origin of the left subclavian artery is involved with ductal tissue and it may become stenotic with time. The ascending aorta, carrying retrograde flow, is an end artery (a common coronary artery) and is frequently 2 mm or less in diameter. This small size is appropriate for the coronary flow required by the newborn heart. However, it must be remembered that coronary blood flow is dependent upon a long unobstructed path from the right ventricle to the ascending aorta via the ductus arteriosus. Shortly after birth, coronary flow, as well as cerebral flow, can be compromised, because the aortic isthmus may include ductal tissue that can constrict and obstruct the aorta.

At birth, when the ductus arteriosus is widely patent and the pulmonary arteriolar resistance is relatively high, a brief "honeymoon" begins. The widely patent ductus arteriosus does not restrict systemic blood flow at a "normal" right ventricular systolic pressure. In the absence of ductal constriction, there is no narrowing of the aortic arch, assuring good coronary and renal perfusion.

A modestly restrictive foramen ovale limits pulmonary blood flow to some extent. More important, in newborns the elevation in pulmonary arteriolar resistance keeps pulmonary blood flow at manageable levels. The moderate limitation in pulmonary blood flow caused by the relatively high resistance is not enough to produce a dangerously low systemic arterial oxygen saturation (Fig. 2).

Unfortunately, this "ideal" state of physiologic palliation is short lived. Although infants diagnosed *in utero* by 2-D echocardiography are seen in this state, the majority of children with the hypoplastic left heart syndrome pass through this "honeymoon" period without recognition. They behave normally and, unless their "duskiness" is questioned, are often thought to be well.

Two normal physiologic events conspire to bring children with a hypoplastic left heart to medical attention: the ductus arteriosus begins to close and pulmonary vascular resistance decreases. Partial closure of the ductus arteriosus has several profound effects. The first, and most obvious, is the alteration in the relative resistances of blood flow to the systemic and pulmonary circulations. The effect on the systemic circuit can be either subtle or dramatic. A decrease in systemic output in a newborn has many manifestations. The child's color may be "poor" despite a rise in the systemic oxygen saturation (see below); peripheral pulses are weak with a narrow pulse pressure; peripheral perfusion can deteriorate; and the child may become lethargic. Concomitant with these changes is an absolute and relative increase in pulmonary blood flow. The major manifestation of this change is tachypnea, with the inevitable inability to breathe and suck at the same time. The "force feeding" of the pulmonary circulation by the closure of the ductus arteriosus is abetted by the normal fall in pulmonary resistance. The relaxation of the pulmonary bed, which may be seen even in the first day of life,[15] may be tempered by the development of acidosis secondary to poor cardiac output.

More often than not, the end result of progressive ductal closure and falling pulmonary vascular resistance is profound cardiogenic shock. The decreased systemic blood flow is accompanied by poor coronary perfusion. Thus, the right ventricle has an increased pressure load (secondary to ductal constriction), an increased volume load (secondary to increased pulmonary blood flow), and, because of poor coronary flow, has less wherewithal to do the work. Right ventricular dysfunction and dilatation with tricuspid regurgitation only exacerbate the volume overload. Finally, the increased pulmonary blood flow, with obstructed outflow from the left atrium, increases pulmonary venous pressure, contributing to the difficulty in breathing. It is no surprise that children with the hypoplastic left heart syndrome often arrive gasping for breath, in a profound low output state, acidotic, and in renal failure (Fig. 3).

Before the introduction of prostaglandins E, a child in profound cardiogenic shock secondary to hypoplastic left heart syndrome died quickly, often before surgical intervention could be organized. Although some children did survive to undergo palliative surgery, they were a select few whose systemic circulation was maintained by persistent patency of the ductus arteriosus. With the use of prostaglandins E, the ductus arteriosus almost invariably reopens. Once an unobstructed pathway from the right ventricle to the aortic arch has been secured, support for the right ventricle is needed. Usually, the ventricle has suffered from a period of relative ischemia secondary to poor coronary

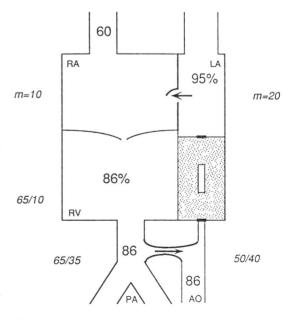

Figure 3. Diagram showing "closing ductus" physiology. There is decreased systemic blood flow, poor coronary perfusion, increased pulmonary blood flow, and the Q_p/Q_s is approximately 3. There is an increase in right ventricular volume overloading, right ventricular end-diastolic pressure, and left atrial pressure. There is right ventricular dysfunction.

perfusion; indeed, right ventricular infarctions have been seen occasionally. In addition, the ventricle has had both a pressure and a volume overload and has probably been deprived of adequate metabolic substrate because of hypoglycemia and hypocalcemia. Renal failure may result in an additional fluid overload and hyperkalemia. Finally, hepatic insufficiency, a frequent finding in the setting of low systemic output, may exacerbate the problems of hypoglycemia and acidosis. Inotropic support of the right ventricle must be given gingerly so that whatever metabolic aberrations are present do not contribute to toxic drug reactions.

The physiologic state following resuscitation is never quite as "ideal" as that seen shortly after birth (Fig. 4). The relative resistance of the pulmonary and systemic circuits will have changed in the days following birth and that change may have been influenced by the infusion of prostaglandins E. The overall pulmonary-to-systemic flow ratio is likely to be at least 2, with resulting systemic arterial oxygen saturation in the range of 85%. Consequently, the right ventricle is volume loaded to the extent that it is pumping three times the normal volume in order to maintain an adequate systemic cardiac output. An increase in right ventricular end-diastolic pressure is a usual finding. The excessive pulmonary blood flow results once again in a volume load to the left atrium. The obstruction to left atrial outflow results in pulmonary venous hypertension.

All of this is relatively acceptable. Unfortu-

nately, the transitional circulation is not stable. With the passage of hours and with, ironically, metabolic improvement, there is a continued decrease in pulmonary vascular resistance. Because the relative resistance of the pulmonary and systemic circulations determines the relative flows to the two circuits, when the maximum volume capacity of the right ventricle is reached (perhaps between four and five times normal, a Qp/Qs of 4), there is a decrease in systemic output. This time, the low output state is not a function of ductal obstruction, but simply a product of the inability of the right ventricle to meet the ever increasing volume demand caused by a decreasing pulmonary vascular resistance. The result of all of this is a continuation of the earlier evolution of the transitional circulatory changes. There is severe right ventricular volume overloading, the right ventricular end-diastolic pressure rises, and there may be right ventricular dilatation with tricuspid regurgitation, making matters worse. Once again, the poor systolic perfusion may result in renal failure and acidosis. Left atrial hypertension will impair gas exchange and, in all probability, necessitate intubation and assisted ventilation (Fig. 5).

Clinical Manifestations

The infant, usually male (67%), seems normal at birth. The incidence of prematurity and associated

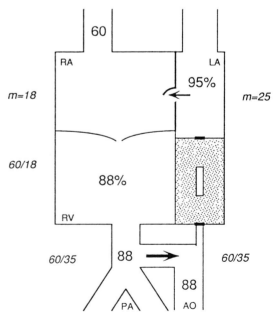

Figure 5. Diagram of the "low pulmonary resistance" physiology. The Q_p/Q_s is approximately 4. There is severe right ventricular volume overloading (approximately 5 × normal), an increase in right ventricular diastolic pressure, an increase in left atrial pressure, poor systemic perfusion, low urine output, acidosis, poor right ventricular performance, right ventricular dilatation, and tricuspid regurgitation.

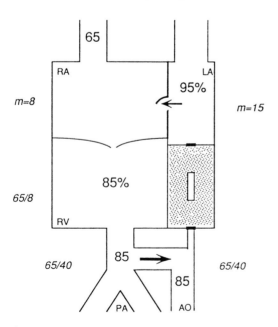

Figure 4. Diagram showing "acceptable" physiology. The Q_p/Q_s is approximately 2. There is mild right ventricular volume overloading (approximately 3 × normal), a mild increase in right ventricular end-diastolic pressure, and a mild increase in left atrial pressure.

extracardiac anomalies is low. No murmur is heard. Within hours, or a day or so, the nursery nurse may notice that the baby, at times, has poor color, is pale, or somehow just "doesn't seem right." These observations are an exception rather than the rule. Most often, without warning, the infant suffers circulatory collapse, becoming ashen, cyanotic, gasping, and near death. There are no palpable pulses. The infant is resuscitated, infusion of prostaglandins E is begun, and the baby is transferred immediately to the nearest pediatric cardiac center.

Electrocardiography

While, statistically, electrocardiograms in infants with hypoplastic left heart syndrome tend to show less than the usual left ventricular voltages for a newborn infant, this feature is not helpful, because many normal newborns also have this pattern. Suffice it to say that the electrocardiogram of an infant with hypoplastic left heart syndrome is rarely interpreted as showing left ventricular hypertrophy and usually shows a little more right ventricular hypertrophy than normal.

Chest X-ray

There is little about the chest x-ray that is specific. The size of the heart and the amount of pul-

monary vasculature are variable; the heart may be very large and the pulmonary vasculature increased.

Echocardiography

The hypoplastic left heart syndrome is recognized in detail at echocardiography. The abnormal mitral and aortic valves, the diminutive left ventricle, and the hypoplastic ascending aorta, as well as the flow of blood from the left atrium to the right, are readily identified and confirm the diagnosis. The coronary arteries are supplied from a tiny ascending aorta, often only a few millimeters in diameter. Doppler imaging may reveal retrograde flow in the ascending aorta. The left atrium is small and the atrial septum bulges toward the right. An absent or hypoplastic mitral valve is recognized and the diminutive left ventricle is often visualized (Fig. 6A). The ductus arteriosus is large and carries blood from the pulmonary artery to the aorta (Fig. 6B).

The atretic or hypoplastic mitral valve and the hypoplastic left ventricle can be seen in subxiphoid or apical views. Doppler examination of the mitral valve is useful to determine if it is atretic. A potential pitfall in evaluating left ventricular size results from the tendency for the left ventricle long-

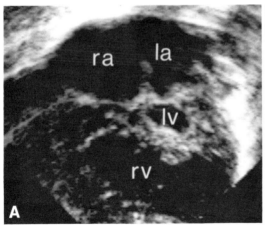
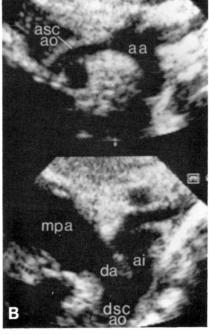

Figure 6. Echocardiogram in patients with the hypoplastic left heart syndrome. **A**, Apical view showing the tiny left ventricular cavity (lv). rv, right ventricle; ra, right atrium; la, left atrium. **B**, Two suprasternal notch views showing the hypoplastic ascending aorta (asc ao), the pulmonary artery (mpa), and the ductus arteriosus (da). ai, aortic isthmus; aa, aortic arch.

axis dimension to be reduced before the short-axis dimension. If the left ventricle is evaluated using either two-dimensional or M-mode echocardiography in short-axis projection only, the severity of hypoplasia can be underestimated.

Parasternal and suprasternal views are best for imaging the hypoplastic ascending aorta and aortic arch. The point of juncture of the ductus arteriosus and the arch is often narrow, with a discrete coarctation being present.

The atrial septum can be imaged using subxiphoid views. Tricuspid valve function should be evaluated with Doppler technique from apical and parasternal views, in that tricuspid regurgitation occurs in a significant proportion of patients. Right ventricular function can be evaluated using subxiphoid views.

Cardiac Catheterization

Cardiac catheterization may not be required in the newborn period, but is required for management later. Virtually all patients come to cardiac catheterization by the age of 6 months and again before a Fontan procedure.

Management

Medical Treatment

Most infants arrive at the cardiac center intubated and receiving prostaglandins E. An attempt must be made to "turn back the clock" and return to the "acceptable" level of pulmonary and systemic blood flow that existed prior to the patient's collapse. Factors that tend to decrease pulmonary vascular resistance (within limits) are needed. The most direct and controllable means of meeting this end is with "controlled hypoventilation." The FiO_2 should be reduced to as close to 0.21 as possible to maintain an arterial pO_2 of 30 torr. The pCO_2 should be allowed to rise to 40 torr in an attempt to maintain a pH of 7.35–7.40. Positive end-expiratory pressure may also be "beneficial" in increasing total pulmonary resistance. Because the intrinsic respiratory drive leads to a lower than desired pCO_2, heavy sedation is often required.

The desired result is reduction of the Qp/Qs from 4 to 2 and reduction of the right ventricular volume load from 5 to 3 times normal. This benefit far exceeds the potential benefit of inotropic medications and, because there are no selective pulmonary vasodilator agents, pharmacologic manipulation of the resistance ratio is unrewarding.

A small subgroup of patients require separate consideration. Rarely, the interatrial communication can be so obstructive that left atrial hypertension limits pulmonary blood flow to levels that do not permit adequate oxygenation for prolonged survival. In this instance, the pO_2 is below 20 torr despite the reverse of the manipulations described above (i.e., high FiO_2, hyperventilation to the

point of hypocarbia, and alkalosis). In this setting, rapid relief of the pulmonary venous obstruction is the only alternative.

Surgical Treatment

Based on the initial attempts to manage the hypoplastic left heart syndrome, the following goals for successful palliation were established. **First** is the need to establish a permanent unobstructed communication between the right ventricle and the aorta with preservation of right ventricular function. **Second** is the necessity of limiting pulmonary blood flow with preservation of pulmonary artery architecture. The **third** goal is to relieve pulmonary venous obstruction.

The surgical procedure developed by Norwood most nearly satisfies the goals for initial palliation and subsequent repair of children with hypoplastic left heart syndrome (Fig. 7).[26] Prosthetic material is avoided in both the systemic and pulmonary circulations, allowing for maximal potential growth. The prosthetic aortopulmonary shunt placed at the time of initial palliation is, of course, removed at the time of reparative surgery. The first-stage operation consists of transection of the distal main pulmonary artery. The aorta, from the takeoff of the left subclavian artery to the ascending aorta, is incised, and a direct anastomosis is established between the proximal main pulmonary artery and the ascending aorta and aortic arch. To provide adequate pulmonary flow, a 4-mm Gore-

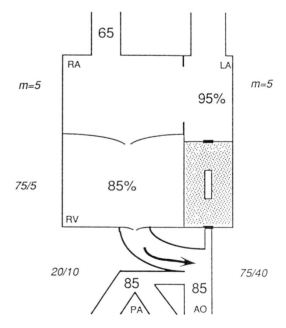

Figure 7. Diagram showing "ideal" postoperative physiology. Widely patent pathway from the right ventricle to the aorta, limitation of pulmonary blood flow without distortion to the pulmonary arteries, unrestricted pulmonary venous return, normal-sized right ventricle, and normal tricuspid valve.

tex shunt is established between the new ascending aorta (formerly the proximal main pulmonary artery) and the distal main pulmonary artery. This stage of the operation is completed by ligating the ductus arteriosus and opening the atrial septum, unless there is an atrial septal defect.

Complications. There are numerous problems following surgery. Some relate primarily to the underlying anatomic defect, some to the physiologic derangements associated with the circulatory collapse that first signaled the presence of heart disease, and some to the surgery.

Atrial Septum. The first level of concern following palliative surgery is the atrial septum (Fig. 8). This structure is thicker and more leftward in orientation than it is in normal individuals. It is not readily amenable to balloon septostomy. In addition, the small cavity size of the left atrium has made the use of blade atrial septostomy unappealing. Therefore, surgical septectomy has become an integral part of the initial palliative surgery. Even with purported generous excision of atrial septal tissue, obstruction to flow has developed. As opposed to initial palliation, subsequent management with blade atrial septostomy can be achieved.[28] Because pulmonary venous hypertension can adversely affect the development of the pulmonary vascular bed, a restrictive atrial septal defect should be treated aggressively.

Postoperative development of obstruction to flow across the interatrial septum may be subtle.

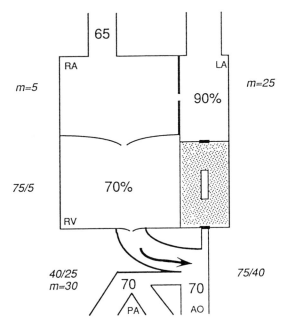

Figure 8. Diagram showing "restrictive atrial septal defect" physiology. The Q_p/Q_s is approximately 1. There is pulmonary artery hypertension due to high left atrial pressure and decreased oxygen saturation caused by low Q_p/Q_s and pulmonary venous desaturation.

Increasing cyanosis before the time when the child should be "outgrowing" the systemic-to-pulmonary shunt might be the first indication that there is a problem. The intensity of the shunt murmur may decrease as pulmonary artery pressure increases subsequent to pulmonary venous hypertension. Luckily, two-dimensional echocardiography usually provides a definitive diagnosis of the problem.

Stenosis of the Pulmonary Veins. Progressive stenosis of the pulmonary veins may be associated with extreme left atrial hypoplasia. Whether this occurs because of ongoing development of the left heart structures, progressive mediastinal fibrosis, or atherogenic difficulties based on the initial surgery remains unclear.

Tricuspid Regurgitation. The next level of concern following palliative surgery is the status of the tricuspid valve. As mentioned earlier, the right ventricle carries an excess volume and may have been subjected to metabolic and ischemic injury prior to palliation. Thus, some degree of tricuspid regurgitation may be expected. The effect of tricuspid regurgitation on early and late mortality is not clear.[7,14] How much tricuspid regurgitation can occur before it is necessary to recommend annuloplasty or valve replacement, or simply to refer these children for allotransplantation, is under discussion.

Right Ventricular Myocardial Problems. The right ventricle may fare poorly regardless of the status of the tricuspid valve. Right ventricular dysfunction secondary to a period of ischemia, acidosis, or severe volume loading may preclude normal (or even adequate) functional status. Ventriculocoronary connections may play a role in poor right ventricular function in the hypoplastic left heart syndrome.[17,18,27,31] Thick-walled coronary arteries and myocardial fibrillar disarray have been demonstrated in a subset of these patients, particularly those with a patent left ventricular inflow and obstructed left ventricular outflow. If these were to have a major effect on survival following palliative surgery, one would think that overall survival would be significantly better for patients with mitral atresia than for those with mitral stenosis. A study comparing those two groups failed to demonstrate a significant difference. Right ventricular dysfunction after palliative surgery has not been a prominent finding.[7,16]

Coarctation of the Reconstructed Aorta. Until patients began to survive with palliative surgery, it was not realized that coarctation of the aorta is a common complication of the hypoplastic left heart syndrome (Fig. 9).[16,34] How much of this is caused by constricting ductal tissue and how much is the result of surgical manipulation is not clear. After testing a variety of ways to avoid this problem, our current practice at the Boston Children's Hospital is to bypass the area of potential coarctation with

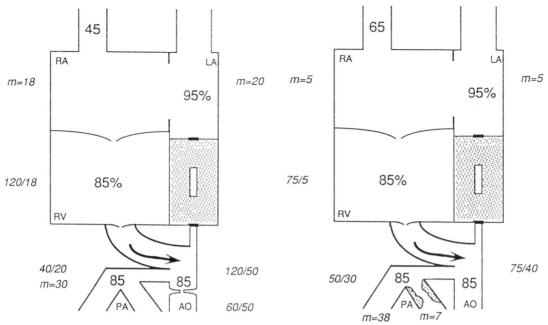

Figure 9. Diagram showing "coarctation" physiology. The Q_p/Q_s is approximately 4. There is increased right ventricular end-diastolic pressure because of decreased right ventricular function and tricuspid regurgitation, pulmonary artery hypertension due to increased pulmonary flow, and increased left atrial pressure.

Figure 10. Diagram showing "distorted pulmonary artery" physiology. The Q_p/Q_s is approximately 2. There is right pulmonary artery hypertension and left pulmonary artery hypotension because of iatrogenic distortion.

a homograft at the time of initial palliation.[15] If coarctation develops, the resulting increase in right ventricular pressure and the increased pulmonary blood flow will produce symptoms; the diminished femoral pulses will provide the diagnosis. Management with balloon dilatation has been successful.[23,32]

Pulmonary Vascular Disease. The pulmonary vascular bed must evolve normally if a successful Fontan operation is to be performed later. The excess of blood volume and pressure to which the pulmonary vasculature is exposed must be kept in mind. Pulmonary vascular disease may be as devastating as right ventricular dysfunction in terms of the subsequent suitability of a patient for a modified Fontan operation.

Peripheral Pulmonary Stenosis. If a later Fontan operation is to be successful, undistorted pulmonary arteries are required (Fig. 10). Three features conspire to deform the pulmonary arteries:

1. If the surgeon uses a long segment of the main pulmonary artery in reconstructing the ascending aorta, central pulmonary artery deformity may be the result.[1,14,29]

2. Constricting ductal tissue may produce obstruction at the point of insertion of the ductus into the origin of the left pulmonary artery. Severe narrowing at the takeoff of the proximal left pulmonary artery may be seen.

3. The point of insertion of the arterial-pulmo-

nary shunt may cause distortion of the pulmonary artery.

Arterial-Pulmonary Shunts. A modified right Blalock-Taussig shunt is the preferred method to supply pulmonary blood flow.[15] Although this provides a more favorable regulation of overall pulmonary blood flow, the distribution to right and left lungs is not symmetrical. The usual 2:1 (ipsilateral:contralateral) distribution of blood flow that occurs following a Blalock-Taussig shunt is exaggerated by whatever degree of proximal left pulmonary artery obstruction is present. This combination of factors can lead to potential right pulmonary artery hypertension and left pulmonary artery hypoplasia. Once again, the adverse effects on a subsequent Fontan operation are apparent.

The Systemic Pulmonary Valve. Concern about the ability of the pulmonary valve to manage the systemic circulation seems to be unwarranted. There have been no recognizable problems.[9]

Management After Palliation

The initial palliation must allow the baby to survive surgery (Exhibit 1), to accommodate to the changes in pulmonary arteriolar resistance that occur during the first weeks of life, and to accommodate to the doubling or tripling of body size. Indeed, cardiopulmonary bypass (with or without a period of circulatory arrest), general anesthesia, and neuromuscular blockade, followed by a period of assisted ventilation, all have profound effects on

Exhibit 1

Boston Children's Hospital Experience 1973–1987

Hypoplastic Left Heart Syndrome

There were 240 patients diagnosed as having the hypoplastic left heart syndrome. Of these, 158 underwent cardiac surgery, mostly in the past 10 years. The initial survival rate improved reaching 65% by 1986. As of 1987, 23 Fontan or variations of Fontan procedures had been undertaken, with 12 survivors.

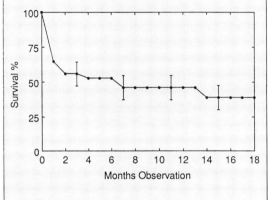

Note the improvement in initial and 18-month survival in recent years.

the pulmonary vasculature. It is not unusual to have an anatomically large shunt appear to be physiologically small immediately following cardiopulmonary bypass. Within hours there may be a profound lowering of the pulmonary arteriolar resistance and the shunt that was "too small" an hour ago has suddenly become "too large." The same modalities of treatment that were employed before surgery are equally important immediately following surgery. Administration of high inspired oxygen, together with hyperventilation and alkalosis, may be necessary in the first hour after surgery, rapidly followed by a decrease in FiO_2 to room air, with controlled hypoventilation for the remainder of the period of assisted ventilation. The right ventricle may require some degree of inotropic support in the days following surgery. Virtually all children require a cardiotonic regimen of digoxin and diuretics for the period during which the shunt is relatively large. If all goes well, it will take several months for the child to "grow into the shunt."

The status of the interatrial septum, right ventricular function, the aortic arch reconstruction, and the pulmonary artery architecture should be monitored using oximetry and two-dimensional echocardiography. Cardiac catheterization should be carried out some time before the child is 6 months of age. Assuming an adequate atrial septectomy, good right ventricular and tricuspid valve function, an unobstructed pathway from the right ventricle around the aortic arch, and normal

growth of the pulmonary arterial bed with a normal pulmonary arteriolar resistance, there is no need for further intervention before the Fontan operation.

However, any and all of the monitored areas may be amiss. Treatment of an obstructed interatrial septum or an aortic arch anomaly is the most straightforward. Therapeutic cardiac catheterizations are the preferable forms of treatment, but, if unsuccessful, surgery may be required. Problems with the pulmonary arteries or the pulmonary arteriolar bed are more complicated. Stenosis of the proximal left pulmonary artery may be a difficult problem. When all pulmonary blood flow is dependent on a right Blalock-Taussig shunt, growth of the left pulmonary artery may be poor. In addition, disadvantageous collateral blood vessels develop in some patients. Recently, a bidirectional Glenn shunt has been used to correct and compensate for distortions in pulmonary artery architecture (see ch. 54). Such an approach has the additional advantage of supplying more effective pulmonary blood flow without any additional load on the right ventricle.

Primary problems of right ventricular function and tricuspid valve abnormalities pose major unanswered questions. Severe tricuspid regurgitation associated with preserved right ventricular function is probably best handled directly. Tricuspid valve annuloplasty or even valve replacement has been performed, although complete heart block is a risk. When tricuspid valve dysfunction is secondary to right ventricular volume overload, an alternative approach has been to reduce the load on the right ventricle. This can also be accomplished, in appropriate patients, with a bidirectional Glenn shunt.

Right ventricular dysfunction as an isolated problem is a more thorny dilemma. If one believes that the right ventricle is unlikely to improve, once the amount it must pump is reduced by a Fontan operation, there are no alternatives short of allotransplantation.

Fontan Operation

Despite the initial success of the Fontan operation following palliative surgery for the hypoplastic left heart syndrome,[26] subsequent procedures met with a number of problems.[11,16] In part, the poor initial results were a function of poor patient selection (Exhibit 1). Many of the problems which adversely affect the outcome of Fontan operations are the result of the near lethal preoperative physiology and the complicated surgical manipulations required for survival. Nowadays, with an eventual Fontan operation in mind, every effort is made to avoid right ventricular injury, to assist the normal evolution of the pulmonary vasculature, and to avoid distortion of the pulmonary arteries. Various modifications of the Fontan operation, classical Glenn procedures, and bidirectional Glenn procedures are helpful. Recent outcomes are much improved.[25]

Cardiac Transplantation

Cardiac transplantation is an alternative form of therapy for infants born with the hypoplastic left heart syndrome.[3-6,19] The technical feasibility of such a procedure has never been seriously questioned. Issues are the availability of donors[19] and the problems of rejection. The results of allotransplantation in newborns with the hypoplastic left heart syndrome remain astonishingly good.[8] If issues of donor availability are resolved, and if the exceptionally low incidence of rejection reactions is confirmed over a longer period of observation, cardiac transplantation will gain favor as an alternative form of treatment.

Ethical Issues

The management of babies with the hypoplastic left heart syndrome, whether by palliation leading to a Fontan procedure or by transplantation, has provoked vigorous ethical discussion. The scientific facts are:

1. Untreated hypoplastic left heart syndrome is rapidly and virtually 100% fatal.

2. Surgical treatment (primary palliation followed by secondary palliation using a Fontan procedure) has a grim but improving mortality and an unknown long-range outcome.

3. The initial mortality for transplantation may be better, provided a donor heart is found, but the long-range outcome is equally unknown.

4. Both approaches have produced a few children who appear and act normal.

It is clear that not all physicians would recommend either surgical route and not all parents would choose to risk the grief and expense associated with either form of treatment. The present-day standard of practice does not require that either form of treatment be recommended by the cardiologist or that the parents should agree.

The only ethical question remaining concerns the adequacy of the information available to all concerned in such decisions. A responsible physician may recommend against either approach, but no responsible physician would withhold his or her opinion, or deny the information to anyone.

MITRAL ATRESIA WITH NORMAL AORTIC ROOT

Patients with mitral atresia and a normal aortic outflow[22] are not properly classified under the hypoplastic left heart syndrome; yet, by convention, this lesion complex appears in the hypoplastic left ventricle file of the Boston Children's Hospital.

Prevalence

In the period from January 1973 to December 1987 there were 44 children with mitral atresia and a normal aortic root seen at the Boston Children's Hospital. There were 19 with unspecified atrioventricular valve atresia and 23 with dextrocardia who were described as having mitral atresia.

Pathophysiology

Mitral atresia with a good-sized left ventricle is associated with a ventricular septal defect if the aorta arises from the left ventricle. Sometimes the tricuspid valve is straddling. There may be a double-outlet right ventricle, the left ventricle being a blind pouch, or there may be inverse ventricles, the physiology being that of tricuspid atresia. The great vessels may be transposed, the aorta arising from the right ventricle. A patent and incompetent foramen ovale is usually present, although egress from the left atrium may take other routes (i.e., via a sino-septal defect). Often the orifice of the foramen ovale is small enough to raise left atrial pressure and the atrial septum is thickened. At the Boston Children's Hospital, most of these patients are classified as having a double-outlet right ventricle, the aorta arising from the right ventricle. Others use different terminology.[33] Sometimes the aorta arises from the left ventricle, in which case the size of the ventricular defect may have important hemodynamic consequences. Roughly half of these patients have pulmonary stenosis and occasionally one sees a patient who has pulmonary valve atresia. Coarctation of the aorta was noted in about 15% of our patients (Exhibit 2). Others have reported similar experience.[25,30]

Whether mitral atresia results from an absence of the mitral valve or represents an imperforate valve[12] is important in understanding these abnormalities but, as yet, has little bearing on the ultimate outcome for these patients.

Clinical Manifestations

All of these patients are cyanotic, though among those with excessive pulmonary blood flow this may not be apparent at first. Tachypnea is common because left atrial pressures are often high, causing pulmonary edema, or there is excessive pulmonary blood flow. When there is limited pulmonary blood flow because of pulmonary stenosis or atresia, cyanosis may be the chief complaint. The majority are symptomatic in the first weeks of life with either tachypnea or cyanosis.

Electrocardiogram

In the majority of cases the electrocardiogram shows right ventricular hypertrophy.

Exhibit 2

**Boston Children's Hospital Experience
1973–1987**

Mitral Atresia

There were 44 patients considered to have mitral atresia with an adequate aortic outflow. Of these, 22 had pulmonary stenosis, 11 had pulmonary atresia, and 9 had coarctation of the aorta. Three had associated total anomalous pulmonary veins.

Twenty-five had banding procedures and 21 had shunting operations. Twenty had surgical atrial defect enlargement and 5 had attempts to enlarge the atrial opening with catheters. Fifteen have had a Fontan operation or one of its variants; 10 survived.

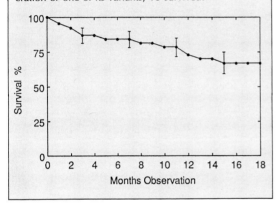

Chest X-ray

The heart size is variably enlarged, depending on the amount of pulmonary blood flow, and the pulmonary vasculature may be prominent because of excess flow or may be diminished because of pulmonary stenosis. In either case there may be evidence of pulmonary edema. Pulmonary edema is possible in the presence of pulmonary stenosis because the size of the foramen ovale determines left atrial pressure, and it may be very small even in the presence of normal or reduced amounts of pulmonary flow.

Echocardiography

The detailed anatomy can be documented by two-dimensional echocardiography using previously described techniques (see ch. 13).

Cardiac Catheterization

Most patients undergo cardiac catheterization because the physiologic data are critical to successful management. A firm sense of the amount of pulmonary blood flow and the degree of obstruction at the foramen ovale is required. Too often an arterial-pulmonary shunt produces more pulmonary flow than an obstructive foramen ovale can accommodate.

Management

With excessive pulmonary blood flow, pulmonary artery banding may be needed, or with diminished flow an arterial shunt may be helpful.[20] Enlargement of the atrial septal defect should be considered in all patients, particularly if a shunt procedure is being considered.[26] Unfortunately, balloon atrial septostomy is rarely successful in newborns, although an angioplasty balloon may suffice, and blade septostomy is difficult when the left atrium is small. Consequently, open atrial septectomy is often the only solution in the neonate. The goal is survival with anatomy and physiology that satisfy the requirements for a Fontan procedure at a later date, a goal not easily attained, but possible (Exhibit 2).

Course

Although a patient has been reported to survive untreated for 20 years,[21] there are too few survivors to give an indication of the long-range quality of life. At the Children's Hospital in Boston, about one-third of the patients survive to undergo a Fontan operation.

AORTIC ATRESIA WITH NORMAL LEFT VENTRICLE

Aortic atresia with right and left ventricles of functionally normal capacity is an extremely rare anomaly (5 in the Boston Children's Hospital experience, 1973–1987) that is sometimes correctable.[2]

REFERENCES

1. Alboliras ET, Chin AJ, Barber G, et al: Pulmonary artery configuration after palliative operations for hypoplastic left heart syndrome. J Thorac Cardiovasc Surg 97:878–885, 1989.
2. Austin EH, Jonas RA, Mayer JE, et al: Aortic atresia with normal left ventricle: single-stage repair in the neonate. J Thorac Cardiovasc Surg 97:392–395, 1989.
3. Bailey LL: Role of cardiac transplant in the neonate. J Heart Transplant 4:506–509, 1985.
4. Bailey LL, Assaad AN, Trim RF, et al: Orthotopic transplantation during early infancy as therapy for incurable congenital heart disease. Ann Surg 208:279–286, 1988.
5. Bailey L, Concepcion W, Shattuck H, et al: Method of heart transplantation for treatment of hypoplastic left heart syndrome. J Thorac Cardiovasc Surg 92:1–5, 1986.
6. Bailey LL, Nehlsen-Cannarella SL, Doroshow RW, et al: Cardiac allotransplantation in newborns as therapy for hypoplastic left heart syndrome. N Engl J Med 315:949–951, 1986.
7. Barber G, Helton JG, Aglira BA, et al: The significance of tricuspid regurgitation in hypoplastic left-heart syndrome. Am Heart J 116:1563–1567, 1988.
8. Boucek MM, Kanakriyeh MS, Mathis CM, et al: Cardiac transplantation in infancy: donors and recipients. J Pediatr 116:171–176, 1990.

9. Chin AJ, Barber G, Helton JG, et al: Fate of the pulmonic valve after proximal pulmonary artery-to-ascending aorta anastomosis for aortic outflow obstruction. Am J Cardiol 62:435–438, 1988.

10. Ehrlich M, Bierman FZ, Ellis K, et al: Hypoplastic left heart syndrome: report of a unique survivor. J Am Coll Cardiol 7:361–365, 1986.

11. Farrell PE, Chang AC, Murdison KA, et al: Outcome and assessment following modified Fontan repair for hypoplastic left heart syndrome (abstract). J Am Coll Cardiol 15:204A, 1990.

12. Gittenberger-de Groot AC, Wenink ACG: Mitral atresia: morphologic details. Br Heart J 51:252–258, 1984.

13. Glauser TA, Rorke LB, Weinberg PM, et al: Congenital brain anomalies associated with the hypoplastic left heart syndrome. Pediatrics 85:984–990, 1990.

14. Helton JG, Aglira BA, Chin AJ, et al: Analysis of potential anatomic and physiologic determinants of palliation surgery for hypoplastic left heart syndrome. Circulation 74(Suppl):I70–76, 1986.

15. Jonas RA, Lang P, Hansen D, et al: First-stage palliation of hypoplastic left heart syndrome. J Thorac Cardiovasc Surg 92:6–13, 1986.

16. Lang P, Norwood WI: Hemodynamic assessment after palliative surgery for hypoplastic left heart syndrome. Circulation 68:104–108, 1983.

17. Lloyd TR, Evans TC, Marvin WJ: Morphologic determinants of coronary blood flow in the hypoplastic left heart syndrome. Am Heart J 112:666–671, 1986.

18. Lloyd TR, Marvin WJ: Age at death in the hypoplastic left heart syndrome: multivariate analysis and importance of the coronary arteries. Am Heart J 117:1337–1343, 1989.

19. Mavroudis C, Willis W, Min D, et al: Orthotopic cardiac transplantation for the neonate: the dilemma of the anencephalic donor. J Thorac Cardiovasc Surg 97:389–391, 1989.

20. Mickell JJ, Mathews RA, Park SC, et al: Left sided atrioventricular valve atresia: clinical management. Circulation 61:123–127, 1980.

21. Mohan JC, Jain RK, Arora R: Mitral atresia with double outlet right ventricle in an asymptomatic adult. Int J Cardiol 27:117–119, 1990.

22. Moreno F, Quero M, Perez-Diaz L: Mitral atresia with normal aortic valve. Circulation 53:1004–1010, 1976.

23. Murphy JD, Sands BL, Norwood WI: Intraoperative balloon angioplasty in aortic coarctation in infants with hypoplastic left heart syndrome. Am J Cardiol 59:949–951, 1987.

24. Noonan JA, Nadas AS: The hypoplastic left heart syndrome: an analysis of 101 cases. Pediatr Clin North Am 5:1029–1056, 1959.

25. Norwood WI: Hypoplastic left heart syndrome: a review. Cardiol Clin 7:377–385, 1989.

26. Norwood WI, Lang P, Hansen DD: Physiologic repair of aortic atresia – hypoplastic left heart syndrome. New Engl J Med 308:23–26, 1983.

27. O'Connor WN, Cash JB, Cottrill CM: Ventriculo-coronary connections in hypoplastic left heart syndrome: autopsy microscopic study. Circulation 66:1078–1086, 1982.

28. Perry SB, Lang P, Keane JF, et al: Creation and maintenance of an adequate interatrial communication in left atrioventricular valve atresia or stenosis. Am J Cardiol 58:622–626, 1986.

29. Pigott JD, Murphy JD, Barber G, et al: Palliative reconstructive surgery for hypoplastic left heart syndrome. Ann Thorac Surg 45:122–128, 1988.

30. Rowe RD, Freedom RM, Mehrizi A, et al: The Neonate with Congenital Heart Disease. Philadelphia, W.B. Saunders, 1981, pp. 602–608.

31. Sauer U, Gittenberger-de Groot AC, Geishauser M, et al: Coronary arteries in the hypoplastic left heart syndrome: histopathologic and histometrical studies and implications for surgery. Circulation 80(Suppl I):I-168–I-176, 1989.

32. Saul JP, Keane JF, Fellow KE, et al: Balloon dilation angioplasty of post-operative aortic obstruction. Am J Cardiol 59:943–948, 1987.

33. Thiene G, Daliento L, Frescura C, et al: Atresia of the left atrial orifice: anatomical investigation in 62 cases. Br Heart J 45:393–401, 1981.

34. Von Rueden TJ, Knight L, Moller JH, et al: Coarctation of the aorta associated with aortic valvular atresia. Circulation 52:951–954, 1975.

35. Weinberg PM, Chin AJ, Murphy JD, et al: Postmortem echocardiography and tomographic anatomy of hypoplastic left heart syndrome after palliative surgery. Am J Cardiol 58:1228–1232, 1986.

Chapter 40

PULMONARY ATRESIA WITH INTACT VENTRICULAR SEPTUM

Donald C. Fyler, M.D.

DEFINITION

In this condition there is complete obstruction of right ventricular outflow, an intact ventricular septum, and variable hypoplasia of the right ventricle and tricuspid valve.

PREVALENCE

In the New England Program[10] pulmonary atresia with intact ventricular septum was the tenth most common defect encountered among sick cardiac infants (0.069–0.074 per 1000 live births), comprising 3% of the case material. Others (see Table 1, ch. 18) have reported similar findings. In the Boston Children's Hospital experience over the past 15 years, it was the 23rd most common lesion, totaling 84 patients (see Table 2, ch. 18). In The Hospital for Sick Children in Toronto, the incidence was found to be 2.5% among neonates[20] and 0.71% of all patients with congenital heart disease.[8]

EMBRYOLOGY

The large pulmonary arteries despite low pulmonary blood flow, the frequent observation of fused, but well-formed, valve leaflets, the absence of arterial collaterals to the pulmonary circulation, the variable size of the right ventricle, and the rarity of associated extracardiac anomalies, as well as the anatomic similarity to newborns with critical pulmonary valvar stenosis, all support the idea that pulmonary atresia with an intact ventricular septum is an acquired disease rather than an aberration of embryologic development. Comparison with patients who have pulmonary atresia and ventricular septal defect tends to support this attractive theory.[15]

ANATOMY

The pulmonary valve is atretic. The valve ring is usually small, rarely tiny; the valve leaflets, although fused, are often identifiable. The main pulmonary artery is present, usually somewhat smaller than normal, but only rarely is represented by a string-like connection as is seen in patients with pulmonary atresia and ventricular septal defect. The right ventricle and right ventricular outflow tract are variably small, varying from minuscule to near normal size. Right ventricular size has been related to survival; the larger the ventricle, the better survival. This concept has been refined by identifying three types of right ventricular hypoplasia.[3] The normal right ventricle is composed of an inlet portion, a trabecular portion and an infundibulum. Type 1 requires the presence of all three; in Type 2 the trabecular portion is absent; in Type 3 both the trabecular and infundibular areas are absent. As might be predicted, Types 1 and 2, usually having the greatest volume, are the most favorable. Although this classification is erudite, we have yet to be convinced that this concept contributes to treatment or survival.

The tricuspid valve is proportionately small and may be deformed. At times a diminutive tricuspid valve appears stenotic, sometimes like that in Ebstein's disease, and is often regurgitant, sometimes grossly incompetent.

Vascular structures (sinusoids) are seen between the right ventricle, the right ventricular myocardium, and the coronary arteries, particularly when the right ventricular pressure is high; these may represent the dominant source of blood flow to a coronary artery.[7,8] As many as 50% of patients (it is nearer to 30% in our experience) have sinusoids communicating with the coronary arteries.[4] There is some evidence that sinusoidal connections increase after birth.[17] At autopsy there is often histologic evidence of myocardial ischemia, which we at the Children's Hospital in Boston relate to myocardial sinusoids, but others[9] are not confident that sinusoids are the only cause of myocardial dysfunction. The poorly oxygenated blood supplied to the coronary artery may influence ventricular function and the coronary arteries supplied by sinusoids may have obstructive lesions, occasionally severe.[4] Coronary perfusion with poorly oxygenated blood from sinusoids and the intracoronary lesions explain the findings of myocardial ischemia and poor myocardial function, but what happens when surgery results in lower right ventricular pressure? Do the coronary-sinusoidal connections allow a coronary-to-right ventricular shunt, in effect, a steal?[12] It seems likely.

Collateral circulation from the descending aorta to the lung via bizarre connecting vessels has been seen but is extremely rare, unlike in patients with pulmonary atresia and ventricular septal defect in whom such structures are relatively common.

Other associated cardiac anomalies are rare. Right aortic arch is virtually unknown. Extracardiac anomalies are rare, as is low birth weight.[10]

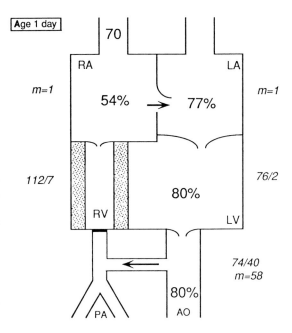

Figure 1. Diagram of the hemodynamics in a patient with pulmonary atresia with intact ventricular septum. The tiny right ventricle most often has a higher pressure than the left ventricle; it is sometimes in excess of 200 mm Hg. The entire venous return (cardiac output) passes through the foramen ovale to the left atrium. The entire pulmonary blood flow is supplied by a patent ductus arteriosus.

PHYSIOLOGY

The possible avenues of egress from the right ventricle are (1) the sinusoids to the coronary circulation, and (2) the return to the right atrium through the tricuspid valve. Depending on available egress, the right ventricle may develop pressures to very high levels during systole, up to 200 mm Hg (Fig. 1). The more opportunity for flow out of the ventricle, the lower the systolic pressure, and in the odd case of free tricuspid regurgitation, the right ventricular systolic pressure may be near normal. With virtual absence of the tricuspid valve, flow in and out of the right ventricle may be sufficient to considerably enlarge the valve ring, the ventricle, and the right atrium (Fig. 2). Estimations of the degree of tricuspid regurgitation are difficult since a 1-ml regurgitant volume from a 1-ml ventricle may be massive regurgitation, whereas 1 ml from a larger ventricle may be inconsequential.

The venous return to the right atrium, except for that passing out of the right ventricle via sinusoids, goes through the foramen ovale to the left atrium and left ventricle. Restrictive foramina ovale have been described, but in our experience it has been rare to measure a pressure gradient between the right and left atrium of more than 2 or 3 mm Hg. After birth, blood flow to the lungs is initially supplied via the patent ductus arteriosus. Having been the source of pulmonary blood flow *in utero*, the ductus arteriosus is small compared with that in normal infants, whose ductus has supplied systemic blood flow to the descending aorta. Because the arterial oxygen saturation is determined by the amount of pulmonary blood flow,

the arterial oxygen may be low. With closure of the ductus in the first few days of life, survival is no longer possible.

CLINICAL MANIFESTATIONS

These infants are cyanotic at birth and because of their blueness they are generally referred to a cardiac hospital within the first days of life. Frequently there is a systolic murmur (tricuspid regurgitation), and rarely a continuous murmur (patent ductus arteriosus), but usually there is no murmur at all. Depending on the level of arterial oxygen, the infant may be in more or less distress with tachypnea or dyspnea.

Electrocardiography

The electrocardiogram shows a QRS axis between 0 and 120 degrees and evidence of left ventricular dominance (Fig. 3). The other forms of right-sided obstruction can largely be distinguished by the electrocardiogram. A QRS axis to the right is most likely associated with pulmonary atresia and a ventricular defect; a QRS axis in the normal range is seen in patients with pulmonary atresia and intact ventricular septum; and a leftward-superior axis is associated with tricuspid atresia (Exhibit 1).

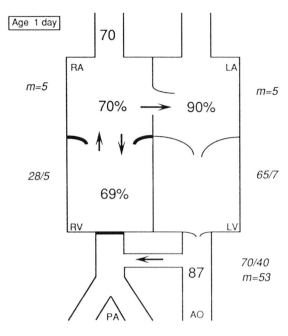

Figure 2. Diagram of the hemodynamics in a patient with pulmonary atresia with intact ventricular septum and a grossly incompetent tricuspid valve. Although most patients with pulmonary atresia and intact ventricular septum have some tricuspid insufficiency, occasionally a patient has a grossly incompetent tricuspid valve incapable of supporting significant elevation of right ventricular pressure. Some of these patients have an Ebstein-like deformity of the tricuspid valve.

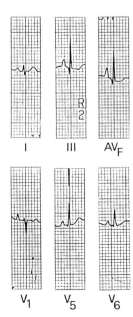

Figure 3. The electrocardiogram of a patient with pulmonary atresia with intact ventricular septum at birth. Note the axis of +60 degrees without the normal degree of right ventricular dominance seen at birth.

Chest X-ray

The heart size is variable, usually not large, with normal or decreased pulmonary vascularity. In the rare situation in which there is free tricuspid regurgitation, the right ventricle and right atrium may both be large, contributing to a huge cardiac silhouette.

Echocardiography

The right ventricle and tricuspid valve can be visualized and the degree of hypoplasia can be estimated.[16,23] The absence of blood flow across the pulmonary valve can be identified using Doppler cardiography, and the source of blood flow to the lungs via the ductus arteriosus can be shown. The size and shape of the pulmonary arteries can be determined, and in many cases coronary fistulae can be detected.

Diagnostic features include (1) thickened, immobile pulmonary valve leaflets without color Doppler evidence for anterograde flow, (2) variable hypoplasia and hypertrophy of the right ventricle, (3) a patent tricuspid valve, (4) right-to-left atrial shunting, (5) well-developed pulmonary arteries, and (6) a tortuous, siphon-shaped ductus arteriosus supplying the pulmonary arteries.

The **pulmonary valve** is best examined in the subxiphoid or parasternal short axis view (Fig. 4). Doppler examination (especially Doppler color flow mapping) of the right ventricular outflow tract should be performed in at least these two views to confidently exclude anterograde flow. Continuous flow into the main pulmonary artery from the ductus arteriosus can be confusing. However, if the valve is not atretic and the right ventricle is hypertensive, a high-velocity jet can be seen crossing the valve. If the right ventricular pressure is low, due to severe tricuspid regurgitation, then the absence of valve motion or anterograde flow is not conclusive evidence of pulmonary valve disease. A syndrome of pseudo pulmonary atresia has been described, with severe anomalies of the tricuspid valve and right ventricular dysfunction *in utero*[2,24] and in neonates.[8] The characteristic feature that distinguishes this syndrome from pulmonary atresia is the presence of pulmonary regurgitation demonstrable by Doppler cardiography or arterial contrast injection at the level of the ductus.

The **right ventricle** is examined most readily in the subxiphoid long- and short-axis views. Right ventricular volume, measured using these views, coupled with the diameter of the tricuspid annulus, derived from subxiphoid long-axis or apical four-chamber views, is very useful for predicting the need for a systemic-to-pulmonary shunt in addition to right ventricle outflow tract plasty.[23] Few infants with an indexed **tricuspid valve** diameter greater than 1.0 cm per cube root of body surface area and a right ventricular volume greater than 10 cc per

Exhibit 1

Boston Children's Hospital Experience
1973–1987

Pulmonary Atresia with Intact Ventricular Septum

There were 83 infants with pulmonary atresia and intact ventricular septum. In five, the tricuspid valve was grossly incompetent. Eight had been first seen in earlier years. Of the 75 new patients, the majority were seen in the first week of life; of the 22 who were seen later, all but two had had prior interventions.

Age First Seen

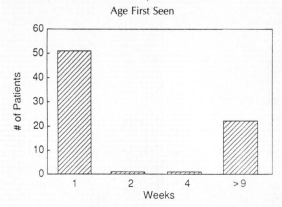

Age of patients with pulmonary atresia and intact ventricular septum when first seen at Boston Children's Hospital. The bimodal distribution results from many infants, especially in recent years, having received their first surgery elsewhere. Thus, virtually all of these infants, whether first seen at Boston Children's Hospital or elsewhere, were first seen by a cardiologist within the first week of life.

Electrocardiographic Frontal Plane Axis

	QRS Axis in degrees					
Diagnosis	Less than 0		0 to 90		90 or More	
	No.	%	No.	%	No.	%
Pulmonary atresia with intact ventricular septum n = 31	0	(0)	24	(77)	7	(23)
Tricuspid atresia n = 44	26	(59)	16	(36)	2	(5)
Pulmonary atresia with ventricular defect n = 81	3	(4)	22	(27)	56	(69)

square meter of body surface area will need a shunt if an adequate outflow tract plasty can be performed.

Another characteristic of the tricuspid valve worthy of noting is the extent of leaflet opening. Even if the diameter of the tricuspid annulus is adequate, decreased leaflet excursion due to fusion of the leaflet edges or closely spaced papillary muscles may limit flow. Doppler color flow mapping may be useful for estimating the size of the effective orifice of the valve.

Tricuspid regurgitation is best evaluated using Doppler color flow mapping in subxiphoid, apical, and parasternal views. The diameter of the regurgitant jet and the size of the right atrium are reasonable indices of the severity of regurgitation. The right ventricular systolic pressure can be estimated from the peak flow velocity of the regurgitant jet using the modified Bernoulli equation

RV peak pressure $= 4 \times v^2 + 10$ mm Hg (or assumed RA pressure).

The **foramen ovale** can be imaged from subxiphoid views, and the right-to-left shunt can be demonstrated using Doppler color flow mapping or contrast echocardiography.

The **pulmonary arteries** are best seen from a high left parasternal, parasagittal, or suprasternal notch view. The main and branch pulmonary arteries should be measured, although more than mild hypoplasia is uncommon. The ductus arteriosus is best imaged in a high left parasternal or parasagittal plane view. The shape of the ductus has been shown to have diagnostic significance in that the ductus in patients with pulmonary atresia is tortuous and S-shaped.

Our preliminary observations indicate that Doppler color flow mapping can detect **right ventricular sinusoids** in many cases.[21] The ventricle, including the epicardial surface, should be scanned carefully in multiple views with Doppler color flow mapping. Fistulous connections are characterized by biphasic flow into and out of an enlarged cor-

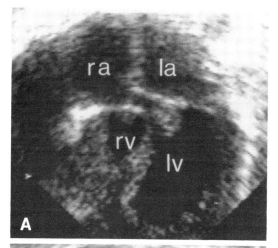

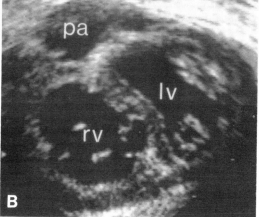

Figure 4. Echocardiograms in patients with pulmonary atresia and intact ventricular septum. **A,** Apical four-chamber view in a patient with severe right ventricular hypoplasia. **B,** Subxiphoid short-axis view in a patient with normal sized right ventricle. Note the posterior bowing of the interventricular septum indicating suprasystemic right ventricular pressure. rv, right ventricle; lv, left ventricle; ra, right atrium; la, left atrium; pa, pulmonary artery.

onary vessel in systole and diastole respectively. However, coronary stenoses have not been detected reliably by echocardiography or Doppler cardiography.

Cardiac Catheterization

The diagnosis is established by echocardiography. Cardiac catheterization is used to further define the size, shape, and function of the right ventricle. Some would catheterize virtually all such children to produce an atrial septal defect with Rashkind balloon septostomy.[8] Perhaps the most useful information obtained at cardiac catheterization is the identification of abnormalities of the coronary circulation that might produce ventricular ischemia and further subsequent dysfunction if the right ventricular pressure were reduced.[11]

A right ventricular angiogram is carried out with a pediatric NIH catheter positioned in the right ventricle. Contrast material (0.3–1.0 cc/kg) is injected carefully by hand during filming in the frontal and lateral positions. Coronary angiograms, or at least retrograde aortic angiography, is used to evaluate suspected coronary fistulas or coronary stenoses (Fig. 5).

MANAGEMENT

Initial Management

Some means of supplying adequate pulmonary blood flow is required for survival. Initially, prostaglandins E satisfy this need and stabilize the patient before surgery. Then pulmonary valvotomy or a systemic artery-pulmonary artery shunt or both provide a more permanent solution.[6]

Pulmonary valvotomy alone has produced the best overall result but this has been successful in less than 10% of our patients at the Children's Hospital in Boston. Others are more enthusiastic, particularly when the ventricular size and type are taken into consideration.[5]

Pulmonary valvotomy combined with a systemic artery–pulmonary artery shunt has been our usual surgical management. In a child with essentially no right ventricle, pulmonary valvectomy may help to decompress the right ventricle, but an aortic-pulmonary shunt is required for survival.

When there are right ventricular sinusoids supplying a coronary artery, the possibility that right ventricular decompression will result in reversal of sinusoidal flow, abruptly diminishing myocardial perfusion, should be kept in mind. Detailed study of the coronary circulation is required to make the required management decision. Our present data suggest that the combination of a coronary artery–right ventricular fistula and coronary stenoses are prerequisites to sudden death with right ventricular decompression.[11]

Later Management

Once a reliable pulmonary blood flow has been established, resulting in an arterial oxygen saturation in the range of 75–85%, the patients tend to grow. Within weeks or months, cardiac catheterization should be undertaken to assess the result of initial surgery. The desirable outcomes include an arterial oxygen saturation of more than 70%, an increase over the initial right ventricular volume, right ventricular pressure that is less than systemic pressure, sufficient flow through the right ventricle to predict probable future growth of the ventricle, undistorted pulmonary arteries, and no suggestion of coronary fistulas, actually or potentially, affecting the delivery of oxygen to the myocardium by the coronary artery.

The best ways to handle coronary stenoses and shunting sinusoids have not been determined. At

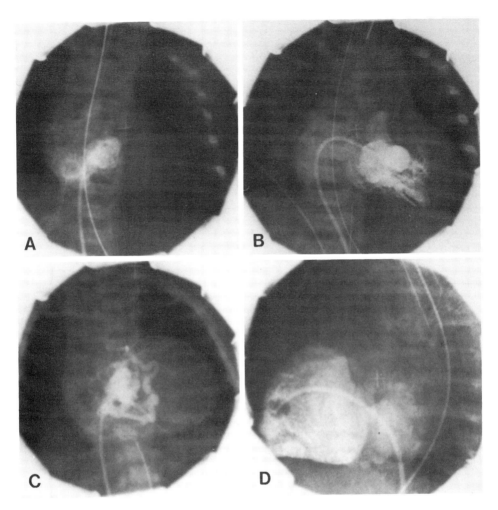

Figure 5. Right ventricular angiograms in four patients with pulmonary atresia and intact septum. Note: **A,** the tiny right ventricle with contrast spilling into the right atrium; **B,** the larger right ventricle with inflow, outflow, and trabecular components; **C,** a small right ventricle with fistulous sinusoids draining into the coronary arteries; and **D,** a large right ventricle with a completely incompetent tricuspid valve.

the Children's Hospital in Boston we have managed each patient individually, basing our decisions on the following presumptions:

1. Coronary abnormalities are present from fetal life.[14]

2. Coronary obstructions may progress.[18]

3. Myocardial ischemia may be the result of poorly oxygenated blood supplied by a right ventricle under high pressure.[13]

4. A right ventricle–coronary artery fistula may be the only source of blood flow to a particular coronary vessel.[22]

5. Reduction of right ventricular pressure may reverse the flow through the fistula, producing a coronary steal.[12]

6. The combination of fistulous communication and coronary stenosis is particularly dangerous.[11]

Obviously, precise catheterization data are needed.

Later, at a suitable time (as yet imprecisely defined), the right ventricular outflow tract and valve should be surgically enlarged if the right ventricle and the tricuspid valve annulus are large enough[1] and if there is no suggestion that a coronary artery steal will be produced.[11] The right ventricle rarely responds with normal function. Even the patients who seem normal years after pulmonary valvotomy as the only operation have evidence of right ventricular dysfunction. This is matter of some interest because a channel that has a diameter more than adequate for a successful Fontan procedure may not provide adequate circulation through the right ventricle. The contracting right ventricle sometimes seems to get in its own way. How much is due to contraction of a valveless ventricle, how much is due to tricuspid and pulmonary valve dysfunction, and how much is due to myocardial dysfunction remain to be determined.

Exhibit 2

Boston Children's Hospital Experience
1973–1987

**Surgical Procedures for Pulmonary Atresia
with Intact Ventricular Septum**

Operative Procedure	First Operation Elsewhere N = 22	First Operation at Children's Hospital N = 61	Total* N = 83
Atrial defect creation	3	6	9
Formalinization of ductus	1	9	10
Tricuspid valvectomy	3	4	7
Fontan procedure	2	7	9
Systemic artery–pulmonary artery shunt	16	35	51
Pulmonary valvotomy	18	49	67

*Some patients had more than one procedure.

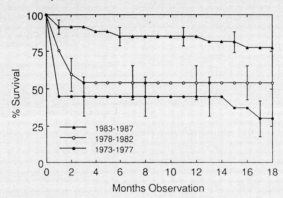

Life table presentation of survival of 52 patients with pulmonary atresia and intact ventricular septum. This figure considers only patients with initial evaluation at Boston Children's Hospital: 1973–77, n = 11; 1978–1982, n = 12; 1983–1987, n = 29. The calculations are based on the day the child was first seen. Note that a major factor in survival was the year the infant was born.

For patients who are not candidates for repair, who have limited pulmonary blood flow and otherwise reasonable physiologic measurements, Fontan procedures should be considered at a later date.[1] If this is not possible, adjustments in the shunting of blood to the lungs through the systemic arterial shunts are all that remain short of transplant surgery.

COURSE

With flow through the right ventricle established, the right ventricle grows,[19] although some abnormality of function is almost always detectable afterward. Few children live to be adults. The three patients we have followed who have reached the age of 21 had valvotomy without a shunting procedure. Others who have had shunts and valvotomies are doing fairly well in their teens, and a few patients are surviving with successful Fontan procedures (Exhibit 2).

VARIATION

The patient with an absent tricuspid valve represents a particular subset of the patients who have pulmonary atresia and intact ventricular septum (5 of 83 cases) (Exhibit 1). Some of these patients have an Ebstein-like deformity of the tricuspid valve, but in others this is not obvious. The right atrium and right ventricle may be large (Fig. 5). The right ventricular systolic pressure is minimally elevated, if at all. Sometimes forward flow through the pulmonary valve after pulmonary valvotomy is not a realistic possibility; indeed, pulmonary valvotomy may result only in pulmonary regurgitation, and if a Blalock shunt is constructed, the flow may be dominantly from the pulmonary artery, retrograde, to the right ventricle. To decide whether it is safe to open the right ventricular outflow tract into the pulmonary arteries, one needs to know the pressure in the right ventricle (if the pressure is quite low and the tricuspid valve leaks, there may be little antegrade flow postoperatively). Survival with a systemic artery–pulmonary artery shunt has been observed. Right ventricular sinusoids are not seen in these patients.

REFERENCES

1. Alboliras ET, Julsrud PR, Danielson GK, et al: Definitive operation for pulmonary atresia with intact ventricular septum. J Thorac Cardiovasc Surg 93:454–464, 1987.
2. Allan LD, Crawford DC, Tynan MJ: Pulmonary atresia in prenatal life: J Am Coll Cardiol 8:1131–1136, 1986.
3. Bull C, de Leval MR, Mercanti C, et al: Pulmonary atresia and intact ventricular septum: a revised classification. Circulation 66:266–280, 1982.
4. Calder AL, Co EE, Sage MD: Coronary arterial abnormalities in pulmonary atresia with intact ventricular septum. Am J Cardiol 59:436–442, 1987.
5. Cobanoglu A, Metzdorff MT, Pinson CW, et al: Valvotomy for pulmonary atresia with intact ventricular septum. J Thorac Cardiovasc Surg 89:482–490, 1985.
6. de Leval MR, Bull C, Stark J, et al: Pulmonary atresia and intact ventricular septum: surgical management based on a revised classification. Circulation 66:272–280, 1982.
7. Freedom RM: The morphologic variations of pulmonary atresia with intact ventricular septum: guidelines for surgical intervention. Pediatr Cardiol 4:183–190, 1983.
8. Freedom R (ed): Pulmonary atresia with intact ventricular septum. Mount Kisco, New York, Futura Publishing Co., 1989.
9. Fyfe DA, Edwards WD, Driscoll DJ: Myocardial ischemia in patients with pulmonary atresia and intact ventricular septum. J Am Coll Cardiol 8:402–406, 1986.
10. Fyler DC, Buckley LP, Hellenbrand WE, et al: Report of the New England Regional Infant Cardiac Program. Pediatrics 65(Suppl):376–460, 1980.
11. Giglia TM, Mandell VS, Connor AR, et al: Right ventricular-dependent coronary circulation in pulmonary atresia with intact ventricular septum. Abstract AHA, November 13–16, 1989.
12. Gittenberger-De Groot AC, Sauer U, Bindl L, et al: Competition of coronary arteries and ventriculo-coronary arterial communication in pulmonary atresia with intact ventricular septum. Int J Cardiol 18:243–258, 1988.
13. Hausdorf G, Gravinghoff L, Keck EW: Effects of persisting myocardial sinusoids on left ventricular performance in pulmonary atresia with intact septum. Eur Heart J 8:291–296, 1987.
14. Kasznica J, Ursell PC, Blanc WA, et al: Abnormalities of the coronary circulation in pulmonary atresia and intact ventricular septum. Am Heart J 114:1415–1420, 1987.
15. Kutsche LM, Van Mierop LHS: Pulmonary atresia with and without ventricular septal defect: a different etiology and pathogenesis for the atresia in the two types? Am J Cardiol 51:932–935, 1983.
16. Leung MP, Mok CK, Hui PW: Echocardiographic assessment of neonates with pulmonary atresia and intact ventricular septum. J Am Coll Cardiol 12:719–725, 1988.
17. O'Connor WN, Cottrill CM, Johnson GL, et al: Pulmonary atresia with intact ventricular septum and ventriculocoronary communications: surgical significance. Circulation 65:805–809, 1982.
18. O'Connor WN, Stahr BJ, Cottrill CM, et al: Ventriculocoronary connections in hypoplastic right heart syndrome: autopsy serial section study of six cases. J Am Coll Cardiol 11:1061–1072, 1988.
19. Patel RG, Freedom RM, Moes CAF, et al: Right ventricular volume determinations in 18 patients with pulmonary atresia and intact ventricular septum: analysis of factors influencing right ventricular growth. Circulation 61:428–440, 1980.
20. Rowe R, Freedom RM, Mehrizi A: The Neonate with Congenital Heart Disease. Philadelphia, W.B. Saunders, 1981.
21. Sanders SP, Parness IA, Colon SD: Recognition of abnormal connections of coronary arteries with the use of Doppler color flow mapping. J Am Coll Cardiol 13:922–926, 1989.
22. Sauer U, Bindl L, Pilossoff V, et al: Pulmonary atresia with intact ventricular septum and right ventricle-coronary artery fistulae: selection of patients for surgery. In Doyle EF, Engle MA, Gersony WM, et al (eds): Pediatric Cardiology. New York, Springer-Verlag, 1986.
23. Trowitzsch E, Colan SD, Sanders SP: Two-dimensional echocardiographic evaluation of right ventricular size and function in newborns with severe right ventricular outflow tract obstruction. J Am Coll Cardiol 6:388–393, 1985.
24. Yeager SB, Parness IA, Sanders SP: Severe tricuspid regurgitation simulating pulmonary atresia in the fetus. Am Heart J 115:906–908, 1988.

Chapter 41

DOUBLE-OUTLET RIGHT VENTRICLE

Donald C. Fyler, M.D.

DEFINITION

Double-outlet right ventricle is said to be present when both great arteries arise completely or nearly completely above the right ventricle.

PREVALENCE

Among critically ill infants seen between 1968 and 1973, double-outlet right ventricle ranked 17th, or 0.032 per 1000 live births.[4] Figures ranging from 0.03 per 1000 to 0.07 per 1000 live births have been reported (see ch. 18). In a recent 15-year period 213 children with double-outlet right ventricle were seen at Children's Hospital in Boston (Exhibit 1).

The diagnosis of double-outlet right ventricle depends greatly on how much one or the other great vessel overrides the right ventricle. The criteria for this diagnosis have varied over the years. The decision to use the term "double-outlet right ventricle" is, therefore, judgmental and its use has varied from time to time. Consequently, variation in prevalence from center to center and within one center over time is inherent in this diagnosis.

PATHOLOGY

Double-outlet right ventricle is not a single cardiac anomaly or even a part of a complex of anomalies. It is a term that is used to describe the position of the great arteries found in association with a variety of cardiac anomalies that can be viewed, physiologically, as ventricular septal defects, tetralogy of Fallot, transposition of the great arteries, single ventricle, or atrioventricular atresia.[1,3,16,17,19] Pulmonary stenosis is common in patients with double-outlet right ventricle of all types. The relation of the great arteries to each other is often side-by-side and parallel, with the aorta on the right or left, anterior or posterior, often resembling transposition of the great arteries. A variety of atrioventricular valvar abnormalities and outflow valve

and subvalvar obstructions are encountered. Interrupted aortic arch and coarctation of the aorta are often seen (Exhibit 1). Hypoplasia or stenosis of the aortic valve is often encountered when there is coarctation of the aorta, although subvalvar aortic stenosis may be seen in the absence of coarctation.

Any malfunction of the atrioventricular or semilunar valves may be present, with various types of pulmonary stenosis being the most common. A defect of the common atrioventricular canal is frequently present, with its associated mitral and tricuspid valve abnormalities (Exhibit 1).

There is a gradation of defects ranging from subaortic ventricular septal defect with pulmonary stenosis, to tetralogy of Fallot, to double-outlet right ventricle with pulmonary stenosis. There is a similar range of clinical problems extending from subpulmonary ventricular septal defect with varying degrees of overriding of the pulmonary artery (transposition of the great arteries) to double-outlet right ventricle. Another anatomic spectrum ranges from a single right ventricle giving rise to both great vessels, to a single right ventricle with a hypoplastic left ventricle, to a double-outlet right ventricle with a small left ventricle that is, nevertheless, of sufficient size to permit a two-ventricle repair.

Ventricular Septal Defect

A ventricular septal defect is almost always present, although rarely there is none, the pulmonary venous blood reaching the right ventricle by shunting left-to-right through an atrial septal opening. The ventricular defect may be subaortic, subpulmonary, uncommitted (both subaortic and subpulmonary), or remote (muscular or endocardial cushion type) (Fig. 1).[13] The subaortic and subpulmonary defects rarely lie immediately below the corresponding semilunar valve without intervening conal tissue. Indeed, the case can be made that the subpulmonary and the subaortic ventricular defects have the same location and that it is the variation in distribution of conal tissue that

Exhibit 1

Boston Children's Hospital Experience
1973–1987

There were 213 patients who were categorized as having double-outlet right ventricle. Additionally, 118 patients were categorized under "malpositions" who also had double-outlet right ventricle. Thirty-eight children listed under the category of "single ventricle" were also listed as having a double-outlet right ventricle. All were considered to be examples of single right ventricle. Forty-seven cases carried codes indicating double-outlet right ventricle but were categorized with the hypoplastic left heart group. Virtually all of these had mitral atresia with an unobstructed aortic outflow and, hence, were not true examples of hypoplastic left heart.

Because this is such a diverse group of patients, survival curves, ages on first admission, and change over the years were not recorded.

Diagnoses Associated with Double-Outlet Right Ventricle (DORV)

Associated Diagnoses	DORV n = 213	Malposition with DORV* n = 118	Single Ventricle with DORV n = 38	Hypoplastic Left Ventricle with DORV* n = 47
Single Ventricle	14	49	38	20
Hypoplastic Left Ventricle	6	18	2	47
D-Transposition Great Arteries	69	39	21	12
L-Transposition Great Arteries	19	32	8	7
Total Anomalous Pulmonary Veins	5	28	2	5
Endocardial Cushion Defect	23	68	7	5
Tetralogy of Fallot	32	14	3	3
Pulmonary Atresia	24	35	8	4
Pulmonary Stenosis	151	94	30	25
Aortic Stenosis	10	7	1	5
Subaortic Stenosis	34	9	3	6
Coarctation of Aorta	37	10	3	16
Mitral Atresia	0	11	2	45

*The majority of those categorized as having double-outlet right ventricle within the context of malposition had asplenia or polysplenia. Almost all of those categorized as having hypoplastic left heart had double-outlet right ventricle and mitral atresia with unobstructed aortic outflow.

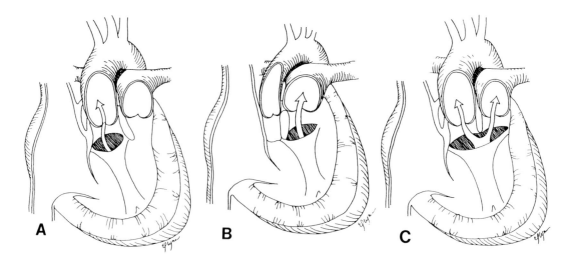

Figure 1. Three drawings of double-outlet right ventricle. **A,** Subaortic ventricular defect. **B,** Subpulmonary ventricular defect. **C,** An uncommitted ventricular defect related equally to both great arteries. Not shown are ventricular defects of the atrioventricular canal type or one or more muscular ventricular defects that may be associated with the above anomalies or exist as the sole communication between the left and right ventricles. Additionally, double-outlet right ventricle with inverse ventricles and ventricular defects of comparable variety are encountered.

determines the great artery with which the ventricular defect is associated. Because of variations in location of infundibular tissue (conal tissue), anteriorly or posteriorly, malalignment of the ventricular septal defect is directly related to the presence of subaortic stenosis on the one hand and pulmonary stenosis on the other.[6] Another factor that determines the relationship between the ventricular defect and the great arteries is the relative rightward or leftward position of the great arteries themselves. However it is explained, the location of the ventricular defect relative to the great arteries determines the surgical possibilities.

As in most other complex groups of cardiac anomalies, some ventricular defects have a tendency to get smaller with time. This must be considered in the clinical management of these children.[9]

Pulmonary Stenosis

Almost three fourths of patients with double-outlet right ventricle have some degree of pulmonary stenosis, even, rarely, pulmonary atresia. The stenosis is usually subvalvar and is derived from conal tissue. Because extreme degrees of aortic override seen in patients with tetralogy of Fallot may resemble the anatomy seen in double-outlet right ventricle, at times it may not be possible to distinguish between the two. Usually, however, the presence of mitral-aortic valvar continuity establishes the diagnosis of tetralogy of Fallot, whereas absence of mitral-aortic continuity characterizes double-outlet right ventricle. The majority of patients in whom this question arises have tetralogy of Fallot, and the diagnosis of double-outlet right ventricle with subaortic ventricular septal defect and subvalvar pulmonary stenosis is most often not correct.

Transposition of the Great Arteries

When there is a subpulmonary ventricular defect that delivers left ventricular blood to the pulmonary artery, the hemodynamics and the anatomy resemble those of transposition of the great arteries. The distinction between double-outlet right ventricle and transposition of the great arteries can be made if there is mitral-pulmonary valvar continuity. When continuity can be confidently said to be present, the patient has transposition of the great arteries; when it is not, the diagnosis is double-outlet right ventricle. Although this distinction is readily described, it not always obvious to the angiographer who may not have obtained the perfect view or to the echocardiographer who was in a hurry.

The **Taussig-Bing anomaly** is a specific variation of this problem, which includes the hemodynamics and usual anatomy of transposed great arteries but in which both arteries arise from the right ventricle. There is a subpulmonary ventricular defect, no pulmonary stenosis, and absence of mitral-pulmonary valvar continuity. The level of the semilunar valves is the same and the great vessels are parallel.[14,18]

Other Associated Anomalies

Virtually every other cardiac anomaly can be found associated with double-outlet right ventricle. Mitral atresia, mitral stenosis, and straddling atrioventricular valves are common. Some babies with mitral atresia and a hypoplastic left ventricle do surprisingly well, because there may be no aortic valve obstruction and an aorta of normal size receives normal amounts of blood flow from the right ventricle.

Supero-inferior ventricles (upstairs-downstairs ventricles) are often associated with the origin of both great arteries from the upper right ventricle. This interesting relationship may become modified with growth, the ventricles assuming a more nearly normal position if the child survives.

Inverse ventricles are common, as are visceral heterotaxy, polysplenia, and asplenia (Exhibit 1).

The great arteries may be normally related to each other, or in a position reminiscent of tetralogy of Fallot, or as situated in D- or L-transposition of the great arteries. Most often the great arteries are side-by-side, with the plane of the valves being identical. Continuity between the mitral valve and the adjacent semilunar valve is absent and is thought by most to represent the sine qua non of this diagnosis. Conal musculature is usually seen under both great arteries, but it may be absent under one or the other, or both. In cases without bilateral conal tissue, there is usually continuity between the adjacent great artery and the tricuspid valve; most of these children have mitral atresia.

PHYSIOLOGY

The relationship between the ventricular defect and the great arteries, the relative outflow obstruction, and the relative systemic-to-pulmonary artery resistance determine the hemodynamic situation. Double-outlet right ventricle may mimic ventricular septal defect, tetralogy of Fallot, single right ventricle, or transposition of the great arteries with or without pulmonary stenosis. Depending on the physiology, the child may have the problems of cyanosis, of congestive heart failure, or both. Some degree of arterial unsaturation is almost always present.

CLINICAL MANIFESTATIONS

The patient may have the symptoms of congestive heart failure, cyanosis, or no symptoms at all.[12]

Electrocardiography

There is no characteristic electrocardiographic pattern, although virtually all have a pattern compatible with right ventricular hypertrophy.

Chest X-ray

Similarly, there is no characteristic chest x-ray. The size of the heart and the amount of pulmonary vascularity are dependent on the hemodynamics and may range from a relatively small heart with decreased pulmonary vascularity to a large heart with increased pulmonary vascular markings.

Echocardiography

The diagnosis is usually apparent from the subxiphoid view. The criterion for diagnosis is alignment of both great arteries, totally or predominantly, with the right ventricle. Bilateral conus is often, but not invariably, present. Parasternal long- and short-axis views are also useful for detecting the alignment of the great arteries and for detecting subarterial conal muscle. Because there are a large number of anatomic variations and associated intracardiac lesions, a thorough examination of all segments of the heart is mandatory.[8,11]

Cardiac Catheterization

Before cardiac surgery is undertaken, cardiac catheterization is scheduled to confirm the echocardiographic findings and the clinical understanding of the hemodynamics. The patients usually have some degree of arterial oxygen unsaturation and have the hemodynamics of tetralogy of Fallot, single right ventricle, transposition of the great arteries, dominant left-to-right shunt, or pulmonary vascular obstructive disease. The wide variety of physiologic possibilities are unraveled by the usual techniques. The information obtained from the echocardiogram may suggest the best positioning of the patient in order to demonstrate the origins of the great vessels and the location of the ventricular defects. Often these are seen best in a biplane angiogram in anteroposterior and straight lateral views, since the great arteries often are side-by-side with the semilunar valves at the same level (Fig. 2).

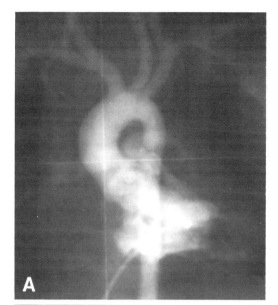

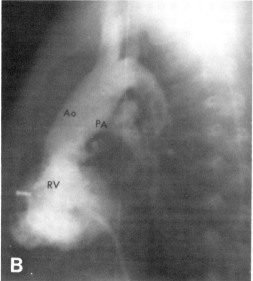

Figure 2. Anteroposterior and lateral angiogram of a patient with double-outlet right ventricle. Note that the semilunar valves are at the same level; the great vessels are side-by-side and both arise from the right ventricle. Ao, aorta; PA, pulmonary artery; RV, right ventricle.

Management[7]

The initial decision in management concerns the ultimate goal. Can a two-ventricle repair be imagined? Are the ventricles of reasonable size? Or is the only realistic possibility a Fontan type of palliation? If a two-ventricle repair is possible, is there pulmonary stenosis and will a conduit be required? In very small infants, because of expected rapid growth, the use of conduits is avoided if reasonably

possible. At the same time, a shunting procedure, which will require surgical takedown later, is scarcely better than a reparative procedure with a conduit that needs replacement later. When the ventricular septal defect is closed, will the circulation be transposed and, if so, will an arterial switch be possible (i.e., is the coronary anatomy favorable for an arterial switch)?[22] Sometimes placement of the ventricular patch can cure the patient and sometime placement of the patch and surgery

Exhibit 2

Boston Children's Hospital Experience 1973–1987
There were 8 patients categorized as having double-outlet left ventricle. Three were first seen in the first week of life, 3 more in the first 6 months, and 2 were 3 years old. Two had pulmonary atresia, 2 had aortic stenosis, 1 had an interrupted aortic arch, 2 had tricuspid valve abnormalities, and 1 had right ventricular hypoplasia. Four had palliative cardiac surgery (1 death) and 4 had reparative operations (1 death).

**Surgical Procedures Used in Patients with
Double-Outlet Right Ventricle (DORV)**

Operative Procedure	DORV n = 199	Malposition with DORV n = 106	Single Ventricle with DORV n = 32	Hypoplastic Left Ventricle with DORV n = 39
Fontan	21	28	18	10
Coarctation Repair*	18	6	2	7
Tetralogy of Fallot Repair	15	3	0	0
Double-outlet Right Ventricle Repair†	51	6	0	0
Transposition of Great Arteries Repair‡	28	0	0	0
Rastelli	5	2	0	0
Arterial-Pulmonary Shunt	64	66	21	22
Pulmonary Artery Band	35	14	8	12

*Includes patients with interrupted aortic arch.
†Repair of double-outlet right ventricle is, unfortunately, an acceptable code in our system that conveys little information and skews the figures in a table of this type.
‡Includes arterial and atrial (e.g., Senning and Mustard) repairs.

for pulmonary stenosis provides a satisfactory result (Exhibit 1).[5]

Immediate survival is dependent on the anatomy.[7,10]

COURSE

The long-range course depends on the anatomy and the surgical procedures used. In general, these patients face shorter survival and more complicating problems than their counterparts without the added feature of double-outlet right ventricle. Rhythm problems are common.[5]

DOUBLE-OUTLET LEFT VENTRICLE

As the name implies, double-outlet left ventricle requires the dominant origin of both great arteries from the left ventricle. This anomaly has little or nothing in common with double-outlet right ventricle but will be briefly mentioned here for lack of a better place.

This is a rare anomaly. At Boston Children's Hospital, the diagnosis was proposed 15 times and was probably correct in 8 patients in the course of 15 years. As with double-outlet right ventricle, any other early congenital cardiac anomaly may be present (Exhibit 2). The patient may or may not have pulmonary stenosis, situs inversus, inverse ventricles, anomalous atrioventricular valves, etc. Many of the possible variations on this theme have

been reported. Few have been seen more than once or twice.

There is one exception to this. A third of the patients have lesions mimicking tetralogy of Fallot. Often, the similarity is so close that the presence of double-outlet left ventricle is only recognized at surgery. Today, one presumes that the vast majority will be recognized by echocardiography. Once it is recognized that the pulmonary artery, as well as the aorta, originates from the left ventricle in a patient who otherwise seems to have tetralogy of Fallot, the diagnosis is made. Often the aorta appears to be overriding, and there may be a right aortic arch.

Management depends on the specific anatomy. If the anatomy is tetralogy-like, a two-ventricle repair connecting the right ventricle to the pulmonary artery with a patch or conduit is possible.

For an exhaustive discussion of all possibilities, see the article by Van Praagh and coworkers.[15]

REFERENCES

1. Anderson RH, Becker AE, Wilcox BR, et al: Surgical anatomy of double-outlet right ventricle—a reappraisal. Am J Cardiol 52:555–559, 1983.
2. Brawn WJ, Mee RBB: Early results for anatomic correction of transposition of the great arteries and for double-outlet right ventricle with subpulmonary ventricular septal defect. J Thorac Cardiovasc Surg 95:230–238, 1988.
3. Cameron AH, Acerete F, Quero M, et al: Double outlet right ventricle: study of 27 cases. Br Heart J 38:1124–1132, 1976.

4. Fyler DC, Buckley LP, Hellenbrand WE, et al: Report of the New England Regional Infant Cardiac Program. Pediatrics 65:375–461, 1980.
5. Judson JP, Danielson GK, Puga FJ, et al: Double-outlet right ventricle: surgical results, 1970–1980. J Thorac Cardiovasc Surg 85:32–40, 1983.
6. Kurosawa H, Van Mierop LHS: Surgical anatomy of the infundibular septum in transposition of the great arteries with ventricular septal defect. J Thorac Cardiovasc Surg 91:123–132, 1986.
7. Luber JM, Castaneda AR, Lang P, et al: Repair of double-outlet right ventricle: early and late results. Circulation 68(Suppl II):144–147, 1983.
8. Macartney FJ, Rigby ML, Anderson RH, et al: Double outlet right ventricle: cross sectional echocardiographic findings, their anatomical explanation, and surgical relevance. Br Heart J 52:164–177, 1984.
9. Marino B, Loperfido F, Sardi CS: Spontaneous closure of ventricular septal defect in a case of double outlet right ventricle. Br Heart J 49:608–611, 1983.
10. Piccoli G, Pacifico AD, Kirklin JW, et al: Changing results and concepts in the surgical treatment of double-outlet right ventricle: analysis of 137 operations in 126 patients. Am J Cardiol 52:549–554, 1983.
11. Sanders SP, Bierman FZ, Wiliams RG: Conotruncal malformations: diagnosis in infancy using subxiphoid 2-dimensional echocardiography. Am J Cardiol 50:1361–1367, 1982.
12. Sondheimer HM, Freedom RM, Olley PM, et al: Double outlet right ventricle: clinical spectrum and prognosis. Am J Cardiol 39:709–714, 1977.
13. Sridaromont S, Feldt RH, Ritter DG, et al: Double outlet right ventricle: hemodynamic and anatomic correlations. Am J Cardiol 38:85–94, 1976.
14. Van Praagh R: What is the Taussig-Bing malformation? Circulation 38:445–449, 1968.
15. Van Praagh RV, Weinberg PM, Srebro JP: Double-outlet left ventricle. In Adams FH, Emmanouilides GC, Riemenschneider TA (eds): Moss' Heart Disease in Infants, Children, and Adolescents. Baltimore, Williams & Wilkins, 1989, pp. 461–485.
16. Wilcox BR, Ho SY, Macartney FJ, et al: Surgical anatomy of double-outlet right ventricle with situs solitus and atrioventricular concordance. J Thorac Cardiovasc Surg 82:405–417, 1981.
17. Williams WG, Freedom RM: Double-outlet right ventricle and double outlet left ventricle. In Glenn WWL, Bane AE, Geha AS, et al (eds): Thoracic and Cardiovascular Surgery, Norwalk, CT, Appleton-Century-Crofts, 1983.
18. Yacoub MH, Radley-Smith R: Anatomic correction of the Taussig-Bing anomaly. J Thorac Cardiovasc Surg 88:380–388, 1984.
19. Zamora R, Moller JH, Edwards JE: Double-outlet right ventricle: anatomic types and associated anomalies. Chest 68:672–677, 1975.

Chapter 42

SINGLE VENTRICLE

Donald C. Fyler, M.D.

DEFINITION

At Boston Children's Hospital a **single ventricle** is defined as the presence of two atrioventricular valves with one ventricular chamber or a large dominant ventricle associated with a diminutive opposing ventricle.[30-32] The term **double-inlet ventricle** is also used to describe this group of anomalies.

While the concept of a **univentricular heart**[2-4] fits the physiologic idea of a common mixing chamber and has pathologic merits as well, lumping patients with mitral atresia, tricuspid atresia, and others into one category adds confusion rather than contributing to classification. The easy distinction between a single atrioventricular valve and two atrioventricular valves has been a reproducible basis for clinical impressions extending over many years. To change nomenclature would require significant benefits that are not apparent at the present time.

PREVALENCE

Using the above definition, single ventricle ranked fifteenth among consecutive infants with critical congenital heart disease in the New England states,[12] with an incidence between 0.054 and 0.103 per 1000 live births. Single ventricle is somewhat more common in the Children's Hospital experience, being the thirteenth most common defect (see Table 2, ch. 18). If the idea of a univentricular heart is employed, there are more than twice as many (Exhibit 1).[3]

Because all patients with malposed hearts are discussed elsewhere (see ch. 37), some patients with dextrocardia or asplenia and single ventricle are not discussed here. Most notable, the patients who have single right ventricle with asplenia are not considered in this section.

EMBRYOLOGY

In early embryologic life, the atrioventricular canal, which later contributes to both the mitral and tricuspid valves, opens into the ventricular portion of the primitive heart tube, which later becomes the left ventricle (see Fig. 6, p. 9). From the ventricular portion of the primitive heart tube, blood passes to the bulbus cordis, which later contributes to the development of the right ventricle. The arterial trunk, later to become both the aorta and the main pulmonary artery, arises from the bulbus cordis. With an arrest or a defect in interventricular septation, a double-inlet single left ventricle with a rudimentary right ventricular outflow chamber results,[29] most often in the context of L looping of the ventricles (see ch. 3).

ANATOMY

A single ventricular chamber can usually be recognized as being most like a left or a right ventricle because of the presence or absence of characteristic trabeculation, as well as the position and anatomy of the atrioventricular valves. The most common form of single ventricle is a single left ventricle with L-transposition of the great arteries, with the aorta arising from a diminutive, leftward right ventricle and following the leftward, ascending pattern characteristic of "corrected transposition." The pulmonary artery usually arises posteriorly; the mitral valve is right sided and the tricuspid valve is to the left (Fig. 1). This form of single ventricle accounts for 74% of autopsied cases[32] and for 68% of our clinical experience (Exhibit 1). In some cases, the ventricular septal defect between the large left ventricle and the rudimentary right ventricular outflow chamber (the bulboventricular foramen) may become progressively smaller with time, producing functional subaortic stenosis.[5,11] There is pulmonary stenosis or atresia in about 50% of patients; the remainder have unfettered flow to the pulmonary circuit. Coarctation of the aorta and

649

Exhibit 1

Boston Children's Hospital Experience 1973–1987

There were 191 patients with single ventricle with the heart located in the left chest and without abdominal heterotaxy. An additional 66 with single ventricle had asplenia, polysplenia, abdominal heterotaxy, or dextrocardia (see ch. 37)

Type of Single Ventricle
n = 191

Single Left Ventricle	129
Single Right Ventricle	28
Holmes' Heart	5
Unspecified	29

Ninety-seven had pulmonary stenosis or atresia and 94 did not. 39 were thought to have coarctation of the aorta or interrupted aortic arch, a relatively serious complication (mortality 16/39 [41%]). Complete heart block developed in 16 individuals; all had single left ventricle. Noncardiac anomalies were a complication in 63 patients (53%) but did not contribute excessively to mortality (30%).

Twelve developed scoliosis, which is 6% of the all patients with single ventricle; the percentage would be much greater if only those surviving long enough to get scoliosis were counted.

Univentricular Hearts
n = 509 patients

	Not Malposed	Malposition	Total
Tricuspid Atresia	155	28	183
Mitral Atresia	43	25	68
Single Ventricle	192	66	258
Total	390	119	509

There were 509 patients who could be categorized as having univentricular hearts.

Surgical Treatment of Single Ventricle

Surgical Procedure	No Pulmonary Stenosis n = 74	With Pulmonary Stenosis n = 82	% Known Dead
Pulmonary Artery Band	61	—	30
Arterial-Pulmonary Shunt	26	55	19
Coarctation Repair	21	5	36
Aortic Outflow Bypass	14	6	35
Fontan	35	50	16
Glenn	13	21	6
Other	5	5	60

One-hundred fifty-six patients underwent surgery. There are 71 survivors with Fontan procedures (including preliminary operations; there were 2.8 operations per patient). Sixteen patients succumbed without surgery and 19 have had no operative procedure.

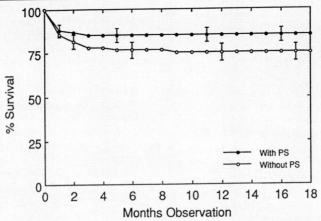

When a comparison of the actuarial survival between those with pulmonary outflow obstruction and those without outflow obstruction was made, those with pulmonary stenosis had better survival.

Exhibit 1 *(continued)*

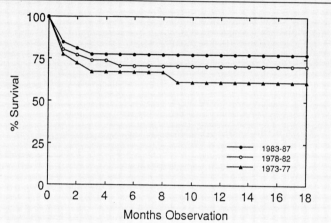

Management	Obstructed Bulboventricular Foramen		
	With No Pulmonary Stenosis n = 29		With Pulmonary Stenosis n = 10
	With pulmonary artery band n = 21	No pulmonary artery band n = 8	
Aortic outflow bypass	9	5	6
No aortic outflow bypass	12	3	4

During the period of observation a restrictive bulboventricular foramen was reported in 39 patients, usually in the absence of pulmonary stenosis. Careful review of the 10 patients with pulmonary stenosis showed that some of these children had minimal degrees of pulmonary stenosis and 2 or 3 could be classified as severe.

Regardless of treatment, survival was poor in the early 1970s. Later survival improved and at the present time most patients survive the early months of life.

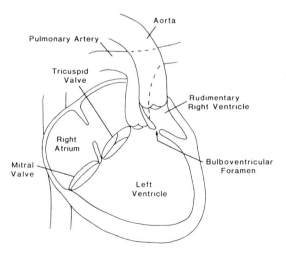

Figure 1. Sketch of a single left ventricle with transposed great arteries. There is a left-sided rudimentary right ventricle under the aortic valve. Entry to this chamber is through a bulboventricular foramen that tends to close spontaneously. The positions of the atrioventricular valves are reversed: the mitral is right-sided; the tricuspid is left-sided. The great vessels are transposed: the aorta is leftward and anterior; the pulmonary artery is rightward and posterior. This is the most common form of single ventricle.

interrupted aortic arch are common (Exhibit 1), as are abnormalities of the mitral or tricuspid valves.

The eponym "Holmes' heart"[14] describes a rare, double-inlet, single left ventricle without transposition and with pulmonary stenosis.

In the remaining patients the types of single ventricle are less homogeneous; sometimes they appear to be derived from an anatomic right ventricle and are necessarily viewed case by case. Asplenia has not been observed in the group of patients with single left ventricle, but it is common among those with single right ventricle.[32]

Until recent times most data about patients with single ventricle were based on pathologic observations; if clinical data are considered (and nowadays a majority of patients are survivors, see Exhibit 1) a somewhat different picture emerges. As might be expected, some of the living patients have not been classified or the classification is debatable. This is particularly true when multiple observers from different disciplines (echocardiographers, angiographers, surgeons) are involved. Still the number of cases about which there is general agreement gradually increases as the years go by.

PHYSIOLOGY

The amount of pulmonary blood flow, as limited by pulmonary stenosis or pulmonary vascular resistance, determines the clinical course of babies with single ventricle. In the absence of pulmonary stenosis and with regression of the fetal pulmonary vascular resistance, the pulmonary blood flow gradually increases, ultimately causing congestive heart failure (Fig. 2). It is not possible for pulmonary resistance to be reduced to normal levels and have the patient survive unless there is pulmonary stenosis. The balance point at which pulmonary resistance stabilizes varies from patient to patient, but usually is sufficiently low to result in congestive failure in a matter of days or weeks after birth.

Infants with single ventricle and pulmonary atresia are cyanotic at birth, the degree of cyanosis being determined by the amount of pulmonary flow supplied by the ductus arteriosus, persistent aortopulmonary collaterals, or bronchial circulation. Patients with severe pulmonary stenosis are comparable to those with pulmonary atresia. Those with moderate pulmonary stenosis may fare quite well (Fig. 3). Indeed, a few patients with pulmonary blood flow limited to about twice the systemic blood flow do very well for years and, despite recognizable cyanosis, grow and seem otherwise normal.

A single ventricle acts as a common mixing cham-

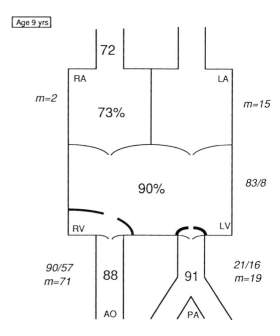

Figure 3. Physiologic diagram of the circulation in a patient with single left ventricle, transposed great arteries, and pulmonary stenosis. Note the low pressure in the pulmonary artery and the similarity of pulmonary and aortic oxygen saturation. Abbreviations as in Figure 2.

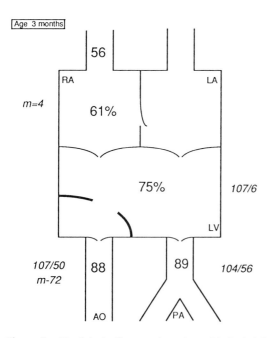

Figure 2. Physiologic diagram of a patient with single left ventricle and transposed great arteries. Note the similarity of pulmonary, arterial and aortic oxygen concentration. In this case the rudimentary right ventricle has a large bulboventricular foramen and, therefore, systemic pressure in the left ventricle is equal to that in the aorta and pulmonary artery. A pulmonary artery band was placed. See later data Figure 4. RA, right atrium; LA, left atrium; AO, aorta; PA, pulmonary artery; %, percent oxygen saturation; italics, pressure in mm Hg.

ber in 80% of the patients, the aorta and pulmonary artery having identical oxygen saturation regardless of their anatomic location. Surprisingly, the remainder may have sufficient streaming of pulmonary and systemic venous return that mixing is incomplete (Fig. 4). It is possible for the pulmonary artery to receive dominantly pulmonary venous return and the aorta to receive dominantly systemic venous return despite the fact that both receive blood from the same ventricle. This is a variation on the circulation of transposition of the great arteries and occasionally, in the past, clinical improvement has occurred following atrial inversion surgery. For the most part, however, whether the great arteries are transposed or not has little influence on the hemodynamics.

An obstructed bulboventricular foramen, most often associated with a pulmonary artery band and rarely with pulmonary stenosis, may cause the single ventricle to pump at suprasystemic pressure (Fig. 5). Abnormalities of the mitral or tricuspid valve are common and occasionally they dominate the clinical picture (Fig. 6). Coarctation of the aorta and interrupted aortic arch cause high ventricular pressure if there is a pulmonary artery band, but, in the absence of pulmonary outflow obstruction, the pulmonary blood flow is forced to intolerable levels.

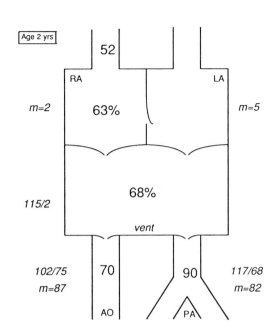

Figure 4. Physiologic diagram of a patient with single ventricle and transposition of the great arteries. Note that the pulmonary artery and aortic saturations are dissimilar. This lack of complete mixing is seen in about 20% of patients with single ventricle. Abbreviations as in Figure 2.

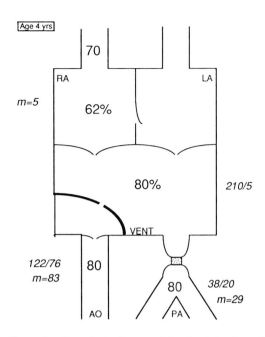

Figure 5. Physiologic diagram of the circulation in an 8-year-old with single left ventricle and transposed great arteries. See prior data on this patient as an infant in Figure 2. Following the pulmonary artery banding procedure, there was spontaneous reduction in the size of the bulboventricular foramen sufficient to raise ventricular pressure to over 200 mm Hg. Abbreviations as in Figure 2.

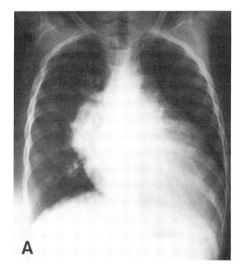

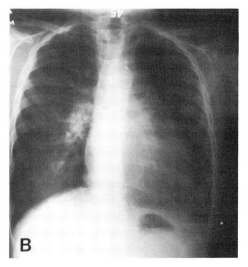

Figure 6. Chest x-ray of a child who has a single left ventricle and developed progressively severe regurgitation of the right-sided mitral valve (**A**). Fortunately, there was an adequate left atrioventricular valve. At Fontan operation the mitral valve was occluded. One year later the heart was much smaller (**B**).

CLINICAL MANIFESTATIONS

The majority of infants with single ventricle are discovered in the first days or weeks of life.[12] They are seen earlier if there is severe pulmonary stenosis, because of cyanosis, and later, in the absence of pulmonary stenosis, with congestive heart failure. Although all patients with single ventricle are cyanotic, among those with a large pulmonary flow, often in congestive heart failure, cyanosis may be so slight it is overlooked.

In patients with pulmonary stenosis there is a

systolic murmur; without a systolic murmur there
can be no pulmonary stenosis. Right or left atrioventricular valvar regurgitation may also be the
source of a systolic murmur. A continuous murmur
suggests a patent ductus arteriosus or aortopulmonary collateral circulation. Coarctation of the
aorta is discovered by a difference between arm
and leg pulses or pressures.

Electrocardiography

The electrocardiogram is not especially helpful
in recognizing ventricular hypertrophy, except that
the tracing usually can be described as abnormal.
Left ventricular hypertrophy is thought to be more
common. Rhythm abnormalities are encountered
in increasing numbers with advancing age; they
include spontaneously occurring complete heart
block and rhythms of junctional origin.[1]

Chest X-ray

If there is no pulmonary stenosis, the heart is
enlarged on the chest x-ray and the pulmonary
vascularity is increased. With pulmonary stenosis,
the heart is of normal size or mildly enlarged and
the pulmonary vasculature is normal or decreased.
The more the pulmonary vascularity is increased,
the more likely will there be gross congestive heart
failure and, contrariwise, the more decreased the
pulmonary vascularity the more cyanotic the patient will be.

Echocardiography

The anatomy can be recognized at echocardiographic examination.[27] Fortunately, most of these
patients are discovered in early infancy when the
most precise examinations by echocardiography
are possible. Virtually every detail can be recognized if sufficient time is taken for a complete examination (Fig. 7). There are no specific views that
will uncover the diagnosis. Rather, a systematic
search must be made for the missing ventricle; the
origins of the great vessels must be documented;
the location, description, and competence of the
atrioventricular valves must be established; the
size of a bulboventricular orifice should be measured; the location and severity of possible pulmonary stenosis should be considered; and possible
associated defects must be documented.

Both long-axis and short-axis views of the ventricle are required to document the entrance of
both atrioventricular valves into the single ventricle without an intervening septum. The type of
single ventricle can be determined from the morphology of the chamber (see ch. 13).

The large muscle bundles seen in a single right
ventricle may mimic a septum, especially in the
long-axis view. In the short axis, however, the muscle bundle is surrounded by a cavity for a significant
part of its length, whereas a true septum should

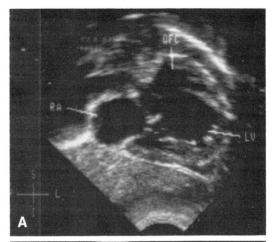

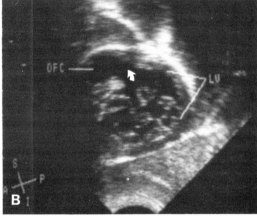

Figure 7. Echocardiograms in the subxiphoid short-axis
view of a patient with a single left ventricle. **A,** The single
left ventricle (LV) and the more superior outflow chamber
(OFC). RA, right atrium. **B,** Both atrioventricular valves are
shown entering the single left ventricle. The superiorly located outflow chamber communicates with the left ventricle
via a large bulboventricular foramen (arrow).

connect with the anterior and/or posterior free wall
for a significant portion of its length.

The size and function of the atrioventricular
valves can be evaluated in an apical or subxiphoid
"four-chamber" view. In patients with an L-loop
single left ventricle, the left atrioventricular (tricuspid) valve is often hypoplastic and stenotic,
whereas in a D-loop single left ventricle, the right
atrioventricular valve (tricuspid) is often regurgitant. Doppler color flow mapping from apical and
parasternal views is ideal for detecting regurgitation, whereas pulsed or continuous-wave Doppler
examination from an apical view is useful for detecting stenosis. In the presence of a large atrial
septal defect, however, a gradient may not be de-
tectible across even a severely stenotic valve.

The great artery alignment is determined as described in chapter 13. With normally related great
arteries, the pulmonary artery is aligned with the

outflow chamber and the aorta with the left ventricle; with transposition, the opposite is true. Rarely, a double-outlet infundibulum may occur when both great arteries are aligned with the outlet chamber.

Pulmonary stenosis is best detected using pulsed or continuous-wave Doppler from an apical or suprasternal notch transducer location. In normally related great arteries it is usually muscular, subvalvar, and/or valvar stenosis. In addition, the ventricular septal defect may be small. When there is transposition of the great arteries, a small ventricular septal defect produces functional subaortic stenosis. In a sick neonate, a gradient may not be detected despite a very small ventricular septal defect. In these very ill infants, the appearance of the defect is more important than the absence of a pressure gradient.

At least two types of ventricular septal defects can be recognized by echocardiography. Subaortic defects are usually associated with hypoplasia and/ or malalignment of the infundibular septum. This defect is immediately below the semilunar valves and often is associated with pulmonary stenosis due to posterior deviation of the infundibular septum. This type of defect is best seen in the long-axis view in a plane that intersects the pulmonary root.

The other type of defect recognizable by echocardiography is a muscular ventricular septal defect closer to the apex of the outflow chamber. Such defects are distant from the semilunar roots and best seen in a more posterior long-axis cut. These defects are commonly obstructive.

Any suggestion of subarterial obstruction should prompt a careful search for coarctation. A high parasternal–parasagittal plane view or a suprasternal notch view is best for examining the arch. When the aorta is leftward, the orientation of the aortic arch may be from left to right, even with a left arch. Therefore, imaging in a sagittal plane view, possibly with counterclockwise rotation, may be necessary to image the arch. Long-segment hypoplasia of the aorta frequently accompanies a discrete juxtaductal coarctation. Consequently, the ascending, transverse, and proximal descending portions of the aorta should be measured. A ductus arteriosus can be sought using the same views that display the arch.

The main pulmonary artery and its branches should be imaged in parasternal and suprasternal notch transverse views, displaying the branches in as much detail as possible. If pulmonary stenosis is present, the pulmonary artery branches should be measured.

Cardiac Catheterization

Every symptomatic patient in whom single ventricle is suspected should undergo cardiac catheterization. Asymptomatic patients (those having mild cyanosis and no congestive heart failure) may be studied some time after the first months of life.

Physiologic information, including the degree and variability of the arterial oxygen saturation, pressure gradients across valves, and the functional effects of obstructive lesions, should be documented in detail. It is important to determine whether there is any pressure gradient across the bulboventricular foramen. Although outflow obstruction may be demonstrable by echocardiography, the degree of obstruction can be determined more precisely by direct pressure measurements, except in a very sick infant whose output is so low that a reliable gradient cannot be measured.

Angiography confirms the anatomy and serves as a good permanent record of the anatomic detail (Fig. 8). This is accomplished best with a balloon angio or pigtail catheter positioned at the apex of the ventricle, antegrade or retrograde. With biplane filming, with the patient in the frontal or hepatoclavicular position, depending on the precatheterization echocardiogram, 2.0–2.5 ml/kg of body weight of contrast are injected as rapidly as possible. The anatomic variability of single ventricle is such that prediction of the anatomy of the great vessel or bulboventricular foramen is difficult. Frequently, subsequent atriograms, ventriculograms, aortograms, and pulmonary arteriograms are needed.

MANAGEMENT

Initially, management is concerned with lifesaving measures. Babies with pulmonary atresia who survive because there is a patent ductus arteriosus may be in grave difficulty when the ductus begins

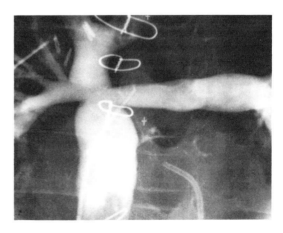

Figure 8. Angiogram in a patient with a functioning bidirectional Glenn procedure showing the anastomosis of the superior vena cava to the right pulmonary artery. There is simultaneous opacification of the proximal and distal superior vena cava and the right and left main pulmonary arteries.

to close on schedule. Prostaglandins are lifesaving in this situation, and usually an early Blalock shunt is necessary. Babies in congestive heart failure may need a pulmonary artery band simply to survive beyond the neonatal period.

With a more stable infant, it may be necessary to deal with noncardiac anomalies and other cardiac anomalies first. A tracheoesophageal fistula may be the major problem and require attention first. Interruption of the aorta or coarctation of the aorta may require surgical attention. If there is any suggestion of a restrictive bulboventricular foramen, a subaortic bypass procedure to provide an unobstructed outlet to the aorta must be contemplated.[6,17,28] The timing and technical details of such a bypass are a matter of debate.[7,16,18,25,26] It is best to deal with any obstruction to the systemic blood flow as soon as possible because it tends to get worse and because severity is often dangerously underestimated in the sick infant with low cardiac output.

The management goal for infants with single ventricle is for them to arrive at a suitable age, with sufficient growth that the Fontan procedure can be performed successfully.[9,13] To be a suitable candidate for a Fontan procedure, the cardiac status must include acceptable pulmonary artery mean pressure and pulmonary resistance (see ch. 54), good ventricular function, competent atrioventricular valves and undistorted pulmonary arteries. Generally, this amounts to providing adequate pulmonary blood flow with the least distortion of the pulmonary arteries. The ideal pulmonary blood flow is approximately twice the systemic flow and produces an arterial saturation averaging in excess of 75% but less than 85%.

It is easier to describe these goals than to accomplish them. Often there is prolonged hospitalization and a difficult struggle to gain a growing and an acceptably well child. Virtually all surviving infants come to cardiac catheterization in the second half of the first year of life to determine how effective the surgical maneuvers have been. Further surgery may be needed to correct residual problems.

The baby who has grown well, who has acceptable pulmonary artery pressures and resistance, and who has undistorted pulmonary arteries and competent atrioventricular valves is a candidate for a Fontan procedure or one of its variants (see ch. 54). Separation of the pulmonary venous and systemic venous circulations at the cavo-atrial level needs to be planned. Whether to leave the patient with two systemic atrioventricular valves or to baffle the pulmonary venous circulation to the best of the two valves, closing an incompetent one, must be decided (Fig. 6). The systemic venous blood is channeled directly to the pulmonary artery, bypassing the ventricle. Occasionally, because of distorted pulmonary arteries, it is easier to connect

the right atrium to the left pulmonary artery while the right lung is connected to the superior vena cava, as in a Glenn procedure, leaving the cava in communication with the right atrium. All of the possible variations on Glenn and Fontan connections are used to direct most of the systemic venous blood into the pulmonary artery in patients with single ventricle (see Fig. 5, p. 744).

Survival with a Fontan procedure is good in patients who meet the criteria for the surgery.[19] For patients in whom the indications are borderline and, nonetheless, surgery is undertaken, the chances for survival are somewhat less. The immediate complications of Fontan surgery are discussed elsewhere (see ch. 54).

At the present time it is not possible to predict the percentage of infants with single ventricle who will be able to survive with anatomy and physiology suitable for Fontan surgery. First-year survival for patients with single ventricle was in the order of 50% in the 1970s; at the present time mortality is substantially better (Exhibit 1).

Intraventricular septation is an innovative surgical management for single ventricle without pulmonary stenosis (51% of children with single ventricle) (Exhibit 1). In the future this operation may come into more general use if satisfactory survival can be documented.[8,15,20,24]

COURSE

Natural survival with single ventricle is poor.[12,22] In the early 1970s, using palliative operations (pulmonary artery band or an arterial–pulmonary artery shunt), survival was not much better (47% mortality).[12,23] At the present time the same palliative surgery is associated with considerably improved mortality (Exhibit 1). Still, as of 1988, less than 40% of the patients first known to us after 1973 have had the Fontan operation and only 50% of the children who have survived beyond the age of 4 years have had this surgery attempted (Exhibit 1). It is clear that the child born with a single ventricle during the 1973–87 era faced not only significant infant mortality but also an outcome from palliative surgery that might prohibit a possible Fontan operation. With the present-day management of infants with single ventricle aiming toward a Fontan operation, greater salvage of these patients is expected and seems likely.

For some patients, the development of increasing restriction to blood flow through the bulboventricular foramen is a matter of serious concern. Usually, this occurs in patients with a pulmonary artery band[10] or, rarely, with pulmonary stenosis, and it results in intolerable, suprasystemic pressure in the single ventricle, excessive hypertrophy, and reduced ventricular compliance.

Atrioventricular valve regurgitation (right- or

left-sided) is encountered and may be progressive.[21] This does not preclude a Fontan operation, because the incompetent valve can be surgically excluded or closed and all pulmonary venous flow baffled toward the other valve (Fig. 6).

Patients with a single left ventricle have had several kinds of problems as they grow older. Complete heart block develops in 12% of patients with single left ventricle (Exhibit 1) and is, fortunately, surprisingly well tolerated. These patients are managed with pacemaker implantation, in the belief that the average systemic venous pressure will be lower with a higher heart rate.

Patients who survive the Fontan procedure do not have normal physical ability. The right atrial pressure is high; the patient exists in the equivalent of mild right-sided congestive heart failure. Despite their ability to engage in vigorous sports and to hold physically demanding jobs, their measured exercise tolerance is less than normal and may progressively lessen with increasing age.

After Fontan operation, atrial arrhythmias have been particularly common (more than 50% of the patients). Inability to maintain the subjectively desired level of exercise has been a problem for some of the males. Nonetheless, the number of pink patients, with stable hemodynamics, who are happily working and supporting themselves is gratifying. So far, pregnancy seems to be tolerated and other major surgical procedures have been undertaken safely.

REFERENCES

1. Alboliras ET, Porter CJ, Danielson GK, et al: Results of the modified Fontan operation for congenital heart lesions in patients without preoperative sinus rhythm. J Am Coll Cardiol 6:228–233, 1985.
2. Anderson RH, Becker AE, Freedom RM, et al: Problems in the nomenclature of the univentricular heart. Herz 4:97–106, 1979.
3. Anderson RH, Macartney FJ, Tynan M, et al: Univentricular atrioventricular connection: the single ventricle trap unsprung. Pediatr Cardiol 4:273–280, 1983.
4. Anderson RH, Becker AE, Tynan M, et al: The univentricular atrioventricular connection: getting to the root of a thorny problem. Am J Cardiol 54:822–828, 1984.
5. Barber G, Hagler DJ, Edwards WD, et al: Surgical repair of univentricular heart (double inlet left ventricle) with obstructed anterior subaortic outlet chamber. J Am Coll Cardiol 4:771–778, 1984.
6. Damus PS: Letter to the editor. Ann Thorac Surg 20:724–725, 1975.
7. DeLeon SY, Idriss FS, Ilbawi MN, et al: The Damus-Stansel-Kaye procedure. Should the aortic valve or subaortic valve region be closed? J Thorac Cardiovasc Surg 91:747–753, 1986.
8. Ebert PA: Staged partitioning of single ventricle. J Thorac Cardiovasc Surg 88:908–913, 1984.
9. Fontan F, Baudet E: Surgical repair of tricuspid atresia. Thorax 26:240–248, 1971.
10. Freedom RM: The dinosaur and banding of the main pulmonary trunk in the heart with functionally one ven-

tricle and transposition of the great arteries: a saga of evolution and caution. J Am Coll Cardiol 10:427–429, 1987.
11. Freedom RM, Benson LN, Smallhorn JF, et al: Subaortic stenosis, the univentricular heart, and banding of the pulmonary artery: an analysis of the courses of 43 patients with univentricular heart palliated by pulmonary artery banding. Circulation 73:758–764, 1986.
12. Fyler DC, Buckley LP, Hellenbrand WE, et al: Report of the New England Regional Infant Cardiac Program. Pediatrics 65(Suppl):376–460, 1980.
13. Gale AW, Danielson GK, McGoon DC, et al: Modified Fontan operation for univentricular heart and complicated congenital lesions. J Thorac Cardiovasc Surg 78:831–838, 1979.
14. Holmes WF: Case of malformation of the heart. Trans Med-Chir Soc Edinburgh 1:252, 1824.
15. Imai Y: Personal communication, September 1, 1989.
16. Jonas RA, Castaneda AR, Lang P: Single ventricle (single- or double-inlet) complicated by subaortic stenosis: surgical options in infancy. Ann Thorac Surg 39:361–366, 1985.
17. Kaye MP: Anatomic correction for transposition of great arteries. Mayo Clin Proc 50:638–640, 1975.
18. Lin AE, Laks H, Barber G, et al: Subaortic obstruction in complex congenital heart disease: management by proximal pulmonary artery to ascending aorta end to side anastomosis. J Am Coll Cardiol 7:617–624, 1986.
19. Mayer JE, Helgason H, Jonas RA, et al: Extending the limits for modified Fontan procedures. J Thorac Cardiovasc Surg 92:1021–1028, 1986.
20. McKay R, Pacifico AD, Blackstone EH, et al: Septation of the univentricular heart with left anterior subaortic outlet chamber. J Thorac Cardiovasc Surg 84:77–87, 1982.
21. Moak JP, Gersony WM: Progressive atrioventricular valvular regurgitation in single ventricle. Am J Cardiol 59:656–658, 1987.
22. Moodie DS, Ritter DG, Tajik AJ, et al: Long-term follow-up in the unoperated univentricular heart. Am J Cardiol 53:1124–1128, 1984.
23. Moodie DS, Ritter DG, Tajik AJ, et al: Long-term follow-up after palliative operation for univentricular heart. Am J Cardiol 53:1648–1651, 1984.
24. Pacifico A, Naftel DC, Kirklin JM, et al: Ventricular septation within the spectrum of surgery for double inlet ventricles. J Jpn Assoc Thorac Surg 33:593–601, 1985.
25. Penkoske PA, Freedom RM, Williams WG, et al: Surgical palliation of subaortic stenosis in the univentricular heart. J Thorac Cardiovasc Surg 87:767–781, 1984.
26. Rothman A, Lang P, Lock JE, et al: Surgical management of subaortic obstruction in single left ventricle and tricuspid atresia. J Am Coll Cardiol 10:421–426, 1987.
27. Sahn DJ, Harder JR, Freedom RM, et al: Cross-sectional echocardiographic diagnosis and subclassification of univentricular hearts: imaging studies of atrioventricular valves, septal structures and rudimentary outflow chambers. Circulation 66:1070–1077, 1982.
28. Stansel HC: A new operation for D-loop transposition of the great vessels. Ann Thorac Surg 19:565–567, 1975.
29. Streeter GL: Quoted by Van Praagh R, Plett JA, Van Praagh S.[32]
30. Van Praagh R, David I, Van Praagh S: What is a ventricle? The single ventricle trap. Pediatr Cardiol 2:79–84, 1982.
31. Van Praagh R, Ongley PA, Swan HJC: Anatomic types of single or common ventricle in man: morphologic and geometric aspects of 60 necropsied cases. Am J Cardiol 13:367–386, 1964.
32. Van Praagh R, Plett JA, Van Praagh S: Single ventricle: pathology, embryology, terminology, and classification. Herz 4:113–150, 1979.

Chapter 43

TRICUSPID ATRESIA

Donald C. Fyler, M.D.

DEFINITION

Tricuspid atresia is characterized by absence of the tricuspid valve and hypoplasia of the right ventricle. By convention, patients are divided into those with or without transposition of the great arteries, and whether or not there is pulmonary stenosis or atresia (Fig. 1).

PREVALENCE

Tricuspid atresia ranked 14th among the 2,251 infants hospitalized for congenital heart disease in New England, ranging from 0.034 to 0.185/1000 live births in several studies (see ch. 18, Table 1).[31] It was the 18th most common congenital heart lesion in the Boston Children's Hospital series (see ch. 18, Table 2) and was found in 1.5% of neonates in The Hospital for Sick Children in Toronto.[33]

ANATOMY

While rarely an atretic tricuspid valve or severely stenotic tricuspid valve is found, in the majority of these children there is no suggestion that a valve ever existed or that the atrium was ever aligned toward the right ventricle.[37] Egress from the right atrium is through an atrial defect or, more often, a patent foramen ovale. In patients with normally related great arteries, entry to the pulmonary circulation occurs either through a ventricular defect and a hypoplastic right ventricle or, rarely, through a patent ductus arteriosus as the sole source of pulmonary blood flow. The right ventricle is variably small; in some patients it consists of no more than a channel from the left ventricle to the pulmonary artery. The passage through the ventricular defect to the pulmonary artery is usually restrictive; there may be pulmonary valvar stenosis, subvalvar obstruction, or pulmonary atresia. Usually, the ventricular defect is small; it tends to

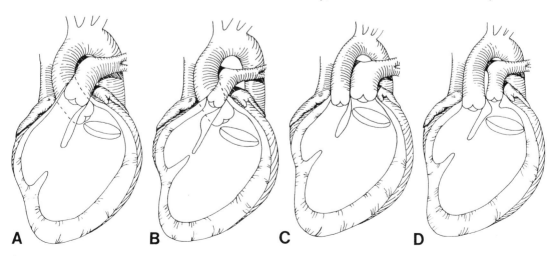

A   **B**   **C**   **D**

Figure 1. Tricuspid atresia is usually classified according to the absence (**A,C**) or the presence (**B,D**) of pulmonary stenosis and the presence of transposition of the great arteries (**C,D**). The ventricular septal defect varies considerably in size, and over time tends to get smaller. It may provide obstruction to pulmonary blood flow (**B**) or in the presence of transposition obstruct outflow to the aorta (functional subaortic stenosis).

get smaller with time and ultimately may close. The ductus arteriosus usually has a small diameter and closes on schedule. In a few individuals (14%) the passage of blood to the main pulmonary artery is completely unobstructed.

When the great arteries are transposed, the ventricular defect carries blood to the aorta and, in some patients with single ventricle, it is directly analogous to the bulboventricular foramen (see ch. 42). A comparatively small ventricular defect suffices for patients without transposition (pulmonary blood flow usually being less than normal), but when there is transposition the entire cardiac output must pass through the ventricular defect to the aorta. Pulmonary stenosis or pulmonary atresia is common (60%). Patients with tricuspid atresia and transposition of the great arteries (40%) are more likely to have excessive pulmonary blood flow than those with normally positioned great arteries.

At Children's Hospital in Boston, about two-thirds of our patients with transposition of the great arteries and tricuspid atresia had pulmonary stenosis or pulmonary atresia (Exhibit 1). The other third may have had, in addition, coarctation of the aorta or an interrupted aortic arch, usually associated with unobstructed pulmonary blood flow.

In some patients with tricuspid atresia the atrial appendages lie immediately side by side (juxtaposition of the atrial appendages), more often toward the left than the right.[26]

A right aortic arch is seen in 9% of patients.[33]

Patients with L-looped ventricles may have left-sided (tricuspid) atrioventricular valve atresia and a diminutive, left-sided right ventricle. This circulatory physiology is comparable to mitral atresia. When there is an L-loop ventricle and mitral atresia with a diminutive, right-sided left ventricle, the circulatory difficulties are comparable to those in patients with tricuspid atresia.

PHYSIOLOGY

The entire cardiac output must pass through the foramen ovale; the adequacy of this passage has been questioned by several observers,[22] but fewer than 6% of our patients with untouched foramina ovale have had pressure gradients of more than a few mm Hg between the two atria. The streams of pulmonary venous return and systemic venous return join in the left atrium, passing to the left ventricle, which functions as a single ventricle. This prompts the terms "functionally single ventricle" or "univentricular" heart.[1] Blood passes from the left ventricle to the aorta and, via the ventricular defect, to the diminutive right ventricle and pulmonary artery (Fig. 2). Obstruction to flow by a restrictive ventricular defect, by right ventricular outflow, by the pulmonary valve and, in early infancy, by persistent elevation of fetal pulmonary

resistance determines the amount of pulmonary blood flow. In general, the course of patients with tricuspid atresia is characterized by increasing cyanosis because of progressively diminishing pulmonary blood flow, most often because the ventricular defect gets smaller. Rarely, mostly in those with transposition of the great arteries, there is little obstruction, and pulmonary blood flow is excessive, to the point of producing congestive failure. The ductus arteriosus provides some blood flow to the pulmonary circulation after birth but most often it closes on schedule.

Infants with transposition of the great arteries also face the problem of "subaortic stenosis" because of an obstructive and closing ventricular defect (Fig. 2). As the ventricular defect gets smaller, there is increasing obstruction to outflow to the aorta. To provide adequate cardiac output, left ventricular pressure must rise. This increases pulmonary blood flow, ultimately resulting in congestive heart failure. This has been proposed as a virtually certain outcome for these children.[11] For unknown reasons the ventricular defect (bulboventricular foramen) becomes more obstructive when the pulmonary artery has been banded.[11]

CLINICAL MANIFESTATIONS

Most patients with tricuspid atresia are discovered in early infancy because of cyanosis or a murmur. A few with excessive pulmonary blood flow have symptoms of congestive failure. The age at presentation depends on the pulmonary blood flow and because it is usually less than optimal, cyanosis is the most common presenting symptom. Those with maximal obstruction who are dependent on ductal blood flow become deeply cyanotic when the ductus closes (50% of infants with tricuspid atresia were first seen in the first week of life).[12] Others gradually become more cyanotic as the months go by. When the cyanosis becomes intense, cyanotic spells may occur.

Hepatomegaly is rarely a notable observation in the more cyanotic children, although occasionally an obstructed foramen ovale is discovered by this means. Hepatomegaly is regularly seen in those with minimal cyanosis, tachypnea, and congestive heart failure because of unfettered pulmonary blood flow. There is usually, but not invariably, a moderate systolic murmur and the second heart sound is single.

Electrocardiography

The electrocardiogram shows a leftward-superior axis with, most often, left dominance. Some patients with transposition of the great arteries show a more nearly normal axis. Left-sided S-T and T wave abnormalities may be present from birth. The contrast among electrocardiograms of

Exhibit 1

Boston Children's Hospital Experience 1973–1987
There were 154 children with tricuspid atresia. Eleven had their initial surgery elsewhere; 10 have had no surgery at all; 44 were first seen prior to 1973. With incomplete follow-up, 33 are known dead.
The age on initial contact, excluding those first seen before 1973 and those first seen in another cardiac institution, ranged from 1 day to 27 years and averaged less than 1 year.

Types of Tricuspid Atresia

Other Lesions	Normal Great Arteries n = 115	Transposed Great Arteries n = 39	Total 154
Coarctation of Aorta	4	13	17
Pulmonary Atresia	30	7	37
Pulmonary Stenosis	47	25	72

Initial Surgery

Type of Operation	Normal Great Arteries n = 108	Transposed Great Arteries n = 35	Total n = 143
Pulmonary Artery Band	16	16	32
Coarctation Repair	2	9	11
Glenn Procedure	23	6	29
Arterial-Pulmonary Shunt	54	17	71
Bypass Subaortic Obstruction	1	7	8

Fontan operation was carried out at Boston Children's Hospital for 89 children with tricuspid atresia, 69 without transposed great arteries, and 20 with transposed great arteries. Some patients had more than one procedure at the initial surgery.

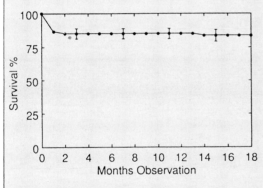

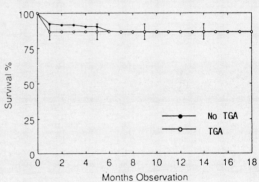

Life-table analysis of the first 18 months survival following Fontan operation. The analysis starts with the time of the Fontan operation.

Life-table analysis of survival of patients with tricuspid atresia with and without transposition of the great arteries, irrespective of treatment. The analysis starts with the first observation at Children's Hospital in Boston.

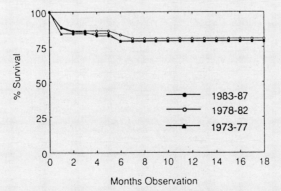

Life-table analysis of survival of patients with tricuspid atresia by year of first contact with patient: 1973–77, n = 20; 1978–82, n = 37; 1983–87, n = 50. For this purpose, 3 patients had flawed data. The remarkable similarity among the time periods was an unexpected result. It is suspected that initial treatment has varied little over the years and that the effect of Fontan operations requires a longer period of observation to affect such an analysis.

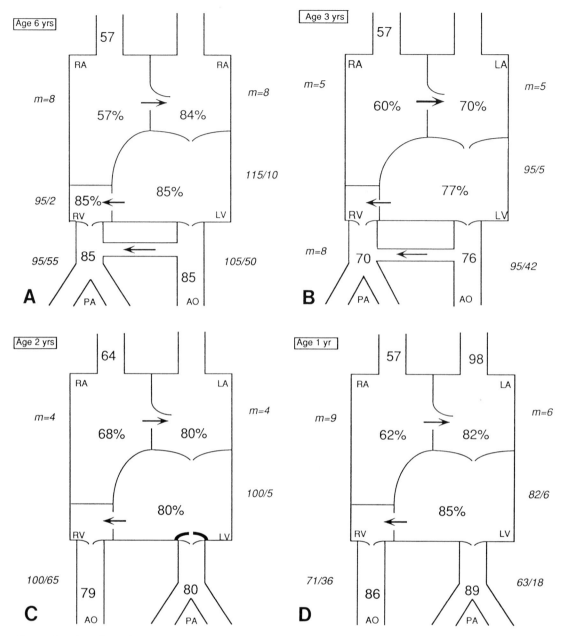

Figure 2. Physiologic diagrams of patients with tricuspid atresia. **A,** Tricuspid atresia with normally positioned great arteries and a pulmonary artery pressure that approaches the systemic level is unusual and may require a pulmonary artery banding operation to control congestive heart failure and prevent pulmonary vascular disease. **B,** Tricuspid atresia with normally related great arteries is usually associated with low pulmonary artery pressure either because of a small ventricular defect or, less often, because of pulmonary stenosis. Tricuspid atresia and transposition of the great arteries may be associated with pulmonary stenosis (**C**) or without pulmonary stenosis (**D**). Italics, mm Hg; %, oxygen saturation; RA, right atrium; RV, right ventricle; LA, left atrium; LV, left ventricle; PA, pulmonary artery; AO, aorta.

patients with tricuspid atresia (leftward-superior axis), pulmonary atresia with intact ventricular septum (normal axis), and pulmonary atresia with ventricular defect (right axis) is clinically useful in arriving at a presumptive diagnosis (see ch. 40).

Chest X-ray

The heart size is proportionate to the pulmonary blood flow. Because the average patient has relatively limited blood flow, the heart size tends to be small or minimally enlarged; the resemblance to patients with tetralogy of Fallot is often striking. With increased pulmonary blood flow, the heart becomes proportionately enlarged.

Echocardiography

The anatomic features of tricuspid atresia are readily documented with modern echocardiographic technique. The absence of a tricuspid orifice, the passage of blood from the right to the left atrium through the atrial septum, a ventricular defect, a diminutive right ventricle, and whether the great vessels are transposed can be documented and any pulmonary stenosis can be observed.

Tricuspid atresia is usually obvious from the initial subxiphoid view. Absence of the tricuspid valve and the marked hypoplasia of the right ventricle can be seen in the long-axis scans as well as the apical views. Usually the atrioventricular junction is filled with fibrous tissue. Occasionally the tricuspid valve is present but imperforate because of leaflet fusion. In such cases the valve leaflets may move with the cardiac cycle so that a Doppler examination is required to determine if the valve is patent. An uncommon cause of tricuspid atresia is complete alignment of a common atrioventricular valve with the left ventricle so that the tricuspid portion of the valve is atretic. The clue to this diagnosis is the presence of a primum atrial septal defect seen in an apical or subxiphoid "four-chamber" view (Fig. 3).

Bulging of the septum primum into the left atrium can be seen in a subxiphoid, short-axis view. The right-to-left atrial shunt can be documented by Doppler examination in this view as well. The hypoplastic right ventricle and the ventricular septal defect can be seen more leftward in the subxiphoid short-axis scan. The ventriculo-arterial alignment can be easily determined from subxiphoid or parasternal views (see ch. 13).

Pulmonary stenosis is common in infants with normally related great arteries and is usually due to subvalvar muscular hypertrophy and/or a small ventricular septal defect. The pulmonary valve is usually well formed and nearly normal in size. The severity of pulmonary stenosis should be assessed with Doppler examination from a subxiphoid or apical transducer location. In patients with transposition of the great arteries, a small ventricular

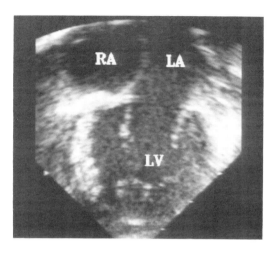

Figure 3. Echocardiogram in a patient with tricuspid atresia, apical view. Note the absence of the right atrioventricular valve and the bowing of the atrial septum into the left atrium. RA, right atrium; LA, left atrium; LV, left ventricle.

septal defect or midcavity obstruction of the outflow chamber produces subaortic stenosis. The ventricular septal defect and subaortic area should be imaged and measured in at least two planes, and Doppler interrogation should be performed from subxiphoid, apical, and parasternal transducer locations. If subaortic obstruction is documented by the Doppler examination or if the ventricular septal defect and outflow chamber appear small by imaging, then coarctation should be suspected.

The aortic arch should be imaged in the suprasternal notch and parasternal-parasagittal planes. If the ductus arteriosus is widely patent, coarctation cannot be completely excluded. Right-to-left shunting in the ductus may indicate a ductus-dependent systemic circulation.

The pulmonary artery branches should be imaged and measured in parasternal and suprasternal notch short-axis views.

Mitral valve prolapse with mitral regurgitation can be seen in some older patients with tricuspid atresia.

Cardiac Catheterization

Usually, the anatomy is well demonstrated by echocardiography, and therefore, cardiac catheterization is rarely needed unless there is concern about the accuracy of the diagnosis. On the other hand, if there is transposition of the great arteries, cardiac catheterization is required because estimates of the degree of obstruction posed by the ventricular septal defect are difficult when the cardiac output is depressed, as is often the case on first examination. The echocardiographic view of the size of the ventricular defect and the pressure measurements should be reconciled because obstruction or potential obstruction will determine the surgical options.

Patients who are being considered for Fontan surgery must have, in addition to good-sized pulmonary arteries, normal pulmonary arteriolar resistance, an adequately functioning atrioventricular valve, and good ventricular function. Because slight differences in pressure and function make a great deal of difference, all patients who are being considered for this operation should undergo cardiac catheterization preoperatively. It is important to demonstrate that the pulmonary arteries are undistorted and that the systemic venous drainage, particularly of the upper torso, will be easily managed. Whether there is a left superior vena cava and whether it is connected to the right vena cava is necessary information. How much drainage occurs by the azygos or hemiazygos veins may influence the decision, as may the location of the atrial appendages. Measurements of pulmonary artery pressure must be carefully repeated. In general, pulmonary artery mean pressure in excess of 19 mm Hg or pulmonary resistance greater than 2.5 units is associated with a greater chance for a poor outcome.[24] In theory, accurate measurement of pulmonary vascular resistance should provide the most reliable guide; the problem is to acquire precise data. Entry to the pulmonary circulation may be limited by the anatomy. Pulmonary vein wedge pressures may be the only available means (albeit indirect) for estimating the pulmonary arterial pressure.

MANAGEMENT

The goal of management for patients with tricuspid atresia is to achieve a successful Fontan operation.[9,19] To do this, it is required that: (1) there is no significant pulmonary arterial distortion from prior surgery (a potential problem because of prior shunting or banding operations), (2) there is normal pulmonary arteriolar vascular resistance (also a potential problem because of prior shunting procedures or inadequate pulmonary artery bands),[17] (3) there is good left ventricular function, and (4) there is a well-functioning mitral valve.

Ideally, a Fontan operation is accomplished as early in life as is possible, but, unfortunately, this operation is not tolerated well in early infancy. In the first months of life, there is pulmonary arteriolar muscle available to constrict and cause undesirable elevation of pulmonary resistance. The venous structures are small, and unobstructed flow to the lungs is difficult to achieve. Problems with recurrent pleural effusion are more common in this age group. The observed difficulties with Fontan surgery in infants seem to decrease with age, so it may be best to put off this intervention until the age of 4 or 5 years if things are going well clinically.

Strictly speaking, the problem may not be age but rather factors associated with age. Multivariate analysis shows that age is not a factor, although elevated pulmonary resistance, distorted pulmonary arteries, and left ventricular dysfunction and hypertrophy are.[24]

Because there are several hurdles between recognizing the diagnosis and a successful Fontan operation, the average patient requires two surgical procedures and only about 52% of the patients reach the intended goal.

Normally Positioned Great Arteries

The average patient with normally positioned great arteries is seen early in infancy because of cyanosis caused by decreased pulmonary blood flow. In the neonatal period, prostaglandin E-1 may be useful to maintain a survivable arterial oxygen level while management is being planned. An arterial shunt is often required, although occasionally patients (14%) can be managed for months and sometimes years without surgery. The shunt should provide sufficient pulmonary blood flow to allow growth, while not promoting pulmonary vascular changes because of excessive flow.[27] An ideal shunt (a Blalock-Taussig procedure), does not deform the pulmonary arteries and is readily accessible for take down and reconstruction at a later date.

Occasionally children (14%) with normally positioned great arteries require pulmonary artery banding because of unrestricted pulmonary blood flow and congestive heart failure. Most patients become increasingly cyanotic, usually because of decreasing size of the ventricular defect.[31]

Babies who do not require surgery until after the first birthday may be managed initially with a Glenn procedure but, even though this is desirable, it is an unlikely possibility because most infants require an operation before then.

Because excessive shunting and pulmonary artery distortion are sometimes progressive and may interfere with a later Fontan operation, the results of surgery should be reevaluated in detail 6 months later even if the patient is doing well. Reoperation to correct pulmonary artery deformities, to adjust the amount of pulmonary blood flow through a shunt, or to adjust a pulmonary band may be needed. Cardiac catheterization to dilate pulmonary arterial obstructions with balloon catheters may be desirable prior to the Fontan operation. Cardiac catheterization is mandatory immediately preceding Fontan surgery to document the precise physiologic circumstances, the size and shape of the pulmonary arteries, and the competency of the mitral valve and the left ventricle. Any suggestion of elevation of pulmonary resistance is a matter of concern (i.e., pulmonary resistance levels of 2.5 units or more). Unrestricted blood flow to both lungs is a major requirement for a successful Fontan operation. Nuclear scanning procedures as part of the pre-Fontan work-up are useful to document the relative flow of blood to both lungs. Although patients with a single functioning lung have had successful Fontan procedures, free flow to both lungs is highly desirable.

Occasionally patients have physiologic findings which are borderline and yet not deemed prohibitive for Fontan surgery. A "bidirectional" Glenn operation (see Fig. 8, ch. 42) the partial equivalent of a Fontan operation but with less than the entire cardiac output passing though the lungs, can be very helpful, particularly as an intermediate operation. Of course, these children remain cyanotic, usually only slightly, and should be considered for further surgery later. If the child has done well and demonstrated good physiologic measurements, redirecting the circulation, based on the Fontan principle, can be completed (see ch. 54).

Transposed Great Vessels

Children with transposition of the great arteries often require pulmonary artery banding (25%). This has a tendency to cause pulmonary artery distortion and occasionally to disrupt the blood flow to one or both lungs. Further, the bulboventricular foramen (ventricular septal defect) tends to become smaller when a pulmonary artery band is in place.[11] Obstruction at the ventricular defect is the equivalent of subaortic stenosis in these children and can represent a major problem (Fig. 4). Enlarging the ventricular defect often leads to complete heart block[32] and, therefore, it is preferable to bypass the restrictive ventricular defect by creating an aortopulmonary window.[5,16,18,23,28-30,32,35] Having established free communication between the ascending aorta and the main pulmonary artery, the distal main pulmonary artery is ligated and pulmonary blood flow is established by an aortopulmonary connection, usually a modified Blalock shunt. Both semilunar valves now serve the systemic circulation. The pulmonary valve functions well in the systemic circuit.[3] If there is a proximal pulmonary artery band, it may be difficult to establish a satisfactory aortopulmonary window. For this reason, when the child is first seen (usually in the neonatal period), it is desirable to decide whether a bypassing procedure should be the first operation or whether a band is likely to be successful without need for a later aortopulmonary window. Because there is inadequate information that allows a prediction that a banding procedure would be best and there is information that pulmonary artery bands tend to promote subaortic obstruction, most borderline patients receive some variant of the aortopulmonary bypassing window at the present time.

Patients with coarctation of the aorta or interrupted aortic arch (one-third of patients with transposition of the great arteries) may need attention to that defect first. These are the very patients who are also likely to need relief from an obstructing subaortic defect.

The possible need for further palliative surgery, before the definitive Fontan procedure, requires close follow-up. Sometime within 6 months of initial surgery, the result should be carefully evaluated. Resting arterial oxygen saturation insufficient for adequate growth and development (less than 75%), objective limitation of growth and development, or congestive heart failure are adequate reasons for even earlier reevaluation with echocardiograms and cardiac catheterization. Based on the echocardiographic findings, it is possible to decide which children should undergo cardiac catheterization ahead of schedule, but echocardiograms cannot be taken as sufficiently accurate to make cardiac catheterization unnecessary if unexplained clinical problems exist. Regardless of the symptoms, cardiac catheterization within 6 months after initial or repeated surgery is appropriate and is required prior to a Fontan operation.

The term Fontan operation is used here, loosely, to describe any redirection of the entire systemic venous return to the pulmonary circulation. One or more connections of the systemic veins to the pulmonary arteries through conduits, homografts, or by direct anastomosis to the right ventricle, main or branch pulmonary arteries, including a combination of Glenn procedures and Fontan operations, may be used. The greater the access of the systemic venous blood to the pulmonary circulation the better. The perceived need for providing artificial caval, tricuspid, or pulmonary valves has not turned out to be as vital as originally suspected and whether the connection is atrioventricular or atriopulmonary does not seem to matter.[21] Combinations of Glenn and Fontan procedures connecting to opposite lungs are as effective as any other modification of the Fontan principle, or may be even more so. Direct connection without conduits or homografts is desirable because the requirement for replacement of conduits or homografts seems to be only a matter of time.

After the Fontan operation in any of its modifications has been accomplished, the patient should be followed for possible obstruction in the venous-to-pulmonary artery connection. Obstruction of a conduit is common; an obstructing inner peel develops within a year in some patients. The high incidence of late appearance of atrial arrhythmias (approximately 50% of patients in the first 10 years) requires that all patients get regular Holter monitoring.

Since the Fontan procedure became available, only 50% of the patients who were initially candidates for this operation have come to definitive surgery. There is a significant loss of patients who

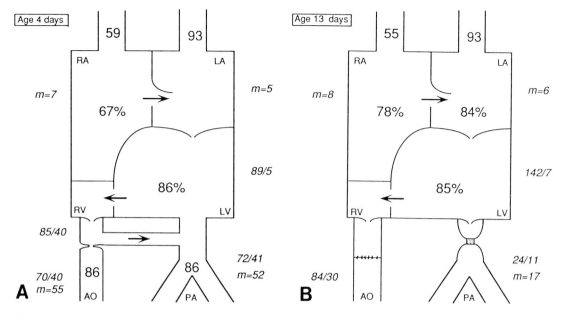

Figure 4. Catheterization data from a patient with tricuspid atresia, transposition of the great arteries, a patent ductus arteriosus, and coarctation of the aorta. **A,** At 4 days. **B,** After repair of the coarctation, ligation of the ductus, and a pulmonary artery banding procedure the infant was not doing well. A second catheterization (age 13 days) was carried out that showed that the ventricular defect was so small that it obstructed blood flow to the aorta. In effect, the infant had subaortic obstruction that had been masked prior to surgery.

started out as likely candidates. Some of these are not candidates for a variety of acquired anatomic or physiologic reasons; others have died. Still others are doing so well with shunting operations that a Fontan operation is not presently considered justifiable. This is a decision the author understands, but believes it is not likely to provide the best outcome for most patients.

COURSE

Survival of untreated patients with tricuspid atresia to the age of 1 year is poor (in the order of 10–20%).[7,33] With shunting procedures or pulmonary artery bands, as needed, the survival is better (53%).[12] Boston's Children's Hospital experience is notably better (Exhibit 1).

While Fontan surgery for these patients is clearly successful, the outcome for the average infant born with tricuspid atresia has not improved as much as might be wished. Of the babies with tricuspid atresia, 85% survive 18 months after being seen and 85% survive the Fontan operation for a similar period (Exhibit 1).[36]

Patients with successful Fontan operations have a nearly normal life;[6,10,13,20,34] most can support themselves with gainful occupations. Recently, with much concern, a young woman was shepherded through an uneventful pregnancy with no obvious difficulty. Some participate in sports, but most find themselves limited by the restricted car-

diac output that is associated with this procedure.[2,8,14] Others have problems of chronic atrial hypertension and, particularly, atrial arrhythmias. Problems with chronic pleural effusions and even ascites are seen.

The operation has been done at all ages. Patients in the third or fourth decades seem to do as well as the young.[15] It is remarkable that these people with the equivalent of mild, chronic, right-sided congestive heart failure do so well for so long. To date, late deaths after Fontan surgery are uncommon.

Without solid information the author recommends that individuals with Fontan operations avoid living at high altitudes because of the dangers of pulmonary hypertension. Transitory episodes at high altitudes seem to be tolerated well and airplane travel has not been a problem. Any measures that will preserve lung function (or prevent pulmonary hypertension) seem justified. Cigarette smoking is to be avoided.

It is well established that, in a small number of patients, the Glenn operation is associated with the development of pulmonary arteriovenous fistulas.[25] The obvious possibility that this may occur in patients with Fontan operations has been suggested.[4]

REFERENCES

1. Anderson RH, Macartney FJ, Tynan M, et al: Univentricular atrioventricular connection: the single ventricle trap unsprung. Pediatr Cardiol 4:273–280, 1983.
2. Ben Shachar G, Fuhrman BP, Wang Y, et al: Rest and

exercise hemodynamics after the Fontan procedure. Circulation 65:1043–1048, 1982.

3. Chin AJ, Barber G, Helton JG, et al: Fate of the pulmonic valve after proximal pulmonary artery-to-ascending aorta anastomosis for aortic outflow obstruction. Am J Cardiol 62:435–438, 1988.

4. Cloutier A, Ash JM, Smallhorn JF, et al: Abnormal distribution of pulmonary blood flow after the Glenn shunt or Fontan procedure: risk of development of arteriovenous fistulae. Circulation 72:471–479, 1985.

5. Damus PS: A proposed operation for transposition of the great vessels. Ann Thorac Surg 20:724–725, 1975.

6. deBrux JL, Zannini L, Binet JP, et al: Tricuspid atresia: results of treatment in 115 children. J Thorac Cardiovasc Surg 85:440–446, 1983.

7. Dick M, Fyler DC, Nadas AS: Tricuspid atresia: the clinical course in 101 patients. Am J Cardiol 36:327–337, 1975.

8. Driscoll DJ, Danielson GK, Puga FJ, et al: Exercise tolerance and cardiorespiratory response to exercise after the Fontan operation for triscuspid atresia or functional single ventricle. J Am Coll Cardiol 7:1087–1094, 1986.

9. Fontan F, Baudet E: Surgical repair of tricuspid atresia. Thorax 26:240–248, 1971.

10. Fontan F, Deville C, Quaegebeur J, et al: Repair of tricuspid atresia in 100 patients. J Thorac Cardiovasc Surg 85:647–660, 1983.

11. Freedom RM, Benson LN, Smallhorn JF, et al: Subaortic stenosis, the univentricular heart, and banding of the pulmonary artery: an analysis of the course of 43 patients with univentricular heart palliated by pulmonary artery banding. Circulation 73:758–764, 1986.

12. Fyler DC, Buckley LP, Hellenbrand WE, et al: Report of the New England Regional Infant Cardiac Program. Pediatrics 65(Suppl):376–460, 1980.

13. Girod DA, Fontan F, Deville C, et al: Long term results after the Fontan procedure for tricuspid atresia. Circulation 75:605–610, 1987.

14. Grant GP, Mansell AL, Garofano RP, et al: Cardiorespiratory response to exercise after the Fontan procedure for tricuspid atresia. Pediatr Res 24:1–5, 1988.

15. Humes RA, Mair DD, Porter CB, et al: Results of modified Fontan operation in adults. Am J Cardiol 61:602–604, 1988.

16. Jonas RA, Castaneda AR, Lang P: Single ventricle (single- or double-inlet) complicated by subaortic stenosis: surgical options in infancy. Ann Thorac Surg 39:361–366, 1985.

17. Juaneda E, Haworth SG: Pulmonary vascular structure in patients dying after Fontan procedure: the lung as a risk factor. Br Heart J 52:575–580, 1984.

18. Kaye MP: Anatomic correction of transposition of the great arteries. Mayo Clin Proc 50:638–640, 1975.

19. Kreutzer G, Galindez E, Bono H, et al: An operation for the correction of tricuspid atresia. J Thorac Cardiovasc Surg 66:613–621, 1973.

20. Laks H, Milliken JC, Perloff JK, et al: Experience with the Fontan procedure. J Thorac Cardiovasc Surg 88:939–951, 1984.

21. Lee CN, Schaff HV, Danielson GK, et al: Comparison of atriopulmonary versus atrioventricular connection for modified Fontan repair of tricuspid atresia. J Thorac Cardiovasc Surg 92:1038–1043, 1986.

22. Lennox CC, Zuberbuhler JR: Balloon septostomy in tricuspid atresia after infancy. Am J Cardiol 25:723–726, 1970.

23. Lin AE, Laks H, Barber G, et al: Subaortic obstruction in complex congenital heart disease: management by proximal pulmonary artery to ascending aorta end to side anastomosis. J Am Coll Cardiol 7:617–624, 1986.

24. Mayer JE, Helgason H, Jonas RA, et al: Extending the limits for modified Fontan procedures. J Thorac Cardiovasc Surg 92:1021–1028, 1986.

25. McFaul RC, Tajik AJ, Mair DD, et al: Development of pulmonary arteriovenous shunt after superior vena cava-right pulmonary artery (Glenn) anastomosis: report of four cases. Circulation 55:212–216, 1977.

26. Melhuish BPP, Van Praagh R: Juxtaposition of the atrial appendages: a sign of severe cyanotic heart disease. Br Heart J 30:269–284, 1968.

27. Mietus-Snyder M, Lang P, Mayer JE, et al: Childhood systemic-pulmonary shunts: subsequent suitability for Fontan operation. Circulation 76(Suppl III):39–44, 1987.

28. Norwood WI, Kirklin JK, Sanders SP: Hypoplastic left heart syndrome experience with palliative surgery. Am J Cardiol 45:87–91, 1980.

29. Park SC, Siewers RD, Neches WH, et al: Surgical management of univentricular heart with subaortic obstruction. Ann Thorac Surg 37:417–421, 1984.

30. Penkoske PA, Freedom RM, Williams WG, et al: Surgical palliation of subaortic stenosis in the univentricular heart. J Thorac Cardiovasc Surg 87:767–781, 1984.

31. Rao PS (ed): Tricuspid Atresia. Mt Kisco, NY, Futura, 1982, pp. 13–24; 210–229.

32. Rothman A, Lang P, Lock JE, et al: Surgical management of subaortic obstruction in single left ventricle and tricuspid atresia. J Am Coll Cardiol 10:421–426, 1987.

33. Rowe RD, Freedom RM, Mehrizi A, et al: The Neonate with Congenital Heart Disease. Philadelphia, W.B. Saunders Co., 1981.

34. Sanders SP, Wright GB, Keane JF, et al: Clinical and hemodynamic results of the Fontan operation for tricuspid atresia. Am J Cardiol 49:1733–1740, 1982.

35. Stansel HC: A new operation for d-loop transposition of the great vessels. Ann Thorac Surg 19:565–567, 1975.

36. Tam CKH, Lightfoot NE, Finlay CD, et al: Course of tricuspid atresia in the Fontan era. Am J Cardiol 63:589–593, 1989.

37. Van Praagh R, Ando M, Dungan WT: Anatomic types of tricuspid atresia: clinical and developmental implications (abstract). Circulation 63(Suppl II):115, 1971.

Chapter 44

TRICUSPID VALVE PROBLEMS

Donald C. Fyler, M.D.

Among terminally ill cardiac patients, tricuspid incompetence is a common phenomenon usually associated with right ventricular hypertension and myocardial dysfunction. On the other hand, congenital tricuspid incompetence or stenosis as an isolated phenomenon is extremely rare. Tricuspid dysfunction in association with hypoplasia of the right ventricle is well documented in patients with pulmonary atresia and intact septum (see ch. 40). How much is simply hypoplasia of the valve relative to the small ventricle and how much is inherently abnormal about the tricuspid valve is often not clear. Tricuspid valve disease is rarely acquired with rheumatic fever (see ch. 22) and very rarely is acquired as part of the carcinoid syndrome.

Occasionally, a patient with functional tricuspid atresia and a nearly atretic valve can be described as having severe tricuspid stenosis with a hypoplastic right ventricle. Rarely, generalized right-sided abnormality involving the tricuspid valve, pulmonary valve, and right ventricular dysfunction are encountered. As a general rule, moderate degrees of tricuspid valve deformity (whether stenosis or regurgitation) or moderate pulmonary valve deformity (whether stenosis or regurgitation) is well tolerated, but moderate abnormalities of both valves may cause symptoms. Symptomatic combinations of these lesions are rare and must be managed on an individual basis. The obvious physiologic question is why a simple connection between the right atrium and pulmonary artery such as in a Fontan procedure functions so well when, at the same level of pulmonary artery pressure, pulmonary valve and tricuspid valve dysfunction allow less forward flow of blood. That the right heart, in some situations, can get in its own way seems obvious. Where and when and why remain for future generations to unravel.

There are several convincing descriptions of transient tricuspid incompetence in newborns.[4,23] The problem is presumed to result from major metabolic and hypoxic insults to the myocardium and is therefore associated with death or complete recovery.

Recognition of tricuspid incompetence depends on the presence of a systolic murmur audible at the lower left sternal border, sometimes loudest at the right lower sternal border, which varies with respiration. Two-dimensional echocardiography will establish the diagnosis.

Tricuspid stenosis is clinically recognizable because of the presence of a diastolic rumbling murmur at the lower left sternal border, seeming to occur somewhat earlier in diastole than a mitral diastolic murmur. The diastolic murmur of tricuspid stenosis has been observed in patients in whom a free-floating foreign object, such as a piece of catheter with a clot, has lodged in the tricuspid valve. Rarely, extension of tumor up the inferior vena cava, such as Wilms' tumor, will obstruct the tricuspid valve sufficiently to cause an audible diastolic rumble.

EBSTEIN'S DISEASE

Definition

Ebstein's disease is a characteristic anomaly involving the septal and posterior leaflets of the tricuspid valve. The leaflets are deformed and variably adherent to the ventricular septum below the atrioventricular junction.

Prevalence

Ebstein's disease is rare: 120 patients were seen between 1973 and 1987 at the Children's Hospital in Boston; 45 had Ebstein's disease in association with other cardiac anomalies (Exhibit 1). The New England Regional Infant Cardiac Program found 13 infants with Ebstein's disease, 0.012/1000 live births (see ch. 18).

Pathology

The septal and posterior leaflets of the tricuspid valve are downwardly displaced and adherent to the right ventricular septum. The leaflets may be redundant, contracted, or thickened, and even rarely atretic.[2,11,25] That portion of the right ventricular wall that is above the adherent valve leaflets is described as the **atrialized** portion of the right ventricle. The distal right ventricular chamber is usually enlarged, but may be normal sized, even small, whereas the right atrium is almost invariably enlarged, sometimes grossly enlarged (Fig. 1).[24] The mechanism of right ventricular dilation is not established, although abnormalities of the muscle fibers may be involved.[1] The tricuspid valve may be incompetent or, less commonly, stenotic. The involved portion of the right ventricular wall is thin and in extreme cases may be paper thin—Uhl's disease.[20,21]

There is virtually always either a patent foramen ovale or an atrial septal defect.

Pulmonary stenosis, pulmonary atresia, tetralogy of Fallot, ventricular septal defect, and other lesions are sometimes associated with Ebstein's deformity of the tricuspid valve. When the ventricles are inverse, the left-sided tricuspid valve may have some of the features of Ebstein's disease (see ch. 49). An unusual form of Ebstein's anomaly in association with an atrioventricular septal defect has been reported.[25]

Physiology

Whether there is tricuspid insufficiency or tricuspid stenosis or both, the practical effect is limitation of passage of blood through the right heart. The right atrial pressure is higher than normal, and right-to-left shunting through a patent foramen ovale is usual. Occasionally, with minimal Ebstein's disease, there is left-to-right shunting through an atrial defect but, as a rule, if there is a left-to-right shunting, the Ebstein's deformity is minor. At birth cyanosis may be extreme, gradually improving as pulmonary arterial resistance and right-to-left shunting decrease over the first days and weeks of life.[17]

Attempts to define relative stenosis or regurgitation are sometimes unsuccessful when limited amounts of blood pass through the right ventricle. How much influence the atrialized ventricular muscle, contracting simultaneously with the rest of the ventricle, disrupts forward flow of blood is not clear, but that right ventricular and atrialized ventricular muscle oppose each other seems likely. It has been proposed that the distal attachments of the tricuspid valve subdivide the right ventricle into two chambers with deleterious effect on function.[13]

Replacement of the valve at or above the valve ring, or valvoplasty, in association with closure of the atrial opening, seems to help, so it is reasonable to suggest that at least some of the problem in Ebstein's disease is the valve itself. Still, much of the symptomatology in patients with Ebstein's disease can be attributed to cyanosis, and raising the average arterial oxygen saturation is usually helpful.[3]

Clinical Manifestations

Infants. Infants with Ebstein's disease are recognized because of cyanosis in the first days of life. This may vary from slight to severe and may be associated with tachypnea in direct proportion to the degree of cyanosis. The liver may be enlarged. There are no characteristic auscultatory findings and often there is no systolic murmur. The presence of a murmur does not exclude the diagnosis because other cardiac lesions are sometimes associated with Ebstein's disease (Exhibit 1).

Children. After infancy, the child may or may

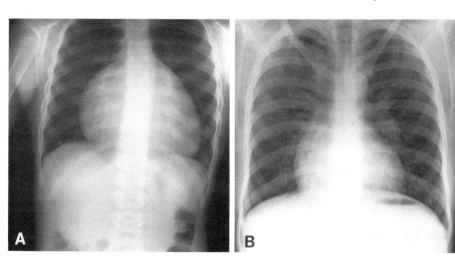

Figure 1. The chest x-rays of two patients with Ebstein's disease showing the great variation in heart size that may be encountered.

Exhibit 1

	Boston Children's Hospital Experience 1973–1987 Ebstein's Disease									
	Proof of Diagnosis					Surgery				
Anatomy	No.	Deaths	Echo	Cath	Clinical	Tri-Valve Replacement	Valvuloplasty	Other	Any Surgery	Arrhythmias
Ebstein's, Primary Dx	75	14	28	49	9	4	4	10	18	32
Ebstein's, Secondary Dx										
Ventricular septal defect	4	0	0	2	1	0	4	2	2	2
Tetralogy of Fallot	4	1	1	4	0	0	0	3	3	1
Pulmonary stenosis	4	1	3	3	3	1	0	2	3	2
Malposition	4	0	2	4	0	2	0	2	4	4
Pulmonary atresia with intact ventricular septum	4	2	1	4	0	0	0	4	4	0
L-transposition of the great arteries	8	2	5	8	0	2	0	4	6	5
Other	17	9	5	15	0	1	0	9	10	8
Total	120	29	45	89	13	10	4	36	50	54

There were 120 individuals with the diagnosis of Ebstein's disease seen in the period 1973–1987: 75 had no other cardiac problem, whereas 45 were labelled as having Ebstein's anomaly as a secondary feature of some other congenital cardiac disease.

Note that rhythm abnormalities were encountered in almost half of the patients with Ebstein's disease as a primary diagnosis and almost half of the patients with Ebstein's as a secondary diagnosis. Note that less than half than patients were examined by echocardiography because the diagnosis was established before echocardiography became available as a diagnostic tool.

Data Source†	No.	Primary Diagnosis		Secondary Diagnosis*	
		No.	Mortality	No.	Mortality
Children's Hospital	120	75	19%	45	33%
Guiliani[8]	67	67	22%	—	—
Radford[17]	35	27	7%	8	50%
Kumar[11]‡	40	40	18%	15	66%
Watson[22]	505	—	12%	—	48%

*Atrial septal defect, patent ductus arteriosus, and patent foramen ovale are considered part of Ebstein's disease.
†In each of these reports patients were observed in different time periods and for different periods of time.
‡As many as 34 of Kumar's patients may be included in The Children's Hospital data.

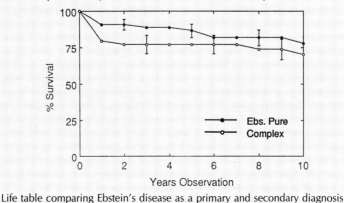

Life table comparing Ebstein's disease as a primary and secondary diagnosis

not be cyanotic and is usually otherwise asymptomatic. Poor growth is rarely an issue. Older children may suffer the limitations of cyanosis and some may develop congestive heart failure.

There are usually more than two heart sounds; there may be a diastolic sound and often a mid-diastolic rumble. Triple and quadruple gallops are common. The second heart sound is often widely split. A systolic murmur usually suggests some associated cardiac anomaly.

Electrocardiography. Characteristically, the electrocardiogram shows right bundle branch block. Bizarre widening of the QRS may not be present at birth only to appear later. The P-waves are often huge, reflecting the grossly enlarged right atrium (Fig. 2). Sometimes the P-R interval is long, although more often Wolff-Parkinson-White syndrome is identifiable. Right-sided preexcitation, localized to the atrialized portion of the right ventricle, is found in most patients.[19] Atrial rhythm abnormalities are common in older children. Because, in general, rhythm problems in patients with congenital heart disease are more common the older the patient, and death, either suddenly or clearly due to rhythm disturbance, is less common in infancy and early childhood, it is not surprising that pediatric patients with Ebstein's disease are not as plagued with rhythm problems as are adult patients with Ebstein's disease.

Chest X-ray. The heart size is variably enlarged in proportion to the severity of the anomaly. The right atrium may be gigantic (Fig. 1) in an otherwise asymptomatic patient. Gross cardiomegaly does not specifically imply congestive heart failure

because the enlargement may be almost entirely the result of a giant right atrium.

Echocardiography. The relative size of the chambers and the deformity of the tricuspid valve are readily visualized and quantified.[18] Downward displacement of the septal leaflet is the best criterion for the diagnosis of Ebstein's disease and is easily assessed by 2-D echocardiography (Fig. 3). Because of this, it is now possible to diagnose minimal forms of Ebstein's abnormality, and because of the problems of distinguishing between normal and abnormal degrees of downward displacement, questions of definition arise. For the present, minimal Ebstein's disease is diagnosed when there is a difference in downward displacement between the mitral and tricuspid valve of more than 15 mm in a child and 20 mm in an adult.[9]

Evidence of tricuspid stenosis or regurgitation can often be documented. Other cardiac lesions can be detected or excluded.

It should be mentioned that, except in the mildest forms of disease, echocardiography is not required to make the diagnosis because the diagnosis is generally otherwise obvious.

Cardiac Catheterization. Even as long ago as the 1960s, cardiac catheterization was not needed for the diagnosis of Ebstein's disease in the average patient. It was, however, undertaken to gain better understanding of the hemodynamic problem posed, and now after some years of attempting to learn more, it is clear that not much was gained. Atrial and ventricular pressure tracing do not clearly establish the location of the tricuspid valve ring because the two pressures curves are similar.

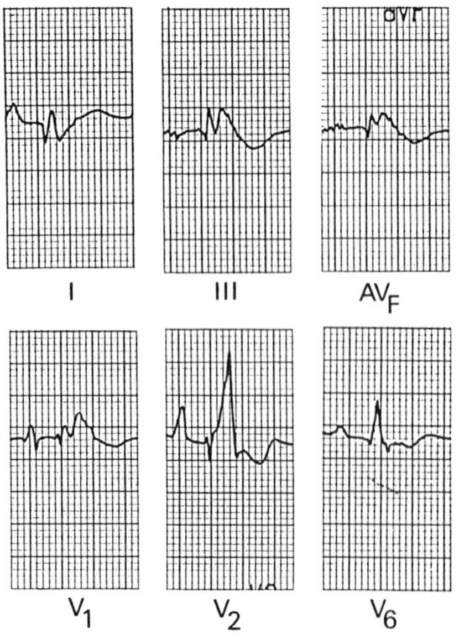

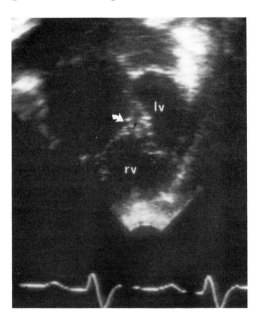

Figure 2. An electrocardiogram from a patient with Ebstein's disease. Note the large and bizarre P-waves and the wide and bizarre QRS complexes.

Figure 3. Echocardiogram from a patient with Ebstein's disease showing apical displacement of the septal tricuspid valve leaflet (arrow).

The presence of atrial pressures where ventricular electrocardiograms are recorded is helpful and should be virtually diagnostic of Ebstein's anomaly. It is generally somewhat difficult to pass a catheter from right ventricle to the pulmonary artery.

The angiographic anatomy is usually characteristic (Fig. 4). Downward displacement of the tricuspid valve ring, an enlarged right atrium, and compartmentalization of the right ventricle are readily recognized. But, occasionally, the problem is to recognize Ebstein's disease in the presence of associated anomalies such as tetralogy of Fallot or ventricular septal defect.

Balloon test occlusion of the atrial opening may provide useful information when surgery is being contemplated.

The high mortality[22] associated with catheterization of patients with Ebstein's disease in the 1950s no longer occurs.

Management

In the newborn period, all efforts to support the infant through the period of transitional circulation are desirable. Prostaglandins will increase pulmonary blood flow when the patient is dangerously cyanotic; oxygen and correction of anemia may be helpful. Still, some infants die.

Older children generally require no treatment. Rhythm problems can be managed as they appear. Generally, heart size (in truth, right atrial size) is not an indication of the severity or potential danger of the lesion. Cyanosis, particularly if it is marked, or the appearance of congestive failure are ominous. The earlier these symptoms appear, the more likely life expectancy will be limited.

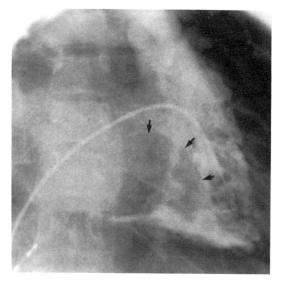

Figure 4. A right ventricular angiogram in a patient with Ebstein's disease. Note the large right atrium, the displaced tricuspid valve (arrows), and relatively small right ventricle.

Generally, surgery is reserved for patients with severe symptoms, deep cyanosis, congestive heart failure, or other complicating cardiac anomalies. Both valvoplasty[6] and replacement of the tricuspid valve[5,16] are reported to be valuable. We have insufficient experience to have an opinion and are waiting for clear evidence of success before embarking on valve surgery as the answer to this disease. For the present, the patient either must be sufficiently cyanotic or have congestive heart failure before considering surgery. Surgery for the relief of rhythm problems is tempting and may be justified if a bypass tract is identified that might be amenable to surgery. Relief provided by valve replacement or valvoplasty represents palliation rather than cure, and what happens later is as yet undefined.

Course

If patients survive the newborn period, the natural history[8,10] of Ebstein's disease favors continued survival if there are no complicating cardiac defects (Exhibit 1). Survival of a deeply cyanotic newborn is problematic, but surprisingly, the infants who do survive the neonatal period improve and can often be described as no longer critically ill.

Because modern echocardiographic techniques have uncovered patients who formerly would have been unrecognized, a cadre of patients with mild forms of Ebstein's disease has been added to the patient pool known to have this disease. These children are expected to have a nearly normal life expectancy.

That the anatomy must determine the outcome seems obvious,[13] but a reliable predicter remains to be identified.[15] The factors that we believe indicate a bad outcome include, in order of importance, (1) congestive heart failure, (2) symptoms, (3) cyanosis, and (4) additional cardiac defects. It is a matter of some interest that serious rhythm problems seem to be much more common among adult patients and often are considered to be the cause of death. This has not been our experience in children. Rhythm problems surely occur and, as the years go by, perhaps become more frequent, but they are not commonly the cause of death.

Brain abscess is a threat; infective endocarditis is rare.

CARCINOID HEART DISEASE

Rarely a young adult or adolescent with a carcinoid tumor, usually located in the bowel, will develop the carcinoid syndrome. Perhaps because of excess secretion of serotonin, there may be diarrhea, flushing, and even cardiac manifestations of tricuspid regurgitation and pulmonary valvar stenosis. High concentration of 5-hydroxyindolacetic acid in the urine is diagnostic, although not all

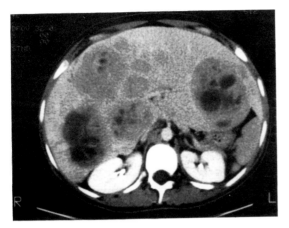

Figure 5. Abdominal computed tomography of a teenager whose problem was severe right heart failure because of the carcinoid syndrome. Note the large metastases in the liver. Some years later, this child is alive and relatively well, although she is still receiving chemotherapy.

patients will show this on first examination.[7] If there are metastases, the liver may be very large and hard (Fig. 5).

The key to recognition of this cardiac problem is the acquired appearance of tricuspid regurgitation and pulmonary stenosis in an adolescent or young adult. Several experimental drugs are being tested in the treatment of this often fatal disease.[12,14]

REFERENCES

1. Anderson KR, Lie JT: The right ventricular myocardium in Ebstein's anomaly: a morphometric histopathologic study. Mayo Clin Proc 54:181–184, 1979.
2. Anderson KR, Zuberbuhler JR, Anderson RH, et al: Morphologic spectrum of Ebstein's anomaly of the heart: a review. Mayo Clin Proc 54:174–180, 1979.
3. Barber G, Danielson GK, Heise CT, et al: Cardiorespiratory response to exercise in Ebstein's anomaly. Am J Cardiol 56:509–514, 1985.
4. Bucciarelli RL, Nelson RM, Egan EA, et al: Transient tricuspid insufficiency of the newborn: a form of myocardial dysfunction in stressed newborns. Pediatrics 59:330–337, 1977.
5. Burakovsky VI, Bukharin VA, Bokeriia LA, et al: Radical surgical correction of Ebstein's anomaly: experience with 54 tricuspid valve protheses. Grudn Khir 6:5, 1984.
6. Danielson GK, Maloney JD, Devloo RAE: Surgical repair of Ebstein's anomaly. Mayo Clin Proc 54:185–192, 1979.
7. Feldman JM: Detection and treatment of carcinoid tumors. Hosp Pract 23:219–226, 233–236, 1988.
8. Giuliani ER, Fuster V, Brandenburg RO, et al: Ebstein's anomaly: the clinical features and natural history of Ebstein's anomaly of the tricuspid valve. Mayo Clin Proc 54:163–173, 1979.
9. Gussenhoven EJ, Stewart PA, Becker AE, et al: "Offsetting" of the septal tricuspid leaflet in normal hearts and in hearts with Ebstein's anomaly: anatomic and echographic correlation. Am J Cardiol 53:172–176, 1984.
10. Kumar AE, Fyler DC, Miettinen OS, et al: Ebstein's anomaly: clinical profile and natural history. Am J Cardiol 28:84–95, 1971.
11. Kumar AE, Gilbert G, Aerichide N, et al: Ebstein's anomaly, Uhl's disease and absence of tricuspid leaflets: a new spectrum. Am J Cardiol 25:111–125, 1970.
12. Kvols LK: Metastastic carcinoid tumors and the carcinoid syndrome: a selective review of chemotherapy and therapy. Am J Med 81:49–55, 1986.
13. Leung MP, Baker EJ, Anderson RH, et al: Cineangiographic spectrum of Ebstein's malformation: its relevance to clinical presentation and outcome. J Am Coll Cardiol 11:154–161, 1988.
14. Moertel CG: Treatment of the carcinoid tumor and the malignant carcinoid syndrome. J Clin Oncol 1:727–740, 1983.
15. Nihoyannopoulos P, McKenna WJ, Smith G, et al: Echocardiographic assessment of the right ventricle in Ebstein's anomaly: relation to clinical outcome. J Am Coll Cardiol 8:627–635, 1986.
16. Pasque M, Williams WG, Coles JG, et al: Tricuspid valve replacement in children. Ann Thorac Surg 44:164–168, 1987.
17. Radford DJ, Graff RF, and Neilson GH: Diagnosis and natural history of Ebstein's anomaly. Br Heart J 54:517–522, 1985.
18. Shiina A, Seward JB, Edwards WD, et al: Two-dimensional echocardiographic spectrum of Ebstein's anomaly: detailed anatomic assessment. J Am Coll Cardiol 3:356–370, 1984.
19. Smith WM, Gallagher JJ, Kerr CR, et al: The electrophysiologic basis and management of symptomatic recurrent tachycardia in patients with Ebstein's anomaly of the tricuspid valve. Am J Cardiol 49:1223–1234, 1982.
20. Uhl HSM: A previously undescribed congenital malformation of the heart: almost total absence of the myocardium of the right ventricle. Bull Johns Hopkins Hosp 91:197–205, 1952.
21. Vecht RJ, Carmichael DJS, Gopal R, et al: Uhl's anomaly. Br Heart J 41:676–682, 1979.
22. Watson H: Natural history of Ebstein's anomaly of tricuspid valve in childhood and adolescence: an international co-operative study of 505 cases. Br Heart J 36:417–427, 1974.
23. Yeager SB, Parness IA, Sanders SP: Severe tricuspid atresia simulating pulmonary atresia in the fetus. Am Heart J 115:906–908, 1988.
24. Zuberbuhler JR, Allwork SP, Anderson RH: The spectrum of Ebstein's anomaly of the tricuspid valve. J Thorac Cardiovasc Surg 77:202–211, 1979.
25. Zuberbuhler JR, Becker AE, Anderson RH, et al: Ebstein's malformation and the embryological development of the tricuspid valve. Pediatr Cardiol 5:289–296, 1984.

Chapter 45

TRUNCUS ARTERIOSUS

Donald C. Fyler, M.D.

DEFINITION

Truncus arteriosus is characterized by a single arterial vessel that originates from the heart, overrides the ventricular septum, and supplies the systemic, coronary, and pulmonary circulations. Confusion arises when a single great artery arises from the heart, but the pulmonary circulation is supplied from the descending aorta by collateral vessels (p. 482) or a ductus arteriosus, in which case the anatomy may be that of tetralogy of Fallot with pulmonary atresia. There must be no remnant of a separate main pulmonary artery connected to the heart and no evidence of a separate pulmonary valve if one is to be confident of the presence of true truncus arteriosus.

Prevalence

The vast majority of patients with truncus arteriosus are symptomatic in the first months of life, so the prevalence of 0.034–0.210 infants per 1000 births (see ch. 18) is a reasonable estimate. Truncus arteriosus represents about 1% of all patients with heart disease seen at the Boston Children's Hospital (see ch. 18) and it ranks 19th among children with cardiac lesions. According to The Hospital for Sick Children in Toronto, truncus arteriosus accounts for 1–4% of their patients with congenital heart disease.[16]

EMBRYOLOGY

The single arterial vessel (truncus arteriosus) arising from the heart begins to separate into an aorta and main pulmonary artery in the third to fourth week of embryonic life. The normal spiraling division of the truncus arteriosus separates into a posterior aorta and an anterior pulmonary artery. Persistence of the truncus arteriosus in a newborn represents an arrest of development of the heart at this point in embryogenesis.[6,10] Whether absence of the normal spiraling division of the truncus, twisting of the dividing truncus because of

looping of the ventricles, atresia of the subinfundibulum, or abnormal location of the anlage of the semilunar valves is responsible, a single arterial vessel is the result.[1,4,18,19] Kirby[12,13] has demonstrated that timely ablation of the neural crest results in a persistent truncus arteriosus. The neural crest is also the origin of the pharyngeal pouches, i.e., is responsible for the development of the thymus and the parathyroid glands, hence the association of truncus arteriosus with DiGeorge syndrome.

ANATOMY

A single arterial trunk, larger in diameter than the normal aorta at a comparable age, arises from the heart. The trunk is positioned above the ventricular septum, being dominantly over either ventricle (the right in 42%, the left in 16%, and equally shared in 42%).[3] The truncal valve is rarely normal, often having thickened and deformed leaflets (72%)[3] that are variably stenotic or, more often, incompetent (50%).[4] The valve may be tricuspid (42%), bicuspid (30%), quadricuspid (24%), or unicuspid (1%).[3] There is almost invariably a malaligned ventricular septal defect in the membranous septum that is rarely small. The aortic arch is right sided in about 21–36% of patients.[3,19] The malaligned ventricular defect, the overriding great artery, and the tendency to have a right aortic arch are reminiscent of tetralogy of Fallot anatomy. The pulmonary arteries usually arise from the truncus within a short distance of the valve, either as a single vessel that divides into right and left pulmonary arteries (Fig. 1),[5,19] or as two vessels from the posterior aspect of the trunk. Some patients have obstruction at the orifice of the pulmonary arteries that is equivalent to pulmonary stenosis. Occasionally, one or the other pulmonary artery may be absent,[8] again reminiscent of tetralogy of Fallot, because the absent pulmonary artery is usually the left (8%).[4] Often there is an interrupted aortic arch (11%).[3] Associated extracardiac anomalies are common (21–40%).[9,19] Evidence of the

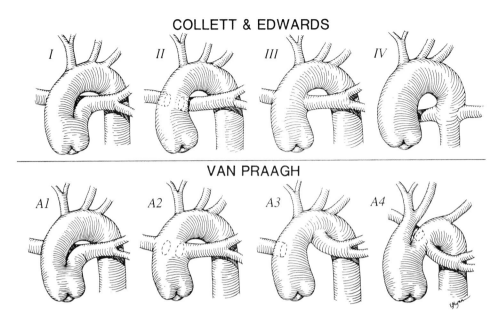

Figure 1. There are similarities between the Collett and Edwards and the Van Praagh classifications of truncus. Type I is the same as A1. Types II and III are grouped as a single type A2, because they are not significantly distinct embryologically or therapeutically. Type A3 denotes unilateral pulmonary artery atresia with collateral supply to the affected lung. Type A4 is truncus associated with an interrupted aortic arch (13% of all cases of truncus arteriosus). (From Hernanz-Schulman M, Fellows KE: Persistent truncus arteriosus: pathologic, diagnostic and therapeutic considerations. Semin Roentgenol 20:121–129, 1985, with permission.)

DiGeorge syndrome is common (33%);[15,17] the serum calcium levels in small infants are generally low. We have yet to uncover sufficient immunologic abnormality to cause a clinical problem.

Hemitruncus is an unrelated anomaly (see p. 697).

PHYSIOLOGY

The truncus receives the output of both ventricles and, within a short distance, the blood destined for pulmonary circulation is diverted to the lungs (Fig. 2). In the absence of pulmonary stenosis, the pulmonary arterial pressure is equal to that in the truncus. The amount of pulmonary blood flow is determined by the presence of pulmonary stenosis or by the level of pulmonary arteriolar resistance. In the absence of pulmonary stenosis, the expected reduction in pulmonary resistance in the first days of life is not well tolerated; survival depends on persistence of some pulmonary arteriolar resistance to prevent flooding of the lungs. Pulmonary blood flows are greater than normal, the exact amount determining the systemic arterial saturation. When a main pulmonary artery arises immediately beyond the truncal valve, the pulmonary circulation may largely derive from the right ventricle, the pulmonary arterial oxygen saturation being less than that observed in the aorta. Truncal regurgitation is present in 50% of patients, and when it is severe, the added burden of the regurgitant flow may be more than can be tolerated. The amount of blood passing through the truncal valve to supply the systemic blood flow and the pulmonary blood flow, as well as the regurgitant blood flow, is greatly excessive and often leads to early congestive heart failure. Because of the large pulmonary blood flow, development of pulmonary vascular obstructive disease is common among survivors who have not undergone surgery. It can occur as early as 6 months of age.

CLINICAL MANIFESTATIONS

The majority of these babies are discovered to have a cardiac problem within the first weeks of life, either because of a murmur or the appearance of tachypnea and/or costosternal retractions. The infants are sometimes visibly cyanotic, although tachypnea, and even costal retractions, are more common presenting symptoms. These evidences of congestive heart failure are usually readily apparent. The peripheral pulses are bounding. There is usually a systolic murmur at the left sternal border, sometimes associated with the diastolic murmur of aortic regurgitation. The second heart sound is single, but this is usually difficult to distinguish in a small sick infant.

Once pulmonary vascular obstructive disease has developed, the clinical features reflect the elevated pulmonary vascular resistance (see ch. 10).

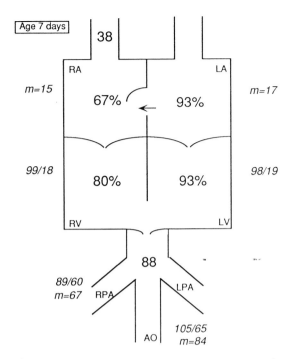

Figure 2. Diagram of the hemodynamics in a patient with truncus arteriosus. Note the equilibration of systemic and pulmonary pressures; the complete mixing of systemic and pulmonary blood as evidenced by similar systemic and pulmonary oxygen concentrations; and the large left-to-right shunt as evidenced by high pulmonary oxygen saturation. There is often selective flow of systemic venous blood to the pulmonary artery with resulting differences in systemic and pulmonary oxygen concentrations when the patient has a Type I (A1) deformity. Ao, aorta; LA, left atrium; LPA, left pulmonary artery; LV, left ventricle; RA, right atrium; RPA, right pulmonary artery; RV, right ventricle.

Electrocardiography

The electrocardiogram may show left or right ventricular hypertrophy, with left or combined ventricular hypertrophy being more common.

Chest X-ray

The heart is large; pulmonary vasculature is increased. There may be a right aortic arch. The high, arching origin of the left pulmonary artery[20] is rarely identifiable in a small baby.

Echocardiography

The diagnosis of truncus arteriosus is usually apparent from the initial subxiphoid long-axis view (Fig. 3). The truncal root can be seen overriding the crest of the ventricular septum through a large conoventricular septal defect. The pulmonary artery is seen arising from the leftward and posterior aspect of the truncal root. A subxiphoid, short-axis scan provides excellent visualization of the atrial and ventricular septa, the atrioventricular valves, and the ventricular septal defect. Additional mus-

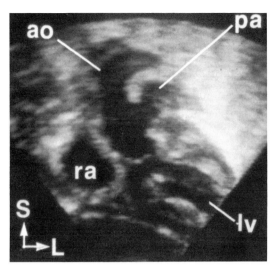

Figure 3. Echocardiogram in a patient with truncus arteriosus. Subxiphoid long-axis view showing the truncal root giving rise to the ascending aorta (AO) and the pulmonary artery (PA). LV, left ventricle; RA, right atrium.

cular defects, although rare, can be sought in this projection using imaging and Doppler color flow mapping.

The truncal valve is best examined in parasternal long- and short-axis views. The thickness and mobility of the leaflets are best appreciated in the long-axis view, whereas the short-axis view is required to determine the number of commissures (usually 2–4). Truncal valve stenosis should be suspected if the leaflets are thick with decreased mobility and systolic doming. Continuous-wave Doppler examination from the apex, suprasternal notch, or right sternal border is used to quantify the severity of stenosis. Truncal valve regurgitation should be sought using pulsed Doppler or Doppler color flow mapping from parasternal and apical transducer locations. The diameter of the jet(s) as it crosses the valve is a useful index of the severity of the regurgitation.

Because coronary artery anomalies are common in truncus arteriosus, the proximal coronary arteries should be examined in parasternal long- and short-axis views. The distance between the coronary artery ostia and the origin of the pulmonary arteries is an important surgical consideration and should be measured.

Then the truncal root should be examined in the parasternal short-axis and suprasternal notch views to determine the size and location of the branch pulmonary arteries. If a main pulmonary artery segment is present (Type I), it can be seen separating from the leftward and posterior aspect of the truncal root while scanning superiorly and rightward in a short-axis view. If no main pulmonary segment is present (Type II), then the pulmonary artery branches are seen originating separately.

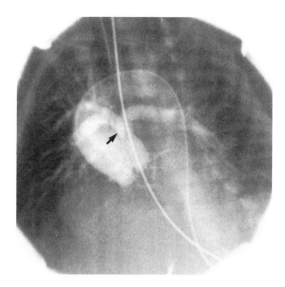

Figure 4. Cineangiogram with injection into the left anterior oblique view showing a truncus arteriosus 1. The main pulmonary artery (arrow) arises from the common trunk and branches into right and left main pulmonary arteries.

The left pulmonary artery invariably arises anterior and slightly superior to the right pulmonary artery, although the orifices are usually immediately adjacent. Rotation or angulation of the transducer, or even relocation to another interspace, often is necessary to adequately image the origins of the pulmonary artery branches. Doppler color flow mapping is useful for identifying and defining the size of these origins. The pulmonary artery branches should be imaged as far distally as possible using parasternal or suprasternal notch views.

If one or the other proximal pulmonary artery branches is absent (Type III, Van Praagh[19]), only one pulmonary artery will be seen joining the truncal root. An attempt should be made to image the distal portion of the other pulmonary artery branch near the hilum of the lung. Doppler color flow mapping is useful for detecting aortopulmonary collaterals to that lung as well.

Interruption of the aortic arch (Type IV, Van Praagh[19]) should be suspected in an infant if the main pulmonary artery segment is larger than the ascending aorta. A suprasternal notch, short-axis view demonstrates the small ascending aorta branching into the brachiocephalic arteries with no transverse arch connecting with the descending aorta. In contrast, a high parasternal position and rotation into a parasagittal plane shows the large main pulmonary artery giving rise to the pulmonary artery branches and continuing with the descending aorta via the ductus arterious. The origins of the ductus arterious and the origins of the brachiocephalic arteries can be determined from this parasternal view and from the suprasternal notch views.

If the aortic arch is intact, the side of the arch (left or right) and the branching pattern should be determined from suprasternal notch views as described in chapter 13.

Cardiac Catheterization

Usually the anatomic details are well described by the echocardiographers and, in the small infant, the physiologic circumstances can be surmised or even measured. Unfortunately, truncal regurgitation, a major determinant of survival, can only be

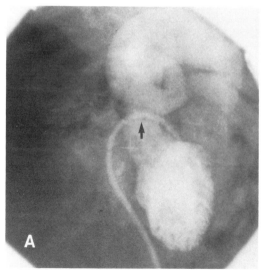

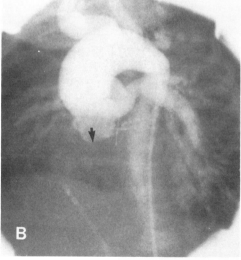

Figure 5. Cineangiogram with injection into the left ventricle **(A)** and the truncus arteriosus **(B)**. Passage of contrast through a ventricular septal defect into the right ventricle can be seen in A. There is a huge truncus type 1. Arrows indicate the truncal valve.

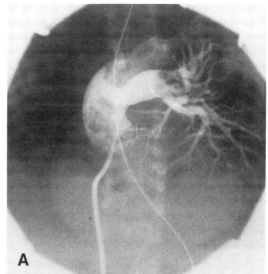

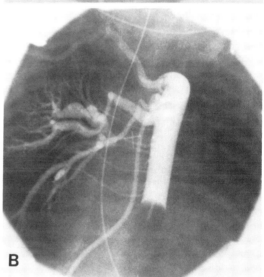

Figure 6. **A,** Cineangiogram in the anteroposterior view. The catheter enters the truncus from the right ventricle. Note that only the left pulmonary artery is opacified. **B,** Injection of contrast in the descending aorta shows that the right pulmonary artery blood arises from collateral vessels, which originate from the descending aorta.

imprecisely evaluated by cardiac catheterization or echocardiography alone, and both techniques are needed to provide the best assessment of semilunar valve function. Largely for this reason these infants undergo cardiac catheterization. An aortogram with good contrast in more than one view, preferably biplane, is required (Figs. 4–8). The problems that occur in the intensive care unit following surgery for truncus arteriosus may require an emergency cardiac catheterization in the immediate postoperative period as well; in that case, baseline preoperative data are particularly valuable. Perhaps the indications for cardiac catheterization are better stated in philosophical terms: When managing cardiac infants with known high mortality and morbidity, to undertake cardiac surgery without examining all obtainable data is foolhardy.

In the older child, evaluation of pulmonary vascular resistance prior to surgery is mandatory. Of course, whenever there is any doubt as to some anatomic or physiologic detail, cardiac catheterization should be performed.

Truncal valve function is seen best with retrograde aortography, and the ventricular septum is evaluated best in the long axial oblique projection.

MANAGEMENT

Infants with truncus arteriosus and congestive heart failure are treated with anticongestive medications. However, survival without surgery is uncommon (Exhibit 1), and the survivors are severely limited. Hence, the decision is not whether to at-

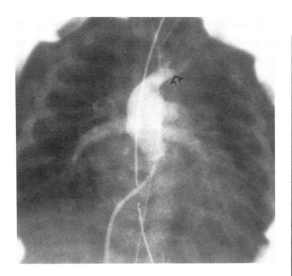

Figure 7. Cineangiogram in the anteroposterior view. Origin of the right and left pulmonary arteries from the truncus can be seen. The ascending aorta tapers and the transverse arch (arrow) is interrupted. The descending aorta is supplied by a patent ductus arteriosus.

tempt surgical correction, but when. It is desirable for these babies to grow, or at least to mature as much as possible, prior to surgery. The trend toward better survival with increasing age has been documented, and although it may be simply a reflection of the truncal anatomy most compatible with survival, survival does improve when the infants are operated on at an older age.[7] Because the median age at death in the untreated patient is about 5 weeks,[19] not much delay is possible except in the most favorable cases. Because pulmonary vascular obstructive disease becomes a threat after the age of 6 months,[11] surgery should be performed before that time. Occasionally, for a patient with truncal regurgitation requiring valve replacement who also has an interrupted aortic arch, the most compassionate treatment may be simply to make the infant comfortable, particularly if there are extracardiac anomalies as well.

Although a few patients survive with pulmonary artery banding procedures, surgical correction in infancy is a more satisfactory plan. The ventricular septal defect is closed and a graft is placed, connecting the right ventricle to the main pulmonary artery.[7,14] Fortunately, the right and left pulmonary arteries almost always arise close enough that a button of aortic tissue can be fashioned to allow anastomosis to a single graft. The main determinants of surgical survival include the patient's age at operation and truncal valve function. The neonate, because of size and immaturity, is at increased risk, as is the infant over the age of 6 months because of pulmonary vascular disease.[7] At Children's Hospital in Boston, our present policy is to attempt to manage the baby medically for the

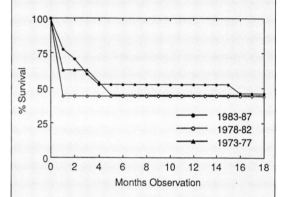

Life table analysis of all children with truncus arteriosus first seen after January 1, 1973, without respect to type of treatment. Fourteen children were first seen between 1973 and 1977; 30, between 1978 and 1982; and 49, between 1983 and 1989. Late survival among all patients with truncus arteriosus (32 did not have reparative surgery) has improved little over the years.

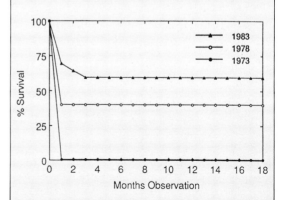

Life table analysis of children ungoing reparative surgery. Six children were repaired between 1973 and 1977; 20, between 1978 and 1982; and 36, between 1983 and 1987. Survival with repair is improving.

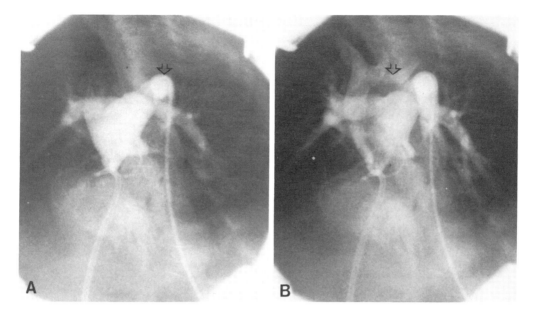

Figure 8. **A,** Cineangiogram in the left anterior oblique view showing a truncus arteriosus 1. The descending aorta is supplied by a ductus arteriosus (arrow), through which the catheter entered the common truncus. **B,** The small transverse arch (arrow) ends in an interrupted aortic arch.

first months of life; thereafter, surgery is performed as soon as there is evidence of failure to thrive and at the latest by 6 months of age.

With survival the problems remaining are those of managing a conduit that will require replacement in early childhood (up to 67% require replacement by 2 years of age).[2] Children with artificial valves require anticoagulation. It is anticipated that the right ventricular incision will produce some ectopy in the long-range follow-up.

REFERENCES

1. Bartelings MM, Gittenberger de Groot AC: The arterial orifice level in the early human embryo. Anat Embryol (Berl) 177:537–542, 1988.
2. Boyce SW, Turley K, Yee ES, et al: The fate of the 12mm porcine valved conduit from the right ventricle to the pulmonary artery: a ten-year experience. J Thorac Cardiovasc Surg 95:201–207, 1988.
3. Butto F, Lucas RV, Edwards JE: Persistent truncus arteriosus: pathologic anatomy in 54 cases. Pediatr Cardiol 7:95–101, 1986.
4. Calder L, Van Praagh R, Van Praagh S, et al: Truncus arteriosus communis: clinical, angiocardiographic, and pathologic findings in 100 patients. Am Heart J 92:23–38, 1976.
5. Collett RW, Edwards JE: Persistent truncus arteriosus: classification according to anatomic types. Surg Clin North Am 29:1245–1270, 1949.
6. De La Cruz MV, Pio da Rocha J: An ontogenetic theory for the explanation of congenital malformations involving the truncus and conus. Am Heart J 51:782–805, 1956.
7. Ebert PA, Turley K, Stanger P, et al: Surgical treatment of truncus arteriosus in the first six months of life. Ann Surg 200:451–456, 1984.
8. Fyfe DA, Driscoll DJ, DiDonato RM, et al: Truncus arteriosus with single pulmonary artery: influence of
pulmonary vascular obstructive disease on early and late operative results. J Am Coll Cardiol 5:1168–1172, 1985.
9. Fyler DC, Buckley LP, Hellenbrand WE, et al: Report of the New England Regional Infant Cardiac Program. Pediatrics 65(Suppl):1–461, 1980.
10. Hernanz-Schulman M, Fellows KE: Persistent truncus arteriosus: pathologic, diagnostic and therapeutic considerations. Semin Roentgenol 20:121–129, 1985.
11. Juaneda E, Haworth SG: Pulmonary vascular disease in children with truncus arteriosus. Am J Cardiol 54:1314–1320, 1984.
12. Kirby ML: Nodose placode provides ectomesenchyme to the developing chick heart in the absence of cardiac neural crest. Cell Tissue Res 252:17–22, 1988.
13. Kirby ML, Gale TF, Stewart DE: Neural crest cells contribute to normal aorticopulmonary septation. Science 220:1059–1061, 1983.
14. McGoon DC, Rastelli GC, Ongley PA: An operation for the correction of truncus arteriosus. JAMA 205:59–63, 1968.
15. Radford DJ, Perkins L, Lachman R, et al: Spectrum of DiGeorge syndrome in patients with truncus arteriosus: expanded DiGeorge syndrome. Pediatr Cardiol 9:95–101, 1988.
16. Rowe RD, Freedom RM, Mehrizi A, et al: The Neonate with Congenital Heart Disease. Philadelphia, W.B. Saunders, 1981.
17. Van Mierop LHS, Kutsche LM: Cardiovascular anomalies in DiGeorge syndrome and importance of the neural crest as a possible pathogenetic factor. Am J Cardiol 58:133–137, 1986.
18. VanMierop LHS, Patterson DF, Schnarr WR: Pathogenesis of persistent truncus arteriosus in the light of observations made in a dog with the anomaly. Am J Cardiol 41:755–762, 1978.
19. Van Praagh R, Van Praagh S: The anatomy of common aorticopulmonary trunk (truncus arteriosus communis) and its embryologic implications. Am J Cardiol 16:406–425, 1965.
20. Victorica BE, Elliott LP: The roentgenologic findings and approach to persistent truncus arteriosus in infancy. Am J Roentgenol 104:440–451, 1968.

Chapter 46

TOTAL ANOMALOUS PULMONARY VENOUS RETURN

Donald C. Fyler, M.D.

DEFINITION

Drainage of the entire pulmonary venous circulation into systemic venous channels characterizes total pulmonary venous anomaly.

PREVALENCE

Total anomalous pulmonary venous return as an isolated problem was the twelfth most common cardiac defect among critically ill infants in the New England states (0.056/1000 live births, 1968–1974), constituting 2.6% of the total experience. This compares to the experience reported by others (see Table 1, p. 274).[7] Because total anomalous pulmonary venous return is a disease of infancy, when it is listed as part of the entire experience of a cardiology department, it is a much less significant entity (21st in diagnostic frequency, see Table 2, p. 276). If patients with asplenia or polysplenia are included, the number of patients with total anomalous pulmonary venous return is increased by 30% (see Exhibit 1).

ANATOMY

Any pulmonary vein, or combination of pulmonary veins, may drain anomalously into the systemic venous or right heart circulation, producing a left-to-right shunt. When all pulmonary veins return to the systemic venous circulation, the patient is said to have total anomalous pulmonary venous return (drainage, connection). There are several anatomic variations (Fig. 1; Exhibit 1).

1. **Supracardiac.** All of the pulmonary veins return to a common pulmonary vein located behind the left atrium, which may then drain upward on the left side of the chest toward the innominate vein, crossing the midline and proceeding down to the right superior vena cava. Sometimes the common pulmonary venous channel drains directly

into the superior vena cava and sometimes into the azygos system.

2. **Cardiac.** All pulmonary veins may drain into a common pulmonary vein, which then drains into the right atrium or more often into the coronary sinus.

3. **Infradiaphragmatic.** After collection by a common pulmonary vein behind the heart, the pulmonary venous blood passes down a venous channel through the diaphragm to the portal system, re-entering the heart through the ductus venosus and inferior vena cava.

4. **Mixed.** Any combination of anatomic entry of the pulmonary veins into the venous circulation is possible. For example, the right-sided veins may enter the right atrium, whereas the left veins travel upward to the innominate.

Except for the uncommon mixed variety, there is a collecting reservoir (common pulmonary vein) behind the left atrium.

The pulmonary venous system may be variably, absolutely, or relatively obstructed.[11] The point of obstruction may be caused by compression by adjacent structures, but may be within the pulmonary venous system, almost always downstream from the common pulmonary vein. Veins draining below the diaphragm are almost always obstructed either at the diaphragm or at the ductus venosus. Those entering the coronary sinus are less often obstructed,[6] whereas all other types may be obstructed in variable locations. Often increased pulmonary flow accentuates the obstruction. When there is obstruction there is pulmonary venous hypertension and reflex pulmonary arterial hypertension, often at suprasystemic pressure levels.

Rarely, other isolated, simple, cardiac anomalies, such as a ventricular septal defect, are associated with total anomalous veins; however, other major cardiac abnormalities are more likely to be present when there is asplenia and polysplenia (see p. 592).

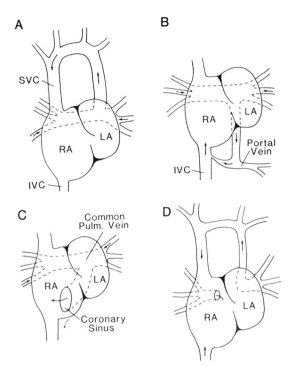

Figure 1. **A**, Supracardiac total anomalous pulmonary venous return. SVC, superior vena cava; IVC, inferior vena cava; RA, right atrium; LA, left atrium. All of the pulmonary veins collect in a common channel behind the left atrium. From there, blood courses upward to the innominate vein, down the superior vena cava, and re-enters the heart at the right atrium. All blood entering the left atrium passes from the right to the left atrium. **B**, Infradiaphragmatic total anomalous veins. All of the pulmonary veins collect behind the left atrium and, via a common channel, proceed through the diaphragm to the portal vein and ductus venosus to the inferior vena cava and back to the right atrium. **C**, Total anomalous pulmonary venous return to the coronary sinus. All of the pulmonary veins collect behind the left atrium and enter the coronary sinus. The pulmonary venous blood with coronary sinus blood drains into the right atrium. **D**, Mixed type of total anomalous pulmonary venous return. There are multiple variations on this anatomy. All pulmonary veins ultimately drain into the right atrium, with all blood entering the left atrium via the foramen ovale. In the example presented, the left veins course upward through the innominate vein, and down the superior vena cava to the right atrium, while the right pulmonary veins drain directly into the right atrium.

Physiology

The entire pulmonary venous blood flow is returned to the systemic venous circulation, where there is mixing of the two venous returns. Characteristically, mixing is virtually complete, each chamber of the heart receiving blood of practically identical oxygen content (Fig. 2). With maximal streaming, the right and left ventricular oxygen saturation may differ as much as 10%, rarely more. The level of arterial oxygen saturation is dependent on the size of the pulmonary blood flow. When there is large pulmonary blood flow, the percent

of arterial oxygen saturation may reach the high eighties, but with limited blood flow it may be much lower (these patients are discovered to have heart disease in the neonatal period because of cyanosis).

The amount of pulmonary blood flow is governed by the pulmonary arteriolar resistance and by obstructions of the pulmonary veins. Although the obstruction may be severe, the entire pulmonary

Exhibit 1

Boston Children's Hospital Experience 1973–1987
Total Anomalous Pulmonary Venous Return

There were 178 patients with total anomalous pulmonary venous return seen after January 1973, and before January 1988. Sixty patients had associated asplenia, polysplenia, malposition, or other major anomaly. When these were excluded, there were 118 patients with total anomalous pulmonary venous return that was uncomplicated except for a small number with ventricular septal defect; two had ventricular defect closure. Of the 118, 23 were survivors from the era before January 1973.

Surgery for Total Anomalous Pulmonary Venous Return by Age—30-Day Mortality

Age (days)	No. of Patients	No. of Deaths	% Mortality
0–14	27	3	11
15–60	25	4	16
61–180	28	1	4
181–	14	1	7
Total	94	9	10

Half of the new patients first seen after January, 1973, underwent corrective surgery before the age of 2 months with an overall initial mortality of 10% which improved over the years. The younger infants had a somewhat higher mortality, as did those with the infradiaphragmatic type.

Surgery for Total Anomalous Pulmonary Venous Return by Years—30-Day Mortality

Years	No. of Patients	No. of Deaths	% Mortality
1973–1976	20	4	20
1977–1982	44	3	7
1983–1987	31	2	6
Total	95	9	10

Surgical mortality has improved over the years.

Surgical Experience with Total Anomalous Pulmonary Venous Return by Type—30-Day Mortality

Type	No. of Patients	No. of Deaths	% Mortality
Supracardiac	43	3	7
Cardiac	23	0	0
Infracardiac	21	4	19
Other + Unspecified	7	2	29
Total	94	9	9

The mixed varieties and the infradiaphragmatic type have the highest surgical mortality.

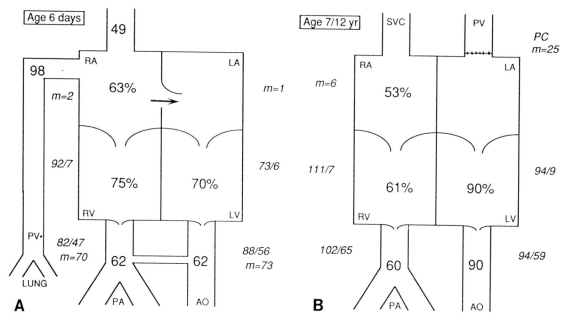

Figure 2. Total anomalous veins below the diaphragm. **A,** At the age of 6 days, this infant had pulmonary hypertension approximately equal to the systemic pressure. The difference in the percent of oxygen saturation within the chambers of the heart and the great arteries was no greater than 13% by any comparison. The source of all blood entering the left heart was via the foramen ovale from the right atrium to the left. **B,** A surgical procedure was carried out and seven months later the infant was recatheterized. On this occasion there was pulmonary hypertension, some arterial oxygen desaturation and an elevated pulmonary wedge pressure of 25 mm Hg. It was discovered that the original anastomotic site was obstructed and this was subsequently repaired with complete recovery. RA, right atrium; LA, left atrium; RV, right ventricle; LV, left ventricle; AO, aorta; PA, pulmonary artery; PV, pulmonary vein; PC, pulmonary capillary wedge pressure; large bold numbers, arterial oxygen saturation; italics, pressure in mm Hg.

venous return is rarely completely obstructed. Surprisingly, this anatomy is compatible with life for a few days or so (Fig. 3). When the obstruction is severe, the amount of pulmonary flow is small; when this is mixed with the systemic venous return, the result is a low arterial oxygen saturation. Pulmonary arterial pressure may be suprasystemic with severe obstruction and, because of this, in the first days of life, the ductus arteriosus may shunt right to left. Detection of the ductal right-to-left shunt is not possible by comparing the arterial oxygen saturation above and below the ductus, because all oxygen saturations in the heart are identical, negating the value of this otherwise useful test.

Total anomalous pulmonary venous return below the diaphragm is characterized by severe obstruction (Fig. 4), the portal system being unable to accommodate multiples of the cardiac output. Less often there is obstruction in the tortuous pulmonary venous channels of the supracardiac types. Asymmetric obstructions in some pulmonary veins and not in others, in certain mixed varieties, forces increased blood flow to the least obstructed area of lung, thereby stimulating persistence of fetal pulmonary arteriolar vasculature, which may help the patient to survive.

With minimal obstruction, the pulmonary blood

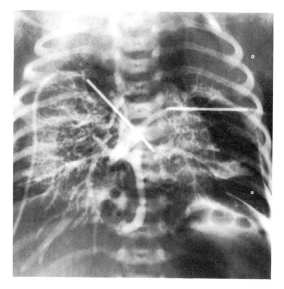

Figure 3. Complete obstruction of infradiaphragmatic total anomalous veins. This shows a postmortem injection of contrast material into the pulmonary venous system. There was no point of egress from the pulmonary veins into the systemic venous circulation at any point. This infant lived 3 days.

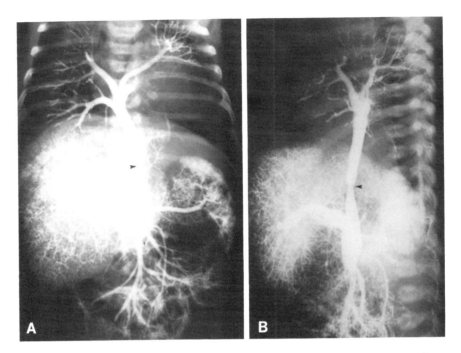

Figure 4. **A** and **B**, Total anomalous veins below the diaphragm. This shows a postmortem injection of contrast material into the portal system, filling the pulmonary veins and portal drainage. Note the point of obstruction at approximately the point where the common pulmonary venous channel pierces the diaphragm.

flow can be enormous; the patient may be pink and in congestive heart failure.

Generally, the left atrium and left ventricle seem to be relatively small compared with the very large right ventricle.[9,13] If the ductus arteriosus is patent, some of the cardiac output may bypass the left heart, further contributing to the impression of a small left ventricle. For some years it was thought that the left ventricle was too small to support life and that operation to salvage these infants was a futile gesture. We have no convincing examples of this.

It is a matter of curiosity that the entry of the pulmonary veins below the diaphragm produces a higher systemic arterial oxygen saturation than entry above the diaphragm because of the selective flow of inferior vena caval blood flow to the left atrium. This difference may be as much as 10–15%. Of somewhat more practical value is the fact that blood from the portal vein has a high oxygen saturation in this condition, a virtually diagnostic feature sometimes accidentally discovered during umbilical vein catheterization.

CLINICAL MANIFESTATIONS

Patients with total anomalous pulmonary venous return range from those with maximally obstructed to those with completely unrestricted pulmonary blood flow. Although the extremes will be described in some detail, it must be recognized that the majority of patients fall some place between them.

Total anomalous pulmonary venous return is not readily recognized by clinical, echocardiographic, or catheterization techniques. Although its former position as the most common, uncomplicated diagnosis to be overlooked, unrecognized, or confused is probably no longer justified, vigilance is still required to avoid error. The key to success (for the pediatrician) is to recognize that there is a cardiac problem and (for the cardiologist) to recognize and demonstrate the anatomic details. The surgeons handle these babies with remarkable success compared with a decade ago.

Obstructed Pulmonary Veins

When there is severe obstruction of the pulmonary venous return, the infant is discovered to be cyanotic in the first days or weeks of life. Usually there is tachypnea and, at times, episodes of paroxysmal tachypnea, gasping, and retractions which suggest pulmonary edema. The more severe the obstruction, the earlier the infant is symptomatic and discovered to have heart disease.

Physical Examination. On physical examination, the infant often appears very ill. There is cyanosis, tachypnea, and hepatomegaly. Often there is no murmur, the only abnormality being a loud second heart sound.

Electrocardiography. The electrocardiogram

shows right ventricular hypertrophy, but because these patients are usually neonates, it is difficult to be certain that the tracing is abnormal. There is usually P pulmonale.

Chest X-ray. On chest x-ray, the heart is of normal size or slightly enlarged. There is evidence of pulmonary edema, sometimes marked (Fig. 5).

Echocardiography. Echocardiography should establish the diagnosis, documenting the collection of all pulmonary veins to a common collecting reservoir behind the heart, with subsequent passage to the systemic venous circulation.[2] Right ventricular and pulmonary hypertension is discovered, and if the ductus is open, right-to-left shunting may be demonstrable. The location of each pulmonary vein should be documented so that the need to search for pulmonary veins in the operating room can be minimized. Doppler techniques can be used to recognize the presence or absence of pulsatile pulmonary venous blood flow. Absence of pulsatile flow suggests pulmonary venous obstruction.[14,16]

The first step in making the diagnosis of total anomalous pulmonary venous return is identifying a separate pulmonary venous confluence behind the left atrium or the common atrium. The confluence and individual pulmonary veins are seen best from the suprasternal notch or high left sternal border. If the venous channel is obstructed, the confluence is usually dilated and the velocity of blood flow is low. A diligent search should be made for at least two individual veins on each side, although there are often three veins on the right side. Transducer positions in the suprasternal notch or high left sternal border, with rotation to the short-axis view, provide the best images of the individual pulmonary veins. The subxiphoid short-axis view, angled to the right, demonstrates at least two right pulmonary veins passing posterior to the superior vena cava (right atrium junction). Leftward angulation in the short-axis view may show the left pulmonary veins as well. If at least four pulmonary veins are not identified, multiple drainage sites should be suspected.

Once the pulmonary venous confluence and individual pulmonary veins have been identified, the site(s) of communication with the systemic venous circuit should be sought. The most common drainage site for obstructed anomalous venous connection is the portal-hepatic system. The descending vertical vein can be seen in a subxiphoid transverse view as a third vascular channel crossing the diaphragm between the inferior vena cava and the descending aorta (Fig. 6). Flow in the channel is directed inferiorly and, using Doppler color flow mapping, can be traced into the liver. Pulmonary venous flow returns to the right atrium via the inferior vena cava. The inferior vena cava is often dilated and flow velocity may be increased depending on the severity of stenosis.

Less commonly, obstruction occurs in supracardiac total anomalous pulmonary venous drainage (Fig. 7). One cause of obstruction in this type of drainage is compression of the vertical vein between the left pulmonary artery and the left main bronchus. The vertical vein can be seen with the transducer in a left parasternal position and rotated to the parasagittal plane. Also with the transducer in the suprasternal notch and rotated to the short-axis view, the vertical vein can be traced by scanning anteriorly from the posterior pulmonary venous confluence to the anterior innominate vein. The innominate vein can be traced to the superior vena cava by scanning to the right. The innominate

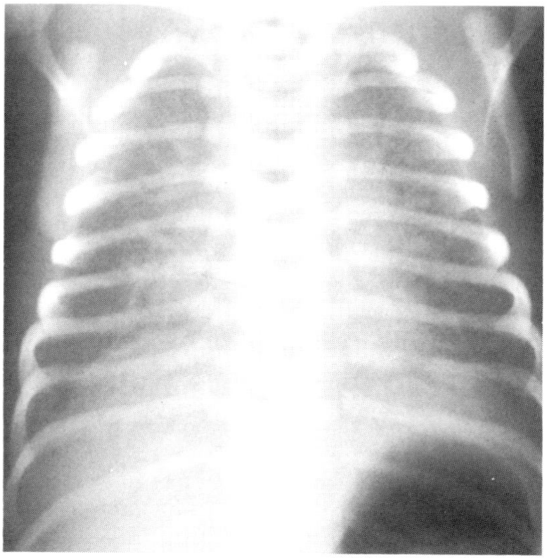

Figure 5. This infant with obstructed total anomalous pulmonary veins has gross pulmonary edema with poorly visible pulmonary structures. The heart is small.

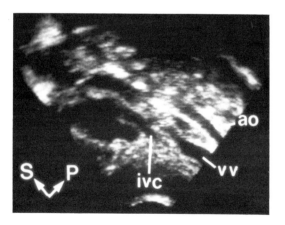

Figure 6. Echocardiogram in a patient with subdiaphragmatic total anomalous pulmonary venous drainage. Subxiphoid sagittal plane view showing the vertical venous connector penetrating the diaphragm between the inferior vena cava and the aorta.

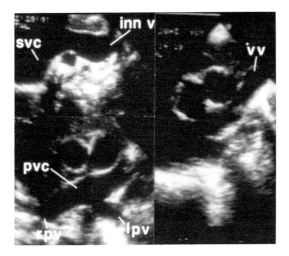

Figure 7. Echocardiograms in the suprasternal notch views in a patient with supracardiac total anomalous pulmonary venous drainage. Upper left panel shows a dilated innominate vein and dilated superior vena cava. Lower left panel shows a pulmonary venous confluence receiving the right and left pulmonary veins. Right panel shows the vertical venous connector draining the venous confluence to the innominate vein. pvc, pulmonary venous confluence; rpv, right pulmonary vein; lpv, left pulmonary vein; svc, superior vena cava; vv, vertical vein.

vein and superior vena cava are more or less dilated, depending on the severity of obstruction to pulmonary venous flow.

Rarely, total anomalous venous return to the coronary sinus is obstructed.[6] The point of obstruction is usually the junction of the individual veins with the coronary sinus or with a short vertical connecting vein. Usually the connection to the coronary sinus is seen best from subxiphoid long- and short-axis views. Alternative views include parasternal and apical views.

Other sites of communication with the systemic venous circuit that can be obstructed include the azygos vein and the right superior vena cava. We know of no example of obstructed pulmonary venous connection directly to the right atrium. These uncommon sites of connection can be identified most easily by locating a vessel leading away from the venous confluence, as demonstrated by Doppler color flow mapping or pulsed Doppler examination, and following it to its termination. Often the channel is small and tortuous, making it difficult to trace. Multiple views may be needed to image the complete course of the channel. Segments passing posterior to the trachea or a bronchus often cannot be imaged due to shadowing by the airway.

Pulsed and continuous-wave Doppler echocardiography are useful for identifying points of obstruction. The flow pattern is nonpulsatile; there is nearly constant peak velocity proximal to a point of obstruction, but disturbed and high velocity at, and just distal to, the obstruction. Using the pulsed Doppler technique, the flow pattern should be sampled in the individual veins, as well as in the venous confluence, because obstruction can occur at multiple sites.

Isolated connection of individual veins directly to the systemic venous circuit should be sought, using combined imaging and Doppler examination. If the vein can be identified near the hilum of the lung, it can be traced with imaging and Doppler color flow mapping to its termination. Otherwise, the usual sites of connection, such as the left innominate vein, the superior vena cava, and the right atrium, should be searched for an abnormal, continuous flow jet, using Doppler color flow mapping or pulsed Doppler.

Other data that support the diagnosis of total anomalous pulmonary venous return, and which should be sought, include a right-to-left flow through the foramen ovale, a small left atrium, and an enlarged amd hypertensive right ventricle. With severe obstruction the right ventricular pressure is often suprasystemic, with posterior bowing of the ventricular septum. If tricuspid regurgitation is present, an effort should be made to estimate the right ventricular pressure (see ch. 13).

Cardiac Catheterization. Cardiac catheterization is not needed to make this diagnosis and does little but delay the surgery.

Unrestricted Pulmonary Blood Flow

With unrestricted pulmonary blood flow, the patient presents at a later age, sometimes in childhood (the oldest person we have seen was 52 years old). The vast majority are first encountered by the age of 2–4 months (Exhibit 1). Discovery is usually a consequence of congestive heart failure.

Physical Examination. On physical examination, the infant has not grown well and is tachypneic. There is minimal or no visible cyanosis. Often there is hepatomegaly. There may be prominence of the left side of the chest; the cardiac impulse is hyperactive. Often there is a gallop rhythm. The second heart sound is accentuated and split, and the splitting does not vary with respiration. There is a systolic murmur, rarely more than grade 3, at the left upper sternal border, and a diastolic rumbling murmur can be heard early in diastole at the lower sternal border. In the uncomplicated situation the physical findings are similar to those of a large atrial septal defect. A loud systolic murmur suggests some additional cardiac anomaly.

Electrocardiography. The electrocardiogram shows right ventricular hypertrophy that can be described as abnormal for age when the infant is more than a few weeks old. P pulmonale is usually present.

Chest X-ray. On chest x-ray, the heart is enlarged and there is pulmonary vascular engorgement. In older children, the common pulmonary vein may be visible but this is rarely discernible in small babies (Fig. 8). Compared with the obstructive type, there is excessive pulmonary blood flow, often marked, but usually without pulmonary edema.

Laboratory Data. The patient has abnormally low arterial pO_2 that rises to unexpectedly high levels with a hyperoxia test (breathing 100% oxygen for 10 minutes). Results as high as 200–250 torr are encountered in patients with torrential pulmonary blood flow.

Echocardiography. The echocardiographic examination demonstrates total anomalous pulmonary venous drainage collecting into a common point behind the left atrium. Generally, each pulmonary vein can be identified and its point of entry noted. Those not entering the common collecting vein must be identified, because they will cause significant problems at surgical correction. The levels of pulmonary hypertension and right ventricular hypertension should be documented and any suggestion of obstruction of pulmonary veins proximal to the collecting vein should be noted.

The examination is carried out as previously described for obstructed total anomalous pulmonary venous return.

Cardiac Catheterization. Usually there is no need for cardiac catheterization in the diagnosis of total anomalous pulmonary venous return. However, any suggestion of incomplete information or atypical features requires physiologic study. Are all pulmonary veins accounted for? Are there other cardiac defects?

Although the precise location of the venous drainage may vary considerably, infants with this condition rarely have associated defects such as ventricular septal defect or valvar abnormalities. Thus, if the clinical and two-dimensional echocardiographic findings are typical, and the infant is unstable, these patients may be served best by referral for complete repair without cardiac catheterization.[5,14]

With a balloon angiocatheter positioned in the right or left main pulmonary artery, 1–2 ml of contrast material per kg of body weight (depending on whether or not obstruction of pulmonary veins is suspected), are injected while filming in the frontal and lateral position (Fig. 9). The opposite pulmonary artery is then injected in similar fashion. When there is torrential pulmonary blood flow, a total of 4 ml/kg may be needed; otherwise, dilution of contrast through the lungs will result in an inadequate levophase. A single main pulmonary artery injection should be avoided, in part because with torrential flow the contrast may be too diluted to provide adequate pictures and, among those with obstruction, reactive pulmonary vasospasm may cause considerable hemodynamic instability. Frequently it is possible to enter the anomalous draining vein directly; if so entered, angiographic contrast should be injected, because this usually provides the most reliable anatomic demonstration. With severely obstructed veins, the ductus should be balloon-occluded during the injection to reduce right-to-left shunting; otherwise, most of the contrast may pass into the aorta.

With a balloon catheter passed through the foramen ovale and positioned in the apex of the left ventricle, and the patient in the long axial oblique and right anterior oblique position, 1 ml/kg of contrast material is injected in one second or less. This

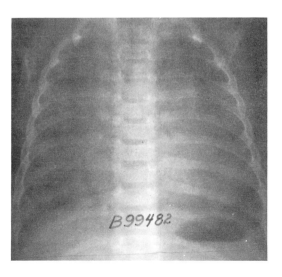

Figure 8. A chest x-ray of a patient with total anomalous pulmonary venous return to the superior vena cava. The heart is enlarged. Compare with Figure 5. Note the relatively large heart and absence of pulmonary edema.

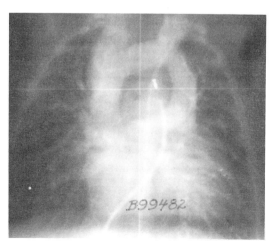

Figure 9. This is the same patient as in Figure 8, showing an angiographic demonstration of the supracardiac drainage of the pulmonary veins upward to an innominate vein and then down the right superior vena cava to the right heart. Note that the upward draining pulmonary veins were not recognizable on the chest x-ray (Fig. 8).

angiogram not only allows measurement of left ventricular volumes, it also identifies any associated ventricular septal defects.

MANAGEMENT

In otherwise uncomplicated total anomalous pulmonary venous return, the cardiac output (the systemic blood flow) passes through the foramen ovale and the ductus arteriosus. With closure of the ductus, the entire cardiac output must pass through the foramen. This is the basis for the belief that the foramen ovale is another point of obstruction to the cardiac output and that opening it may contribute to survival. We have not accepted this line of thinking because (1) there is rarely a significant gradient across the foramen, and (2) measured outputs are in the expected range. This is not to say that perhaps a few older patients may not experience obstruction at this point, but rather to express the belief that, in the majority of patients, this is an unnecessary concern that we have ignored without recognized detriment to our patients.

Most patients with total anomalous pulmonary venous return have neither maximally obstructed nor completely unrestricted pulmonary blood flow. They present clinical problems ranging from one extreme to the other. Usually, complicating cardiac defects associated with asplenia and polysplenia can be readily identified, and recognition of complicated heterotaxy is easy. These patients have special problems (see p. 592).

When the anatomy of the pulmonary veins is identified, the entry point of all pulmonary veins is located and surgical repair can be planned. If there is more than one place where the pulmonary veins enter the systemic venous circuit, a plan to connect all, or virtually all, pulmonary veins to the left atrium is devised.

We do not find significant improvement in surgical mortality with increasing age or larger size, although others disagree.[1,3,12,15] For this reason, in our institution, infants with total anomalous pulmonary venous return are referred for surgery on discovery (Exhibit 1).

At surgery a large anastomosis is made between the pulmonary venous confluence and the left atrium. The larger the anastomosis, the better. The mortality with this surgery has been improving over the years (Exhibit 1),[10] and at the present time is quite acceptable. Most often, late follow-up shows a good result.

COURSE

We now have survivors who had surgical corrections more than 20 years ago and continue to do well. It is our impression that, barring rare problems in the first few years after surgery, these patients are cured.

About 10% of the survivors have residual pulmonary venous obstruction that may occur at the anastomotic site, or rarely, it may be located proximal to the surgical suture line. At times it is located at the entry point of individual pulmonary veins. Re-operation for relief of obstruction at the anastomotic site is often successful, but surgical relief of obstruction at the orifices of the pulmonary veins, or within the pulmonary veins, whether this is inherent[4] or acquired, is rarely successfully accomplished.[8] This complication of surgery for total anomalous pulmonary venous return seems to occur irrespective of the type of total anomalous veins. In patients in whom individual pulmonary vein obstruction occurs, it is a progressive lesion much like that seen in acquired pulmonary venous obstruction in other circumstances (see ch. 38).[8]

TOTAL ANOMALOUS PULMONARY VENOUS RETURN WITH ASPLENIA OR POLYSPLENIA

Total anomalous pulmonary venous return is either an isolated phenomenon or is associated with the complex cardiac abnormalities found in the asplenia-polysplenia syndromes (see ch. 37). It is associated with these syndromes in 25–30% of these patients.

The physiologic effect of total anomalous pulmonary venous return may be negligible in this situation, in that these syndromes usually include other cardiac defects that allow common mixing, such as single ventricle, common atria, and common atrioventricular canal. Occasionally, obstructive total anomalous pulmonary veins, in the presence of pulmonary stenosis or pulmonary atresia, are a major problem when planning shunt surgery. (Can additional pulmonary blood flow be forced past the obstructive point?) Otherwise, total anomalous pulmonary veins present a problem to be reckoned with when considering possible repair or Fontan surgery. In these children it often comes down to repairing the total anomalous veins first, without notable functional or symptomatic gain, before further surgery can be undertaken (see ch. 37).

REFERENCES

1. Byrum CJ, Dick M, Behrendt DM, et al: Repair of total anomalous pulmonary venous connection in patients younger than 6 months old: late postoperative hemodynamic and electrophysiologic status. Circulation 66 (Supp I):I-208–213, 1982.
2. Chin AJ, Sanders SP, Sherman F, et al: Accuracy of subcostal two-dimensional echocardiography in prospective diagnosis of total anomalous pulmonary venous connection. Am Heart J 113:1153–1159, 1987.

3. Hawkins JA, Clark EB, and Doty DB: Total anomalous pulmonary venous connection. Ann Thorac Surg 36:548–560, 1983.
4. Haworth SG: Total anomalous pulmonary venous return. Prenatal damage to pulmonary vascular bed and extrapulmonary veins. Br Heart J 48:513–524, 1982.
5. Huhta JC, Gutgesell HP, Nihill MR: Cross-sectional echocardiographic diagnosis of total anomalous pulmonary venous connection. Br Heart J 53: 525–534, 1985.
6. Jonas RA, Smolinsky A, Mayer JE, et al: Obstructed pulmonary venous drainage with total anomalous pulmonary venous connection to the coronary sinus. Am J Cardiol 59:431–435, 1987.
7. Keith JC, Rowe RD, and Vlad P: Heart Disease in Infancy and Childhood, 3rd ed. Toronto, Macmillan, 1978.
8. Kelley LM, Cheatham JP, Kugler JD, et al: Postnatal atresia of extraparenchymal pulmonary veins, fulminant necrotizing pulmonary arteritis and elevated circulating immune complexes. J Am Coll Cardiol 9:1043–1048, 1987.
9. Lima CO, Valdes-Cruz LM, Allen HD, et al: Prognostic value of left ventricular size measured by echocardiography in infants with total anomalous pulmonary venous drainage. Am J Cardiol 51:1155–1159, 1983.
10. Lincoln CR, Rigby ML, Mercanti C, et al: Surgical risk factors in total anomalous pulmonary venous connection. Am J Cardiol 61:608–611, 1988.
11. Lucas RV, Lock JE, Tandon R, et al: Gross and histologic anatomy of total anomalous pulmonary venous connections. Am J Cardiol 62:292–300, 1988.
12. Reardon MJ, Cooley DA, Kubrusly L, et al: Total anomalous pulmonary venous return: report of 201 patients treated surgically. Texas Heart Inst J 12:131–141, 1985.
13. Rosenquist GC, Kelly JL, Chandra R, et al: Small left atrium and change in contour of the ventricular septum in total anomalous pulmonary venous connection: a morphometric analysis of 22 infant hearts. Am J Cardiol 55:777–782, 1985.
14. Smallhorn JF, Freedom RM: Pulsed Doppler echocardiography in the preoperative evaluation of total anomalous pulmonary venous connection. J Am Coll Cardiol 8:1413–1420, 1986.
15. Turley K, Tucker WY, Ullyot DJ, et al: Total anomalous pulmonary venous connection in infancy: influence of age and type of lesion. Am J Cardiol 45:92–97, 1980.
16. Vick GW, Murphy DJ, Ludomirsky A, et al: Pulmonary venous and systemic ventricular inflow obstruction in patients with congenital heart disease: detection by combined two-dimensional and Doppler echocardiography. J Am Coll Cardiol 9:580–587, 1987.

Chapter 47

AORTOPULMONARY WINDOW

Donald C. Fyler, M.D.

DEFINITION

An aortopulmonary window (aortopulmonary fenestration, aortopulmonary septal defect) is a hole between the ascending aorta and the main pulmonary artery. There must be two distinct and separate semilunar valves before this diagnosis can be made. The opening of variable size is located adjacent to the semilunar valves or closer to the origin of the right pulmonary artery.

PREVALENCE

Aortopulmonary window is a rare anomaly; 19 patients have been seen in the past 15 years at the Children's Hospital in Boston (Exhibit 1). The Toronto group has reported 23 instances of aortopulmonary septal defect in a series of 15,100 patients.[3] These experiences result in a figure of 0.13–0.15% of patients referred to them with congenital heart disease.

EMBRYOLOGY

There is failure of aortopulmonary septation which, although in many ways reminiscent of truncus arteriosus communis, probably develops by a different mechanism.[4] Fifty percent of the patients have no associated cardiac defect. Pulmonary atresia, tetralogy of Fallot,[4,5] interrupted aortic arch, and coarctation of the aorta are seen in association with aortopulmonary window (Exhibit 1).

ANATOMY

An aortopulmonary window consists of an opening usually between the ascending aorta and the main pulmonary artery close to the aortic valve. Occasionally, the opening is more distal in the aorta and connects to the origin of the right pulmonary artery.[2,3,6,7] The orifice varies in size, but commonly is large enough to be associated with pulmonary hypertension.

Exhibit 1

Boston Children's Hospital Experience
1973–1987

Aortopulmonary Window

There were 19 children who had aortopulmonary window. The associated cardiac defects included ventricular septal defect (8), pulmonary atresia (4), coarctation (2), interrupted aortic arch (1), double-outlet right ventricle (2), and tricuspid atresia (1). Seventeen underwent surgical repair. One 30-year-old woman has advanced pulmonary vascular disease and one infant has yet to undergo surgery. Two infants died during surgery: one was a premature infant with the respiratory distress syndrome who died at surgery at the age of 44 days; another did not survive closure of the aortopulmonary window and a ventricular septal defect at the age of 29 days.

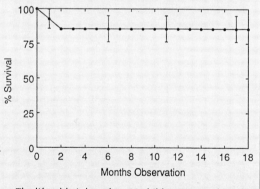

The life table is based on 19 children starting from the time of first observation.

PHYSIOLOGY

The physiologic effects are those of a left-to-right shunt, such as with ventricular septal defect or persistent patent ductus arteriosus. As pulmonary resistance drops in the days and weeks after birth, there is increasing left-to-right shunting and, ultimately, if the window is big, congestive heart failure develops in the first weeks of life. Because these defects are most often large, there is usually pulmonary hypertension at systemic levels.[1] With-

693

out repair, pulmonary vascular disease develops later, possibly as early as the end of the first year of life.

CLINICAL MANIFESTATIONS

The clinical features are indistinguishable from those seen in a patient with a persistently patent ductus arteriosus. With a smaller opening the murmurs are those of a classical patent ductus arteriosus (see ch. 33). With larger defects the murmurs are not necessarily continuous, and evidence of congestive heart failure[6] or pulmonary hypertension may dominate the auscultatory findings. In the past, the typical auscultatory findings of a patent ductus arteriosus resulted in ligation of the ductus without further workup, with an acceptable error rate attributable to aortopulmonary window. Nowadays, the diagnosis of aortopulmonary window can be readily made preoperatively by echocardiography.

Electrocardiography

The electrocardiographic patterns are the same as those seen in patients with patent ductus arteriosus.

Chest X-ray

The chest x-ray shows evidence of left-to-right shunting and pulmonary hypertension indistinguishable from that seen in patients with patent ductus arteriosus.

Echocardiography

The hyperdynamic function and the enlarged chambers provide useful clues to the presence and location of a left-to-right shunt. The defect itself can be visualized and the shunting can be documented by Doppler examination.

The diagnosis is made by scanning the aortopulmonary septum in multiple views,[7] including the subxiphoid (Fig. 1), parasternal, and suprasternal notch. The ability to image the defect in multiple views and to detect the flow through the defect by Doppler color flow mapping makes it possible to distinguish true defects from false dropout. At the level of the defect the joined vessels are elliptical in cross-section, whereas in contrast, false dropout is characterized by persistence of the normal circular contour of each vessel.

The distinguishing feature between aortopulmonary window and truncus arteriosus is the presence of two separate semilunar valves in the former. The aortopulmonary window is proximal to, and/or at the level of, the pulmonary artery branches, whereas a persistent ductus arteriosus is more distal and usually has some length.

Surgically important information that is readily derived from the echocardiogram includes the distance between the proximal border of the defect and the semilunar valves and coronary arteries, as well as the distance between the distal border and the pulmonary arteries.

Cardiac Catheterization

Although a patient with typical clinical features and unequivocal echocardiographic findings is reasonably sent to surgery without further workup, these patients are rare enough and the possibility

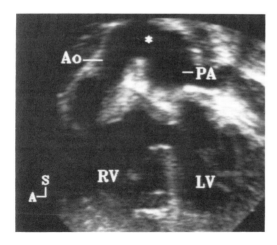

Figure 1. Subxiphoid short-axis view in an infant with double-outlet right ventricle and aortopulmonary window. *, Aortopulmonary window; Ao, ascending aorta; LV, left ventricle; PA, pulmonary artery; RV, right ventricle; S, superior; A, anterior.

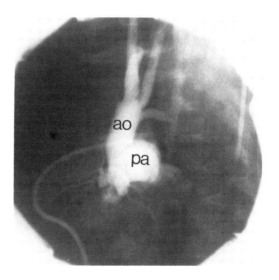

Figure 2. Cineangiogram in the left anterior oblique view. Separate aortic and pulmonary valves were identified. Note simultaneous opacification of the main pulmonary artery (pa) and ascending aorta (ao), similar to that in truncus arteriosus. Note the very small transverse arch; there was a severe coarctation of the aorta.

of associated cardiac defects is high enough (Exhibit 1) that most come to cardiac catheterization. The *sine qua non* in establishing this diagnosis at cardiac catheterization is cineangiographic filming of contrast material in the ascending aorta in more than one view (Fig. 2).

MANAGEMENT

Ideally, the discovery of an aortopulmonary window does not lead directly to surgical correction in the first weeks of life. Generally, an attempt to gain the advantage of anticongestive medications and the advantage of avoiding surgery in the immediate newborn period are worthwhile, although not vital. Depending on possible associated extracardiac anomalies and associated additional cardiac defects, as well as on the response to medication, surgery should be performed as early as needed, (rarely later than the age of 2 months). Surgery amounts to patch closure of the defect. Surgical results are good; we are unaware of late problems.

REFERENCES

1. Blieden LC, Moller JH: Aorticopulmonary septal defect: an experience with 17 patients. Br Heart J 36:630–635, 1974.
2. Doty DB, Richardson JV, Falkovsky GE, et al: Aortopulmonary septal defect: hemodynamics, angiography, and operation. Ann Thorac Surg 32:244–250, 1981.
3. Keith JC, Rowe RD, Vlad P: Heart Disease in Infancy and Childhood, 3rd ed. New York, Macmillan, 1978.
4. Kutsche LM, Van Mierop LHS: Anatomy and pathogenesis of aorticopulmonary septal defect: analysis of 286 reported cases. Am J Cardiol 59:443–447, 1987.
5. Lau KC, Calcaterra G, Miller GAH, et al: Aorto-pulmonary window. J Cardiovasc Surg 23:21–27, 1982.
6. Richardson JV, Doty DB, Rossi NP, et al: The spectrum of anomalies of aortopulmonary septation. J Thorac Cardiovasc Surg 78:21–25, 1979.
7. Satomi G, Nakamura K, Imai Y, et al: Two-dimensional echocardiographic diagnosis of aorticopulmonary window. Br Heart J 43:351–356, 1980.

Chapter 48

ORIGIN OF A PULMONARY ARTERY FROM THE AORTA (HEMITRUNCUS)

Donald C. Fyler, M.D.

DEFINITION

The term hemitruncus is used when either pulmonary artery originates from the aorta in the presence of a pulmonary valve and main pulmonary artery. The terminology "origin of the right (left) pulmonary artery from the aorta" may be more precise, because there is no known relation of hemitruncus to true truncus arteriosus.

PREVALENCE

This is a rare anomaly, having been seen four times in 2,251 critically ill infants with cardiac disease.[2] Ten infants with this diagnosis were seen at the Boston Children's Hospital between 1973 and 1987 (Exhibit 1).

PATHOLOGY

The pathology is as defined. Either the right or the left pulmonary artery arises from the aorta, while the other pulmonary artery arises from the main pulmonary trunk. Origin of the right pulmonary artery from the aorta is much more common than origin of the left pulmonary artery from the aorta.[6] A single case of origin of both the right and left pulmonary arteries from the aorta in the presence of a pulmonary valve and main pulmonary artery has been described.[5] In the usual case, a

patent ductus arteriosus communicates with the pulmonary artery that derives its blood flow from the right ventricle. Tetralogy of Fallot is a relatively common concomitant when the left pulmonary artery arises from the aorta.[4] Evidence has been presented that anomalous origin of the right pulmonary artery and anomalous origin of the left pulmonary artery have different pathogenetic mechanism and that neither is related to the pathogenesis of truncus arteriosus.[4]

PHYSIOLOGY

Before birth, one lung is supplied from the left ventricle and the ascending aorta, while the contralateral lung is supplied from the right ventricle and the main pulmonary artery. After birth, with falling pulmonary resistance, there is opportunity for excessive pulmonary flow into the lung supplied by the aorta. Blood flow to the opposite lung is excessive to the extent that it receives the entire venous return (cardiac output). The pulmonary artery pressure in both lungs is elevated, often equally (Fig. 1). A persistently patent ductus arteriosus may shunt left to right into the left lung. Congestive heart failure (a nearly universal phenomenon) occurs within the first weeks of life and is often severe.

CLINICAL MANIFESTATIONS

A systolic murmur is heard at birth. Within days or a week or so after birth, tachypnea, dyspnea, and the clinical syndrome of congestive heart failure become evident. The infant has the clinical picture of a large left-to-right shunt without cyanosis.

Electrocardiography

The electrocardiogram shows right ventricular hypertrophy.

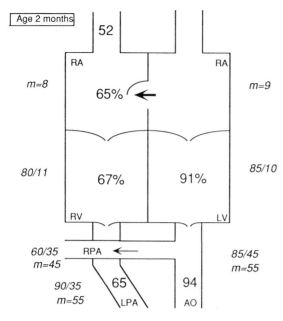

Figure 1. Diagram of the hemodynamics in a patient with origin of the right pulmonary artery from the aorta. Note pulmonary hypertension in both lungs. The left lung receives the entire systemic venous return plus possible minimal left-to-right shunting through an atrial opening. The right lung carries greatly increased blood flow derived entirely from the ascending aorta.

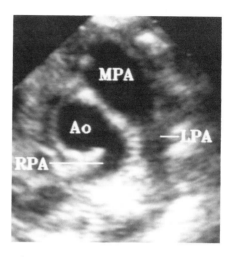

Figure 2. Parasternal short-axis view in an infant with hemitruncus. Note the right pulmonary artery (RPA) arising from the posterior aspect of the ascending aorta (AO). The left pulmonary artery (LPA) arises normally from the main pulmonary artery (MPA).

Chest X-ray

The heart is large and the pulmonary vasculature is increased bilaterally. Sometimes the difference in vascularity between the right and left lung is distinguishable, but usually only in retrospect.

Echocardiography

Hemitruncus, or origin of a pulmonary artery branch from the ascending aorta, is a rare anomaly. The most difficult part of making the diagnosis is thinking of it.[3] The pulmonary artery branch arising from the aorta (usually the right pulmonary artery) can be seen in a parasternal long- or short-axis view (Fig. 2).[1]

The point of connection with the aorta is usually posterior and leftward. Doppler color flow mapping or the pulsed Doppler examination demonstrates continuous flow into the pulmonary artery branch from the aorta. The other artery branch (usually the left pulmonary artery) connects normally with the main pulmonary trunk.

A persistent ductus arteriosus is commonly associated with hemitruncus. If the ductus is large, the pulmonary trunk may appear to bifurcate normally. This potential diagnostic pitfall is especially important if the left pulmonary artery connects abnormally with the aorta. It is essential to identify unequivocally both pulmonary artery branches and the ductus arteriosus or ligamentum arteriosum. If the ductus is small, a moderately high-velocity flow (>1.5–2 m/sec) may be detected from the pulmonary trunk to the aorta, because the pressure in the pulmonary trunk and the normally connecting pulmonary artery branch are often suprasystemic.

Cardiac Catheterization

Unless there is reason to believe that some other cardiac defect is present, there is little to be gained from a cardiac catheterization, once a confident echo diagnosis has been made. In former times, the diagnosis was readily demonstrated with a left ventricular or ascending aorta angiogram (Fig. 3).

MANAGEMENT

As soon as the diagnosis is established, the infant is stabilized on anticongestive medications and cardiac surgery is carried out.[5] A variety of operations have been proposed in the past, but the anastomosis of the pulmonary artery arising from the aorta to the contralateral pulmonary artery best normalizes the circulation. Surgical mortality is negligible. Later, if right peripheral pulmonary stenosis develops at the site of anastomosis, it can be dealt with by surgery or with balloon catheter techniques as needed (see ch. 14).

The biggest difficulty in these children has been recognition of a very rare diagnosis. Now that modern echocardiographic techniques are available, it seems likely that most patients will be discovered, diagnosed, and referred for surgery.

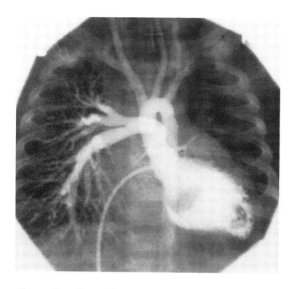

Figure 3. Cineangiogram in anteroposterior view. The catheter enters the left ventricle via a patent foramen ovale. Origin of the right pulmonary artery from the aorta is well demonstrated. The left pulmonary artery had earlier been entered from the right ventricle and the main pulmonary artery.

REFERENCES

1. Duncan WJ, Freedom RM, Olley PM, et al: Two-dimensional echocardiographic identification of hemitruncus: anomalous origin of one pulmonary artery from the ascending aorta with the other pulmonary artery arising normally from the right ventricle. Am Heart J 102:892–896, 1981.
2. Fyler DC, Buckley LP, Hellenbrand WE, et al: Report of the New England regional infant cardiac program. Pediatrics 65:376–461, 1980.
3. King DH, Huhta JC, Gutgesell HP, et al: Two-dimensional echocardiographic diagnosis of anomalous origin of the right pulmonary artery from the aorta: differentiation from aortopulmonary window. J Am Coll Cardiol 4:351–355, 1984.
4. Kutsche LM, Van Mierop LHS: Anomalous origin of a pulmonary artery from the ascending aorta: associated anomalies and pathogenesis. Am J Cardiol 61:850–856, 1988.
5. Penkoske PA, Castaneda AR, Fyler DC, et al: Origin of pulmonary artery branch from ascending aorta: primary surgical repair in infancy. J Thorac Cardiovasc Surg 85:537–545, 1983.
6. Richardson JV, Doty DB, Rossi NP, et al: The spectrum of anomalies of aortopulmonary septation. J Thorac Cardiovasc Surg 78:21–27, 1979.

Chapter 49

"CORRECTED" TRANSPOSITION OF THE GREAT ARTERIES

Donald C. Fyler, M.D.

DEFINITION

"Corrected" transposition of the great arteries is characterized by inverted ventricles and transposition of the great arteries. Systemic venous blood passes from the right atrium through a mitral valve into a left ventricle and then to the main pulmonary artery. Pulmonary venous blood passes from the left atrium through a tricuspid valve to a right ventricle and then to the aorta. This combination of ventricular inversion (atrioventricular discordance) and transposition of the great arteries (ventriculoarterial discordance) without cardiac anomalies results in normal arterial oxygen content, hence the term "corrected." Unfortunately, the condition rarely exists without other major cardiac anomalies. Patients with a single ventricle or with one atrioventricular valve are discussed elsewhere (see chs. 39, 42, 44). In this chapter, only patients with two ventricles are considered.

PREVALENCE

Transposition of the great arteries with two functionally adequate but inverted ventricles is a rare anomaly, occurring in approximately 0.7% of infants with congenital heart disease or 0.02 per 1000 live births (see ch. 18). At The Children's Hospital in Boston over the 15-year period from 1973 through 1987, there were 89 patients with this anomaly, or 0.6% of those with congenital heart disease.

ANATOMY[1,11]

The right atrium empties through a morphologic mitral valve, which has two papillary muscles, into a morphologically left ventricle that is rightward and anterior. The ventricle is finely trabeculated and empties into an outflow tract that leads posteriorly to the pulmonary valve. The left atrium empties through a morphologic tricuspid valve into a coarsely trabeculated right ventricle. The right ventricular outflow is anterior, emptying through an aortic valve into an anterior and leftward ascending aorta (Figs. 1 and 2). The segmental analysis of this is SLL (see ch. 4). Compared with the crossing of outflow tracts in a normal heart, the outflow tracts in patients with "corrected" transposition are parallel and the ventricular septum lies in a more anteroposterior position.

Rarely, there are no associated cardiac defects, and the patients survive as long as 70 years.[10] More often, however, there are other cardiac anomalies that determine the outcome.[17]

Tricuspid abnormalities are frequently described and tricuspid incompetence is often a clinical problem (30–70% of cases). This is usually, but not always, based on an Ebstein-like deformity (see ch. 44); the septal leaflet is downwardly displaced and some of the left ventricle seems atrialized. Obstructive, left-sided inflow and outflow lesions are found in 10–15% of the patients.[12]

Pulmonary outflow obstruction is common and is usually subpulmonary, with some associated valvar deformity. Subpulmonary stenosis may consist of a diaphragm or bits of fibrous tissue apparently arising from the mitral valve, with added obstruction caused by muscular hypertrophy. Rarely, isolated valvar stenosis is encountered.

Ventricular septal defects may occur anywhere in the septum but are most commonly located in the membranous portion of the septum and adjacent areas. The pulmonary trunk may be substantially overriding. The tricuspid or mitral valve may be straddling and associated with varying degrees of underdevelopment of either ventricle.

Conduction System

Over the years, the anatomy and course of the conduction system have been a matter of some debate. The sinus node is in its usual location at

701

NORMAL   **CORRECTED TRANSPOSITION**

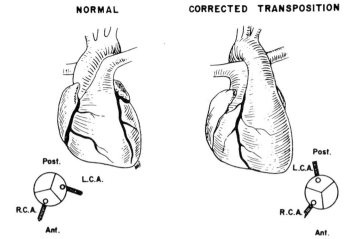

Figure 1. External view of the heart and great vessels in a normal person and in one with corrected transposition of the great arteries. Note that the left border of the heart in the patient with corrected transposition is occupied by the aorta, not the pulmonary artery. Note also the anterior position of the aorta. The origin of the coronary arteries is illustrated in the insert. The left coronary originates from the posterior sinus and the right coronary from the right anterior sinus. (From Nadas AS, Fyler DC: Pediatric Cardiology. Philadelphia, W.B. Saunders, 1972, with permission.)

the right atrial–superior vena caval junction, and the septum (the ventricles being reversed) depolarizes in the reverse of normal. Discussion centers around the location and number of atrioventricular nodes and the distal conduction system. The location of the conduction bundles is dependent on the associated defects, particularly ventricular septal defects.

Coronary Anatomy

The coronary arteries are reversed; that is, the right coronary supplies the anterior descending branch, which follows the course of the septum and gives rise to a circumflex, which encircles the

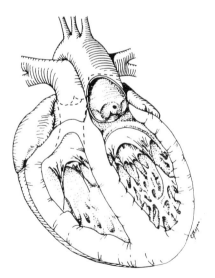

Figure 2. Drawing of corrected transposition viewed in an anteroposterior view. The finely trabeculated right-sided left ventricle supplies a posterior main pulmonary artery. The mitral valve is right-sided and has the usual two papillary muscles. The tricuspid valve is left-sided, inserts lower on the septum, and a papillary muscle attaches to the ventricular septum. There is a coarsely trabeculated, left-sided right ventricle that supplies an anterior positioned aorta.

mitral valve. The left-sided coronary artery resembles a right coronary artery. Generally, if this anatomy is not present, a diagnosis of "corrected" transposition is suspect.[4]

Atrioventricular and ventriculoarterial discordance ("corrected" transposition) is also present in dextrocardia (IDD) (see ch. 4) and is a feature of patients with single ventricle, tricuspid atresia, mitral atresia, and double-outlet right ventricle (Exhibit 1).

PHYSIOLOGY

The physiologic problems presented by patients with "corrected" transposition of the great arteries are directly related to the associated defects.

The myocardial function of the systemic, but anatomic right, ventricle has been a matter of interest. Because the two ventricles have different geometric configuration, it is postulated that the right ventricle may not perform systemic pumping as well as an anatomic left ventricle. Although the situation is not clear, the performance of the right ventricle as a systemic ventricle is suspect.[3,7,15]

CLINICAL MANIFESTATIONS

The clinical features are, similarly, a direct function of the associated cardiac anatomy. The infant may suffer cyanosis or congestive heart failure, be discovered because of a murmur, or be found because of an abnormality on a chest x-ray taken for some reason unrelated to the heart.

Electrocardiography

With the first depolarization of the ventricular septum there may be a Q wave in the right-sided chest leads and absence of a Q wave in the left. Varying degrees of heart block, usually with a QRS complex of normal duration, may be recorded. As many as 32% of these patients are born with, or

Exhibit 1

The Boston Children's Hospital Experience
1973–87

Corrected Transposition of the Great Arteries

There were 90 children who were categorized as having corrected transposition of the great arteries as their primary problem: 53 were males (59%) and 37 (41%) were females; 56 patients had cardiac surgery; 9 had tricuspid valve replacement. Complete heart block developed in 29 patients.

Corrected transposition, or segmental description SLL, was mentioned in 311 patients listed under other diagnostic categories, mainly single ventricle and malposition. Of these, 52 developed complete heart block (17%) at some time.

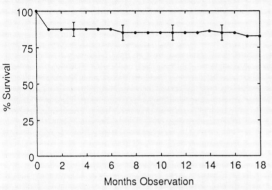

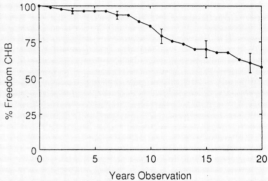

Life table plotted from date of first surgery of any type. There were 36 children who did not undergo cardiac surgery. None of these patients is known to have died.

This curve is based on experience with 90 patients. It is calculated beginning with the date of birth and using the date of first-documented complete heart block (CHB) at Boston Children's Hospital as the end-point. Because complete heart block could have been present for several years at the time of the first contact, the curve may underestimate the presence of heart block at any given age. Because heart block may have precipitated referral, the true incidence may be overestimated. It is doubtful that either of these considerations actually confuses this curve. Six patients developed heart block in association with cardiac surgery.

Other Cardiac Problems Associated with "Corrected" Transposition of The Great Arteries

Other Diagnosis	Number
Pulmonary Stenosis	68
(11 with Pulmonary Atresia)	
Ventricular Septal Defect	70
Tricuspid Valve Problems	50
(7 with Ebstein's Anomaly)	
Atrial Septal Defect	33
Mitral Valve Disease	33
Patent Ductus Arteriosus	10
Aortic Stenosis	12
Pulmonary Vascular Disease	11
Endocardial Cushion Defect	3
Coarctation of the Aorta	3
Complete Heart Block	29

develop, complete heart block (Exhibit 1).[5,21] The appearance of complete heart block seems to be unrelated to associated anomalies.[5]

Chest X-ray

The anterior and leftward ascending aorta can often be recognized on the plain chest x-ray (Fig. 3).

Echocardiography

As in most patients with congenital heart disease, echocardiography is a highly reliable means of describing the anatomy. Inversion of the ventricles can be recognized by identification of the right-sided mitral valve and left-sided tricuspid valve. The tricuspid valve attaches to the septal surface of the right ventricle, while the papillary muscles of the bicuspid mitral valve attach only to the free wall of the left ventricle. The fine trabeculations of the left ventricle may distinguish it from the coarse trabeculations of the right ventricle. Usually, the transposed aortic valve and main pulmonary artery are readily recognized. The function of the tricuspid valve should be evaluated because incompetence is common.[12,18]

The diagnosis is generally apparent from the initial subxiphoid long- and short-axis scans (Fig. 4). The anterior and right-sided morphologically left ventricle is seen aligned with the pulmonary artery. Scanning more anteriorly displays the anterior and left-sided aorta aligned with the right ventricle. Because a ventricular septal defect is common, the septum should be scanned in multiple views with and without Doppler color flow mapping. The tricuspid valve should be imaged using apical views to assess the location of the septal leaflet and a Doppler examination should be performed to de-

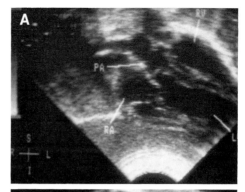

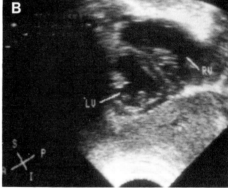

Figure 4. Echocardiograms in patients with corrected transposition of the great arteries. **A,** subxiphoid long-axis view demonstrating alignment of the pulmonary artery (PA) with the anterior left ventricle (LV). RA, right atrium; RV, right ventricle. **B,** Subxiphoid short-axis view. Note the smooth septal surface and the papillary muscles attached to the free wall of the anterior left ventricle (LV). The right ventricle (RV) is posterior.

tect and grade regurgitation. A careful Doppler examination of the pulmonary outflow tract should be performed from subxiphoid and apical transducer locations because pulmonary stenosis is often present.

Cardiac Catheterization

The need for cardiac catheterization is dependent on the available data. Generally, there are enough questions about valvar problems, outflow abnormalities, and associated defects to warrant further documentation by cardiac catheterization prior to surgery, to confirm details that might influence the outcome or affect the surgical and postoperative management.

Because the ventricular septum is usually oriented in an anteroposterior plane, many angiograms are satisfactorily taken from the anteroposterior view. Occasionally, a right anterior oblique position projects the septum more tangentially and provides a better examination of the right-sided, left ventricular outflow. For angiography, entry of the left-sided, right ventricle is best accomplished

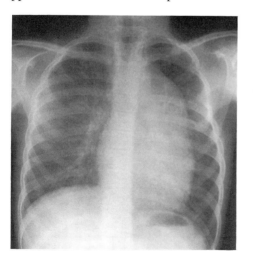

Figure 3. Anteroposterior chest x-ray. The left-sided ascending aorta is recognizable in this patient with corrected transposition of the great arteries.

via the aortic valve, since tricuspid regurgitation is so common in this condition (Figs. 5 and 6).[6]

MANAGEMENT

Management is primarily influenced by the underlying cardiac defects.[2] Complete heart block that is not associated with surgery is managed expectantly unless there is a history suggestive of circulatory collapse with cardiac rhythm problems. The author is aware of 2 patients who developed permanent complete heart block during cardiac catheterization. When surgery is being contemplated, operation is often delayed because of the risk of inducing complete heart block; if it occurs it must be considered as surgically induced and is managed as any other surgical heart block, including the use of permanent pacemakers.[21] The risk

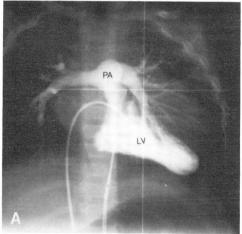

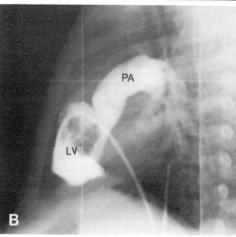

Figure 5. Anteroposterior (A) and lateral (B) views of a left ventricular (pulmonary ventricle) angiogram in a child with corrected transposition of the great arteries. The finely trabeculated, right-sided, anatomic left ventricle empties into a rightward, posterior pulmonary artery. PA, pulmonary artery; LV, left ventricle.

is high enough[13,21] that all patients with corrected transposition should have temporary pacing wires at time of surgery and postoperatively. Whether surgery stimulates an earlier appearance of predestined complete heart block or induces block which otherwise would not have occurred is unknown. The former seems more likely. Still, pursuit of ways to avoid the conduction bundle during surgery (i.e., closing a ventricular defect through the aortic valve) is of more than academic interest.[20]

Decisions about the timing of surgery are further influenced by the lack of progression of associated defects (such as pulmonary stenosis) in these patients. Severe pulmonary stenosis is not amenable to direct surgery because of the adjacent structures that may be injured, and often requires a conduit bypass from the anatomic left ventricle to the pulmonary artery.[21] Conduits, whether homografts or of plastic materials, imply further surgery in the future. Tricuspid (left-sided) atrioventricular valves require replacement in as many as 17% of patients.[13]

When needed, surgery is undertaken despite the possible need of a conduit or artificial tricuspid valve, or despite the risk of complete heart block, because all of these complications can be managed. Reported mortalities are acceptable but are higher than mortalities following surgery for comparable defects not confounded by inverted ventricles (see Exhibit 1).[9,13,14,21]

COURSE

Tricuspid incompetence can be progressive in these patients. Whether this is simply because tricuspid incompetence begets further tricuspid incompetence as the years go by, or whether some other mechanism is involved, is not clear. In any case, this problem can become progressively more severe and significantly affects long-term survival.[8]

Presumably, complete heart block occurs because of the abnormal anatomic location of the conduction system. Varying degrees of heart block are encountered. Often third-degree heart block is presaged by transient first- or second-degree block. Complete heart block may appear before or after birth or develop many years later. After 20 years of observation, actuarial tables suggest that as many as 55% of patients remain free of complete heart block (Exhibit 1).

ANATOMICALLY CORRECTED TRANSPOSITION OF THE GREAT ARTERIES

Very rarely the spatial position of the great arteries will be that of "corrected" transposition when the connections between the atria and ventricles and between the ventricles and great arter-

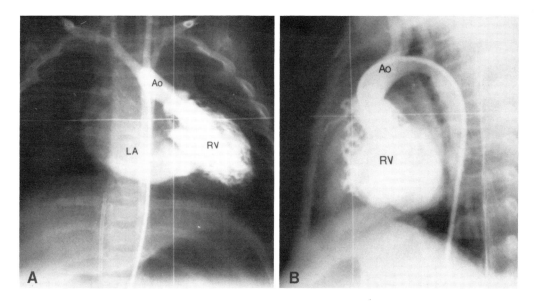

Figure 6. Anteroposterior (A) and lateral (B) views of a right ventricular (systemic ventricle) angiogram in the same child as in Figure 4. Note that the coarsely trabeculated, posterior, anatomic right ventricle empties into an anterior, leftward aorta. There is tricuspid incompetence with regurgitation of contrast material from the ventricle into an enlarged left atrium. Ao, aorta; LA, left atrium; RV, right ventricle.

ies are otherwise appropriate.[19] Associated congenital cardiac defects can be surgically repaired.[16]

REFERENCES

1. Allwork SP, Bentall HH, Becker AE, et al: Congenitally corrected transposition of the great arteries: morphologic study of 32 cases. Am J Cardiol 38:910–922, 1976.
2. Attie F, Ovseyevitz J, Llamas G, et al: The clinical features and diagnosis of a discordant atrioventricular connexion. Int J Cardiol 8:395–419, 1985.
3. Benson LN, Burns R, Schwaiger M, et al: Radionuclide angiographic evaluation of ventricular function in isolated congenitally corrected transposition of the great arteries. Am J Cardiol 58:319–324, 1986.
4. Dabizzi RP, Barletta GA, Caprioli G, et al: Coronary artery anatomy in corrected transposition of the great arteries. J Am Coll Cardiol 12:486–491, 1988.
5. Daliento L, Corrado D, Buja G, et al: Rhythm and conduction disturbances in isolated, congenitally corrected transposition of the great arteries. Am J Cardiol 58:314–318, 1986.
6. Freedom RM, Culhara JAG, Moes CAF: Angiocardiography of Congenital Heart Disease. New York, Macmillan, 1984, pp. 536–554.
7. Graham TP, Parrish MD, Boucek RJ, et al: Assessment of ventricular size and function in congenitally corrected transposition of the great arteries. Am J Cardiol 51:244–251, 1983.
8. Huhta JC, Danielson GK, Ritter DG, et al: Survival in atrioventricular discordance. Pediatr Cardiol 6:57–60, 1985.
9. Hwang B, Bowman F, Malm J, et al: Surgical repair of congenitally corrected transposition of the great arteries: results and follow-up. Am J Cardiol 50:781–785, 1982.
10. Lieberson AD, Schumacher RR, Childress RH, et al: Corrected transposition of the great arteries in a 73 year old man. Circulation 36(Suppl I):96–100, 1969.
11. Losekoot TC, Anderson RH, Becker AE: Congenitally

Corrected Transposition. Edinburgh, Churchill Livingstone, 1983.
12. Marino B, Sanders SP, Parness IA, et al: Obstruction of right ventricular inflow and outflow in corrected transposition of the great arteries {S,L,L}: two-dimensional echocardiographic diagnosis. J Am Coll Cardiol 8:407–411, 1986.
13. McGrath LB, Kirklin JW, Blackstone EH, et al: Death and other events after cardiac repair in discordant atrioventricular connection. J Thorac Cardiovasc Surg 90:711–728, 1985.
14. Metcalfe J, Somerville J: Surgical repair of lesions associated with corrected transposition: late results. Br Heart J 50:476–482, 1983.
15. Parrish MD, Graham TP, Bender HW, et al: Radionuclide angiographic evaluation of right and left ventricular function during exercise after repair of transposition of the great arteries. Comparison with normal subjects and patients with congenitally corrected transposition. Circulation 67:178–183, 1983.
16. Rittenhouse EA, Tenckhoff L, Kawabori I, et al: Surgical repair of anatomically corrected malposition of the great arteries. Ann Thorac Surg 42:220–228, 1986.
17. Ross-Ascuitto NT, Ascuitto RJ, Kopf GS, et al: Discrete subaortic obstruction in a patient with corrected transposition of the great arteries. Pediatr Cardiol 8:147–149, 1987.
18. Sutherland GR, Smallhorn JF, Anderson RH et al: Atrioventricular discordance: cross-sectional echocardiographic-morphological correlative study. Br Heart J 50:8–20, 1983.
19. Van Praagh R, Van Praagh S: Anatomically corrected transposition of the great arteries. Br Heart J 29:112–119, 1967.
20. Vargas F, Kreutzer GO, Schlichter AJ, et al: Repair of corrected transposition associated with ventricular septal defect and pulmonary stenosis. Ann Thorac Surg 40:509–511, 1985.
21. Westerman GR, Lang P, Castaneda AR, et al: Corrected transposition and repair of associated intracardiac defects. Circulation 66(Suppl I):I197–I201, 1982.

Chapter 50

CONGENITAL VASCULAR FISTULAS

Donald C. Fyler, M.D.

SYSTEMIC ARTERIOVENOUS FISTULAS

Definition

Any systemic arteriovenous connection bypassing the capillary circulation is an arteriovenous fistula. Clinical cardiology experience is readily classified into (1) cerebral arteriovenous fistulas, (2) hepatic fistulas, and (3) fistulas in other parts of the body.

Prevalence

Although hemangiomas are common and many short-circuit the local capillary circulation, hemangiomas that shunt enough blood to cause cardiac embarrassment are rare. Fistulas composed of large vessel arteriovenous connections are rare but are more likely to cause congestive heart failure. In Boston Children's Hospital experience, from 1973–87 there were 7 cerebral, 26 coronary, 5 hepatic, 6 pulmonary, 3 ruptured sinus of Valsalva, 3 aorto–left ventricular tunnels, and 10 systemic arteriovenous fistulas.

Pathophysiology

Cerebral fistulas may connect any cerebral artery to a nearby vein and are often multiple; there may be multiple feeding arteries or multiple draining veins. The most common variety involves the vein of Galen (Fig. 1). The hepatic arteriovenous fistulas usually have many shunting channels and are often described as hemangiomas or hemangioendotheliomas.

All systemic arteriovenous fistulas allow left-to-right shunting, which adds to the volume of blood being handled by all chambers of the heart as well as the pulmonary circulation. When the shunt is very large, intrauterine congestive heart failure, manifested by fetal hydrops, may develop.[12,15,23] Somewhat smaller shunts are associated with normal intrauterine growth, yet following a normal delivery there is the rapid development of gross congestive heart failure and death within a few days

of birth. One explanation for this remarkable occurrence is that the infant had congestive heart failure in utero. This ignores the obvious question of how it was possible for the child to grow so well

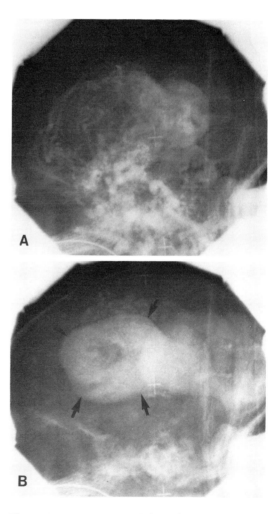

Figure 1. Angiograms in a baby with a large intracranial arteriovenous fistula. **A,** Multiple arterial feeding vessels. **B,** Grossly enlarged vein of Galen (arrows).

in utero and why there was no hydrops. An alternate theory is that an intrauterine shunt that can be tolerated becomes intolerable with conversion from parallel to serial circulation because there is a sudden overloading of already overloaded cardiac chambers at a time when the left ventricle must normally struggle to cope (Fig. 2). The author suspects that this mechanism accounts for the rapid onset of fatal congestive heart failure in the first days of life in a well-nourished newborn without signs of growth failure.

Many of these patients are cyanotic. In some cases this is due to lack of peripheral perfusion; in others, large right-to-left shunts through a ductus arteriosus or a foramen ovale are found.[5] Retrograde flow through the aortic arch has been demonstrated in prenatal and postnatal patients. The relative blood flow to a cerebral fistula may be so much greater than that to the rest of the systemic circulation[19,20] that a misdiagnosis of coarctation of the aorta is made.[6,20,27]

Clinical Manifestations

A large systemic arteriovenous fistula should be suspected in a normal-sized newborn in gross con-

gestive heart failure in the first days of life. Smaller shunts may cause cardiac enlargement but, otherwise, cause no difficulty and, if the child survives the first few months, further cardiac embarrassment is unlikely. Depending on the location of the fistula, there may be symptoms referrable to structures that are adjacent to the enlarged, tortuous, fistulous vessels, i.e., convulsions with a fistula in the central nervous system.

The sickest infants may be cyanotic, tachypneic, and shocky in the first hours of life. The heart is hyperactive and the peripheral pulses are prominent unless the infant is in terminal cardiovascular shock. Prominent pulsations may remain in the arteries feeding the fistula, whereas other peripheral vessels may have diminished pulsations. Thus, the carotid pulsations may be prominent while the femoral pulsations are absent. Understandably diagnostic confusion with coarctation of the aorta has been reported. The liver and spleen are usually enlarged.

Electrocardiography. In this situation, an electrocardiogram may show right or left ventricular hypertrophy, depending somewhat on the distri-

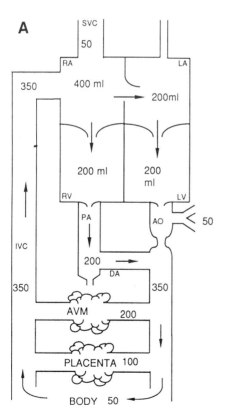
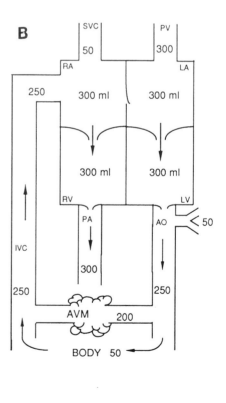

Figure 2. A hypothetical comparison of the volumes of blood pumped before and after birth in a baby with a large systemic arteriovenous fistula. The combined output of the two ventricles in the fetus (**A**) is twice the combined placental and body flow, a tolerable amount. After birth (**B**) there is a sudden increase in the amount of blood pumped by the two ventricles resulting from the switch from parallel to serial intracardiac circulation. The schema presupposes that the fistula carries as much blood before as after birth. It is proposed that this sudden increase in cardiac work accounts for normal intrauterine growth, despite the fistula, and, yet, sudden death within days of birth.

bution of blood flow through the various chambers of the heart prior to birth.

Chest X-ray. On chest x-ray, the sick newborn usually has gross cardiomegaly with increased pulmonary vascularity. Later cardiomegaly in proportion to the size of the shunt is demonstrable.

Echocardiography. Generalized enlargement of all chambers may be recognized. Enlargement of the superior vena cava suggests a shunt in the upper part of the body,[20,25] specifically a cerebral arteriovenous fistula, whereas enlargement of the inferior vena cava and hepatic vessels suggests a hepatic hemangioma or other fistula in the lower torso. A fistula involving the vein of Galen can be directly visualized[25] and evaluated using Doppler echocardiography (Fig. 1).[26]

Cardiac Catheterization. Usually cardiac catheterization is not needed to make this diagnosis. However, in a confused situation, cardiac catheterization provides evidences of high cardiac output (small arteriovenous oxygen difference), congestive heart failure, an enlarged ascending aorta, an enlarged cava (depending on the location of the fistula), generalized enlargement of the cardiac chambers, and evidence of a large runoff (wide pulse pressure).

Imaging Techniques. Any of the imaging techniques—ultrasound, magnetic resonance or computer assisted tomography—may demonstrate the fistula.

Management

The only way to salvage infants in gross congestive heart failure is to reduce the amount of shunting. Any means may be considered to occlude the feeding arteries. Surgical intervention or catheter manipulation to extrude occluding objects into feeding vessels have been successfully used.[3]

A hepatic hemangioendothelioma is likely to be influenced by the use of steroids.[13,32] Alpha interferon is a promising new agent.[31] Most hepatic hemangiomas regress with time; hence, controlling the congestive heart failure and giving the hemangiomas time to regress may be lifesaving in these patients.

PULMONARY ARTERIOVENOUS FISTULAS

Definition

Arteriovenous connections which bypass the pulmonary capillary circulation may take the form of multiple tiny angiomatous intercommunications (telangiectases) or may consist of large pulmonary artery-to-pulmonary vein communications.

Prevalence

Pulmonary arteriovenous fistulas are rare. The files of the Children's Hospital in Boston list 4 patients with this diagnosis in the years 1973–1987.

Pathology

Multiple tiny arteriovenous fistulas (Osler-Weber-Rendu syndrome) are often diffusely spread throughout both lung fields. Whether this is an acquired or congenital anomaly is not clear. In any case, the number of shunting fistulas seems to increase as the child grows older. Telangiectases in other parts of the body, especially on the skin, are a feature of this disease. It is reasonable to think of this as generalized telangiectasia, even though some patients have only pulmonary manifestations.

Arteriovenous connections between large vessels are also encountered. Depending on the number and the location of the fistulous aneurysm, excision or occlusion is possible, sometimes with complete cure. While the anatomy suggests a lesion of fixed size, the fact is that these lesions (as all other arteriovenous malformations except for hepatic hemangioma) get larger with time.

The mechanism by which pulmonary arteriovenous fistulas produce cyanosis in children with cirrhosis of the liver is an enigma.[4]

Physiology

The effect of a pulmonary arteriovenous fistula is to bypass the pulmonary capillaries. The consequence is that pulmonary venous oxygen content is less than normal in direct relation to the size of the shunt. Otherwise, there is little, if any, effect on the circulation. Pulmonary artery pressures are normal and pulmonary arteriolar resistance is very low in the fistula itself, but calculates to a higher than normal number in that part of the lung which supplies the capillaries. There is no accompanying histologic abnormality in these "high" resistance vessels.[8]

The mechanism of increased shunting as the child grows older is not understood. Whether there is an increasing number of shunting connections or dilatation of an existing connection,[16] these patients tend to become more cyanotic with time.

Clinical Manifestations

The patient is cyanotic in proportion to the amount of blood bypassing the pulmonary capillaries. There may be a continuous murmur over the fistula, although if multiple small lesions are present, murmurs are only rarely heard.

The **electrocardiogram** is normal.

The **chest x-ray** may reveal an isolated lesion. When there are multiple, tiny defects these can sometimes be identified.

Echocardiography has little place in evaluating pulmonary parenchymal problems. A normal echocardiographic examination in a cyanotic child should suggest the possibility of this diagnosis.

Cardiac catheterization shows a normal cardiac output and normal pressures. The arterial oxygen unsaturation can be traced to the pulmonary venous circulation, sometimes to the specific lobe involved. Angiography in multiple views identifies the defect and provides the anatomic detail needed to plan treatment. It is important to identify all intrapulmonary shunts. Balloon occlusion of pulmonary artery branches may provide clues as to the extent and location of the fistulas (Fig. 3).

Management

Isolated fistulas can be managed by placing catheter extruded devices into the feeding artery.[29] Multiple defects in a single lobe can be managed by lobectomy. Whether catheter occlusion of multiple small arterial vessels will ever be a successful form of treatment remains to be established. In some patients this may be all that is possible.

Course

Removal of a large, single fistula, by whatever means, is likely to be successful permanently. Management of multiple tiny fistulas has been unsuccessful. Brain abscess is a well-known complication![11]

CORONARY FISTULAS

Definition

Fistulous connections between the coronary arteries and coronary veins, between coronary arteries and chambers of the right heart, and between coronary arterial and pulmonary vessels have been described.[1,17,28] Fistulous connections between the coronary arteries and the left ventricle have been described most often as aorto–left ventricular tunnels (see p. 711).

Prevalence

Coronary artery fistulas are rare. There were 26 patients seen at Boston Children's Hospital between 1973 and 1987 (Exhibit 1).

Pathology

The most common coronary fistula arises from the right coronary artery and enters the right ventricle. Other points of entry are the right atrium, the cava, or the pulmonary arteries. Most often the entry point is a single orifice but, rarely, it may be multiple. The connecting structures are dilated, tortuous, and sometimes seem aneurysmal. These structures are thought of as having a congenital origin and enlarging gradually throughout life. Consequently, these defects are more common in older patients.

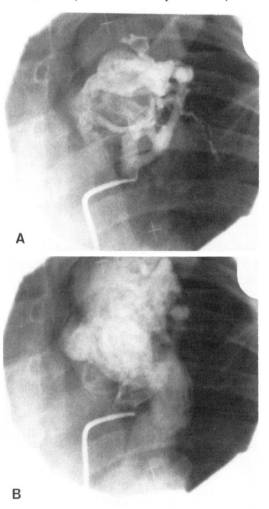

A

B

Figure 3. Angiogram showing a pulmonary arteriovenous fistula in the left upper lobe. ART, arterial phase; VEN, venous phase.

Exhibit 1

Boston Children's Hospital Experience 1973–1987		
Arteriovenous Fistulas*		
Type of Fistula	As a Primary Diagnosis	As a Secondary Diagnosis
Coronary	14	12
Cerebral	5	2
Systemic	5	5
Pulmonary	4	2
Hepatic	3	2
Ruptured Sinus of Valsalva	1	2
Aorto-Left Ventricular Tunnel†	2	1
Descending Aorta–Pulmonary Arterial Connections	0	23

*The data included here are based on echocardiography, cardiac catheterization, and notations made at surgery.

†Fistulas into the left ventricle are not strictly arteriovenous fistulas. There was 1 patient with a subclavian artery-to-pulmonary vein fistula.

Physiology

The fistula acts as a shunt from the coronary artery to the right heart chambers. It is unusual for it to carry a shunt large enough to cause symptoms, although this occurs occasionally and may even be noticed in infancy.[26] Because the fistula is present from an early stage and only gradually changes, it rarely steals blood from the myocardium. Therefore, evidences of myocardial ischemia and underperfusion are not common. Encroachment of an aneurysm on an adjacent structure is an imaginable consequence but is rarely reported. Infective endocarditis is thought to occur in the fistula in as many as 5% of patients.

Clinical Manifestations

These patients are almost invariably discovered through routine auscultation of an otherwise well child. A continuous murmur is present, usually maximal over the precordium. Rarely, it is heard at the second intercostal space, where it may be confused with a patent ductus arteriosus. Fortunately, the murmur is usually loudest elsewhere, often at the lower sternal border to the right or the left of the sternum. The shunt is rarely sufficient to affect the pulse pressure.

Electrocardiography. Generally, there is no abnormality recognizable on the electrocardiogram unless the shunt is sufficiently large to overload the right heart circulation.

Chest X-ray. Often, the chest x-ray shows a normal-sized heart. Occasionally, with appropriate views, a bulge, representing the fistula, can be seen on the surface of the heart.

Echocardiography. The fistulous structures are recognizable at echocardiography.[9,21] Doppler color flow mapping is especially useful for documenting the connections with heart chambers.[22] Aortic root contrast echocardiography may be useful for clarifying the connections of the fistula as well.[18] Indirect evidence of shunt size can be recognized through chamber enlargement.

Cardiac Catheterization. It is important to confirm, in detail, the echocardiographic impression of the origin and entry point of the fistula when preparing for surgery. More than one set of biplane angiograms may be needed in various views to best display the anatomy for surgical planning (Fig. 4).

Management

Because these fistulas rarely close spontaneously, because infective endocarditis is a significant risk, and because these fistulas tend to become larger with time, all are referred for surgery. Using cardiopulmonary bypass, the surgical plan is to interrupt the fistula without compromise to the coronary circulation. This is best accomplished with closure of the fistulous point nearest to the entry

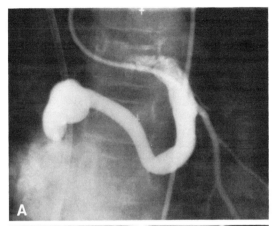

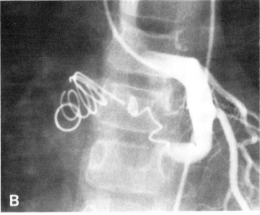

Figure 4. Angiogram with injection into a coronary artery (**A**), which has a fistulous connection shunting into the right atrium. This fistula was later embolized using a coil. After embolization (**B**) there was no further shunting.

into the right heart chambers. In recent years, mortality with this problem has been negligible.

Course

Recurrence is described and sometimes requires reoperation but, fortunately, this is rare. Otherwise, late problems have not been reported.

AORTO–LEFT VENTRICULAR TUNNEL

Definition

An aorto–left ventricular tunnel is a rare, congenital tunnel communication between the aortic root and the left ventricle beneath the right side of the aortic valve.[2,7] Thirty-seven cases were reported in the literature by 1988.[14]

Anatomy

The nature of this lesion is a matter of controversy. Proposed theories include the suggestions that the defect is an abnormal coronary artery or that the defect is a variation of ruptured sinus of Valsalva that must have occurred in utero. The majority of infants with this condition are known to have a cardiac lesion at birth; hence the impression that the lesion is congenital rather than acquired. The majority are known to have aortic regurgitation, which is thought not to be an anomaly, but rather to be caused by displacement of the adjacent aortic sinus by the progressively enlarging, sometimes aneurysmal, tunnel (Fig. 5).

Physiology

The physiologic effect of this left-to-left shunt is comparable to aortic regurgitation. The burden on the circulation is proportionate to the amount of blood that flows retrograde from the aorta to the left ventricle.

Clinical Manifestations

In at least 50% of the cases a murmur is known to have been present at birth. The murmur is dominantly diastolic, although a systolic component may be present. The diastolic part of this murmur may be so loud and coarse that it is initially thought to be a systolic murmur. Sooner or later congestive heart failure develops in most patients.

Electrocardiograms show left ventricular hypertrophy.

On **chest x-ray** the heart is enlarged but the pulmonary vasculature is not engorged.

Echocardiography[10] or cardiac catheterization establishes this diagnosis, but, with casual review of even the best data, the diagnosis may be missed, because it is not a common problem. Evidence suggesting aortic regurgitation associated with an abnormal structure between the septum and the right aortic sinus when there is no ventricular de-

fect should raise the possibility of this diagnosis. Probably all patients should be catheterized until it is clear that a precise diagnosis can be made using echocardiographic techniques.

Management

Surgical interruption of the aortic runoff is the treatment of choice.[30] Whether this should be done by closing the aortic end or the ventricular end of the tunnel, or simply by interrupting it at its most accessible point is a matter of debate. The majority of these patients have aortic regurgitation that is not necessarily relieved by the surgery. Ultimately, aortic valve replacement is often needed.[24]

Course

Apparently, untreated patients have died. The oldest untreated survivor known to have this disease was 25 years old.

DESCENDING AORTOPULMONARY ARTERIAL CONNECTIONS

In addition to patients with pulmonary atresia and ventricular septal defect who have large bizarre collateral vessels that supply pulmonary blood flow, there are, occasionally, patients with small arterial vessels arising from the lower thoracic aorta, above or below the diaphragm, which connect with the arterial supply to the lower lungs. Often, this is associated with sequestration of a section of lung, hypoplasia of a lung, or with some other pulmonary abnormality. Of the 23 patients noted (Exhibit 1), all had congenital heart disease, such as ventricular septal defect, scimitar syndrome, or endocardial cushion defect. The anomaly is almost always discovered accidentally when an aortogram is made for some other problem. For this reason it seems likely that the numbers presented here are underestimated. These vessels are rarely considered enough of a problem to undertake surgery; in 2 of the 23 patients the fistulas were ligated.

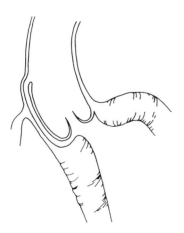

Figure 5. A drawing of an aorta–left ventricular tunnel. Note that the tunnel runs through the adjacent ventricular septum. (After Tuna IC, Edwards JE: Aortico–left ventricular tunnel and aortic insufficiency. Ann Thorac Surg 45:5–6, 1988, with permission.)

REFERENCES

1. Baim DS, Kline H, Silverman JF: Bilateral coronary artery–pulmonary artery fistulas: report of five cases and review of the literature. Circulation 65:810–815, 1982.
2. Bernhard WF, Plauth W, Fyler D: Unusual abnormalities of the aortic root or valve necessitating surgical correction in early childhood. N Engl J Med 282:68–71, 1970.
3. Burrows PE, Lasjaunias PL, Ter Brugge KG, et al: Urgent and emergent embolization of lesions of the head and neck in children: indications and results. Pediatrics 80:386–394, 1987.
4. Crary GS, Burke BA, Alford BA, et al: Pulmonary arteriovenous shunting in a child with cirrhosis of the liver. Am J Dis Child 143:749–751, 1989.

5. Cummings GR: Circulation in neonates with intracranial arteriovenous fistula and cardiac failure. Am J Cardiol 45:1019–1024, 1980.

6. Deverall PB, Taylor JF, Sturrock GS, et al: Coarctation-like physiology with cerebral arteriovenous fistula. Pediatrics 44:1024–1028, 1969.

7. Diamant S, Luber JM Jr, Gootman N: Successful repair of aortico-left ventricular tunnel associated with severe aortic stenosis in a newborn. Pediatr Cardiol 6:171–173, 1985.

8. Friedlich A, Bing RJ, Blount SG: Physiological studies in congenital heart disease. IX. Circulatory dynamics in the anomalies of venous return to the heart including pulmonary arteriovenous fistula. Bull Johns Hopkins Hosp 86:20–57, 1950.

9. Friedman DM, and Rutkowski M: Coronary artery fistula: a pulsed Doppler/two-dimensional echocardiographic study. Am J Cardiol 55:1652–1654, 1985.

10. Fripp RP, Werner JC, Whitman V, et al: Pulsed Doppler and two-dimensional echocardiographic findings in aortico-left ventricular tunnel. J Am Coll Cardiol 4:1012–1014, 1984.

11. Gelfand MS, Stephens DS, Howell EI, et al: Brain abscess: association with pulmonary arteriovenous fistula and hereditary hemorrhagic telangiectasia: report of three cases. Am J Med 85:718–720, 1988.

12. Griscom NT, Colodny AH, Rosenberg HK, et al: Diagnostic aspects of neonatal ascites: report of 27 cases. AJR 128:961–970, 1977.

13. Holcomb GW, Oneill JA, Mahboubi S, et al: Experience with hepatic hemangioendothelioma in infancy and childhood. J Pediatr Surg 23:661–666, 1988.

14. Hovaguimian H, Cobanoglu A, Starr A: Aortico-left ventricular tunnel: a clinical review and new surgical classification. Ann Thorac Surg 45:106–112, 1988.

15. Johnson W, Berry JM, Einzig S, et al: Doppler findings in nonimmune hydrops fetalis and cerebral arteriovenous malformation. Am Heart J 115:1138–1140, 1988.

16. Knight WB, Bush A, Busst CM, et al: Multiple pulmonary arteriovenous fistulas in childhood. Int J Cardiol 23:105–166, 1989.

17. Liberthson RR, Sagar K, Berkoben JP, et al: Cogenital coronary arteriovenous fistula: report of 13 patients, review of the literature and delineation of management. Circulation 59:849–854, 1979.

18. Martin GR, Cooper MJ, Silverman NH, et al: Contrast echocardiography in the diagnosis of anomalous left coronary artery arising from the pulmonary artery. Pediatr Cardiol 6:203–205, 1986.

19. Moller JM: Arteriovenous fistula in the neonate. J Am Coll Cardiol 12:1536–1537, 1988.

20. Musewe NN, Smallhorn JF, Burrows PE, et al: Echocardiographic and Doppler evaluation of the aortic arch and brachiocephalic vessels in cerebral and systemic arteriovenous fistulas. J Am Coll Cardiol 12:1529–1535, 1988.

21. Pickoff AS, Wolff GS, Bennett VL, et al: Pulsed Doppler echocardiographic detection of coronary artery to right ventricle fistula. Pediatr Cardiol 2:145–149, 1982.

22. Sanders SP, Parness IA, Colan SD: Recognition of abnormal connections of coronary arteries with the use of Doppler color flow mapping. J Am Coll Cardiol 13:922–926, 1989.

23. Schmidt KG, Silverman NH, Harrison MR, et al: High-output cardiac failure in fetuses with large sacrococcygeal teratoma: diagnosis by echocardiography and Doppler ultrasound. J Pediatr 114:1023–1028, 1989.

24. Serino W, Andrade JL, Ross D, et al: Aorto-left ventricular communication after closure: late postoperative problems. Br Heart J 49:501–506, 1983.

25. Snider AR, Soifer SJ, Silverman NH: Detection of intracranial arteriovenous fistula by two-dimensional ultrasonography. Circulation 63:1179–1185, 1981.

26. Starc TJ, Bowman FO, Hordof AJ: Congestive heart failure in a newborn secondary to coronary artery-left ventricular fistula. Am J Cardiol 58:366–367, 1986.

27. Starc TJ, Krongrad E, Bierman FZ: Two-dimensional echocardiography and Doppler findings in cerebral arteriovenous malformation. Am J Cardiol 64:252–254, 1989.

28. Takahashi M, and Lurie PR: Abnormalities and diseases of the coronary vessels. In Adams, FH, Emmanouilides GC (eds): Moss' Heart Disease in Infants, Children, and Adolescents, 4th ed. Baltimore, Williams & Wilkins, 1989.

29. Taylor BG, Cockerill EM, Manfredi F, et al: Therapeutic embolization of the pulmonary artery in pulmonary arteriovenous fistula. Am J Med 64:360–365, 1978.

30. Turley K, Silverman NH, Teital D, et al: Repair of aortico-left ventricular tunnel in the neonate: surgical, anatomic and echocardiographic considerations. Circulation 65:1015–1020, 1982.

31. White CW, Sondheimer HM, Crouch EC, et al: Treatment of pulmonary hemangiomatosis with recombinant interferon alfa-2a. N Engl J Med 320:1197–1200, 1989.

32. Wisnicki JL: Hemangiomas and vascular malformations. Ann Plast Surg 12:41–59, 1984.

Chapter 51

ANOMALOUS ORIGIN OF THE LEFT CORONARY ARTERY

Donald C. Fyler, M.D.

DEFINITION

Origin of the left coronary artery from the pulmonary artery is a rare, but important anomaly because early death is often the natural outcome. At present, with early diagnosis and surgery, it appears that the child may be completely cured.

PREVALENCE

This anomaly was encountered 29 times in the series of patients seen at the Children's Hospital in Boston between 1973 and 1987 (Exhibit 1).

PATHOLOGY

The left coronary artery arises from the low-pressure main pulmonary artery and follows its usual course over the heart. Because the high-pressure right coronary artery is the source of perfusion for the myocardium, it is bigger than the left and takes over the left coronary circulation through collateral connections and may flow retrograde to the pulmonary artery. Because the myocardium is generally poorly perfused, the heart may be dilated and histologic evidence of inadequate myocardial perfusion may be found. At postmortem examination there may be obvious myocardial infarction.

PHYSIOLOGY

Before birth, the pulmonary artery pressure equals systemic pressure, allowing for satisfactory myocardial perfusion from the pulmonary artery via the anomalous coronary. With birth and falling pulmonary artery pressure, the antegrade perfusion of the left coronary gradually falls, the circulation being taken over by collateral vessels from the right coronary. In many patients the flow in the left coronary artery reverses and, effectively, a coronary artery steal develops from the myocar-

Exhibit 1

The Children's Hospital Experience
1973–1987

Anomalous Coronary Artery Arising from the Pulmonary Artery

There were 29 patients categorized as having an anomalous coronary arising from the pulmonary artery. One of these was associated with a patent ductus arteriosus and pulmonary vascular disease; two older individuals were asymptomatic. There were 13 males and 16 females. The age distribution was unexpected. Ten patients were first seen after their first birthday and seven were older than 10 years. Twenty-six underwent coronary surgery; in five the left coronary was ligated (one death), and 21 had either Takeuchi operations or reimplantation of the left coronary directly into the aorta (two deaths). There were no late deaths.

dium to the pulmonary artery. The size of this left-to-right shunt is rarely enough to be a significant hemodynamic burden except that it deprives the myocardium of perfusion. Sometime in the first weeks of reversed coronary flow, myocardial ischemia becomes sufficient to be recognizable on an electrocardiogram. The heart enlarges and congestive heart failure becomes manifest. With ischemic damage to the left papillary muscles, mitral regurgitation is often added to an already deteriorating situation.

If, for any reason, the patient maintains systemic pressure in the pulmonary arteries, this sequence of events will not occur and the left coronary will be perfused by blood originating from the pulmonary artery. Despite the fact that this blood may have substantially lower oxygen saturation than that from the right coronary, evidences of myocardial ischemia are not seen.

Some patients with uncorrected anomalous origin of the left coronary from the main pulmonary artery survive to adulthood.[9] Rarely, the right coronary artery arises from the pulmonary artery[17]

715

and, even more rarely, both coronary arteries arise from the pulmonary artery.[3,12]

CLINICAL MANIFESTATIONS

These patients seem to be normal at birth; approximately 60% of the patients seen at the Boston Children's Hospital developed congestive heart failure weeks later. Occasionally, a history of irritability, perhaps related to angina, is elicited. But this is more of a retrospective explanation than a useful fact. Older patients are discovered because of the systolic murmur of mitral regurgitation or because of chest x-ray showing cardiomegaly.

Electrocardiography

The electrocardiogram almost always shows evidence of anterolateral myocardial infarction in the symptomatic patient (Fig. 1).

Chest X-ray

The heart is enlarged, sometimes grossly enlarged, without an increase in pulmonary vascularity. The x-ray is characteristic of primary myocardial disease and, in the past, caused frequent confusion with other forms of primary myocardial disease (Fig. 2).

Echocardiography

An enlarged, poorly functioning left ventricle is characteristic. Evidences of mitral regurgitation may be documented and differential enlargement of the right coronary versus the left may be demonstrable. In recent years, identification of the origin of the left coronary artery from the pulmonary artery has usually been possible.[4,5,10,13,14] As a rule, all patients with unexplained myocardial disease should have the origin of the coronary arteries identified.

Parasternal short-axis view best demonstrates the origins of the coronary arteries from the aorta (Fig. 3). An anomalously connecting left coronary artery passes near to the usual left sinus of Valsalva of the aortic root before connecting with the pulmonary root. The closer the vessel passes to the aorta, the more difficult it may be to establish the diagnosis by imaging alone. Scanning in a parasternal, long-axis view may demonstrate more clearly the orifice of the coronary artery in the pulmonary root.

Doppler color flow mapping has proved to be extremely valuable for demonstrating both the flow from the left coronary into the pulmonary root and the direction of flow in the left coronary artery. At the Boston Children's Hospital, we require clear imaging of the coronary ostium in the pulmonary root, demonstration of flow from the coronary artery into the pulmonary root, and documentation of retrograde flow in the left coronary artery and branches for the diagnosis of anomalous left coronary artery. Similarly, documentation of anterograde flow in the left coronary artery and branches by Doppler color flow mapping excludes anomalous left coronary artery. With careful imaging,

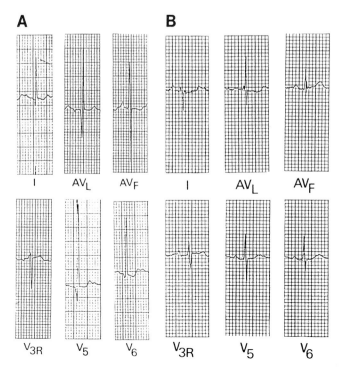

A   **B**

I   AV$_L$ AV$_F$ I   AV$_L$ AV$_F$

V$_{3R}$ V$_5$ V$_6$ V$_{3R}$ V$_5$ V$_6$

Figure 1. Electrocardiograms from the same patient before (**A**) and after (**B**) a Takeuchi operation. Note the wide and deep Q waves in the left chest leads and in aV$_L$ before surgery and their disappearance afterward.

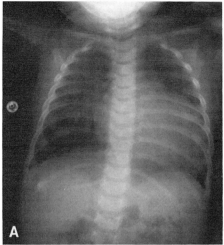

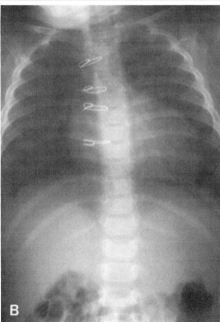

Figure 2. Chest x-ray before **(A)** and after **(B)** a Takeuchi operation in the same patient presented in Figure 1. Note the decrease in heart size.

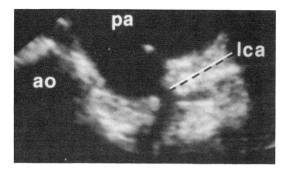

Figure 3. Echocardiogram in a patient with origin of the left coronary from the pulmonary artery. This is a parasternal, short-axis view showing origin of the left coronary artery from the pulmonary artery root. pa, pulmonary artery; lca, left coronary artery; ao, aorta.

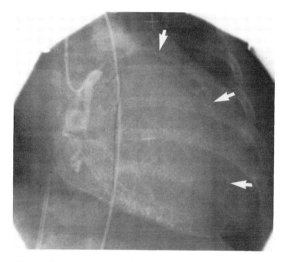

Figure 4. Angiogram with injection into the right coronary artery showing opacification of a large right coronary system and subsequent retrograde filling of the left coronary system (arrows). Some dye reaches the pulmonary artery.

coupled with Doppler color flow mapping, a highly accurate diagnosis or exclusion of the diagnosis is possible. In the past two to three years, patients with a confident echocardiographic diagnosis of anomalous left coronary artery have undergone surgical bypass without cardiac catheterization.

Cardiac Catheterization

At cardiac catheterization, the findings are those of a dilated cardiomyopathy. Left ventricular dysfunction, as evidenced by an elevated left ventricular end-diastolic pressure and elevated left atrial pressure, is usually demonstrable. The diagnosis is established when an angiogram of the aortic root shows a large right coronary artery with opacification of the left coronary system, and even of the main pulmonary artery (Fig. 4).[6] Angiograms with the contrast injected into the pulmonary artery have not been successful unless a balloon is inflated in the pulmonary artery and contrast material is injected proximal to the balloon.[15]

MANAGEMENT

Delaying surgery while waiting for the child to grow[2] is no longer justifiable. Once the diagnosis has been recognized and the infant stabilized with anticongestive medications, surgery is undertaken to correct the coronary circulation. Formerly, ligation of the left coronary artery at its source from the pulmonary artery was used to eliminate the left-to-right shunt and prevent a steal from the myocardium. Although this surgery was often successful, the initial and late mortality were significant. A variety of methods to connect the left coronary artery to the aorta have been tried with varying success. One of the most satisfactory has been the operation proposed by Takeuchi.[16] However it is accomplished, the desired effect is perfusion of the left coronary from the aorta.[1,7,8] With survival, the evidences of myocardial infarction may disappear (Fig. 1), the heart size may return to normal (Fig. 2), the child becomes asymptomatic, and measures of myocardial function improve.[11] Revision of the operative connections may be needed. Close follow-up of these patients is necessary until the long-term outcome is established.

COURSE

The remarkable improvements in the electrocardiogram, the echocardiographic measures of function, and the patient are surprisingly impressive, suggesting that the infant myocardium has a capacity for repair after ischemia and infarction that exceeds that seen in the adult. It is too early to be confident that these patients are truly cured. At present, the future seems promising.

Among older patients any evidence of cardiac embarrassment may be a reason to connect the coronary artery to the aorta. The reports of sudden death in these patients are sufficient to encourage surgery to provide a two-coronary system wherever possible.[9]

REFERENCES

1. Bunton R, Jonas RA, Lang P, et al: Anomalous origin of left coronary artery from pulmonary artery: ligation versus establishment of a two coronary artery system. J Thorac Cardiovasc Surg 93:103–108, 1987.
2. Driscoll DJ, Nihill MR, Mullins CE, et al: Management of symptomatic infants with anomalous origin of the left coronary artery from the pulmonary artery. Am J Cardiol 47:642–648, 1981.
3. Heifetz SA, Robinowitz M, Mueller KH, et al: Total anomalous origin of the coronary arteries from the pulmonary artery. Pediatr Cardiol 7:11–18, 1986.
4. Jureidini SB, Nouri S, Pennington DG: Anomalous origin of the left coronary artery from the pulmonary trunk: repair after diagnostic cross sectional echocardiography. Br Heart J 58:173–175, 1987.
5. King DH, Danford DA, Huhta JC, et al: Noninvasive detection of anomalous origin of the left main coronary artery from the pulmonary trunk by pulsed Doppler echocardiography. Am J Cardiol 55:608–609, 1985.
6. Levin DC, Fellows KE, Abrams HL: Hemodynamically significant primary anomalies of the coronary arteries: angiographic aspects. Circulation 58:25–33, 1978.
7. Menahem S, and Venables AW: Anomalous left coronary artery from the pulmonary artery: a 15 year sample. Br Heart J 58:378–384, 1987.
8. Midgley FM, Watson DC, Scott LP, et al: Repair of anomalous origin of the left coronary artery in the infant and small child. J Am Coll Cardiol 4:1231–1234, 1984.
9. Moodie DS, Fyfe D, Gill CC, et al: Anomalous origin of the left coronary artery from the pulmonary artery (Bland-White-Garland syndrome) in adult patients: long-term follow-up after surgery. Am Heart J 106:381–388, 1983.
10. Peerenboom PJHA, van Tellingen C, Plokker HWM: Echocardiographic features after surgical treatment for Bland-White-Garland syndrome. Int J Cardiol 7:69–71, 1985.
11. Rein AJJT, Colan SD, Parness IA, et al: Regional and global left ventricular function in infants with anomalous origin of the left coronary artery from the pulmonary trunk: preoperative and postoperative assessment. Circulation 75:115–123, 1987.
12. Roberts WC: Anomalous origin of both coronary arteries from the pulmonary artery. Am J Cardiol 10:595–600, 1962.
13. Robinson PJ, Sullivan ID, Kumpeng V, et al: Anomalous origin of the left coronary artery from the pulmonary trunk: potential for false-negative diagnosis with cross sectional echocardiography. Br Heart J 52:272–277, 1984.
14. Sanders SP, Parness IA, Colan SD: Recognition of abnormal connections of coronary arteries with the use of Doppler color flow mapping. J Am Coll Cardiol 13:922–926, 1989.
15. Shem-Tov AA, Hegesh J, Schneeweiss A, et al: Visualization of left coronary artery in anomalous origin of left coronary artery from pulmonary artery. Am Heart J 108:621–622, 1984.
16. Takeuchi S, Imamura H, Katsumoto K, et al: New surgical method for repair of anomalous left coronary artery from pulmonary artery. J Thorac Cardiovasc Surg 78:1–11, 1979.
17. Worsham C, Sanders SP, Burger BM: Origin of the right coronary artery from the pulmonary trunk: diagnosis by two-dimensional echocardiography. Am J Cardiol 55:232–233, 1985.

Chapter 52

VASCULAR RINGS AND SLINGS

Valerie S. Mandell, M.D., and Richard M. Braverman, M.D.

In an effort to be complete, many discussions of vascular rings and slings are long and cumbersome. They include so many malformations, both real and theoretical, that the reader finds it difficult to learn about the few lesions that are significant. The most important of these uncommon malformations are those causing tracheal and esophageal compression due to complete or partial encirclement by vascular elements (Exhibit 1). The three major lesions are: (1) the double aortic arch, (2) the right aortic arch with an aberrant left subclavian and (short) left ductus or ligamentum, and (3) the anomalous left pulmonary artery, or pulmonary artery sling.

DEFINITION

A vascular ring (double aortic arch or right aortic arch with a left subclavian and a left ductus arteriosus) encircles the trachea and the esophagus (Figs. 1 and 2). Pulmonary artery sling consists of a left pulmonary artery passing to the right and behind the trachea before supplying the left lung (Fig. 3).

EMBRYOLOGIC ANATOMY

Vascular rings result from abnormal development of the primitive paired arch system in the first three weeks after conception.[2,19] Six paired arches, and paired, segmental dorsal aortas join at the ninth segment into a single descending aorta (Fig. 4). The first and second arches regress completely. The third arches contribute to the formation of the carotid arteries bilaterally. The left fourth arch forms that part of the definitive left aortic arch between the left carotid and left subclavian arteries. The right fourth arch is incorporated into the right subclavian. The fifth arches regress. The proximal parts of the sixth arches form the pulmonary arteries, while the distal portions join the pulmonary vascular tree to the descending aorta via bilateral ductus, the right typically regressing to leave a left ductus arteriosus. Between the sixth arch (the ductus) and the descending aorta are the paired dorsal aortic segments three through eight, which join the descending (dorsal) aorta at segment nine. The seventh segment of the dorsal arch is the embryonic subclavian artery. When the eighth segment of the right dorsal aorta regresses, as is usual, the definitive left aortic arch is formed.

The theoretical double arch model originally introduced by Edwards, and modified, simplified and redrawn multiple times since, helps one to understand various arch anomalies (Fig. 5).[8,19] In this model, which includes both a right and a left ductus, the ascending aorta divides into two arches, one passing to the right of the trachea and esophagus and the other to the left. These arches join posteriorly to form the descending aorta. From each arch there is a segment that gives rise to the right and left common carotids as the first branches on either side, and the right and left subclavian arteries as the second branches on either side. A

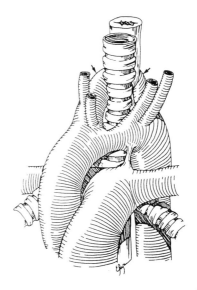

Figure 1. Drawing of ring around trachea and esophagus caused by double aortic arch. Right arch (arrows) is the higher and larger of the two in most cases.

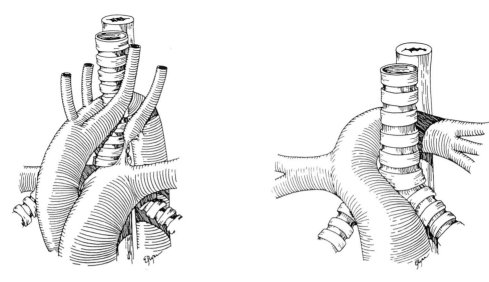

Figure 2. Drawing of ring around the trachea and esophagus caused by a right arch with an aberrant left subclavian and left ductus or ligamentum.

Figure 3. Drawing of anomalous left pulmonary artery as seen from the front, depicting its course between the esophagus and trachea as it courses to the left lung.

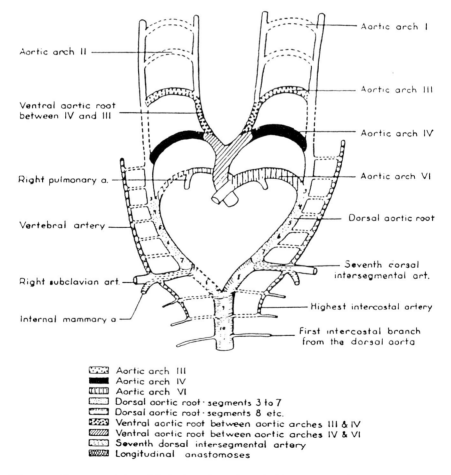

Figure 4. Diagrammatic representation of the embryonic aortic arch. Those portions that are not normally present after fetal life are represented by broken lines. Roman numerals represent the embryonic arches, whereas arabic numbers represent segments of the dorsal aorta. (From Barry A: The aortic derivatives in the human adult. Anat Rec 111:221–238, © 1951, reprinted with permission of Wiley-Liss, a division of John Wiley and Sons, Inc.)

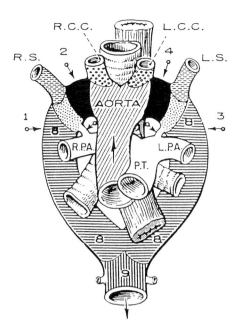

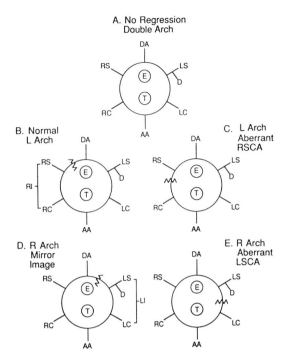

Figure 5. Edwards' hypothetical double aortic arch with bilateral ducti. Arrows indicate the four locations at which regression may occur. Arrow 1, the eighth segment of the right dorsal aortic root; arrow 2, the right fourth arch; arrow 3, the eighth segment of the left dorsal aortic root; and arrow 4, the left fourth arch. R.S., right subclavian; R.C.C., right common carotid; L.C.C., left common carotid; L.S., left subclavian; P.T., pulmonary trunk; R.P.A., right pulmonary artery; L.P.A., left pulmonary artery. (From Stewart JR, Kincaid OW, Edwards JE: An Atlas of Vascular Rings and Related Malformations of the Aortic Arch System. Springfield, IL, Charles C Thomas, 1964, with permission.)

Figure 6. **A,** Simple line drawing of the hypothetical double arch with a left ductus. **B,** The break (jagged line) between the right subclavian and the descending aorta indicates the pattern of the normal left arch and left ductus. **C,** The break (jagged line) between the right carotid and the right subclavian indicates the pattern of a left arch with an aberrant right subclavian (no ring). **D,** The break (jagged line) between the left subclavian and the descending aorta indicates the pattern of a right arch with mirror image branching (no ring). **E,** The break (jagged line) between the left subclavian and the left carotid indicates the pattern of a right arch with aberrant left subclavian and left ductus (ring is present). AA, ascending aorta; DA, descending aorta; RC, right carotid; RS; right subclavian, LC, left carotid; LS, left subclavian; D, ductus; T, trachea; E, esophagus. (Adapted from VanZandt TF, courtesy of the author, personal communication.)

ductus arises from the proximal aspect of each subclavian segment.

This model allows anomalies of the aortic arch to be conceptualized as variations in regression of segments of the primitive double arch. For example, beginning with the further simplified line drawing in Figure 6A,[22] a number of anatomic situations can be visualized and illustrated. A normal left arch develops when the regression occurs between the right subclavian and the descending aorta (Fig. 6B). Likewise, regression of the right arch between the right carotid artery and the origin of the right subclavian results in a left arch with an aberrant right subclavian artery arising as the fourth vessel from the arch (Fig. 6C). Similarly, when regression occurs between the left subclavian and the descending aorta, a right arch with mirror image branching is formed (Fig. 6D). Regression between the left carotid and the left subclavian arteries results in a right arch with an aberrant left subclavian (Fig. 6E). In the last instance, when the ductus arteriosus originates from the aberrant left subclavian artery (as it usually does), its insertion into the pulmonary artery creates a vascular ring. This model is easily sketched and can be used in

daily practice to conceptualize virtually every known arch anomaly, as well as to hypothesize some that have not yet been reported.

VASCULAR RINGS

Prevalence

The two most common vascular rings, double aortic arch and right aortic arch with an aberrant left subclavian artery and a left ligamentum (ductus), will be considered together because their symptoms, radiographic findings, and management are so similar. These two anomalies compose more than 95% of all complete vascular rings. However, vascular rings represent less than 1% of congenital cardiovascular anomalies (see ch. 18).[12]

Usually, double aortic arch is an isolated anomaly, although it does occur with congenital heart disease (Exhibit 1).[13] A right aortic arch with an aberrant left subclavian artery and a left ductus is the most common type of right arch anomaly[16] and usually is an isolated defect, although it has been reported to occur with congenital cardiac anomalies, including tetralogy of Fallot.[20] In contrast, right arch with mirror image branching, occurs almost exclusively with congenital heart anomalies, most often with tetralogy of Fallot, but with some other lesions as well (Exhibit 1).[9] In right arch with mirror image branching, the ductus or ligamentum arises from the left innominate anteriorly and, thus, does not form a ring (Fig. 6D).

Anatomy

Double Aortic Arch. Double aortic arch is due to failure of regression of any part of either the right or left arch. Both arches persist and the trachea and esophagus are completely encircled (Fig. 6A). There are four great vessels, two from each arch. The ligamentum (ductus) is most often left-sided. Usually, both arches are patent, the right arch being higher and larger than the left in 90% (Fig. 1). Occasionally, the left arch is merely an atretic fibrous cord either between the carotid and subclavian arteries, or distal to the left subclavian artery. Atresia of the right arch is a theoretical possibility but was not found in Edwards' review.[19]

Right Arch with Aberrant Left Subclavian Artery. A right arch with an aberrant left subclavian artery is thought to occur as an independent error in arch development[19] and, thus, it is not often associated with congenital cardiac defects.[9] Regression of the left aortic arch between the left common carotid and subclavian segments results in the development of the right aortic arch with an aberrant left subclavian artery (Fig. 6). The left subclavian is the fourth branch from the aorta and originates from a relatively posterior location, coursing behind the esophagus to the left arm. The left ductus originates from a bulbous dilatation at the base of the left subclavian (the diverticulum of Kommerel) and, attached to the left pulmonary artery, it effectively pulls the aorta and the diverticulum forward, compressing the esophagus and

Exhibit 1

Boston Children's Hospital Experience 1973–1987
Vascular Rings and Slings
There were 33 children with vascular ring or pulmonary artery sling as the major diagnosis, 20 of whom underwent surgical correction with no deaths. There were 50 children who had a vascular ring or sling associated with another important cardiac defect. Most commonly this was tetralogy of Fallot (16) or ventricular septal defect (13). Miscellaneous other congenital cardiac defects were associated with vascular rings.

trachea and forming a ring (Fig. 2). Usually, this ring is loose and causes no symptoms; however, in a small percentage of individuals, the ductus or ligamentum may be short and, thus, the ring may be tight. These infants have symptoms identical to those of patients with a double aortic arch.

Clinical Manifestations

Symptoms. The symptoms of vascular rings are due to tracheal compression and, to a lesser degree, to esophageal compression. Patients with double aortic arch tend to be seen in early infancy and often are severely symptomatic.[17,23] Symptoms include stridor, dyspnea, and a barking cough, all of which are worse during feeding or exertion. "Reflex" apnea lasting seconds or even minutes may be triggered by feeding. Older children may have a history of wheezing misdiagnosed as asthma. Recurrent respiratory infections may be a result of aspiration or inadequate clearing of secretions. Symptoms related to esophageal compression are less frequent and less well defined. They include vomiting, choking, and nonspecific feeding difficulties in infants, and dysphagia in older children.

As mentioned earlier, the majority of patients with a right aortic arch and an aberrant left subclavian are asymptomatic and the right arch is discovered when radiographic studies are performed for other reasons. Occasionally, an older individual will complain of mild dysphagia as the aorta and left subclavian become larger and more tortuous, and impinge upon the posterior aspect of the esophagus because of tethering by the ligamentum. Similar symptoms may occur in older patients with a left arch and a retroesophageal aberrant right subclavian artery, even without a right-sided ligamentum. The latter condition has been referred to as "dysphagia lusoria" (Fig. 6).

When patients with a right arch and an aberrant left subclavian have a very short ductus or ligamentum, or when the diverticulum of Kommerel is especially large, a tight vascular ring can be produced (Fig. 2), causing the same symptoms of wheezing, stridor, recurrent infections, apneic spells and feeding difficulties as are produced by a double aortic arch.

Physical Examination. Auscultation may reveal coarse upper airway sounds and wheezing. Mild intermittent cyanosis may be present. Infants show signs of increased respiratory work such as intercostal retractions. Sometimes they lie with the back arched and the neck extended, which probably minimizes tracheal narrowing. Extending the neck may visibly relieve respiratory effort. In patients with a right arch, an aberrant left subclavian and a left ligamentum in whom the ring is loose, the physical examination will be completely normal.

Chest X-ray. A valuable clue to the presence of a vascular ring is the finding of a right aortic arch on the chest x-ray. However, because the thymus is large in infancy, identification of the arch may be difficult. One clue may be a midline trachea (Fig. 7). Usually, the trachea is displaced slightly to the right when only a left arch is present. The left component of a double aortic arch seldom is evident, because, usually, the left arch is the smaller one and is hidden by the thymus. There may be anterior displacement and narrowing of the trachea. This narrowing makes the trachea difficult to identify on a frontal film. Other, more nonspecific radiographic signs of obstruction include air trapping, focal atelectasis, or pneumonitis. Finally, the chest x-ray may be normal.[15] Plain films seldom distinguish between a double arch and a right arch with an aberrant left subclavian artery and a left ligamentum.

The barium esophagram is simple, inexpensive, and diagnostic of the presence of a vascular ring, although usually it will not discriminate between the two lesions discussed above. Characteristically, it shows an indentation on the right side, due to the right arch, and a smaller indentation on the left, due to the left component of a double arch, to the diverticulum of Kommerel, or to the ligamentum in a right arch with an aberrant left subclavian and left ligamentum (Fig. 8). The posterior indentation on the esophagus, seen in the lateral view (Fig. 9), may be slightly larger in patients with a double arch than in those with a right arch and an aberrant left subclavian and left ligamentum. It can be seen by comparing Figures 1 and 2 that the anatomic elements of these rings are similar and, thus, can easily produce similar radiographic findings.

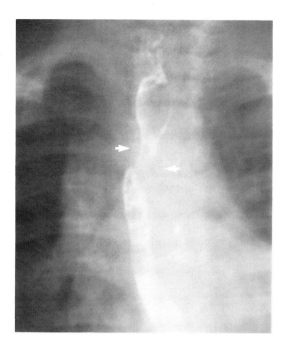

Figure 8. Barium esophagram of a patient with double aortic arch. Note the right-sided indentation (arrow) caused by the right arch and the left-sided, slightly lower indentation (arrow) caused by the left arch.

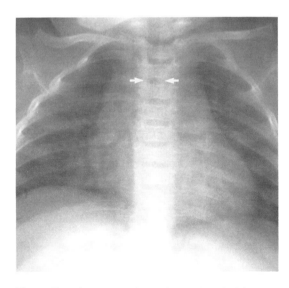

Figure 7. Chest x-ray of an infant with a double aortic arch. Note the midline position of the trachea (arrows). The thymus is large and the arches themselves cannot be outlined.

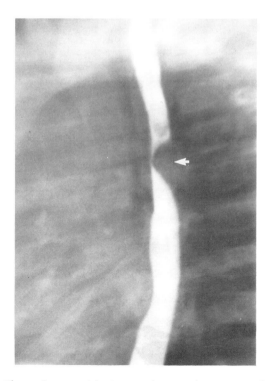

Figure 9. Lateral barium esophagram of a patient with double aortic arch. Note the large posterior indentation caused by the double arch (arrow).

Angiography is seldom necessary, unless it is performed for associated cardiac defects, which are rare in patients with vascular rings. The vast majority of vascular rings are shown satisfactorily on chest x-rays and barium esophagrams.

Echocardiography. Most patients suspected of having a vascular ring should have an echocardiogram, which usually confirms the diagnosis. In fact, it may be able to distinguish between a double arch and a right arch with an aberrant left subclavian artery and a left ligamentum.

Other Diagnostic Methods. Recently, magnetic resonance imaging has been used to demonstrate cardiac and vascular abnormalities in the infant and child. Vascular rings are particularly well displayed by this technology, which shows the anatomy in several planes.[4]

Management

Surgical intervention is considered for all symptomatic patients,[1,17,23] but the timing of operation may be problematical when symptoms wax and wane. A conservative approach might include careful feeding of soft foods and aggressive treatment of pulmonary infections. Many would say that prompt operation is warranted whenever a ring produces symptoms in infants. Operation is clearly indicated when there is repeated respiratory distress, particularly apneic spells and a history of recurrent infections.

The surgical approach for double arch, if the right arch is larger (as is usual), and for all cases of right arch with an aberrant left subclavian and a left ligamentum, is a left thoracotomy.[23] In patients with a double aortic arch, division of the smaller of the two arches (usually the left) is performed. In patients with a right arch and an aberrant left subclavian artery and a left ligamentum, the ligamentum is divided, severing the ring and freeing the trachea and esophagus. Operative mortality is reported to be less than 5%.[3,17,23] Although late follow-up usually reveals significant relief of symptoms, studies of persistently abnormal pulmonary function in some patients have indicated residual obstruction of the central airway, which is thought to be due to an intrinsic tracheal abnormality.[14]

Asymptomatic patients with a right arch and an aberrant left subclavian artery (those found incidentally) need no treatment at all. However, those discovered in infancy are usually symptomatic and often are indistinguishable from patients with double arch and, thus, will be surgically corrected. Occasionally, patients without compression of the airway may develop dysphagia later in life, and may be diagnosed in adulthood by esophagography. When esophageal symptoms are severe, surgical treatment may be warranted.

PULMONARY ARTERY SLING

Definition

"Pulmonary artery sling" and "anomalous left pulmonary artery" are terms that have been applied to the anomaly in which the left pulmonary artery arises aberrantly from the proximal part of the right pulmonary artery and courses to the left, behind the trachea, and anterior to the esophagus. This places the airway in a "vascular sling" (Fig. 3).[6,11,24] Additional cardiovascular anomalies, including patency of the ductus, atrial septal defect, ventricular septal defect, and persistence of the left superior vena cava, occur in about half of the affected infants.[21] Gastrointestinal, genitourinary, and endocrine defects have also been described.[11] The left pulmonary artery sling syndrome has been repaired in asymptomatic adults.[7]

Embryology and Anatomy

It is thought the anomaly occurs when the proximal part of the left sixth arch regresses or fails to develop its normal connections to the left lung bud.[11] Consequently, a "collateral" vessel to the left lung develops. This vessel originates from the transverse portion of the right pulmonary artery, just to the right of the trachea. The vessel then curves posteriorly and sharply to the left, above and behind the right main bronchus, behind the trachea, but anterior to the esophagus in its course to the left hilum. The branches of the left pulmonary artery then take a normal anatomic course.[24] This anatomic course causes constriction of the right main bronchus or trachea, or both. Hypoplasia or stenosis of the bronchus or distal portion of the trachea, usually due to completeness of the cartilaginous rings, occurs frequently either above or near the sling, or even in the distal bronchi, and these may be a more important source of airway symptoms than the sling itself.

Clinical Manifestations

Symptoms. Usually infants are seen in the first weeks or months of life with respiratory stridor that is most marked in expiration. Often, compromise of the airway is severe, and untreated infants have a substantial mortality rate. If an infant escapes early diagnosis, recurrent respiratory infections are likely.

Physical Examination. An affected infant will have stridor, dyspnea, and expiratory wheezing and may be intermittently cyanotic. Because the respiratory obstruction may be due to the artery, to the intrinsic airway abnormalities, or both, the airway obstruction may manifest itself variably. The right lung may be either hyperinflated (and thus hyperresonant) or partly atelectatic. If there is intrinsic bronchial abnormality on the left as well, the aeration abnormality may involve the left lung (Fig. 10). Peripheral breath sounds may be decreased, and there may be signs of a mediastinal shift.

Chest X-ray. A chest x-ray frequently shows abnormal aeration (hyperinflation, atelectasis) of either lung (Fig. 10). On a well-penetrated frontal film, there may be an unusually low level of branching of the left pulmonary artery. On a perfectly lateral chest x-ray, there may be anterior bowing of the lower trachea or right main bronchus, caused by the aberrant left pulmonary artery posterior to it. There may be a round density just posterior to the trachea, which is the aberrant left pulmonary artery, on end, as it courses toward the left lung. This same shadow is more clearly seen on a barium esophagram as an anterior indentation on the esophagus (Fig. 11).[5,24] Computer tomography shows the severity and length of the tracheal narrowing well.

In the absence of any other cardiac defect, angiography probably is not necessary. If performed, a frontal projection with cranial angulation of the tube will demonstrate the anomalous course of the left pulmonary artery clearly (Fig. 12). When problems of aeration are present, as is usual, bronchography can clarify the extent of peripheral bronchial abnormalities that may be present, in addition to the narrowing in the area of the sling itself.

Echocardiography. Usually, echocardiography

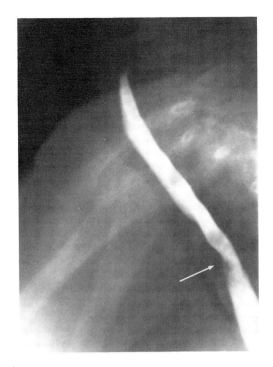

Figure 11. Lateral esophagram in patient with anomalous left pulmonary artery. Note the soft tissue shadow (arrow) of the left pulmonary artery as it courses between the tracheal air shadow and the esophagus. Sometimes this shadow can be seen behind the tracheal air shadow on the plain film.

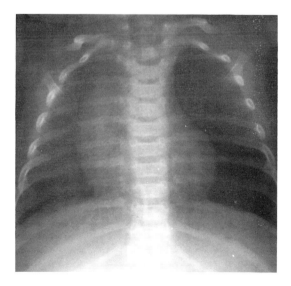

Figure 10. Chest x-ray of patient with anomalous left pulmonary artery showing a mediastinal shift to the right and hyperlucency of the left lung. This suggests trapping of air on the left, associated with some loss of volume on the right. Although the right main bronchus is compressed by the pulmonary sling, the aeration abnormality on the left suggests that intrinsic bronchial obstruction on the left side may be present as well, as is often the case in patients with this abnormality.

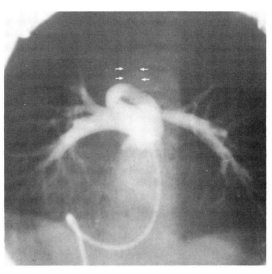

Figure 12. Pulmonary angiogram demonstrating the anomalous left pulmonary artery, which has arisen from the right pulmonary artery and coursed behind the trachea (arrows) to reach the left lung.

can demonstrate the abnormal origin of the left pulmonary artery.[25]

Other Diagnostic Methods. Magnetic resonance imaging affords a sectional means of displaying the origin of the left pulmonary artery and may demonstrate any additional cardiac defects as well.

Management and Course

Because mortality without surgical repair is high, prompt surgical intervention usually is indicated. The most commonly performed procedure involves detaching the left pulmonary artery from its right-sided origin and anastomosing it to the main pulmonary artery on the left. This procedure carries a discouragingly high mortality rate, reported as high as 50% in one large review.[18] This is due largely to residual tracheal or bronchial stenosis. Also, there is a fairly high incidence of postoperative left pulmonary artery obstruction.

In an attempt to solve the problem of tracheobronchial stenosis, a newer technique involves resection of the stenotic segment of the airway. The left pulmonary artery is pulled forward to its usual anterior location before the airway is reanastomosed. This technique involves no vascular anastomosis and, thus, seldom causes left pulmonary artery occlusion. Preliminary experience has been encouraging.[10]

REFERENCES

1. Arciniegas E, Hakini M, Hertzler JH, et al: Surgical management of congenital vascular rings. J Thorac Cardiovasc Surg 77:721–730, 1974.
2. Barry A: The aortic derivatives in the human adult. Anat Rec 111:221–238, 1951.
3. Binet JP, Langlois J: Aortic arch anomalies in children and infants. J Thorac Cardiovasc Surg 73:248–252, 1977.
4. Bissett GS, Strife JL, Kirks DR, et al: Vascular rings: MR imaging. AJR 149:251–256, 1987.
5. Capitanio MA, Ramos R, Kirkpatrick JA: Pulmonary artery sling: roentgen observations. AJR 112:28–34, 1971.
6. Contro S, Miller R, White H, et al: Bronchial obstruction due to pulmonary artery anomalies. I. Vascular sling. Circulation 17:418–423, 1958.
7. Dupuis C, Vaksmon G, Pernot C, et al: Asymptomatic form of left pulmonary artery sling. Am J Cardiol 61:177–181, 1988.
8. Edwards JE: Anomalies of the derivatives of the aortic arch system. Med Clin North Am 52:925–949, 1948.
9. Felson B, Palayew MJ: The two types of right aortic arch. Radiology 81:745–759, 1963.
10. Jonas RA, Spevak PJ, McGill T, et al: Pulmonary artery sling: primary repair by tracheal resection in infancy. J Thorac Cardiovasc Surg 97:548–550, 1989.
11. Jue KL, Raghib G, Amplatz K, et al: Anomalous origin of the left pulmonary artery from the right pulmonary artery. AJR 95:598–610, 1965.
12. Keith JD, Rowe RD, Vlad P: Heart Disease in Infancy and Childhood, 2nd ed. New York, Macmillan, 1967.
13. Keith JD, Rowe RD, Vlad P: Heart Disease in Infancy and Childhood, 3rd ed. New York, Macmillan, 1978.
14. Marmon LM, Bye MR, Haas JM, et al: Vascular rings and slings: long-term follow-up of pulmonary function. Journal of Ped Surg 19:683–690, 1984.
15. Newhauser EBD: The roentgen diagnosis of double aortic arch and other anomalies of the great vessels. AJR 56:1–12, 1946.
16. Poynter CWM: Arterial anomalies pertaining to the aortic arches and the branches arising from them. University Studies of the University of Nebraska 16:229–345, 1916.
17. Roesler M, deLeval M, Chrispin A, et al: Surgical management of vascular ring. Ann Surg 197:139–146, 1963.
18. Sade RM, Rosenthal A, Fellows K, et al: Pulmonary artery sling. J Thorac Cardiovasc Surg 69:333–346, 1975.
19. Stewart JR, Kincaid OW, Edwards JE: An atlas of vascular rings and related malformations of the aortic arch system. Springfield, IL, Charles C Thomas, 1964.
20. Stewart JR, Kincaid OW, Titus JL: Right aortic arch: plain film diagnosis and significance. AJR 97:377–389, 1966.
21. Telser VF, Balsara RH, Niguidular FN: Aberrant left pulmonary artery (vascular sling): report of five cases. Chest 66:402–407, 1974.
22. VanZandt TF, Columbo CA, Danahy SA: Aortic arches simplified. Radiographics 10:126, 1990.
23. Wychulis AR, Kincaid OW, Weidman WH, et al: Congenital vascular rings: surgical considerations and results of operation. Mayo Clin Proc 46:182–188, 1971.
24. Wittenborg MH, Tantiwongse T, Rosenberg BF: Anomalous course of left pulmonary artery with respiratory obstruction. Radiology 67:339–345, 1956.
25. Yeager SB, Chin AJ, Sanders SP: Two-dimensional echocardiographic diagnosis of pulmonary artery sling in infancy. J Am Coll Cardiol 7:625–629, 1986.

Chapter 53

CARDIAC TUMORS

Donald C. Fyler, M.D.

PREVALENCE

Cardiac tumors are rare in infants and children. Although a variety of tumors has been reported in the pediatric age group,[5-7,9,12] rhabdomyomas are by far the most common, with myxomas, sarcomas, and teratomas being seen less frequently (Exhibit 1).

PATHOLOGY

Cardiac tumors are rare, whether primary or metastatic. The most common are as follows:

Rhabdomyoma

Rhabdomyomas may be large (Fig. 1) or small, and are usually multiple nodules involving the ventricular and septal walls. Extensive involvement of the ventricular septum may compromise the ventricular cavities. Histologically, these circumscribed tumors contain large vacuoles of glycogen and strands of cytoplasm extending from the nucleus to the cell membrane, producing a "spider cell."[2] As many as 50% of these children have tuberous sclerosis; 50% of children with tuberous sclerosis have rhabdomyomas.[3]

Fibroma

Fibromas are usually single, occasionally large, and most often arise in the left ventricular myocardium. Unlike the rhabdomyoma, they only rarely involve the septum. The tumor is circumscribed, firm, and fibrous and is composed of fibroblasts and bits of cardiac muscle.

Myxoma

Myxomas are most commonly seen in the adult population in the 30- to 50-year age group; however, they have been described in children, including neonates. Because these tumors become increasingly frequent with advancing age, in a pediatric practice they are most commonly found in teenagers. Myxomas may be seen anywhere in the heart but are predominantly seen in the left atrium, less frequently in the right atrium, and they can occur in the ventricle. The myxomas are thought to be derived from mesenchymal tissue and, as such, they may include histologic evidence of a variety of structures. The histologic similarity to endocardial cushion tissue and the fact that the tumors arise from areas derived from endocardial tissue are noteworthy.[13] The tumors are covered with endothelium, which distinguishes them from thrombi. The stalk of the myxoma often arises from the atrial septum, and when there are right and left atrial myxomas, the stalks of the two tumors rise from the same region of the atrial septum. Rarely metastases have been reported.

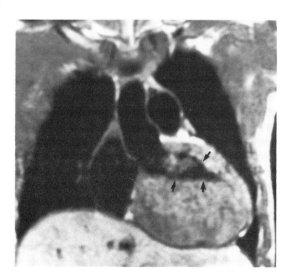

Figure 1. Magnetic resonance imaging of a rhabdomyoma. This baby has a large intracardial tumor almost completely occluding the left ventricle. The ventricular cavity visible on this film is the largest; all other frames showed an even smaller left ventricular cavity. Arrows indicate the left ventricle.

Sarcoma

Rhabdomyosarcoma is, fortunately, a very rare tumor arising from cardiac muscle cells.

Teratoma

Intrapericardial teratomas arise within the pericardium from a pedicle at the base of the great vessels and, although benign, they are nonetheless space-occupying and, more important, cause the production of dangerously excessive pericardial fluid.[10]

Valvar Excrescences

Excrescences of tissue attached to valves are encountered occasionally and, nowadays, are recognized at echocardiography. Usually, these lesions are small and inconsequential, but rarely they may be large enough to threaten obstruction of the circulation (Fig. 2).

Thrombi and Vegetations

Since the advent of 2-D echocardiography, the most common intracavitary tumors are thrombi and vegetations associated with infective endocarditis. Most are found as part of an examination of patients with previously known heart disease, following cardiac surgery, or sometimes because embolic phenomenon have led to a search for a source.

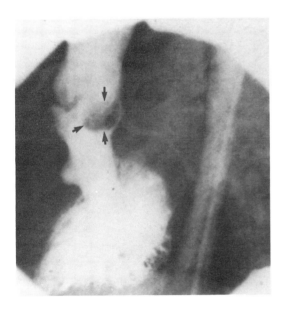

Figure 2. Left ventricular cineangiogram showing a mitral valve excrescence. The tumor was mobile, moving 1–2 cm with systole and diastole. When the child was 6 years old, the tumor was removed to avoid aortic valve damage. It was found to be attached to a stalk arising from the insertion of the septal mitral valve leaflet.

CLINICAL MANIFESTATIONS

Cardiac tumors are discovered because of:

1. **Murmurs.** A murmur is heard because an intracavitary tumor is partially obstructing blood flow.

2. **Ectopy.** Intracavitary and mural tumors are sometimes associated with ectopy or episodes of tachycardia.

3. **Congestive heart failure.** The onset of congestive heart failure is not a common presenting cause for tumor but can occur when the tumor is large.

4. **Embolic phenomena.** Bits of atrial myxoma are known to break loose and produce embolic episodes that are sometimes the first sign that the tumor is present.

5. **Syncope.** Mobile tumors, particularly atrial myxomas, are known to obstruct the circulation suddenly, producing fainting episodes and even sudden death.

6. **Tamponade.** Intrapericardial teratomas are characteristically discovered because of the sudden appearance of cardiac tamponade.

7. **X-ray abnormalities.** Occasionally a cardiac tumor is discovered because of an abnormal cardiac contour on a chest x-ray taken for other reasons.

8. **Echocardiography.** Nowadays, some cardiac tumors are discovered because of systematic examination during echocardiography for some other reason. Routine examination of patients with tuberous sclerosis is now a matter of practice; some rhabdomyomas are found by this mechanism.

Electrocardiography

The electrocardiogram is often abnormal when there is an intracardiac tumor; rhythm problems, bundle branch block, complete heart block, and infarct patterns may be encountered. Most patients show some abnormality.

Chest X-ray

The cardiac contour may be irregular if there is a tumor distorting the outer surface of the heart. Pericardial effusion may be suspected when the heart is very large (Fig. 3).

Echocardiography

Since the use of 2-D echocardiography became routine, the number of intracavitary and intramural tumor masses discovered in the hearts of children has risen substantially (Exhibit 1).[8,11] Intracavitary tumors of relatively small size are readily identified on routine scanning; intramural tumors are identified by differences in echo density between the tumor and the surrounding myocardium (see Fig. 30, p. 181).

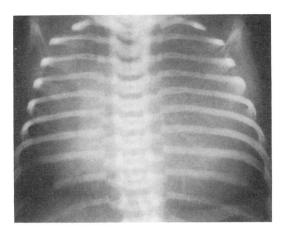

Figure 3. Posteroanterior chest film of a patient with an intrapericardial teratoma. This 2-week-old infant had had multiple pericardial taps because of tamponade. An intrapericardial teratoma arising from the root of the great vessels was removed. Now, many years later, the child continues to be well.

Cardiac Catheterization

When considering excision of a cardiac tumor, cardiac catheterization and angiography should be carried out to provide the maximal amount of information prior to operation. Occasionally, a patient is referred to the cardiac catheterization laboratory because of an obstructive lesion which, on angiography, turns out to be a tumor obstructing the outflow of the heart.

MANAGEMENT

Tumors that are obstructing the circulation, or potentially may obstruct the circulation, should be surgically removed if possible. Surely, all intrapericardial teratomas should be removed as a lifesaving measure.[1,10] Atrial myxomas should be surgically removed on discovery,[4] because they tend to get larger and have the potential for causing embolic episodes, occlusion of the circulation, and even sudden death. Any suggestion of transitory obstruction to the circulation makes immediate removal of an atrial myxoma imperative. Often, an obstructing rhabdomyoma may be usefully excised. Otherwise, benign cardiac tumors are best left alone. Ectopy and arrhythmia are managed well with modern medications, although occasionally a patient will require surgery for a rhythm problem, at which time the tumor may be removed.

Now that 2-D echocardiography regularly reveals thrombi or vegetations within the heart, the cardiologist must decide what to do about them. When a large clot or vegetation in the left heart has caused even one embolic episode, the decision to ask the cardiac surgeons to remove the remaining clot is usually easy. When there are small

Exhibit 1

Boston Children's Hospital Experience 1973–1987 **Cardiac Tumors**	
Type of Tumor	*No. of Patients*
Rhabdomyoma	21
10 Tuberous sclerosis	
1 Congenital heart disease	
Fibroma	2
Myxoma	4
Pericardial	4
3 Adjacent mediastinal or pulmonary tumor	
1 Intrapericardial teratoma	
Sarcoma	1
Valvar excrescences	5
3 Mitral	
1 Tricuspid	
1 Pulmonary	
Hematoma of atrial septum (later healed)	1
Carcinoid (see ch. 44)	1
Unspecified	2
Thrombus	44

Cardiac Tumors and Intracardiac Thrombi
(excludes vegetations associated with infective endocarditis)

	–1972	1973–77	1978–82	1983–87	Total
Cardiac tumors	5	10	8	18	41
Cardiac thrombi	5	5	5	29	44

The increase in tumors and thrombi since 1983 is almost certainly a consequence of newer echocardiographic techniques.

thrombi or vegetations in the right heart and no possibility of right-to-left shunting, it is equally easy to decide merely to keep the patient under observation. The use of anticoagulants is recommended to prevent further formation of thrombi; this may even help existing thrombi to regress, regardless of where they are located. However, when the thrombi have developed in low-pressure venous structures, for example, following postoperative Fontan-type procedures, anticoagulation is mandatory. Indeed, the use of anticoagulants for some weeks to prevent postoperative clots from developing is now becoming routine practice for patients who have undergone operations based on the Fontan principle. The difficult decisions arise when there are thrombi or vegetations that may have the potential for causing emboli to the brain or other major organs but have not yet done so. With trepidation, the clinician, with the help of the surgeon, weighs all available information and hopes to make the right decision.

REFERENCES

1. Aldousany AW, Joyner JC, Price RA, et al: Diagnosis and treatment of intrapericardial teratoma. Pediatr Cardiol 8:51–53, 1987.
2. Arey JB: Cardiovascular Pathology in Infants and Children. Philadelphia, W.B. Saunders, 1984.
3. Bass JL, Breningstall GN, Swaiman KF: Echocardiographic incidence of cardiac rhabdomyoma in tuberous sclerosis. Am J Cardiol 55:1379–1382, 1985.
4. Hanson EC, Gill CC, Razavi M, et al: The surgical treatment of atrial myxomas: clinical experience and late results in 33 patients. J Thorac Cardiovasc Surg 89:298–303, 1985.
5. Keith JD, Rowe RD, Vlad P: Heart Disease in Infancy and Childhood, 3rd ed. New York, Macmillan, 1979, p. 1040.
6. Kissane JM: Pathology of infancy and childhood. St. Louis, C.V. Mosby, 1975, pp. 420–425.
7. Larrieu AJ, Jamieson WRE, Tyers GFO, et al: Primary cardiac tumors: experience with 25 cases. J Thorac Cardiovasc Surg 83:339–348, 1982.
8. Marx GR, Bierman FZ, Matthews E, et al: Two-dimensional echocardiographic diagnosis of intracardiac masses in infancy. J Am Coll Cardiol 3:827–832, 1984.
9. Nadas AS, Ellison RC: Cardiac tumors in infancy. Am J Cardiol 21:363, 1968.
10. Reynolds JR, Donahue JK, Pearce CW: Intrapericardial teratoma. Pediatrics 43:71, 1969.
11. Sharratt CP, Lacson AG, Cornel G, et al: Echocardiography of intracardiac filling defects in infants and children. Pediatr Cardiol 7:189–194, 1986.
12. Van der Hauwaert LG: Cardiac tumours in infancy and childhood. Br Heart J 33:125–132, 1971.
13. Van Praagh R: Personal communication.

Section X

Surgical Considerations

Chapter 54

SURGERY FOR INFANTS WITH CONGENITAL HEART DISEASE

Aldo R. Castaneda, M.D., R.A. Jonas, M.D., and John E. Mayer, Jr., M.D.

Surgery for congenital heart disease has undergone rapid changes in recent years. Improved operative survival rates and encouraging mid-term and late-term hemodynamic and electrophysiologic results have been achieved for many defects. These improved surgical results are related to (1) developments in preoperative diagnosis of congenital heart defects, (2) the development of new surgical techniques, and (3) improvements in postoperative management.

Areas of interest include (1) the philosophy of primary repair early in life (including neonates) rather than palliation followed by secondary repair of congenital heart defects, (2) aggressive open heart, palliative procedures for nonreparable lesions (in neonates), including the use of valved homografts and prosthetic materials, (3) the broadened clinical application of various systemic venous-to-pulmonary artery bypass procedures for the treatment of complex congenital heart defects (such as single ventricle, hypoplastic left heart syndrome, and heterotaxy syndromes with anomalies of pulmonary and systemic venous return), and (4) heart and heart/lung transplantation in the pediatric age group.

At Boston Children's Hospital, over the past 15 years we have experienced a steady increase in babies undergoing surgery (Exhibit 1).

PRIMARY REPAIR OF CONGENITAL CARDIAC DEFECTS IN INFANTS, INCLUDING NEONATES

Approximately a third of all children born with congenital heart defects become ill during the first year of life and require surgical treatment. If they are not treated, death occurs, mostly during the first few months of life; survivors experience progressive and potentially irreversible secondary organ damage, principally to the heart, but also to the lungs and the central nervous system. Congenital heart disease may interfere also with normal postnatal changes, such as myocardial hyperplasia and its accompanying coronary angiogenesis (mostly during the first three months of life),[10] and with the development of pulmonary vascular and alveolar structures (alveologenesis). Although more difficult to quantitate, the presence of cyanosis, congestive heart failure, and failure to thrive cause psychomotor and cognitive abnormalities that also may limit the development of a child significantly.[32] Primary reparative surgery offers the opportunity to decrease the mortality caused by the primary defect and also to prevent secondary morbid effects on the development of other organ systems.[4]

Generally, in the past, critically ill neonates were subjected to a first-stage palliative procedure, followed years later by reparative surgery. These palliative operations, albeit lifesaving in many instances, cause damage to the circulation. For example, systemic-to-pulmonary artery shunts impose a significant volume/pressure overload on the pulmonary circulation, and banding of the pulmonary artery induces a significant pressure overload upon the right (or single) ventricle which, over time, can cause structural abnormalities within the heart, such as narrowing of a bulboventricular foramen. Equally aggravating can be the effects of

Exhibit 1

Repair of Congenital Heart Disease in Neonates from January 1983 through December 1988*

Lesion	No. of Patients	Hospital Mortality n (%)
Transposition of the Great Arteries	201	15 (7.4)
Intact interventricular septum		
Arterial switch	158	13 (8.2)
Senning procedure	16	2 (12.5)
Ventricular septal defect		
Arterial switch	27	0 (0.0)
Pulmonary Stenosis	21	0
Total Anomalous Pulmonary Venous Connection	19	3 (15.7)
Tetralogy of Fallot	19	2 (10.5)
Ventricular Septal Defect	18	2 (11.1)
Truncus Arteriosus	18	3 (16.5)
Interrupted Aortic Arch	19	3 (15.5)
Pulmonary Atresia + Intact Ventricular Septum	12	3 (25.0)
Aortic Stenosis	10	1 (16.6)
Atrioventricular Canal	6	1 (16.6)
Truncus Arteriosus + Interrupted Aortic Arch	4	2 (50.0)
Tumor	1	0
Ebstein's Disease	1	1 (100)
	304	36 (11.8)

*Some patients had more than one lesion.

Age at First Operation in Three Time Periods

Age	Year 1973–77	1978–82	1983–87
1–30 days	190	383	597
31–180 days	150	343	435
181–364 days	122	263	303
1–5 years	291	496	587
5–10 years	286	226	238
> 10 years	278	260	201
Subtotal	1,317	1,971	2,361
First operation before 1973 or elsewhere	383	105	69
Total	1,700	2,076	2,430

these palliative operations on the architecture of the pulmonary arteries. Distortions or interruption of a pulmonary artery branch caused by shunts or pulmonary artery bands can, in certain instances, render a patient unsuitable for a right atrial-pulmonary artery bypass operation. Influenced by these considerations, the authors have discontinued the use of palliative operations whenever possible, and, instead, have adopted a policy of primary reparative operations in infants, including neonates with the following cardiac defects: transposition of the great arteries, total anomalous pulmonary venous connection, tetralogy of Fallot, ventricular septal defect, truncus arteriosus, interrupted aortic arch and ventricular septal defect, complete atrioventricular canal, congenital aortic stenosis, and critical pulmonary stenosis. See Exhibit 1 for experience at Children's Hospital in Boston with primary repair of complex congenital heart lesions in neonates. The anatomic repair of trans-

position of the great arteries in neonates will be discussed as an example of this treatment philosophy.

ANATOMIC REPAIR OF TRANSPOSITION OF THE GREAT ARTERIES IN NEONATES

The first attempts to repair transposition of the great arteries consisted of switching the great arteries, either with or without simultaneous transfer of one or both of the coronary arteries. None of the patients survived. Subsequently, because of impressive results, atrial inversion operations (Mustard or Senning procedures) rapidly gained worldwide acceptance. However, these operations were eventually plagued by (1) a high incidence of late atrial arrhythmias, such as the sick sinus syndrome and/or junctional rhythm, and (2) a less clearly established incidence of late right ventricular (systemic ventricle) dysfunction. A number of theoretical considerations support the assumption that the left ventricle is more suitable than the right to serve the systemic circulation. The right ventricle, with its crescent-shaped cavity, its large internal surface area to volume ratio, its bellows-like contraction pattern, and its separated inlet and outlet segments seems better suited to serve as a volume pump rather than a pressure pump.

In 1975 Jatene reported the first successful arterial switching operation in a patient with transposition of the great arteries and a large ventricular septal defect.[18] He recognized the need for a "prepared" left ventricle and therefore selected patients with left ventricular pressure at systemic levels, usually resulting from the presence of a large ventricular septal defect. Not surprisingly, the early operative mortality was high. Also, because approximately 75% of all patients with transposition of the great arteries have an intact ventricular septum, the application of the switching principle to this larger subset of patients demanded a different approach. To prepare the left ventricle for systemic pressure work, Yacoub, in 1977, introduced a two-stage approach for transposition of the great arteries with an intact ventricular septum by first banding the main pulmonary artery (sometimes adding a systemic-pulmonary artery shunt) to stimulate the development of left ventricular muscle mass, followed by an arterial switching operation many months later.[45] This staged approach had the disadvantage of requiring two operations, with the concomitant risk of added mortality and morbidity.

In patients with transposition of the great arteries and an intact ventricular septum the thickness of the left ventricular wall is normal at birth. However, the rapidly decreasing pulmonary vascular resistance causes a fall in peak left ventricular pressure and wall stress and, hence, decreased stimulus for the development of left ventricular muscle mass. By 1 month of age, most of these patients have a peak left ventricle/right ventricle pressure ratio equal to or less than 65%. Furthermore, the increased left ventricular volume load due to augmented pulmonary blood flow causes progressive left ventricular dilatation. The authors, therefore, reasoned that an arterial switching operation for babies with transposition of the great arteries and intact ventricular septum had to be done during the first few weeks of life when the left ventricle is still "prepared" by the intrauterine physiology to support the systemic circulation.[5] Ideally, the repair should be performed within the first 2 weeks of life. Because this is not always practical, some empirical criteria for predicting postoperative left ventricular performance have been developed. For all patients with transposition of the great arteries with intact ventricular septum, repair should be carried out before the age of 2 weeks, regardless

of preoperative left ventricular pressure measurements. After this age a left ventricle/right ventricle pressure ratio of 0.6 is the lowest limit of acceptable left ventricular pressure. Helpful, but not yet clearly defined, are two-dimensional (2-D) echocardiographic indications of a left ventricle suitable for an arterial switching operation, including the ventricular septal position, thickness of the left ventricular wall, and the muscle mass/volume ration of the left ventricle.

The origin and trajectory of the coronary arteries influence the possibility of an arterial switching operation. In transposition of the great arteries the coronary arteries almost invariably originate from the left- and right-facing sinuses. The most common types of coronary anatomy in transposition of the great arteries are illustrated in Figure 1. Preoperative visualization of the coronary arteries in neonates with transposition of the great arteries is obtained by aortic root angiography and by 2-D echocardiography. Most coronary arterial patterns in transposition of the great arteries lend themselves to the arterial switching operation; however, in a few instances the outcome of coronary transfer is doubtful. For example, coronary arteries with an intramural course (within the aortic wall) are more difficult to transfer without causing distortion.

Ventricular Septal Defect

The presence of a large ventricular septal defect, and the consequent relatively acceptable level of oxygen saturation, allows more time before a switching operation becomes necessary. However, because of the threat of accelerated development of pulmonary vascular obstructive disease in these patients, elective repair of transposition of the great arteries with ventricular septal defect should be carried out by the age of 2 months.

Preoperative Management

All patients are evaluated preoperatively by 2-D echocardiography, cardiac catheterization, and angiography, including aortic root injection (see p. 566). Generally, balloon atrial septostomy is carried out during cardiac catheterization unless the surgery is to be performed immediately. When severe hypoxia and/or metabolic acidosis are present, prostaglandin E1 may be added to maintain ductal patency and improve oxygenation.

Operative Technique

The salient features of the operation include:
1. Deep hypothermia to rectal temperatures of 20°C is used with or without circulatory arrest and cold cardioplegia (20 cc/kg/body weight, St. Thomas solution).
2. After transection of the ascending aorta and pulmonary artery, the left and right coronary ar-

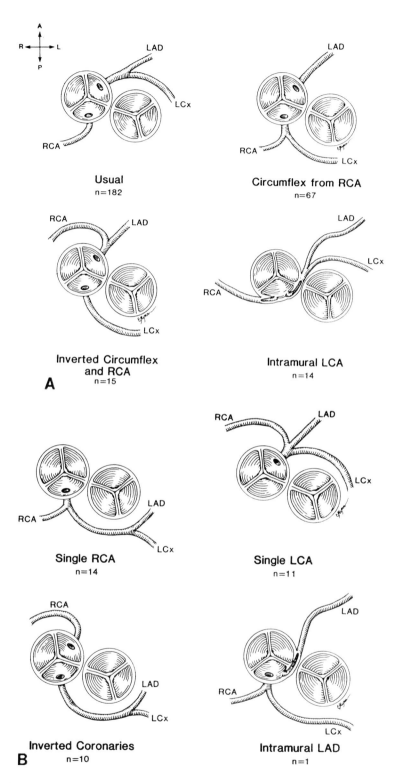

Figure 1. **A** and **B,** Drawings showing the coronary anatomy in patients with transposition of the great arteries. LAD, left anterior descending coronary artery; LCx, circumflex coronary artery; RCA, right coronary artery, n, the number of patients with each type of coronary anatomy.

teries are explanted along with a generous flap of surrounding aortic wall (Fig. 2). After an equivalent V-shaped excision of the proximal pulmonary arterial wall, the coronary flaps are sewn into these incisions with continuous 7-0 absorbable, monofilament suture.

3. Then the distal pulmonary artery is brought anterior to the aorta, the distal aorta is anastomosed to the proximal neo-aorta, and after filling the explanted area of the proximal neopulmonary artery with pericardial patches, the pulmonary artery anastomosis is accomplished.

If a ventricular septal defect is present, it is closed through either the pulmonary artery or the right atrium.

Any abnormality of cardiac rhythm or myocardial performance must be considered suggestive of a coronary perfusion problem. Should this be the case, the cause must be identified and corrected immediately.

Postoperative Management

Postoperative management is similar to that for other neonates or infants undergoing repair of complex cardiac lesions. Mechanical ventilation, sedation, and moderate inotropic support (when necessary) should be provided during the first 24–48 hours or until hemodynamic stability is achieved.

Results

From January, 1983 through December, 1988, 243 patients had arterial switching operations at The Children's Hospital in Boston; 146 of these had transposition of the great arteries with intact ventricular septum, with a total mortality of 9%.[44]

However, among the last 80 consecutive arterial switching operations for transposition of the great arteries with intact ventricular septum, there was only one death (1.2%). Ninety-seven patients had transposition of the great arteries with ventricular septal defect or double-outlet right ventricle, with a mortality of 4.1%.

Clinical Data. None of the surviving patients is receiving cardiac medications and all are following a normal growth pattern.

Hemodynamic Data. The only significant late postoperative complication was supravalvar pulmonary stenosis. A right ventricle-to-pulmonary artery gradient greater than 50 mm Hg developed in 7 patients. Stenosis at the pulmonary artery anastomosis occurred early in our experience and prompted some modifications of the technique, including extensive dissection of the distal pulmonary arteries and enlargement of the explanted coronary donor areas with large patches of autologous pericardium, which helps to enlarge, and to decrease tension on, the pulmonary artery anastomosis. Since adopting this technique, supravalvar pulmonary stenosis has virtually disappeared as a postoperative complication.

Late Occlusion of Coronary Arteries. Occlusion of the left anterior descending coronary artery occurred in 3 patients, 1 with the usual pattern of coronary anatomy and 2 with a circumflex coronary artery arising from the right coronary artery and only a small anterior descending coronary artery arising from the left facing sinus. Postoperatively, all 3 patients had adequate retrograde perfusion through collaterals and showed no left ventricular dysfunction at 2-D echocardiography or cardiac catheterization. A late sudden death in a patient

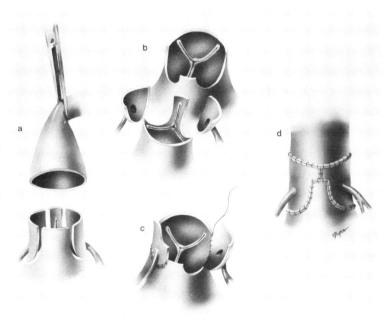

Figure 2. Surgical technique of the arterial switching operation. **a,** After transection of the great arteries, the coronary arterial flaps are excised from the free edge of the aorta to the base of the sinus of Valsalva. **b,** An equivalent segment of pulmonary artery wall is excised. **c,** The coronary arterial flaps are anastomosed to the V-shaped excisions made in the pulmonary (neo-aortic) wall. **d,** Anastomosis of the proximal neo-aorta to the distal aorta.

with transposition of the great arteries with ventricular septal defect, although not confirmed by autopsy, may have been caused by myocardial infarction.

Left Ventricular Function. 2-D echocardiographic analysis as late as 15 months after the arterial switching operation has shown normal left ventricular function. Regional wall motion (viewed in both long and short axes), preload dependent left ventricular function (end-systolic wall stress versus fractional shortening), left ventricle contractility (end-systolic wall stress versus velocity of fiber shortening), and also analysis of diastolic function (both peak thinning and peak filling rate) were normal in all patients.

Electrophysiologic Data. Normal sinus rhythm was present in 98% of the patients as long as 15 months after surgery. Only 1 patient had late sinus node dysfunction. Five patients with transposition of the great arteries and ventricular septal defect had persistent complete heart block.

Palliative Surgery for Nonreparable Lesions

The ultimate goal of the cardiac surgeon dealing with congenital heart disease is to achieve a physiologically normal circulation with a biventricular heart. However, in many patients this cannot be achieved. There is a large subset of patients who have a single ventricular chamber with either one or two inlet valves and either one or two outlet valves. Our present understanding is that the best that can be offered to such patients is application of the **Fontan principle,**[11] namely, diversion of systemic veneous return directly into the pulmonary arteries with separation of pulmonary and systemic venous blood. This principle can be applied only where (1) left ventricular function is excellent, (2) the pulmonary arteries are adequate, and, most important, (3) pulmonary vascular resistance is low. Although the first two criteria can be met in the neonate, the pulmonary vascular resistance is neither low enough (less than 2 units/m² of body surface area) nor stable enough to allow a successful Fontan procedure. Therefore, the neonate must be palliated by a procedure that will achieve and maintain the three essential criteria for successful outcome of the Fontan procedure.

Although originally Fontan recommended 4 years of age to be the youngest at which his principle should be applied, if appropriate hemodynamic and anatomic criteria are met, the operation can be performed safely any time beyond early infancy. In fact, the longer one waits beyond infancy the more likely it is that ventricular function will deteriorate and the child will be at higher risk. Fontan operations have been successfully performed in infants as young as 3 months of age.

There are a wide variety of anatomic entities amenable to the Fontan principle (Exhibit 2). Children with a single right or left ventricle and those with hypoplasia of either ventricle sufficient to prohibit a biventricular repair may be candidates. While the dividing line between ventricles that are large enough to contribute to a biventricular circulation and ventricles that are too small is presently being defined, present data suggest that the critical size is approximately 20 ml/m² of body surface area. If either ventricle is smaller than 20 ml, a biventricular repair will not succeed; if larger than 20, success is likely, and around 20 the outcome is debatable.

Natural History of Infants with Single Ventricle Physiology

The systemic and pulmonary venous returns become mixed in the single ventricle. Blood flow is then distributed between the pulmonary and systemic vascular beds according to the ratio of pulmonary-to-aortic outflow resistance and the ratio of pulmonary-to-systemic vascular resistance.

No Pulmonary Outflow Obstruction. Pulmonary resistance decreases rapidly during early infancy and becomes much lower than systemic resistance; therefore, in the absence of pulmonary outflow obstruction, massive pulmonary blood flow will occur. The volume load on the single ventricle, particularly in the presence of diminished arterial oxygen saturation, is likely to result in congestive heart failure. Or, if the child should survive this, pulmonary vascular disease is likely to develop.

Severe Pulmonary Outflow Obstruction. Severe pulmonary stenosis with hypoplasia of the pulmonary annulus results in inadequate pulmonary blood flow as soon after birth as the ductus arteriosus closes. Muscular subpulmonary stenosis can progress during early infancy, resulting in gradually worsening cyanosis.

Moderate Pulmonary Outflow Obstruction. Some children have pulmonary stenosis sufficient to result in ideal distribution of blood flow between the systemic and pulmonary vascular beds. With complete mixing of one part systemic and two parts of pulmonary venous blood, their arterial oxygen saturation will be approximately 80–85%. Ventricular function is likely to be well preserved and the child grows and is relatively well.

Systemic Outflow Obstruction. Obstruction to the systemic outflow is potentially the most serious complication for the child with single ventricle physiology. Obstruction to the systemic outflow results in increased pulmonary blood flow and an increased risk of pulmonary vascular disease. In addition, ventricular hypertrophy develops because of the increased pressure load. Ventricular hypertrophy is an important risk factor for children undergoing a Fontan procedure because hypertrophy decreases ventricular compliance. After the

Exhibit 2

Boston Children's Hospital Experience 1986–1988 Anatomic Diagnosis and Outcome of Fontan Operation			
Diagnosis	*Number*	*Deaths*	*% Mortality*
Tricuspid Atresia	19	2	10.5
Single Left Ventricle	32	3	9.5
Single Right Ventricle	16	3	18.7
Hypoplastic Right Ventricle with Ventricular Septal Defect	13	2	15.3
Pulmonary Atresia with intact Ventricular Septum	6	1	16.7
Other	22	11	50.0
	108	22	20

Fontan procedure, the resultant, higher left atrial pressures will require right atrial pressure to rise to unacceptable levels.

Neonatal Palliative Surgery

Pulmonary Artery Band. The child with a functionally single ventricle and no pulmonary outflow obstruction requires a pulmonary artery band to control pulmonary artery blood flow and pressure. Otherwise, even if the child survives, either pulmonary vascular disease or chronic congestive heart failure will develop. With banding, the anatomic integrity of the central pulmonary arteries must be preserved. This necessitates careful preoperative assessment of the pulmonary arteries by 2-D echocardiography and pulmonary angiography. It is essential that the anatomic details of the entire pulmonary tree be visualized well enough that a long-term plan that leads to an eventual Fontan procedure can be formulated.

Surgical Technique. Although traditionally the application of a pulmonary artery band is through a left anterolateral thoracotomy, this approach has the disadvantage that access to the right side of the main pulmonary artery for placement of sutures to anchor the band is difficult. Distal migration of the band with impingement on the origin of the right pulmonary artery is by far the most frequent complication of banding. Not only does this cause scarring and stenosis at the origin of the right pulmonary artery, with distal hypoplasia of that vessel, but, in addition, excessive flow tends to be directed to the left pulmonary artery, which may result in pulmonary vascular disease in that lung. An alternative approach is to use a median sternotomy. Dissection between the aorta and main pulmonary artery is minimized, which also helps to decrease the tendency for band migration.

Judging the tightness of the band is more of an art than a science. The effects of anesthesia, mechanical ventilation, variable infolding of the redundant pulmonary artery wall, and the natural lability of the neonate's pulmonary vascular resist-

ance mean that strict objective criteria cannot be relied upon. In general a 50% reduction in diameter results in a fall in arterial oxygen saturation to 80–85% and a transient increase in systolic blood pressure of 15–20 mm. Generally, if distal pulmonary artery pressure is measured, it will be decreased to between 25 and 50% of systemic pressure. The band must be anchored to the proximal main pulmonary artery by a number of sutures to prevent distal migration.

Systemic-to-Pulmonary Shunts. The child with severe pulmonary outflow obstruction that results in a systemic oxygen saturation of less than 70–75% requires augmentation of pulmonary blood flow. Although the decision regarding need for a shunt is easy for the child with pulmonary atresia, children with muscular subpulmonary stenosis may have adequate pulmonary blood in the neonatal period, but over the early months of infancy may become sufficiently cyanotic to require placement of a shunt.

The type of shunt selected will influence the subsequent suitability of the child for a Fontan procedure. Waterston's and Potts' shunts require direct anastomosis of the aorta to the right or left pulmonary artery, respectively. These shunts almost always enlarge with time, resulting in a high risk of pulmonary vascular disease and ventricular dysfunction, as well as distortion of the pulmonary artery. Frequently, differences in growth of the ascending aorta and right pulmonary artery result in excessive flow from a Waterston shunt into the right pulmonary artery and inadequate flow into the left pulmonary artery. Thus, a common result of the Waterston shunt is pulmonary vascular disease in the right lung, severe distortion of the central pulmonary artery, and a hypoplastic left pulmonary artery. Both the Waterston and Potts anastomoses are difficult to take down at the time of repair. For these reasons, probably there is no place for these shunts today.

Surgical Technique. Generally, the classical Blalock shunt performed on the side opposite the aortic arch (i.e., usually on the right) results in satisfactory palliation. However, distal branching of the innominate artery or early multiple branches of the right subclavian artery can result in inadequate length and, therefore, excessive tension at the anastomosis. This can cause narrowing at the anastomosis. Furthermore, because there is tissue-to-tissue continuity, there is a small possibility of the shunt becoming aneurysmal, with a dilated distal anastomosis and excessive shunting.

The modified Blalock shunt involves placement of a synthetic tube between the side of the subclavian artery and the side of the right or left pulmonary artery. This has the advantage of not requiring sacrifice of the subclavian artery as with the classical Blalock shunt. Anastomoses can be performed without tension and have no possibility of enlarging with time. Placement of a 4-mm tube in a neonate with accurate anastomoses results in satisfactory palliation for 12–18 months in more than 90% of infants. Although there was initial enthusiasm for placement of this shunt on the same side as the aortic arch (i.e., usually on the left), the side for the shunt should be dictated by the side of the superior vena cava (which determines the side of the systemic venous-to-pulmonary artery anastomosis of the later Fontan procedure) and, therefore, usually, it should be the right side.[31] Takedown of the left modified Blalock shunt is considerably more difficult than the right, with a high risk of injury to the left phrenic nerve. Most important, if there is any stenosis of the pulmonary artery adjacent to the shunt anastomosis, this can be easily dealt with on the right, usually by inclusion of the stenotic area in the Fontan anastomosis, or by excision. In contrast, stenosis of a distal left pulmonary artery can be extremely difficult to relieve.

Bypass of a Systemic Outflow Obstruction Using the Proximal Pulmonary Artery. To bypass severe obstruction to the systemic outflow from the single ventricle, a new outflow from the ventricle to the aorta must be fashioned or the pulmonary artery must be converted to a neo-aorta. Although the former technique was applied enthusiastically in the 1970s, following introduction of synthetic valved conduits, multiple late problems of such conduits have led to the current popularity of conversion of the proximal pulmonary artery to a neo-aorta. The proximal main pulmonary artery is divided and the end is anastomosed to the side of the ascending aorta. A modified Blalock shunt provides pulmonary blood flow. The use of a pulmonary-to-aortic anastomosis to circumvent systemic outflow obstruction in patients with single ventricle has become increasingly widely used.[8,25,40]

One of the major difficulties with systemic outflow obstruction is its progressive nature. This may be due to natural narrowing of a ventricular septal defect (bulboventricular foramen) (Figs. 3 and 4A) or to hypertrophy of muscle within a subaortic

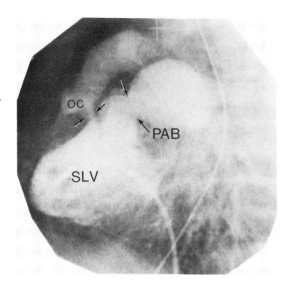

Figure 3. Lateral view of a ventricular angiogram in a patient with double-inlet single left ventricle (SLV) and subaortic outflow chamber (OC) after pulmonary artery banding (PAB). Arrows indicate "subaortic stenosis" has developed due to restrictive bulboventricular foramina. (From Jonas RA, Castaneda AR, Lang P: Single ventricle (single or double inlet) complicated by subaortic stenosis: surgical options in infancy. Ann Thorac Surg 39:361–366, 1985, with permission.)

conus. Placement of a pulmonary artery band may accelerate this process.[13] Thus, for example, when a neonate with tricuspid atresia and transposition presents with a potentially restrictive ventricular septal defect between the single left ventricle and the subaortic infundibular outflow chamber, a decision must be made whether to place a pulmonary artery band (a relatively low risk procedure) or to perform a pulmonary-aortic anastomosis (a moderately high-risk procedure). Probable predictors of subsequent development of a restrictive ventricular septal defect (functional subaortic stenosis) are the presence of coarctation and/or hypoplasia of the aortic arch. Certainly, if the ventricular septal defect is less than the diameter of the aortic annulus in the neonatal period, it is likely that "subaortic stenosis" will develop.

Technique of Pulmonary-to-Aortic Anastomosis. Unlike placement of a pulmonary artery band or a systemic-to-pulmonary shunt, pulmonary-to-aortic anastomosis must be performed with the aid of cardiopulmonary bypass and, frequently, deep hypothermic circulatory arrest. When the child has been cooled to a rectal temperature of 18°C and a tympanic temperature of 15–18°C, bypass is stopped and the cannulas are removed. The proximal main pulmonary artery is divided. The distal main pulmonary artery is closed with a patch of autologous pericardium or pulmonary homograft tissue. A longitudinal arteriotomy is made in the

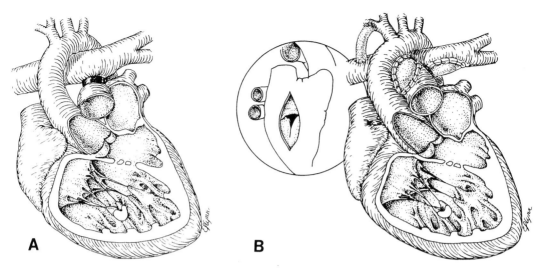

Figure 4. **A,** Drawing of the anatomy of a patient with mitral atresia and normally related great vessels after pulmonary artery banding. Subaortic stenosis has developed because of restrictive multiple muscular ventricular septal defects. **B,** Surgical management of the same patient included division of the main pulmonary artery with pulmonary-aortic anastomosis to bypass subaortic stenosis. Because this child was an infant with high pulmonary vascular resistance, pulmonary blood flow was supplied by a modified right Blalock shunt. An atrial septectomy (inset) must also be performed because of atresia of the left atrioventricular valve. (From Jonas RA, Castaneda AR, Lang P: Single ventricle (single or double inlet) complicated by subaortic stenosis: surgical options in infancy. Ann Thorac Surg 39:361–366, 1985, with permission.)

ascending aorta and the transverse aortic arch. Frequently, it is necessary to extend the aortotomy into the proximal descending aorta beyond the juxtaductal area of potential coarctation formation. The anastomosis of the proximal pulmonary artery to the aorta is fashioned, using a running suture. It is important to supplement the anastomosis with a patch of autologous pericardium or pulmonary homograft tissue. Failure to do so will result in excessive tension and distortion of the anastomosis, resulting in a high risk of bleeding and anastomotic stenosis.

In the neonate or infant, pulmonary blood flow must be supplied at high pressure because of the naturally high pulmonary vascular resistance. This can take the form of either a modified 4-mm right Blalock shunt or a central shunt using a 4-mm Gore-Tex tube from the posterior wall of the neo-aorta to the pulmonary bifurcation area (Fig. 4B).

In the older child, with lower pulmonary vascular resistance, it may be possible to proceed directly to a Fontan procedure. However, this should be done with a great deal of caution, as even a mild degree of ventricular hypertrophy and decreased compliance increases the risk of a Fontan procedure. A safer intermediate step in this setting can be the performance of a bidirectional superior vena cava–pulmonary anastomosis (bidirectional Glenn shunt).[9]

The neonate with aortic atresia and a diminutive ascending aorta represents the most challenging reconstructive problem requiring a pulmonary-aortic anastomosis. When the ascending aorta is less than 2 mm in diameter, it can be particularly difficult to achieve unobstructed retrograde coronary blood flow from the proximal pulmonary artery down the ascending aorta. Under these circumstances, it may be safer to place a complete tube of pulmonary homograft from the proximal pulmonary artery to the undersurface of the arch and the proximal descending aorta, with the distal anastomosis straddling the area of coarctation. Because coarctation is present in at least 80% of children with the hypoplastic left heart syndrome, it should be routine to incorporate this area in the reconstruction.

Another essential component of the neonatal palliative procedure where there is atresia or stenosis of the left atrioventricular valve, as with hypoplastic left heart syndrome, is a wide atrial septectomy. This ensures that pulmonary venous blood can pass unobstructed through the resulting atrial septal defect and through the right atrioventricular valve to the single ventricle.

Perioperative Management of the Child Requiring Pulmonary-Aortic Anastomosis. Because the pulmonary and systemic vascular beds are supplied in parallel from the single ventricle, blood flow is distributed according to the relative resistances of these two vascular beds. This can present a challenge in the perioperative management where both resistances may be very labile. There is a tendency for pulmonary blood flow to be excessive. Therefore, it is important, temporarily, to maintain high levels of pulmonary vascular resistance by exposing the child to a low level of inspired oxygen (generally room air), avoiding hyperventilation, and attempting to maintain pCO_2 close to

40 mm Hg. A low dose of dopamine (5 μg/kg/min) is useful to improve total cardiac output and improve renal blood flow.

Management During the Interval Between Operations. Any neonate who has a palliative surgical procedure, whether a pulmonary artery band, systemic-to-pulmonary shunt, or pulmonary-aortic anastomosis with a shunt and atrial septectomy, requires meticulous follow-up to ensure that growth and development proceed appropriately for the child to become an optimal candidate for the planned Fontan procedure. The most serious, and unfortunately the most common, problem with all these procedures has been the development of **pulmonary artery distortion.** In general, the right and left central pulmonary arteries should be carefully reassessed by angiography and 2-D echocardiography by 6 months of age. If there is evidence of distortion, serious consideration should be given to balloon dilatation or the performance of a patch arterioplasty, possibly combined with placement of a bidirectional superior cava-to-pulmonary anastomosis. For example, failure to deal with stenosis of the central pulmonary artery in the presence of a right Blalock shunt can result in underdevelopment of the left pulmonary arterial tree, excessive flow into the right lung, and the risk of promoting pulmonary vascular disease.

Other problems that have been observed during this interval include the **development of a restrictive atrial septal defect.** This risk can be minimized by extensive septectomy at the time of the initial procedure. The risk of **systemic outflow obstruction in the neo-aorta** can be decreased by avoiding the use of synthetic material in the reconstruction and taking care to straddle the coarctation with the distal anastomosis.

Preservation of ventricular function is vital also during this period. It is rare to achieve a perfect ratio between systemic and pulmonary blood flow. The combination of a moderate volume load and at least a moderate degree of oxygen desaturation (approximately 80%) may result in ultimate deterioration of ventricular function. This argues for earlier rather than later Fontan repair. In general, as soon as one can be confident that pulmonary vascular resistance is sufficiently low and stable, usually by 12–18 months of age, a Fontan procedure should be recommended.

Results. In the current era, both pulmonary artery bands and systemic-to-pulmonary shunts can be placed with an early mortality of less than 5%. Between 1985 and 1988, there were 3 deaths among 24 children having pulmonary-aortic anastomosis at The Children's Hospital in Boston for subaortic stenosis with single ventricle (12.5%). First-stage palliative surgery for hypoplastic left heart syndrome continues to carry a high mortality (approximately 33%).[21] Actuarial survival for these infants declines to between 40 and 50% in the interval before the Fontan procedure.

CONDUITS

One of the goals of any cardiac reconstructive procedure should be to achieve continuity of the child's own tissues in such a fashion that growth is guaranteed. At present, this is not possible in a number of anatomic situations, most commonly long-segment discontinuity of the main pulmonary artery (long-segment pulmonary atresia). This may be associated with a number of intracardiac malformations including tetralogy of Fallot, double-outlet right ventricle, and transposition of the great arteries. In such children reconstruction requires placement of a conduit from the appropriate ventricle (usually the right) to the central pulmonary arteries.

In 1966, Ross and Barratt-Boyes[1,35] independently introduced the use of valved homograft (allograft) conduits. The ascending aorta and aortic valve are harvested from a cadavar or multiple organ donor. Following dissection, the homograft is immersed in antibiotics with tissue culture medium for 48 hours. Subsequently it is either stored at 4°C for 4–6 weeks maximum, or frozen in a controlled-rate liquid nitrogen freezer in the presence of a cryoprotectant, such as dimethyl sulfoxide, to prevent the formation of intracellular ice crystals.

Homografts collected, treated, and stored in these ways have made it possible to achieve excellent results over many years in just a few centers where the original methods were consistently applied. In many centers, however, logistic difficulties with storage and collection and concerns about the sterility of homografts treated with antibiotics alone have led to alternative methods. In the United States, in the late 1960s, irradiation and freeze drying became popular methods of sterilization and storage, respectively. Unfortunately, it was a number of years before it became clear that both these techniques resulted in damage to both the cellular elements and the collagen within the homograft and, particularly, to the delicate valve leaflets. This damage led to accelerated calcification of the valve leaflets with resultant stenosis of the homograft.

In the early 1970s when the poor performance of irradiated and freeze-dried homografts was realized, a new conduit became available and was enthusiastically applied through the remainder of the 1970s. This was the woven dacron conduit containing a glutaraldehyde-treated xenograft (pig aortic valve).[23] Although these conduits had the advantage of ready availability in a wide range of sizes, they suffered from a number of important disadvantages:

1. The woven dacron was stiff and difficult to suture, particularly to delicate pulmonary arteries.

2. The rigid valve ring could result in compression of important structures, particularly the left coronary artery in tetralogy of Fallot.

3. Finally, it became clear that the long-term performance of these conduits was far from satisfactory.[30,36,38]

Children rapidly calcify xenograft tissue which has been treated with glutaraldehyde; this results in the same accelerated valvar stenosis that had been observed with irradiated homografts. In addition, woven dacron has a very low porosity, necessary to prevent blood loss at the time the conduit is inserted when the patient is on cardiopulmonary bypass and fully anticoagulated. The tight weave does not allow fibrous anchoring of the pseudointima, which forms on the internal surface. Repeated dissection deep to the pseudointima can result in an accelerated rate of pseudointima accumulation. Other important factors in pseudointima accumulation probably include the shear stress imposed by the noncompliant nature of the dacron and the chronic inflammatory reaction provoked by dacron. Probably, endothelially-derived growth factor[7] also contributes to fibroblastic proliferation and hypertrophy of the smooth muscle.

The combination of valvar stenosis and pseudointima accumulation resulted in early failure of many synthetic-valved conduits. This led to a re-examination of the results achieved with the early methods of homograft treatment and storage. Since approximately 1985, homografts have reemerged as the conduit of choice in the United States for cardiac reconstructive procedures. Previous logistic difficulties have been lessened by public awareness of the benefits of transplantion and the organization of regional organ banks devoted to the collection and distribution of organs and tissues for transplantation.

Avoidance of Conduits

During the 1970s when the poor long-term performance of conduits had not been appreciated, a number of operations were devised that incorporated a conduit. The original description of the Fontan operation included a connection between the right atrium and the left pulmonary artery, using a conduit. Early descriptions of the technique of arterial switching for transposition included a conduit to achieve continuity from the right ventricle to the pulmonary artery. Today, such operations are rarely undertaken despite the improved availability and better performance of the homograft conduit. Homografts probably do not grow under most circumstances and, with the general trend toward corrective surgery in the first year or two of life, it is inevitable that replacement surgery will be required. Also, it is possible in cases

of moderately long-segment pulmonary atresia, where there is some main pulmonary artery present, to achieve direct right ventricular-to-pulmonary artery anastomosis. This is accomplished by wide mobilization of the pulmonary arteries. Similarly, wide mobilization of the pulmonary arteries combined with the "Lecompte maneuver,"[28] (bringing the bifurcation of the pulmonary artery anterior to the ascending aorta) makes the use of a conduit unnecessary in the arterial switch operation.

VALVE REPLACEMENT IN CHILDREN

The palliative nature of valve replacement in adults, and particularly in children, has become widely appreciated over the last decade. Carpentier[3] has popularized numerous important valvuloplasty techniques which, although primarily designed for rheumatic and degenerative valve disease, can also be applied to congenital malformations. Thus the incidence of mitral valve replacement following atrioventricular canal repair, or of aortic valve replacement for aortic regurgitation associated with ventricular septal defect has decreased dramatically.

Unfortunately, a number of congenital valvar malformations cannot be dealt with by valvuloplasty techniques, necessitating valve replacement. Usually, congenitally incompetent valves can be replaced more easily than stenotic valves because of the annular dilatation often associated with incompetence. If an aortic valve replacement is required in the setting of a hypoplastic left ventricular outflow tract, an annular enlarging procedure such as the Konno operation[27] will be needed in addition to the aortic valve replacement. There are no practical annular enlarging procedures for the mitral valve. However, placement of a prosthesis in the left atrium in the supraannular mitral position can achieve acceptable palliation.[22]

There have been important advances in prosthetic valve design over the last 10–15 years. Today, valves have better hemodynamic characteristics as well as a lower "profile" (e.g., St. Jude Medical valve).[39] This is of particular importance in the small child, in whom a higher-profile valve (e.g., Starr-Edwards ball valve) can cause significant obstruction (e.g., of left ventricular outflow tract following mitral valve replacement for atrioventricular canal).[37] Bioprosthetic valves present a particular problem in children because of their accelerated calcium metabolism. The glutaraldehyde-treated porcine valve mounted on a plastic or metal stent performs well in the adult population, with the advantages of a low risk of thromboembolism and a decreased need for anticoagulants (with their attendant complications) relative to mechanical valves.[17] However, shortly after their introduction it was clear that bioprosthetic valves rapidly calcify and thereby become stenotic in children less than 18–25 years of age.[15,38]

Homografts treated with antibiotics represent a suitable option for some children requiring aortic valve replacement and can be combined with annular enlarging procedures. However, as with any bioprosthesis, homografts have limited durability and, with the possible exception of pulmonary autografts,[16,34] ultimately require replacement because of tissue failure. Undoubtedly the future of surgery on valves in children lies in further refinements of valvuloplasty techniques, with the avoidance of prostheses where at all possible.

APPLICATION OF THE FONTAN PRINCIPLE

Operations based on the concept that the systemic venous return can be made to flow through the lungs without the assistance of a ventricular pump have become known as Fontan procedures in recognition of Dr. Francis Fontan's first successful surgical application of this concept in a patient with tricuspid atresia.[12] Since Fontan's report in 1971, operations based on this principle have been carried out for an increasing variety of congenital cardiac defects in addition to tricuspid atresia, all of which have the common feature that there is only one functional ventricle. A partial list includes: the hypoplastic left heart syndrome, tricuspid atresia with transposition of the great arteries, mitral atresia with normal aortic root, and most patients with single ventricle. Conceptually, the Fontan operation involves separation of the systemic venous return from the pulmonary venous return and the rerouting of the systemic venous blood directly into the pulmonary arteries, bypassing the ventricular cavity. The technical details have been modified in several ways from the original operation described by Fontan, and the criteria by which patients are selected for this type of operation have evolved as well.

Anatomic Factors

Although the Fontan operation was initially performed for tricuspid atresia, patients with a variety of defects (including single ventricle, hypoplastic left heart syndrome, mitral atresia with ventricular septal defect, hypoplastic right ventricle associated with pulmonary valvar atresia and intact ventricular septum, hypoplastic right ventricle associated with transposition or double-outlet right ventricle and straddling tricuspid valve, and double-outlet right ventricle with noncommitted ventricular septal defects) have been physiologically "corrected" by a Fontan type of approach. The results do not appear to be dependent on the anatomic diagnosis when other physiologic and anatomic features are considered,[29] and nearly the same results have been achieved for other defects as for tricuspid atresia (Exhibit 2). In the Boston Children's Hospital series, an anatomic factor that did appear significant was the presence of a left-sided mitral valve as the systemic atrioventricular valve (as is found in tricuspid atresia or pulmonary atresia with an intact ventricular septum, for example). This anatomy was associated with a reduced risk for the Fontan operation, although the reasons for this remain speculative.[29] Another potentially important anatomic variation involves an anomalous connective of either the systemic or pulmonary venous return; however, frequently these anomalies can be managed successfully and they do not appear to be an independent risk factor for the Fontan operation in properly selected patients.[29,43] On the other hand, an anatomic feature of greater importance has been the presence of unreparable distortion of the pulmonary arterial tree by prior palliative operations, such as shunts or pulmonary artery bands; in these cases survival has been relatively poor.[29]

Physiologic Factors

In addition to these anatomic considerations, several physiologic variables measured at preoperative catheterization appear to be important in the subsequent outcome of a Fontan operation. Because the entire cardiac output must pass through the lungs, propelled only by the systemic venous pressure, the resistance of blood flow through the lungs and into the systemic ventricle should (obviously) be as low as possible. Among the initial physiologic criteria suggested by Fontan and Choussat was a preoperative mean pulmonary artery pressure of less than 15 mm Hg.[6] However, pulmonary arteriolar resistance (mean PA pressure minus mean LA pressure/pulmonary blood flow) appears to be a more predictive variable for the outcome of a Fontan operation than the mean pulmonary artery pressure alone.[29] No absolute limit for these physiologic variables can be defined, but when pulmonary arteriolar resistance is greater than 2 Woods units (indexed), there is an increased mortality risk.[29] A patient with pulmonary arteriolar resistance less than 2 units, even though the mean pulmonary artery pressure is greater than 15 mm Hg does not appear to have an increased risk for a Fontan procedure.[29] Downstream from the pulmonary vascular bed, the systemic atrioventricular valve and systemic ventricle are also potential sources of resistance to pulmonary blood flow in the Fontan circulation. The atrioventricular valve should function normally, but, in selected cases, this valve can be either repaired or replaced at the time of the Fontan operation.[43] Ventricular compliance, although more difficult to measure quantitatively, appears to be of great importance in the outcome of Fontan operations, and others[26] have found that hypertrophied (and presumably non-compliant) ventricles are associated with an increased risk for this type of operation.

Many of these risk factors for Fontan operations are influenced greatly by prior surgical interventions. Pulmonary artery distortion frequently results from prior palliative operations such as systemic-to-pulmonary shunts or pulmonary artery bands, and severe ventricular hypertrophy has been associated with pulmonary artery banding in certain forms of single ventricle. Chronic volume overload of a single ventricle, such as may result after systemic-to-pulmonary artery shunts, can lead to depressed systolic ventricular function and atrioventricular valve regurgitation. Finally, pulmonary vascular resistance can become elevated as a result of either inadequate prior limitation of pulmonary blood flow (inadequate pulmonary artery band) or excessive pulmonary blood flow through a systemic-to-pulmonary artery shunt. These findings have led to the conclusion that initial palliative operations should be minimized for patents who are candidates for a Fontan operation.

This requires that Fontan operations can be undertaken with low risk in patients younger than 4 years, the age previously suggested by Fontan and Choussat. Young age alone is not associated with an increased risk for a Fontan operation;[43] successful Fontan procedures have been carried out in infants less than 1 year old. Also, it can be documented that second palliative operations[29] in patients more than 1 year of age may result in a number of them becoming unsuitable candidates for a Fontan operation.[32] If the anatomic or physiologic status of the patient is unsuitable, preliminary operations to attempt to restore the anatomy and physiology to more "ideal" status are needed. Distorted pulmonary arteries may be reconstructed utilizing homograft patches, and excessive pulmonary blood flow through shunts can be reduced by narrowing or replacing the shunt. Regurgitant atrioventricular valves have been replaced or repaired prior to Fontan operations, and restrictive outflow from a single ventricle has been bypassed with a proximal pulmonary artery-to-aortic anastomosis and restoration of the pulmonary blood flow with a systemic-to-pulmonary artery shunt. A newer approach that the authors and others[24] have employed for patients who are not ideal candidates for the Fontan operation is the direct connection of the superior vena cava to the pulmonary arteries by either a classic or bidirectional Glenn procedure. This preliminary Glenn type of operation has the advantages of providing improved arterial saturation, reducing the volume load on the systemic ventricle and, therefore, potentially reducing the amount of atrioventricular valvar regurgitation and ventricular end-diastolic pressure. It is unclear whether or not this approach

will ultimately allow these patients to become Fontan candidates, but it appears to provide relatively good palliation in any event, with arterial saturations ranging between 80 and 85%.

Technical Modifications

As noted previously, the operative technique to achieve a connection between the systemic venous return and the pulmonary artery has been modified in a number of important ways since the original description by Fontan. Conceptually, the most important departure from the original Fontan approach was the recognition that the atrium probably plays no more than a minor role in augmenting pulmonary blood flow after a Fontan type of operation. This conclusion was reached after finding that the use of direct cavo-pulmonary anastomoses to deal with anomalies of systemic venous drainage did not adversely affect the outcome of the modified Fontan procedure.[42] The authors have extended this principle to the intracardiac portion of the repair by creating an intra-atrial "tunnel" from the inferior vena cava to the superior caval orifice in order to separate the systemic and pulmonary venous returns (Fig. 5).[19] Then, the connection of the systemic venous return to the pulmonary arteries can be made outside the heart by direct cavo-pulmonary anastomosis. One major advantage of this approach is that by making the "baffle" relatively small in the creation of this "tunnel," the chances of "baffle" distortion and resulting pulmonary venous obstruction are virtually eliminated. The problem of baffle distortion and pulmonary venous obstruction is most serious when the right atrioventricular valve is the major valve in the pulmonary venous return to the ventricle (as in mitral atresia, hypoplastic left heart syndrome, etc.).

A second potential advantage of this approach is that an atrial incision near the sinus node artery is avoided, and the incidence of atrial arrhythmias following the Fontan procedure may be reduced. In addition, the cavo-pulmonary connection may be utilized to deal with distortion of the central pulmonary arteries caused by prior palliative procedures by incorporating stenotic areas into the cavo-pulmonary connection. Also, extracardiac prosthetic conduits are totally avoided. Finally, the intra-atrial tubular pathway between the inferior and superior vena cava may reduce the turbulence in the systemic venous blood. It is possible that a reduction in turbulence would mean that more total fluid energy would be retained in the venous return, which would the propel the blood through the pulmonary circulation more effectively. However, this latter advantage remains only theoretical at present.

A second conceptual departure from Fontan's original procedure has been the recognition that a

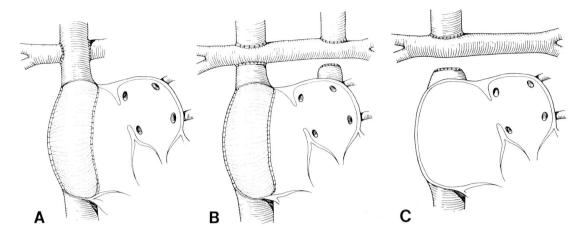

A   **B**   **C**

Figure 5. **A** and **B** are two modifications of the Fontan procedure: **A,** when there is one vena cava; **B,** when there are bilateral venae cavae. In each case the right atrial baffle may be fenestrated to limit the level of pressure inside the baffle while providing some additional cardiac output (albeit blood of low oxygen saturation). **C,** A bidirectional Glenn procedure is used for patients with borderline physiology for a Fontan operation. Note that inferior vena caval blood enters the systemic circulation and the patient remains cyanotic, though arterial oxygen is improved. (Bridges N, Lock JE, Castaneda AR: Baffle fenestration with subsequent transcatheter closure: modification of the Fontan operation for patients at increased risk. Circulation 82:1681–1689, 1990. Bridges N, Jonas R, Mayer JE, et al: Bidirectional cavopulmonary anastomosis as interim palliation for high-risk Fontan candidates. Circulation 82(Suppl): IV-171–176, 1990, by permission of the American Heart Association, Inc.)

valve in the venous-to-pulmonary pathway provides no physiologic advantage in the usual Fontan circulation. In addition to the lack of a physiologic advantage, virtually all the bioprosthetic valves which were used in these connections have become stenotic with time and have required additional surgery to replace them. Therefore, the use of valves in the systemic venous-to-pulmonary artery pathway is now avoided in almost all cases.

Results

Results of modified Fontan procedures have continued to improve, based on the previously described modifications in both patient selection criteria and altered operative techniques. Between 1986 and 1988, 86 of 108 patients undergoing modified Fontan procedures survived surgery and were discharged. Only 19 of these patients had tricuspid atresia (Exhibit 2).

A frequent postoperative problem which occurs in nearly a third of patients undergoing Fontan operations is persistent pleural and/or pericardial effusion. Frequently, these effusions require chest-tube drainage or repeated aspiration, and they can lead to prolonged hospitalization. The etiology of these effusions is not completely understood, but it is related to the extent to which right atrial pressures are elevated after Fontan procedures.[20] Other factors that are statistically related to increased risk of persistent pleural effusion are young age and non-tricuspid atresia defects.[2] The reasons why young age may be associated with an increased risk are speculative, but interestingly, data from experimental animals suggest that the capillary permeability–surface area product is increased in young animals compared with older animals and, therefore, more transudation of fluid out of the vascular space may occur for a given intravascular pressure. The reasons for the relationship between anatomic diagnosis and occurrence of effusion formation are unknown.

A second postoperative problem following Fontan procedures is atrial tachyarrhythmias or sinus node dysfunction. Two possible mechanisms for these arrhythmias are atrial distention and injury to the artery of the sinus node. The exact incidence is unknown, but these concerns were part of the motivation to alter the operative techniques as previously described. No data exist as to whether the incidence of arrhythmias has been reduced by the use of these techniques.

Data are beginning to accumulate on the long-range follow-up of these patients. Many older patients are gainfully employed and at least one woman is safely a mother. Several have undergone major noncardiac surgical operations, including two spinal fusions for scoliosis. Concerns that high altitude might be poorly tolerated have not materialized, though one boy collapsed on Mount Washington (6000 ft) after ascending on foot with his father. Each patient is allowed to set his or her own limits. Several have become involved in sports, although evidence of persistent involvement in aggressive physical sports is lacking. Some patients, who were relatively well before the procedure, with arterial oxygen saturation in the 80s, have remarked that they did not notice a great difference after this surgery. In the soul searching following such discussions, the authors have been satisfied that the patient no longer faces the risks of cyanosis and the functioning ventricle is required to do less work. This conclusion has led to the conviction that all asymptomatic patients with suitable anatomy and physiology should undergo a Fontan type of operation as early as is compatible with a likely good outcome.

CARDIAC TRANSPLANTATION

In contrast to the Fontan approach, the implantation of a structurally normal heart offers the opportunity to restore relatively normal cardiovascular physiology. Unfortunately, transplantation remains a palliative operation because of the current status of immunosuppressive therapy. Despite the widespread use of cyclosporine A, rejection of the transplanted organ has not been eliminated and the patients remain more susceptible to infection than non-immunosuppressed patients. Concerns remain over the long-term renal toxicity of cyclosporine and the effects of chronic steroids on growth in children. The experience in the pediatric age group has been small,[33,41] and there has been the impression that rejection has been more difficult to control than in adults.[14] The question of whether long-term survival (for a lifetime) for pediatric patients is possible remains unknown.

Despite these uncertainties, cardiac transplantation has been undertaken for pediatric patients in a few centers, including The Children's Hospital in Boston. In the initial reports the majority of patients were in their teens[41] and generally had idiopathic cardiomyopathy as their end-stage heart failure. In our own patient population, ventricular dysfunction complicating underlying structural heart disease has accounted for more than half of the patients and transplantation has been carried out as early as the first year of life.

The current survival rates for pediatric patients undergoing cardiac transplantation appear to be equivalent to those for adults, with 84% alive 1 year after operation. In our own small experience 16 of 19 patients remain alive, with follow-up ranging from 6 months to 5 years. There was no 30-day mortality; 2 died in the first 6 months after surgery; 1 died of chronic rejection 2½ years after transplantation.

Rejection has been frequent early after surgery, requiring treatment with corticosteroids and antithymocyte globulin or monoclonal antibodies. However, in several patients it has been possible to markedly reduce corticosteroid doses after the first year. Also, in the younger children there has been a frequent requirement for much higher total daily doses of cyclosporine and for a more frequent dosing schedule in order to achieve therapeutic cyclosporine levels.

Early results have been encouraging but long-term outcome clearly remains unknown. We remain cautiously optimistic about the long-term outlook for this "palliative" approach to selected children with end-stage heart disease.

REFERENCES

1. Barratt-Boyes BG, Roche AHG, Whitlock RML: Six year review of the results of free-hand aortic valve replacements using antibiotic sterilized homograft valve. Circulation 55:353–361, 1977.
2. Britton LW, Mayer JE, Galinanes M, et al: Effusive complications of Fontan procedures (abstract). Circulation 74(Suppl II):II-49, 1986.
3. Carpentier A, Chauvaud S, Fabiani JN, et al: Reconstructive surgery of mitral valve incompetence: ten-year appraisal. J Thorac Cardiovasc Surg 79:338–748, 1980.
4. Castaneda AR, Mayer JE, Jonas RA, et al: Neonates with critical congenital heart disease: repair—a surgical challenge. J Thorac Cardiovasc Surg 98:869–875, 1989.
5. Castaneda AR, Norwood WJ, Jonas RA, et al: Transposition of the great arteries and intact ventricular septum: anatomical repair in the neonate. Ann Thorac Surg 38:438–443, 1984.
6. Choussat A, Fontan F, Besse P, et al: Selection criteria for Fontan's procedure. In Anderson RH, Shinebourne EA (eds): Pediatric Cardiology. Edinburgh, Churchill Livingstone, 1978, pp. 559–566.
7. Clowes AW, Keileman TR, Clowes MM: Mechanisms of arterial graft failure. II. Chronic endothelial and smooth muscle cell proliferation in healing polytetrafluoroethylene prosthesis. J Vasc Surg 3:877–884, 1988.
8. Damus PS: A proposed operation for transposition of the great vessels. Ann Thorac Surg 20:724–725, 1975.
9. DiDonato R, DiCarlo DC, Giannico S, et al: Palliation of complex cardiac anomalies with subaortic obstruction: new operation approach. J Am Coll Cardiol 13:406–412, 1989.
10. Flanagan MF, Fujii AM, Colan SD, et al: Inhibitory effects on myocardial perfusion in pressure overload hypertrophy in immature lambs (abstract). Pediatr Res 23:218A, 1988.
11. Fontan F, Baudet E: Surgical repair of tricuspid atresia. Thorax 26:240–248, 1971.
12. Fontan F, Mournicot FB, Baudet E, et al: Correction de l'atresia tricuspidienne. Rapport de deux cas corriges par l'utilization d'un technique chirugical novelle. Ann Chir Thorac Cardiovasc 10:39–47, 1971.
13. Freedom RM, Benson LN, Smallhorn JF: Subaortic stenosis, the univentricular heart, and banding of the pulmonary artery: an analysis of the courses of 43 patients with univentricular heart palliated by pulmonary artery banding. Circulation 73:758–764, 1986.
14. Fricker F, Trento AB, Griffith B, et al: Cardiac allograft rejection is more frequent in children than in adults (abstract). Am J Cardiol 60:642, 1987.
15. Geha AS, Laks H, Stansel HC, et al: Late failure of porcine valve heterografts in children. J Thorac Cardiovasc Surg 78:351–364, 1979.
16. Gula G, Wain WH, Ross DN: Ten years' experience with pulmonary autograft replacements for aortic valve disease. Ann Thorac Surg 28:392–396, 1979.
17. Heng MK, Barratt-Boyes BG, Agnew TM, et al: Isolated mitral valve replacement with stent mounted antibiotic-treated aortic allograft valves. J Thorac Cardiovasc Surg 74:230–237, 1977.
18. Jatene AD, Fontes VF, Souza ICB, et al: Anatomic

correction of transposition of the great vessels. J Thorac Cardiovasc Surg 83:20–26, 1982.

19. Jonas RA, Castaneda AR: Modified Fontan procedure: atrial baffle and systemic venous to pulmonary artery anastomotic techniques. J Cardiac Surg 3:91–96, 1988.

20. Jonas RA, Freed MD, Mayer JE, et al: Long term followup of patients with synthetic right heart conduits. Circulation 72(Suppl II): 77–83, 1985.

21. Jonas RA, Lang P, Hansen D, et al: First stage palliation of hypoplastic left heart syndrome: the importance of coarctation and shunt size. J Thorac Cardiovasc Surg 92:6–13, 1986.

22. Kadoba K, Jonas RA, Mayer JE, et al: Mitral valve replacement in the first year of life. J Thorac Cardiovasc Surg 100:762–768, 1990.

23. Kaiser GA, Hancock WD, Lukban SB, et al: Clinical use of a new design stented xenograft heart valve prosthesis. Surg Forum 20:137–138, 1969.

24. Kawashima Y, Kitamura S, Mitsuda H, et al: Total cavopulmonary shunt operation in complex cardiac anomalies. J Thorac Cardiovasc Surg 87:74–81, 1984.

25. Kaye MP: Anatomic correction of transposition of the great arteries. Mayo Clin Proc 50:638–649, 1975.

26. Kirklin JK, Blackstone EH, Kirklin JW et al: The Fontan operation: ventricular hypertrophy, age and date of operation as risk factors. J Thorac Cardiovasc Surg 92:1049–1064, 1986.

27. Konno S, Imai Y, Iida Y, et al: A new method for prosthetic valve replacement in congenital aortic stenosis associated with hypoplasia of the aortic valve ring. J Thorac Cardiovasc Surg 70:909–917, 1975.

28. Lecompte Y, Neveux JY, Leca F, et al: Reconstruction of the pulmonary outflow tract without a prosthetic conduit. J Thorac Cardiovasc Surg 84:727–733, 1982.

29. Mayer JE, Helgason H, Jonas RA, et al: Extending the limits for modified Fontan procedures. J Thorac Cardiovasc Surg 92:1021–1028, 1986.

30. McGoon DC, Danielson GK, Puga FJ, et al: Results after extracardiac conduit repair for congenital cardiac defects. J Thorac Cardiovasc Surg 83:569–576, 1982.

31. Mietus-Snyder M, Lang P, Mayer JE, et al: Childhood systemic-pulmonary shunts: subsequent suitability for Fontan operation. Circulation 76(Suppl III):III-39–44, 1987.

32. Newburger JW, Silbert AR, Buckley LP, et al: Cognitive function and age at repair of transposition of the great arteries in children. N Engl J Med 310:1495–1499, 1984.

33. Parness IA, Nadas AS: Cardiac transplantation in children. Pediatr Rev 10:111–118, 1988.

34. Ross DN: Replacement of aortic and mitral valve with a pulmonary valve autograft. Lancet 2:956–958, 1967.

35. Ross DN, Somerville J: Correction of pulmonary atresia with a homograft aortic valve. Lancet 2:1446–1447, 1967.

36. Sanders SP, Levy RJ, Freed MD, et al: Use of Hancock porcine xenografts in children and adolescents. Am J Cardiol 46:429–438, 1980.

37. Schaff HV, Danielson GK, DiDonato RM, et al: Late results after Starr-Edwards valve replacement in children. J Thorac Cardiovasc Surg 88:583–589, 1984.

38. Schaff HV, DiDonato RM, Danielson GK, et al: Reoperation for obstructed pulmonary ventricle-pulmonary artery conduits. J Thorac Cardiovasc Surg 88:334–343, 1984.

39. Spevak PJ, Freed MD, Castaneda AR, et al: Valve replacement in children less than 5 years of age. J Am Coll Cardiol 8:901–908, 1986.

40. Stansel HC: A new operation for d-loop transposition of the great vessels. Ann Thorac Surg 19:565–567, 1975.

41. Starnes VA, Stenson EB, Oyer PE, et al: Cardiac transplantation in children and adolescents. Circulation 76(Suppl V):43–47, 1987.

42. Vargas FJ, Mayer JE, Jonas RA, et al: Anomalous systemic and pulmonary venous connection in conjunction with atrio-pulmonary anastomosis (Fontan-Kreutzer) technical considerations. J Thorac Cardiovasc Surg 93:523–532, 1987.

43. Vargas FJ, Mayer JE, Jonas RA, et al: Atrioventricular valve repair or replacement in atrio-pulmonary anastomosis: surgical considerations. Ann Thorac Surg 43:403–405, 1987.

44. Wernovsky G, Hougen TJ, Walsh EP, et al: Mid-term results following the arterial switch operation for transposition of the great arteries with intact ventricular septum: clinical, hemodynamics, echocardiographic, and electrophysiologic data. Circulation 77:1333–1344, 1988.

45. Yacoub MH, Radley-Smith R, MacLaurin R: Two stage operation for anatomic correction of transposition of the great arteries with intact interventricular septum. Lancet 1:1275–1278, 1977.

Section XI

THE FUTURE

Chapter 55

A CELLULAR AND MOLECULAR
APPROACH TO PEDIATRIC CARDIOLOGY

Bernardo Nadal-Ginard, M.D., Ph.D., and Vijak Mahdavi, Ph.D.

As is the case for other organ systems, the development, structure, and physiology of the cardiovascular system depend on the proper development and function of its constituent cellular elements. Derangement of these cellular functions during development or in the adult is the basis of all congenital and acquired cardiopathies. However, each and every relevant developmental and physiologic process at the cellular and organ level is the product of complex biochemical reactions. These biochemical reactions are carried out by proteins, which in turn are the product of specific genes. At some point in the near future, it should be possible to describe cardiovascular physiology as well as congenital and acquired pathologic cardiovascular processes at cellular, molecular, and genetic levels. Unfortunately, however, for congenital malformations this is still an elusive goal. Because of the lack of a basic mechanistic understanding, the pathogenesis of most congenital malformations, as well as most diagnostic and therapeutic approaches, is based on empirical observation rather than on the precise cellular and molecular dysfunction underlying the disease.

Although the physiologic properties of the myocardium and their dynamic character have been the focus of intense research during the past three decades, the biochemical and molecular correlates underlying cardiac development and performance remain poorly understood. The central role of the myocardium in the maintenance of the cardiac output notwithstanding, until very recently, the prevailing view of the heart was that of a biochemically very static organ. Therefore, it did not seem particularly interesting or suitable to address major questions of cellular and molecular biology affecting normal and pathologic states. As a consequence, the effect of the newly developed techniques of recombinant DNA and genetic manipulation in transgenic animals on the understanding of cardiac cellular and molecular biology has been slower and to a certain extent less significant than in other fields in the biomedical sciences. The power of these new techniques and approaches is just beginning to be felt in the field of cardiovascular biology and is lagging farther behind in its application to cardiac development and the pathogenesis of cardiac malformations. This state of affairs is surprising, given the biomedical importance of the cardiovascular system in general and the myocardium in particular, as well as the large number of investigators dedicated to its study. This situation is due, at least in part, to the characteristics of the myocardium that, until recently, have made this organ less than ideal for a molecular and genetic approach.

The development of modern cellular and molecular biology has provided the necessary tools for dissecting the cardiovascular system and its associated diseases at the cellular and molecular level. These techniques hold great promise for identifying the mechanisms involved in cardiac development and their disturbances, as well as for studying important clinical and experimental problems in cardiovascular physiology. At the same time, these techniques already provide, or will provide in the future, means to devise rational diagnostic and therapeutic approaches that are based on detailed cellular and molecular understanding of the long-term physiological alteration produced by congenital malformations, such as pulmonary vascular obstructive disease or irreversible cardiac failure.

The main reason for the slow development of a molecular and genetic approach to cardiac development and pathogenesis of cardiac malformations is because of the essential role of the myocardium in the survival of the organism. Although this statement seems paradoxical, the fact remains that for the genetic dissection of a developmental pathway and its alterations, it is essential to have access to mutations affecting the organ under study. Most genetic mutations that significantly affect the development and/or function of the cardiovascular system are lethal early in fetal life and, therefore, are not available for study. This feature explains the very small number of mutations described so far affecting the myocardium in human or animal models. This is in contrast to the large number of mutations affecting blood cells, the endocrine system, and metabolic pathways, among others. The existence of these mutations has provided the port of entry for the molecular dissection of these systems. In addition to the unavailability of mutations, the difficulty of obtaining repeated samples of the myocardium from the same animal that are suitable for biochemical and molecular analysis has also slowed progress. Furthermore, the existence of well-characterized cell lines that can be grown in homogeneous populations and mutated at will is almost essential for the exploitation of recombinant DNA technology to elucidate regulatory pathways. Given that the cardiac myocyte is a terminally differentiated cell that has lost its ability to replicate in vivo or in vitro shortly after birth,[77] no cell lines with well-defined characteristics of cardiac myocytes have been available until now. This combination of characteristics, broadly outlined above, has played an important role in delaying the dissection of the cellular and molecular basis of cardiac development and its performance in physiologic and pathologic states. Yet, it is clear that the modern techniques of cellular and molecular biology hold great promise to elucidate some of the major problems in clinical and experimental cardiovascular medicine. In addition, it is becoming increasingly clear that the cardiovascular system in general and the myocardium in particular are excellent model systems for addressing not only particular cardiovascular problems but also some broad biologic questions that have general significance and are of import to a large number of organs and systems.

One of the major determinants of long-term outcome for most congenital and acquired cardiac diseases in children as well as adults is the contractile state of the myocardium. During the past several years significant progress has been made in un-

derstanding the developmental and physiologic changes of the myocardium that affect cardiac performance. This chapter reviews some of these recent advances. Particular emphasis is on the contractile apparatus in order to highlight the extraordinary plasticity of myocardial tissue at the biochemical level and its ability to respond to different pathologic and physiologic stimuli.

THE CARDIAC CONTRACTILE APPARATUS

The unit of contraction in the myocardium, as well as in the skeletal muscle, is the sarcomere (Fig. 1).[69] The contractile properties of the myocardium, both in terms of force generated and velocity of contraction, depend on the number and biochemical composition of its sarcomeres. The sarcomere is composed of seven major proteins and several minor ones organized into thin and thick filaments. The thin filaments, anchored at the Z lines, are formed by a double helix of polymerized sarcomeric actin molecules. In the major groove of this double helix is located a continuous head-to-tail coiled-coil of tropomyosin (TM) dimers. Every tropomyosin dimer interacts with seven actins and is associated with a troponin (Tn) complex. Each

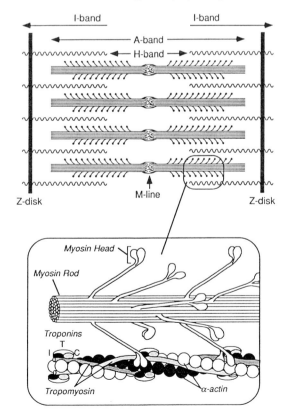

Figure 1. Structural organization of a sarcomere. Each sarcomere (top panel) is constituted by sets of parallel thick and thin filaments (bottom panel) that partially overlap and are interconnected.

complex is composed of one molecule of each of the three troponins—T, C, and I. This tropomyosin-troponin complex is responsible for the calcium sensitivity of the contractile apparatus. It regulates the interaction between the heads of the myosin molecule, located in the thick filament, and actin, the main constituent of the thin filament. Although most is known about this interaction, the precise molecular mechanisms responsible for the biochemical-mechanical transduction have not yet been fully elucidated. The thick filament contains the molecular motor of contraction, the myosin heavy chain (MHC). This is a bifunctional molecule that exists in a dimeric form. The two functional domains are constituted by the rod portion and the head. The rod is constituted by the carboxyl-terminal half of the molecule and is a regular coiled-coil α-helix responsible for the assembly of myosin into an organized anti-parallel thick filament with heads regularly spaced every 14.3 A at both ends with a bare zone in the middle. The rod carries the load during contraction and, because of its anti-parallel organization, makes possible the shortening of the sarcomere by pulling together two thin filaments pointing in opposite orientation and attached to two neighboring Z lines. During the contraction cycle, the head of MHC, which is constituted by the amino-terminal half of the molecule, interacts directly with the actin molecules in the thin filament and carries the ATPase activity required to produce the physical translocation needed for fiber shortening. The ATPase activity of MHC is modulated by two smaller protein subunits bound to each MHC head—the alkali and essential myosin light chains (MLC). As originally pointed out by Barany,[2] there is a direct correlation between the unloaded maximum velocity of shortening of a muscle fiber and the actin-activated ATPase activity of its MHC. Although there are some apparent exceptions to this rule, fibers with an MHC with high ATPase activity shorten faster than ones with lower enzymatic activity.[59,62] Interestingly, there is an inverse correlation between ATPase activity of the MHC in a fiber and the energy cost to perform a given workload.[1,59] The faster the fiber, the higher the energy cost to produce the same amount of work. It is clear, therefore, that the type of MHC present in the sarcomeres is physiologically significant and has a profound effect on the contractile properties of the myocardium.

In addition to the seven major protein mentioned above, the sarcomere contains a number of proteins, such as α-actinin, C protein, titin, and nebulin,[15,52] that are present in lower amounts and are thought to play an important role in its organization or in modulation of function. However, with the exception of α-actinin, which is the main constituent of the Z line and serves to anchor the actin filament,[52] the precise physiologic function of these

minor components of the sarcomere remains to be determined.

Although the intrinsic properties of the sarcomere are the main determinants of the contractile state, a number of other molecules, such as adrenergic receptors,[68] ion channels,[8] Na, K ATPase, sarcolemmal and sarcoplasmic calcium pump, and sarcoplasmic calcium release channel,[4,24,45] are also involved in its modulation. Most of these molecules exert their effect on contractility by directly or indirectly modulating either the availability or the response to calcium of the contractile proteins.

Cardiac Contractile Proteins

Each of the cardiac contractile proteins is a member of a family of isoforms that is specific to the cell type and stage of development. The regulated expression of structurally distinct, developmentally regulated, and cell-type–specific protein isoforms is a fundamental characteristic of higher organisms. The molecular mechanisms responsible for the generation of this protein diversity can be broadly categorized into two main systems: those that select a particular gene among the members of a multigene family for expression in a particular cell and those that generate several different isoforms from a single gene. This latter mechanism includes DNA rearrangement and alternative pre-mRNA splicing. Both mechanisms involve the differential use of intragenic sequences that lead to the production of multiple protein isoforms from a single gene. DNA rearrangement appears to be restricted to a very limited set of genes coding for immunoglobulins and T-cell receptors.[27,66] In contrast, increasing number of genes in organisms ranging from insects to human, including their DNA and RNA viruses, are known to be alternatively spliced.

Alternative pre-mRNA splicing is particularly prevalent in striated muscle tissues, including the myocardium. Among the contractile protein genes, this mode of gene regulation has been documented for α- and β-tropomyosin, troponin T, and the myosin light chains, in addition to a number of other genes (reviewed in refs. 6, 67). Furthermore, the major constituents of the thick filaments (MHC and MLCs) and thin filaments (actin, TMs, and troponins [C, T, and I]) of mammalian sarcomeres are each encoded by a multigene family of moderate size, ranging from four to eight members.[15,35,69] The expression of each member of these multigene families is regulated at the transcriptional level in a tissue-specific and developmentally regulated manner. The different isoforms of sarcomeric contractile proteins, generated either through the transcription of different genes or from the same gene by alternative pre-mRNA splicing, are able to substitute for each other and to assemble combinatorially when present in the same cell. The restricted combined use of the different members of these multigene families allows for the generation of a moderate number of qualitatively different sarcomere types that, at least in some cases, exhibit significantly different physiologic characteristics.[15,35,53,68] This potential for the production of different sarcomeres is highly increased by the generation of multiple protein isoforms by individual MLC, TM, and TnT genes. Therefore, in order to understand the mechanisms involved in generating myocardial protein diversity, it is necessary to elucidate both the elements responsible for the selective transcription of a given gene in a particular cell type at a particular time in development or physiologic state as well as the factors that regulate alternative pre-mRNA splicing in the same cell.

During the past 6 or 7 years, most of the genes coding for contractile proteins have been identified, cDNA and genomic sequences have been obtained, mapped to the human genome, and characterized for their potential to generate multiple protein isoform by alternative splicing. Although some of these genes are closely clustered on the same chromosome, as is the case for the cardiac and skeletal MHCs,[40,57] most other contractile protein gene families are not linked but rather are scattered on several chromosomes.[11,26] Therefore, although the contractile proteins are assembled in the sarcomere in very precise stoichiometric amounts, their regulation is by necessity complex, because it involves multiple genes that are located in different regions of the genome that, with very few exceptions, do not seem to have common regulatory sequences.

Some of the contractile protein isoforms expressed in the myocardium are shared with the skeletal muscle, whereas others are expressed exclusively in the myocardium (Table 1).[15,35,69] Moreover, for several of these proteins, the atrial and ventricular isoforms are different from each other and both differ from the ones expressed in the conduction system. Although the physiologic basis for the selective advantage that has produced this isoform distribution is not apparent from our present understanding of contractility, two main general trends are obvious. In general, the myocardial genes are more likely to be shared with slow than with fast skeletal muscle. Embryonic and fetal isoforms are shared more often with striated muscle than with their adult counterparts.

Because the MHC isoform switches in the myocardium are physiologically the most relevant and are better understood at the molecular level, they will be used to illustrate some of the regulatory mechanisms involved. The processes regulating the expression of these genes appear to be broadly used and, in general terms, are likely to apply to isoform switches in the myocardium.

The cardiac proteins undergo isoform switches in response to physiologic and pathologic stimuli.

In the cardiac ventricles of most mammalian species, including humans, three myosin isoforms have been identified based on their electrophoretic mobility—V1, V2, V3.[26,54] However, these three myosins are composed of only two distinct types of MHCs, referred to as α and β. V1 and V3 are composed of αα and ββ homodimers, respectively, whereas V2 is an αβ heterodimer (Fig. 2). These two myosins are produced by two different genes that are closely linked[40,46] and are located on chromosomes 14 and 3 in mouse and human, respectively.[46]

As for all muscle types, the myosin composition of the myocardium is of physiologic importance, since the relative distribution of α- and β-MHC is directly correlated with the contractile properties of the heart. The α-MHC, which has high Ca2 + and actin-activated ATPase activity,[54,62] is associated with an increased shortening velocity of the cardiac fibers.[44,62] In contrast, the β-MHC, which has lower ATPase activity,[54,62] is associated with slower shortening velocity (Fig. 2).[44,62] It is interesting, therefore, that the ratio of these two different cardiac isoforms is developmentally regulated. In the ventricles of all mammalian species studied so far, β-MHC is the most abundant isoform in utero until late fetal life.[45] In small mammals, such as rat and mouse, α-MHC increases immediately prior to birth and becomes the predominant form throughout perinatal and adult life.[42,43] In contrast, in large mammals, such as man, α-MHC is only transiently predominant shortly after birth, with β-MHC becoming the most abundant isoform in the adult.[42,43] The situation is different in the atria, in which α-MHC is the predominant isoform throughout life in both small and large species.[10,42,69] In addition, in all species studied, including man, the distribution of the cardiac MHC isoforms changes in response to certain pathologic and experimental conditions such as work overload,[44,50,60] diabetes,[14] gonadectomy,[48] and, more importantly, changes in thyroid hormone levels (Figs. 3 and 4).[18,26,31,42,62] These changes are regulated at the level of transcription of the respective genes, since there is a direct correlation between the levels of α- and β-MHC and the corresponding mRNAs[31,42] and between these and the rate of transcription.[73]

THYROID HORMONE

It is clear now that thyroid hormone plays a fundamental role in the regulation of the MHC phenotype both in the myocardium and in skeletal muscle.[31] In mammals at least, all the genes of the striated MHC multigene family are, without exception, responsive to thyroid hormone. Surprisingly, however, whether the hormone induces or represses the expression of a given MHC depends

Table 1. Expression of Contractile Protein Genes in Striated Skeletal and Cardiac Muscles of Small Mammals[15,35,69]

| Gene | Skeletal Muscles | | | Cardiac Ventricle | | | Cardiac Atrium |
	Embryonic/ Neonatal	Adult Fast	Adult Slow	Embryonic	Adult	Pressure Overload Adult	Adult
Myosin heavy chain (MHC)	Embryonic MHC Neonatal MHC	Fast II A MHC Fast II B MHC	Slow 1-βMHC	Slow/βMHC	αMHC +βMHC	Slow/βMHC + αMHC	α MHC
Myosin light chain (LC)	LC1e LC1f	LC1f LC3f	LC1 slow/cardiac	LC1e	LC1 slow/cardiac	LC1 slow/cardiac + LCe	LC1e LC1 slow/cardiac
Myosin light chain 2	LC2sk	LC2sk	LC2sk	LC2 cardiac	LC2 cardiac	LC2 cardiac	LC2 cardiac
Tropomyosin	ββ	α/β α/α	α/β	β/α	α/α	α/β	α/α
Troponins T	Fast TnT Slow TnT	Fast TNT	Slow TNT	(emb)cardiac TNT	(adult)cardiac TNT		Cardiac TNT
C	cTNC(slow/ cardiac)	skTNC(skeletal)	cTNC	cTNC	cTNC	cTNC	cTNC
I	Fast TNI	Fast TNI	slow/cardiac TNI	slow/cardiac TNI	slow/cardiac TNI		slow/cardiac
Actin	c α-actin sk α-actin	sk α-actin	sk α-actin	sk α-actin c α-actin	c α-actin	c α-actin sk α-actin	c α-actin
Creatine kinase	BB ck BM ck	MM ck	MM ck	BB ck MM ck	MM ck	MM ck BB ck	

MHC = myosin heavy chain; each member of this gene family is indicated by a prefix indicating the most common nomenclature used to duplicate the gene. MLC = myosin light chain gene products: LC1e = light chain 1 embryonic, LC1 slow/cardiac = light chain specific for slow and cardiac tissues. LC1f and LC3f are the two products for the myosin light chain 1/3 that is predominantly expressed in fast muscle. LC2sk and LC2 cardiac denote the light chain 2 characteristic of skeletal (sk) and cardiac muscle, respectively. Tropomyosin α and β designate these products of these two genes. α-TM is characteristic of differentiated striated muscle while β is characteristic of the undifferentiated cells. TNC, TNT, TNI indicate troponin C, T, and I, respectively. The prefix cardiac, skeletal, slow, embryonic, etc. indicate the tissue and or developmental stage where this gene product is predominantly expressed. cα-actin and skα-actin indicate the isoform characteristic of adult normal cardiac and skeletal muscle, respectively. Creatine kinase B and M isoform indicate the muscle-specific (M) and non-muscle (B) isoforms.

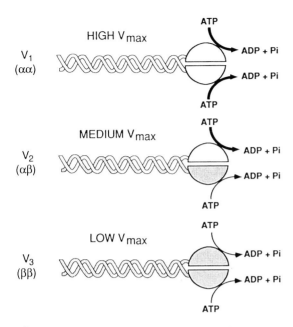

Figure 2. The relative distribution of α and β myosin heavy chains is correlated to the shortening velocity of the cardiac myofibers.

on the gene itself and the muscle in which it is expressed. The same gene can be induced by the hormone in one muscle and repressed in another,[31] indicating that the regulation of this gene family by thyroid hormone is likely to be more complex than described so far for a variety of steroid hormones.[73] In the heart, there is a precise correlation between the levels of circulating thyroid hormone and the relative levels of α- and β-MHC in the ventricles.[42] The expression of α-MHC is dependent on the presence of thyroid hormone; in its absence, the α-MHC gene is not transcribed. The converse is true for β-MHC. The expression of this gene is repressed by thyroid hormone and it is induced in hypothyroid states.[31,42] The induction of α-MHC at the time of birth directly correlates with the surge in the circulating thyroid hormone that occurs at this time.[42] This effect of thyroid hormone on cardiac MHC expression can be directly demonstrated in experimental animals by manipulating their thyroid state. After surgical or chemical (5-thiouracil) thyroidectomy, the expression of α-MHC is completely suppressed and only β-MHC is expressed in the myocardium. Replacement therapy restores the normal phenotype. On the other hand, hyperthyroid states repress the expression of the β-MHC gene both at the mRNA and protein levels and produces a myocardium constituted exclusively by α-MHC (Fig. 4).[18,42] That these results are not indirect and produced by changes in metabolic state, circulating catecholamines, innervation, etc. due to the general effects of changes in thyroid hormone status is demonstrated by the fact that they can be reproduced in isolated tissue slices and cells in culture.[73]

The thyroid hormone receptors are transcriptional factors that interact directly with the cardiac MHC genes. The molecular mechanism of thyroid hormone action has been elucidated, at least in part, by the demonstration that the c-erb proto-oncogenes are the nuclear receptor for this hormone.[30,58,71,74] At least two genes with well-defined, tissue-specific expression encode this receptor,[58,71,74] and each one can generate several different isoforms by alternative splicing.[71] The functional properties of some of these alternatively spliced isoforms are very different and some have lost their ability to bind T3.[30] It has been recently proposed that the isoforms that are impaired in their ability to bind ligand might function as anti-oncogenes and/or anti-receptor molecules.[12,36] This

CARDIAC MYOSIN HEAVY CHAIN ISOFORMS

	ATPase ACTIVITY	SHORTENING VELOCITY	EFFICIENCY of FORCE PRODUCTION
α-MHC (V1)	HIGH	FAST	LOW
β-MHC (V3)	LOW	SLOW	HIGH

ISOFORM SWITCHES

	THYROID HORMONE	EXERCISE	WORK OVERLOAD	AGING
α-MHC (V1)	↑	↑	↓	↓
β-MHC (V3)	↓	↓	↑	↑

Figure 3. Correlation of the ventricular myosin heavy chain phenotype and contractile performance of the myocardium in response to physiologic, pathologic, and developmental stimuli.

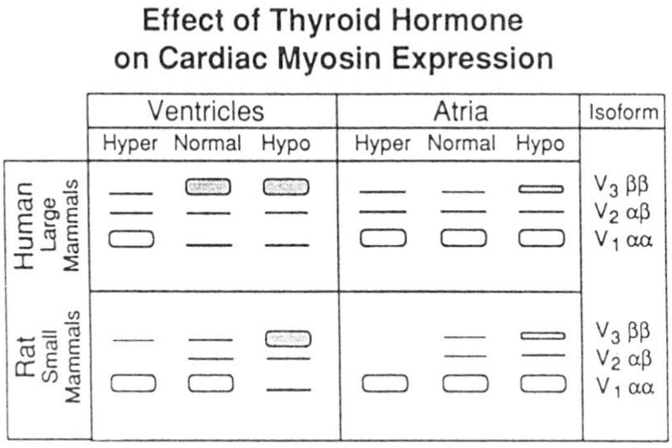

Effect of Thyroid Hormone on Cardiac Myosin Expression

	Ventricles			Atria			Isoform
	Hyper	Normal	Hypo	Hyper	Normal	Hypo	
Human Large Mammals	—	▭	▭	—	—	▭	V_3 ββ
	—	—	—	—	—	—	V_2 αβ
	▭	—	—	▭	▭	▭	V_1 αα
Rat Small Mammals	—	—	▭	—	—	▭	V_3 ββ
	—	—	—	—	—	—	V_2 αβ
	▭	▭	—	▭	▭	▭	V_1 αα

Figure 4. Distribution of myosin heavy chain isoforms in the ventricular and atrial myocardium of large and small mammals in response to change in the level of thyroid hormones. Note the species- and tissue-specific differences in the relative distribution of the MHC isoforms.

is so because of their ability to compete for DNA binding sites, but due to their absence of ligand binding, they are unable to stimulate transcription. Whether this is a general phenomenon remains to be demonstrated.

The functional T3 receptors are hormone-dependent transcriptional factors that exercise their effect through binding to a thyroid hormone responsive element (TRE) in the responsive gene.[20,30,36] The TRE for the human and rat α-MHC genes has been determined by a combination of deletion mapping, site-directed mutagenesis and in vitro and in vivo hormone receptor binding assays.[30,47,72] The two genes have a TRE with identical sequence and both are able to confer thyroid hormone sensitivity to heterologous genes.[30,47,72] Therefore, the sequence containing the TRE is both required and sufficient to confer T3 responsiveness to a gene.

The mechanism of T3 repression of MHC gene expression is less understood. Both human and rat β-MHC genes have sequences with a high degree of homology to the TRE of the α-MHC genes.[47,72] These sequences do not have an effect on the heterologous gene promoters so far tested, and it is not clear whether or not they are specifically recognized by the thyroid hormone receptor. Since these putative TRE sequences in the β-MHC genes are overlapping with the CAAT box sequences,[47] an essential promoter element in these genes, the possibility that T3 exerts its negative regulatory role by sterically hindering the binding of an essential transcription factor is presently being investigated.

The results summarized above demonstrate that thyroid hormone plays an important role in regulating cardiac MHC expression and raise the question of whether this hormone is solely responsible for the regulation of these genes. Several lines of evidence indicate that this is not the case. First, it is clear that the α- and β-MHC genes respond

to thyroid hormone in a tissue-dependent manner. For example, in the ventricle, the α-MHC gene is exquisitely sensitive to T3 and it is not expressed at all in the hypothyroid state. However, in the atria of the same heart, this gene is practically unresponsive to the hormone. The different behavior in the two tissues is not due to the lack of functional thyroid hormone receptors in the atria, since other genes in this structure are readily responsive to the hormone. A similar phenomenon is apparent for the β-MHC gene. As indicated above, in the ventricle the expression of this gene is repressed by thyroid hormone. Yet, in the same animals, its expression continues at almost normal level in the slow muscle fibers of skeletal muscle. Moreover, the TRE of these genes does not explain their tissue specificity because they act as positive regulators of transcription in the presence of receptor and T3, irrespective of the cell type where they are expressed. In fact, the tissue specificity of these genes is conferred by a combination of positive and negative transcriptional regulatory elements.[72] These other regulatory elements are likely to be responsible for the species-specific differences in the expression of these genes. There are some differences in the organization of the 5′ flanking sequences between rat and human. Although the TRE in the α-MHC gene of the two species is identical in sequence, in co-transfection experiments, the human gene is less responsive to the hormone.[72] Taken together, these results indicate that, in addition to thyroid hormone and its receptors, other factors that are specific to different muscles also play an important role. The nature of these factors is not yet known.

WORK OVERLOAD HYPERTROPHY

Work overload hypertrophy induces MHC gene isoform switches in the myocardium. The involvement of different regulatory pathways in the expression of the cardiac MHC genes becomes more evident when the changes produced by work overload hypertrophy are analyzed. In small mammals, and particularly in rats, in response to a moderate increase in mean aortic pressure (~30 mm Hg) produced by aortic coarctation[29] or by other means, there is a rapid induction of β-MHC mRNA followed by the appearance of comparable levels of β-MHC protein, in parallel with an increase in left ventricular weight. A similar change is not detectable in larger mammals, including humans, because β-MHC is the predominant isoform expressed in the normal ventricle. However, in the human atria, which normally expresses α-MHC, a switch to β-MHC is readily apparent in response to increased pressure.[49] Therefore, the hypertrophic myocardium induces the expression of β-MHC and represses the expression of the α-gene. Therefore, with respect to the MHC phenotype, it resembles the fetal and hypothyroid state. Yet, in these animals, the circulating level of thyroid hormone remains normal and their metabolic state argues against hypothyroidism. Other features argue persuasively that this isoform switch produced in response to work overload hypertrophy is not regulated through the thyroid hormone pathway.[29]

Work overload hypertrophy induces the re-expression of many fetal isoforms in the postnatal myocardium. The isoform switches produced in response to increased afterload are not limited to MHC. In fact, a general myocardial response to work overload occurs rapidly and affects a multitude of cellular compartments.[32] This response is characterized by the re-expression of the protein isoforms normally expressed in fetal life but normally suppressed in adulthood (Fig. 5). To the best of our knowledge, this phenomenon has been demonstrated for all the gene phenotypes analyzed so far, including other contractile proteins such as skeletal α-actin,[32,63] myosin light chain 1,[25] and β-tropomyosin;[32] membrane proteins such as Na,K ATPase (the cardiac glycoside receptor);[7] secreted molecules such as atrial natriuretic factor (ANF);[32] and those involved in ATP regeneration such as creatine kinase.[28] With the exception of ANF, all the above examples represent the re-expression of an isoform normally expressed only during fetal and early postnatal life that is later replaced by the corresponding adult isoform. ANF expression in the ventricles is normally suppressed after birth and it is not replaced by another isoform. Its expression, however, is rapidly re-induced in response to the hypertrophic stimulus.

From the above observations it is clear that from a molecular perspective, myocardial hypertrophy is not only a quantitative phenomenon that results in an increase in cardiac mass, but, more importantly, it results in a significant qualitative change in important constituents of the myocardium. In general, these changes produce a muscle that has many of the biochemical characteristics of the fetal myocardium.

What is the stimulus for this dramatic and concerted change in myocardial gene expression in response to work overload? A potential candidate would be thyroid hormone itself. However, as already indicated above, no changes in thyroid hormone levels are detected in these animals. Furthermore, if thyroid hormone were responsible, it should be possible to re-establish the normal phenotype in response to thyroid hormone therapy. Yet, this is not the case. Thyroid hormone can overcome the effect of pressure overload on MHC gene expression, but has no effect on the other phenotypic changes.[29,32] Administration of high doses of T3 in hypertrophic animals produces a rapid re-induction of the β-MHC gene with concomitant induction of the α-gene, despite the fact that these animals have a higher degree of hypertrophy than those with simple hemodynamic overload.[29,32] None of the changes in the expression of other genes is affected by the hormone. These results further support the contention that the changes induced by hemodynamic overload are not secondary to thyroid hormone changes. However, in the case of the MHC genes, T3 has a dominant effect and can overcome the regulatory mechanisms induced by the hypotrophic stimulus. This behavior highlights the complex interplay that exists between hemodynamic and hormonal stimuli in myocardial gene expression.

It is noteworthy that in coarctected animals, the most commonly used model system, increased afterload is not the only consequence of the manipulation. It might produce a rise in circulating catecholamine levels and/or activation of the reinin-angiotensin system secondary to decreased renal blood flow. Norepinephrine[38,65] and possibly angiotensin II could, in principle, directly stimulate myocardial cell hypertrophy independently of the hemodynamic effects. The effect of norepinephrine on cardiac cell growth in culture has been shown to be mediated by stimulation of the α1-adrenergic receptor,[65] which couples the hydrolysis of membrane phosphatidylinositol followed by

GENE SWITCHES IN CARDIAC VENTRICLES

	FETUS & NEONATES	NORMAL ADULT	WORK OVERLOAD	HYPO-THYROID	HYPER-THYROID
MYOSIN HEAVY CHAIN	β, α	α	β α	β	α
α-ACTIN	Skeletal Cardiac	Cardiac	Cardiac Skeletal		
TROPOMYOSIN	α, β	α	α, β	Same as Normal Adult	
Na, K-ATPase	α₁, α₂	α₁	α₁, α₂		
ANF	+	−	+ +		

Figure 5. Effect of different stimuli on the relative distribution of fetal and adult isoforms in the ventricular myocardium. Overload hypertrophy induces re-expression of several fetal protein genes. In contrast, thyroid hormones affect mainly the expression of the myosin heavy chain genes.

the release of IP3[3] and activation of protein kinase C.[51] Furthermore, phorbol esters, direct activators of protein kinase C, can produce hypertrophy and isoform switches when administered to cultured neonatal cardiac cells.[64] However, the fact that the atria and the right ventricle of the coarctected animals do not exhibit the isoform's transitions described above, strongly suggests that these humoral mechanisms do not play an important role, if they are involved at all, in the processes described here.

Hypertrophic Cardiomyopathy

The molecular basis for certain forms of hypertrophic cardiomyopathy is an altered cardiac myosin heavy chain gene expression. A surprising feature of the genes coding for contractile proteins is that until recently not a single mutation for any of them had been identified in vertebrates. This is in contrast to the large number of mutations with impaired function detected in lower organisms such as *C. elegans* and *D. melanogaster*. The lack of phenotypic mutants in vertebrates could be explained by assuming that either most mutations are lethal or that they lack a distinctive phenotype because the mutant isoform is replaced by another from the same multigene family. The latter hypothesis was given credence by the finding of a mouse strain that lacks a functional cardiac α-actin gene. These animals, which have a normal life-span and apparently normal cardiac performance, express the skeletal α-actin gene in the myocardium at all stages of development and physiologic states. This phenotype, together with the changes induced by thyroid hormone and work overload hypertrophy, strongly supports the concept that different isoforms are interchangeable, although they might result in subtle changes in cardiac performance. For this reason it has come as a surprise that the mutation responsible for certain forms of familial hypertrophic cardiomyopathy maps to the cardiac myosin genes. This disease is a dominant disorder characterized by cardiac hypertrophy, a wide spectrum of clinical symptoms, and sudden death. Pathologic findings include increased myocardial mass with myocyte and myofibrillar disarray. Recent results have demonstrated that at least two different mutations can produce the disease. In one case there is a novel α/β cardiac MHC hybrid,[70] whereas in the other a single base pair mutation produces a missense mutation in the β-MHC.[19] From the sequence, it appears that both mutant MHCs should be functional, although the mutation maps to an amino acid residue that is conserved in all MHCs sequenced so far, ranging from unicellular organisms to man. Although the molecular mechanisms responsible for the production of the anatomic changes in familial hypertrophic cardiomyopathy remain to be elucidated, the dominant character of the phenotype suggests that the assembly of the thick filament is affected by the mutation. Because not all cases of this disease map to the MHC locus, it is likely that mutations in other genes encoding contractile proteins can also produce the same clinical syndrome.

Proto-oncogenes in Cell Growth

Work overload and stretch produce the rapid expression of a set of proto-oncogenes involved in normal cell growth. The cardiac response to normal growth requirements, as well as to work overload, is dependent on the developmental state of the organ. During fetal and early postnatal life, the demand for an increased cardiac mass is fulfilled mainly by an increase in the number of myocytes (hyperplasia). However, soon after birth, cardiac myocytes lose their ability to divide.[77] Later in life, demand for increased mass is fulfilled exclusively through an increase in the size of a fixed number of preexisting myocytes. The molecular mechanisms responsible for the loss of replicative ability (terminal differentiation) remain completely unknown. Genes involved in determining the myogenic lineage and terminal differentiation in skeletal muscle, such as MyoD,[39] myogenin,[76] and Myf5,[5] which function as tissue-specific transcriptional factors, are not involved in the determination and differentiation of the cardiac myocytes, because they are not expressed in these cells. It is likely that a family of genes with functional similarities but with significant sequence divergence from the ones identified in skeletal muscle is responsible for the cardiac phenotype.

What is the mechanism involved in inducing cell growth and isoform switches in response to work overload? The observed re-expression of fetal isoforms in cardiac hypertrophy is reminiscent of the mitogenic response of many differentiated cell types, such as hepatocytes, which often involves the suppression of the adult phenotype and re-expression of the fetal pattern, such as the inhibition of albumin and induction of α-protein expression during liver regeneration.[56] In a general biologic context, cardiac hypertrophy could be considered the equivalent of the growth response exhibited by most cell types in response to mitogens. In this particular case, the growth response is carried out by terminally differentiated cells (myocytes) that are unable to undergo cell division and have only the hypertrophic response open to them. If this hypothesis were correct, it would be expected that the initial response to the hypertrophic stimuli would mimic early events of cell division induced by growth factors in a large variety of cell types.

One of the early responses of stationary cells to growth stimuli is the induction of a series of proto-oncogenes, such as c-fos and c-myc, among others, that directly or indirectly turn on the cascade of events that lead to cell division. These molecules owe their name to the fact that they are the cellular counterpart of viral oncogenes and their regulation is usually altered in neoplastic cells. Recently, however, it has been demonstrated that these proto-oncogenes are bona fide transcriptional factors that, in most cases, form part of the normal growth induction machinery of the cell in response to growth stimuli.[34] Furthermore, c-myc is able to induce a family of heat shock or stress proteins that is involved in protecting the viability of cells under adverse conditions by mechanisms that are not fully elucidated but might affect proper protein folding[55] and/or modulation of gene transcription.[61]

Not surprisingly, therefore, c-fos and c-myc mRNAs begin to accumulate within 1 hour after the increase in afterload, reach high levels within 3 hours, and return to the basal levels in less than 24 hours. Similarly, the mRNA for one of the major stress proteins, HSP 70, is also increased within 30 minutes of increasing aortic pressure.[32] Thus, similar to the mitogenic response of a variety of cell types induction of the cellular proto-oncogenes and major stress protein genes reflect early changes occurring in the nuclei of myocardial cells in response to acute pressure overload and appear to play an important role in mediating the hypertrophic response. That this factor plays a causative role in the hypertrophic response is suggested because the overexpression of c-myc in the myocardium of transgenic animals induces cardiac enlargement and cellular hyperplasia.[33] Recently, it has been demonstrated that several growth factors, including transforming growth factor β (TGFβ) and basic fibroblast growth factor (bFGF), applied to cardiocytes in culture induce a pattern of contractile protein and proto-oncogene expression that is very similar to the one produced by work overload in the intact heart.[61] These results demonstrate that the lack of mitogenic response by the cardiac myocytes is not due to a loss of receptors for growth factors. They also give further support to the hypothesis that work overload affects gene expression through mechanisms similar or shared by the growth factor receptors. The inability of the cardiocytes to mount a full mitogenic response in response to work overload or growth factors remains an important challenge that also applies to all other terminally differentiated cells, such as neuron and certain epithelial cells. On one hand, these cells could have irreversibly lost the expression of some of the genes required to traverse the cell cycle. In that case it should be impossible for them to re-enter the cell cycle in response to any stimulus. On the other hand, as part of the terminally differentiated program, an inhibitor of the cell cycle could be induced. In that case, repression or neutralization of the inhibitor should enable the cells to cycle again. Recently, recessive cellular onco-

genes with many of the properties required for this role have been described. One of them, the product of the retinoblastoma (Rb) gene, has been shown to belong to this class. The activity of this gene product is neutralized by certain viral oncogenes—SV40 T antigen[13] and adenovirus E1A.[75] Based on the finding that SV40 T antigen is able to re-induce the ability to cycle to terminally differentiated myotubes,[16] it has been possible to re-induce the cell cycle in terminally differentiated cardiocytes and to create cell lines that express many of the differentiated characteristics (W.R. Thompson et al., unpublished observations). These results suggest the presence of inhibitors in the differentiated cardiocytes. Identification of the molecule(s) involved could provide the tool required to induce cardiac muscle regeneration.

In various models of cardiac hypertrophy, systolic and diastolic wall stress have both been implicated as major determinants of the degree and pattern of hypertrophy during pressure and volume overload.[22] In addition, studies using isolated heart preparations have demonstrated that increased wall tension alone can directly stimulate protein synthesis.[69,77] Although the precise molecular mechanisms by which wall stress is communicated to the myocyte nucleus remains to be elucidated, the recently discovered stretch-sensitive ion channels[23] provide a likely candidate for the sensor mechanism. These channels could provide a very sensitive measure of wall stress. The ionic changes produced by their opening or closing could trigger a second messenger cascade (perhaps involving IP3) that results in the changes in gene expression described above. The recent demonstration that stretch of isolated cardiocytes in culture induces the changes of contractile gene and proto-oncogene expression[37] described for work overload and growth factors is in agreement with this hypothesis.

In physiologic terms, the re-expression of the fetal isogenes might be a beneficial adaptation to hemodynamic overload. As a consequence of the changes induced in the thin and thick filaments during cardiac hypertrophy, sarcomeres with significantly different functional properties are produced. For the myocardium, the fetal isoform of MHC has been shown to be bioenergetically more efficient than that of the adult. Moreover, because ANF has potent natriuretic, diuretic, and vasodilatory effects, the marked induction of this molecule in the ventricle in response to increased blood pressure might be interpreted as an adaptational response to reduce hemodynamic load imposed on the ventricle.

CONCLUSION

The results summarized in this chapter are a limited sample of the insights that cellular and molecular biology can provide to further our understanding of the developmental, physiologic, and pathologic biology of the myocardium. Despite the limited nature of the survey presented, the examples used are sufficient to demonstrate that the myocardium is biochemically very plastic. Despite its peculiar biologic characteristics, it is amenable to cellular and molecular dissection. Moreover, as shown by some of the examples presented, the myocardium can serve as a good experimental model to address some important questions that not only are relevant to the cardiovascular system but are of general biologic significance. In addition, it is clear that cardiac development and hypertrophy are simple quantitative processes leading to an increase in ventricular mass. They are qualitatively different and heterogeneous processes that are highly influenced by the nature of the hypertrophic stimulus and the developmental stage of the myocardium. Induction of cellular proto-oncogenes that play a role in cell growth in the very early stages of work overload hypertrophy mimics the mitogenic response to growth factors by a variety of cells. The quantitative and qualitative changes in the expression of contractile and regulatory genes that occur later most likely represent but a small sample of the changes produced in the myocardium in response to the hypertrophic stimuli. The fact that each fetal gene examined so far is re-expressed in response to pressure overload hypertrophy suggests that re-induction of the fetal program might be a general adaptive process to hemodynamic stress. Further work is needed, however, to elucidate the precise mechanisms by which the hemodynamic and/or mechanic stimuli are converted into biochemical signals that lead to quantitative as well as qualitative changes in gene expression. A better understanding of the genes involved in converting precursor mesenchymal cell into the cardiogenic pathway, the cell-specific transcriptional factors responsible for the expression of the cardiac specific genes, as well as the genes involved in blocking these cells in the terminally differentiate phenotype is also required. Without this information it will be difficult to prevent the development of end-stage cardiac failure in patients with long-standing congenital cardiac malformations or their sequelae. Therefore, it is imperative to obtain this information in order to manipulate the process of cardiac hypertrophy and changes of contractile state to physiologic advantage.

REFERENCES

1. Alpert NR, Mulieri LA: Increased myothermal economy of isometric force generation in compensated cardiac hypertrophy induced by pulmonary artery constriction in the rabbit: a characterization of head liberation in normal and hypertrophied right ventricular papillary muscles. Circ Res 50:491–500, 1982.
2. Barany M: ATPase activity of myosin correlated with speed of muscle shortening. J Gen Physiol 50 (Suppl):197–218, 1967.
3. Berridge MJ, Irvine RF: Inositol trisphosphate, a novel second messenger in cellular signal transduction. Nature 312:315–321, 1984.
4. Brandl CJ, Green NM, Korczak B, MacLennan DH: Two Ca^{2+} ATPase genes: homologies and mechanistic implications of deduced amino acid sequences. Cell 44:597–607, 1986.
5. Braun T, Buschhausen-Denker G, Bober E, et al: A novel human muscle factor related to but distinct from MyoD1 induces myogenic conversion in 10T1/2 fibroblasts. EMBO J 8:701–709, 1989.
6. Breitbart RE, Andreadis A, Nadal-Ginard B: Alternative splicing: a ubiquitous mechanism for the generation of multiple protein isoforms from single genes. Annu Rev Biochem 56:467–495, 1987.
7. Cantley LC: Structure and mechanism of the (Na,K)-ATPase. Curr Top Bioenergetics 11:201–237, 1981.
8. Catteral WA: Molecular properties of voltage-sensitive sodium channels. Annu Rev Biochem 55:953–985, 1986.
9. Chizzonite RA, Everett AW, Clark WA, et al: Isolation and characterization of two molecular variants of myosin heavy chain from rabbit ventricle: change in their content during normal growth and after treatment with thyroid hormone. J Biol Chem 257:2056–2065, 1982.
10. Chizzonite RA, Zak R: Regulation of myosin isoenzyme composition in fetal and neonatal rat ventricle by endogenous thyroid hormones. J Biol Chem 259:12628–12632, 1984.
11. Czosnek H, Nudel U, Shani M, et al: The genes coding for the muscle contractile proteins, myosin heavy chain, myosin light chain 2, and skeletal muscle actin are located on three different mouse chromosomes. EMBO J 1:1299–1305, 1982.
12. Damm K, Thompson CC, Evans RM: Protein encoded by c-erbA functions as a thyroid hormone receptor antagonist. Nature 339:593–597, 1989.
13. DeCaprio JA, Ludlow JW, Figge J, et al: SV40 large tumor antigen forms a specific complex with the product of the retinoblastoma susceptibility gene. Cell 54:275–283, 1988.
14. Dillmann WH: Diabetes mellitus induces changes in cardiac myosin of the rat. Diabetes 29:579–582, 1980.
15. Emerson C, Fischman DA, Nadal-Ginard B, Siddiqui MAQ (eds): Molecular Biology of Muscle Development. UCLA Symposia on Molecular and Cellular Biology. New Series, 29. New York, Alan R. Liss, 1986.
16. Endo T, Nadal-Ginard B: In Kedes LH, Stockdale FE (eds): UCLA Symposia on Molecular and Cellular Biology. New Series, vol. 93. New York, Alan R. Liss, 1989, pp. 95–104.
17. Evans RM: The steroid and thyroid hormone receptor superfamily. Science 240:889–895, 1988.
18. Everett AW, Clark WA, Chizzonite RA, Zak R: Change in synthesis rates of α and β myosin heavy chains in rabbit heart after treatment with thyroid hormone. J Biol Chem 258:2421–2425, 1983.
19. Geisterfer-Lowrance AAT, Kass S, Tanigawa G, et al: A molecular basis of familial hypertrophic cardiomyopathy: a β cardiac myosin heavy chain missense mutation. Cell 62:999–1006.
20. Glass CK, Franco R, Weinberger C, et al: A c-erb-A binding site in rat growth hormone gene mediates transactivation by thyroid hormone. Nature 329:738–741, 1987.

21. Gorza L, Pauletto P, Pessina AC, et al: Isomyosin distribution in normal and pressure-overloaded rat ventricular myocardium: an immunohistochemical study. Circ Res 49:1003–1009, 1981.

22. Grossman W: Cardiac hypertrophy: useful adaptation or pathologic process? Am J Med 69:576–584, 1980.

23. Guharay F, Sachs F: Stretch-activated single ion channel currents in tissue-cultured embryonic chick skeletal muscle. J Physiol (Lond) 352:685–701, 1984.

24. Herrera VL, Emanuel JR, Ruiz-Opazo N, et al: Three differentially expressed Na, K-APTase α subunit isoforms: structural and functional implications. J Cell Biol 105:1855–1865, 1987.

25. Hirzel HO, Tuckschmid CR, Schneider J, et al: Relationship between myosin isoenzyme composition, hemodynamics, and myocardial structure in various forms of human cardiac hypertrophy. Circ Res 57:729–740, 1985.

26. Hoh JF, McGrath PA, Hale PT: Electrophoretic analysis of multiple forms of rat cardiac myosin: effects of hypophysectomy and thyroxine replacement. J Mol Cell Cardiol 10:1053–1076, 1978.

27. Honjo T, Habu S: Origin of immune diversity: genetic variation and selection. Annu Rev Biochem 54:803–830, 1985.

28. Ingwall JS, Kramer MF, Fifer MA, et al: The creatine kinase system in normal and diseased human myocardium. N Engl J Med 313:1050–1054, 1985.

29. Izumo S, Lompre AM, Matsuoka R, et al: Myosin heavy chain messenger RNA and protein isoform transitions during cardiac hypertrophy: interaction between hemodynamic and thyroid hormone-induced signals. J Clin Invest 79:970–977, 1987.

30. Izumo S, Mahdavi V: Thyroid hormone receptor isoforms generated by alternative splicing differentially activate myosin HC gene transcription. Nature 334:539–542, 1988.

31. Izumo S, Mahdavi V, Nadal-Ginard B: All members of the MHC multigene family respond to thyroid hormone in a highly tissue-specific manner. Science 231:597–600, 1986.

32. Izumo S, Mahdavi V, Nadal-Ginard B: Protooncogene induction and reprogramming of cardiac gene expression produced by pressure overload. Proc Natl Acad Sci USA 85:339–343, 1988.

33. Jackson T, Allard MF, Sreenan CM, et al: The c-myc proto-oncogene regulates cardiac development in transgenic mice. J Mol Cell Biol 22:3709–3716, 1990.

34. Johnson PF, McKnight SL: Eukaryotic transcriptional regulatory proteins. Annu Rev Biochem 58:799–839, 1989.

35. Kedes LH, Stockdale FE (eds): UCLA Symposia on Molecular and Cellular Biology of Muscle Development. New York, Alan R. Liss, 1988.

36. Koenig RJ, Lazar MA, Hodin RA, et al: Inhibition of thyroid hormone action by a non-hormone binding c-erbA protein generated by alternative mRNA splicing. Nature 337:659–661, 1989.

37. Komuro I, Kurabayashi M, Takaku F, Yazaki Y: Expression of cellular oncogenes in the myocardium during the developmental stage and pressure-overloaded hypertrophy of the rat hearts. Circ Res 62:1075–1079, 1988.

38. Lacks MM, Morandy F: Norepinephrine-Hre myocardial hypertrophy hormone. Am Heart J 91:674–675, 1976.

39. Lassar AB, Paterson BM, Weintraub H: Transfection of a DNA locus that mediates the conversion of 10T1/2 fibroblasts to myoblasts. Cell 47:649–656, 1986.

40. Leinwand LA, Fournier RE, Nadal-Ginard B: Shows TB Multigene family for sarcomeric myosin heavy chain in mouse and human DNA: localization on a single chromosome. Science 221:766–769, 1983.

41. Litten RZ III, Martin BJ, Low RB, Alpert NR: Altered myosin isozyme patterns from pressure-overloaded and thyrotoxic hypertrophied rabbit hearts. Circ Res 50:856–864, 1982.

42. Lompre AM, Mahdavi V, Nadal-Ginard B: Expression of the cardiac ventricular α and β myosin heavy chain genes is developmentally and hormonally regulated. J Biol Chem 259:6437–6446, 1984.

43. Lompre AM, Mercadier JJ, Wisnewsky C, et al: Species- and age-dependent changes in the amounts of cardiac isoenzymes in mammals. Dev Biol 84:286–291, 1981.

44. Lompre AM, Schwartz K, d'Albis A, et al: Myosin isoenzyme redistribution in chronic heart overload. Nature 282:105–107, 1979.

45. MacLennan DH, Brandl CJ, Korczak B, Green NM: Amino-acid sequence of a Ca^{2+} + Mg^{2+}-dependent ATPase from rabbit muscle sarcoplasmic reticulum, deduced from its complementary DNA sequence. Nature 316:696–700, 1985.

46. Mahdavi V, Chambers AP, Nadal-Ginard B: Cardiac α and β myosin heavy chain genes are organized in tandem. Proc Natl Acad Sci USA 81:2626–2630, 1984.

47. Mahdavi V, Koren G, Michaud S, et al: In Cellular and Molecular Biology of Muscle Development. Kedes LH, Stockdale FE (eds): New York, Alan R. Liss, 1989, pp. 369–379.

48. Malhotra A, Penpargkul S, Fein FS, et al: The effect of streptozotocin-induced diabetes in rats on cardiac contractile proteins. Circ Res 49:1243–1250, 1981.

49. Mercadier JJ, Bouveret P, Gorza L, et al: Myosin isoenzymes in normal and hypertrophied human ventricular myocardium. Circ Res 53:52–62, 1983.

50. Mercadier JJ, Lompre AM, Wisnewsky C, et al: Myosin isoenzyme changes in several models of rat cardiac hypertrophy. Circ Res 49:525–532, 1981.

51. Nishizuka Y: The role of protein kinase C in cell surface signal transduction and tumour promotion. Nature 308:693–698, 1984.

52. Obinata T, Maruyama K, Sugita H, et al: Dynamic aspects of structural proteins in vertebrate skeletal muscle. Muscle Nerve 4:456–488, 1981.

53. Pette D, Vrbova G: Neural control of phenotypic expression in mammalian muscle fibers. Muscle Nerve 8:676–689, 1985.

54. Pope B, Hoh JF, Weeds A: The ATPase activities of rat cardiac myosin isoenzymes. FEBS Lett 118:205–208, 1980.

55. Rothman JE: Signal-peptide recognition: GTP and methionine bristles (news). Nature 340:433–434, 1989.

56. Ruoslahti E, Pihko H, Seppala M: Alpha-fetoprotein: immunochemical purification and chemical properties. Expression in normal state in malignant and non-malignant liver disease. Transplant Rev 20:38–60, 1974.

57. Saez LJ, Gianola KM, McNally EM, et al: Human cardiac myosin heavy chain genes and their linkage in the genome. Nucleic Acids Res 15:5443–5459, 1987.

58. Sap J, Munoz A, Damm K, et al: The c-erb-A protein is a high-affinity receptor for thyroid hormone. Nature 324:635–640, 1986.

59. Scheuer J, Bhan AK: Cardiac contractile proteins. Adenosine triphosphatase activity and physiological function. Circ Res 45:1–12, 1979.

60. Scheuer J, Malhotra A, Hirsch C, et al: Physiologic cardiac hypertrophy corrects contractile protein abnormalities associated with pathologic hypertrophy in rats. J Clin Invest 70:1300–1305, 1982.

61. Schneider MD, Shih HT, Parker TG: Peptide growth factors and activated oncogenes can selectively induce

expression of "fetal" contractile protein genes. J Mol Cell Cardiol 21:(Suppl III) abstract 67, 1989.

62. Schwartz K, Lecarpentier Y, Martin AF, et al: Myosin isoenzymic distribution correlates with speed of myocardial contraction. J Mol Cell Cardiol 13:1071–1075, 1981.

63. Schwartz K, Lompre AM, Bouveret P, et al: Accumulation of skeletal actin mRNA in experimental cardiac hypertrophy. J Mol Cell Cardiol 17:(Suppl 3) abstract 22, 1985.

64. Simpson PC, Karliner JS: Regulation of Cardiac Myocyte Hypertrophy by a tumor-promoting phorbol ester. Clin Res 33:229A (abstract), 1985.

65. Simpson P: Norepinephrine-stimulated hypertrophy of cultured rat myocardial cells is an α1 adrenergic response. J Clin Invest 72:732–738, 1983.

66. Siu G, Kronenberg M, Strauss E, et al: The structure, rearrangement and expression of Dβ gene segments of the murine T-cell antigen receptor. Nature 311:344–350, 1984.

67. Smith CWJ, Patton JG, Nadal-Ginard B: Alternative splicing in the control of gene expression. Annu Rev Genet 23:527–577, 1989.

68. Stiles GL, Lefkowitz RJ: Cardiac adrenergic receptors. Annu Rev Med 35:149–164, 1984.

69. Swynghedauw B: Developmental and functional adaptation of contractile proteins in cardiac and skeletal muscles. Physiol Rev 66:710–771, 1986.

70. Tanigawa G, Jarcho JA, Kass S, et al: A molecular basis for familial hypertrophic cardiomyopathy: an α-β cardiac myosin heavy chain gene. Cell 62:991–998, 1990.

71. Thompson CC, Weinberger C, Lebo R, Evans RM: Identification of a novel thyroid hormone receptor expressed in the mammalian central nervous system. Science 237:1610–1614, 1987.

72. Thompson WR, Koren G, Izumo S, et al: Molecular regulation of myosin heavy chain switches: a model for study of cardiac gene expression. In Clarck EB, Takao A (eds): Developmental Cardiology: Morphogenesis and Function. Mount Kisco, NY, Futura, 1990, pp. 13–25.

73. Umeda PK, Levin JE, Shinha AM, et al: In Emerson C, Fischman D, Nadal-Ginard B, Siddiqui MAW (eds): Molecular Biology of Muscle Development. New York, Alan R. Liss, 1986, pp. 809–823.

74. Weinberger C, Thompson CC, Ong ES, et al: The c-erb-A gene encodes a thyroid hormone receptor. Nature 324:641–646, 1986.

75. Whyte P, Buchkovich KJ, Horowitz JM, et al: Association between an oncogene and an anti-oncogene: the adenovirus E1A proteins bind to the retinoblastoma gene product. Nature 334:124–129, 1988.

76. Wright WE, Sassoon DA, Lin VK: Myogenin, a factor regulating myogenesis, has a domain homologous to MyoD. Cell 56:607–617, 1989.

77. Zak R: Development and proliferative capacity of cardiac muscle cells. Circ Res 35(Suppl III):17–26, 1974.

APPENDIX

Principal Drugs Used in Pediatric Cardiology

ANTICONGESTIVES

Drug	Route	Initial Dose	Maintenance Dose	Indication	Therapeutic Blood Level	Side Effects and Toxicity	Drug Interactions
Digoxin (Lanoxin)	PO	Digitalizing dose Premie 20 µg/kg Neonate 30 µg/kg Child 40 µg/kg In 3 doses over 24 hours Adult 0.75–1.25 mg divided in 2–3 doses first 24 hours	8 µg/kg/day bid 10 µg/kg/day bid 10 µg/kg/day qd 0.125–0.250 mg qd	Congestive failure, supraventricular arrhythmias	0.5–2.0 ng/ml Toxic >2.2 ng/ml	Nausea, vomiting, arrhythmias, prolonged P-R Toxicity greater with low calcium	Quinidine Verapamil Amiodarone
	IV	80% of above					
Furosemide (Lasix)	IV	1.0 mg/kg/dose		Congestive failure, fluid retention		Dermatitis, nausea, vomiting, electrolyte depletion, hyperglycemia, azotemia, anemia, hearing loss Use with care in presence of renal or hepatic disease	
	PO	2.0 mg/kg/day in 3–4 doses	Same as initial, may increase by 1–2 mg/kg/day Max 6 mg/kg/day				
Chlorothiazide (Diuril)	PO	20 mg/kg/day in 2 doses	Same as initial Max 2.0 g/day	Congestive failure, systemic hypertension, alone or in combination with spironolactone		Potassium depletion, low-salt syndrome	

Drug	Route	Dose	Administration	Indication	Therapeutic level	Side effects	Comments
Aminophylline	Slow IV diluted in 5% D/W	1–2 mg/kg	Slow IV diluted in 5% D/W 0.7–1.4 mg/kg/hr	Diuretic, pulmonary edema, bronchospasm	10–20 µg/ml Toxic >20 µg/ml	Headaches, low blood pressure, palpitation	
Spironolactone (Aldactone)	PO	2.0–3.5 mg/kg/day	Same dose qd	Commonly used with furosemide or chlorothiazide		Electrolyte imbalance	
Bumetanide (Bumex)	PO / IV	Adult dose: 0.5–2.0 mg (PO); 0.5–1.0 mg (IV)	Same dose qd	Loop diuretic, rapid onset, short mechanism of action		Volume and electrolyte depletion	
Dopamine (Intropin)	IV	2–20 µg/kg/min in dilute nonalkaline IV solutions	5–10 µg/kg/min	Shock, hypotension			
Amrinone (Inocor)	IV	Loading dose: 1.0 mg/kg/15 min		Congestive heart failure		Do not mix with solutions containing dextrose or furosemide	

ANTIARRHYTHMICS

Class 1A

Drug	Route	Dose	Administration	Indication	Therapeutic level	Side effects	Comments
Quinidine sulfate	PO	15–60 mg/kg/day	q6h	Supravent. and vent. arrhythmias	2–5 µg/ml Toxic >7.0	Widened QRS complexes, ventricular arrhythmias, thrombocytopenia, anemia, nausea, diarrhea, long Q-T	Reduce digoxin dose by ½
Quinidine gluconate (Quinaglute)	PO	Test dose for idiosyncrasy then 15–60 mg/kg/day	Effective dose q8h	Same		See above	See above

Principal Drugs Used in Pediatric Cardiology *(Continued)*

Drug	Route	Initial Dose	Maintenance Dose	Indication	Therapeutic Blood Level	Side Effects and Toxicity	Drug Interactions
Procainamide (Pronestyl)	PO	15–50 mg/kg/day	Divided q4h or q6h with slow release	Supravent. and vent. arrhythmias	4–10 µg/ml	Hypotension, ventricular arrhythmias, wide QRS, long Q-T	
	IV	Loading dose: 5–15 mg/kg/30 min	Then drip 20–60 µg/kg/min		Product (NAPA) 1–10 µg/ml Toxic >15 µg/ml	Fever, lupus syndrome	
Disopyramide (Norpace)	PO	Infants: 20–30 mg/kg/day Children: 10–20 mg/kg/day Teenagers: 5–15 mg/kg/day	q6h q12h with slow-release form	Supravent. and vent. arrhythmias	2–5.0 µg/ml Toxic >8 µg	Negative inotrope, wide QRS, long Q-T, ventricular arrhythmias, dry mouth	
Class IB							
Lidocaine (Xylocaine)	IV	Load: 1 mg/kg/dose May repeat q10 min × 3	Drip 20–50 µg/kg/min	Ventricular arrhythmias	2–5 µg/ml Toxic 8 µg/ml	Nausea, seizures	
Phenytoin (Dilantin)	IV	10 mg/kg over 30–60 min	5 mg/kg/day q12h	Digitalis toxicity	10–20 µg/ml Toxicity is variable	Blood dyscrasias, ataxia, rash	
	PO	10–15 mg/kg/day in 4 doses	5 mg/kg/day q12h	Selected supravent. and vent. arrhythmias			
Mexiletine (Mexitil)	PO	5–15 mg/kg/day in 3 doses	Divided q8–12h	Ventricular arrhythmias	0.5–2.0 µg/ml	Proarrhythmia, rash, nausea	
Tocainide (Tonocard)	PO	20–40 mg/kg/day 1–2 gm/day for adults	Divided q8h	Ventricular arrhythmias	4–10 µg/ml	Similar to mexiletine	

Drug	Route	Dose	Schedule	Indication	Level	Side effects	Interactions
Class IC Flecainide (Tambocor)	PO	2–5 mg/kg/day (adult 50–150 mg bid)	Divided q8–12h	Life-threatening supravent. and vent. arrhythmias	0.2–1.0 µg/ml	Negative inotrope, proarrhythmia, rash	Avoid using with verapamil
Encainide (Enkaid)	PO	1–4 mg/kg/day (adult 25–35 mg tid)	Divided q6–8h	Life-threatening supravent. and vent. arrhythmias		Negative inotrope, proarrhythmia	
Propanfenone	IV	Investigational					
Class II Propranolol (Inderal) (β₁ + β₂ blocker)	IV	Load: .02–.10 mg/kg Repeat q6h as needed	1–4 mg/kg/day q6h	Atrial arrhythmias, selected vent. tachycardias, long Q-T syndrome		Negative inotrope, heart block, sinus bradycardia	Avoid using with verapamil
	PO	0.5–1.0 mg/kg/dose q6h	q24h for slow-release form				
Nadolol (Corgard) B₁ blocker	PO	1 mg/kg/day	Divided into 1 or 2 doses/day	See propranolol		See propranolol	Avoid using with verapamil
Atenolol (Tenormin) B₁ blocker	PO	1 mg/kg/day	Divided into 1 or 2 doses/day	? Less bronchoconstrictor effect		See propranolol	Avoid using with verapamil
Esmolol (Brevibloc) B₁ blocker	IV	Loading dose 0.5 mg/kg/dose over 1 min	Intravenous drip 50–100 µg/kg/min	Rapid onset, short duration		See propranolol	Avoid using with verapamil
Class III Amiodarone (Cordarone)	PO	10 mg/kg/day q12h for 7 days as a loading dose	5 mg/kg/day q day	Life-threatening atrial or ventricular arrhythmias	1–2 µg/ml reverse T3 4 × normal	Proarrhythmia, multiple noncardiac toxicities, hypothyroidism, long duration of action	Digoxin: reduce digoxin dose by ½ Phenytoin: reduce dose

Principal Drugs Used in Pediatric Cardiology (Continued)

Drug	Route	Initial Dose	Maintenance Dose	Indication	Therapeutic Blood Level	Side Effects and Toxicity	Drug Interactions
Sotalol	PO	Investigational				Proarrhythmia, negative inotrope	
Bretylium tosylate (Bretylol)	IV	5 mg/kg slowly over 15 min	Intravenous drip: 20–50 µg/kg/min	Ventricular arrhythmias		Proarrhythmia, hypotension	
Class IV							
Verapamil (Isoptin)	PO	1–10 mg/kg/day	Divided q8h or q24h slow release	Reentry SVT		Unsafe for infants Extreme caution in WPW	Avoid beta blockers Reduce digoxin dose ⅓ to ½
	IV	0.05–0.1 mg/kg rapid injection	Repeat in 15 min ×2	Infants 6–12 months may have hypotension bradycardia		Bradycardia, negative inotrope, constipation	
Miscellaneous							
Adenosine	IV	0.05–0.25 mg/kg rapid injection		Reentry SVT		Transient bradycardia, AV block	
HYPERTENSIVES							
Phenylephrine hydrochloride (Neo-Synephrine)	IV	0.1–0.5 µg/kg/min or 10 mg (1 ml of 1% solution) in 100 ml in constant drip		Hypotensive states, paroxysmal atrial tachycardia		Bradycardia, hypertension, arrhythmias	
Epinephrine	IV	0.5 mg (0.5 ml of 1:1000 solution) in 100 ml in constant drip		Hypotension		Tachycardia, hypertension, arrhythmia	
Calcium chloride	IV or intracardiac	0.1–0.3 mg/kg 10% solution	Repeat q30–60 min PRN	Slow and weak cardiac action		Cardiac arrest	
Calcium gluconate	IV or intracardiac	0.5–1.0 mg/kg 10% solution	Repeat q30 min				

ANTIHYPERTENSIVES

Drug	Route	Dose		Use	Side Effects
Hydralazine (Apresoline)	PO	0.75–3 mg/kg/day in 2–4 doses	Same	Mild hypertension, chronic atrial or sinus tachycardia	Hypotension, headaches, vomiting tachycardia
	IV	0.1–0.5 mg/kg/dose			
Magnesium sulfate	IM	25% solution: 0.1 ml/lb	Repeat q4–6 h	Hypertensive crisis	Paralysis, respiratory failure, bradycardia, hypotension
	IV	3% solution: 0.5–100 mg/lb/1 hr	Repeat PRN		
Methyldopa (Aldomet)	IV	20–40 mg/kg/day in 3–4 doses	Same	Hypertensive crisis, mild to moderate hypertension	Postural hypotension, liver damage, positive Coombs' test, headache
	PO	10 mg/kg/day in 2–4 doses mg/day if needed	Same		
Diazoxide (Hyperstat)	IV	2–5 mg/kg/dose	Titrate. Can repeat q4–12h	Hypertension	Nausea, vomiting, flushing, hypotension
Captopril (Capoten)	PO	0.5–3.0 mg/kg/day divided in 3 doses	Repeat	Hypertension, afterload reduction	Hypotension
Prazosin (Minipres)	PO	25–40 µg/kg/dose	Titrate q12h	Hypertension	Postural hypotension, syncope
Labetalol (Normodyne)	IV	0.25 mg/kg/2 min 1.0 mg/kg max bolus Total dose 4 mg/kg		Smooth blood pressure drop	Postural hypotension, syncope

Principal Drugs Used in Pediatric Cardiology (Continued)

Drug	Route	Initial Dose	Maintenance Dose	Indication	Therapeutic Blood Level	Side Effects and Toxicity	Drug Interactions
Propranolol (Inderal)	IV	0.01–0.1 mg/kg/dose		Arrhythmia, tetralogy spells			
	PO	0.5 mg/kg/day not to exceed 1.5 mg	0.5–4.0 mg/kg/day q6h	Arrhythmia			
Sodium nitroprusside (Nipride)	IV in 5% DW	0.3–6 µg/kg/min		Thiocyanate blood levels measured every 48 hours	Thiocyanate 50–100 mg/L	Nausea, vomiting, muscle twitching, sweating, thiocyanate intoxication, apprehension	Decomposes on exposure to light
Clonidine (Catapres)	PO	Adult dose 0.1–0.2 mg bid	q8–12h	Hypertension			
MISCELLANEOUS							
Morphine sulfate	SC	0.1 mg/kg/dose to max 10 mg/dose	Repeat PRN q4h	Anoxic spells, congestive failure, pulmonary edema, excitement		Central nervous system depression, respiratory failure, vomiting	
Meperidine (Demerol)	PO or IM	1.0 mg/kg/dose	Repeat PRN q4h	Anoxic spells, congestive failure, pulmonary edema, excitement		Central nervous system depression, respiratory failure, vomiting	

Naloxone (Narcan)	IV	0.01 mg/kg/dose q2 min to ×10	Morphine over-dose	Short duration of action
Chloral hydrate	PO	25 mg/kg/dose	Sedation for pro-cedures	Avoid large doses in compromised cardiacs
Potassium chloride	IV	2 mEq/ml	2–4 times daily	To replace potas-sium loss, digi-talis intoxication	Watch, particularly in renal disease, for potassium intoxi-cation
	PO	300 mg/tablet (en-teric coated)		
Heparin sodium (Liquaemen sodium)	IV	50–100 units/kg loading dose	20 units/kg/hr	Keep partial thromboplastin time at 1.5–2.0 times normal	Bleeding
Warfarin sodium (Coumadin sodium, Panwarfin)	PO	2–10 mg/day until prothrombin time prolonged	2–10 mg/day	To keep pro-thrombin time at 1.25–1.5 normal	Bleeding
Protamine	IV	1 mg neutralizes 100 units heparin Max dose 5 mg/min		To reverse heparin	Hypotension
Prostaglandins E1	IV	0.5 µg/kg/min up to 0.4 mg/kg/min		To maintain patency of duc-tus arteriosus	Apnea Seizures

INDEX

Page numbers in **boldface type** indicate complete chapters.

Abdominal pain, with rheumatic fever, 311
Accessory pathway, concealed, orthodromic tachycardia
  due to, 405
Accutane, teratogenic effects on embryo, 39
Acidosis. *See also* Metabolic acidosis
  cardiac catheterization and, 189
Acquired immunodeficiency syndrome (AIDS), 276
Adenosine, 424, 764
Adrenal hypertension, 301
Adriamycin, and cardiomyopathy. *See* Doxorubicin
  cardiomyopathy
Aerobic exercise, cardiovascular changes with, 252
Afterload, 228–231, 234
A-H interval, 119–120
AICD (autonomic implantable cardioverter defibrillator),
  426, 427
Air emboli, cardiac catheterization and, 190
Alveolar hypoxemia, pulmonary hypertension associated
  with, 94–95
Aminophylline, 761
Aminorex, pulmonary hypertension and, 95
Amiodarone, 422–423, 763
Amrinone, 71, 761
Anaerobic exercise, cardiovascular changes with, 252
Anaerobic threshold, as index of cardiovascular fitness,
  251–252
Anatomy, morphologic, **17–26**
  importance of understanding normal, 25–26
  of atria, 17–20
  of ventricles, 20–25
Angiographic views, of congenital heart lesions, 202, 206
Angiography, 187, 197–202
  cineangiographic film and processing, 199
  contrast agents, 200–202
  digital processing, 199
  for anomalous origin of left coronary artery, 717
  for atrioventricular canal defects, 584–585
  for corrected transposition of great arteries, 705–706
  for single ventricle, 655
  for tetralogy of Fallot, 477
  for tetralogy of Fallot with pulmonary atresia, 484
  for vascular ring, 724
  for ventricular septal defect, 444–445
  for visceral heterotaxy, 605–606
  image production, 197–199
  image recording, 199
  radiation exposure and protection, 199–200
Anthracycline antibiotics, and cardiomyopathy. *See*
  Doxorubicin cardiomyopathy
Antiarrhythmic drugs, 419–424, 761–764
  adenosine, 424
  class IA drugs (quinidine, procainamide,
    disopyramide), 420, 761–762
  class IB drugs (lidocaine, mexiletine, tocainide,
    phenytoin), 420, 762
  class IC drugs (flecainide, encainide, propafenone),
    420–421, 763
  class II drugs (propranolol, nadolol, atenolol, esmolol),
    421–422, 763

Antiarrhythmic drugs (*Continued*)
  class III drugs (amiodarone, sotalol, bretylium),
    422–423, 763–764
  class IV drugs, 423, 764
  digoxin, 423–424
  for hypertrophic cardiomyopathy, 343
  verapamil, 423
Antibiotics, for prevention of infective endocarditis,
  371–373
Antidromic reciprocating tachycardia, and Wolff-
  Parkinson-White syndrome, 402–403
Antimicrobial therapy, for infective endocarditis,
  373–374
Antithrombotic therapy, management of Kawasaki
  syndrome with, 322–323
Aorta, coarctation of. *See* Coarctation of the aorta
Aortic arch, development of, 15–16
  double, producing vascular ring, 722, 723
  flow in, echocardiographic examination of, 171
  interruption of, 549–553
  right, producing vascular ring, 722, 723
Aortic atresia, with normal left ventricle, 633
Aortic outflow abnormalities, **493–512**
Aortic pressure, cardiac catheterization and, 193
Aortic regurgitation, 507–510
  ventricular septal defect and, 451–452
  with tetralogy of Fallot, 480
Aortic stenosis. *See also* Subaortic stenosis
  balloon valvotomy for, 207–210
  coarctation of the aorta with, 548–549
  supravalvar, 506–507
  valvar, 493–501
    clinical manifestations of, 495–498
    course of, 500–501
    definition of, 493
    infants with, 501–502
    management of, 498–500
    pathology of, 493–494
    physiology of, 494–495
    prevalence of, 493
  valve replacement for, 501
Aortic valve, bicuspid, 510–511
Aorto-left ventricular tunnel, 711–712
Aortopulmonary collaterals, coil embolization of, 217
Aortopulmonary fenestration, 693
Aortopulmonary septal defect, 693
Aortopulmonary window, **693–695**
Apnea, cardiac catheterization and, 189–190
Arm ergometer, exercise testing with, 253–254
Arrhythmias. *See* Cardiac arrhythmias
Arterial complications, cardiac catheterization and, 189
Arterial pressure, examination of, 104–105
Arterial-pulmonary shunts, for hypoplastic left heart
  syndrome, 630, 631
Arterial pulses, examination of, 103–104
Arterial switching procedure, for transposition of the
  great arteries, 567, 568, 571, 572, 732–733
Arteriovenous fistulas, pulmonary, 709–710
  systemic, 707–709
Arteriovenous malformations, coil embolization of, 218

Arthritis, monoarticular, 313
  rheumatoid, 313
Aschoff bodies, in rheumatic fever, 308
Ashman's phenomenon, 393, 394
Asplenia, 20, 590–607
  anatomic findings in, 602
  clinical manifestations of, 602–606
  diagnosis of, 606
  pathology of, 591–602
  total anomalous pulmonary venous return with, 690
Ataxia, Friedreich's, 348
Atenolol, 421–422, 763
Atresia, tricuspid. *See* Tricuspid atresia
Atria, morphologic anatomy of, 17–20
Atrial arrhythmias, atrial septal defects and, 519
Atrial enlargement, electrocardiogram showing, 129–131
Atrial fibrillation, 385, 393–394, 403–405
Atrial flutter, 385, 391–393
Atrial inversion, dilation of obstructed venous baffle
    following, 214–216
Atrial isomerism, 20
Atrial premature beats, evaluation and management of,
    380–382
Atrial septal defect, anatomy of, 513–514
  arrhythmia with, 519
  clinical manifestations of, 516–518
  course of, 519–520
  definition of, 513
  hypoplastic left heart syndrome and, 629
  management of, 518–519
  ostium primum type of, 581–584
  physiology of, 514–516
  prevalence of, 513
  pulmonary vascular obstruction with, 88, 519–520
  secundum, **513–524**
    anatomy of, 514
    ventricular septal defect and, 453
  sinoseptal defects with, 514, 515, 521–523
  transcatheter closure of, 219–220
  variations of, 520–523
  with cyanosis, 523
Atrial septostomy, balloon and blade, 216–217
Atrial septum, abnormality involving, and visceral
    heterotaxy, 597, 599
Atrial sinus, 20
Atrial situs, with visceral heterotaxy, 597–598
Atrioventricular block, acquired complete, 419
  congenital complete, 418–419
  first-degree, 417
  Mobitz I (Wenckebach), 417
  Mobitz II, 417–418
  second-degree, 417–418
  third-degree (complete), 418–419
Atrioventricular bundle, 18
Atrioventricular canal, defects in, 584–586
  echocardiographic examination of, 173
  tetralogy of Fallot with common, 488–489
Atrioventricular canal septum, abnormality involving,
    and visceral heterotaxy, 597, 599
Atrioventricular conduction, disorders of, 417–419
Atrioventricular node, 18
Atrioventricular valve anomalies, in visceral heterotaxy,
    600
Atrioventricular valve regurgitation, echocardiography
    for diagnosis of, 177–178
Atrioventricular valve stenosis, echocardiography for
    diagnosis of, 178
Atrioventricular valves, flow through, echocardiographic
    examination of, 171

Atrium, common, 514
  left, in visceral heterotaxy, 599–600
  right, in visceral heterotaxy, 598–599
  single, 514
Auscultation, 106–112
Automaticity, abnormal, 377
  triggered, 377–378
Autonomic implantable cardioverter defibrillator
    (AICD), 426, 427
Autonomic testing, 144
AV node, functional characteristics of, 153
AV-nodal reentrant tachycardia, 394–396

Bacterial endocarditis. *See also* Infective endocarditis
  associated with brain abscess, 79
  ventricular septal defect and, 448, 449
Balloon angioplasty,
  management of coarctation of the aorta with, 213–214,
    541–543
  management of obstructed venous baffles with,
    214–216
  management of pulmonary venous obstructions with,
    216
  pulmonary arterial, 210–213
Balloon atrial septostomy, for transposition of the great
    arteries, 565
Balloon valvotomy, for mitral valvar stenosis, 210
  for prosthetic valve stenosis, 210
  for subaortic stenosis, 210
  for valvar aortic stenosis, 207–210
  for valvar pulmonary stenosis, 204–207
Balloon valvuloplasty, for infant aortic stenosis, 501
  for valvar pulmonary stenosis, 465–468
  for valvar aortic stenosis, 498–500
Becker's muscular dystrophy, 349–351
Bernoulli equation, simplified, in Doppler analysis, 175
Beta-adrenergic blockade, for hypertrophic
    cardiomyopathy, 343
Bicycle, exercise testing with, 253
Bifascicular block, electrocardiogram of, 135–136
  ventricular septal defect and, 448
Bilateral ventricular hypertrophy, electrocardiogram of,
    133
Bile-acid binding resins, treatment of dyslipidemia with,
    292
Bjork-Shiley valve prosthesis, 180
Blalock-Taussig shunt, 737–738, 740
  coil embolization of, 217–218
  for hypoplastic left heart syndrome, 630, 631
  for tricuspid atresia, 664
Blood cell count, 114
Blood chemistries, 115
Blood cultures, 115
Blood gases, monitoring of, 115
Blood pressure, abnormal, 295–298
  changes in, with exercise, 254–255
  measurement of, 295–297
  normal, 295–298
  regulation of, 298–299
Bradycardia, 379–381
  due to depressed pacemaker function, 415–417
  sinus, 415, 416
Brain, anomalies of, hypoplastic left heart syndrome
    and, 623
Brain abscess, with hypoxemia, 76
  with tetralogy of Fallot, 482
Brain infection, with cyanotic heart disease, 79–89
Branchial arch disorders, 51–53
Bretylium, 422–423, 764

Bronchoscopy, prevention of infective endocarditis with, 371–372
Bruce treadmill protocol, 254, 255
Bruit, supraclavicular arterial, 283
Bulboventricular foramen, 502–503
Bumetanide, 69, 761
Bundle branch block, complete left, electrocardiogram of, 135
  complete right, electrocardiogram of, 134, 135–136
  incomplete right, electrocardiogram of, 133
Bypass. *See* Cardiopulmonary bypass

Calcium blockers, for hypertrophic cardiomyopathy, 343
Calcium chloride, 764
Calcium gluconate, 764
Cantrell's syndrome, 607
Captopril, 765
Carcinoid heart disease, 673, 674
Cardiac action potentials, 117–118
Cardiac arrhythmias, **377–433**. *See also* Antiarrhythmic drugs *and* Tachycardias
  atrial septal defects and, 519
  cardiac catheterization and, 189
  pacemaker therapy for, 424–426
  pathophysiology of, 377–380
    bradycardia and block, 379–381
  premature beats, 377–382
  surgical therapy for, 426–428
  transcatheter therapy for, 429–430
  with tetralogy of Fallot, 480
Cardiac catheterization, 78, **187–223**, 497–498
  calculations in, 194–197
    cardiac output, 195–197
    shunts, 194–195
    valve areas, 197
    vascular resistance, 197
  changing trends in, 277–279
  closure of atrial septal defects with, 519
  closure of patent ductus arteriosus with, 529–530
  exercise testing with, 253
  for anomalous origin of left coronary artery, 717
  for aortic regurgitation, 510
  for aortopulmonary window, 694–695
  for atrial septal defects, 518
  for atrioventricular canal defects, 584–585
  for cardiac tumors, 729
  for cardiomyopathies, 333–334
  for coarctation of the aorta, 539, 544–545, 548–549
  for cor triatriatum, 618
  for coronary fistulas, 711
  for corrected transposition of great arteries, 704–706
  for D-transposition of great arteries, 565
  for double-outlet right ventricle, 646
  for Ebstein's disease, 672–673
  for hemitruncus, 698, 699
  for hypertrophic cardiomyopathy, 342
  for hypoplastic left heart syndrome, 628
  for interrupted aortic arch, 553
  for Kawasaki syndrome, 321
  for mitral atresia, 633
  for mitral regurgitation, 611
  for mitral stenosis, 612–613
  for mitral valve prolapse, 616
  for ostium primum defects, 582
  for patent ductus arteriosus, 529, 532
  for pericardial disease, 365
  for pulmonary arteriovenous fistulas, 709–710
  for pulmonary atresia with intact ventricular septum, 639

Cardiac catheterization *(Continued)*
  for rheumatic fever, 311
  for single ventricle, 655
  for subaortic stenosis, 504, 505
  for supravalvar aortic stenosis, 507
  for systemic arteriovenous fistulas, 709
  for tetralogy of Fallot, 477, 479, 484, 487
  for tricuspid atresia, 663–664
  for truncus arteriosus, 678–679
  for valvar pulmonary stenosis, 465–466
  for ventricular septal defect, 444–445
  for visceral heterotaxy, 605–606
  hemodynamic evaluation with, 190–194
    aortic pressure, 193
    left atrial pressure, 191
    left ventricular pressure, 192–193
    pressure gradients, 193
    pressure measurements, 190–191
    pulmonary artery pressure, 193
    pulmonary artery "wedge" pressure, 191–192
    pulmonary vein pressure, 192
    pulmonary vein "wedge" pressure, 192
    right atrial pressure, 191
    right ventricular pressure, 192
    superior and inferior vena caval pressure, 191
  in Duchenne's and Becker's muscular dystrophy, 350
  indications for, 187–188
  interventional, 202–221
    balloon and blade atrial septostomy, 216–217
    balloon angioplasty, 210–216
    balloon valvotomy, 204–210
    closure techniques, 217–221
    myocardial biopsy, 203–204
  pulmonary hypertension and, 91
  risks of, 188–190
Cardiac defects, incidence of, 273, 276, 277
  of postnatal onset, 42
  of prenatal onset, 40–42
Cardiac deformations, 40
Cardiac disruptions, 40–41
Cardiac impulse, observations and palpation of, 106
Cardiac lesions, congenital, pulmonary hypertension with, 87–90
Cardiac malformation syndrome, 42–45
Cardiac malformations, 40
  caused by teratogens, 39, 42, 43, 48–49
  congenital, 43–45
  infective endocarditis and, 369
  multiple defects, 40, 41–42
  single versus multiple, 40–42
  with genetic etiology, 41–42
Cardiac malpositions, **589–608**. *See also* Visceral heterotaxy
  classification of, 589
  clinical manifestations, of, 590
  definition of, 589
  electrocardiogram of, 129, 130
  pathology of, 589–590
  physiology of, 590
  prevalence of, 589
Cardiac output, cardiac catheterization for measuring, 195–197
  changes in, with exercise, 249
  Fick method of measuring, 196–197
Cardiac segments, 27–34
Cardiac transplantation, for hypoplastic left heart syndrome, 632
Cardiac tumors, **727–730**
Cardiomyopathies, **329–361**. *See also* Hypertrophic cardiomyopathy
  Becker's muscular dystrophy, 349–351

Cardiomyopathies (Continued)
  classification of, 329
  clinical manifestations of, 331–334
  course of, 334–335
  definition of, 329
  dilated, electrocardiographic findings in, 138
  doxorubicin cardiomyopathy, 344–347
  Duchenne's muscular dystrophy, 349–351
  etiology of, 329–331
  Friedreich's ataxia, 348
  management of, 334
  myocarditis and, 335–337
  pathology of, 330–331
  prevalence of, 329
Cardiopulmonary bypass, 77–78
Cardiovascular development. See Embryology
Cardiovascular fitness, indices for measuring, 251–252
Cardiovascular surgery, 77–78
Carditis, with rheumatic fever, 309–310
Carnitine deficiency, 337–338
Carnitine transferase enzyme disorders, 338
Carotid pulses, examination of, 103–104
Cat eye syndrome, 41
Catheter, placement of, using echocardiography, 182
Catheterization. See Cardiac catheterization
Cellular action potential, 117–118
Cellular approach to pediatric cardiology, **747–759**
Central nervous system, injury to, with D-transposition
    of the great arteries, 569–570
  infection, with cyanotic heart disease, 79–89
Central nervous system-mediated hypertension, 301
Cerebrovascular accidents, 76, 78, 482
Cervical venous hum, 282–283
CHARGE association, 53
Chest deformity, and congenital heart disease, 105
Chest pain, 102
  in hypertrophic cardiomyopathy, 341
Chest x-ray, 115
  for anomalous origin of left coronary artery, 716, 717
  for aortic regurgitation, 509
  for aorto-left ventricular tunnel, 712
  for aortopulmonary window, 694
  for atrial septal defects, 516
  for atrioventricular canal defects, 584
  for bicuspid aortic valve, 510
  for cardiac tumors, 728, 729
  for cardiomyopathies, 332
  for coarctation of the aorta, 538, 544, 546–548
  for cor triatriatum, 618
  for coronary fistulas, 711
  for corrected transposition of great arteries, 704
  for D-transposition of great arteries, 562–563
  for double-outlet right ventricle, 646
  for Ebstein's disease, 672
  for hemitruncus, 698
  for hypertrophic cardiomyopathy, 342
  for hypoplastic left heart syndrome, 627
  for interrupted aortic arch, 551
  for Kawasaki syndrome, 321
  for mitral atresia, 633
  for mitral regurgitation, 610
  for mitral stenosis, 612
  for mitral valve prolapse, 615
  for ostium primum defects, 582
  for patent ductus arteriosus, 527, 532
  for pericardial disease, 364
  for pulmonary arteriovenous fistulas, 709
  for pulmonary artery sling, 725
  for pulmonary atresia with intact ventricular septum,
    637
  for rheumatic fever, 311, 312

Chest x-ray (Continued)
  for single ventricle, 654
  for subaortic stenosis, 504
  for supravalvar aortic stenosis, 506
  for systemic arteriovenous fistulas, 709
  for tetralogy of Fallot, 475–476, 484, 487
  for tricuspid atresia, 663
  for truncus arteriosus, 677
  for valvar aortic stenosis, 496
  for valvar pulmonary stenosis, 464
  for vascular ring, 722–724
  for ventricular septal defect, 442
  for visceral heterotaxy, 604
Chloral hydrate, 767
Chlorothiazide, 69, 760
Cholesterol, modification of, in childhood, 287
Chondroectodermal dysplasia, 37, 38, 49–50
Chorea, with rheumatic fever, 310–311, 312
Chromosomal abnormalities, and cardiac defects, 41
Chylomicrons, 285
Cineangiographic film, for medical imaging, 199
Circulation, fetal and transitional, **57–61**
Circulatory arrest, in open heart surgery for infants,
    77–78
Clicks, 108, 109–110
Clonidine, 766
Clubbing, 74, 103
Coarctation of the aorta, **535–556**
  anatomy of, 536–537
  atypical, 553–554
  balloon angioplasty for, 213–214, 541–543
  clinical manifestations of, 537–539
  course of, 542–543
  definition of, 535
  echocardiographic examination of, 171–172
  embryology of, 535
  hypertension and, 301
  management of, 539–542
  physiology of, 537
  postoperative, balloon angioplasty for, 213–214,
    542–543
  prevalence of, 535
  surgical repair of, 540–541
  transposition of great arteries and, 571
  unrepaired, balloon angioplasty for, 213
  with aortic stenosis, 548–549
  with complex heart disease, 549
  with intact ventricular septum, in infants, 543–545
  with mitral valve abnormalities, 547–548
  with single ventricle, 649, 651, 654
  with ventricular septal defect, 545–547
Coarctation of the reconstructed aorta, hypoplastic left
    heart syndrome and, 629–630
Coeur en sabot, 476
Coil embolization, of aortopulmonary collaterals, 217,
    485
  of other vessels, 217–218
Collagen disease, pericardial disease and, 367
  pulmonary hypertension and, 95
Color flow mapping, Doppler, 164–165
Computerized tomography, 116
Computing, in cardiology, **265–271**
Conduction, cell-to-cell, 118–119
  through intact heart, 119–121
Conduits, 740–741
Congenital heart disease, central nervous system
    sequelae of, **77–82**
  chest deformity and, 105
  genetic counseling for, 43–44
  prenatal diagnosis of, 45
  prevalence of, 273–275

Congenital heart disease (Continued)
  recurrence of, 44–45
  S-T segment changes and, 256, 258–259
  surgery for infants with, **731–746**
  survival with, 279–280
  ventricular tachycardia and, 413–414
Congenital heart lesions, views of, 202, 206
Congestive heart failure, **63–72**
  cardiomyopathies and, 331
  causes of, 63–65
  clinical manifestations of, 65–66
  treatment of, 66–72
Connective tissue disorders, 50–51
Continuous murmurs, 112, 114
Contractile apparatus, 748–750
Contractile proteins, 749–750, 751
Contractility, 231–237
Conus arteriosus, 22
Cor triatriatum, 617–618
Coronary arteries, aneurysms of, in Kawasaki syndrome,
    321, 324
  status of, Kawasaki syndrome and, 325
Coronary fistulas, 710–711
Coronary sinus, 17, 18
  electrophysiologic study of, 150
  unroofed, 20, 514, 521
Coronary sinus septum, abnormality involving, and
    visceral heterotaxy, 593
Coxsackie virus myocarditis, 335–336
Crista terminalis, 18
Cushing's syndrome, 301
Cyanosis, 73–76, 78. See also Hypoxemia
  and transposition of the great arteries, 562
  atrial septal defect with, 523
  brain abscess with, 79–80
  cerebrovascular accident with, 482
  depressed intelligence quotient with, 482
  examination for, 103
  gallstones with, 482
  gout with, 482
  polycythemia with, 482
  scoliosis with, 76, 103, 482
  taking history of patient with, 102
  with single ventricle, 653
  with tetralogy of Fallot, 473–475, 477–479
Cyanotic spells, 75–76
  with tetralogy of Fallot, 474–475, 477–479
Cyclooxygenase inhibitors, pulmonary hypertension and,
    95

Data management, computerized, for cardiology
    patients, **265–271**
Death. See Sudden death
Dental diseases and procedures, infective endocarditis
    and, 369–372
Dextrocardia, 129, 130, 589
  with visceroatrial situs solitus, 607
Diagnosis, segmental approach to, **27–35**
  value of tests in, 258
Diastolic dysfunction, in hypertrophic cardiomyopathy,
    341
Diastolic filling, 241–242
  and myocardial properties, relation between, 243–244
Diastolic mitral inflow, 242–243
Diastolic murmurs, 111–112, 113
Diastolic performance, assessment of, 237–244
  diastolic filling, 241–242
  diastolic mitral inflow, 242–243
  overlap of active and passive periods of diastole, 241

Diastolic performance (Continued)
  relation between diastolic filling and myocardial
      properties, 243–244
  ventricular and myocardial compliance, 240–241
  ventricular relaxation, 238–240
Diazoxide, 765
DiGeorge sequence, 51–52
DiGeorge syndrome, 675, 676
Digitalis, treatment of congestive heart failure with,
    67–69
Digitalis intoxication, 69
Digoxin, 423–424, 760
  toxicity of, 69
  treatment of congestive heart failure with, 68–69
Dilated cardiomyopathies, 138, 329, 331
Dinamap, in blood pressure monitoring, 295, 296
Disopyramide, 420, 762
Diuretic therapy, for congestive heart failure, 69–70,
    761
  for hypertrophic cardiomyopathy, 342–343
Dobutamine, 71
Dopamine, 71, 761
Doppler echocardiography, 159, 311
  color flow mapping, 164–165
  continuous wave, 162
  diagnosis of structural heart defects with, 176–177
  diagnosis of valvar heart disease with, 177–180
  equipment for, 164, 166
  evaluating ventricular function with, 180–181
  for anomalous origin of left coronary artery, 716–717
  for aortic regurgitation, 509–510
  for atrial septal defects, 516–517
  for atrioventricular canal defects, 584
  for cardiomyopathies, 332–333
  for coarctation of the aorta, 539, 540
  for cor triatriatum, 618
  for coronary fistulas, 711
  for corrected transposition of great arteries, 704
  for D-transposition of great arteries, 563–565
  for hemitruncus, 698
  for hypoplastic left heart syndrome, 627–628
  for Kawasaki syndrome, 321
  for mitral regurgitation, 611
  for mitral stenosis, 612
  for mitral valve prolapse, 616
  for ostium primum defects, 582
  for pulmonary arteriovenous fistulas, 709
  for pulmonary atresia with intact ventricular septum,
      637–639
  for single ventricle, 654–655
  for subaortic stenosis, 504
  for supravalvar aortic stenosis, 507
  for systemic arteriovenous fistulas, 709
  for tetralogy of Fallot, 476–477, 484, 487
  for tricuspid atresia, 663
  for truncus arteriosus, 677–678
  for valvar aortic stenosis, 496–497
  for valvar pulmonary stenosis, 464–465
  for ventricular septal defect, 442–444
  for visceral heterotaxy, 605
  principles of, 161–164
  pulsed Doppler, 162, 164
  quantitative analysis of, 175–176
  with 2-D echocardiography, 171–172, 176–177
Double-inlet ventricle, 649
Double-outlet left ventricle, 647
Double-outlet right ventricle 34, 472–473, **643–648**
  clinical manifestations of, 645–646
  course of, 647
  definition of, 643
  management of, 646–647

Double-outlet right ventricle (Continued)
  pathology of, 643–645
  physiology of, 645
  prevalence of, 643
  pulmonary stenosis and, 645
  transposition of great arteries and, 645
  ventricular septal defect with, 643, 645
Down syndrome, 41, 46–47
  endocardial cushion defects and, 579–581, 583,
    584–586
Doxorubicin cardiomyopathy, 344–347
Drug addiction, infective endocarditis and, 370
Duchenne's muscular dystrophy, 349–351
Ductus arteriosus. See also Patent ductus arteriosus
  aneurysm of, 532
Dyslipidemia, **285–293**
  familial, 290–291
  management of, 291–292
  screening for, 288
  secondary causes of, 289
Dysmorphology, **37–55**
Dysphagia lusoria, 722

Ebstein's disease, 136, 407, 669–673
Echocardiography, **159–186**, 496–497, 506–507. See also
    Doppler echocardiography
  anatomic analysis of, 172–175
    atrioventricular canal, 173
    great arteries, 174
    infundibulum, 174
    veno-atrial segment, 173
    ventricles, 173–174
    ventriculoarterial alignments, 174–175
  catheter placement using, 182
  changing trends in, 276–278
  clinical applications of, 176–183
  contrast, 159
  diagnosis of structural heart defects with, 176–177
  diagnosis of valvar heart disease with, 177–180
  echocardiographic views, 167–171
    apical views, 168–169
    parasternal views, 169–170
    subxiphoid views, 167–168
    suprasternal notch views, 170–171
  equipment for, 164, 166
  evaluating ventricular function with, 180–181
  examination room for, 167
  examination technique with, 164, 166–171
  fetal, 182–183, 267
  for anomalous origin of left coronary artery, 716–717
  for aortic regurgitation, 509–510
  for aorto-left ventricular tunnel, 712
  for aortopulmonary window, 694
  for atrial septal defects, 516–519
  for atrioventricular canal defects, 584
  for bicuspid aortic valve, 510
  for cardiac tumors, 728
  for cardiomyopathies, 332–333
  for coarctation of the aorta, 538–539, 540, 544,
    546–549
  for cor triatriatum, 618
  for coronary fistulas, 711
  for corrected transposition of great arteries, 704
  for D-transposition of great arteries, 563–565
  for diagnosis of rheumatic fever, 311
  for double-outlet right ventricle, 646
  for Duchenne's and Becker's muscular dystrophy,
    349–350
  for Ebstein's disease, 672
  for Friedreich's ataxia, 348

Echocardiography (Continued)
  for hemitruncus, 698
  for hypertrophic cardiomyopathy, 342
  for hypoplastic left heart syndrome, 627–628
  for interrupted aortic arch, 551–553
  for Kawasaki syndrome, 321
  for mitral atresia, 633
  for mitral regurgitation, 610–611
  for mitral stenosis, 612
  for mitral valve prolapse, 615–616
  for ostium primum defects, 582
  for patent ductus arteriosus, 527, 529, 532
  for pericardial disease, 364–365
  for Pompe's disease, 338
  for pulmonary arteriovenous fistulas, 709
  for pulmonary artery sling, 725–726
  for pulmonary atresia with intact ventricular septum,
    637–639
  for single ventricle, 654–655
  for subaortic stenosis, 504, 505
  for systemic arteriovenous fistulas, 709
  for tetralogy of Fallot, 476–477, 484, 487
  for transposition of great arteries, 733
  for tricuspid atresia, 663
  for truncus arteriosus, 677–678
  for valvar pulmonary stenosis, 464–465
  for vascular ring, 724
  for ventricular septal defect, 442–444
  for visceral heterotaxy, 604–605
  interpretation of, 172–176
  intraoperative, 183
  M-mode, 159–161
  of cardiac masses, 181
  of pericardial effusion, 181
  physical principles of, 160–164
  preparation of patient for, 167
  quantitative analysis of, 175–176
  two-dimensional, 159, 161
    with Doppler echocardiography, 171–172, 176–177
  who should perform examination, 172
Ectopia cordis, 607
Ectopic atrial tachycardia, 384, 387–389
Edema, examination for, 103
Eisenmenger syndrome, 90, 449–451
Ejection fraction, changes in, with exercise, 259
Ejection murmurs, 110, 111
Electrical alternans, 137, 138
Electrocardiogram. See also Electrocardiography
  abnormal, atrial enlargement, 129–131
    cardiac malpositions, 129, 130
    ventricular hypertrophy, 130–142
  diagnosis of tachycardia with, 383–387
  exercise testing and autonomic studies, 144–145
  intracardiac electrophysiologic testing, 148–15
  lead systems and recording techniques, 124–125
  normal, 125–129
    axes, 125–127
    clinical correlation, 129
    P wave, 127
    P-R interval, 127
    Q-T interval, 128
    QRS complex, 127–128
    rhythm and rate, 127
    S-T segment, 128
    T wave, 127–128
    U wave, 128–129
  rhythm monitoring (Holter) and event recording,
    142–144
  surface, 123–142
  surface averaging of, 145, 146

Electrocardiogram *(Continued)*
  syndromes and diseases of childhood with distinctive
    findings, 142, 143
  transesophageal recording and pacing, 145, 147–150
Electrocardiography, **117–158**
  for anomalous origin of left coronary artery, 716
  for aortic regurgitation, 509
  for aorto-left ventricular tunnel, 712
  for aortopulmonary window, 694
  for atrial septal defects, 516
  for atrioventricular canal defects, 584
  for bicuspid aortic valve, 510
  for cardiac tumors, 728
  for cardiomyopathies, 332
  for coarctation of the aorta, 538, 544, 546–548
  for cor triatriatum, 618
  for coronary fistulas, 711
  for corrected transposition of great arteries, 702, 704
  for D-transposition of great arteries, 562
  for double-outlet right ventricle, 646
  for Duchenne's muscular dystrophy, 349
  for Ebstein's disease, 671–672
  for Friedreich's ataxia, 348
  for hemitruncus, 697
  for hypertrophic cardiomyopathy, 342
  for hypoplastic left heart syndrome, 627
  for interrupted aortic arch, 551
  for Kawasaki syndrome, 321
  for mitral atresia, 632
  for mitral regurgitation, 610
  for mitral stenosis, 612, 613
  for mitral valve prolapse, 615
  for ostium primum defects, 582
  for patent ductus arteriosus, 527, 532
  for pericardial disease, 364
  for pulmonary arteriovenous fistulas, 709
  for pulmonary atresia with intact ventricular septum,
    636
  for rheumatic fever, 311
  for single ventricle, 654
  for subaortic stenosis, 504
  for supravalvar aortic stenosis, 506
  for systemic arteriovenous fistulas, 708–709
  for tetralogy of Fallot, 475, 484, 487
  for tricuspid atresia, 660, 663
  for truncus arteriosus, 677
  for valvar aortic stenosis, 496
  for valvar pulmonary stenosis, 464
  for ventricular septal defect, 442
  for visceral heterotaxy, 604
Electrolyte abnormality, electrocardiographic findings
  in, 140–142
Electrophysiologic studies, changing trends in, 279
Electrophysiologic techniques, introduction to, **117–158**
Electrophysiology, 117–125
  cell-to-cell conduction, 118–119
  cellular action potential, 117–118
  conduction through intact heart, 119–121
  graphic recording of cardiac electrical activity,
    121–125
Ellis-van Creveld syndrome, 37, 38, 50
Embryology,
  and cardiovascular development, **5–16**
    development of aortic arches, 15–16
    fifth week of life, 8, 12–14
    first week of life, 5, 6
    fourth week of life, 5–6, 8, 9–11
    second week of life, 5, 7
    sixth and seventh weeks of life, 14, 15
    third week of life, 5, 7–9
  definition of, 5

Encainide, 420–421, 763
End-diastolic fiber length, 227–228, 230–231, 234
End-diastolic pressure, 227
End-diastolic stress, 227
End-diastolic volume, 227
End-systolic pressure-volume relation and contractility,
  232–233
End-systolic stress, and afterload, 229–231
End-systolic wall stress, 230–231
Endocardial cushion defects, 438, **577–587**
  anatomy of, 577–580
  atrioventricular canal defects, 584—586
  clinical manifestations of, 581–586
  definition of, 577
  Down syndrome and, 579–581, 583, 584–586
  embryology of, 577
  ostium primum defects, 580, 581–584
  physiology of, 580–581
Endocardial cushion tissue, accessory, subaortic stenosis
  with, 503, 505
Endocarditis. *See also* Bacterial endocarditis *and*
  Infective endocarditis
  cardiac catheterization and, 190
Endocrine hypertension, 301
Endomyocardial biopsy, 203–204
Epinephrine, 71, 764
Erythema marginatum, with rheumatic fever, 310
Esmolol, 421–422, 763
Esophageal echocardiography, 278
Esophageal electrogram, 145, 147–150
Ethacrynic acid, 69
Event recorders, 142
Excrescences, valvar, 728
Exercise, changes in blood pressure with, 254–255
  changes in ejection fraction with, 259
  changes in S-T segment with, 255–259
  physiology of, 249–253
    cardiovascular adaptation to chronic exercise,
      252–253
    changes in cardiac output, 249
    exercise response of pulmonary circulation, 250–251
    indices for measuring cardiovascular fitness,
      251–252
    myocardial oxygen consumption, 250
    neurohumoral changes, 250
    peripheral factors, 250
  sudden death during, 252–253
Exercise fitness, indices for measuring, 251–252
Exercise intolerance, with hypoxemia, 76
Exercise programs, for cardiac patients, 252
Exercise testing, 115–116, 144–145, **249–263**
  exercise protocols, 254
  safety of, 259–260
  types of, 253–254
Exercise tolerance, evaluation of, 101–102
Extracardiac anomalies, examination for, 103

Facioauriculovertebral spectrum, 52–53
Fallot's tetralogy. *See* Tetralogy of Fallot
Familial combined hyperlipidemia, 289
Familial dysbetalipoproteinemia hyperlipoproteinemia,
  289, 291
Familial dyslipidemia, 290–291
Familial hypercholesterolemia, 289
Familial hypertriglyceridemia, 291
Familial hypoalphalipoproteinemia, 291
Fatty acid metabolism, 337
Femoral pulses, examination of, 103–104
Fetal alcohol syndrome, 48

Fetal anticonvulsant syndromes, 48–49
Fetal circulation, 57–59
Fetal echocardiography, 182–183, 267
Fibrillation, atrial. *See* Atrial fibrillation
Fibroma, 727, 729
Fick method of measuring cardiac output, 196–197
Fistulas, congenital vascular, **707–713**
   coronary, 710–711
   pulmonary arteriovenous, 709–710
   systemic arteriovenous, 707–709
Flecainide, 420–421, 763
Flutter, atrial. *See* Atrial flutter
Fontan procedure, 736, 737, 739–744
   for hypoplastic left heart syndrome, 631–632
   for pulmonary atresia with intact ventricular septum,
    641
   for single ventricle, 656–657
   for tricuspid atresia, 664–666
Foramen ovale, patent, 521
Frank-Starling mechanism, 249
Friedreich's ataxia, 348
Furosemide, 69, 760

Gallium scanning, for cardiomyopathies, 334
Gallstones, with cyanosis, 482
Gamma globulin, intravenous, management of Kawasaki
   syndrome with, 322
Gastrointestinal tract surgery, prevention of infective
   endocarditis after, 372–373
Genetic counseling, for congenital heart defects, 43–44
Genitourinary surgery, prevention of infective
   endocarditis after, 372–373
Glenn procedure, for single ventricle, 655, 656
   for tricuspid atresia, 664–666
Glenn shunt, 739
Glomerulonephritis, with hypertension, 299
Glycogen storage disease type 2, 338
Gorlin's formula, 197, 612
Gout, with cyanosis, 482
Great arteries, anatomically corrected transposition of,
   33–34, 706
   "corrected" transposition of, **701–706**
    anatomy of, 701–703
    clinical manifestations of, 702, 704–705
    course of, 705
    definition of, 701
    management of, 705
    physiology of, 702
    prevalence of, 701
   D-transposition of, **557–575**
    anatomy of, 558–559
    classification of, 557
    clinical manifestations of, 562–565
    course of, 569–570
    definition of, 557
    embryology of, 557–558
    management of, 565–569
    overriding tricuspid valve and, 559, 572–573
    physiology of, 559–562
    prevalence of, 557
    pulmonary stenosis with, 560–561
    pulmonary vascular disease with, 562
    surgical management of, 567–569
    ventricular defects with, 559–561, 567–568
    with intact ventricular septum and pulmonary
     stenosis, 571
    with intact ventricular septum, 559, 566, 568
   echocardiographic examination of, 174

Great arteries *(Continued)*
   transposition of, 32–33
    anatomic repair in neonate, 732–740
    coarctation of the aorta and, 571
    double-outlet right ventricle with, 645
    tricuspid atresia with, 665–666
    with ventricular defect and pulmonary stenosis,
     571–572
    with ventricular septal defect, 733, 735–736
Growth, assessment of, in physical examination, 101,
   102–103

Heart. *See also* under Cardiac
   inverted normal, 31
   solitus normal, 31
Heart block, 18, 379–381. *See also* Atrioventricular
   block
   ventricular septal defect and, 448
   with D-transposition of the great arteries, 569
   with tetralogy of Fallot, 482
Heart defects, structural, echocardiography for diagnosis
   of, 176–177
Heart disease congenital. *See* Congenital heart disease
   pediatric, prevalence of, 273–275
Heart murmurs. *See also* Heart sounds
   cervical venous hum, 282–283
   continuous, 112, 114
   diastolic, 111–112, 113
   ejection, 110, 111
   in coarctation of the aorta, 537–538, 539
   innocent, **281–284**
    clinical manifestations of, 281–283
    laboratory tests for, 283
    management of, 283
    prevalence of, 281
    prognosis with, 283
   innocent pulmonic systolic, 282
   regurgitant, 110, 112
   Still's murmur, 281–282
   supraclavicular arterial bruit, 283
   systolic, 110–111, 112
Heart rate, changes in, with exercise, 249–251, 254
Heart size, estimation of, 106
Heart sounds. *See also* Heart murmers
   clicks, 108, 109–110
   first, 107, 108, 109
   fourth, 109, 111
   opening snap, 109, 110
   second, 107–108, 109, 110
   squeaks and honks, 112
   third, 109, 110
Hematocrit, 114
Hemiblock, left anterior, electrocardiogram of, 134–135
   left posterior, electrocardiogram of, 135
Hemitruncus, 676, **697–699**
Hemoptysis, with tetralogy of Fallot, 486
Hemorrhage, intracranial, 79
Heparin sodium, 767
Hepatic veins, abnormality involving, 592–593
Hepatomegaly, 113–114
Heterotaxy. *See* Visceral heterotaxy
High right atrium, electrophysiologic testing of, 149
His bundle electrogram, 149–150
His-Purkinje conduction, 119–121
   atrioventricular block and, 417–419
   depolarization within, 145, 146
   functional characteristics of, 153–154
History, taking pediatric, **101–102**
Holmes' heart, 651
Holt-Oram syndrome, 49, 50
Holter monitors, 142–144

Hurler syndrome, 39, 42
Hydralazine, 71, 765
Hypercholesterolemia, dietary treatment of, 291
  familial, 289
  polygenic, 289
Hyperkalemia, electrocardiographic findings in, 140–141
Hyperlipidemia, dietary treatment of, 291
  familial combined, 289
Hyperlipoproteinemia, familial dysbetalipoproteinemia,
    289, 291
Hypertension, accelerated, 301
  acute, 301, 302
  causes of, 299–302
  central nervous system-mediated, 301
  coarctation of the aorta and, 301
  diagnostic studies of child with, 302–303
  endocrine, 301
  glomerulonephritis with, 299
  iatrogenic and other forms of, 300, 301
  obstructive uropathy with, 299
  polycystic kidney disease with, 299–300
  pulmonary, **83–100**
  pyelonephritis with, 299
  renal parenchymal disease with, 299–300
  renovascular disease and, 300–301
  sustained, therapy for, 303
  systemic arterial, **295–304**
Hypertensive crisis, 301
Hyperthyroidism, 301
Hypertriglyceridemia, 291
Hypertrophic cardiomyopathy, 329, 338–344
  clinical manifestations of, 137–139, 341–342
  course of, 343–344
  definition of, 338–339
  genetic transmission of, 339
  management of, 342–343
  molecular basis for, 755
  pathology of, 339–340
  physiology of, 340–341
  prevalence of, 339
  sudden death in, 343
Hyperuricemia, diuretics and, 70
Hypoalphalipoproteinemia, familial, 291
Hypokalemia, diuretics and, 70
  electrocardiographic findings in, 140
Hyponatremia, diuretics and, 70
Hypoplastic left heart syndrome, **623–632**
  anatomy of, 624, 624
  arterial-pulmonary shunts for, 630, 631
  atrial septal defects and, 629
  cardiac transplantation for, 632
  clinical manifestations of, 626–628
  coarctation of the reconstructed aorta and, 629–630
  definition of, 623
  Fontan operation for, 631–632
  management of, 628–632
    after palliation, 630–631
    ethical issues in, 632
  peripheral pulmonary stenosis and, 630
  physiology of, 623–626
  prevalence of, 623
  pulmonary vascular disease and, 630
  right ventricular myocardial problems and, 629
  stenosis of pulmonary veins and, 629
  surgical management of, 628–630, 739, 740
  tricuspid regurgitation and, 629
Hypothermia, deep, in cardiopulmonary bypass, 77
Hypoxemia, **73–76**. See also Cyanosis
  chronic, 78–79

Hypoxemia (*Continued*)
  clinical correlates of, 73–76
    brain abscess, 76
    cerebrovascular accidents, 76
    clubbing, 74, 103
    cyanosis, 73–74
    exercise intolerance, 76
    hypoxic spells, 75–76
    polycythemia, 73, 74
    scoliosis, 76
    squatting, 74–75
Hypoxia, cardiac catheterization and, 189
Hypoxic spells, 75–76
  with tetralogy of Fallot, 474–475, 477–479

Idiopathic ventricular tachycardia, 415
Immunosuppressive therapy, for myocarditis, 336–337
Indomethacin, and closure of patent ductus arteriosus,
    526
Infective endocarditis, **369–375**. See also Bacterial
    endocarditis
  complications of, 371
  diagnosis of, 370–371
  differential diagnosis between rheumatic fever and,
    313
  involving prosthetic materials, 374
  microbiology of, 370
  predisposing factors for, 369–370
  prevention of, 371–373
  therapy for, 373–374
  with tetralogy of Fallot, 482
Inferior vena cava, abnormality involving, 592–593
Infundibuloarterial inversion, isolated, 32
Infundibulum, 22
  echocardiographic examination of, 174
Innocent murmurs. See Heart murmurs, innocent
Intelligence quotient, depressed, with cyanosis, 482
Interatrial septum, echocardiographic examination of,
    171
Interrupted aortic arch, 549–553
Interventricular septum, echocardiographic examination
    of, 171
Intracardiac electrophysiologic testing, 148–158
  applications of, 151–158
    baseline recording, 151, 152
    evaluation of supraventricular tachycardia, 154–157
    evaluation of ventricular arrhythmias, 157–158
    functional characteristics of AV node, 153
    functional characteristics of His-Purkinje
      conduction, 153–154
    functional characteristics of SA node, 151–153
    functional characteristics of ventricular tissue, 154
  coronary sinus, 150
  equipment and technique for, 148–149, 151
  high right atrium, 149
  His bundle electrogram, 149–150
  right ventricular apex, 150–151
Intraventricular conduction abnormalities,
    electrocardiogram of, 133
Inverted normal heart, 31
Ischemia, electrocardiographic findings in, 138–141
  S-T segment changes and, 256, 258–259
Isomeric atrial appendages, 20
Isoproterenol, treatment of congestive heart failure
  with, 71

James fibers, 397
Jantene procedure, for transposition of great arteries,
    567, 568, 571, 572, 732–733
Jones criteria, for rheumatic fever, 312

Junctional ectopic tachycardia, 384–385, 389–390
Junctional premature beats, evaluation and management
    of, 381
Junctional reciprocating tachycardia, permanent form of,
    405–407

Kartagener's syndrome, 607
Kawasaki syndrome, 276, **319–327**
    clinical manifestations of, 140, 320–324
    course of, 324–325
    definition of, 319
    etiology and pathogenesis of, 319
    management of, 322–324
    pathology of, 319–320
    prevalence of, 319
    surgical management of, 323–324
Kidney disease, polycystic, hypertension in, 299–300

Labetalol, 765
Laboratory tests, for cardiomyopathies, 334
    for Kawasaki syndrome, 321
    for rheumatic fever, 311
    for ventricular septal defect, 445
    routine, **114–116**
Laplace, law of, 228
Late potentials, 145, 146
Left anterior hemiblock, electrocardiogram of, 134–135
Left atrial pressure, cardiac catheterization and, 191
Left atrial problems, 617–619
    cor triatriatum, 617–618
    pulmonary venous stenosis, 619
    supravalvar mitral membrane, 618–619
Left atrium, in visceral heterotaxy, 599–600
    morphologic anatomy of, 19–20
Left bundle branch block, complete, electrocardiogram
    of, 135
Left coronary artery, anomalous origin of, **715–718**
Left posterior hemiblock, electrocardiogram of, 135
Left pulmonary artery, anomalous, 724
Left ventricle, double-outlet, 34, 647
    echocardiographic examination of, 173–174
    morphologic anatomy of, 22–25
Left ventricular hypertrophy, electrocardiogram of,
    132–133
Left ventricular outflow gradient, in hypertrophic
    cardiomyopathy, 340
Left ventricular pressure, cardiac catheterization and,
    192–193
LEOPARD syndrome, 339
Levocardia, 129, 589
Lidocaine, 420, 762
Limbic ledge, 17
Lipid biochemistry, 285–287
Lipid modification, in childhood, 287
Lipid-lowering drugs, 291–292
Lipids, measurement of, 287–288
Lipoprotein levels, plasma lipid and, 289, 290
Lipoproteins, high-density, 285–287
    low-density, 285–287
    very low density, 285–287
Liver, abnormality involving, and visceral heterotaxy,
    592
    examination of, 113–114
Long Q-T syndrome, 413–414
Long-segment pulmonary atresia, 740
Lovastatin, treatment of dyslipidemia with, 292
Lown classification, for ventricular ectopy, 383
Lown-Ganong-Levine syndrome, 137, 151, 397

Lungs, abnormality involving, and visceral heterotaxy,
    592
    biopsy of, and pulmonary vascular resistance, 89
    examination of, 112–113
Lutembacher's syndrome, 523

Magnesium sulfate, 765
Magnetic resonance imaging, 116
    for coarctation of the aorta, 539
    for pulmonary artery sling, 726
    for supravalvar aortic stenosis, 507
    for tetralogy of Fallot with pulmonary atresia, 484
    for vascular ring, 724
    for ventricular septal defect, 444
Mahaim fibers, 136–138, 151, 387, 397, 407–409
Maladie de Roger, 442
Marfan syndrome, 51, 614, 616
Masses, echocardiographic evaluation of, 181
Meperidine, 766
Mesenteric abnormalities, and visceral heterotaxy, 592
Mesocardia, 589
Metabolic acidosis, interrupted aortic arch and, 551
Metabolic alkalosis, diuretics and, 70
Methyldopa, 765
Mexiletine, 420, 762
Mitral atresia, with normal aortic root, 632–633
Mitral regurgitation, 609–611
    ventricular septal defect and, 455–456
Mitral stenosis, 611–614
    balloon valvotomy for, 210
    opening snap with, 109
    ventricular septal defect and, 455–456
Mitral valve, 23–25
    abnormalities of, coarctation of the aorta with,
        547–548
    disease of, **609–617**
        mitral regurgitation, 609–611
        mitral stenosis, 611–614
        mitral valve prolapse, 110, 349, 523, 614–616
        pathology of, 609
        physiology of, 609
        prevalence of, 609
        ventricular septal defect and, 455–456
    prolapse of, 523, 614–616
        in Duchenne's muscular dystrophy, 349
        midsystolic click with, 110
Mobitz block. *See* Atrioventricular block
Moderator bands, 459, 471, 489
Molecular approach to pediatric cardiology, **747–759**
Morphine sulfate, 766
Mullins' technique, for closure of patent ductus
    arteriosus, 218–219
Multifocal atrial tachycardia, 384, 389
Multiple malformation syndrome, 40, 41–42
Murmurs. *See* Heart murmurs
Muscular dystrophy, Becker's, 349–351
    Duchenne's, 349–351
Musculi pectinati, 18
Mustard procedure, for transposition of great arteries,
    567, 568, 569, 732
Myocardial abnormalities, with D-transposition of great
    arteries, 570–571
Myocardial biopsy, 203–204
Myocardial compliance, 240–241
Myocardial disease, differential diagnosis between
    rheumatic fever and, 313
    prevalence of, 273, 276, 277
Myocardial dysfunction, with tetralogy of Fallot,
    481–482

Myocardial energy metabolism, defects of, 337–338
Myocardial function, in Duchenne's and Becker's muscular dystrophy, 350
  Kawasaki syndrome and, 325
Myocardial infarction, Kawasaki syndrome and, 324
Myocardial ischemia, electrocardiographic findings in, 138–141
Myocardial oxygen consumption, during exercise testing, 250
Myocardial performance, assessment of, **225–248**
Myocarditis, cardiomyopathies and, 335–337
  Coxsackie virus, 335–336
  electrocardiographic findings in, 137, 139
  immunosuppressive therapy for, 336–337
  viral, 335
Myocardium, contractile properties of, 748–749
Myopathy, ventricular tachycardia and, 414–415
Myxoma, 727, 729

Nadas, Alexander Sandor, **1–4**
Nadolol, 421–422, 763
Naloxone, 767
Niacin, treatment of dyslipidemia with, 292
Nitroprusside, 70–71, 766
Nodules, subcutaneous, with rheumatic fever, 310
Noonan syndrome, 469
Nuclear scans, for cardiomyopathies, 344

Opening snap, 109–110
Oral contraceptives, pulmonary hypertension and, 95
Orthodromic tachycardia, 405
  due to Wolff-Parkinson-White syndrome, 398–402
Ostium primum defects, 580, 581–584
Ototoxicity, diuretics and, 70
Oxygen consumption, maximum, as measure of cardiovascular fitness, 251
Oxygen content, 194
Oxygen saturation, 115, 194

P-R interval, normal, 127
P-wave, normal, 127
P-wave axis, normal, 127
Pacemaker therapy, for arrhythmias, 424–426
Palpitations, 102
Papillary muscles, of left ventricle, 24
Partial anomalous venous return, 514, 521–522
Patent ductus arteriosus, **525–534**
  anatomy of, 525–526
  clinical manifestations of, 166, 171, 527–529
  closure of, 218–219, 526
  course of, 530–531
  definition of, 525
  in premature infants, 531–532
  management of, 218–219, 529–530
  maternal rubella and, 533
  physiology of, 526–527
  prevalence of, 525
  umbrella closure of, 218–219
  variations of, 531–533
  ventricular septal defect and, 453–454
Patent foramen ovale, 521
Premature beats, evaluation and management of, 380–382
Pericardial disease, **363–368**
  absence of pericardium, 367–368
  bacterial pericarditis, 365–366
  causes of pericardial effusion, 367

Pericardial disease (Continued)
  clinical manifestations of, 364–365
  collagen disease and, 367
  constrictive pericarditis, 366–367
  definition of, 363
  idiopathic pericarditis, 367
  intrapericardial teratoma, 367
  physiology of, 363–364
  postpericardiotomy effusions, 366
  prevalence of, 363
  rheumatic fever and, 367
  tuberculous pericarditis, 367
  viral pericarditis, 366
Pericardial effusion, causes of, 367
  echocardiographic evaluation of, 137, 138, 181
Pericardial tamponade, 104, 105
Pericardiocentesis, 365
Pericarditis, bacterial, 365–366
  constrictive, 366–367
  electrocardiogram of, 137, 138
  idiopathic, 367
  rheumatic, 367
  tuberculous, 367
  viral, 366
Pericardium, absence of, 367–368
Persistent pulmonary hypertension of the newborn, 93–94
Pharyngitis, group A streptococcal, and rheumatic fever, 306–307, 308
Phenylephrine, 764
Phenytoin, 420, 762
Physical examination, **102–104**
  for atrial septal defects, 516
  for atrioventricular canal defects, 584
  for cardiomyopathies, 331–332
  for D-transposition of great arteries, 562
  for hypertrophic cardiomyopathy, 341–342
  for pulmonary artery sling, 724–725
  for tetralogy of Fallot, 475, 476
  for vascular ring, 722
  for ventricular septal defect, 441–442
  for visceral heterotaxy, 602–604
Plasma lipid, and lipoprotein levels, 289, 290
Polyarthritis, with rheumatic fever, 308–309
Polycythemia, 73, 74
  with cyanosis, 482
Polygenic hypercholesterolemia, 289
Polysplenia syndrome, 20, 590–607
  anatomic findings in, 602
  clinical manifestations of, 602–606
  diagnosis of, 606
  pathology of, 591–602
  total anomalous pulmonary venous return with, 690
Pompe's disease, 338
Potassium chloride, 767
Potts shunt, 737
Prazosin, 71, 765
Predictive value of a test, 258
Preexcitation, electrocardiogram of, 136–137
Preexcitation syndrome, 151
Preload, 227–228, 231, 233–235
Premature beats, 377–379
Pressure gradients, cardiac catheterization and, 193
Pressure recordings, during cardiac catheterization, 190–191
Prevalence of pediatric heart disease, 273–275
Procainamide, 420, 762
Propafenone, 420–421, 763
Propranolol, 343, 421–422, 763, 766
Prostaglandin E1, and closure of patent ductus arteriosus, 526, 767
  for D-transposition of the great arteries, 566

Prostaglandins E, for hypoplastic left heart syndrome, 625, 627
Prosthetic valve endocarditis, 374
Prosthetic valve stenosis, balloon valvotomy for, 210
Prosthetic valves, echocardiographic imaging of, 179–180
    in children, 741
Protamine, 767
Proto-oncogenes, in cell growth, 755–756
Pulmonary arterial angioplasty, 210–213
Pulmonary arterial flow, decreased, 88
    echocardiographic examination of, 166, 171
    increased, 88
Pulmonary artery, congenital absence of, 468
    originating from aorta, **697–699**
Pulmonary artery band, 736–737
    for D-transposition of the great arteries, 567
Pulmonary artery pressure, cardiac catheterization and, 193
    and flow, increased, 88
Pulmonary artery sling, 724–726
Pulmonary artery stenosis, with tetralogy of Fallot, 480
Pulmonary artery "wedge" pressure, cardiac catheterization and, 191–192
Pulmonary atresia. *See also* Tetralogy of Fallot, with pulmonary atresia
    single ventricle and, 649, 655
    with intact ventricular septum, **635–642**
        anatomy of, 635–636
        clinical manifestations of, 636–639
        course of, 641
        definition of, 635
        embryology of, 635
        management of, 639–641
        physiology of, 636
        prevalence of, 635
        variation of, 641–642
Pulmonary blood flow, unrestricted, 688–690
Pulmonary circulation, exercise response of, 250–251
Pulmonary hypertension, **83–100**
    associated with alveolar hypoxemia, 94–95
    other causes of, 95
    persistent, of the newborn, 93–94
    primary, 90–93
    ventricular septal defect and, 450
    with congenital cardiac lesions, 87–90
Pulmonary regurgitation, 469
Pulmonary stenosis, **459–470**
    anatomy of, 459–461
    balloon valvotomy for, 204–207
    critical, in the neonate, 467–468
    D-transposition of the great arteries with, 560–561
    definition of, 459
    double-outlet right ventricle with, 645
    infundibular, anatomy of, 460
    peripheral, 460, 461, 468–469
        hypoplastic left heart syndrome and, 630
    physiology of, 460, 462
    prevalence of, 459
    single ventricle and, 649, 652–655
    transposition of great arteries and, 571
    valvar, 462–467
    variations of, 467–469
    ventricular defects with, 454–455
Pulmonary valve, absent, tetralogy of Fallot with, 486–488
    systemic, hypoplastic left heart syndrome and, 630
Pulmonary vascular development, normal, 83

Pulmonary vascular disease, D-transposition of great arteries with, 562
    hypoplastic left heart syndrome and, 630
    ventricular septal defect and, 449–451
Pulmonary vascular obstruction, associated with congenital heart defects, therapy for, 88–89
    atrial septal defects and, 88, 519–520
    patent ductus arteriosus and, 530
    with tetralogy of Fallot, 480
Pulmonary vascular resistance, increased, pathophysiology of, 85–87
    increased, repair of congenital heart defects with, 89
    measurement of, 83–84
    normal values of, 84–85
Pulmonary vascular structure, pathologic changes in, with pulmonary hypertension, 85–87
Pulmonary vein pressure, cardiac catheterization and, 192
Pulmonary vein "wedge" pressure, cardiac catheterization and, 192
Pulmonary veins, 19
    flow from, echocardiographic examination of, 171
    obstructed, 686–688
    stenosis of, hypoplastic left heart syndrome and, 629
Pulmonary veno-occlusive disease, pulmonary hypertension and, 95
Pulmonary venous connections, in visceral heterotaxy with congenital heart disease, 595–597
Pulmonary venous obstructions, balloon angioplasty for, 216
Pulmonary venous return. *See* Total anomalous pulmonary venous return
Pulmonary venous stenosis, 619
Pulmonary-to-aortic anastomosis, 738–740
Pulse pressure, examination of, 105
Pulsus alternans, 105
Pulsus paradoxus, 104, 105
Pyelonephritis, with hypertension, 299

Q-T interval, normal, 128
    prolonged, syndrome of, 413–414
QRS axis, normal, 127
QRS complex, 121, 123–124
    normal, 127–128
Quinidine, 420, 761

Radial pulses, examination of, 103–104
Radiation exposure and protection, 199–200
Radioisotope scans, 115
Rastelli operation, for D-transposition of the great arteries, 568, 572
Reentry, 378–379
    and narrow QRS tachycardia, 385
    AV-nodal reentrant tachycardia, 394–396
    sinus node, 390–391
Refractory periods, 118–119
Regurgitant murmurs, 110, 112
Relative risk, in diagnostic value of a test, 258
Renal artery stenosis, hypertension due to, 301
Renal parenchymal hypertension, 300
Renovascular disease, hypertension and, 300–301
Repolarization, early, 128
Respiration, assessment of, in physical examination, 102
Respirophasic sinus arrhythmia, 127
Restrictive cardiomyopathies, 329
Retinoic acid embryopathy, 39
Rhabdomyoma, 727, 729

Rheumatic fever, **305–318**
   clinical manifestations of, 308–312
      polyarthritis, 308–309
   course of, 314–315
   diagnosis of, 312–313
   differential diagnosis of, 313
   management of, 313–317
   pancarditis with, 335
   pathogenesis of, 306–307
   pathology of, 307–308
   prevalence of, 305–306
   prevention of, 316–317
   recurrent, 315–316
Rheumatic pericarditis, 367
Rheumatoid arthritis, differential diagnosis between
      rheumatic fever and, 313
Rhythm, normal, 127
   monitoring of, 142–144
   problems, with D-transposition of great arteries, 569
Right atrial pressure, cardiac catheterization and, 191
Right atrium, in visceral heterotaxy, 598–599
   morphologic anatomy of, 17–18
Right bundle branch block, complete, electrocardiogram
      of, 134, 135–136
   incomplete, electrocardiogram of, 133
   ventricular septal defect and, 448
Right ventricle. *See also* Double-outlet right ventricle
   double-chambered, ventricular septal defect and, 455
   echocardiographic examination of, 173–174
   morphologic anatomy of, 21–23
Right ventricular apex, electrophysiologic study of,
      150–151
Right ventricular failure, with D-transposition of great
      arteries, 569
Right ventricular hypertrophy, electrocardiogram of,
      130–132
Right ventricular myocardial problems, hypoplastic left
      heart syndrome and, 629
Right ventricular outflow tract, echocardiographic
      examination of, 174
Right ventricular pressure, cardiac catheterization and,
      192
   suprasystemic, with tetralogy of Fallot, 480
Rubella, maternal, and patent ductus arteriosus, 533
   and pulmonary stenosis, 468

S-T segment, changes in, with exercise, 255–259
   normal, 128
   pathologic changes in, electrocardiogram of, 137
SA nodes, functional characteristics of, 151–153
St. Jude valve prosthesis, 179
St. Vitus' dance, 310
Salicylates, management of Kawasaki syndrome with,
      322
Sarcoma, 728, 729
Sarcomeres, 748–750
Scimitar syndrome, 514, 522, 590
Scoliosis, with cyanotic heart disease, 103, 482
   with hypoxemia, 76
Segmental approach to diagnosis of congenital heart
      disease, **27–35**
Segmental combinations, in visceral heterotaxy, 601
Semilunar valve regurgitation, echocardiographic
      examination of, 171, 178–179
Semilunar valve stenosis, echocardiography for diagnosis
      of, 179
Senning procedure, for transposition of great arteries,
      567, 568, 569, 572, 732
Sensitivity of a test, determining, 258

Septal defects, atrial, pulmonary vascular obstruction
      with, 88
   congenital, pulmonary hypertension and, 85–87
   ventricular, echocardiographic examination of, 174
Septal myotomy or myectomy, for hypertrophic
      cardiomyopathy, 343
Septostomy, balloon and blade atrial, 216–217
   balloon atrial, for transposition of the great arteries,
      565
Septum secundum, 17, 18
Shunts, 194–195. *See also* Blalock-Taussig shunt
   arterial-pulmonary, for hypoplastic left heart
      syndrome, 630, 631
   Glenn, 739
   left-to-right, 194–195
   Potts, 737
   right-to-left, 194–195
   systemic-to-pulmonary, 737–738
   Waterston, 737
Siamese twins, 607
Sick sinus syndrome, 18, 415–417
Sickle cell disease, differential diagnosis between
      rheumatic fever and, 313
Signal averaging, of surface cardiogram, 145, 146
Single ventricle, **649–657,** 736–738
   anatomy of, 649–651
   clinical manifestations of, 653–655
   course of, 656–657
   definition of, 649
   embryology of, 649
   management of, 655–656
   physiology of, 651–653
   prevalence of, 649
   pulmonary artery band for, 736–737
Single ventricular hypertrophy, electrocardiogram of,
      133
Sino-atrial conduction time, 153
Sinoatrial node, 18
Sinoseptal defects, inferior vena caval, 514, 521
   with atrial septal defect, 514, 515, 521–523
Sinus bradycardia, 415, 416
Sinus node recovery time, 152–153
Sinus node reentry tachycardia, 390–391
Sinus tachycardia, 383–384
Sinus venous defects, 514, 521
Situs ambiguus, 20
Situs inversus totalis, 607
Snap, opening, 109–110
Sodium nitroprusside, 70–71, 766
Solitus normal heart, 31
Sotalol, 422–423, 764
Spinal fusion, in Duchenne's muscular dystrophy, 351
Spironolactone, 69, 761
Spleen, abnormality involving, and visceral heterotaxy,
      591–592
   examination of, 114
Squatting, and cyanotic heart disease, 74–75
Squeaks and honks, 112
Stethoscopes, 106
Still's murmur, 281–282
Streeter's horizons, 6, 8, 9, 11–14
Stress testing, 144–145. *See also* Exercise testing
   for valvar aortic stenosis, 497
Stress-shortening, contractility and, 233–237
Stress-velocity analysis, contractility and, 233–237
Stroke volume, changes in, with exercise, 249
Subaortic stenosis, 502–506
   accessory endocardial cushion tissue with, 503, 505
   balloon valvotomy for, 210

Subaortic stenosis (*Continued*)
    clinical manifestations of, 504
    course of, 505–506
    definition of, 502
    hypertrophic, 502
    management of, 504–505
    pathogenesis of, 503
    pathology of, 502–503
    physiology of, 503–504
    prevalence of, 502
    tunnel type, 502, 505
    ventricular septal defect and, 452–453
Sudden death, aortic stenosis and, 500–501
    during exercise, 252–253
    in hypertrophic cardiomyopathy, 343
Superior vena cava. *See* Vena cava
Supraclavicular arterial bruit, 283
Supravalvar mitral membrane, 618–619
Supraventricular tachycardia. *See* Tachycardia,
    supraventricular
Surgery, changing trends in, 279
Survival, with congenital heart disease, 279–280
Switch, arterial, for TGA, 567, 568, 571, 572, 732–733
Sydenham's chorea, 310
Syncope, 102, 341
Systemic arterial hypertension, **295–304**
Systemic outflow obstruction, bypass of, using proximal
    pulmonary artery, 738
Systemic venous connections, in visceral heterotaxy with
    congenital heart disease, 593
Systemic-to-pulmonary shunts, 737–738
Systolic fiber shortening, factors influencing, 226–227
Systolic murmurs, 110–111, 112
Systolic performance, assessment of, 226–237
    afterload, 228–231, 234
    contractility, 231–237
    factors influencing fiber shortening, 226
    preload, 227–228, 231, 233–235

T-wave, normal, 127, 128
    normal axis, 127
    pathologic changes in, electrocardiogram of, 137
Tachycardias, 377–379, 382–415. *See also* Ventricular
    tachycardia
    antidromic reciprocating, and Wolff-Parkinson-White
      syndrome, 402–403
    automatic supraventricular, management of, 387–390
    AV-nodal reentrant, 394–396
    ectopic atrial, 384, 387–389
    evaluation and management of, 382–415
    junctional ectopic, 384–385, 389–390
    junctional reciprocating, permanent form of, 405–407
    Mahaim fiber, 407–409
    multifocal atrial, 384, 389
    narrow QRS, differential diagnosis of, 383–385, 386
      reentry and, 385
    orthodromic reciprocating, due to Wolff-Parkinson-
      White syndrome, 398–402
    reentrant supraventricular, management of, 390–396
    sinus, 383–384
    sinus node reentry, 390–391
    supraventricular, 382
      due to accessory pathways, 396–409
      electrophysiologic evaluation of, 154–157
    terminology and classification of, 382–383
    wide QRS, differential diagnosis of, 385–387
Taussig-Bing anomaly, 645
Tendon of Todaro, 18

Teratogens, cardiac malformations caused by, 39, 42, 43,
    48–49
Teratoma, 728, 729
Test. *See also* specific names
    diagnostic value of, how to determine, 258
Testing, exercise, 115–116, 144–145, **249–263**
Tetralogy of Fallot, 74–76, 88, **471–491**
    acyanotic, 454
    anatomy of, 471–473
    aortic regurgitation with, 480
    arrhythmias with, 480
    brain abscess with, 482
    clinical manifestations of, 474–477
    course of, 480–486
    cyanosis with, 473–475
      management of, 477–479
    definition of, 471
    embryology of, 471
    heart block with, 482
    hemoptysis with, 486
    infective endocarditis with, 482
    late death following repair of, 482
    management of, 477–480
    myocardial dysfunction with, 481–482
    physiology of, 473–474
    prevalence of, 471
    progression of, 480
    pulmonary artery stenosis with, 480, 481
    pulmonary regurgitation and, 469
    pulmonary stenosis with, surgical management of, 479
    pulmonary vascular obstructive disease with, 480
    reoperation for, 482
    suprasystemic right ventricular pressure with, 480
    surgical management of, 479–480
    with absent pulmonary valve, 486–488
    with common atrioventricular canal, 488–489
    with obstructive moderator bands, 489
    with pulmonary atresia, 472–473, 480–486
      anatomy of, 483
      clinical manifestations of, 484
      course of, 486
      definition of, 482
      embryology of, 483
      management of, 484–486
      physiology of, 483–484
      prevalence of, 482–483
Thoracoabdominal ectopia cordis, 607
Thoracophagus twins, 607
Thrills, presence of, in physical examination, 106
Thrombi, intracardiac, 728, 729
Thromboembolism, chronic, pulmonary hypertension
    and, 95
Thrombolytic therapy, management of Kawasaki
    syndrome with, 323
Thrombosis, cerebral venous, with cyanotic heart
    disease, 78
Thyroid hormone, 750, 752–753
Tinea sagittalis, 18
Tocainide, 420, 762
Tonsillectomy, prevention of infective endocarditis with,
    371–372
Total anomalous pulmonary venous return, **683–691**
    anatomy of, 683–684
    clinical manifestations of, 686–690
    course of, 690
    definition of, 683
    management of, 690
    physiology of, 684–686
    prevalence of, 683
    with asplenia or polysplenia, 690
Transcatheter ablation, for cardiac arrhythmia, 429–430

Transcatheter closure, of atrial septal defects, 219–220
  of ventricular septal defects, 220–221
Transcutaneous oxygen, 114–115
Transesophageal recording and pacing, 145, 147–150
Transient neurological deficits, cardiac catheterization
  and, 190
Transitional circulation, 60–61
Transplantation, cardiac, 744–745
Treadmill, exercise testing with, 253, 254
Trends in cardiology, **273–280**
Triangle of Koch, 18
Tricuspid atresia, **659–667**
  anatomy of, 659–660
  clinical manifestations of, 660, 663–664
  course of, 666
  definition of, 659
  management of, 664–666
  physiology of, 660, 662
  prevalence of, 659
  transposition of great arteries with, 665–666
Tricuspid incompetence, with D-transposition of great
  arteries, 569
Tricuspid regurgitation, hypoplastic left heart syndrome
  and, 629
Tricuspid valve, 22
  overriding or straddling, and D-transposition of great
    arteries, 559, 572–573
    and endocardial cushion defects, 578
  problems with, **669–674**
Trisomy 13 syndrome, 41, 47
Trisomy 18 syndrome, 37, 38, 41, 47
Trisomy 21 syndrome, 41, 46–47
Truncus arteriosus, **675–682**
  anatomy of, 675–676
  clinical manifestations of, 676–679
  definition of, 675
  embryology of, 675
  management of, 679–681
  physiology of, 676, 677
  prevalence of, 675
Tuberculous pericarditis, 367
Tumors, cardiac, **727–730**
  clinical manifestations of, 728
  fibroma, 727, 729
  management of, 729
  myxoma, 727, 729
  pathology of, 727–728
  prevalence of, 727
  rhabdomyoma, 727, 729
  sarcoma, 728, 729
  teratoma, 728, 729
  thrombi, 728, 729
  valvar excrescences, 728
  vegetations, 728, 729
Turner syndrome, 41, 47–48

U wave, normal, 128–129
Ultrasound, cardiovascular. *See* Echocardiography
Umbrella closure, of patent ductus arteriosus, 218–219
Unifocalization, treatment of tetralogy of Fallot with
  pulmonary atresia with, 486
Univentricular heart, 649
Unroofed coronary sinus, 200, 514, 521
Urinalysis, 114
Uropathy, obstructive, with hypertension, 299

Valproic acid, prenatal exposure to, 49
Valvar heart disease, echocardiography for diagnosis of,
  177–180

Valvar regurgitation, Kawasaki syndrome and, 325
Valve areas, cardiac catheterization for measuring, 197
Valve prosthesis, echocardiographic imaging of, 179–180
Valve replacement, 741
  treatment of aortic stenosis with, 501
Valvotomy. *See* Balloon valvotomy
Valvuloplasty, 741. *See also* Balloon valvuloplasty
  treatment of valvar aortic stenosis with, 498–500
Vascular resistance, cardiac catheterization for
  measuring, 197
Vascular rings, **719–726**
  anatomy of, 722
  clinical manifestations of, 722–724
  definition of, 719
  embryologic anatomy of, 719–721
  management of, 724
  prevalence of, 721–722
Vascular slings, **719–726**
  definition of, 719
  embryologic anatomy of, 719–721
Vasodilator therapy, treatment of congestive heart
  failure with, 70–71
VATER association, 53
Vegetations, associated with infective endocarditis, 728,
  729
Vena cava, inferior and superior, 17, 18
  pressures, superior and inferior, cardiac
    catheterization and, 191
  superior, and visceral heterotaxy, 593–595
Veno-atrial segment, echocardiographic examination of,
  173
Venous baffles, obstructed, balloon angioplasty for,
  214–216
Venous complications, cardiac catheterization and, 189
Venous hum, 112, 114
Venous pressure, examination of, 105
Ventricle, single. *See* Single ventricle
Ventricles, echocardiographic examination of, 173–174
  morphologic anatomy of, 20–25
Ventricular arrhythmias, electrophysiologic evaluation
  of, 157–158
Ventricular compliance, 240
Ventricular ectopy, exercise testing for, 144
  Lown classification for, 383
Ventricular function, echocardiographic evaluation of,
  180–181
Ventricular hypertrophy, electrocardiogram showing,
  130–142
Ventricular inversion, isolated, 32
Ventricular noninversion, isolated, 32
Ventricular outflow tract obstructions, in visceral
  heterotaxy, 600–601
Ventricular performance, assessment of, **225–248**
Ventricular premature beats, evaluation and
  management of, 381–382
Ventricular relaxation, 238–240
  factors affecting, 239–240
  indices of, 238–239
Ventricular septal defect, 22, **435–457**
  anatomy of, 437–438
  aortic regurgitation with, 451–452
  bacterial endocarditis and, 448, 449
  clinical manifestations of, 440–445
  closure of, 446–447
  coarctation of the aorta with, 545–547
  course of, 448–453
  definition of, 435
  discovery of, 440
  double-chambered right ventricle with, 455
  double-outlet right ventricle with, 643, 645

Ventricular septal defect *(Continued)*
  echocardiographic examination of, 174
  embryology of, 436–437
  heart block with, 448
  management of, 445–448
  mitral valve disease and, 455–456
  patent ductus arteriosus and, 453–454
  physiology of, 438–440
  prevalence of, 435–436
  pulmonary stenosis and, 454–455
  pulmonary vascular disease with, 449–451
  secundum atrial septal defect with, 453
  spontaneous diminution in size of, 449
  subaortic stenosis with, 452–453
  survival after, 448
  symptoms of, 440–441
  transcatheter closure of, 220–221
  transposition of great arteries with, 733, 735–736
  valvar pulmonary stenosis with, 454–455
  variations of, 453–456
Ventricular tachycardia, 382, 409–415
  and congenital heart disease, 413–414
  and myopathy, 414–415
  exercise testing for, 144, 145
  late potentials and, 145, 146
Ventricular tissue, functional characteristics of, 154
Ventriculoarterial alignment, in visceral heterotaxy, 601

echocardiographic examination of, 174–175
Verapamil, 423, 764
Visceral heterotaxy, **590–607**
  clinical manifestations of, 602–606
  management of, 606–607
  noncardiac anomalies in, 606
  pathology of, 591–602
  prevalence of, 273, 591
Visceroatrial situs solitus, ventricular inversion with
    inverted normally related great arteries in, 31–32
Volume depletion, diuretics and, 70

Warfarin sodium, 767
Waterston shunt, 737
Williams syndrome, 50, 469, 506
Wolff-Parkinson-White syndrome, 151, 385–387,
    396–397
  antidromic reciprocating tachycardia and, 402–403
  atrial fibrillation in, 403–405
  digoxin for, 424
  electrocardiogram of, 136–138
  exercise testing for, 144, 145
  orthodromic tachycardia and, 398–402, 405
Work overload hypertrophy, 753–756

X-ray. *See* Chest x-ray